AIIMS-MAMC-PGI IMAGING SERIES

DIAGNOSTIC RADIOLOGY

Chest and Cardiovascular Imaging

Pioneers of AIIMS-MAMC-PGI Imaging Series

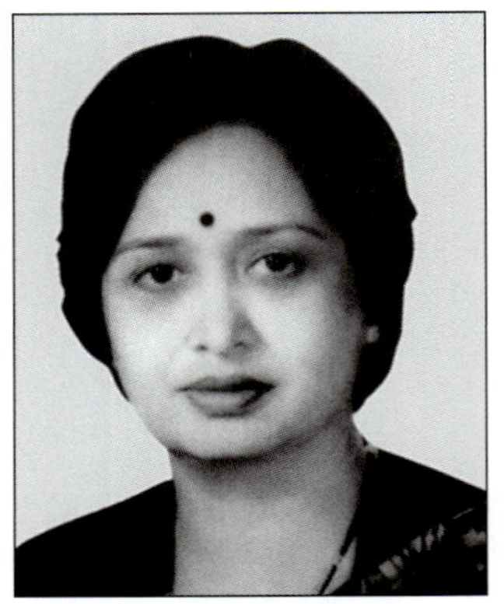

Manorama Berry

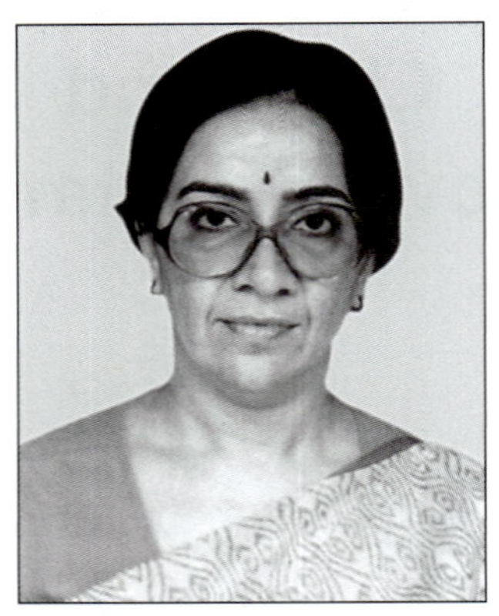

Veena Chowdhury

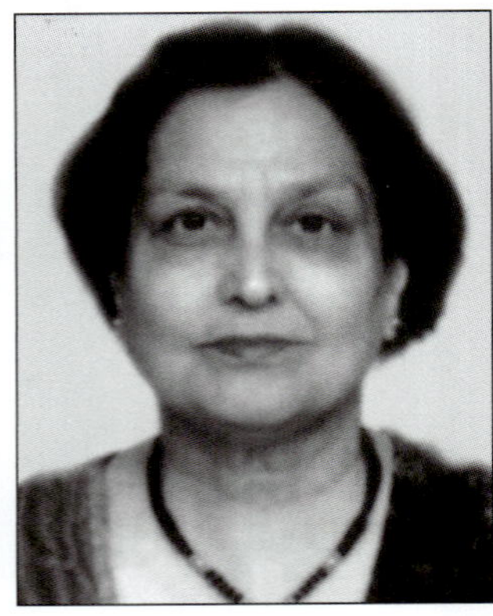

Sudha Suri

Past Editors

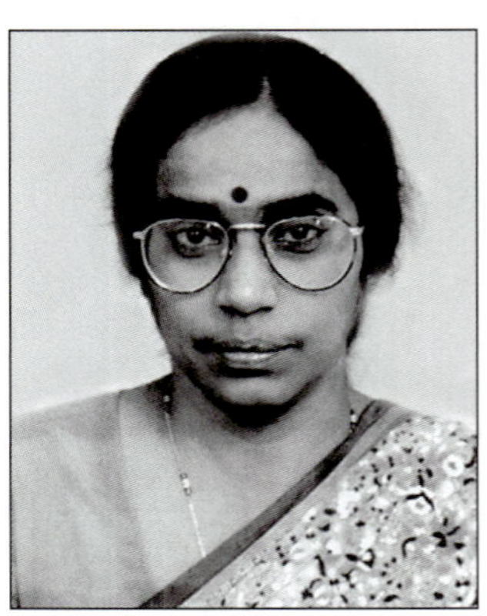

Sima Mukhopadhyay

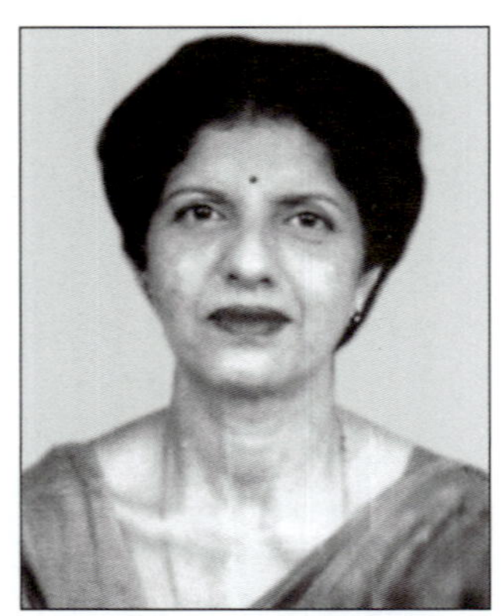

Sushma Vashisht

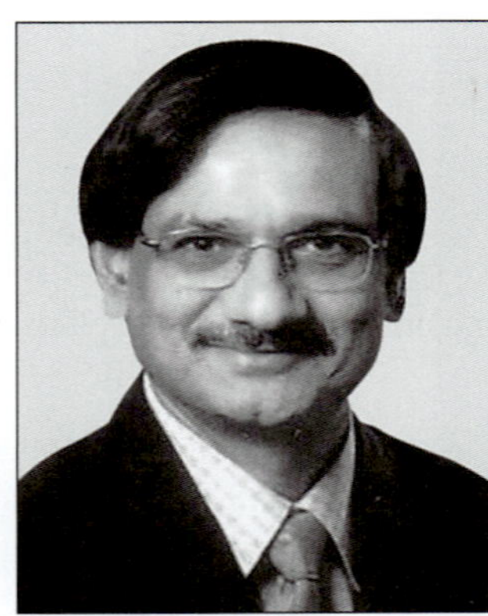

Niranjan Khandelwal

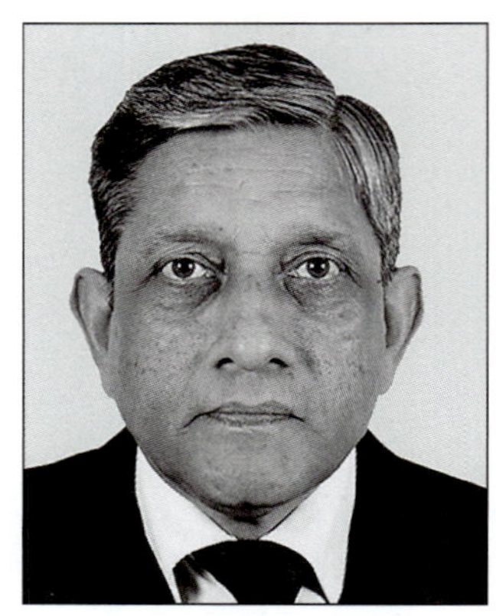

Arun Kumar Gupta

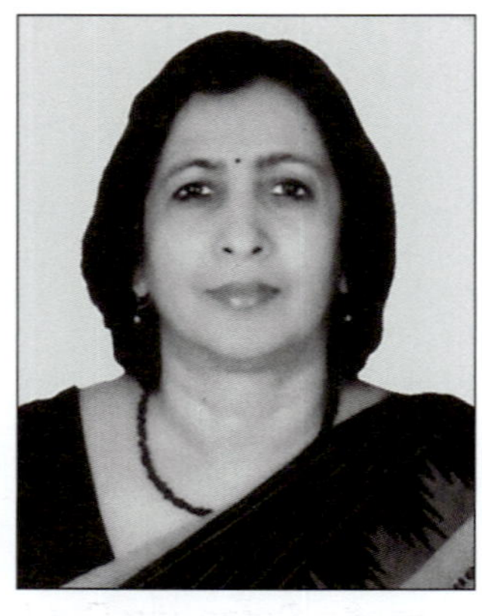

Anju Garg

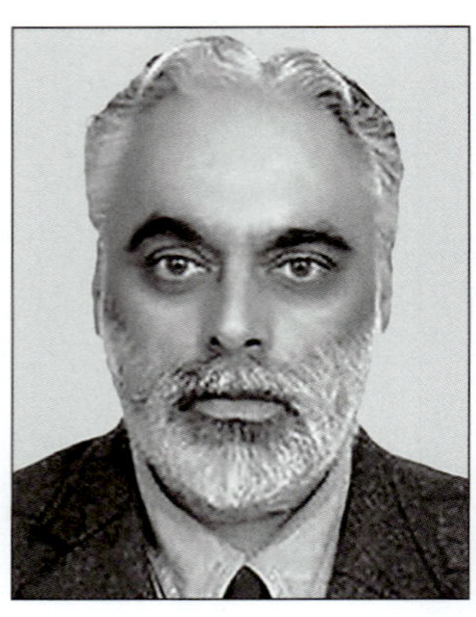

Manavjit Singh Sandhu

AIIMS-MAMC-PGI IMAGING SERIES

DIAGNOSTIC RADIOLOGY

Chest and Cardiovascular Imaging

Fifth Edition

Editors

Gaurav Shanker Pradhan DMRD DNB
Director Professor and Head
Department of Radiodiagnosis
Maulana Azad Medical College (MAMC)
and Lok Nayak Hospital
New Delhi, India

Raju Sharma MD MAMS FICR
Professor and Head
Department of Radiodiagnosis and
Interventional Radiology
All India Institute of Medical
Sciences (AIIMS)
New Delhi, India

Paramjeet Singh MD FICR CCST(UK)
Professor and Head
Department of Neuroimaging and
Interventional Neuroradiology
Postgraduate Institute of Medical Education
and Research (PGIMER)
Chandigarh, India
Convenor DM (NIINR)

Associate Editors

Alpana Manchanda MD
Director Professor
Department of Radiodiagnosis
Maulana Azad Medical College (MAMC)
New Delhi, India

Ashu Seith Bhalla MD FICR MAMS
Professor
Department of Radiodiagnosis and
Interventional Radiology
All India Institute of Medical Sciences
(AIIMS)
New Delhi, India

Mandeep Garg MD FRCR
Professor
Department of Radiodiagnosis and
Imaging
Postgraduate Institute of Medical
Education and Research (PGIMER)
Chandigarh, India

Jyoti Kumar MD DNB MNAMS FICR
Director Professor
Department of Radiodiagnosis
Maulana Azad Medical College
(MAMC)
New Delhi, India

Priya Jagia MD DNB
Professor and Head
Department of Cardiovascular Imaging and
Endovascular Interventions
Cardiothoracic Sciences Centre
All India Institute of Medical Sciences
(AIIMS)
New Delhi, India

Manphool Singhal MD DNB MAMS FICR
FSCCT FSCMR
Professor
Department of Radiodiagnosis and
Imaging
Postgraduate Institute of Medical
Education and Research (PGIMER)
Chandigarh, India

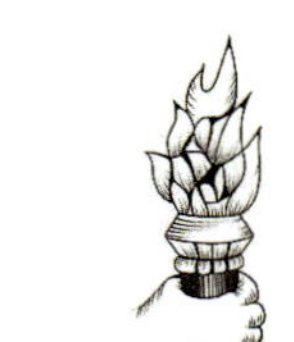

JAYPEE BROTHERS MEDICAL PUBLISHERS
The Health Sciences Publisher
New Delhi | London

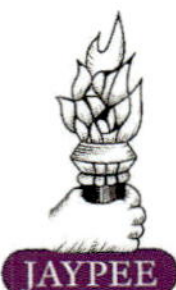

Jaypee Brothers Medical Publishers (P) Ltd

Headquarters
EMCA House
23/23-B, Ansari Road, Daryaganj
New Delhi 110 002, India
Landline: +91-11-23272143, +91-11-23272703
+91-11-23282021, +91-11-23245672
E-mail: jaypee@jaypeebrothers.com

Corporate Office
Jaypee Brothers Medical Publishers (P) Ltd.
4838/24, Ansari Road, Daryaganj
New Delhi 110 002, India
Phone: +91-11-43574357
Fax: +91-11-43574314
E-mail: jaypee@jaypeebrothers.com

Overseas Office
JP Medical Ltd.
83, Victoria Street, London
SW1H 0HW (UK)
Phone: +44-20 3170 8910
Fax: +44(0)20 3008 6180
E-mail: info@jpmedpub.com

Website: www.jaypeebrothers.com

Website: www.jaypeedigital.com

Inquiries for bulk sales may be solicited at: jaypee@jaypeebrothers.com

***Diagnostic Radiology: Chest and Cardiovascular Imaging* / Gaurav Shanker Pradhan, Raju Sharma, Paramjeet Singh**

First Edition: 1996

Fifth Edition: **2025**

ISBN: 978-93-6616-667-4

Printed at: Samrat Offset Pvt. Ltd.

Contributors

Ajay Gulati MD MAMS FICR Fellowship Abdominal Imaging(Canada)
Professor
Department of Radiodiagnosis and Imaging
Postgraduate Institute of Medical Education and Research (PGIMER)
Chandigarh, India

Akshay Kumar Saxena MD DNB FICR
Professor
Department of Radiodiagnosis and Imaging
Postgraduate Institute of Medical Education and Research (PGIMER)
Chandigarh, India

Akshit Kumar MD
Senior Resident
Department of Cardiovascular Radiology and Endovascular Interventions
Cardiothoracic Sciences Center
All India Institute of Medical Sciences (AIIMS)
New Delhi, India

Alpana Manchanda MD
Director Professor
Department of Radiodiagnosis
Maulana Azad Medical College (MAMC)
New Delhi, India

Amarinder Singh Malhi MD DM(Cardiovascular Radiology and Endovascular Interventions)
Assistant Professor
Department of Radiodiagnosis and Interventional Radiology
All India Institute of Medical Sciences (AIIMS)
New Delhi, India

Amit Gupta MD FRCR EDiR
Consultant Radiologist
AI Center of Excellence for Healthcare
All India Institute of Medical Sciences (AIIMS)
New Delhi, India

Anindita Sinha MD MAMS
Professor
Department of Radiodiagnosis and Imaging
Postgraduate Institute of Medical Education and Research (PGIMER)
Chandigarh, India

Anjali Prakash DMRD DNB MNAMS FICR
Director Professor
Department of Radiodiagnosis
Maulana Azad Medical College (MAMC) and Associated Hospitals
New Delhi, India

Anju Garg MD
Director Professor
Department of Radiodiagnosis
Maulana Azad Medical College (MAMC)
New Delhi, India

Ankita Aggarwal MD
Assistant Professor
Department of Radiodiagnosis and Interventional Radiology
All India Institute of Medical Sciences (AIIMS)
New Delhi, India

Ankur Goyal MD DNB MNAMS FICR FESUR(Europe)
Additional Professor
Department of Radiodiagnosis and Interventional Radiology, All India Institute of Medical Sciences (AIIMS)
New Delhi, India

Anmol Bhatia MD(Radiodiagnosis) and Fellowship PGI(Pediatric Radiology)
Additional Professor
Department of Radiodiagnosis and Imaging
Postgraduate Institute of Medical Education and Research (PGIMER)
Chandigarh, India

Anupam Lal MD
Professor
Department of Radiodiagnosis and Imaging
Postgraduate Institute of Medical Education and Research (PGIMER)
Chandigarh, India

Aprateem Mukherjee MD DM
Senior Resident
Department of Cardiovascular Radiology and Endovascular Interventions
Cardiothoracic Sciences Center
All India Institute of Medical Sciences (AIIMS)
New Delhi, India

Arun Sharma DM
Assistant Professor
Department of Radiodiagnosis and Imaging
Postgraduate Institute of Medical Education and Research (PGIMER)
Chandigarh, India

Ashu Seith Bhalla MD FICR MAMS
Professor
Department of Radiodiagnosis and Interventional Radiology
All India Institute of Medical Sciences (AIIMS)
New Delhi, India

Atin Kumar MD DNB MNAMS FICR
Professor
Department of Radiodiagnosis and Interventional Radiology
Jai Prakash Narayan Apex Trauma Center
All India Institute of Medical Sciences (AIIMS)
New Delhi, India

Chandan Jyoti Das MD DNB PhD MAMS FICR FRCP
Professor
Department of Radiodiagnosis and Interventional Radiology
All India Institute of Medical Sciences (AIIMS)
New Delhi, India

Chandrashekhara SH MD DM DNB
Professor
Department of Radiodiagnosis and Interventional Radiology
Dr BR Ambedkar Institute Rotary Cancer Hospital (IRCH)
All India Institute of Medical Sciences (AIIMS)
New Delhi, India

Devasenathipathy Kandasamy MD DNB FRCR
Professor
Department of Radiodiagnosis and Interventional Radiology
All India Institute of Medical Sciences (AIIMS)
New Delhi, India

Ekta Dhamija MD
Additional Professor
Department of Radiodiagnosis and Interventional Radiology
Dr BR Ambedkar Institute Rotary Cancer Hospital (IRCH)
All India Institute of Medical Sciences (AIIMS)
New Delhi, India

Gaurav Shanker Pradhan DMRD DNB
Director Professor and Head
Department of Radiodiagnosis
Maulana Azad Medical College (MAMC) and Lok Nayak Hospital
New Delhi, India

Harish Bhujade MD FVIR(PGI)
Assistant Professor
Department of Radiodiagnosis and Imaging
Postgraduate Institute of Medical Education and Research (PGIMER)
Chandigarh, India

Jyoti Kumar MD DNB MNAMS FICR
Director Professor
Department of Radiodiagnosis
Maulana Azad Medical College (MAMC)
New Delhi, India

Krithika Rangarajan MD DNB FRCR PhD
Associate Professor
Department of Diagnostic and Interventional Onco-Radiology
Dr BR Ambedkar Institute Rotary Cancer Hospital (IRCH)
All India Institute of Medical Sciences (AIIMS)
New Delhi, India

Kushaljit Singh Sodhi MD PhD MAMS FICR
Professor
Department of Radiodiagnosis and Imaging
Postgraduate Institute of Medical Education and Research (PGIMER)
Chandigarh, India

Madhurima Sharma MD DNB
Assistant Professor
Department of Radiodiagnosis and Imaging
Postgraduate Institute of Medical Education and Research (PGIMER)
Chandigarh, India

Mahesh Prakash MD MAMS FIACM FICR
Professor
Department of Radiodiagnosis and Imaging
Postgraduate Institute of Medical Education and Research (PGIMER)
Chandigarh, India

Mandeep Garg MD FRCR
Professor
Department of Radiodiagnosis and Imaging
Postgraduate Institute of Medical Education and Research (PGIMER)
Chandigarh, India

Mandeep Kang MD MAMS FICR
Professor
Department of Radiodiagnosis and Imaging
Postgraduate Institute of Medical Education and Research (PGIMER)
Chandigarh, India

Manisha Jana MD DNB FRCR
Professor
Department of Radiodiagnosis and Interventional Radiology, All India Institute of Medical Sciences (AIIMS)
New Delhi, India

Manphool Singhal MD DNB MAMS FICR FSCCT FSCMR
Professor
Department of Radiodiagnosis and Imaging
Postgraduate Institute of Medical Education and Research (PGIMER)
Chandigarh, India

Mukesh Kumar Yadav MD
Additional Professor
Department of Radiodiagnosis and Interventional Radiology
Dr BR Ambedkar Institute Rotary Cancer Hospital (IRCH), All India Institute of Medical Sciences (AIIMS)
New Delhi, India

Naveen Kalra MD FAMS FICR FINASL
Professor
Department of Radiodiagnosis and Imaging
Postgraduate Institute of Medical Education and Research (PGIMER)
Chandigarh, India

Nidhi Prabhakar MD DNB
Assistant Professor
Department of Radiodiagnosis and Imaging
Postgraduate Institute of Medical Education and Research (PGIMER)
Chandigarh, India

Niraj Nirmal Pandey MD DM
Assistant Professor
Department of Cardiovascular Imaging and Endovascular Interventions, All India Institute of Medical Sciences (AIIMS)
New Delhi, India

Pankaj Gupta MD
Associate Professor
Department of Radiodiagnosis and Imaging
Postgraduate Institute of Medical Education and Research (PGIMER)
Chandigarh, India

Priya Jagia MD DNB
Professor and Head
Department of Cardiovascular Imaging and Endovascular Interventions
Cardiothoracic Sciences Centre
All India Institute of Medical Sciences (AIIMS)
New Delhi, India

Priyanka Naranje MD DNB MNAMS EBIR
Additional Professor
Department of Radiodiagnosis and Interventional Radiology
All India Institute of Medical Sciences (AIIMS)
New Delhi, India

Radhika Batra MD DNB
Professor
Department of Radiodiagnosis
Maulana Azad Medical College (MAMC)
New Delhi, India

Rajendra Kumar Behera MD Fellow(GI Radiology)
Assistant Professor
Department of Radiodiagnosis and Interventional Radiology
All India Institute of Medical Sciences (AIIMS)
New Delhi, India

Raju Sharma MD MAMS FICR
Professor and Head
Department of Radiodiagnosis and Interventional Radiology
All India Institute of Medical Sciences (AIIMS)
New Delhi, India

Rashmi Dixit MD
Director Professor
Department of Radiodiagnosis
Maulana Azad Medical College (MAMC)
New Delhi, India

Sanjeev Kumar MD
Additional Professor
Department of Cardiovascular Radiology and Endovascular Interventions
Cardiothoracic Sciences Center
All India Institute of Medical Sciences (AIIMS)
New Delhi, India

Sapna Singh MD DNB MNAMS
Director Professor
Department of Radiodiagnosis
Maulana Azad Medical College (MAMC)
New Delhi, India

Satyam DNB MNAMS
Senior Specialist
Department of Radiodiagnosis
Lok Nayak Hospital and Associated Maulana Azad Medical College (MAMC)
New Delhi, India

Shivanand Gamanagatti MD MAMS FICR
Professor
Department of Radiodiagnosis and Interventional Radiology
Jai Prakash Narayan Apex Trauma Center, All India Institute of Medical Sciences (AIIMS)
New Delhi, India

Smita Manchanda MD DNB MNAMS
Additional Professor
Department of Radiodiagnosis and Interventional Radiology
All India Institute of Medical Sciences (AIIMS)
New Delhi, India

Smriti Hari MD MAMS
Professor
Department of Radiodiagnosis and Interventional Radiology
All India Institute of Medical Sciences (AIIMS)
New Delhi, India

Stanzin Spalkit MD DNB EDiR
Assistant Professor
Department of Radiodiagnosis and Interventional Radiology
All India Institute of Medical Sciences (AIIMS)
New Delhi, India

Surabhi Vyas MD DNB MNAMS
Professor
Department of Radiodiagnosis and Interventional Radiology
All India Institute of Medical Sciences (AIIMS)
New Delhi, India

Swati Gupta MD DNB FRCR
Professor
Department of Radiodiagnosis
Maulana Azad Medical College (MAMC)
New Delhi, India

Tulika Singh MD
Professor
Department of Radiodiagnosis and Imaging
Postgraduate Institute of Medical Education and Research (PGIMER)
Chandigarh, India

Ujjwal Gorsi MD DM
Additional Professor
Department of Radiodiagnosis and Imaging
Postgraduate Institute of Medical Education and Research (PGIMER)
Chandigarh, India

Uma Debi MD
Additional Professor
Department of Radiodiagnosis and Imaging
Postgraduate Institute of Medical Education and Research (PGIMER)
Chandigarh, India

Veenu Singla MD
Professor
Department of Radiodiagnosis and Imaging
Postgraduate Institute of Medical Education and Research (PGIMER)
Chandigarh, India

Vineeta Ojha MD DM
Assistant Professor
Department of Cardiovascular Radiology and Endovascular Interventions
Cardiothoracic Sciences Center
All India Institute of Medical Sciences (AIIMS)
New Delhi, India

Preface to the Fifth Edition

It is with great pleasure that we present the 5th edition of "*Diagnostic Radiology: Chest and Cardiovascular Imaging*", an integral part of the AIIMS-MAMC-PGI Imaging Course Series 2025. This updated edition builds upon the foundation of its predecessors, incorporating the latest advancements in imaging techniques, clinical applications, and technological innovations to enhance diagnostic accuracy and patient care.

Radiology plays a crucial role in the evaluation of thoracic and cardiovascular disorders, bridging the gap between clinical assessment and definitive diagnosis. The past few years have witnessed significant progress in CT, MRI, PET-CT, and AI-assisted imaging, revolutionizing the way chest and cardiovascular diseases are diagnosed and managed. This edition reflects these developments with revised content and updated imaging protocols to provide a comprehensive and practical learning experience.

This book is designed to cater to postgraduate students, radiology residents, and practicing radiologists, offering a structured approach to chest and cardiovascular imaging. Each chapter has been contributed by esteemed faculty from AIIMS (New Delhi), MAMC (New Delhi), and PGI (Chandigarh), ensuring a blend of academic and clinical relevance. Highlights of this edition include:

- Expanded sections on radiographic techniques and normal anatomy pertaining to chest and cardiovascular System
- Latest guidelines on imaging in pulmonary infections, vascular pathologies, and oncologic conditions
- New chapters on AI applications in thoracic imaging, and advanced cardiac MRI techniques
- Updated high-quality images and schematic diagrams for better interpretation

We express our sincere gratitude to all contributors who have enriched this book with their expertise. Without their active support, this endeavor would not have been possible. We also acknowledge the unwavering support of our students and readers, whose feedback has been instrumental in shaping this edition.

We hope this book serves as a valuable resource in your academic and professional journey, fostering a deeper understanding of chest and cardiovascular imaging and its critical role in modern medicine.

Gaurav Shanker Pradhan
Raju Sharma
Paramjeet Singh

Preface to the First Edition

It is with great pleasure the faculty of Department of Radiodiagnosis at All India Institute of Medical Sciences, New Delhi; Maulana Azad Medical College, New Delhi, and Postgraduate Institute of Medical Education and Research, Chandigarh present the second book in the series on *Diagnostic Radiology*. This book is devoted to *Emergency and Chest Radiology* and has been written to provide the radiologist in training, in practice or teaching, physician and surgeon, an integrated review of the role of various imaging modalities and roentgen features seen in diseases of the chest and in acute emergency situations, both medical and surgical, including trauma.

The plain chest radiograph remains the initial imaging modality for various chest diseases and its interpretation continues to be a great challenge. Importance of chest radiograph in the diagnosis of various diseases has been dealt with in depth in all the chapters. Technique of CT and its recent advances in the evaluation of chest diseases and potential of MRI for evaluation of thoracic lesions are covered in separate chapters. Detailed discussion on the clinicopathological aspects and radiology in common thoracic diseases like tuberculosis, nontubercular infections and malignancy, role of HRCT in specific conditions and infections in immunocompromised hosts are included. All the chapters provide information about the recent developments in various fields.

Importance of having diagnostic technical facilities and role of a radiologist in handling the patient in acute emergency are highlighted. The increasing use of US and CT as an initial examination in the assessment of acute abdominal conditions has tended to diminish awareness of the value of plain radiography. The role of plain radiograph, US and CT in nontraumatic acute abdomen are covered in separate chapters.

Trauma is one of the leading cause of morbidity and mortality. The incidence and severity have sharply increased during the past few decades, primarily because of the increased use of high speed travel. A disciplined approach to the assessment of trauma provides confident interpretation and avoids errors of misdiagnosis. Computed tomography has revolutionized evaluation of a patient with head injury and it remains the first modality of choice. The diagnostic evaluation of patient with craniofacial injury remains problematic because of anatomic complexity of this region, wide spectrum of fracture types, and diversity of soft tissue complication. The proper approach to radiographic diagnosis of appendicular trauma begins by obtaining the appropriate radiographs of each site. Awareness of the common, the often missed and the probable associated injuries improve interpretation and make assessment of radiographs much easier.

The role of the radiologist in the management of abdominal trauma has expanded considerably in the recent years. Earlier urography, scintigraphy and angiography played an important role in trauma care. The modalities of CT and interventional radiology have improved the assessment of an injured patient and facilitated nonoperative therapy for some injuries.

The proliferation of imaging modalities has increased the possibility of performing inappropriate and unnecessary investigations. The comprehensive discussion on the indications and importance of various imaging techniques in the practice of emergency and chest radiology, a systematic approach for imaging a patient with trauma affecting different organ system are covered in this book.

We hope that the reader may find this book both instructive and informative for the improved use of radiological resources which in turn will serve the common goal of good health care for the benefit of patients everywhere.

We wish to take this opportunity to thank our faculty colleagues from AIIMS, MAMC, and PGI for their active support, cooperation and timely submission of the manuscripts. We owe immense gratitude to Professor K Subbarao and Professor Ratni B Gujral, who have been kind enough to submit their contributions well in time.

Manorama Berry
Veena Chowdhury
Sudha Suri
Sima Mukhopadhyay

Contents

Gaurav Shanker Pradhan, Radhika Batra, Rashmi Dixit

CHAPTER 1

The Chest Radiograph: Techniques, Anatomy and Interpretation

INTRODUCTION

Chest radiography is the mainstay of chest imaging despite the increasing availability and diagnostic superiority of cross-sectional imaging techniques. The chest radiograph is the first examination that is performed in patients with complaints of cough, shortness of breath or chest pain. The advantages of chest radiographs include quick acquisition and interpretation, low cost and low radiation exposure. The chest radiograph plays a vital role in the diagnosis of various conditions, to check the position of monitoring and support devices, prior to surgical procedures and in health check-ups. Portable chest radiography is used to monitor sick patients in intensive care units.[1]

Chest radiographs allow visualization of chest wall, mediastinum, hila, heart, great vessels, airways, lungs, pleural surfaces including the fissures and the diaphragm. The overlap of various radiographic densities (air, fat, soft tissue, calcification and bone) can make interpretation of chest radiographs challenging.

There are many technical challenges in chest radiography which include capturing the attenuation difference between mediastinum and lung, depiction of small contrast differences and fine structural detail, therefore, a radiographic system should have a wide dynamic range to display the mediastinal and retrocardiac abnormalities but should have a high local contrast for detection of focal lesions with subtle contrast and a high spatial resolution for imaging interstitial lung disease. The introduction of digital radiography has improved image quality and reduced radiation exposure in patients.[2]

CHEST RADIOGRAPHY: TECHNIQUES

Chest radiographs are performed with the patient in an erect position and with full suspended respiration, ideally at total lung capacity. Conventional film screen radiography uses kilovoltage (kV) range between 50–85. The advantages of conventional radiography include high spatial resolution, good uniformity over a large area, high sensitivity, operational simplicity and low cost but these systems are limited by the small exposure range of the film. A low-kV radiograph can help visualize the skeleton or detect calcifications such as calcified hilar or mediastinal lymph nodes, pleural plaques and pulmonary nodules. The drawbacks of conventional chest radiography include poor visualization of the mediastinum and retrocardiac regions, inadequate detail of airway and lung apices, obscuration of lung details from bones. A high-kV technique is generally recommended, with a minimum of 120 kV. Additionally, the use of a grid or air gap between the patient and the film is advised. A high-kV technique improves lung visibility by reducing the contrast of the bony thorax and allows better penetration of the mediastinum.

Beam equalization radiography is an imaging technique used to optimize the quality of radiographic images, particularly in areas with significant variations in tissue density, such as the chest. This technique involves the use of compensating filters that help equalize the X-ray beam intensity across the image field, reducing the impact of tissue density differences (e.g., between the heart, lungs, and chest wall) on image quality. By improving uniformity in image exposure, beam equalization enhances diagnostic accuracy, especially for structures with varying radiopacity, and minimizes image artifacts caused by over- or underexposure. It plays an important role in areas like thoracic imaging, where variations in tissue density are common.

Digital Chest Radiography

Computed Radiography

Computed radiography (CR) systems rely on storage phosphor technology. These systems are cost-effective and versatile, offering portability with cassette-based options for bedside imaging or integration into a dedicated Bucky system for chest radiography. Traditional CR systems utilize a single laser beam and a detector screen with an amorphous (powder-based) detector material. The required exposure for these systems is similar to that of a 400-speed film/screen system, with a detector dose of 2.5 μGy. Recently, several improvements in detector materials and read-out technologies have been introduced. Dual-reading CR systems are based on transparent detector material and employ light collection optics in the front and the back side of the detector. Combining these signals improves quantum detection and has only a minimum deteriorating effect on spatial resolution. Parallel reading uses a linear array of laser diodes (linear-line laser diode) to simultaneously read all pixels in a single line, significantly accelerating the process. Additionally, a light collection system equipped with specialized optics and multiple linear asymmetric charged coupled devices (CCDs) enhances the efficiency of the read-out process by improving photon collection.[3] A new crystalline detector material ($CsBr:Eu^{2+}$) for storage phosphor systems allows for creating a thicker detector layer [better detective quantum efficiency (DQE)] without deteriorating spatial resolution. This is possible because of the structure of the detector material: Crystalline needles serve as light pipes and substantially reduce lateral diffusion of photons.[4,5]

The disadvantages of CR include slower image processing time compared to direct digital radiography (DDR), the need to physically handle and insert imaging plates into a reader, potential for image artifacts from improper handling of the plates, higher radiation dose compared to some DDR systems, and a lower image quality due to the limitations of the phosphor plate technology, which can lead to increased noise and decreased detail.

Direct Digital Radiography

Electronic flat panel detector systems provide superior image quality as compared to CR and no external read out is required, the image is available instantly. Two DDR techniques are available both of which are based on thin-film transistors (TFT) matrix arrays. Indirect conversion systems, also known as Opto-direct systems, incorporate a scintillator [such as cesium iodide (CsI), or gadolinium oxysulfide (GOS), also known as "Gadox"] placed atop an array of light-sensitive photodiodes with TFTs. The scintillator converts incoming radiation into light, which is then detected by the photodiode/TFT array. Crystalline scintillators like CsI direct the scintillation light through needle-like crystals, enabling the use of thicker detector layers without compromising modulation transfer function (MTF). CsI-photodiode/TFT systems are commonly used in chest radiography and offer improved the DQE compared to traditional computed radiography or Gadox-TFT systems.[6,7]

Direct conversion systems, or electro-direct systems, use a photoconductive layer (such as amorphous selenium), where absorbed X-ray energy is directly converted into charge on top of a TFT array. These systems are particularly well-suited for the high spatial frequencies needed in mammography. However, because they absorb less X-ray energy, they have lower dose efficiency for structures like vascular or interstitial patterns, or lung infiltrates. This results in a DQE that is about half that of CsI-photodiode/TFT systems, making direct conversion systems less ideal for chest radiography.[6,8]

Digital radiography of the chest provides a wide dynamic range which allows better visualization of soft tissue and bony structures. It also has better contrast and sharper images. The image acquisition is quick. DDR can achieve high quality images with lower radiation exposure. Image manipulation can be done, such as adjustment of contrast and brightness. The images are stored in electronic format and can be retrieved. They can also be transferred via picture archiving and communication system (PACS). DDR allows for the use of advanced processing algorithms such as computer aided diagnosis (CAD), dual energy subtraction, temporal subtraction and digital tomosynthesis.

Computer aided diagnosis programs aim to help the radiologist in detecting or differentiating various disease entities in the chest. The system suggests an abnormality which is verified by the radiologist. Increased sensitivity for small lung nodules (5–15 mm) has been reported. CAD can, therefore, alert the radiologist to potential abnormalities.

Dual-energy subtraction radiography involves capturing two chest images at different X-ray energies. By exploiting the difference in energy dependence of attenuation between bone and soft tissue, either bone or soft tissues can be eliminated by locally weighted subtraction of the two images. To achieve optimal separation of bone and soft tissue, correction for scatter and beam hardening is necessary. While subtraction can significantly increase image noise, this effect is reduced when energy separation is more effective. Dual-energy subtraction has been shown to improve the detection of intrapulmonary nodules by eliminating overlying rib structures that could obscure or distract from the nodules.

There are two acquisition methods for dual-energy subtraction. The single-exposure technique uses a stack of two detectors (typically storage phosphor screens) with a beam-hardening filter (usually copper) in between. This method results in modest energy separation between the low-energy front and high-energy back images, leading to higher image noise but no misregistration issues. The dual-exposure technique, on the other hand, captures two separate chest images in quick succession (200 ms) at low and high kVp settings, offering better energy separation but introducing slight misregistration artifacts. Dual-energy subtraction allows for better differentiation of calcified and non-calcified lesions, enhanced detection of nodules and masses, and improved identification of rib lesions.[2]

Temporal subtraction is a processing method that involves matching and subtracting a follow-up radiograph from a baseline image. As the rib cage moves differently from the lungs, the matching process can be complex and may induce misregistration artifacts. However, this technique is highly effective in identifying subtle changes over time and enhancing the detection of nodules and hazy infiltrates.[2]

Digital tomosynthesis developed from conventional tomography, where multiple projection images of the patient are captured as the X-ray tube moves. These images are then shifted and combined to focus on objects in a specific plane, while other structures are spread out across the image and appear with varying degrees of blur. Tomosynthesis has been shown to enhance the visibility of intrapulmonary nodules.[9]

Advances in Chest Radiography

Dynamic Chest Radiography

Dynamic chest radiography (DCR) is a real-time, high resolution, digital X-ray imaging technique that captures sequential images of the thorax in motion, typically over a span of 10–20 seconds. It uses pulsed image exposure and offers a wider field of view than fluoroscopy, while maintaining a low radiation dose. A high-resolution flat panel detector (FPD) produces both temporal and spatial digital images with a wide field of view (FOV) that encompasses the entire thorax. DCR can achieve a temporal resolution of up to 15 frames per second (fps), sufficient to capture rapid movements. Recent advancements in hardware and segmentation-based proprietary image processing software enable automatic identification of moving structures, such as the diaphragm and the visible posteroanterior lung area, as well as the detection of changes in pixel intensity in lung tissue during the respiratory cycle. When applied to lung parenchyma and vasculature segmentation, pixel density changes can be used to infer ventilation and perfusion, eliminating the need for intravenous contrast agents or inhaled tracers.

Depending on the exposure settings, a single DCR image can often serve diagnostic purposes and closely resembles a standard chest radiograph PA view. DCR offers several advantages as an imaging technology: it has the same footprint as a standard chest radiography unit, and the image acquisition process exposes patients to a lower radiation dose compared to CT or traditional fluoroscopy. DCR is usually performed with the patient in an upright position, though it can also be done supine, and it does not require the forced maneuvers or mouthpieces typically needed for airflow-based lung function tests like spirometry or plethysmography, which can disrupt normal respiratory or cardiovascular function. The image capture is quick, taking only slightly longer than a standard chest radiograph.

A single DCR image series can provide information about diaphragmatic motion, chest wall motion, large airways diameter and ventilation/perfusion. Information on these parameters is important in conditions such as diaphragmatic palsy, restrictive and obstructive lung diseases and pulmonary vascular diseases.[10]

Dark-field Radiography

Dark-field radiography is an advanced imaging technique in chest radiography to enhance visualization of fine details and subtle abnormalities, however it is an evolving technology with limited clinical applications. Unlike traditional X-ray imagers, dark-field X-ray equipment requires additional hardware components that are complex and challenging to manufacture. The alveolar structure of the lungs with its multitude of water-air transitions is a main contributor to the type of small-angle scattering effects detected with dark-field X-ray imaging. As the signal is generated by multiple water air transitions in the lung, healthy lung tissues with unaltered alveoli and a higher density of such interfaces produces relatively high signal levels compared to diseased lung tissue. Dark-field radiography exploits the wave aspect of photons in addition to their particle aspect which results in an image contrast that is both different from and complementary to that of conventional X-ray imaging. Strong signals are detected from healthy lung parenchyma against a dark background yielding an image contrast different from that attained with conventional chest radiography. Bronchi and hila show lower signal levels due to reduced amounts of lung tissue and tissue-air interfaces. While its use is limited by the need for specialized equipment and higher radiation dose, this technique may be useful in assessing diseases such as emphysema and fibrosis. It may also be valuable in detecting small nodules and tumors.[11]

RADIOGRAPHIC PROJECTIONS

Posteroanterior View

The posteroanterior (PA) view is the standard frontal chest view for evaluation of the chest. The patient is made to stand straight with the weight equally distributed on both feet and positioned to face the image detector so as to minimize magnification of the anteriorly positioned heart and consequent obscuration of lungs, and the X-ray beam passes through in the posterior to anterior direction, i.e., PA. The upright position is preferred as it prevents engorgement of pulmonary vessels, allows full expansion of lungs, helps in detection of possible air-fluid levels in the chest and is helpful for the diagnosis of pneumoperitoneum. The patient is asked to move the shoulders forward and downward so that the chest wall and both shoulders are in contact with the detector. The dorsal wrists should be placed on the waist with elbows oriented anteriorly, and the scapulae are rotated anteriorly so that they are projected away from the lungs. The neck, chin and head are extended upward to avoid superimposition with the trachea and upper regions of lungs.

The central ray should be directed at the level of T7 vertebra which corresponds to the inferior angle of scapula. The focal film distance should be at least 180 cm. The radiograph should be acquired at full inspiration.

On a properly positioned frontal chest radiograph the spinous processes of the dorsal vertebrae should be along a straight imaginary line drawn midway between the clavicular heads. Radiographic penetration should allow faint visualization of vertebral bodies and intervening disk spaces, the lung parenchyma should be at mid-gray level and the pulmonary vessels should be easily seen. Motion is detected by assessing the sharpness of the outline of the superior ribs, margins of vessels and diaphragm. Adequate inspiratory effort is indicated by noting the position of top of right hemidiaphragm with respect to the ribs, this should correspond to the sixth anterior rib or tenth posterior rib in mid clavicular line **(Fig. 1)**.[1]

For the chest radiograph PA view the exposure time should not exceed 40 msec.[12] A high-kV technique (120–150 kVp) should be employed. As the coefficients of X-ray absorption of bone and soft tissue approximate each other in the higher kV ranges, radiographic visibility of the bony thorax is reduced with only a slight change in the overall visibility of lung. The penetration of the mediastinum is also better allowing better visualization of the retrocardiac region and the mediastinal lines and interfaces. A high-kV also results in lower radiation exposure as compared to lower voltage. The disadvantage of high-kV technique is the reduced visibility of calcium due to the lower coefficient of X-ray absorption. An anti-scatter technique, i.e., grid or air gap should be used which reduces scatter at least as much as a 10:1 grid (preferably 12:1 grid). In the air gap technique, a space of 15 cm is interposed between the patient and image detector, allowing the scattered radiation to dissipate in the air. The focal film distance should be 10 feet when this technique is used. The effective radiation dose for a digital chest radiograph is 0.1 mSv while the effective radiation dose for a conventional chest radiograph is 0.02 mSv.

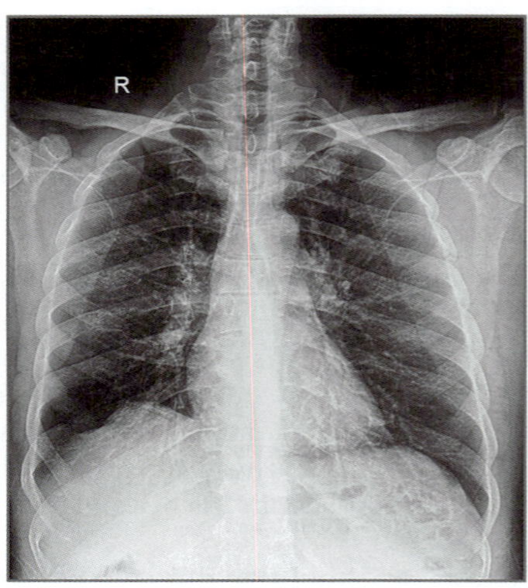

FIG. 1: Normal chest radiograph: Posteroanterior (PA) view, note made of diaphragmatic hump: normal variant.

Anteroposterior View

If a patient is unable to stand erect such as critically ill patients, those in emergency department, elderly frail patients and small children, an anteroposterior (AP) chest radiograph is obtained. The AP view should be interpreted with caution as the mediastinum and cardiac shadow are magnified, patient is unable to take a full inspiration in supine position and there may be rotation. The magnification in the AP view occurs as there is a shortened distance between the X-ray tube and the image detector compared to the standard 180 cm for the PA view. This results in a diverging X-ray beam at the margins of the heart, and the heart and mediastinum are situated further from the image detector than in a PA view **(Fig. 2)**. The differences between PA and AP chest radiographs are listed in **Table 1**.

The other radiographic projections include the lateral view, decubitus view, lordotic view and oblique view. With the wide availability of ultrasonography and cross-sectional imaging techniques, these views are seldom performed in current practice.

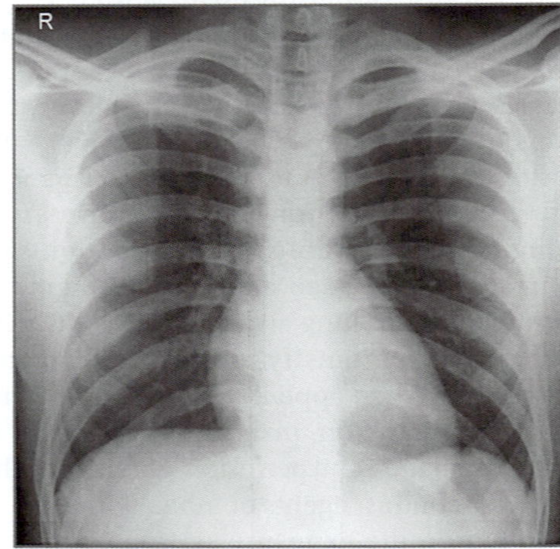

FIG. 2: Chest radiograph: Anteroposterior (AP) view, note the scapulae projecting over the lung fields.

TABLE 1: Difference between the posteroanterior (PA) and anteroposterior (AP) chest radiographs.

PA view	AP view
Scapulae seen in the periphery of thorax	Scapulae project over lung fields
Clavicles project over lung fields	Clavicles are above the apex of lung fields
Posterior ribs are distinct	Anterior ribs are distinct
Fundic air fluid level is seen	Fundic air fluid level is not seen
Cardiac magnification is less	Cardiac magnification is more
Body of vertebrae better visible	Spinous processes are better visible

Lateral View

The lateral view helps in localization of different lobes and segments of the lung. A right or left lateral view may be performed depending upon the area of interest. To obtain the lateral radiograph the arms are held high and away from the patient, if the patient is frail or elderly the arms can be positioned in front of the chest. The side of the patient is turned toward the image detector.

On a lateral chest radiograph, the vertebral bodies should become blacker from above downwards. Both domes of diaphragm should be well-defined and clearly visible, the right dome is seen from front to back, while the left dome disappears anteriorly as it merges with the heart. The diaphragm of the side closer to the detector is more sharply defined. The outline of the overlapping hila should be well defined. There should not be any abrupt change in density across the cardiac shadow. The retrosternal and retrocardiac areas show increased translucency **(Figs. 3A and B)**. The lateral view should always be assessed along with the frontal chest radiograph.[13]

Oblique View

Pleural-pulmonary interfaces that differ from the direction of the projecting X-rays in the PA and lateral views are not properly visualized and oblique views may be needed in such cases. The optimal oblique projection for visualizing the interface in question (tangential view) can be assessed by means of fluoroscopy. The left posteroanterior oblique view is useful in demonstration of trachea and its divisions.[13] **Figure 4** shows a right oblique view of the chest.

Lordotic View

Apical lesions, right middle lobe and lingular abnormalities may be better demonstrated on a lordotic view than on a normal PA projection. This view is obtained by making the patient lean backwards in lordotic position or more commonly with cranial tilt of X-ray tube. **Figure 5A** shows a lordotic view of the chest.

Apicogram

An apicogram was used to evaluate the upper lung fields, particularly the apices. It was commonly used to diagnose conditions like tuberculosis, lung tumors (e.g., Pancoast tumor), and other diseases affecting the upper lobes of the lungs. It can be done in the AP or PA projection. **Figure 5B** shows an apicogram of the chest.

Decubitus View

In a lateral decubitus view, the patient is positioned with one side of the thorax (right or left) in a dependent position.

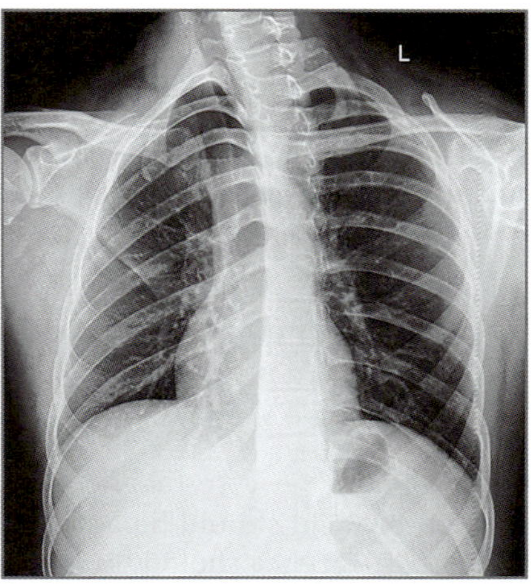

FIG. 4: Right oblique view of normal chest.

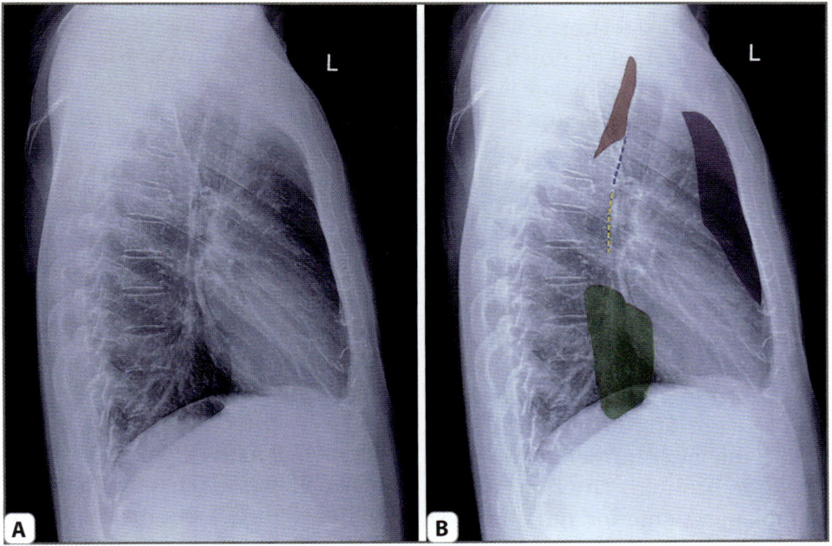

FIGS. 3A AND B: Left lateral radiograph of the chest (A), retrosternal, retrotracheal and retrocardiac spaces marked in purple, red and green, posterior tracheal stripe and posterior wall of bronchus intermedius marked in blue and yellow doted lines respectively (B).

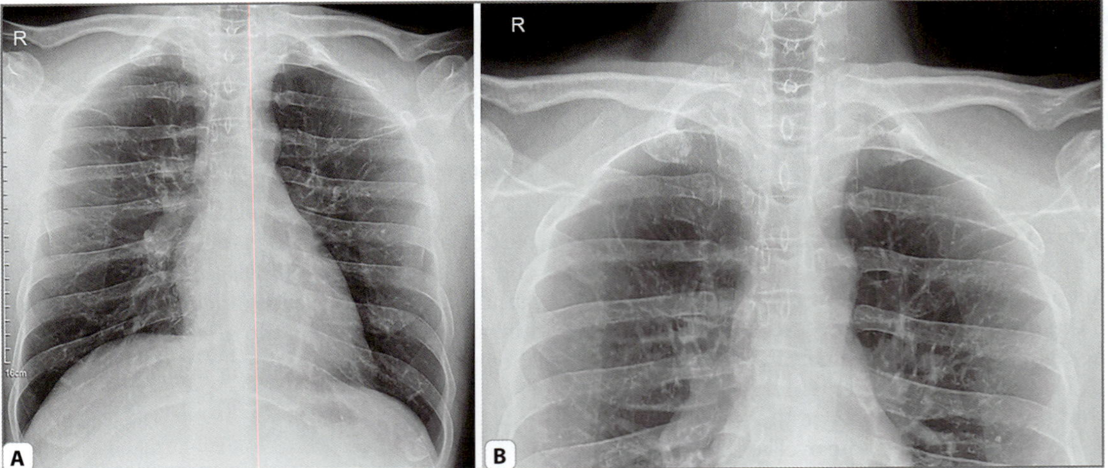

FIGS. 5A AND B: Lordotic view of chest (A) and apicogram (B).

The view is labeled based on the side of the chest that is dependent. Thus, an X-ray obtained with the patient positioned with the left side of the thorax in a dependent position is a "left lateral decubitus" view. The cross-table lateral decubitus views are helpful in visualization of small pleural effusions or pneumothorax.[13]

NORMAL ANATOMY ON THE CHEST RADIOGRAPH

Airways

The trachea and bronchi should be assessed for size, patency and course. Trachea should be seen in midline in the upper part and can be deviated to the right side around the aortic knuckle. In adults the coronal diameters of the trachea are 21 and 25 mm in females and males respectively and sagittal diameters are 23 and 27 mm in females and males respectively.[14] The right tracheal margin (right paratracheal stripe) can be tracked down to the right main bronchus, it is 4 mm or less in thickness and is measured above the azygos vein. The left paratracheal line is rarely visualized. Tracheal narrowing may be focal (after prolonged intubation) or diffuse [can be seen with chronic obstructive pulmonary disease (COPD), saber-sheath trachea where there is narrowing of the transverse diameter of the tracheal lumen].

The trachea divides into the right and left main bronchi at the level of D5 vertebra in adults. The left main bronchus is longer and has a more acute angle with the trachea as compared to the right main bronchus. The right main bronchus divides into the right upper lobe bronchus and bronchus intermedius, the latter further divides into right middle and lower lobe bronchi. The right upper lobe bronchus divides into apical, anterior and posterior segmental bronchi. The middle lobe bronchus divides into medial and lateral branches while the lower lobe bronchus divides into superior, anterior basal, lateral basal, medial basal and posterior basal segmental bronchi. The left main bronchus divides into the upper and lower lobe bronchi. The left upper lobe bronchus has two divisions, the upper division divides into the apicoposterior and anterior branches while the lower division divides into superior and inferior branches which supply the lingula. The left lower lobe bronchus divides into the superior, anteromedial basal, lateral basal and posterior basal segments.

Lungs

The right lung is divided into three lobes and the left lung is divided into two lobes, separated by the interlobar fissures. The major (oblique) fissures on both sides are similar in structure. These fissures run obliquely, slanting forward and downward, with the upper portion facing forward and laterally, and the lower portion facing backward and medially, passing through the hilum. In a lateral view, the fissure begins at the level of the fourth or fifth thoracic vertebra and extends down to the diaphragm, about 5 cm behind the costophrenic angle on the left side and just behind the costophrenic angle on the right side. The right lung has an additional fissure, the minor (horizontal) fissure which separates the middle lobe from the right upper lobe and can be traced on a chest PA film from the right hilum to the sixth rib in the axillary line **(Figs. 6 and 7)**.

Occasionally, accessory fissures can be observed. The azygos lobe fissure is commonly seen on the right side, with an incidence of around 0.4%. This fissure appears as a fine line with slight lateral convexity running across the right upper zone, ending in a comma-like expansion (the azygos vein) near the hilum. The azygos lobe refers to the lung area medial to this fissure. On the left side, the horizontal fissure, similar to the minor fissure on the right, separates the lingula from the rest of the upper lobe segments. Additionally, the superior accessory fissure divides the apical from the basal segments of the lower lobes, while

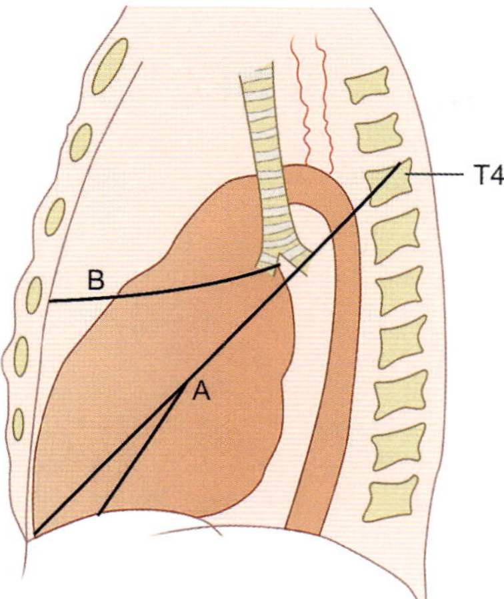

FIG. 6: Diagram showing major (A) and minor (B) fissure on lateral projection of the chest.

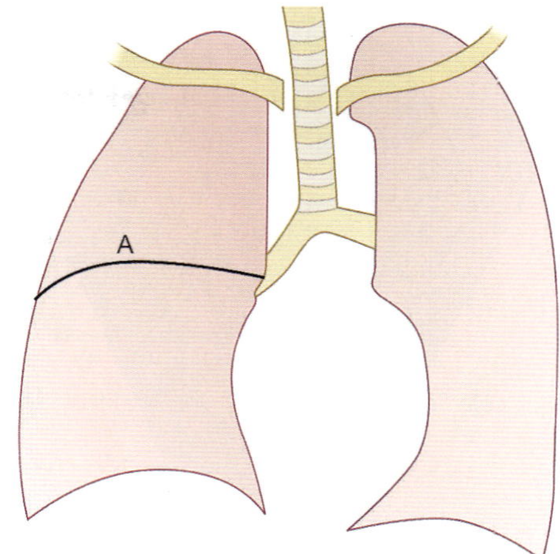

FIG. 7: Diagram showing minor fissure (A) on frontal projection of the chest.

the inferior accessory fissure separates the medial basal segment from the other basal segments.

The lung is divided into lobes and subsequently into multiple bronchopulmonary segments. These segments are functionally independent unit of the lung supplied by their own segmental bronchus and pulmonary artery and have their own venous and lymphatic drainage **(Fig. 8)**. The bronchopulmonary segments may be affected by diseases or be resected during surgical procedures. Knowledge about these anatomical divisions of lungs is essential for detection and localization of pathology and communication to pulmonologists or surgeons. **Table 2** lists the bronchopulmonary segments of the lungs. The lung can be divided into upper, mid and lower zones on the frontal chest radiograph by drawing lines along the anterior ends of 2nd and 4th ribs, the zone above the 2nd rib is taken as upper zone, mid zone is between 2nd and 4th ribs and lower zone is below the 4th rib **(Fig. 9)**.

Hila and Pulmonary Vasculature

The hilum is formed by the pulmonary artery and its main branches, upper lobe pulmonary veins, major bronchi and lymph glands, although only the pulmonary artery and upper lobe veins significantly contribute to the radiographic density of the hilum. In normal chest radiographs, the right hilum is lower than the left in 97% of cases, while the hila may be at the same level in 3% of cases.[1] Any deviation from this expected relationship may indicate volume loss on the affected side, which could be due to atelectasis, scarring, or previous lung resection. Both the hila are of equal density and show a concave lateral border.

The normal diameter of the descending branch of the right pulmonary artery ranges from 10–16 mm in males and 9–15 mm in females. Pulmonary vessels can be categorized into three zones based on their location in the lungs: hilar, mid-lung, and peripheral. The mid-lung vessels extend from the hilum to about 2 cm from the chest wall, while peripheral vessels occupy the remaining 2 cm of the lung fields and are typically not visible on a normal chest radiograph. Pulmonary veins have fewer branches and follow a straighter path. The distinction between intrapulmonary arteries and veins is often challenging and generally not clinically significant, so both are referred to collectively as the pulmonary vasculature. As the vessels extend peripherally, they gradually taper. On upright PA chest radiographs, vessels in the upper lung zones appear narrower than those in the lower zones due to the effects of gravity. Bronchial vessels are normally not visible on a chest radiograph.

Pleura

The normal pleura is not visualized on chest radiographs. Occasionally, the mediastinal surface of the pleura may be seen near the midline in a well-penetrated chest radiograph. The costophrenic and cardiophrenic angles should be sharp and well-defined. Pleural abnormalities manifest radiographically as pneumothorax or pleural effusion in the pleural space, or as abnormalities of the pleural surfaces, including thickening (pleural plaques, neoplasms) and calcification (pleural plaques, fibrothorax).[1]

Mediastinum

The mediastinum is the space located between the pleural reflections of the mediastinal pleura, bounded anteriorly by the sternum and posteriorly by the thoracic vertebrae. It extends from the thoracic inlet superiorly to the diaphragm inferiorly. This area contains the heart, pericardium, major central vessels, esophagus, trachea, carina, proximal main stem bronchi, thoracic duct, lymph nodes, and mediastinal fat. For accurate detection of mediastinal abnormalities on radiographs, the radiologist must be well-acquainted with the normal anatomy of the mediastinal structures, their contours and the mediastinal lines, stripes and interfaces.

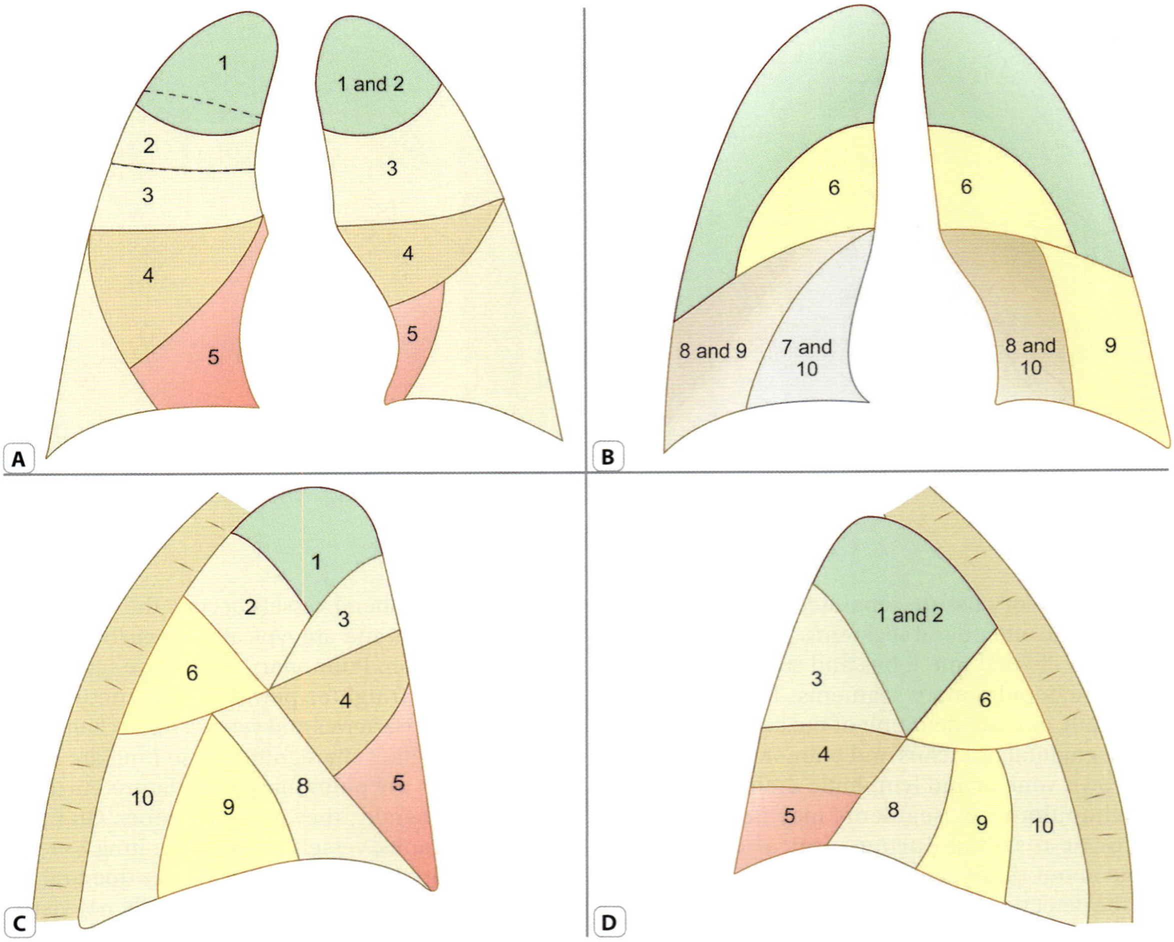

FIGS. 8A TO D: Diagram showing the bronchopulmonary segments on frontal (A and B) and right lateral (C) and left lateral (D) projections of the chest.

TABLE 2: Bronchopulmonary segments.

Right lung		Left lung	
Upper lobe	• Apical • Posterior • Anterior	Upper lobe	• Apicoposterior • Anterior
Middle lobe	• Lateral • Medial	Lingula	• Superior • Inferior
Lower lobe	• Superior • Medial basal • Anterior basal • Lateral basal • Posterior basal	Lower lobe	• Superior • Anteromedial basal • Lateral basal • Posterior basal

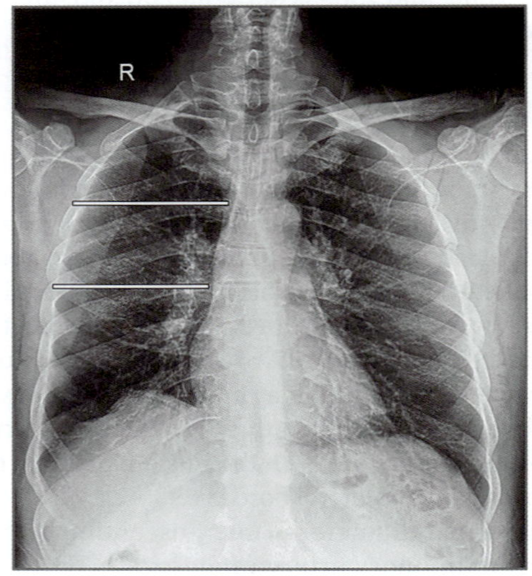

FIG. 9: Division of the lung fields into upper, mid and lower zones by drawing lines along the anterior aspect of 2nd and 4th ribs.

On lateral chest radiograph, the mediastinum can be divided into anterior, middle and posterior compartments. The anterior and middle compartments can be separated by an imaginary line anterior to the trachea and posterior to the heart and inferior vena cava. The middle and posterior compartments are separated by an imaginary line passing 1 cm posterior to the anterior border of the vertebral bodies. This division helps to localize the disease process and narrow the differential diagnosis.

In neonates and young children, the normal thymus can be seen as a triangular sail shaped structure in the mediastinum which may show wavy outline.

Interface Lines and Stripes

The air in the lung abuts various structures in the mediastinum, where the interface is long and vertical it results in a long or slightly angled line on the chest radiograph.

- *Right paratracheal stripe* is formed by contact of the visceral and parietal pleurae of the right upper lobe with the right lateral border of the trachea. The thickness of the stripe is usually 1–4 mm. On a frontal radiograph, it extends from the level of the right clavicle to the right tracheobronchial angle. It is seen in approximately 60% of normal radiographs.
- *Left paratracheal stripe* is formed by contact between left upper lobe visceral and parietal pleurae and structures adjacent to left tracheal wall. The aortic arch and left subclavian artery with their surrounding fat are the structures in this space. It extends from the level of the aortic arch to the reflection of left subclavian artery.
- *Anterior junctional line* is formed where the two lungs abut each other anterior to the heart and pericardium, below the level of the manubrium. This line is made of four layers of pleura (i.e., the parietal and visceral layers covering both lungs).
- *Posterior junctional line* is formed where the two lungs abut each other posterior to the trachea and esophagus and extends from above the clavicles to the level of the aortic arch. This line is also made of four layers of pleura.
- *Aortopulmonary window* is formed where the left lung pleura contacts the aortic arch and left subclavian artery which results in a concave contour along the left mediastinum between the aorta and pulmonary artery silhouettes. Normal structures in the aortopulmonary window include fat, lymph nodes, left bronchial arteries, left phrenic nerve, left vagus nerve and left recurrent laryngeal nerve.
- *Descending aorta line* refers to the interface between left lateral border of descending aorta and pleural layers of left lung. This line may merge with the left paraspinal line in some patients. It extends along the length of the intrathoracic descending aorta and is noted to project over the heart inferiorly.
- *The left paraspinal line* is formed when the left lung parietal and visceral pleurae contact the posterior mediastinal fat, paraspinal muscles and soft tissues. The right paraspinal line is the interface of the paravertebral mediastinum which projects at the level of T8 through T12. The paraspinal lines are often visualized partially or sometimes not at all due to the lateral displacement of mediastinal structures like the aorta, the presence of mediastinal fat or osteophytes.
- *The azygoesophageal recess* refers to the indentation of the right lower lobe into a space bordered by the esophagus and the azygos vein. On a frontal radiograph, the boundary between the lung in the recess and the right lateral border of the esophagus forms a slightly concave, diagonal line that extends from near the midline in the subcarinal region toward the diaphragmatic hiatus on the left.[15] **Figure 10** shows the various lines and stripes on a frontal chest radiograph.

Heart

The right cardiac border is formed by the right atrium with the superior vena cava entering superiorly and the inferior vena cava at the lower margin of the right atrium, while the left cardiac border is formed by the left ventricle and a small part of the left atrial appendage, from inferior to superior, the pulmonary artery and aortic notch extend superiorly. On a lateral chest radiograph, the right ventricle appears to project anteriorly and inferiorly, while the posterior cardiac border is made up of the left ventricle inferiorly and the left atrium superiorly. Normally, two-thirds of the cardiac shadow lies to the left of midline and one-third to the right.[1]

Diaphragm

The diaphragm is a smooth domed structure, with the right hemidiaphragm slightly higher than the left

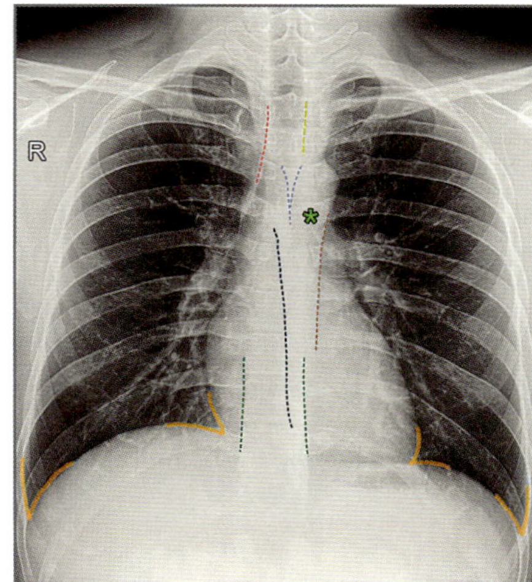

FIG. 10: Lines and stripes on a chest radiograph PA view – anterior junctional line in blue, right and left paratracheal stripes in red and yellow respectively, aortopulmonary window (green asterisk), descending aorta line in brown, azygoesophageal recess in black and paraspinal lines in green, the costophrenic and cardiophrenic angles are highlighted in yellow.

hemidiaphragm owing to the position of the heart on the left. Flattening of the dome can be assessed on a PA view by drawing a perpendicular line from the midpoint of the dome to the line connecting the costophrenic and cardiophrenic angles on the same side. Normally, this distance is greater than 1.5 cm. In about 90% of healthy individuals, the right hemidiaphragm is 1.5–2.5 cm higher than the left. In the remaining cases, the domes are at the same level, or the right diaphragm may be slightly higher. This difference in diaphragm levels is due to the position of the cardiac apex, rather than the position of the liver. A discrepancy of more than 3 cm between the two hemidiaphragms is considered significant.

EVALUATION OF THE CHEST RADIOGRAPH

The evaluation of a chest radiograph is the first step in the diagnostic process for a wide range of thoracic conditions. A systematic approach is essential to accurately assess the various structures of the chest, including the lungs, heart, mediastinum, diaphragm, and chest wall. A thorough evaluation includes assessing the overall quality and technical aspects of the image, followed by the examination of anatomical structures for signs of disease or abnormalities. The radiograph is often used to support clinical findings and guide further diagnostic testing or management. A careful and systematic analysis can reveal various pathologies, making chest radiography an invaluable tool in the diagnosis of respiratory, cardiovascular and systemic diseases.

Technical Factors

The evaluation of the chest radiograph should begin with assessment of technical factors which include patient positioning, mediastinal penetration, sharpness of structures, lung volumes and presence of any artifacts.[1] **Table 3** lists the factors for evaluating the technical adequacy of a chest radiograph.

Airways

The trachea and bronchi should be evaluated for size, patency, and alignment. Tracheal narrowing can be either focal or diffuse. Focal narrowing or stenosis is most commonly caused by mucosal or cartilaginous damage resulting from prolonged intubation while diffuse tracheal narrowing is frequently seen in patients with COPD, where there is narrowing of the transverse diameter of the tracheal lumen leading to a "saber-sheath" appearance. Tracheal dilation, as seen in Mounier–Kuhn syndrome, is a rare congenital condition characterized by the dilation of the trachea and main bronchi due to atrophy of the muscular and elastic tissues.[1]

TABLE 3: Factors for evaluating the technical adequacy of a chest radiograph.

Technical parameter	Assessment
Positioning	Rotation, scoliosis
Penetration	Visualization of intervertebral disk spaces
Motion	Sharpness of hemidiaphragm, ribs, vessels
Lung volumes	Position of diaphragm relative to ribs
Artifacts	Detector drops, grid lines

Primary or metastatic airway tumors may present as endoluminal soft tissue nodules, sometimes associated with volume loss. Endotracheal tumors can grow large enough to obstruct up to 75% of the airway lumen before symptoms develop.

The trachea may be displaced toward an area of upper lobe volume loss, such as in upper lobe fibrosis, or pushed aside by a mass in the thoracic inlet, like an enlarged thyroid. The normal carinal angle is acute, widening of the carinal angle can be seen due to enlargement of the left atrium and lymphadenopathy.

Bronchiectasis refers to the abnormal, irreversible dilation of the bronchi, which can result from infections, cystic fibrosis, primary ciliary dyskinesia, or allergic bronchopulmonary fungal disease. On radiographs, bronchiectasis appears as tram-track signs, indicating thickened bronchial walls in cylindrical bronchiectasis, and clustered, thin-walled cystic lesions in cystic bronchiectasis **(Fig. 11)**.

Lungs

Volume

The lung volume may be increased in obstructive diseases such as emphysema and reduced in restrictive diseases like pulmonary fibrosis. Reduced volume may also be seen in patients with neuromuscular diseases (myasthenia gravis, diaphragmatic dysfunction) or extrathoracic disorders (ascites, obesity).

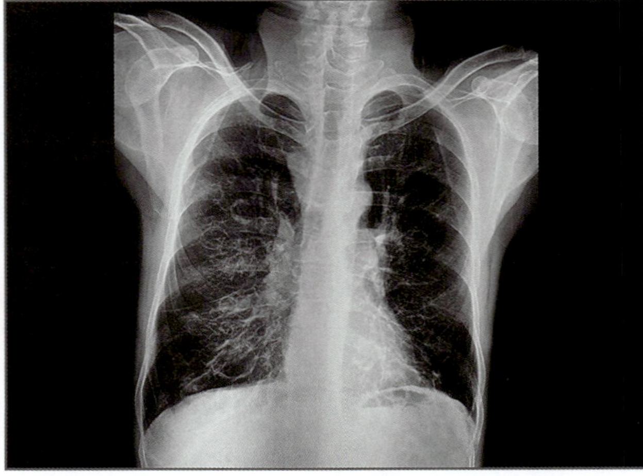

FIG. 11: Frontal chest radiograph shows cystic bronchiectatic changes in bilateral lungs.

Atelectasis

Atelectasis is a partial or complete collapse of the lung. It can be caused by loss of negative pressure in the pleural space and/or by compression of lung parenchyma, by resorption of air following obstruction, or by an increase in alveolar surface tension. The natural tendency of the lung to collapse is opposed by the recoil of the chest wall outwards caused by the contraction of inspiratory muscles and diaphragm. Atelectasis can result due to mechanisms that interfere directly or indirectly with lung expansion. It can be divided into six types: (1) resorptive, (2) adhesive, (3) compressive, (4) passive, (5) cicatrization, and (6) gravity dependent.[16]

When the lung is compressed by any space occupying lesion in the thorax such as pneumothorax, pleural effusion or a mass lesion in the pleural cavity, compressive atelectasis results. The distinction between compressive and passive atelectasis is not well-defined, any space occupying lesion in the thorax may compress the lung or lead to passive retraction of the lung.

The most common form of atelectasis is caused by the resorption of gas from the alveoli.[17] When there is partial or total obstruction to flow of air from tracheobronchial tree to the alveoli, with inadequate air filling by collateral pathways, resorption atelectasis results. The lung becomes devoid of air within 24 hours of bronchial obstruction. Resorption atelectasis occurs rapidly when the patient is breathing pure oxygen as it is quickly absorbed from the alveoli. Mucous impaction in subsegmental bronchus and bronchiolitis obliterans due to repeated infections in early life can result in resorption atelectasis. It is also seen commonly after surgery and general anesthesia.[18]

When the compliance of the lung decreases because of it being diseased due to fibrosis, cicatrization atelectasis can develop. It is often associated with bronchiectasis. Cicatrization atelectasis can be seen with many conditions such as idiopathic pulmonary fibrosis, sarcoidosis, chronic tubercular and fungal infections and collagen vascular diseases.

When there is deficiency of alveolar surfactant along with other coexistent factors, then even in the presence of a patent airway, atelectasis can occur. This is referred to as "non-obstructive" atelectasis or adhesive atelectasis. It is characteristically seen in respiratory distress syndrome of the newborn. It may also be seen in acute respiratory distress syndrome (ARDS), acute radiation pneumonitis and in postoperative patients.[18]

Gravity dependent atelectasis can occur in bedridden patients with shallow breathing. Gravity dependent alterations in alveolar volume may aggravate atelectasis in dependent parts of the lung.

"Plate like atelectasis" are the common linear opacities seen on a chest radiograph. These are usually 1–3 mm in thickness, 4–10 cm in length and are seen in the mid and lower lung zones. These shadows may be horizontal or oblique, single or multiple, unilateral or bilateral. These linear opacities are associated with diseases that limit diaphragmatic excursion, a frequent contributing factor being intra-abdominal disease (such as inflammatory conditions, ascites, etc.).

Direct and Indirect Signs of Collapse

The signs of lobar atelectasis are seen due to the opacity of a given lobe and the volume loss that results.[19-21] There can be direct and indirect signs. Direct evidence of presence of collapse can be inferred by displacement of lobar fissures which is the most reliable sign. Crowding of vessels and bronchi in a lobe can help in diagnosis if displacement of fissures is not apparent. Increased density of an atelectatic part of the lung usually becomes apparent when the collapse is almost complete.

Other indirect signs that may help us to suspect underlying collapse include elevation of part of diaphragm or hemidiaphragm usually seen in lower lobe collapse, whereas upper lobe collapse may be inferred by tracheal or upper mediastinal displacement. Lower lobe collapse may also be associated with cardiac displacement **(Fig. 12)**. Hilar displacement may also point to underlying collapse of lung. This is usually more evident with upper lobe collapse than with lower lobe collapse **(Fig. 13)**. Reduction of intercostal spaces with resultant rib crowding may occasionally be seen with chronic processes and old collapse. A change in the site of a parenchymal lesion, as seen after comparison with previous images, may result from atelectasis and is referred to as the "shifting granuloma sign".

Compensatory hyperinflation of adjoining lung can also be seen with collapsed lung. The hyperinflation may occur over a prolonged period of time and may involve adjacent lobe or entire lung. There is resultant mediastinal displacement with paucity and spread-out vascular markings when compared to contralateral lung. When a large portion of a lung becomes atelectatic, the tendency is greater for overinflation to involve the contralateral lung; this may progress to the stage in which the opposite

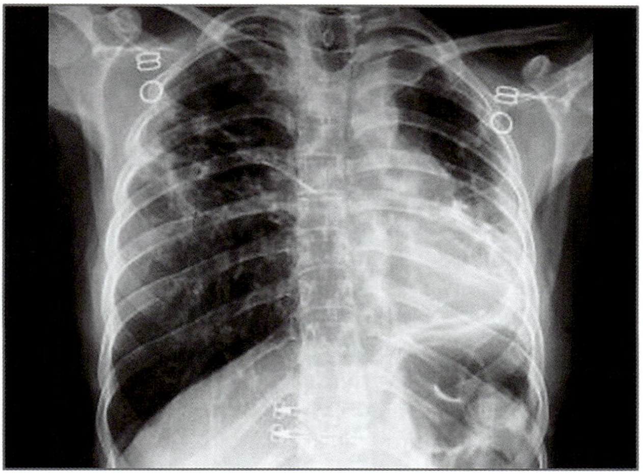

FIG. 12: Left lower lobe collapse with elevated left hemidiaphragm and ipsilateral mediastinal shift along with nodular and few fibronodular opacities in right lung field.

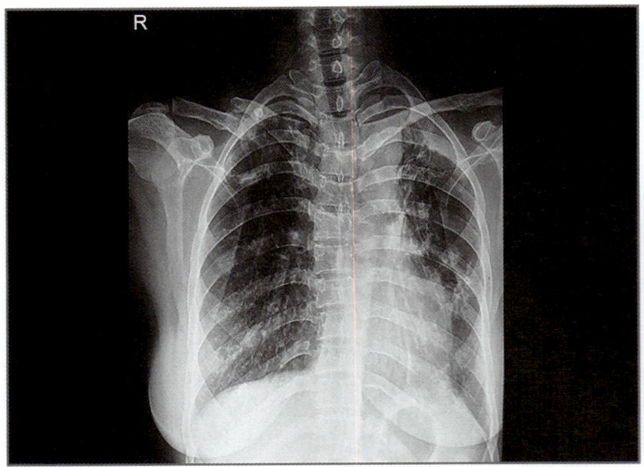

FIG. 13: Left upper lobe collapse with mild ipsilateral tracheal shift, pulled up left hilum and juxtaphrenic peak of left hemidiaphragm, note made of old clavicular fractures bilaterally.

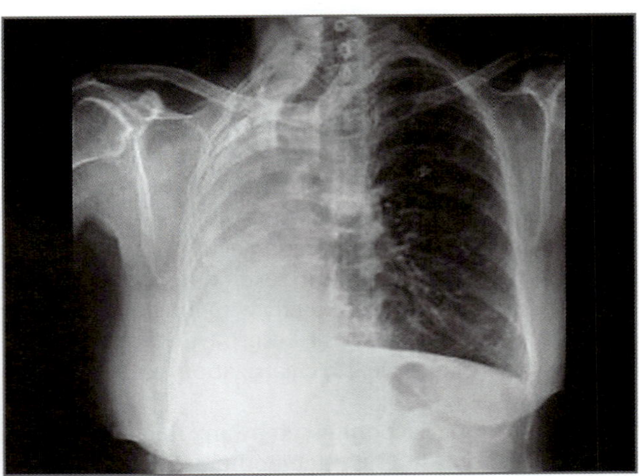

FIG. 14: Opaque right hemithorax with ipsilateral tracheo-mediastinal shift and compensatory hyperinflation of left lung—Complete right lung collapse.

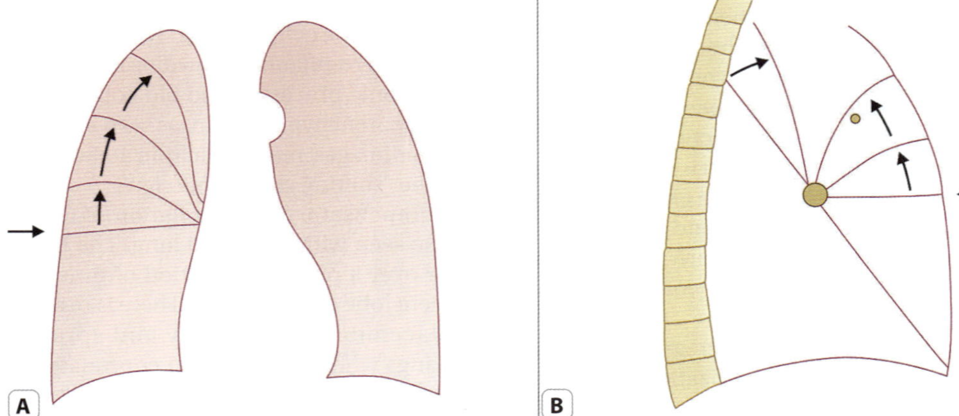

FIGS. 15A AND B: Right upper lobe collapse PA (A) and lateral (B) views: Horizontal fissure is drawn upward and curves toward the apex and mediastinum on PA view. On the lateral view there is upward displacement of the horizontal fissure with forward displacement of the oblique fissure above the hilum.

lung displaces the mediastinum either generally or locally **(Fig. 14)**.

Local displacements occur in the three areas of the mediastinum, where the two lungs are separated only by loose connective tissue: (1) the anterior mediastinal compartment, at the level of the first three or four costal cartilages, limited anteriorly by the sternum and posteriorly by the great vessels; (2) the posterosuperior mediastinum, at the level of the third to fifth thoracic vertebrae, limited anteriorly by the esophagus and trachea and posteriorly by the vertebral column; and (3) the posteroinferior mediastinum, limited anteriorly by the heart and posteriorly by the vertebral column and aorta.

Lobar Atelectasis

Right upper lobe collapse: As the right upper lobe collapses, the lateral end of the horizontal fissure moves upward and medially toward the superior mediastinum and the anterior end moves upward toward the apex. The upper half of the oblique fissure moves anteriorly **(Figs. 15A and B)**.[22] Other radiographic findings associated with right upper lobe collapse include increased density in the upper thorax, silhouetting of the upper mediastinum, mediastinal widening, ipsilateral tracheal shift, elevated hilum, outward rotation of hilum or bronchus and juxtaphrenic peak **(Fig. 16)**. The "Golden's S sign" is seen with right upper lobe collapse due to a centrally located mass **(Fig. 17)**. The superiorly displaced, lateral and concave aspect of the "S" is formed by the minor fissure, while the inferiorly and medially located convex part is formed by the margin of the mass.[23]

Right middle lobe collapse: It is seen as an increased density of the lung silhouetting the right heart border and the minor

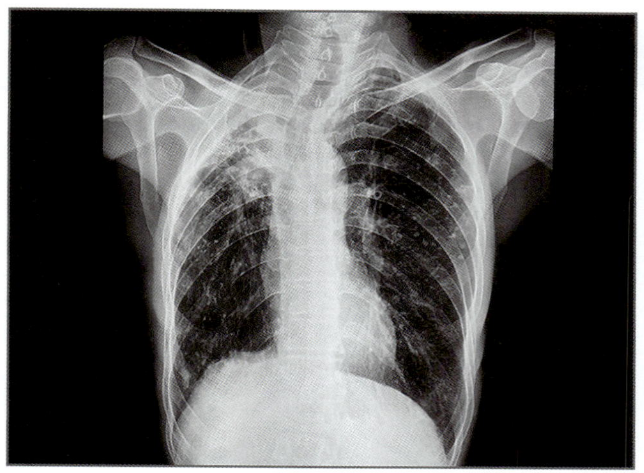

FIG. 16: Right upper lobe collapse with ipsilateral tracheal shift and pulled up right hilum. Multiple nodular calcific opacities are seen in bilateral lungs.

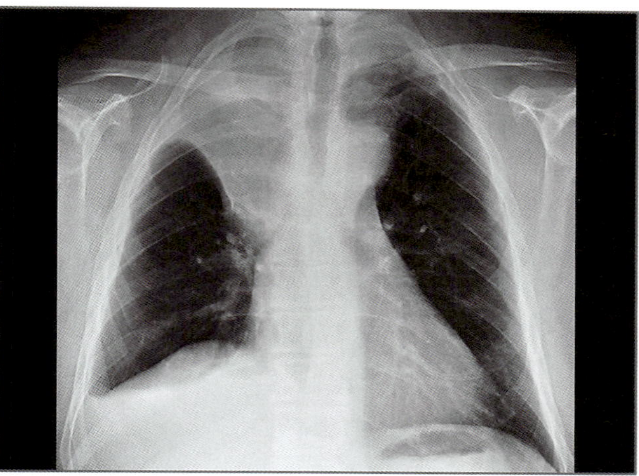

FIG. 17: Golden's S sign—centrally located mass causing right upper lobe collapse.

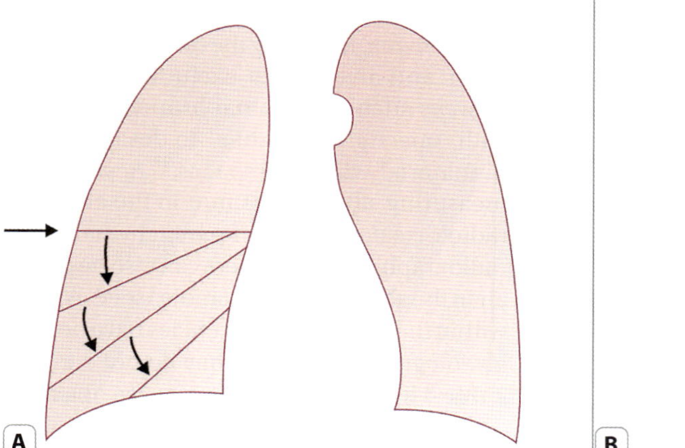

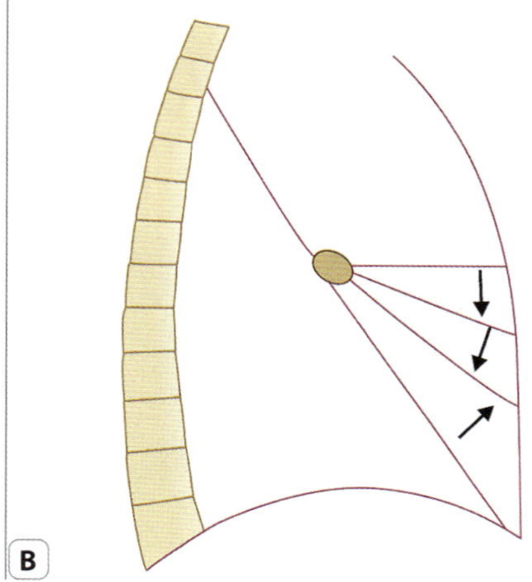

FIGS. 18A AND B: Right middle lobe collapse PA (A) and lateral (B) views: The horizontal fissure is displaced downwards on both views, on the lateral view there is forward displacement of the lower part of the oblique fissure.

fissure is invisible. In this condition, the horizontal fissure and lower half of the oblique fissure move toward each other (**Figs. 18A and B**).

Left upper lobe collapse: It is seen as a hazy opacity in upper, mid and sometimes lower zones. Pulmonary vessels in the hyperinflated lower lobe are seen through the haze. On the lateral radiograph, it is seen as an elongated opacity extending from the apex and reaching the diaphragm. In left upper lobe collapse, there is vertical positioning and anterior and medial displacement of the major fissure (**Figs. 19A and B**). Migration of the superior segment of the left lower lobe superiorly and anteriorly between the arch of the aorta and the collapsed lobe causes a crescent-shaped radiolucency around the aortic arch which is known as the "**Luftsichel sign**" (**Fig. 20**).[24]

Lower lobe collapse: In lower lobe collapse, there is posterior and medial displacement of the oblique fissure. It is seen as a triangular density in the retrocardiac location on a frontal radiograph, downward displacement of the hilum is seen (**Figs. 21 and 22**).[25] The lower lobe pulmonary artery is also obscured on the frontal radiographs. The diaphragmatic contour is obscured, and shift of the heart or mediastinum becomes apparent (**Fig. 23**). The "flat waist sign"[26] can be seen with left lower lobe collapse where there is straightening of the left heart margin, aorta and pulmonary artery. With severe left lower lobe collapse the outline of the superior aortic knuckle may not be seen. On the lateral radiograph, lower lobe collapse may cause partial obscuration of the hemidiaphragm in its posterior aspect and the vertebral column appears to be progressively dense inferiorly.

Parenchymal Opacities

Parenchymal opacities include air space and interstitial opacities.

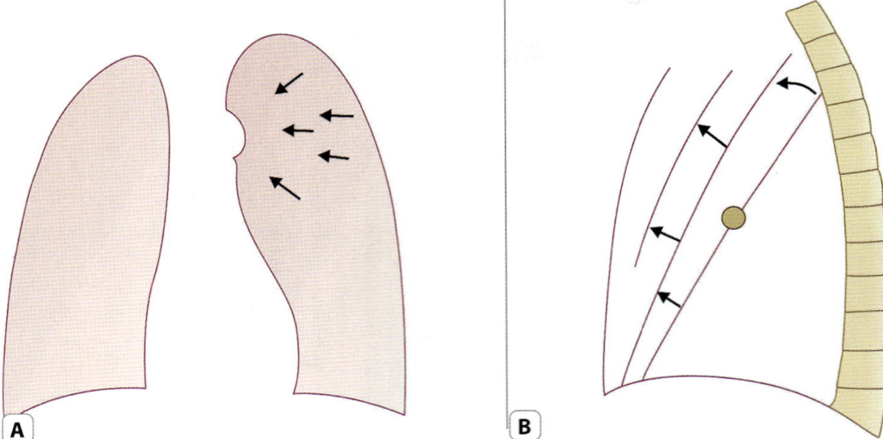

FIGS. 19A AND B: Left upper lobe collapse on PA (A) and lateral (B) views: Increased density is seen with increasing severity of collapse on PA view. The fissure moves forward on lateral view.

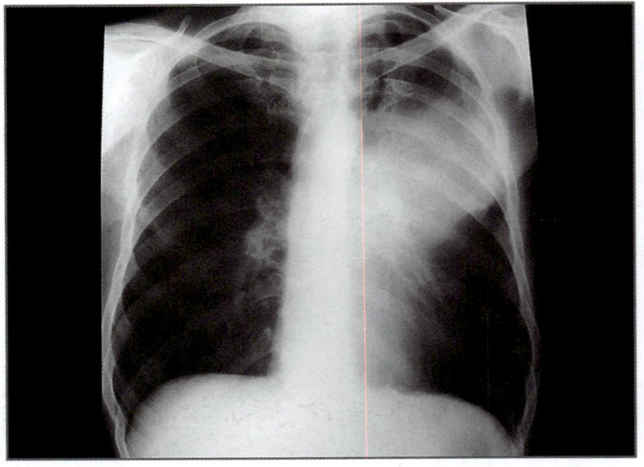

FIG. 20: Luftsichel sign—crescent of hyperlucency seen in para-aortic location in left upper lobe collapse.

Airspace Opacity

Air space is the air- or gas-containing part of the lung parenchyma, including the respiratory bronchioles, alveolar ducts and alveoli, but excluding the purely conductive airways such as terminal bronchioles. This term is used with "opacity" or "nodule" to designate the accumulation of material within airspaces.[27] A small nodular opacity measuring about 4–10 mm in the alveoli may be the first radiological evidence of parenchymal pathology on chest radiograph (**Fig. 24**). There can also be presence of remnant air in the alveoli and bronchioles seen as tiny radiolucencies within the nodule. The lucencies have been referred to as air alveolograms, although they do not correspond to alveoli. **Table 4** lists the causes of air space opacification.

Coalescence

Rapid dissemination of fluid through the collateral pathways of the lung into adjacent airspaces results in ill-defined

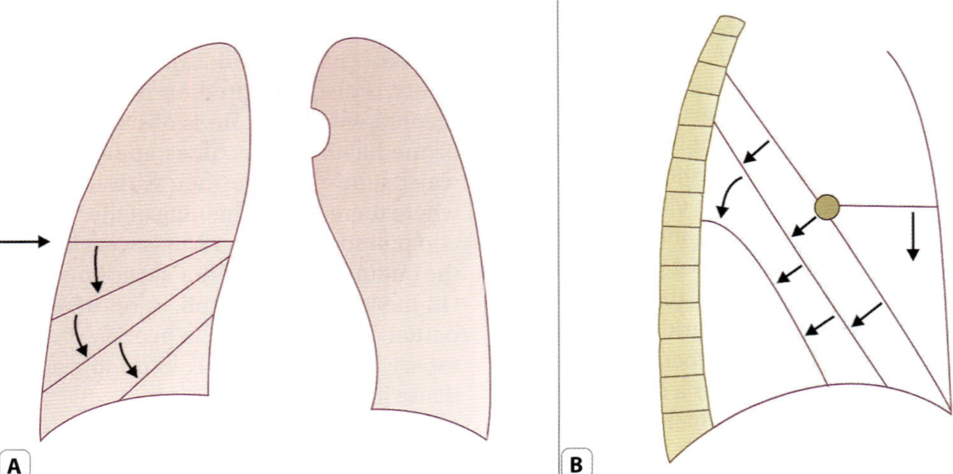

FIGS. 21A AND B: Right lower lobe collapse on PA (A) and lateral (B) views: Downward displacement of horizontal fissure is noted on PA view. The oblique fissure is displaced backwards on lateral view.

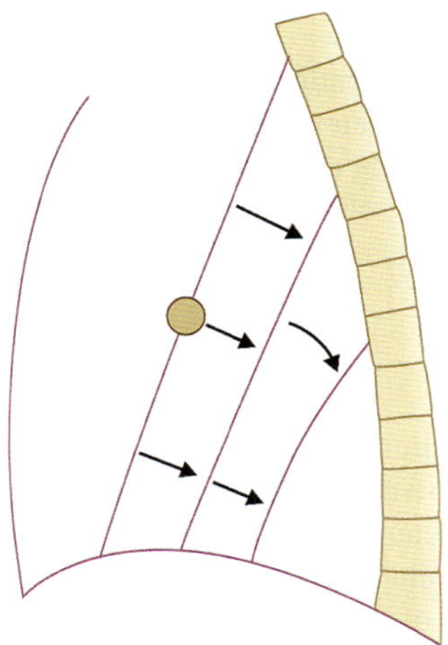

FIG. 22: Left lower lobe collapse on lateral view: No fissure is seen on the PA projection. Lateral view shows the oblique fissure to be displaced posteriorly.

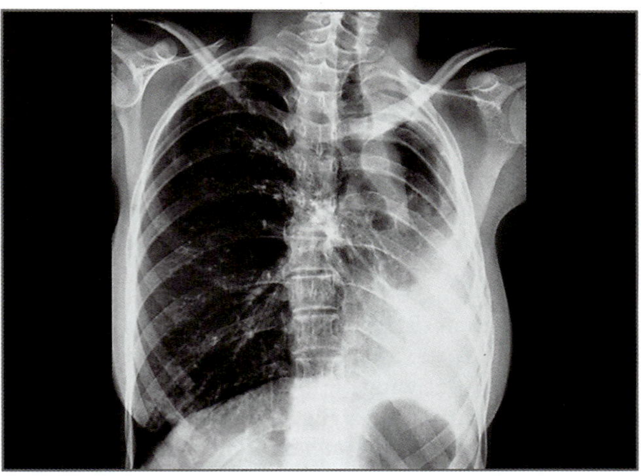

FIG. 23: Near complete collapse of the left lung with ipsilateral tracheomediastinal shift, obscured cardiac margins and left hemidiaphragm. Compensatory hyperinflation of right lung is seen which appears hyperlucent, few calcified granulomas are also seen in right lung.

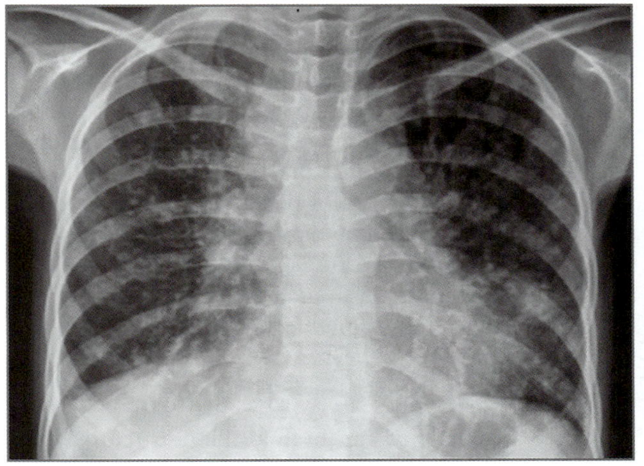

FIG. 24: Multiple nodular air space opacities in bilateral lungs with areas of coalescence in left lower zone.

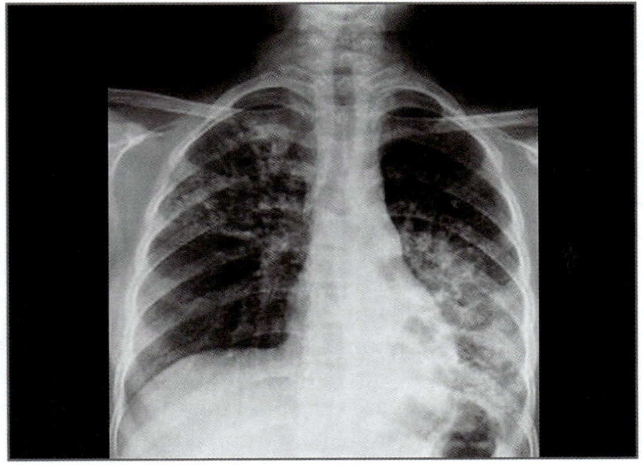

FIG. 25: Confluent air space opacities in right upper, bilateral mid and left lower zones with areas of breakdown in left retrocardiac region.

TABLE 4: Differential diagnosis of air space opacification.

Air space opacification	Disease
Focal or segmental	Pneumonia, contusion, infarct, lung adenocarcinoma
Lobar	Pneumonia, lung adenocarcinoma
Diffuse	Pulmonary edema, hemorrhage, pneumonia
Perihilar	Pulmonary edema, hemorrhage
Peripheral	Eosinophilic pneumonia, organizing pneumonia, acute respiratory distress syndrome, contusions
Rapidly changing/ resolving	Edema, eosinophilic pneumonia, hemorrhage

margins of air space opacities. Asymmetric involvement of the lung results in an irregular area of consolidation with ill-defined margins (**Fig. 25**).

Distribution Characteristics

Rapid spread of fluid or infection results in early coalescence of airspace opacities leading to widespread consolidation, which is characteristically non-segmental in distribution, seen typically in pyogenic infections. Lack of segmental distribution is also seen with acute pulmonary edema. This is in stark contrast to segmental distribution observed in diseases spread through tracheobronchial route like aspiration pneumonias or those through hematogenous route like infarcts. The area of lung involvement in aspiration pneumonias depends on the patient's position at the time of aspiration.

Only certain diseases and not others appear to respect acinar boundaries. This is likely due to the viscosity of the consolidating medium. The inflammatory edema caused by some organisms, e.g., *Streptococcus pneumoniae*, is of low viscosity and therefore spreads rapidly via interalveolar pores, whereas that of others, such as *Mycobacterium tuberculosis*, may be of sufficient viscosity to prevent such ready dissemination.

Margination

The edge characteristics of airspace processes show poor margination. An example of the phenomenon is the "butterfly" or "bat wing" appearance of acute airspace edema or hemorrhage (**Fig. 26**). However, in acute diplococcal or *Klebsiella pneumoniae*, as the infection is propagated by centrifugal spread, the advancing margin of consolidation is sometimes smooth and sharply defined (**Fig. 27**). When consolidation extends up to a pleural surface it may appear lobar.

Air Bronchogram

Presence of remnant air within the bronchi and its branches within the parenchymal opacity gives the radiologically important "air-bronchogram" sign. These bronchi stand out in contrast to opacified lung due to fluid or tissue filled alveolar spaces. It is important to remember that for air-bronchogram to be present, the bronchi need to be patent. The parenchyma may be airless when its air has been replaced by liquid or tissue (consolidation) or when it has been absorbed and not replaced (atelectasis). This sign originally described by Fleischner in 1927, was named the air bronchogram sign by Felson. It is most frequently encountered in pneumonia and pulmonary edema. Lung adenocarcinoma, lymphoma, alveolar hemorrhage, fibrosis due to radiation and sarcoidosis can also present with this sign. In some diseases like pulmonary infarction, air bronchogram may be only temporary because of early filling of airway by blood or exudate.

Time Factor

The airspace opacification persisting for prolonged periods of time usually indicates persistent pathologies like infection and neoplasm (lung adenocarcinoma and lymphoma) as opposed to rapidly clearing or evolving opacities as seen in pulmonary edema, which clear with treatment of underlying heart failure.

Nodule

A **nodule** is a circumscribed, typically round opacity, less than or equal to 3 cm in average diameter. A rounded lesion <6 mm in diameter is a micronodule. Nodules can be round, ovoid or polygonal in shape. The margin of the nodule can be well defined or ill defined, depending on the appearance of the interface with the surrounding lung. Irregular borders can be lobulated with lobule like projections or spiculated with multiple radiating small sharp projections. Linear components extending from the nodule to a pleural surface are called pleural tags.[27]

Mass

A mass is any circumscribed lesion > 3 cm in diameter. The term refers to a predominantly solid soft tissue structure but cavitary, cystic or calcified components may present to various degrees. There may be distortion or invasion of adjacent structures.[27] An intrapulmonary mass tends to be more sharply defined and forms an acute angle with the surrounding lung parenchyma while a mass originating from the pleural space or extrapleurally displaces the pleura and underlying lung inward, such that the angle formed by the margins of the mass and the chest wall is obtuse.

Cavitation

A cavity is an abnormal gas- or fluid-filled structure with a typically thick and often irregular wall, usually produced

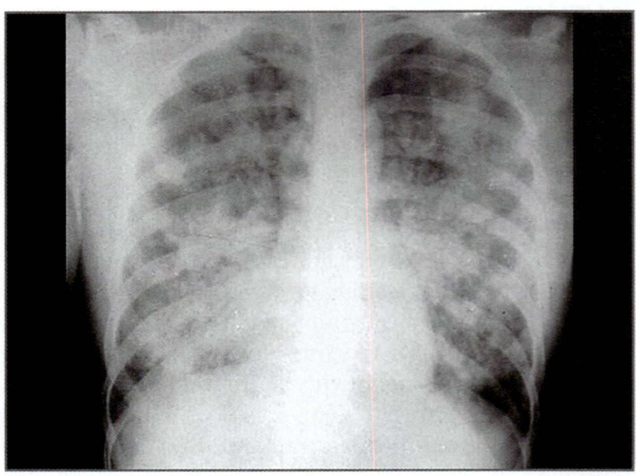

FIG. 26: Chest radiograph showing multiple patchy airspace opacities in bilateral lung fields giving rise to "Bat wing" appearance in a case of pulmonary edema.

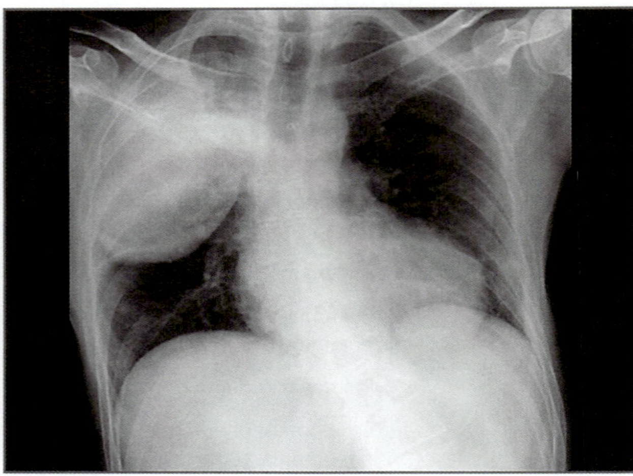

FIG. 27: Bulging fissure sign in *Klebsiella* pneumonia, note made of scoliosis of spine.

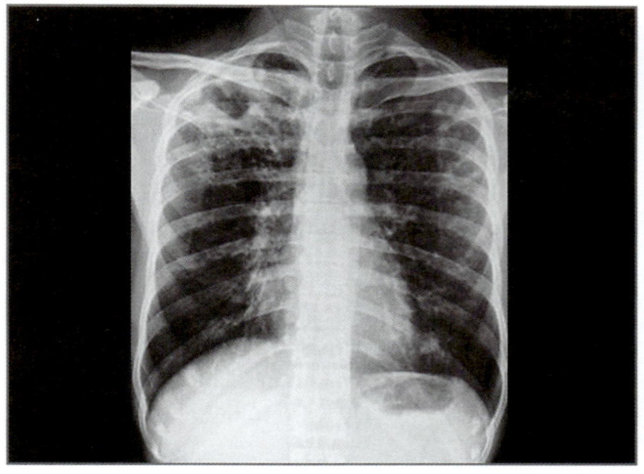

FIG. 28: Cavity in right upper lobe with surrounding consolidation. Multiple nodular opacities seen in bilateral upper and left mid zones.

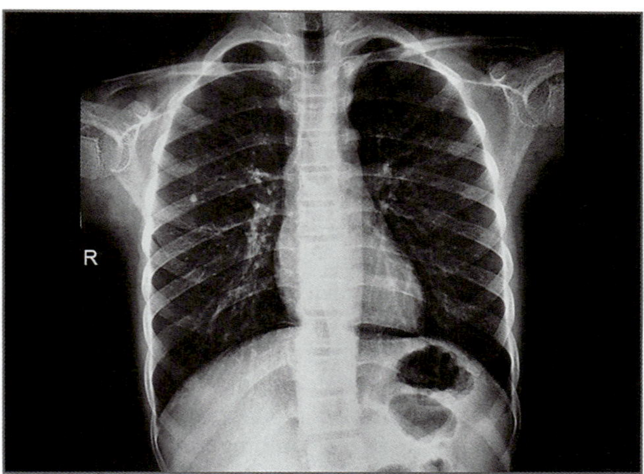

FIG. 29: Calcified granuloma in right mid zone.

by the expulsion or drainage of a necrotic part of the lesion via the bronchial tree. It may be isolated or associated with adjacent lung pathology, and a gas-fluid level may be present in the cavity (**Fig. 28**).[27] Rupture of a bronchogenic cyst or an *Echinococcus* cyst are exceptions where contents were originally fluid; as is infection of an existing cystic space, such as a bulla.

Wall thickness of the cavity, especially at its thickest part, can point to underlying disease process as being benign or malignant. Malignant lesions show a thick, asymmetrical, nodular wall whereas benign lesions tend to have a thin, smooth wall. Nearly 85% of cavities with a wall measuring > 15 mm in its thickest portion are malignant. If the thickest part of the wall is less than 5 mm, 95% are benign.[18] Presence of internal contents like aspergilloma, blood clot or floating membranes as seen with ruptured echinococcal disease giving rise to the "water lily sign" help in narrowing down the differential diagnosis.

FIG. 30: Multiple calcified nodular opacities in bilateral lung fields with volume loss of left lung and an area of cavitation in left upper zone.

Calcification

Presence of parenchymal lung calcification is a helpful indicator, usually pointing toward a benign process. Deposition of calcium in dead or non-vital tissue is referred to as dystrophic calcification, as is commonly seen in India in tubercular afflictions of the lung. Rarely calcification or ossification may occur in healthy lung as in metastasis from osteosarcoma. This is referred to as metastatic calcification.

Dystrophic calcification is fairly common in Ghon's focus as well as healed or old pulmonary tuberculosis and it may be solitary (**Fig. 29**), localized or widespread (**Fig. 30**). Popcorn or speckled calcification can also be seen in benign hamartomas. Calcification may be seen in other infective processes like histoplasmosis, post-chickenpox sequelae and miscellaneous conditions like arteriovenous malformations (phleboliths). Multiple ossific densities due to repeated hemorrhage can often be seen in patients of mitral stenosis. In patients with alveolar microlithiasis and hyperparathyroidism cloudlike punctate calcification of the lung is seen.[28,29]

Interstitial Pattern

Pulmonary interstitium encompasses support tissues within the lung and includes alveolar epithelium, pulmonary capillary endothelium, perivascular and perilymphatic tissues. It can be divided into the axial, parenchymal and peripheral interstitial spaces. The axial interstitial space is constituted by sheath of loose connective tissue around the bronchovascular bundles, the blood vessels, nerves and lymphatics lie in this space. Parenchymal interstitial space is a small space in the walls of the alveoli. Peripheral interstitial space is adjacent to the pleura. The interstitial involvement can be in the form of reticular, nodular, reticulonodular and linear opacities. Inhomogeneous radiographic density can result because of primarily interstitial involvement. It is important to remember that alveolar air may be less but is not significantly compromised in interstitial disease and volume loss is not a feature of interstitial involvement as opposed to diseases with alveolar involvement.

Reticular Pattern

Reticular involvement is characterized by the development of thickening of interstitium around air containing cystic spaces. It can be further subdivided as fine, medium or coarse depending on the size. Fine reticulation implies a slender delicate mesh giving rise to ground glass type of opacity. Medium reticular opacities enclose around 3–10 mm size of air spaces, whilst coarse reticulation encompass large cystic spaces of 1 cm or more. Honeycombing can result as a result of both medium and coarse reticulation and is seen in many conditions afflicting lung interstitium such as fibrosing alveolitis, systemic sclerosis, rheumatoid lung, sarcoidosis, etc. (**Figs. 31 and 32**). There is upper lobe predilection in sarcoidosis and eosinophilic granuloma while most of other disease entities displaying honeycombing have lower lobe preponderance.

Nodular Pattern

Formation of various sized nodules in the interstitium can also occur. These nodules can be of varying sizes but are rounded and usually homogenous in density. The sizes may vary from micronodular (< 1 mm), small (1–3 mm), medium (3–5 mm) to large (> 5 mm). Miliary tuberculosis is a classic example of widespread nodular interstitial involvement occurring as a result of blood-borne spread (**Fig. 33**). Similar appearance can also result in other conditions like miliary carcinomatosis, sarcoidosis and inhalational diseases like silicosis. **Box 1** lists the causes of miliary pattern on chest radiograph.

Reticular as well as Nodular Pattern

Reticular pattern may coexist with nodular pattern due to disease etiology as well as progression. The disease may be interstitial to begin with and may have both nodular as

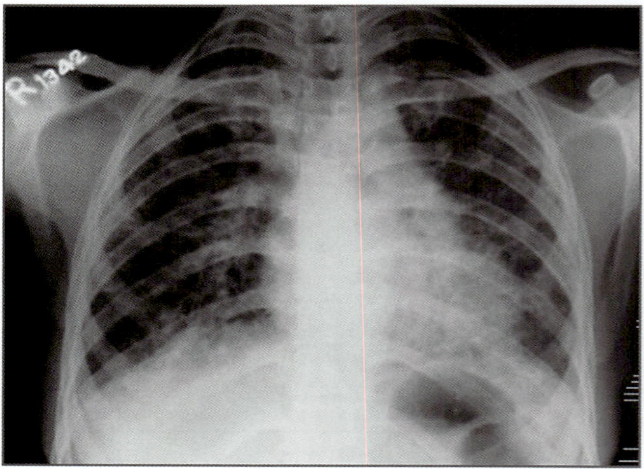

FIG. 31: Chest radiograph showing coarse reticular pattern in a patient with Idiopathic pulmonary fibrosis.

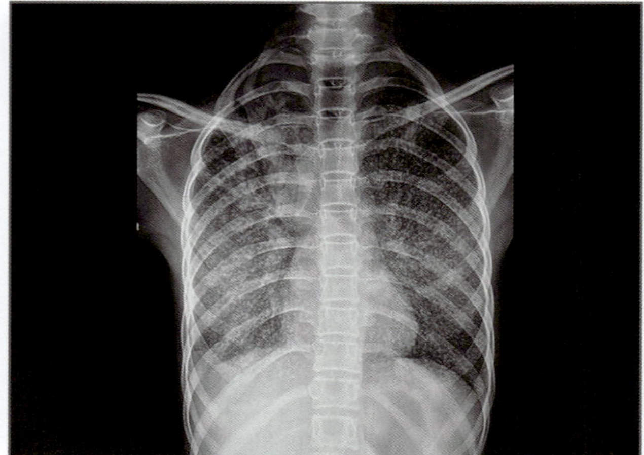

FIG. 33: Multiple small nodules seen scattered in bilateral lungs suggestive of miliary tuberculosis, subsegmental collapse of right upper lobe is noted.

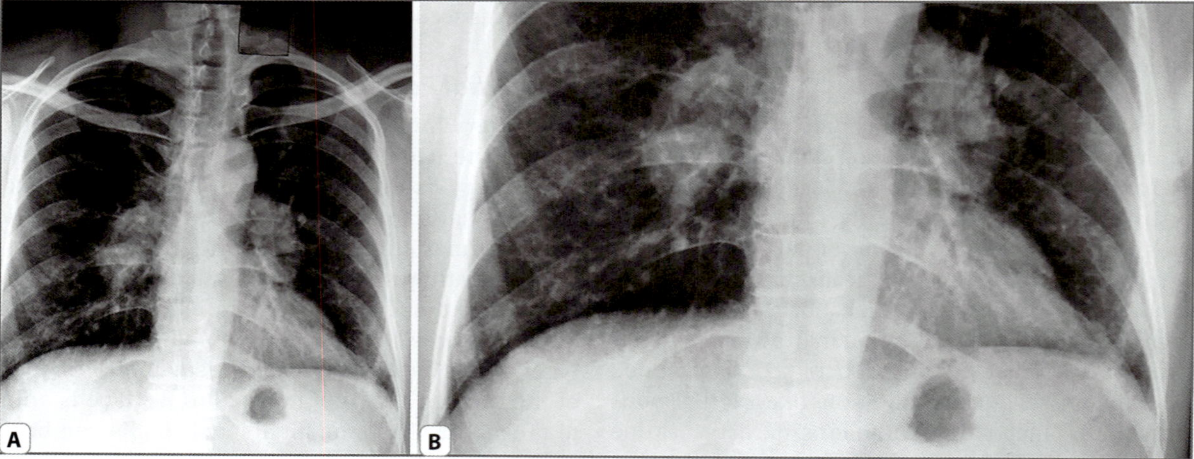

FIGS. 32A AND B: Bilateral hilar lymphadenopathy and reticular opacitites in bilateral lower zones in a case of sarcoidosis.

BOX 1: Causes of miliary pattern on chest radiograph.

- Miliary tuberculosis
- Histoplasmosis
- Coccidioidomycosis
- Cryptococcosis
- Nocardiosis
- Viral infections
- Sarcoidosis
- Silicosis
- Siderosis
- Berylliosis
- Metastases
- Amyloidosis
- Alveolar microlithiasis

BOX 2: Causes of reticulonodular opacities in bilateral lungs on chest radiograph.

- Idiopathic pulmonary fibrosis
- Rheumatic lung disease
- Scleroderma, systemic lupus erythematosus
- Hypersensitivity pneumonitis
- Pneumoconiosis (Coal worker's pneumoconiosis, silicosis, asbestosis)
- Sarcoidosis
- Amyloidosis
- Mycoplasma, viral pneumonia
- Pulmonary edema
- Lymphangitic spread of carcinoma
- Hemosiderosis
- Lymphoid interstitial pneumonitis

well as reticular components as can be seen in sarcoidosis. **Box 2** lists the causes of reticulonodular opacities in bilateral lungs on chest radiograph.

Combination of Airspace Opacities and Interstitial Pattern

Combined involvement of alveolar and interstitial compartments is commonly seen histologically. A similar pattern may be evident radiographically.[30] The disease affecting one compartment may spread to adjoining area with progression of disease. The disease may be interstitial to start with as seen with pulmonary edema, but with further rise of pulmonary venous pressures there is outpouring of fluid in alveolar spaces giving fluffy appearances. Similarly, in infective processes like staphylococcal pneumonias the disease initially involves the bronchial walls with resultant inflammation referred to as bronchiolitis. This leads to narrowing of smaller airways with consequent collapse and consolidation involving alveolar spaces.

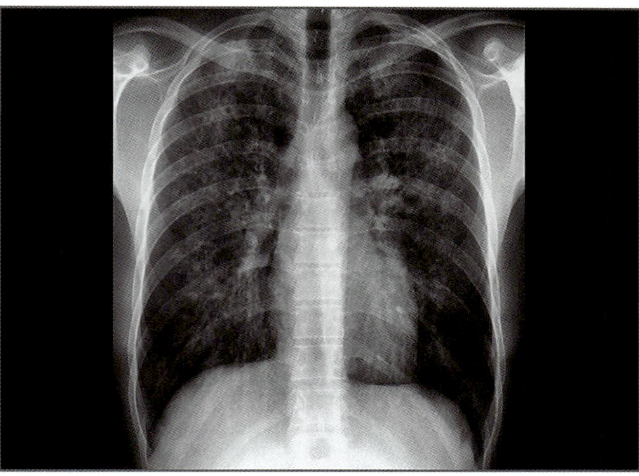

FIG. 34: *Pneumocystis jirovecii* pneumonia: Reticular interstitial pulmonary pattern with few areas of air space opacification, changes are more marked in perihilar location.

This combination is also characteristic of certain infectious diseases of the lung—*Pneumocystis jirovecii* and cytomegalovirus. These two infections are characterized by diffuse interstitial pneumonitis, the disease then spreads into parenchymal airspaces, producing widespread alveolar consolidation (**Fig. 34**). So, the diseases frequently coexist in interstitial as well as alveolar compartment.

Ring Shadows

Ring shadows can be seen in many conditions on chest radiography such as congenital causes including sequestered segment, bronchogenic cysts; infectious causes such as bacterial abscesses, tuberculosis and *Pneumocystis jirovecii* pneumonia; connective tissue diseases such as rheumatoid nodules, Wegener granulomatosis; neoplasms and bronchiectasis. The lesions may be single or multiple and of varying sizes.

Line and Band Shadows

Linear opacities with a diameter of > 5 mm are referred to as band shadows whereas those with a diameter of < 5 mm are called line shadows.[31]

Parenchymal Scarring

Linear shadows can be seen in a segment of lung that was the site of infectious disease and has healed through fibrosis. This may be seen in cases of healed upper lobe post-primary tuberculosis. It can also be seen in healed pulmonary infarction resulting in fibrous scarring secondary to lung necrosis. These linear shadows always extend to a pleural surface, and this may be caused in part by an indrawing of the pleura by the scar.

Mucoid Impaction

Branching bandlike opacities pointing toward the hilum can be seen due to mucoid impaction and give rise to the "gloved finger" shadow. These are characteristically seen in allergic bronchopulmonary aspergillosis but can also be seen in many obstructive conditions such as bronchial carcinoid, carcinoma lung, metastases, bronchial atresia, foreign body aspiration and benign strictures.

Septal Lines

Interstitial thickening involving the interlobular septae and bronchovascular bundle can lead to the development of primarily linear opacities.

Kerley first described septal lines on chest radiographs in cases of pulmonary edema.[32] They were named A, B and C lines as their anatomical basis was uncertain. Septal lines are a more appropriate term as increased fluid or tissue in the interstitium can result in linear opacities called Kerley B lines or rarely Kerley A or C lines.[33]

Kerley B lines are horizontal, peripheral nonbranching fine lines less than 2 cm long, seen typically at lung bases. These linear opacities are less than 1 mm thick, and lie roughly perpendicular to the pleural surface. They are commonly seen as a result of interstitial edema secondary to increase of pulmonary venous pressures, as in rheumatic heart disease and left ventricular failure **(Fig. 35)**.

Kerley A and C lines are rare. Overlapping of Kerley B lines especially near pleural surfaces give rise to interlacing network of fine linear opacities referred to as Kerley C lines. Kerley A lines on the other hand, are slightly thicker than Kerley B lines and about 6 cm long, coursing from pleural interfaces to the lung hilum.

The Kerley B lines may be reversible in early stage of interstitial edema, with treatment of underlying cardiac pathology. However, these lines would persist if interstitial tissue pathology is irreversible, as in lymphangitic carcinomatosis, pneumoconiosis. **Box 3** lists the causes of septal lines on chest radiograph.

Position of Fissures and Hila

Frequently, displacement of the interlobar fissures and hila toward an area of increased density point to the presence of disease nearby like lung collapse (**Fig. 36**). Displacement away from a lesion may be rarely seen because of volume expansion as in Friedlander's pneumonia (*Klebsiella*) where bulging fissure can be seen. This is due to the abundant exudates produced by the organism. It may also be seen with *Streptococcus pneumoniae, Mycobacterium tuberculosis* and plague pneumonia. Expansion of a lobe may also be seen with acute lung abscess, when air trapping by a check valve mechanism in the communicating airway distends the abscess cavity.

The interlobar fissures are an efficient barrier to the interlobar spread of parenchymal disease. A few diseases have a propensity for crossing pleural boundaries which is commonly seen with mycotic or actinomycotic infection of the lungs. In the latter, the organisms pass across visceral and parietal pleural layers, and they may form abscesses leading to osteomyelitis in the chest wall.

BOX 3: Causes of septal lines on chest radiograph.

- Pulmonary edema
- Lymphangitis carcinomatosa
- Malignant lymphoma
- Sarcoidosis
- Pneumoconiosis
- Lymphoid interstitial pneumonitis
- Idiopathic pulmonary hemorrhage (late stages)

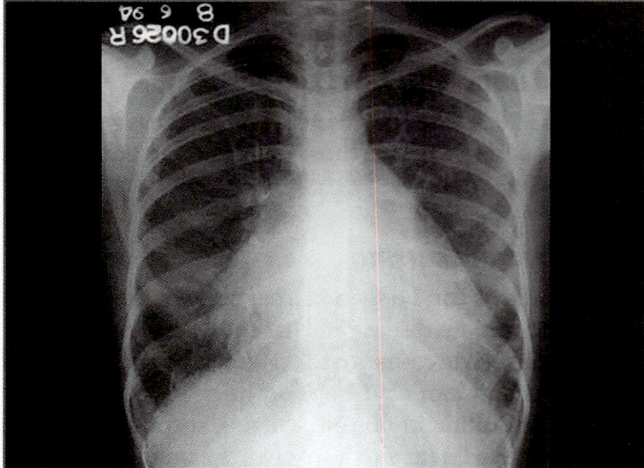

FIG. 35: Septal (Kerley B) lines seen in a case of mitral valve disease.

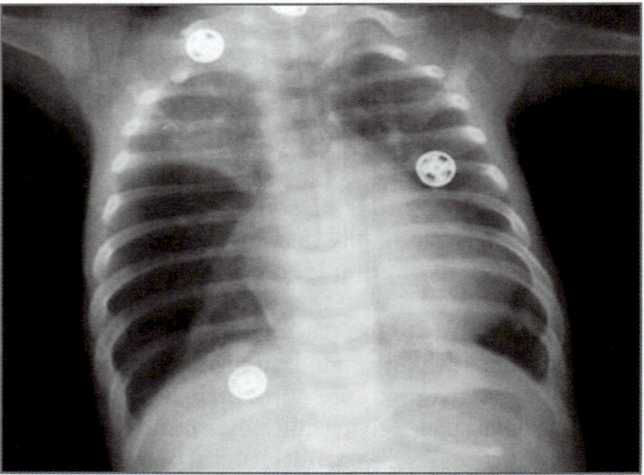

FIG. 36: Right upper lobe atelectasis showing increased density with upper displacement of transverse fissure with compensatory hyperinflation.

Anatomical Basis of Disease

The site of involvement by a particular disease process in the lungs is influenced by certain physiological factors. The ventilation: perfusion ratio is different throughout the lung, primarily because of the influence of gravity. Gravity largely establishes the distribution of disease in aspiration pneumonia. The upper lobes are involved if aspiration occurs when the patient is supine, their posterior portions more frequently than the anterior. If the patient is erect, involvement of the lower lobes predominates. Aspiration occurs more readily into the right than left lung because the right main bronchus is more in line with the trachea. Blood-borne diseases predominate at the lung bases due to the greater perfusion of the lung bases in the upright patient. The hemodynamics of blood flow within the lungs causes embolic phenomena to also produce a peripheral distribution of disease. Pulmonary infarction occurs much more frequently in lower lobes than in upper lobes. Metastatic lesions occur more frequently in lower lobes. In bedridden patients, metastatic deposits do not show the usual anatomic bias and may predominate in upper zones. Pulmonary sequestration occurs almost exclusively in the lower lobes, most commonly in the posterior basal segment and on the left side than the right. The ground-glass opacity and reticulation of asbestosis shows basal distribution. Chronic idiopathic interstitial fibrosis and interstitial fibrosis of progressive systemic sclerosis are also predominantly basal in distribution.

Primary pulmonary carcinoma has an unexplained predilection for upper lung zones. The decrease in perfusion of the well-ventilated lung apices causes the apices to have a higher partial pressure of oxygen (PO_2) than the remainder of the lungs. The predilection of tuberculosis for the lung apices has been attributed to this difference in oxygen pressures. Upper lobe predilection is shown by silicosis, sarcoidosis, eosinophilic granuloma, and the conglomerate shadows of complicated silicosis and coal workers' pneumoconiosis.

Signs on the Chest Radiograph

The *"Silhouette Sign"* was described by Felson and helps in the localization and at times recognition of pulmonary disease. "An intrathoracic lesion touching a border of the heart, aorta or diaphragm will obliterate that border on the roentgenogram. An intrathoracic lesion not anatomically contiguous with a border of one of these structures will not obliterate that border". The sign is produced when the juxtaposed borders are of similar density. On a frontal radiograph, obscuration of specific contours indicates abnormalities in specific lobes, for instance if right superior mediastinum (superior vena cava) is obscured, the pathology is in the right upper lobe. Right heart border is obscured in right middle lobe involvement **(Fig. 37)** and right hemidiaphragm is obscured in right lower lobe involvement. The left superior mediastinum (aortic arch) is obscured in left upper lobe pathology, the left heart border in lingular involvement and the left hemidiaphragm or descending aorta in left lower lobe disease **(Fig. 38)**.[18]

The *"hilum" overlay sign* was described by Felson and helps in determining whether an opacity is within the hilum or anterior or posterior to it **(Fig. 39)**. If the opacity is situated within the hilum, it will be obscured by the opacity from the proximal pulmonary artery and will appear inseparable from hilar structures. If hilar vessels are clearly seen through an opacity, then it can be situated anterior or posterior to the hilum.[34]

The *"hilum convergence sign"* is useful in differentiating between a large pulmonary artery and a hilar mass. As the pulmonary artery branches arise from the main pulmonary artery trunk, an enlarged pulmonary artery will have branches that arise from its lateral margin and its vessels

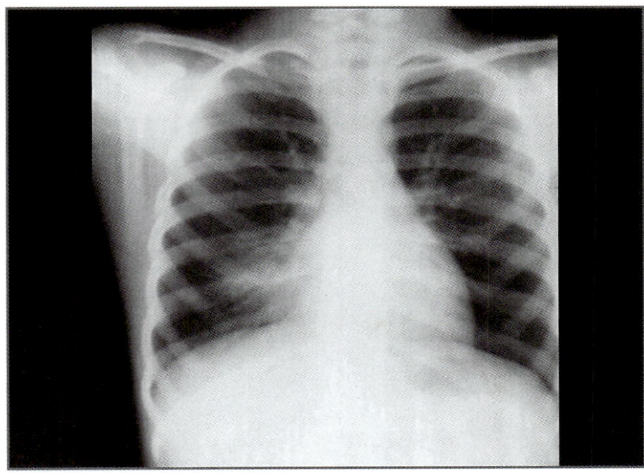

FIG. 37: "Silhouette sign"—right middle lobe consolidation obscuring the right cardiac border.

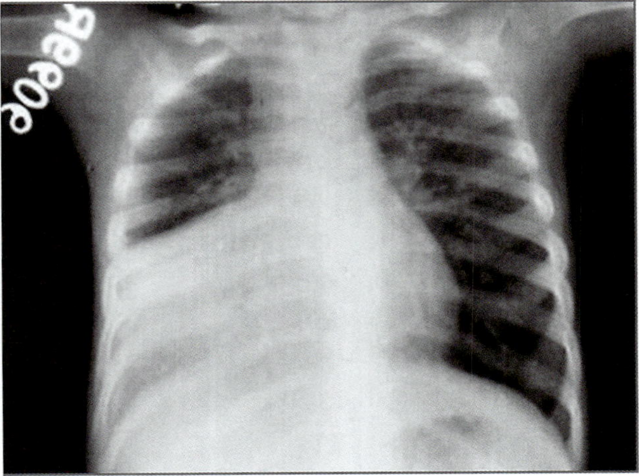

FIG. 38: Consolidation of right middle and lower lobes with smooth and sharply marginated upper border by the horizontal fissure. The right cardiac border and dome of diaphragm are silhouetted.

will appear to converge toward the main pulmonary artery. In case of a hilar mass, the vessels will not arise from its lateral margin but seem to pass through the margin as they converge on the true pulmonary artery. If the convergence of pulmonary arteries appears behind the apparent hilar mass or appears to arise from the heart, a mediastinal mass is more likely.[35]

The *"cervicothoracic sign"* is used to differentiate between an anterior and posterior mass in the superior mediastinum. A posterior mediastinal mass is surrounded by lung tissue from all sides as the posterior part of the lung extends superior to the clavicle at the level of the thoracic inlet. Anterior mediastinal masses show ill-defined superior margins due to their anatomical contact with the soft tissues of the neck, either at or below the clavicle.[36]

Increased Density on Chest Radiograph

Complete opacification of a hemithorax on a chest radiograph is termed as opaque hemithorax. The differential diagnosis is based on the volume of the affected hemithorax. If there is an opaque hemithorax with ipsilateral mediastinal shift, differential diagnosis includes pulmonary agenesis, atelectasis or pneumonectomy. Bronchial obstruction leading to atelectasis may be seen due to foreign bodies in children and tumors in adults. The differential diagnosis for an opaque hemithorax with contralateral mediastinal shift includes large pleural effusion and large thoracic masses. If there is an opaque hemithorax with no tracheomediastinal shift the differential diagnosis includes extensive pneumonia or bronchial carcinoma associated with pleural effusion and atelectasis.

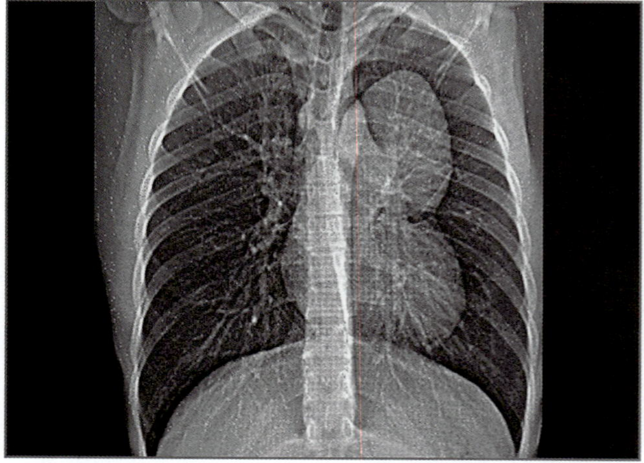

FIG. 39: Hilum overlay sign in anterior mediastinal mass, the hilar vessels are seen through the lesion.

Decreased Density on Chest Radiograph

Diffuse increase in transradiancy of both lungs is seen in airway disease, constrictive bronchiolitis, asthma, emphysema, right to lung cardiac shunts like tetralogy of Fallot, Eisenmenger physiology or severe peripheral pulmonary arterial stenoses.

A focal increase in transradiancy can be seen in emphysema and bullous diseases, cysts, pneumatoceles and cavities. A bulla is a circumscribed air-containing cystic structure in the lung parenchyma lined by a thin layer of collapsed lung parenchyma. It is caused by dilatation, destruction, and confluence of airspaces distal to terminal bronchioles. At imaging, a bulla typically appears as a rounded lucency, with a very fine and usually smooth wall.[27] Multiple bullae may often be seen and are associated with other signs of pulmonary emphysema. A cyst appears as a round parenchymal lucency with a well-defined interface with normal lung. Cysts have variable wall thickness but are usually thin-walled (2 mm) and occur without associated pulmonary emphysema. Cysts in the lung usually contain air but occasionally contain fluid or solid material. Air cysts that develop following infections are known as "pneumatoceles" and are seen following *Pneumocystis jirovecii* or staphylococcal pneumonia **(Figs. 40A and B)** and hydrocarbon fluid aspiration.[31]

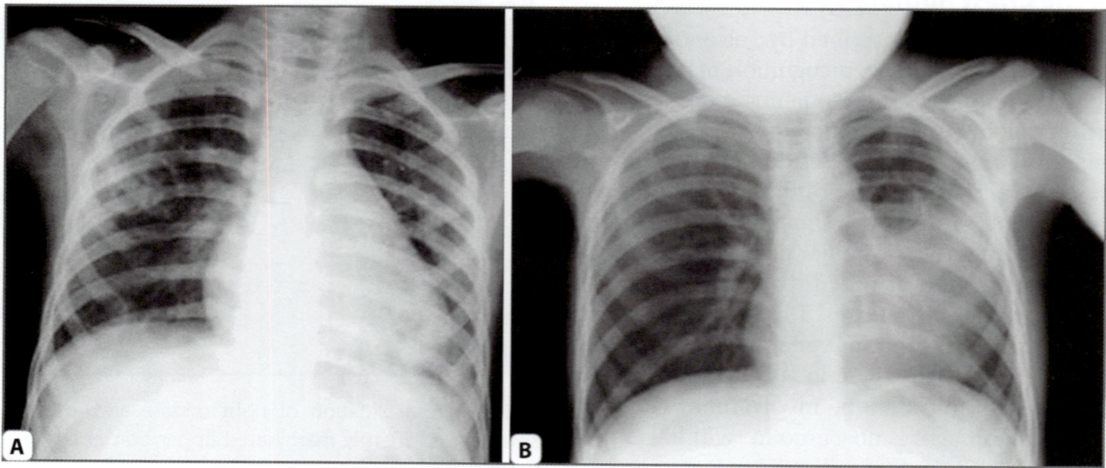

FIGS. 40A AND B: (A) Pneumatoceles in right lung field; and (B) Resolving staphylococcal pneumonia in left lung with pneumatocele.

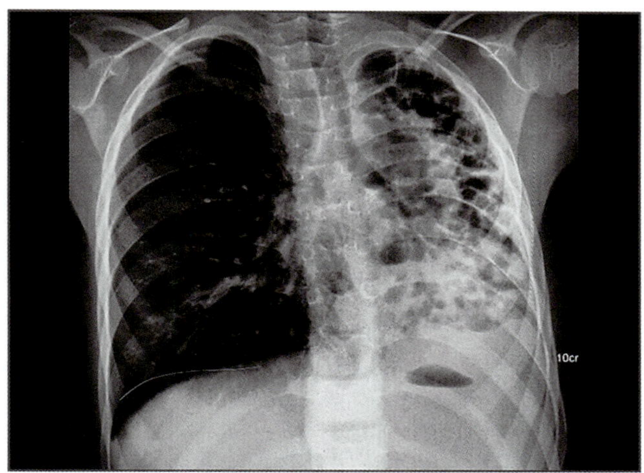

FIG. 41: Multiple cystic bronchiectatic opacities with air fluid levels suggestive of superimposed infection in left lung field with marked volume loss on left side and compensatory hyperinflation of right lung which appears hyperlucent.

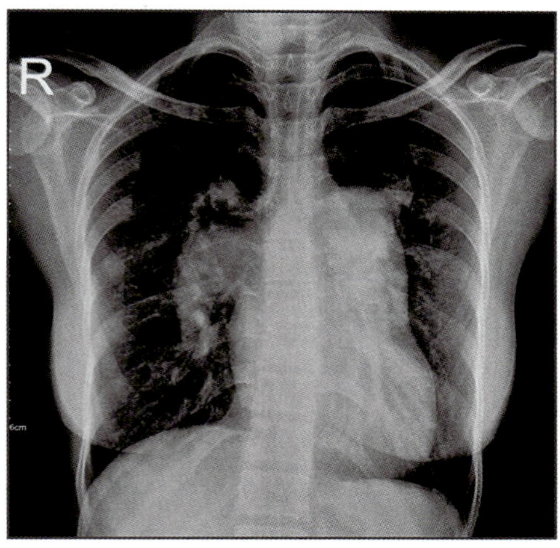

FIG. 42: Bilateral hilar enlargement due to dilated central pulmonary arteries in a case of primary pulmonary arterial hypertension.

Cavities are gas-filled areas of the lung within a nodule, mass or area of consolidation.

Unilateral hyperlucent lung can be seen with thoracic wall and soft tissue abnormalities, diminished perfusion of lung, compensatory hyperinflation of lung associated with collapse (**Fig. 41**) and foreign body impaction with obstructive emphysema.[31] Decrease in pulmonary blood volume may be associated with congenital defects such as agenesis or hypoplasia of pulmonary arteries or acquired reasons such as thromboembolism.[37]

Hila and Pulmonary Vasculature

Hilar abnormalities on radiographs may present as changes in size (increase or decrease), density, or the shape of the hilum. Hilar enlargement is typically caused by a central neoplasm, lymph node enlargement, or dilated central pulmonary arteries, as seen in pulmonary hypertension (**Fig. 42**).

Irregular calcification in lymph nodes is frequently encountered in healing or healed tubercular infections. Rarely calcification results not in the substance but around the margins resulting in what is described as "Egg shell" calcification (**Fig. 43**). This is seen in occupational lung diseases like silicosis and coal workers pneumoconiosis. **Table 5** lists the causes of unilateral and bilateral hilar enlargement.

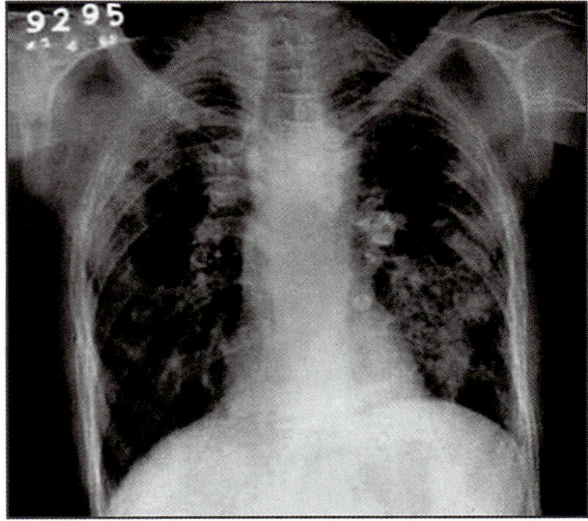

FIG. 43: In a case of sarcoidosis, chest radiograph shows multiple reticulonodular opacities and egg shell calcifications in the hilar lymph nodes.

TABLE 5: Causes of Hilar enlargement.

Unilateral hilar enlargement	Bilateral hilar enlargement
Granulomatous infections	Sarcoidosis
Lung cancer	Granulomatous infections
Metastatic lymphadenopathy	Pulmonary arterial hypertension
Lymphoma	Metastatic lymphadenopathy
Valvular pulmonic stenosis	Lymphoma

Pleura

On erect chest radiographs, pneumothorax appears as a region of increased lucency at the apex, running parallel to the chest wall and outlining the curvilinear visceral pleural line, which is displaced inward from the chest wall (**Fig. 44**). Pneumothorax can be either spontaneous or traumatic. Spontaneous pneumothorax is further classified as primary (without underlying lung disease) or secondary (associated with underlying lung disease).

The radiographic appearance of pleural effusion depends on factors such as the volume of fluid, whether it is free-flowing or loculated, and the positioning of the

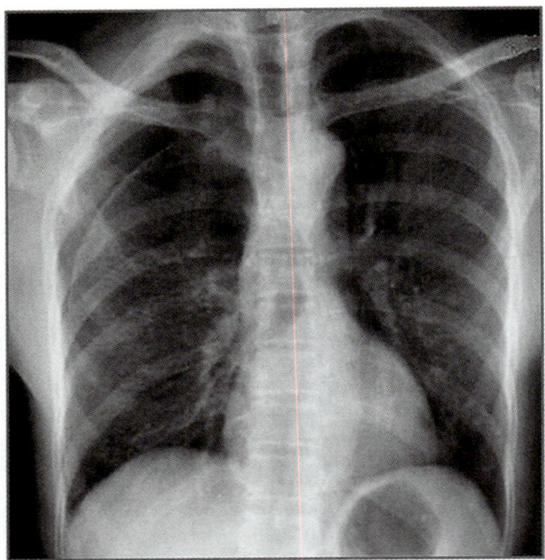

FIG. 44: Right sided pneumothorax with passive atelectasis of right lung. Visceral pleural line is seen. Fractures of third to sixth ribs on right side.

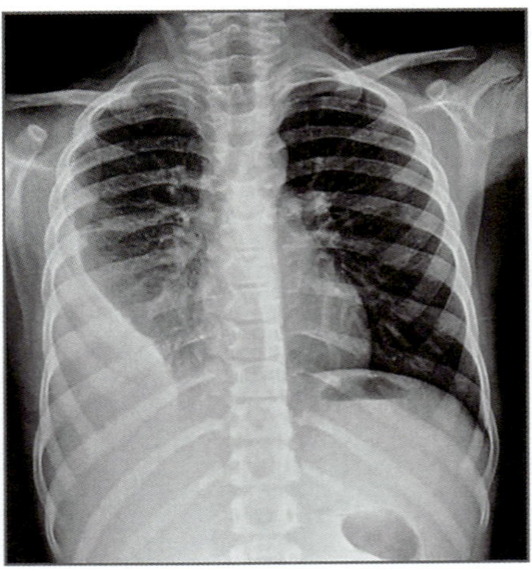

FIG. 45: Right pleural effusion obscuring the right costophrenic angle and forming a meniscus.

patient during the radiograph. A small, free-flowing pleural effusion in an upright patient typically shows a meniscus that blunts the posterior costophrenic angle on lateral views. Larger effusions may blunt the lateral costophrenic angle on frontal views, and effusions over 500 mL can obscure the hemidiaphragm (**Fig. 45**). Loculated pleural effusions, often associated with infection (such as parapneumonic effusions or empyemas), appear as biconvex, mass-like opacities along the dependent costal pleural surfaces. Massive pleural effusions and pleural effusions with associated pleural nodules should suggest malignancy. Presence of circumferential nodular pleural thickening is highly suggestive of malignancy including metastatic disease, malignant pleural mesothelioma, and lymphoma.[1]

Calcification of the pleura may occur and may be seen as a focal plaque of calcification or a long and broad sheet of calcification involving the visceral pleura. This can follow blood, purulent collections in the pleural cavity or tuberculous effusion. Rarely, parietal pleural calcification may be seen, typically involving diaphragmatic pleura as in asbestosis.

Mediastinum

Mediastinal masses include primary and secondary neoplasms, mediastinal cysts, thyroid lesions, thymic masses, vascular lesions and hernias. Focal unilateral mediastinal masses may be due to primary neoplasms, enlarged lymph nodes, cysts, or vascular aneurysms and anomalous vessels. Diffuse, symmetric mediastinal widening without mass effect can be seen in mediastinal lipomatosis, lobulated or asymmetric widening may indicate lymphadenopathy in metastatic disease, lymphoma or a mediastinal hematoma in patients with chest trauma.

Mediastinal masses may be localized on the lateral chest radiograph as described previously, however, with the wide use of cross-sectional imaging techniques, this is seldom done in current practice. Clinical factors such as age, gender and symptoms aid the radiologist in narrowing down the differential diagnosis.[1]

TABLE 6: Differential diagnosis for lines and stripes on chest radiograph.

Lines and stripes	Differential diagnosis
Anterior junctional line	Thymus, thyroid mass, lymphoma, germ cell tumors
Posterior junctional line	Esophageal masses, lymphadenopathy, aortic disease, neurogenic tumors
Right and left paratracheal stripes	Lymphadenopathy, thyroid mass, duplication cyst, right sided aortic arch, vascular injuries
Aortopulmonary window	Lymphadenopathy, aortic aneurysms, enlarged pulmonary artery
Descending aorta line	Aortic aneurysm
Paraspinal line	Osteophytes, paravertebral mediastinal fat, extramedullary hematopoiesis, nerve sheath tumors, tortuous descending thoracic aorta
Azygoesophageal recess	Lymphadenopathy, hiatal hernias, bronchopulmonary-foregut malformations, esophageal neoplasms, esophageal varices, cardiomegaly with left atrial enlargement

Widening, effacement or displacement of lines and stripes on chest radiograph can help in recognizing various disease processes.[15] **Table 6** lists the differential diagnosis for abnormal outline of the various lines and stripes.

Heart

The heart should be evaluated for its shape, size, and position. The cardiac silhouette is considered enlarged if the cardiothoracic ratio is greater than 50% on the PA view **(Fig. 46)**. The cardiothoracic ratio may be upto 60% in neonates. Abnormal shifts in the cardiac silhouette may indicate ipsilateral volume loss (such as lobar atelectasis) or contralateral volume increase (such as a large pneumothorax). The pericardium itself is not visible on standard radiographs. An enlarged cardiac silhouette can be caused by cardiac enlargement or pericardial effusion, with large effusions sometimes presenting as a "water bottle heart" on frontal radiographs. Constrictive pericarditis may be identified by linear pericardial calcifications. Cardiac calcifications can indicate coronary artery disease, valvular or annular calcifications, or curvilinear calcifications in a left ventricular aneurysm following a prior myocardial infarction.[1]

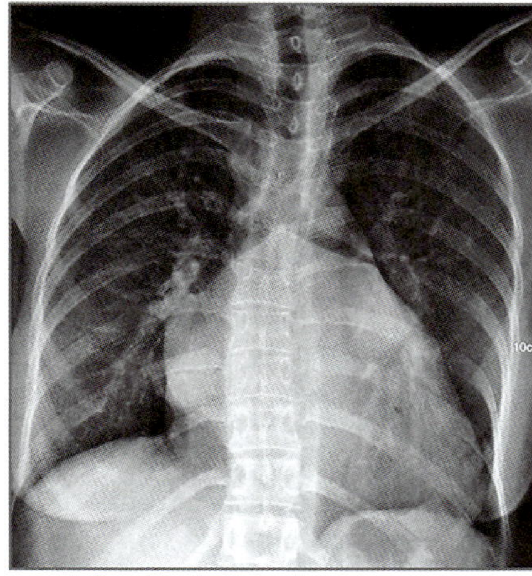

FIG. 46: Cardiomegaly in mitral valvular heart disease, left atrial enlargement is seen with widening of carinal angle.

Diaphragm

A uniformly elevated diaphragm most often results from weakness or paralysis of the diaphragm, while focal bulges in the diaphragmatic contour are typically due to eventration (thinning) of the diaphragm or diaphragmatic hernia through a congenital or acquired diaphragmatic defect (**Fig. 47**).

Chest Wall

Bony structures such as spine, ribs and shoulders should be analyzed. Bony destruction involving ribs or vertebral bodies may indicate an underlying malignancy. Pectus excavatum may mimic right middle lobe disease. Pressure erosions of the rib may be seen with neurogenic neoplasms or chest wall vascular abnormalities such as dilated intercostal arteries in coarctation of aorta. Chest wall masses can produce an incomplete border sign as the mass creates a visible interface with atmospheric air. Soft tissue calcification can be seen in diseases such as myositis ossificans, dermatomyositis or hemangiomas. Poland syndrome is characterized by unilateral underdevelopment of chest wall musculature. The breast shadow should also be analyzed.[1]

Monitoring Devices

Chest radiograph should be assessed for presence of venous catheters, cardiac pacemakers/defibrillators, drainage tubes and endotracheal tubes.

CONCLUSION

Chest radiography is an integral part of the diagnostic work-up of patients with respiratory disease and is a quick,

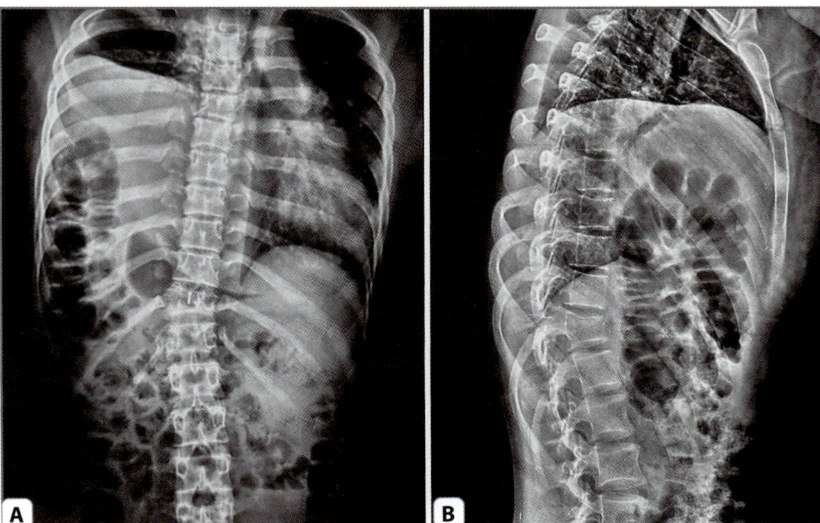

FIGS. 47A AND B: Frontal and lateral radiograph of chest and abdomen shows loss of outline of right hemidiaphragm with soft tissue density and large bowel loops in right hemithorax in a case of right diaphragmatic rupture following blunt trauma abdomen, note made of fracture of D11 vertebral body.

non-invasive, and cost-effective way to assess a wide range of conditions. They are an essential first step in clinical evaluation, especially for respiratory, cardiovascular, and trauma-related issues. The natural contrast of the air containing pulmonary tissue provides a window which allows radiographic evaluation of diseases involving the lungs, tracheobronchial tree, and pleura. Chest radiography is not only valuable for diagnosis of various conditions it is also useful in the follow up of many diseases. It is essential to evaluate the chest radiograph in a systematic way. Computed tomography serves as an important adjunct to the plain film for the purposes of diagnosis and characterization of pathologies affecting the chest including lung parenchymal, pleural, vascular and cardiac abnormalities **(Box 4)**.

BOX 4: Checklist for frontal chest radiograph.

- PA or AP view
- Presence of rotation
- Satisfactory inspiratory effort
- Lung fields
- Cardiac size
- Well delineated domes of diaphragm
- Clearly defined heart borders
- Normal position of hila
- Bones
- Careful assessment of hidden areas—lung apex, retrocardiac region, around each hilum and below the diaphragm

REFRENCES

1. Klein JS, Rosado-de-Christenson ML. A Systematic Approach to Chest Radiographic Analysis. 2019. In: Hodler J, Kubik-Huch RA, von Schulthess GK, (Eds). Diseases of the Chest, Breast, Heart and Vessels 2019-2022: Diagnostic and Interventional Imaging [Internet]. Cham (CH): Springer; 2019.
2. Schaefer-Prokop C, Neitzel U, Venema HW, Uffmann M, Prokop M. Digital chest radiography: an update on modern technology, dose containment and control of image quality. Eur Radiol. 2008;18(9):1818-30.
3. Schaetzing R, Fasbender R, Kersten P. New high-speed scanning technique for computed radiography. SPIE. 2002;4682:511-20.
4. Leblans P, Struye L, Willems P. A new needle-crystalline computed radiography detector. J Digit Imaging. 2000;13(2 Suppl 1):117-20.
5. Frankenberger J, Mair S, Herrmann C, et al. Reflective and transmissive CR scan head technology on needle image plates. In: Flynn MJ (Ed) Medical imaging. Physics of Medical Imaging. 2005;5745(1):499-510.
6. Samei E, Flynn MJ. An experimental comparison of detector performance for direct and indirect digital radiography systems. Med Phys. 2003;30(4):608-22.
7. Metz S, Damoser P, Hollweck R, Roggel R, Engelke C, Woertler K, et al. Chest radiography with a digital flat-panel detector: experimental receiver operating characteristic analysis. Radiology. 2005;234(3):776-84.
8. Bacher K, Smeets P, Vereecken L, Hauwere AD, Philippe Duyck P, Man RD, et al. Image quality and radiation dose in digital chest imaging: comparison of an amorphous silicon and an amorphous selenium flat-panel system. AJR. 2006;187(3):630-7.
9. Dobbins JT, Godfrey DJ, McAdams HP. Chest tomosynthesis. Syllabus RSNA 2003, Advances in digital radiography: RSNA categorical course in diagnostic radiology physics. 2003:211-7.
10. Fyles F, FitzMaurice TS, Robinson RE, Bedi R, Burhan H, Walshaw MJ. Dynamic chest radiography: a state-of-the-art review. Insights Imaging. 2023;14(1):107.
11. Hatabu H, Madore B. Dark-Field Chest X-ray Imaging: An Evolving Technique in the Century-Old History of Chest X-ray Imaging. Radiology. 2021;301(2):396-7.
12. McComb BL, Chung JH, Crabtree TD, Heitkamp DE, Iannettoni MD, Jokerst C, et al. ACR Appropriateness Criteria® Routine Chest Radiography. J Thorac Imaging. 2016;31(2):W13-5.
13. Broder J. Imaging the Chest: The Chest Radiograph. Diagnostic Imaging for the Emergency Physician. 2011:185-296.
14. Breatnach E, Abbott GC, Fraser RE. Dimensions of the normal human trachea. AJR. 1984;142:903-6.
15. Jiao A, Nadim B, Hammer M, Jhala K. 3D Visual Guide to Lines and Stripes in Chest Radiography. Radiographics. 2023;43(9):e230017.
16. Collins J. Chest Radiology: The Essentials (3rd edn). Philadelphia: Wolters Kluwer, 2015.
17. Fraser RG, Pare JAP, Pare PD, et al. Diagnosis of Diseases of the Chest (3rd edn). Vol I: WB Saunders, 1988.
18. Webb WR. Thoracic Imaging: Pulmonary and Cardiovascular Radiology (3rd edn). Philadelphia: Wolters Kluwer, 2017.
19. Woodring JH, Reed JC. Types and mechanisms of pulmonary atelectasis. J Thorac Imaging. 1996;11:92-108.
20. Proto AV, Tocino I. Radiographic manifestations of lobar collapse. Semin Roentgenol. 1980;15:117-73.
21. Woodring JH, Reed JC. Radiographic manifestations of lobar atelectasis. J Thorac Imaging. 1996;11:10944.
22. Sutton D. Textbook of Radiology & Imaging. (7th edn). Edinburgh: Churchill Livingstone, 2009.
23. Golden R. The effect of bronchostenosis upon the roentgen-ray shadows in carcinoma of the bronchus. AJR Am J Roentgenol. 1925;13:21-30.
24. Algın O, Gökalp G, Topa U. Signs in chest imaging. Diagn Interv Radiol. 2011;17:1829.
25. Adam Grainger & Allison's Diagnostic Radiology (6th edn). Philadelphia: Elsevier, 2014.
26. Kattan KR, Wlot JF. Cardiac rotation in left lower lobe collapse. 'The flat waist sign.' Radiology. 1976;118:275-9.
27. Bankier AA, MacMahon H, Colby T, Gevenois PA, Goo JM, Leung ANC, et al. Fleischner Society: Glossary of Terms for Thoracic Imaging. Radiology. 2024;310(2):e232558.
28. Brown K, Mund DF, Aberle DR, Batra P, Young DA. Intrathoracic calcifications: radiographic features and differential diagnoses. Radiographics. 1994;14:1247-61.

29. Chai JL, Patz EF Jr. CT of the lung: patterns of calcification and other highattenuation abnormalities. AJR Am J Roentgenol. 1994;162:1063-6.
30. Felson B. A new look at pattern recognition of diffuse pulmonary disease. AJR Am J Roentgenol. 1979;133:83.
31. Hansell DM. Imaging of Diseases of the Chest (5th edn). St. Louis: Mosby Elsevier, 2009.
32. Kerley P. Radiology in heart disease. BMJ. 1933;2:594-7.
33. Trapnell DH. The differential diagnosis of linear shadows in chest radiographs. Radiol Clin North Am. 1973;11:77-92.
34. Felson B, Felson H. Localization of intrathoracic lesions by means of the posteroanterior roentgenogram; The silhouette sign. Radiology. 1950;55:363-74.
35. Parker MS, Chasen MH, Paul N. Radiologic signs in thoracic imaging: case-based review and self-assessment module. AJR Am J Roentgenol. 2009 Mar;192(3 Suppl):S34-48.
36. Kumaresh A, Kumar M, Dev B, Gorantla R, Venkata Sai PM, Thanasekaraan V. Back to Basics—'Must Know' Classical Signs in Thoracic Radiology. J Clin Imaging. Sci. 2015;5:43.
37. Altinsoy B, Altintas N. Diagnostic approach to unilateral hyperlucent lung. JRSM Short Rep. 2011;2:95.

Madhurima Sharma, Mahesh Prakash, Anindita Sinha, Ajay Gulati

CHAPTER

2

The Essentials of Thoracic Ultrasound

INTRODUCTION

Transthoracic ultrasonography (USG) is a well-established imaging modality in the respiratory medicine. In recent years, its popularity has dramatically increased, and it is now routinely performed in the intensive care unit (ICU) and emergency department. Thoracic USG is a portable, rapid, cost-effective, and radiation-free modality that allows real-time evaluation of thoracic structures. Bedside lung USG in emergency (BLUE) protocol has been adopted as a standardized approach to lung USG in the ICU by the critical care providers and has a diagnostic accuracy >90% for asthma and/or chronic obstructive pulmonary disease, pneumonia, pneumothorax, and pulmonary edema.[1-3] Routine use of lung USG in the ICU has been advocated to decrease the use of chest radiography, which is associated with cumulative radiation exposure (especially in pediatric patients). It is especially useful in pediatric population due to small thoracic diameter and improved acoustic window. Thoracic USG also has a well-established role in guiding various interventional procedures such as fine-needle aspiration cytology (FNAC), biopsy, thoracocentesis, and drainage of chest wall collections. However, it is limited by certain factors such as operator dependence and patient habitus. As compared to chest radiography, lung USG is more time-consuming, as a complete lung USG examination may take up to 20 minutes to perform.[3] Only peripheral abnormalities abutting the pleural surface can be visualized on USG, thereby limiting its utility in the evaluation of deeper structures.

The major indications of chest ultrasound (US) are given as follows:

- Evaluation of pleural pathologies (effusion, hemothorax, empyema, pleural thickening, calcification, pleural mass, etc.)
- Diagnosis of pneumothorax
- Evaluation of opaque hemithorax
- Assessment of chest wall diseases (such as neoplasms, hematoma, abscess, and rib fracture)
- Assessment of diaphragmatic mobility
- To differentiate subpulmonic effusion with subphrenic collection
- Evaluation of peripheral lung parenchymal pathologies (consolidation, collapse, abscess, and tumors)
- Evaluation of mediastinum [anterior mediastinal mass, lymphadenopathy, inferior vena cava (IVC) thrombosis, and pericardial effusion]
- Guidance for interventional procedures

PHYSICS OF LUNG ULTRASONOGRAPHY

In contrast to other USG examinations, in which anatomy is directly visualized, lung USG is predominantly artifact based. The complicated physics of lung USG has been briefly described in this chapter. Pleural interface between chest wall and air-filled lung parenchyma acts as a specular reflector, resulting in pleural line. The pleural line is a bright echogenic line, seen approximately 0.5–1.0 cm below the ribs, corresponding to the apposition of the parietal and visceral pleura.[4] Due to huge difference in the acoustic impedance between these two tissues, whole of US energy is reflected back with very little penetration into the lung parenchyma. A few US waves, which penetrate the lung, are absorbed due to the unfavorable attenuation coefficient of air.[5] As a result, the sonographic depiction of structures deep to pleura is artifactual. Thus, lung abnormalities that are not in direct contact with the pleura are obscured by overlying normal lung artifact. It should be noted that US waves keep reflecting multiple times between pleural surface and overlying structures before returning to the probe, resulting in multiple horizontal lines, known as reverberation artifact. Normal lung artifact comprises of these reverberation artifacts, resulting in horizontal lines known as A lines **(Fig. 1A)**.[3,5] B-line artifacts are hyperechoic vertical lines **(Fig. 1B)**, below the pleural line, which are seen in cases where lung interstitium is thickened. It should

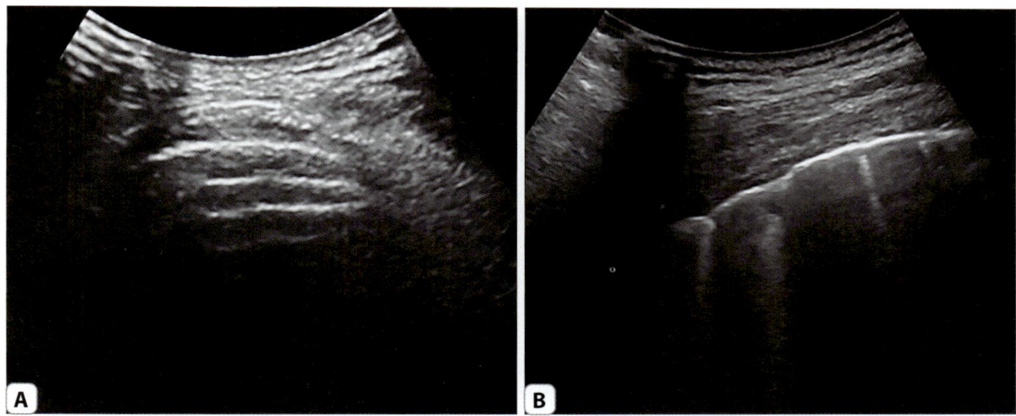

FIGS. 1A AND B: Ultrasound chest image in two different patients demonstrating (A) A lines and (B) B lines.

be noted that solitary B line can be a normal finding in up to 28% of the patients and is seen in lower dependent areas of the lung. Collapse/consolidation of lung parenchyma allows for direct visualization of the parenchyma. Pleural effusions and collections are also directly visualized.[3]

ULTRASOUND TECHNIQUE

Appropriate US probe, proper patient positioning, and placement of probe are the important factors to get good quality images while doing chest US. Ultrasound of chest can be performed with any modern US machine equipped with curvilinear (3–5 MHz) and high-resolution linear array probe (5–13 MHz). Curvilinear transducers' convex shape has a wider field of view and provides visualization of deeper structures. Higher frequency probe results in better resolution at the cost of reduced penetration. Initially, quick look of chest wall, pleura, and lung can be done by curvilinear probe, and once abnormality detected, then detailed depiction of lesion should be done by high-resolution linear probe.[6,7] The lesion can be assessed by both gray scale and color Doppler imaging. Before doing chest US, it is important to review previous imaging, including chest X-ray, to localize the area of interest. It is useful to increase the rib space to facilitate the examination by asking the patient to elevate his/her arm above the head.[6] Folding the patient's arms across their chest displaces the scapulae when scanning the upper posterior thorax.

Liberal application of USG gel should be done to provide smooth slide to the probe and airless interface. Scanning should be done in quite respiration to know the normal lung movement. The detailed assessment of lesion should be done in breath hold, particularly when using color Doppler. The various useful positions/methods are given as follows:

- *Sitting position*: Posterior chest is best imaged with patient sitting upright and putting probe in the intercostal space **(Fig. 2)**. It is useful to detect pleural effusion, which gravitates to dependent position.

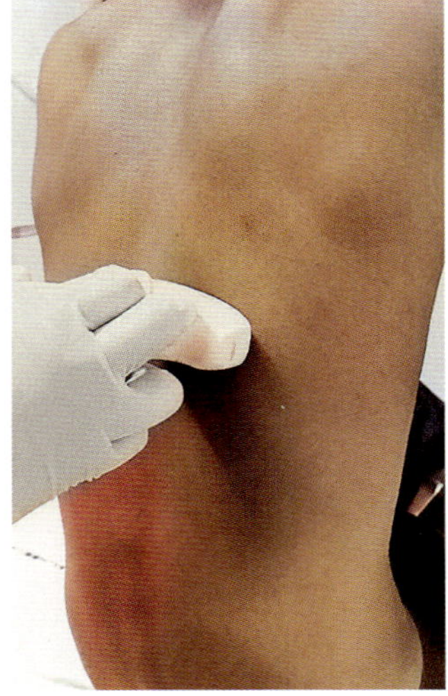

FIG. 2: Ultrasound probe and patient position for the examination of posterolateral chest wall.

- *Lateral decubitus position*: The anterior and lateral chest may be assessed in the lateral decubitus position **(Fig. 3)**.
- *Suprasternal and parasternal position*: It is useful to evaluate superior and anterior mediastinum **(Fig. 4)**.
- *Supraclavicular access*: It allows the visualization of apex of lung and brachial plexus **(Fig. 5)**.
- *Subcostal position*: It is useful to examine diaphragm.
- *Subxiphoid position*: Good to evaluate pericardial effusion and cardiac chambers **(Figs. 6A and B)**.

Complete lung USG comprises of evaluation of lungs in anterior, lateral, and posterior zones. All zones should be examined in both sagittal and transverse planes. Changing to various positions may be difficult to critically ill patients who are usually in supine position with multiple leads/support devices.[8] In this situation, US should be done in supine position.

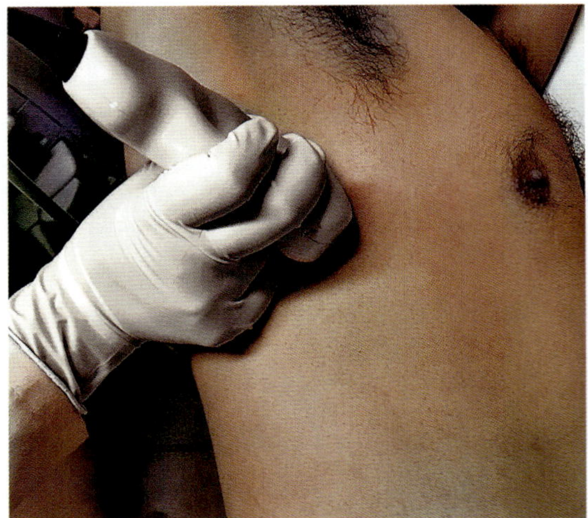

FIG. 3: Anterolateral chest ultrasound in decubitus position.

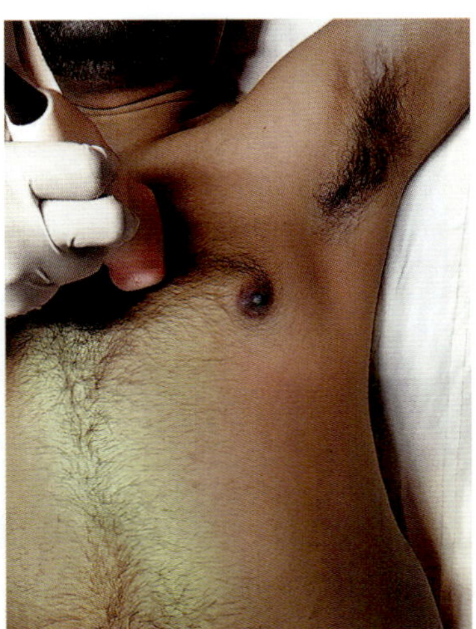

FIG. 4: Parasternal positioning of probe to evaluate anterior mediastinum, pleura, and heart.

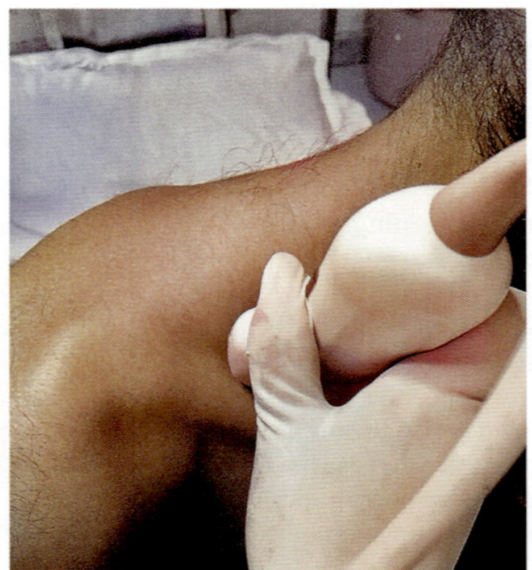

FIG. 5: Evaluation of lung apex by putting probe in supraclavicular location.

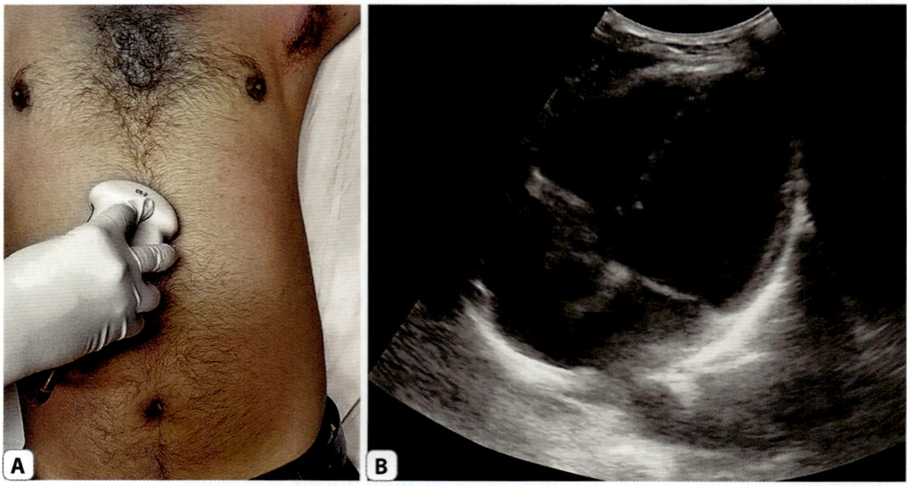

FIGS. 6A AND B: Subxiphoid position of (A) ultrasound probe and (B) corresponding ultrasonography (USG) image.

NORMAL ANATOMY

Familiarity with normal sonographic appearance of the chest components is essential for the correct interpretation of sonographic findings and diagnosis of any abnormal pathology.

Chest Wall

Four components form the chest wall: (1) Skin, (2) subcutaneous fat, (3) muscles, and (4) bones (ribs, sternum, clavicles, and sternoclavicular joints). Skin is most superficial hyperechoic layer. Subcutaneous fat consists of hypoechoic lobules separated by connective tissue septa. The normal chest wall muscles appear as a series of hypoechoic layers separated by echogenic bands.[9-11] Below the chest wall, the ribs appear curvilinear echogenic continuous structure with posterior acoustic shadowing **(Fig. 7)**.

Pleura

Posterior to the rib, the pleura appears as thick approximately 2 mm echogenic line when imaged with curvilinear probe. The high-resolution linear US probe is needed to differentiate parietal and visceral pleura, which are seen as echogenic lines deep to ribs. Both layers of pleura can be seen sliding over each other during real-time USG imaging. It should be noted that pleural sliding is more prominent as one scans caudally down the chest wall, whereas there is less sliding near the apex of the lung.[4]

Diaphragm

The diaphragm is seen as approximately 1–2 mm thick echogenic line, which shows movement during respiration. Usually, the diaphragm is located inferior to 9th rib when patient is in sitting position. Apart from the location of diaphragm, subdiaphragmatic recesses should be evaluated **(Fig. 8)**.

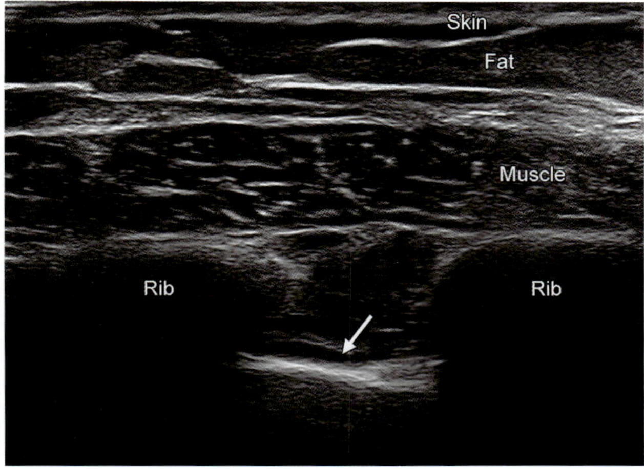

FIG. 7: High-resolution ultrasound image demonstrating normal chest wall anatomy.

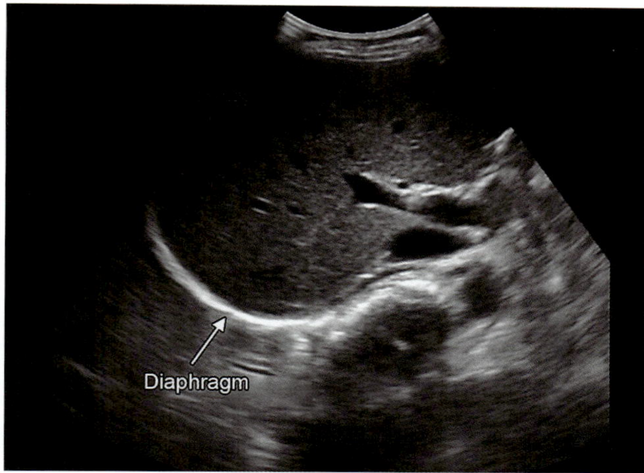

FIG. 8: Subcostal view ultrasound image shows echogenic (arrow) diaphragm.

Lung

The lung is air-filled and cannot be visualized deep to pleural lung interface. There are gross changes of acoustic impedance at this interface, leading to horizontal artifacts, which are seen as echogenic parallel lines, known as A lines **(Fig. 1A)**. Additionally, comet-tail artifacts, which are vertically oriented, can be seen in normal healthy individual. These artifacts are usually seen at the level of just above the diaphragm.

Heart

Identification of heart is important when planning for thoracentesis in left anterolateral aspect for safe puncture. The imaging features of heart on US depend upon axis and position of probe.

THORACIC ULTRASOUND IN SPECIFIC DISEASE ENTITIES

Chest Wall Pathology

Sonography can be used in initial evaluation of focal chest wall lesions, which can arise from the soft tissue or bones. Soft-tissue masses arising from the chest wall can be easily detected by using high-resolution US. Lipoma is commonly encountered chest wall mass and appears as a well-defined focal lesion with echogenicity similar to adjacent fat **(Fig. 9)**. However, sonographic features are nonspecific to differentiate between various other soft-tissue masses.[6,12,13] Lymphatic and vascular malformations can be assessed

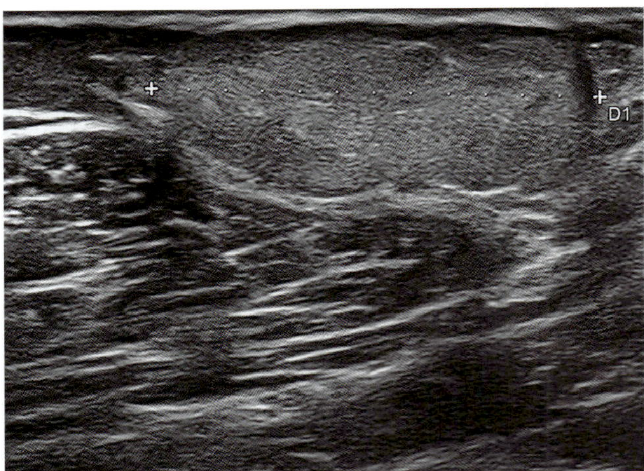

FIG. 9: Ultrasound image demonstrating chest wall lipoma as a lobulated echogenic lesion along the subcutaneous planes (marked by calipers).

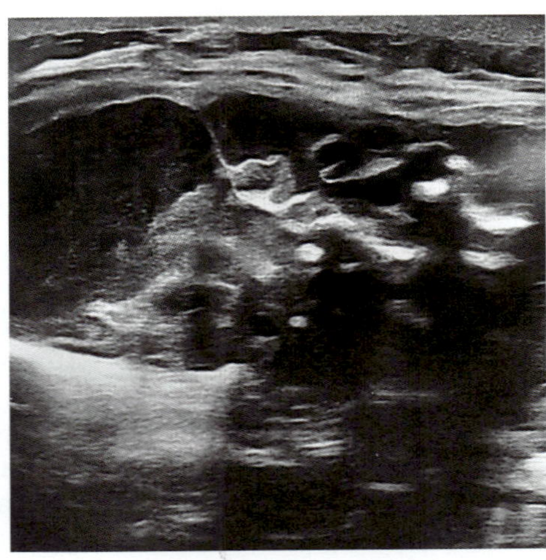

FIG. 10: Ultrasound image in a case of focal rib lesion demonstrating a hypoechoic lesion with multiple calcific foci. Ultrasound-guided biopsy was done from the lesion, which revealed chondrosarcoma.

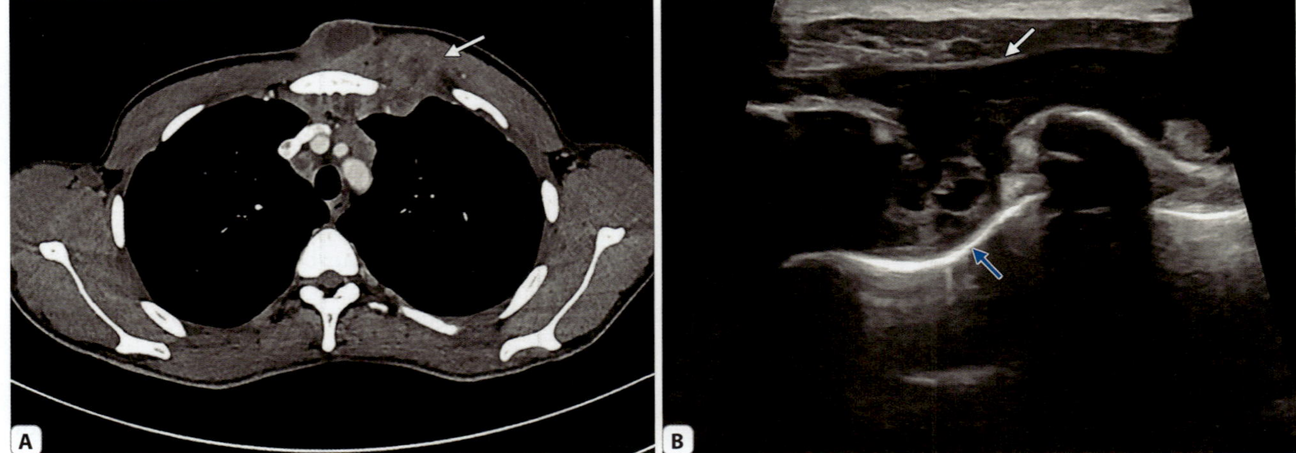

FIGS. 11A AND B: (A) Axial computed tomography (CT) image of chest showing multiloculated chest wall collection in a case of tuberculosis (white arrow). (B) Ultrasound image showing the collection to be predominantly organized (white arrow) with extension till pleural line. Note the indentation caused by the collection on parietal pleura (blue arrow).

for the presence of lymphatic and vascular component using the US. Focal bony lesions can be detected on US if there is associated cortical breach and soft tissue **(Fig. 10)**. Metastases are most commonly encountered rib lesion, which appears as irregular disruption of anterior cortex of rib on USG with associated soft-tissue component. US-guided FNAC or biopsy can be readily performed. Any chest wall collections can also be assessed for extent and intrathoracic extension on USG **(Figs. 11A and B)**. Rib fractures can also be visualized with US, which might even be more sensitive than radiography.[14] Fractures appear as linear cortical discontinuity, which can be associated with a very slight, step-like dislocation **(Fig. 12)**. Associated hematoma can be seen at the anterior contour of the break. USG can also detect coexisting injuries, such as hemothorax, pneumothorax, or pulmonary contusion.[14-18] US is more efficient than conventional radiography in the detection of sternal fractures.[18]

Pleural Pathology

Pleural Effusion

Thoracic USG is ideal for the detection, characterization, and quantification of pleural fluid. It is more sensitive than decubitus films in identifying minimal or loculated effusions. A pleural effusion appears as homogeneous, anechoic space between the parietal and visceral pleura **(Fig. 13A)**. USG can detect as little as 20 cc of pleural fluid.[19] There are two scanning methods to detect the pleural effusion: One is simply sliding the probe cephalad to right or left upper quadrant [as an extension of focused assessment with sonography in trauma (FAST) examination]. Second method is to simply put the probe in posterolateral aspect of thorax.[4,20] Two signs have also been described for the detection of pleural effusion. The static sharp sign (or quad sign) refers to the four borders delineating the anechoic pleural effusion: Superior and inferior rib shadows on either side of the screen, superficial boundary formed by parietal pleura, and the deep boundary by the lung **(Fig. 13B)**. Another sign is the dynamic sinusoidal sign, which refers to the sinusoidal pattern of the effusion seen on M-mode and corresponds to the centrifugal movement of the visceral pleura during respiration.[4] However, adhesions between the two pleural surfaces may result in the absence of lung motion above the effusion. Pleural effusion should be differentiated from pleural thickening **(Figs. 14A and B)**. Absent sinusoidal pattern on M-mode helps to differentiate pleural thickening from effusion. Also, on color Doppler, pleural effusion shows the presence of color signal due to the movement of fluid, which is not seen in pleural thickening.

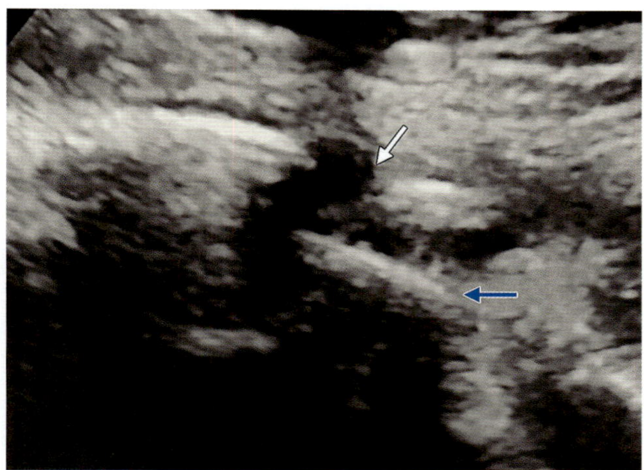

FIG. 12: Ultrasound image in a case of blunt chest trauma showing discontinuity in the echogenic rib shadow (white arrow), suggestive of fracture with displaced bony fragment lying deep to the chest wall (blue arrow).

Depending upon the internal echogenicity, four sonographic appearances of pleural effusions are recognized: (1) Anechoic **(Fig. 15A)**, (2) homogeneously hyperechoic, (3) complex nonseptated, or (4) complex septated.[21] Anechoic nonseptated effusions are usually transudates, while complex effusions with septations or internal echoes are exudative in nature.[22,23] Echogenic strands or septa within the effusion indicate an inflammatory process **(Figs. 15B and C)**. It has been shown that patients with septated effusions need longer chest tube drainage and are more likely to require fibrinolytic therapy or surgery compared to those with nonseptated effusions.[24,25] Pleural effusions associated with pleural thickening of 10 mm or more and pleural and diaphragmatic nodularity are highly suggestive of malignant effusion.[26] Hemothorax in cases of trauma requires urgent diagnosis. Chest radiography has a poor sensitivity for the detection of hemothorax. USG of the chest has been included in extended FAST protocol. The sensitivity of US to diagnose a hemothorax ranges between 92 and 96% and has a specificity of over 99%.[27-29]

Various methods have been described in literature for the quantification of pleural fluid. One method is to

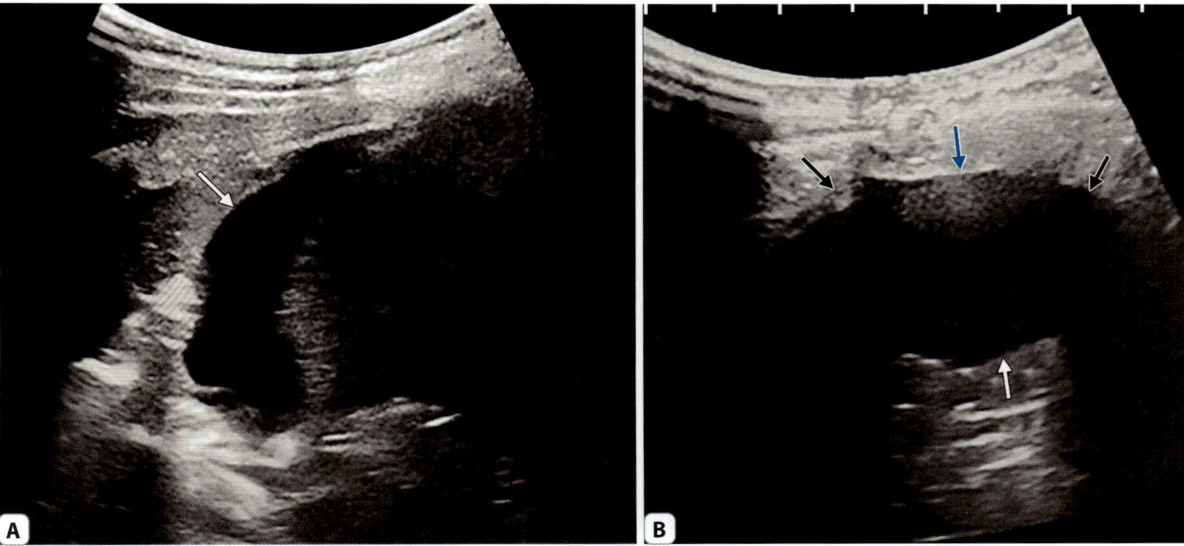

FIGS. 13A AND B: (A) Ultrasound chest image showing uncomplicated pleural effusion as anechoic area between parietal and visceral pleura (white arrow). (B) Ultrasound image showing quad sign in a case of pleural effusion showing four boundaries of pleural effusion: Superior and inferior rib shadows on either side (black arrows), parietal pleura forming superficial boundary (blue arrow), and lung forming deep boundary (white arrow).

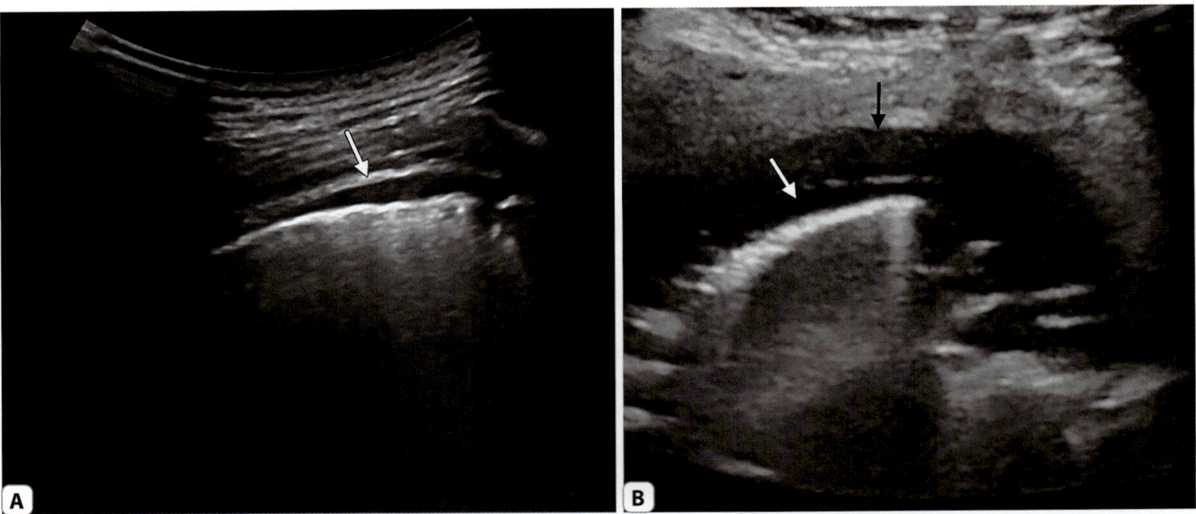

FIGS. 14A AND B: (A) Ultrasound image demonstrating minimal pleural effusion as small anechoic layer between parietal and visceral pleura (white arrow). (B) Ultrasound image in another patient shows thickened parietal pleura (black arrow) with minimal pleural effusion (white arrow).

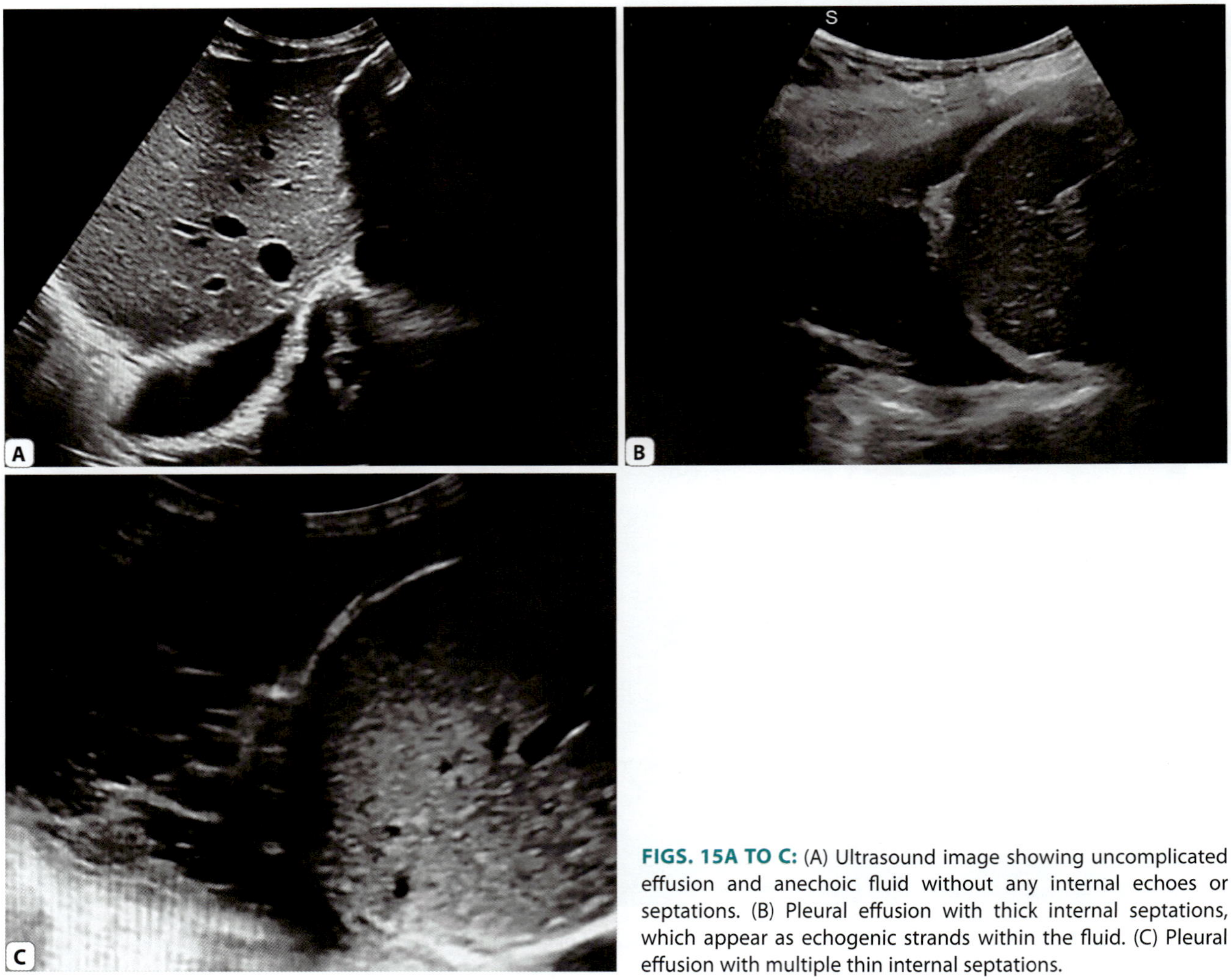

FIGS. 15A TO C: (A) Ultrasound image showing uncomplicated effusion and anechoic fluid without any internal echoes or septations. (B) Pleural effusion with thick internal septations, which appear as echogenic strands within the fluid. (C) Pleural effusion with multiple thin internal septations.

multiply the lateral height of the effusion in centimeters (with the patient in upright position) by a factor of 90, which gives estimated fluid volume (in mL).[30] However, this formula is applicable to free effusion. Another practical method is simply to classify effusions as: (1) Minimal, if anechoic space is limited to the costophrenic angle; (2) small, if the effusion is greater than the costophrenic angle but within the range of the area covered with curvilinear probe; (3) moderate, if the effusion extends the range of one probe but still within a two-probe range; and (4) large, if the space is greater than a two-probe range.[6,12,13,21] Quantification of pleural effusion can be useful in making a decision that whether volume of fluid is enough to warrant drainage for relief of dyspnea.

Ultrasonography guidance can also be used for the guidance for pleural fluid and drainage. There is high-level evidence of improved clinical outcome with USG-guided pleurocentesis.[5] USG is also ideal to identify the safe site for intercostal drainage. USG can be used to mark the appropriate site for drainage or alternatively drainage catheter can be placed by the interventional radiology team under real-time sonographic guidance.

Pneumothorax

Sensitivity of bedside chest radiography for the detection of pneumothorax ranges from 50 to 90%. A meta-analysis concluded that bedside USG performed by clinicians had a higher sensitivity and similar specificity for the diagnosis of a pneumothorax when compared to the chest radiography.[31]

As pneumothorax occurs in nondependent location, sonographic assessment of the lungs begins from the most anterior portion in supine position, usually at the 3rd and 4th intercostal space, at the parasternal-midclavicular line. The most important sign to look for pneumothorax is lung sliding, which is the gliding movement of echogenic parietal and visceral pleura occurring during respiration. The confirmation of lung sliding has a 100% negative predictive value for the absence of pneumothorax.[32] It should be noted that lung sliding can be abolished by breath hold. Power Doppler may help in confirming pleural movement in case lung sliding is not clearly appreciated on gray scale USG.[33] The presence or absence of lung sliding can be confirmed by M-mode. In normal lung, the tissue superficial to the pleural line remains stationary, resulting in smooth horizontal lines at M-mode imaging. Deep to the pleural line, the lung motion interrupts these lines, creating a fine granular pattern. This normal pattern is called the *seashore sign* **(Fig. 16)** as it depicts the boundary between the stationary chest wall (horizontal lines on M-mode resembling the "ocean") and the moving lung (granular pattern resembling the "sand"). In case of a pneumothorax, the chest wall and air deep to the pleura are both stationary, resulting in smooth uninterrupted horizontal lines. This appearance of pneumothorax at M-mode examination has been termed as the *barcode sign* **(Figs. 17A and B)**.[3] "Lung point" refers to the sonographic transition point between normal lung

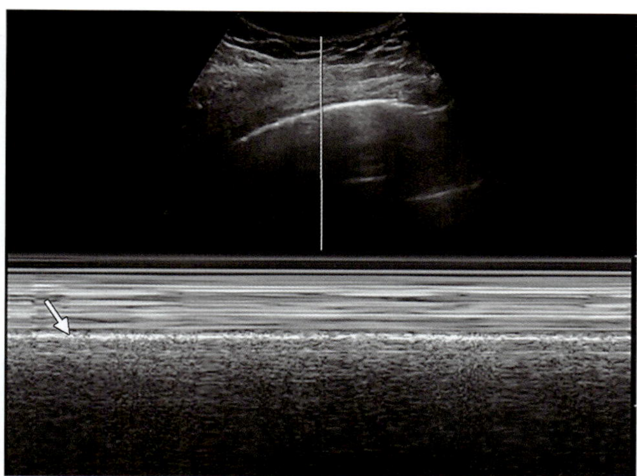

FIG. 16: M-mode sonography demonstrating normal lung motion as fine granular pattern (white arrow): *Seashore sign.*

sliding and absent lung sliding. It indicates the point on the chest wall where the visceral pleura has separated from the parietal pleura and, therefore, delineates the boundary of pneumothorax. Visualization of the lung point is 100% specific for the diagnosis of pneumothorax.[34] It should be noted that in case of complete lung collapse, lung point would not be visualized. Exaggerated A lines and absent B lines in the absence of lung sliding are reliable indicators of pneumothorax.

There are a few pitfalls of US in the diagnosis of pneumothorax. First, lung sliding can be absent in conditions other than pneumothorax such as hyperinflation in airway disease and pleural adhesions. These can mimic pneumothorax on USG. Thus, proceeding to chest tube drainage based on sonographic findings alone in such case can lead to disastrous consequences. Second, US cannot quantify the size of pneumothorax. This is a major limitation of USG as treatment decisions are often based on the size of pneumothorax.[5]

Lung Pathology

Infection

Lung US can be utilized to evaluate and monitor known or suspected pulmonary infection. In several studies, lung US was found to accurately detect the characteristic findings of a consolidation.[35,36] In a prospective study of ICU patients, US was found to have a sensitivity of 90% and a specificity of 98% in diagnosing consolidation when compared with computed tomography (CT) scan.[37] Completely consolidated lung parenchyma mimics the solid, hypoechoic appearance of the liver, known as hepatization **(Figs. 18A and B)**. Superficial boundary of consolidated lung parenchyma corresponds to the pleural line. Deeper boundary is formed by an irregular hyperechoic line, seen at the interface of normal and consolidated lung parenchyma, termed as the shred sign. Air bronchograms

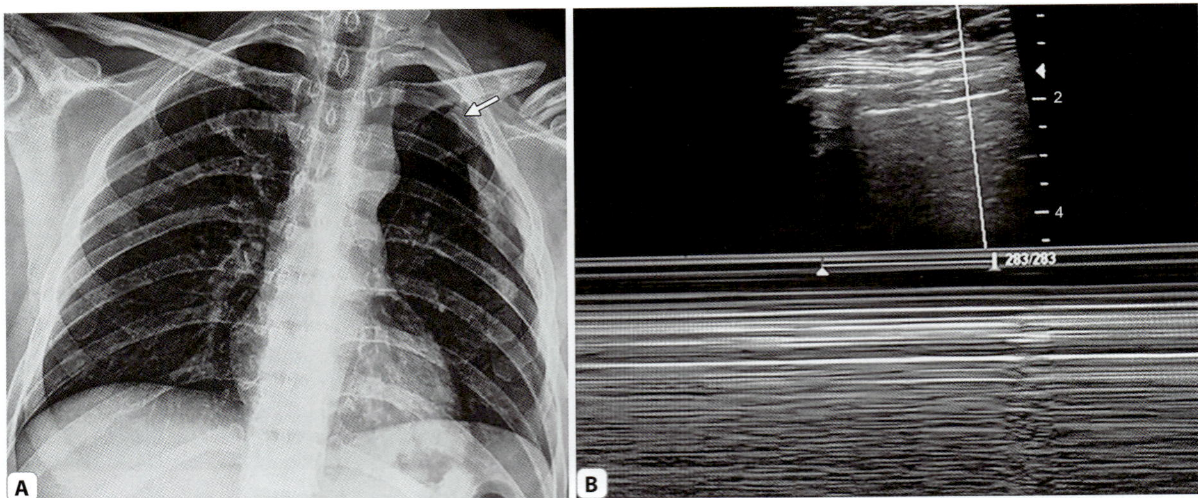

FIGS. 17A AND B: (A) Chest radiograph showing pneumothorax (white arrow) in a case of blunt chest trauma. (B) M-mode sonography showed smooth horizontal lines due to absence of lung motion: *Barcode sign.*

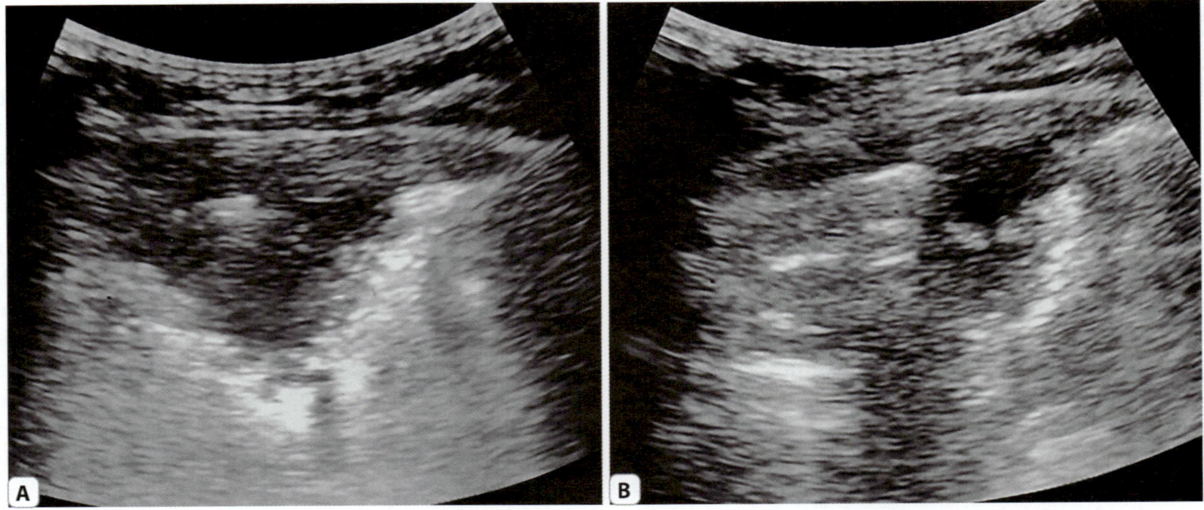

FIGS. 18A AND B: Subpleural patches of consolidation in a case of bronchopneumonia on lung ultrasonography (USG).

are seen as hyperechoic foci within the consolidated lung **(Fig. 19)**. Centrifugal movement of air foci can be seen during respiration (known as dynamic air bronchogram sign), which differentiates consolidation from atelectasis (static air bronchogram).[38] Due to replacement of alveolar air by fluid or cells in consolidation, the normal A lines are lost. Focal B lines may be seen in early infection **(Figs. 20A and B)**, indicating interstitial thickening or inflammation.

Lung abscess if abutting the pleura appears as hypoechoic lesion with a well-defined or irregular wall and anechoic center. Internal echogenic foci can be seen representing the air within the abscess cavity. Color Doppler imaging can prove useful in differentiating lung abscesses from empyema. Due to residual lung parenchyma, a lung abscess demonstrates internal vascularity, while no color flow is seen in empyema. However, air foci within the collection may demonstrate twinkle artifact on color Doppler USG.

Viral infections, including COVID-19 and bronchiolitis, can also be assessed and monitored using lung US.[39-42] Consolidations, B lines, and pleural irregularities have all been visualized in COVID-19 infection. Diffuse confluent B lines are present in focal areas of ground-glass opacification. During the recovery phase, the B lines gradually decrease with reappearance of A lines.

Pulmonary Edema

The presence of multiple comet-tail artifacts (more than four to six per costal space) is suggestive of acute pulmonary edema.[37] Pulmonary edema and acute respiratory distress syndrome (ARDS) are characterized by increase in extracellular lung volume, which manifest on USG as multiple confluent B lines. While confluent B lines can be seen in both entities, abnormalities of pleural line with reduced or absent lung sliding, consolidations, and intervening normal lung parenchyma point toward a diagnosis of ARDS. On the other hand, more diffused involvement with smooth pleural line and associated pleural effusions point toward a diagnosis of pulmonary edema.[43]

Pulmonary Embolism

The use of lung USG for the diagnosis of pulmonary embolism is a relatively new concept. A subpleural wedge-shaped hypoechoic area is the most common sonographic finding in pulmonary embolism. These have been referred to as C lines by Lichtenstein.[44] A localized fluid collection may also develop adjacent to the affected lung. A localized subpleural effusion can be seen in around 40% of patients, while basal pleural effusions can be seen in up to 60% of cases.[5] However, lung USG has limitations in the diagnosis of pulmonary embolism as only peripheral lesions can be visualized, and there are no standardized criteria for diagnosis. However, ability to perform concurrent bedside compression USG for deep venous thrombosis and echocardiography to evaluate right heart strain greatly improves the diagnostic performance of USG in the diagnosis of pulmonary embolism.

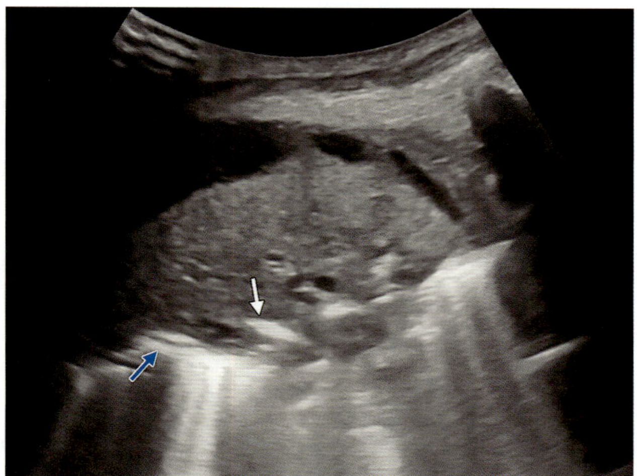

FIG. 19: Ultrasonography (USG) image showing consolidation with air bronchogram (white arrow) and associated pleural effusion. Irregular hyperechoic line is seen at the interface of normal and consolidated lung parenchyma (blue arrow): *Shred sign*. Also, note B lines in underlying lung parenchyma.

Interstitial Lung Disease

Like other diseases involving alveoli or interstitium, B lines can be seen in interstitial lung disease (ILD). Other findings include irregular thickening of pleural line, which is more prominent in the lower lobes. Physiological lung sliding may be decreased. Immobility of the diaphragm can be seen in end-stage disease.[45-47]

Lung Mass

Lung tumors appear as nodular hypoechoic area on USG with irregular blurred margins **(Figs. 21A and B)**. Hyperechoic and anechoic appearances have also been described. Visceral pleural line is interrupted in case of infiltration. Once the mass extends beyond the parietal pleura, there is loss of movement with respiration. It has been shown that high-resolution USG of chest is superior to CT for evaluation of tumor infiltration of pleura and chest wall.[48,49] Contrast-enhanced USG has shown promising results with recent studies showing its ability to characterize peripheral lung masses.[50,51] In addition, USG can provide guidance of FNAC and biopsy of peripheral lung lesions.

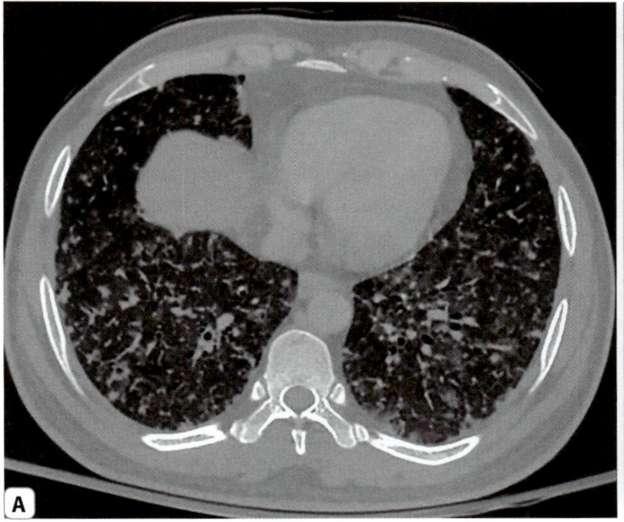

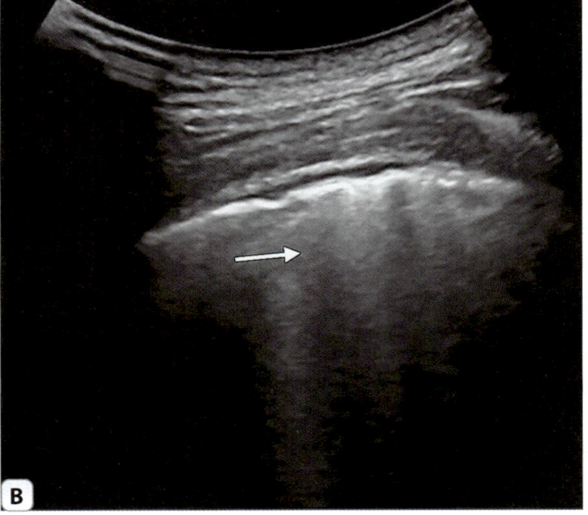

FIGS. 20A AND B: (A) Axial CT image showing multiple air space and interstitial opacities in a case of viral pneumonia. (B) On USG, loss of A lines was seen with presence of B lines (white arrow).

(CT: computed tomography; USG: ultrasonography)

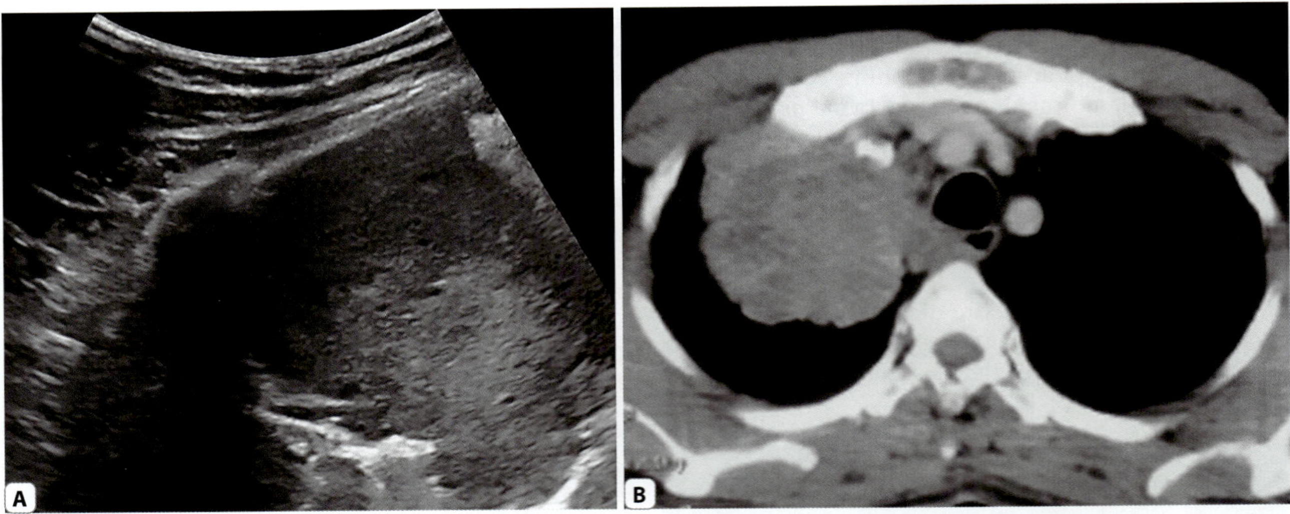

FIGS. 21A AND B: (A) USG of the chest in a case of carcinoma lung showing large hypoechoic mass with lobulated margins abutting the visceral pleura. (B) CT image shows a heterogeneously enhancing mass in right upper lobe, abutting the mediastinal and costal pleura.
(CT: computed tomography; USG: ultrasonography)

CONCLUSION

Thoracic sonography is a rapid, portable, and safe imaging modality that can be performed at the bedside. In recent years, it has become an imaging staple among chest and critical care physicians. Thus, the radiologist should be adept at performing and interpreting the thoracic US to stay relevant and help the clinician.

REFERENCES

1. Lichtenstein DA. Lung ultrasound in the critically ill. Ann Intensive Care. 2014;4(1):1.
2. Lichtenstein DA. BLUE-protocol and FALLS-protocol: two applications of lung ultrasound in the critically ill. Chest. 2015;147(6):1659-70.
3. Marini TJ, Rubens DJ, Zhao YT, Weis J, O'Connor TP, Novak WH, et al. Lung ultrasound: the essentials. Radiol Cardiothorac Imaging. 2021;3(2):e200564.
4. Turner JP, Dankoff J. Thoracic ultrasound. Emerg Med Clin North Am. 2012;30(2):451-73.
5. Hew M, Heinze S. Chest ultrasound in practice: a review of utility in the clinical setting. Intern Med J. 2012;42(8):856-65.
6. Koh DM, Burke S, Davies N, Padley SPG. Transthoracic US of the chest: clinical uses and applications. Radiographics. 2002;22(1):e1.
7. Havelock T, Teoh R, Laws D, Gleeson F; BTS Pleural Disease Guideline Group. Pleural procedures and thoracic ultrasound: British Thoracic Society pleural disease guideline 2010. Thorax. 2010;65 Suppl 2:ii61-76.
8. Feller-Kopman D. Ultrasound-guided thoracentesis. Chest. 2006;129(6):1709-14.
9. Diacon AH, Theron J, Bolliger CT. Transthoracic ultrasound for the pulmonologist. Curr Opin Pulm Med. 2005;11(4):307-12.
10. Tsai TH, Yang PC. Ultrasound in the diagnosis and management of pleural disease. Curr Opin Pulm Med. 2003;9(4):282-90.
11. Smereczyński A, Kołaczyk K, Bernatowicz E. Chest wall–underappreciated structure in sonography. Part I: examination methodology and ultrasound anatomy. J Ultrason. 2017;17(70):197-205.
12. Koegelenberg CFN, Bolliger CT, Diacon AH. Radiology: Pleural ultrasound. In: Light RW, Lee YCG (Eds). Textbook of Pleural Diseases, 2nd edition. London: CRC Press; 2008. pp. 271-84.
13. Koegelenberg CFN, Diacon AH, Bolliger CT. Transthoracic ultrasound of the chest wall, pleura, and the peripheral lung. In: Bolliger CT, Herth FJF, Mayo PH, Miyazawa T, Beamis JF (Eds). Progress in Respiratory Research. Clinical Chest Ultrasound: From the ICU to the Bronchoscopy Suite, 1st edition. Basel: Karger; 2009. pp. 22-33.
14. Mathis G. Thoraxsonography—Part I: chest wall and pleura. Ultrasound Med Biol. 1997;23(8):1131-9.
15. Meuwly JY, Gudinchet F. Sonography of the thoracic and abdominal walls. J Clin Ultrasound. 2004;32(9):500-10.
16. Dietrich CF, Mathis G, Cui XW, Ignee A, Hocke M, Hirche TO. Ultrasound of the pleurae and lungs. Ultrasound Med Biol. 2015;41(2):351-65.
17. Lee RKL, Griffith JF, Ng AWH, Sitt JCM. Sonography of the chest wall: a pictorial essay. J Clin Ultrasound. 2015;43(9):525-37.
18. Smereczyński A, Kołaczyk K, Bernatowicz E. Chest wall–underappreciated structure in sonography. Part II: non-cancerous lesions. J Ultrason. 2017;17(71):275-80.

19. Röthlin MA, Näf R, Amgwerd M, Candinas D, Frick T, Trentz O. Ultrasound in blunt abdominal and thoracic trauma. J Trauma. 1993;34(4):488-95.
20. Lichtenstein D. Lung ultrasound in the critically ill. In:Vincent JL (Ed). Yearbook of Intensive Care and Emergency Medicine. Heidelberg, Germany: Springer; 2004. pp. 624-44.
21. von Groote-Bidlingmaier F, Koegelenberg CFN. A practical guide to transthoracic ultrasound. Breathe. 2012;9(2):132-42.
22. Yang PC, Luh KT, Chang DB, Wu HD, Yu CJ, Kuo SH. Value of sonography in determining the nature of pleural effusion: analysis of 320 cases. Am J Roentgenol. 1992;159(1):29-33.
23. Hirsch JH, Rogers JV, Mack LA. Real-time sonography of pleural opacities. Am J Roentgenol. 1981;136(2):297-301.
24. Chen KY, Liaw YS, Wang HC, Luh KT, Yang PC. Sonographic septation: a useful prognostic indicator of acute thoracic empyema. J Ultrasound Med. 2000;19(12):837-43.
25. Tu CY, Hsu WH, Hsia TC, Chen HJ, Tsai KD, Hung CW, et al. Pleural effusions in febrile medical ICU patients: chest ultrasound study. Chest. 2004;126(4):1274-80.
26. Qureshi NR, Rahman NM, Gleeson FV. Thoracic ultrasound in the diagnosis of malignant pleural effusion. Thorax. 2009;64(2):139-43.
27. Ma OJ, Mateer JR. Trauma ultrasound examination versus chest radiography in the detection of hemothorax. Ann Emerg Med. 1997;29(3):312-5.
28. Brooks A, Davies B, Smethhurst M, Connolly J. Emergency ultrasound in the acute assessment of haemothorax. Emerg Med J. 2004;21(1):44-6.
29. Rocco M, Carbone I, Morelli A, Bertoletti L, Rossi S, Vitale M, et al. Diagnostic accuracy of bedside ultrasonography in the ICU: feasibility of detecting pulmonary effusion and lung contusion in patients on respiratory support after severe blunt thoracic trauma. Acta Anaesthesiol Scand. 2008;52(6):776-84.
30. Goecke W, Schwerk WB. Die real-time-snographie in der diagnostik von pleuraergüssen. In: Gebhardt J, Hackelöer BJ, von Klinggräff G, Seitz K (Eds). Ultraschall-diagnostik'89. Berlin: Springer; 1990. pp. 385-7.
31. Ding W, Shen Y, Yang J, He X, Zhang M. Diagnosis of pneumothorax by radiography and ultrasonography: a meta-analysis. Chest. 2011;140(4):859-66.
32. Lichtenstein DA, Menu Y. A bedside ultrasound sign ruling out pneumothorax in the critically ill. Lung sliding. Chest. 1995;108(5):1345-8.
33. Cunningham J, Kirkpatrick AW, Nicolaou S, Liu D, Hamilton DR, Lawless B, et al. Enhanced recognition of "lung sliding" with power color Doppler imaging in the diagnosis of pneumothorax. J Trauma. 2002;52(4):769-71.
34. Lichtenstein D, Mezière G, Biderman P, Gepner A. The "lung point": an ultrasound sign specific to pneumothorax. Intensive Care Med. 2000;26(10):1434-40.
35. Targhetta R, Chavagneux R, Bourgeois JM, Dauzat M, Balmes P, Pourcelot L. Sonographic approach to diagnosing pulmonary consolidation. J Ultrasound Med. 1992;11(12):667-72.
36. Yang PC, Luh KT, Chang DB, Yu CJ, Kuo SH, Wu HD. Ultrasonographic evaluation of pulmonary consolidation. Am Rev Respir Dis. 1992;146(3):757-62.
37. Lichtenstein DA, Lascols N, Mezière G, Gepner A. Ultrasound diagnosis of alveolar consolidation in the critically ill. Intensive Care Med. 2004;30(2):276-81.
38. Weinberg B, Diakoumakis EE, Kass EG, Seife B, Zvi ZB. The air bronchogram: sonographic demonstration. AJR Am J Roentgenol. 1986;147(3):593-5.
39. Gargani L, Soliman-Aboumarie H, Volpicelli G, Corradi F, Pastore MC, Cameli M. Why, when, and how to use lung ultrasound during the COVID-19 pandemic: enthusiasm and caution. Eur Heart J Cardiovasc Imaging. 2020;21(9):941-8.
40. Peng QY, Wang XT, Zhang LN; Chinese Critical Care Ultrasound Study Group (CCUSG). Findings of lung ultrasonography of novel corona virus pneumonia during the 2019-2020 epidemic. Intensive Care Med. 2020;46(5):849-50.
41. Sultan LR, Sehgal CM. A review of early experience in lung ultrasound in the diagnosis and management of COVID-19. Ultrasound Med Biol. 2020;46(9):2530-45.
42. Volpicelli G, Lamorte A, Villén T. What's new in lung ultrasound during the COVID-19 pandemic. Intensive Care Med. 2020;46(7):1445-8.
43. Copetti R, Soldati G, Copetti P. Chest sonography: a useful tool to differentiate acute cardiogenic pulmonary edema from acute respiratory distress syndrome. Cardiovasc Ultrasound. 2008;6:16.
44. Lichtenstein DA, Loubières Y. Lung sonography in pulmonary embolism. Chest. 2003;123(6):2154.
45. Sperandeo M, Filabozzi P, Varriale A, Carnevale V, Piattelli ML, Sperandeo G, et al. Role of thoracic ultrasound in the assessment of pleural and pulmonary diseases. J Ultrasound. 2008;11(2):39-46.
46. Sperandeo M, Varriale A, Sperandeo G, Filabozzi P, Piattelli ML, Carnevale V, et al. Transthoracic ultrasound in the evaluation of pulmonary fibrosis. our experience. Ultrasound Med Biol. 2009;35(5):723-9.
47. Lichtenstein D, Mézière G, Biderman P, Gepner A, Barré O. The comet-tail artifact. An ultrasound sign of alveolar-interstitial syndrome. Am J Respir Crit Care Med. 1997;156(5):1640-6.
48. Sugama Y, Tamaki S, Kitamura S, Kira S. Ultrasonographic evaluation of pleural and chest wall invasion of lung cancer. Chest. 1988;93(2):275-9.
49. Suzuki N, Saitoh T, Kitamura S. Tumor invasion of the chest wall in lung cancer: diagnosis with US. Radiology. 1993;187(1):39-42.
50. Herth FJF, Becker HD. Transthoracic ultrasound. Respiration. 2003;70(1):87-94.
51. Sperandeo M, Sperandeo G, Varriale A, Filabozzi P, Decuzzi M, Dimitri L, et al. Contrast-enhanced ultrasound (CEUS) for the study of peripheral lung lesions: a preliminary study. Ultrasound Med Biol. 2006;32(10):1467-72.

Rashmi Dixit, Anjali Prakash, Alpana Manchanda

CHAPTER

3

Cross-sectional Imaging of Chest: Techniques and Anatomy

INTRODUCTION

Imaging evaluation of thoracic disease invariably begins with a chest radiograph. Cross-sectional imaging is indicated not only for detailed evaluation of abnormalities seen on the radiograph but also to detect occult lesions not apparent on the radiograph, especially when there is strong clinical suspicion of thoracic disease. Multidetector computed tomography (MDCT) remains the imaging method most widely used for the study of thoracic diseases due to its high spatial and temporal resolution, ease of performance, and widespread availability. Magnetic resonance (MR) is mainly a problem-solving modality with emerging applications.

MULTIDETECTOR COMPUTED TOMOGRAPHY OF THORAX

COMPUTED TOMOGRAPHY TECHNOLOGY

Spiral CT systems introduced in the 1990s represented a significant advancement in CT technology, allowing volumetric data acquisition as opposed to the discontinuous data acquisition in conventional CT.[1] In 1998, the first MDCT scanners were introduced, allowing simultaneous acquisition of four slices (or sections) with gantry rotation times, which were as low as 0.55 seconds.[1] These scanners resulted in improvement in acquisition speed, Z-axis coverage, and temporal and spatial resolution over the single-slice spiral or helical CT scanners. Thus, high-resolution, single breath-hold imaging of the entire thorax became feasible.

Thereon, MDCT technology has developed at a breath-taking pace, with increasing detector rows and decreasing tube rotation times. Currently, scanners with >128 active detector rows and gantry rotation times as low as 0.33–0.25 seconds per rotation are available. These scanners are able to scan the entire thorax in 2–3 seconds, dramatically reducing motion artifacts.[1,2] The best temporal resolution that is achievable in a single-source CT scan is half the rotation time of the scanner, as this is the minimum data needed for image reconstruction close to the isocenter, with gantry rotation time of 0.3 seconds. The best possible temporal resolution is 125–150 ms.

In subsequent years, further increase in spatial and temporal resolution has been made possible by the use of either wide-area detectors or dual-source CT (DSCT) systems.[2] *An area detector* is a CT detector that is wide enough in the Z-axis to cover an entire organ such as the heart, kidney, or brain without table movement. Area detector systems have the ability to acquire dynamic volume data by scanning the same anatomic range repeatedly without table movement. This is useful for perfusion scanning of pulmonary nodules.[2] *DSCT* systems use two X-ray tubes and detector systems positioned at 90° to each other, which can simultaneously acquire data at the same Z-position. DSCT systems allow a significant improvement of temporal resolution below 100 ms.[3] Due to two X-ray tubes, the best temporal resolution achievable in these CT systems is quarter of a gantry rotation, as the two 90° segments acquired can be put together to give the required minimum 180° of scan data at the isocenter. Thus, with DSCT scanners, the entire thorax can be scanned within 0.3 seconds, almost eliminating respiratory and even cardiac motion artifacts.[1,4] They also allow a reduction in contrast dose. DSCT systems also provide dual energy applications, which are discussed later. *Photon-counting detector CT* is the most recent advancement in CT technology. It uses semiconductors that convert X-ray photons directly to electronic pulses (not to light as scintillation detectors do), resulting in improved spatial resolution and noise as well as radiation dose reduction. In-plane spatial resolution is high at 0.125 mm (vs. 0.3–0.5 mm for MDCT), with improved visibility of interstitial abnormalities and pulmonary nodules. Superior spectral CT capabilities, allowing reconstruction at a variety of photon energies, can be useful in perfusion imaging, radiation dose, metal artifact, and contrast dose reduction.[5,6]

COMPUTED TOMOGRAPHY ACQUISITION AND RECONSTRUCTION PROTOCOLS

Routinely, scans are acquired in the supine position in full inspiration to fully expand the lungs. This optimizes the contrast between the aerated lung and other normal high attenuation structures (e.g., vessels) and various abnormalities. Full inspiration also minimizes the occurrence of transient atelectasis. Scanning is generally done with thin collimation, while images are reconstructed at a thickness slightly greater than the collimation to reduce noise in the reconstructed image. For example, in a 64 detector row scanner, the collimation is 64 × 0.625 or 64 × 0.5 (depending on the vendor), while images can be reconstructed at 1, 3, and 5 mm thickness from the same dataset.

The clinical indication dictates the choice of reconstruction. While 1 mm sections provide higher spatial resolution, a 3-mm thick slice has a better signal-to-noise ratio (SNR) for the same acquisition dose. Thin-section reconstructions are used for volumetric assessment and characterization of pulmonary nodules, pulmonary embolism, and for the evaluation of interstitial lung disease (ILD). Thin sections with 20–25% overlap are also used for three-dimensional (3D) reconstructions. Thicker 3–5 mm sections are generally adequate for the assessment of mediastinal masses, lung cancer staging, quick review, and archiving.[1,2,7]

Use of Iodinated Contrast Medium

Most thoracic CT examinations, except high-resolution computed tomography (HRCT) scans, are routinely performed with intravenous contrast. The aim of contrast administration is to opacify organs and delineate vessels within the area of interest. For most indications such as lung cancer staging, evaluation of mediastinal masses, or lymphadenopathy, a small-to-moderate amount of contrast medium, i.e., 60–120 mL of 300 mg I/mL at a slow injection rate of 1.5–3 mL/second with a long injection duration and scan delay of about 25 seconds produces adequate opacification of thoracic vessels. The contrast injection should ideally end about 5 seconds before the MDCT acquisition and should be followed by a saline flush to reduce perivenous artifacts and improve the contrast bolus. A caudocranial direction of acquisition also minimizes perivenous artifacts.[7,8]

Window Settings and Reconstruction Algorithms[1,7]

Organs in the thorax have a wide range of densities or Hounsfield unit (HU) values ranging from –800 for aerated lungs to +700 for osseous structures such as the ribs. A single window setting would be unable to represent these. A minimum of two window settings is required, one to display the lung parenchyma and another to display the soft-tissue structures of the mediastinum. Although the exact window settings may vary between institutions, a window width of 300–500 HU and center of +40 HU are used for the mediastinum; while for the lungs, a wide window of 1,200–1,500 HU with a center of –600 HU is more appropriate. For the evaluation of osseous structures, bone window settings at a window width of around 1,500 HU and center of 450 HU are used in addition.

The choice of window settings is important, as it can affect the approximate size of normal structures and pathology. The most accurate size measurement is done when the window level is halfway between the density of the structure to be measured and density of the surrounding tissue. Thus, the diameter of a pulmonary nodule will be underestimated if measured at soft-tissue settings appropriate for the mediastinum. The smaller structures, e.g., peripheral pulmonary vessels, are more affected by inappropriate window settings than larger structures. Some authors recommend the use of specific window settings for certain conditions such as the use of wide window settings (600 HU – WW and 100–150 HU window level) while interpreting routine CT scans of the chest to improve detection of unsuspected pulmonary embolism. Specific window settings have also been described for the evaluation of airways and emphysema.

Each manufacturer provides several *reconstruction algorithms* to optimize the visualization of various structures. The high frequency algorithm provides the best visualization of lung architecture, while a standard smooth algorithm gives best soft-tissue resolution and lowest noise for the mediastinum.

HIGH-RESOLUTION COMPUTED TOMOGRAPHY

High-resolution computed tomography is the use of thin-section CT images (0.625–1.5 mm) with high spatial frequency reconstruction algorithm to detect and characterize diseases of pulmonary parenchyma and small airways.

Before the advent of MDCT, routine CT of the chest and HRCT were strongly differentiated. The traditional HRCT protocol consisted of thin-section CT obtained with 1 mm slice thickness at intervals of 10 or even 20 mm and reconstructed using high spatial frequency algorithms. The logic behind this protocol was that analysis of a diffuse parenchymal process did not require continuous coverage.

The other reason is that the relatively higher doses required to achieve excellent SNR and image quality did not result in an exponential increase in patient dose with discontinuous scanning. With the current MDCT scanners, each CT of the chest is an HRCT as the whole chest can be covered with a narrow detector width of 0.5–1.25 mm at sufficiently low radiation dose and images reconstructed at 1–1.5 mm thickness with a high spatial frequency algorithm—the two essential factors that constitute an HRCT. Thus, in the past few years, discontinuous HRCT acquisition has been largely replaced by volumetric HRCT.[1,7,9]

Volumetric scan allows easier and more precise delineation of disease distribution and comparison in follow-up studies. Subtle focal disease can also be detected, which may be missed on the discontinuous scan. This may be especially useful when the diagnosis of ILD versus focal lung disease is not apparent clinically.

Modifications in Scanning Technique for High-resolution Computed Tomography[7,10,11]

Intravenous contrast is not required and, in fact, should be avoided, as it may cause fallacious parenchymal opacification and interfere with interpretation.

Images are usually obtained in the *supine position in full inspiration* such as routine scanning. In the normal lung effects of gravity on blood flow and gas volume as well as some nongravity, dependent effects can result in increase in attenuation and vessel size from anterior to posterior portion of the lung and may produce appearances similar to subpleural lines or atelectasis. In the *prone position*, these hydrostatic densities will disappear, while true pathology will persist. The older publications with scans obtained on slower scanners with discontinuous technique reported the utility of prone scans in around 20% of patients. This, however, is not the case with the current fast scanning technique. Prone scanning may be useful in a few selected patients with questionable subtle disease in dorsobasal area only, which would be critical in deciding the presence or absence of early disease, e.g., in a patient with asbestosis.

Addition of *expiratory scans* may be useful in the detection of focal or diffuse air trapping. In most cases with clinically significant small airway disease, mosaic attenuation may be visible on inspiratory scans, though much less conspicuous than expiratory scans. Diseases of the larger airways such as tracheobronchomalacia, however, will not be detected if only end-inspiratory images are obtained.

High-quality HRCT examinations provide a spatial resolution of 0.5 mm and due to the high contrast within the lung parenchyma, even structures as small as 0.2 mm can be seen well. Certain *modifications in reconstruction techniques* are important for achieving this given as follows:

- Use of *thin collimation* of 1 mm slice improves resolution and allows detection of important morphological features such as septal thickening, dilatation of airways, and detection of small nodules. However, a slice thickness below 1 mm does not result in any significant improvement in spatial resolution while increasing image noise.
- Application of *high-spatial frequency reconstruction algorithm*: Standard reconstruction algorithms result in smoothening of the image by reducing visible image noise and increasing the contrast resolution. High-spatial frequency or "sharp" high-resolution algorithms reduce image smoothening and increase spatial resolution. Tissue interfaces and anatomic margins, e.g., the pleura, fissures, or septae, appear sharper, and small vessels and bronchi are better seen **(Figs. 1A and B)**.
- Use of a *suitably small field of view (FOV)* decreases pixel size and, thus, increases spatial resolution. The FOV should be adjusted to the outer cortex of the ribs—this ensures that the field is restricted to the size of the lungs while no portion of the lung is cutoff. This results in a spatial resolution of 0.5–0.3 mm. Sometimes, targeted reconstruction of a particular lung or lobe may be done to further increase the spatial resolution for the evaluation of minute abnormalities. However, the resolution is limited by the intrinsic resolution of the detectors. Targeted reconstruction is generally a matter of personal preference, and there is no definitive literature recommending its use.

ACQUISITION PROTOCOL AND CONTRAST OPACIFICATION FOR COMPUTED TOMOGRAPHY PULMONARY ANGIOGRAPHY[1,8,12]

The major factor to be considered for the technical success of a computed tomography pulmonary angiography (CTPA) examination is excellent opacification of pulmonary vessels. The attenuation within the pulmonary arteries should be at least 250 HU to allow detection of filling defects and thrombi. A caudocranial acquisition is preferred; as with this, the basal portion will not show motion artifacts even in severely dyspneic patients. This is a common region for pulmonary emboli to lodge. Caudocranial acquisition also reduces perivenous streak artifacts. With the older generation of scanners, which took about 20–25 seconds to scan the thorax, 120–140 mL of 350–380 mg/mL iodine was required; however, with the latest MDCT scanners, injected volume and iodine dose can be reduced markedly, and 50 mL of contrast may be sufficient **(Figs. 2A and B)**. Scanners with capability of scanning at 70 kV are now available where the dose of iodine may be reduced to as low as 20 mL. In order to reduce radiation and optimize the contrast dose during CTPA, the following should be done:

- Reduce kV from the routine 120 to 100 kV or even 80 kV especially in thin patients to take advantage of the K-edge absorption of iodine.

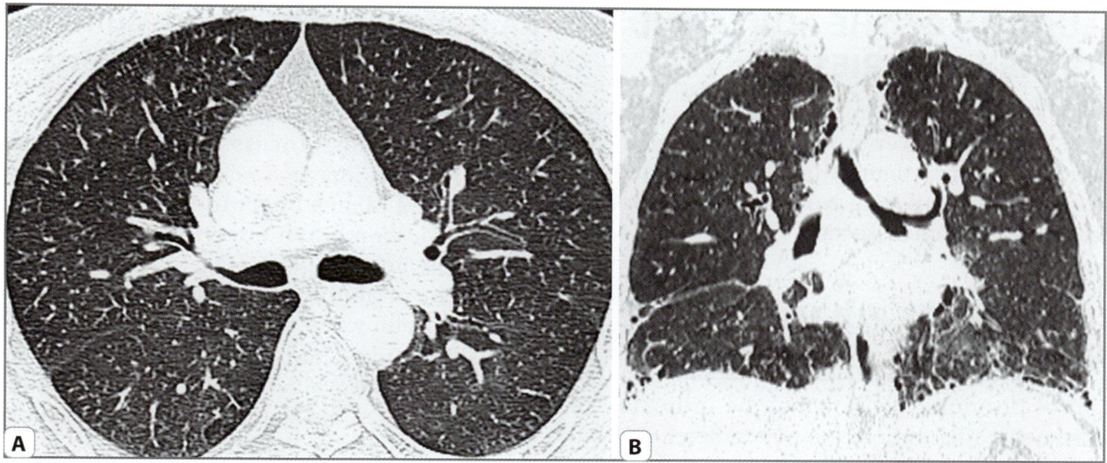

FIGS. 1A AND B: Normal HRCT. (A) 1 mm axial section from a volumetric spiral acquisition on a 128-slice MDCT scanner shows small vessels and bronchi in exquisite detail. (B) Coronal reconstruction in another patient shows the apicobasal gradient of interstitial lung disease.

(HRCT: high-resolution computed tomography; MDCT: multidetector computed tomography)

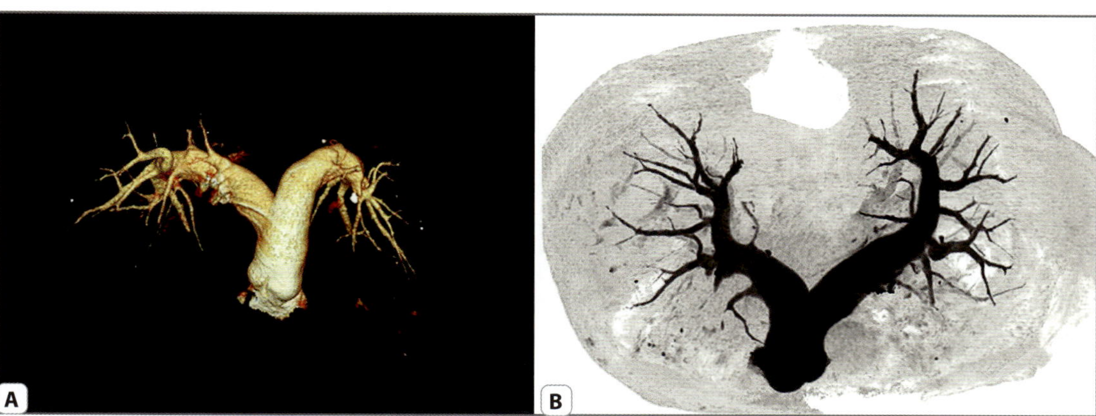

FIGS. 2A AND B: Normal CT pulmonary angiogram. (A and B) Volume-rendered and MIP imaging displayed in the negative or angiographic mode obtained with 30 mL of 350 mg I/mL contrast.

(CT: computed tomography; MIP: maximum intensity projection)

- Optimize flow rates to patient physiology, e.g., for old patients with possible altered left ventricular function, flow rate of 3 mL/second with high iodine concentration of 350–400 mg/mL is needed, while in a young patient or a pregnant patient, a much higher flow rate of 5–6 mL/second will be required.[12]
- *Calculate the correct contrast volume required*: The acquisition time should be noted by setting the acquisition box in the scout. For a 128-slice scanner, this is about 2 seconds. Acquisition time is added to time for breath-hold instruction (generally 5 seconds) and a reserve time of 5 seconds, which equals 12 seconds (2 + 5 + 5) in this case. Using a flow rate of 4 cc/second, total volume can be calculated as total time × flow rate (12 × 4 = 48 cc) for perfect vessel opacification. Scan should be triggered by bolus-tracking region of interest (ROI) in the main pulmonary artery (MPA) or right ventricle with a trigger threshold of 80–120 HU.
- Holding of breath in deep inspiration or Valsalva maneuver is to be avoided to prevent *transient interruption of contrast medium*. This results in poor opacification of the pulmonary artery, while the superior vena cava (SVC) and aorta are well opacified. Various mechanisms have been proposed for this, which include increased venous return of unopacified blood from inferior vena cava (IVC) to right atrium (RA), resulting in poor opacification of pulmonary arteries. Opening of patent foramen ovale due to Valsalva maneuver is thought to be the other reason. Hence, the patient should be asked simply to hold his breath and not to take deep inspiration during acquisition.

EVALUATION OF THE AORTA AND CORONARY ARTERIES

Evaluation of the aorta and coronary arteries is discussed elsewhere in this book; however, electrocardiogram (ECG) gating is mandatory for coronary artery evaluation and can also help to eliminate confusing artifacts at the aortic root in patients with suspected dissection.

EVALUATION OF PULMONARY VEINS

Evaluation of pulmonary veins may be indicated in suspected stenosis after radiofrequency catheter ablation treatment of chronic atrial fibrillation. A preprocedure CT is also indicated to map variant venous anatomy to enhance the success rate of the procedure and to exclude atrial thrombi, which are an absolute contraindication for the procedure. This requires 70–85 mL of 300–370 mg I/mL contrast to be administrated at 4–5 mL/second, acquisition being triggered by bolus-tracking ROI placed in the left atrium (LA). ECG gating is not routinely required as the atria move much less compared with coronary arteries with cardiac motion, and the pulmonary veins are much larger structures.[13]

EXTENDED CHEST PAIN PROTOCOL OR TRIPLE RULE-OUT COMPUTED TOMOGRAPHY

In this case, the aim of contrast injection is to achieve opacification of the aorta, coronary arteries, and pulmonary arteries. The details are discussed elsewhere.[14]

POSTPROCESSING TECHNIQUES[1,11,15,16]

The goal of true isotropic imaging, i.e., each voxel with equal dimensions in all three axes, was achieved with the introduction of modern MDCT scanners. This allows high-quality two-dimensional (2D) and 3D reconstructions, converting CT from a 2D imaging modality to a volumetric or 3D imaging technique. Although axial images remain critical to establishing the diagnosis, these reconstructions are extremely useful for the display of airways (including complex congenital abnormalities), vascular structures, and distribution of pulmonary disease. Isotropic imaging has also helped the development of computer-aided detection and diagnosis programs. They increase diagnostic confidence, allow preprocedural planning for surgery or bronchoscopy, and improve communication with clinicians and patients.

Multiplanar and Curved Multiplanar Reconstruction or Curved Planar Reconstruction

These are 2D postprocessing techniques that can be used to obtain images in coronal, sagittal, oblique, or even curved planes by reordering voxels into a single voxel thick tomographic section, excluding the voxels outside the imaging plane **(Fig. 3)**. They allow viewing of a structure or abnormality in alternative planes; hence, they are useful when there are interpretative difficulties on axial sections. Multiplanar reconstructions (MPRs) are useful for the evaluation of large airways and vascular structures and to distinguish periarteriolar peribronchial lesions from endoluminal ones. They are especially valuable for determining the craniocaudal length of airway stenosis, which may be underestimated on axial images alone. They also allow accurate delineation of structures that run obliquely to the axial imaging plane. Demonstration of centrilobular emphysema is facilitated as well. Coronal reformation helps to display of the distribution of parenchymal lung disease, e.g., the craniocaudal gradient in ILD. Sagittal images can sharply delineate fissures and help to assess transfissural extension of disease.

Maximum Intensity Projection

Maximum intensity projection (MIP) is a 3D reconstruction technique in which a ray is passed through the dataset, and only pixels above a certain assigned value are used, reducing the data to a single plane (this lacks depth information). Slabs of 5–10 mm for thin MIPs or the entire dataset may be used for thick MIPs. In the thorax, it is used mainly for vascular imaging and for evaluation of small pulmonary nodules where it may help to distinguish small nodules from vessels and in the precise delineation of nodule distribution

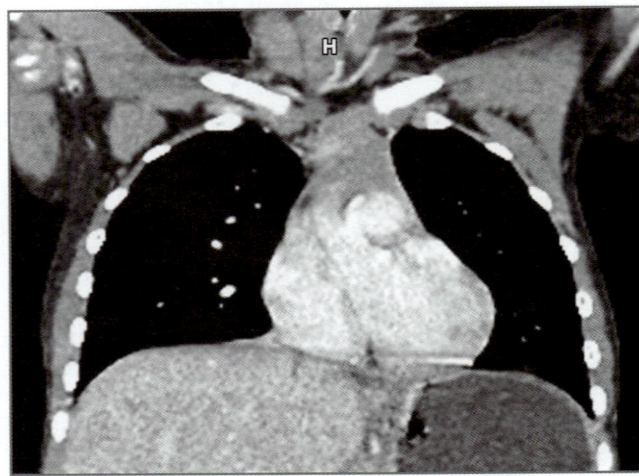

FIG. 3: Coronal multiplanar reconstruction at mediastinal window setting depicting the normal cardiac chambers.

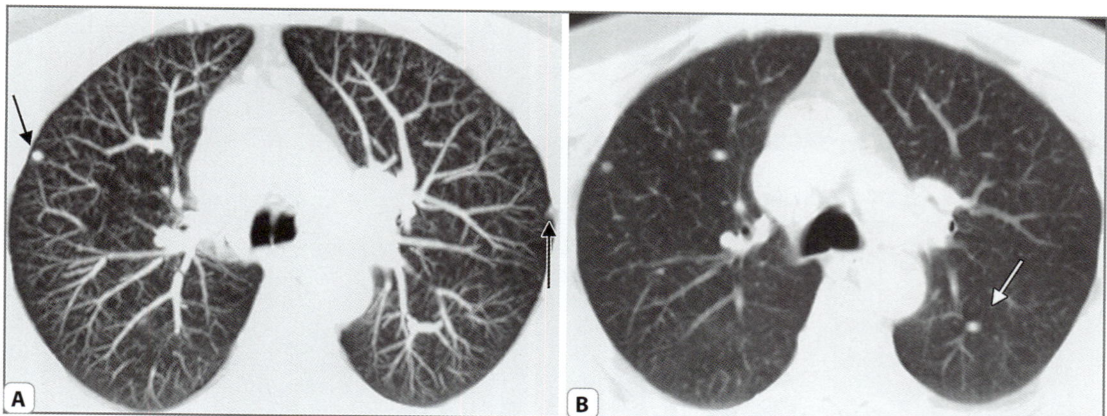

FIGS. 4A AND B: Axial MIP image at lung window settings (A) showing small nodules in the subpleural location on both sides (black arrows), which are easily discerned from vessels. Note that one lesion that appears to be a small nodule in the apical segment of the left lower lobe (white arrow) on the 3 mm axial CT section (B) is actually a vessel on the MIP image.

(CT: computed tomography; MIP: maximum intensity projection)

(Figs. 4A and B). In patients with mosaic attenuation, it can help in the differentiation of ground-glass attenuation (normal vascular diameter) and mosaic perfusion (altered vascular diameter).

Minimum Intensity Projection

This is similar to MIP, but only data below a certain value are displayed. It is useful to increase the conspicuity of low attenuation areas such as emphysema, air trapping, or cystic changes **(Fig. 5)**. It is also useful for the detection of ground-glass and linear attenuation patterns. Some authors have also found it useful to distinguish between bronchiectasis and honeycombing and for demonstrating bronchopleural fistula.

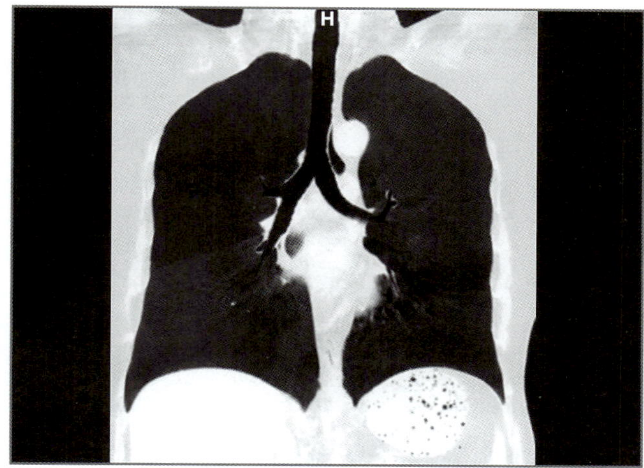

FIG. 5: Coronal minimum intensity projection (MinIP) image demonstrating not only the trachea, carina, and central bronchi but also the smaller segmental bronchi.

Shaded Surface Display

Shaded surface display (SSD) is a 3D surface-rendering technique that defines the surface of tissue but does not provide any internal details. It is used in the evaluation of airway abnormalities.

Volume Rendering

This is a unique 3D postprocessing technique, which displays depth information and 3D spatial relationships. A histogram representation of the entire dataset is done based on attenuation values. Voxels that are only partially filled with density of interest are also included. This is then manipulated to display internal and external perspectives. The CT attenuation data can be mapped to brightness, color, and opacity to display a particular structure of interest. Volume-rendered imaging can provide invaluable information because it preserves the 3D interrelationships of data. This is used extensively in the thorax for angiographic examinations and airway evaluation, allowing evaluation of both central and peripheral airways and chest wall abnormalities **(Figs. 6A and B)**. Volume-rendering (VR) technique is extremely useful for the evaluation of aneurysms and pseudoaneurysms, dissection, vascular slings, and anomalous vessels. These images are valuable for preoperative planning. Imaging of the chest wall and thoracic cage benefits from VR because of the extremely complex anatomy of this region with a number of overlapping structures such as the shoulder girdle.

Virtual Bronchoscopy

Virtual endoscopic images of the airway are produced akin to bronchoscopy using surface and VR techniques. The major advantage over conventional bronchoscopy is the ability to visualize the airway distal to an obstructing lesion **(Figs. 7A and B)**.

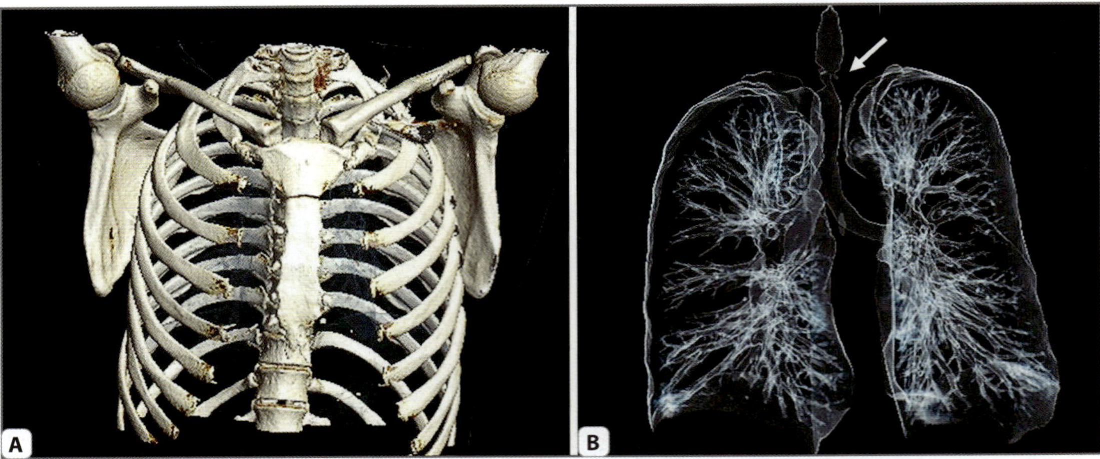

FIGS. 6A AND B: Volume-rendering technique (VRT) images demonstrating the complex interrelationship between thoracic structures forming the thoracic cage. (A and B) VRT image (transparency rendering) to show the central and peripheral airways. Note the area of narrowing in the trachea (white arrow).

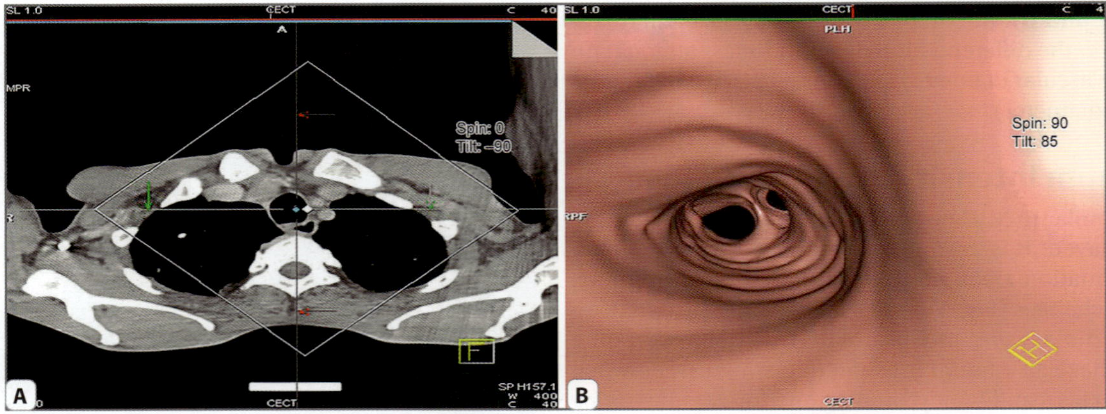

FIGS. 7A AND B: Virtual bronchoscopy image along with a source image showing the normal inner surface of the trachea and carina.
(CECT: contrast-enhanced computed tomography)

Dual-energy Computed Tomography/ Spectral Computed Tomography: Thoracic Applications

Dual-energy computed tomography (DECT) allows differentiation of materials due to their different attenuation properties at different photon energies.[1] DECT requires simultaneous acquisition of data at two different kilovoltages, generally 100 and 140 kVp. This can be achieved using a DSCT scanner with two X-ray tubes positioned at 90° to each other operating at two different kVs (Siemens) or a single-source CT with rapid kVs switching (GE) or a dual-layer detector with different detectors absorbing different energies (Philips). A single-source twin-beam DECT, which uses two filters one of tin (Sn) and the other of gold (Au) to split a 120-kV beam into a high-energy and low-energy beams, respectively, allowing DE acquisition is also available. Most modern scanners allow analysis at multiple kVs, also referred to as spectral CT. Photon-counting detector CT is the latest advancement allowing spectral evaluations.

Thoracic applications are based on the fact that the need for pre- and postcontrast images is eliminated with the computation of pseudomonoenergetic images. For pulmonary nodule characterization, the generation of virtual noncontrast images, thus, allows exact enhancement to be measured. Iodine maps of the lung parenchyma can also be generated to get a map of pulmonary blood volume and lung perfusion. This can help detect perfusion defects in acute and chronic thromboembolism, providing a new functional aspect independent of thrombus visualization **(Figs. 8A and B)**.[17]

Four-dimensional Scanning[18,19]

Dynamic four-dimensional (4D) images to gain functional information on breathing mechanisms can be obtained using physiologic respiratory triggers. Retrospective gating can be done using a cine mode where the table is still in one

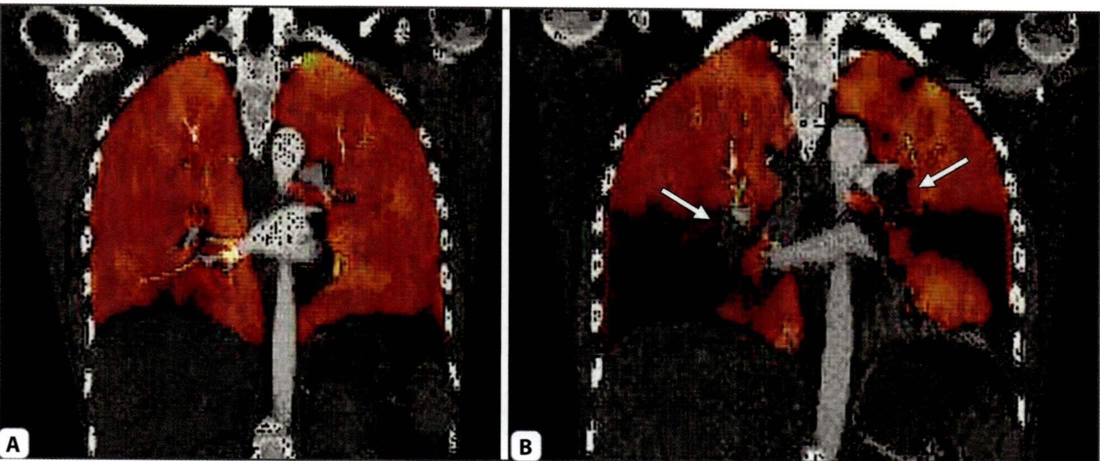

FIGS. 8A AND B: (A) Normal lung perfusion with dual-energy (DE) acquisition displayed in a coronal format. (B) Large wedge-shaped perfusion defects due to pulmonary emboli in another patient (white arrows).

breathing cycle and then it is moved to cover a subsequent portion of the lung. All the pieces of each respiratory phase are then put together to create a volume dataset of the lung or tracheobronchial tree. The other technique is continuous acquisition of the whole chest in free shallow breathing. These can be acquired at low-dose protocols with iterative reconstruction algorithms, so that the radiation dose is not higher than an average low-dose CT. Prospective gating similar to cardiac step-and-shoot is also becoming available.

Artificial Intelligence and Radiomics[5,6]

Artificial intelligence (AI) tools are being used for the detection of pulmonary nodules and pulmonary emboli. They have also been used for identifying pneumothorax, position of various lines and tubes, and rib fractures. AI is expected to streamline time-consuming processes, allowing automated volumetric measurements and grading the severity of parenchymal lung diseases.

Radiomics, which uses imaging features extracted by computer-generated algorithms to predict characteristics of disease, has been used to further decode the molecular features and prognostic implications of lung cancers, especially early-stage tumors treated by surgery.

DOSE CONSIDERATIONS AND DOSE REDUCTION TECHNIQUES IN THORACIC COMPUTED TOMOGRAPHY[1,2,20]

In the past few decades, the utilization of CT for diagnostic purposes has increased exponentially, raising concerns related to radiation exposure. With MDCT, the dose profile is trapezoidal along the Z-axis; only the central or umbral portion of the beam contributes to the image, while the penumbral dose is wasted (also referred to as *overbeaming*) **(Fig. 9)**. In a single-slice CT, on the other hand, the entire

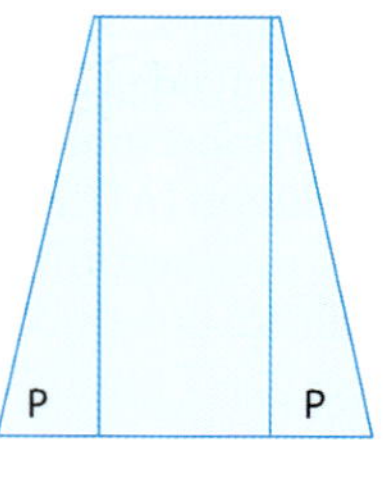

FIG. 9: Line diagram to show the trapezoidal dose profile along the Z-axis. The area outside the rectangle (P) on both sides represents the penumbra.

dose contributes to image formation. However, the relative contribution of the penumbral region decreases as the number of simultaneously acquired slices increases; thus, a 128-slice CT results in less wasted radiation than a four-slice CT. Gaps between detector elements in MDCT are another reason for decreased geometric efficiency and wasted dose, as the photons falling in these regions do not contribute to image formation. Another problem with helical scanners is *overranging*, i.e., irradiation beyond the imaged length is necessary for helical scanning for the reconstruction of first and last images. This is larger with wider Z-beam collimation (or larger number of detectors) offsetting improvement in dose efficiency of overbeaming for shorter scan lengths. Modern CT systems now have *dynamic collimation diaphragms* such that the collimator opens asymmetrically at the beginning and end of acquisition to eliminate radiation of tissues outside the range, reducing this problem.

Dose Reduction Strategies

The first and foremost step in dose reduction is assessment of need. No CT should be performed without a valid indication, and each study should be tailored to answer the specific clinical question at hand. Several technological advancements and modifications in technique can result in significant dose reduction. These are given as follows:

- *Tube current modulation using automatic exposure control (AEC)*: Essentially, there are three methods available: (1) patient size-based modulation, (2) Z-axis AEC, and (3) angular or X-Y-axis AEC. For patient size AEC, the appropriate current is selected by the system for the given patient size. Scanners assess the X-ray absorption profile over the patient's thorax during the topogram or scout acquisition and automatically choose the lowest tube potential for the patient and selected protocol. In the Z-axis or longitudinal modulation, the tube current is adjusted as the patient attenuation changes in the longitudinal direction or Z-axis to ensure a constant image quality at each anatomical level. The angular tube current modulation adjusts the tube current, as the tube rotates around the patient to compensate for attenuation changes as the view angle changes. The tube current is reduced at angles that are of less diagnostic importance. In most modern scanners, automatic tube current modulation (ATCM) adapts the tube current in all three X-Y-Z-axes according to patient weight and can result in significant dose reduction while maintaining image quality.

  There are, however, two important considerations: (1) determination of an acceptable level of image noise (this is generally preset by the manufacturer) and (2) optimal patient position. The patient should be positioned centrally on the CT table ideally close to the isocenter prior to acquisition. This is because the use of automatic dose modulation software in patients who are off the isocenter may result in a higher dose.
- *Tube current reduction in low-dose examinations*: A 50% reduction in the tube current can reduce the effective radiation dose to half the original level. Several studies have demonstrated that the tube current time product or mAS may be reduced to levels as low as 40–70 mAS in chest CT without significantly affecting image quality since the lung is a high-contrast organ. Most of these have been studied to detect pulmonary nodules in a screening setting. Some authors have demonstrated that common patterns of pulmonary diseases such as solid nodules, airspace consolidation, and airway and pleural diseases could be adequately demonstrated at 120 kV/40 mAS protocol using thin slices, high-spatial frequency reconstruction kernel, and standard filtered back projection (FBP) reconstruction. However, ground-glass opacities and interstitial opacities require higher tube current or iterative noise reconstruction.
- *Tube potential reduction or low kilovoltage examinations*: The standard chest protocol is usually acquired at 120 kV. A low tube potential of 70–80 kV is useful in children and small adults due to the lower X-ray absorption profile. A tube potential of 80–100 kVp is also beneficial in adults when the area of interest is enhanced by iodinated contrast for the thoracic aorta or pulmonary arteries. This is because the X-ray attenuation of iodine increases with the use of lower kilovoltage due to the K edge of iodine at 33 keV. The X-ray attenuation of soft tissue depends only weakly on tube potential; hence, the contrast of vessels and tissues that take up iodinated contrast increases with respect to surrounding tissue, increasing the contrast-to-noise ratio (CNR) at the same dose. This effect can be utilized to either reduce radiation dose to the patient or reduce the amount of iodinated contrast administered. A trade-off while decreasing tube potential or voltage is that the milliampere-seconds have to, thus, be significantly increased. Because of the lack of tube power reserves, low kilovoltage scanning was limited to children and small patients. New X-ray tubes with increased milliampere reserves and increased power at low kilovoltage have been introduced, which can extend this advantage to adults and obese patients. This may reduce radiation dose by as much as 52%. Technologies that automatically adapt the tube voltage to the size and shape of the patient keeping in mind the power reserves of the tube are also available. This automatic tube voltage selection may reduce radiation dose in CT chest angiographies by as much at 38% compared to the 120 kV protocol.
- *Use of a higher pitch*: Pitch is defined as table feed per rotation divided by the total width of the collimated beam. Using a higher table speed for a given collimation can significantly reduce patient dose if all other acquisition parameters are the same. An important factor to take into account, however, is that in some scanners, e.g., Siemens and Philips, an increase in table feed is automatically compensated by an increase in tube current to maintain the same effective tube current time product or *mAS effective* (defined as mAS/pitch).
- *Use of filters*: These are of two types given as follows:
  1. Beam-shaping filters: Filters such as bowtie filters reduce ray intensity in the peripheral parts reducing radiation dose, especially skin radiation dose.
  2. Spectral shaping: Spectral shaping by using a tin filter in the prepatient tube collimator box can significantly reduce patient dose in noncontrast lung examinations. The filter makes the beam "harder" removing lower energy photons, which would be absorbed by the patient without contributing to the image. This provision is available in the third-generation DSCT system. Low-dose CT with spectral shaping and iterative reconstruction can reduce patient dose in quantitative lung CT and nonenhanced CT of the chest for pulmonary nodule detection to as low as 0.06 mSv when using 100 kV. This effect is, however, not valid for contrast-enhanced examinations, as increased X-ray absorption of iodine at lower energies

overcompensates this. It also needs to be determined how well subtle features of lung parenchyma can be evaluated at such low doses.

- The length of coverage should be carefully planned, so as not to extend beyond the area of interest.
- Newer detector systems such as the solid-state detectors have much higher detector efficiency than the conventional ionization chamber-based detectors, helping to reduce radiation dose.
- *Patient shielding*: Use of lead or lead-free shields to protect areas outside the scan zone may help to reduce radiation exposure (e.g., thyroid and gonads). However, the use of bismuth to reduce radiation exposure to breast tissue during chest CT is not recommended, as this increases image noise and artifacts. A similar breast dose reduction can be achieved by the methods already mentioned, such as tube current modulation.
- *Newer reconstruction techniques*: These help to reduce image noise, making it possible to obtain diagnostic images with low-dose examinations. CT images were traditionally reconstructed using the *FBP* technique. However, this requires a large amount of X-ray data to produce diagnostic quality images. The introduction of *iterative reconstruction (IR)* techniques into routine CT, made possible by the increased computational power of computers, greatly enhances image resolution and reduces noise. In FBP, increased spatial resolution is directly correlated with increased image noise, while IR allows for decoupling of spatial resolution and image noise to a certain extent (it maintains or enhances spatial resolution for high-contrast objects while reducing noise in low-contrast areas). The first-generation IR algorithms are image-based IR, the second-generation IR algorithms are statistical weight-based IR, and the latest third-generation IR algorithms are model-based IR. It is reported that with the use of IR, radiation dose could be reduced to <2 mSv for contrast-enhanced chest CT and to sub-mSv levels for noncontrast CT of the chest.
- Prospective ECG gating rather than retrospective gating for ECG-gated examinations also reduces radiation exposure.

MAGNETIC RESONANCE IMAGING

INTRODUCTION

The superior soft-tissue contrast of magnetic resonance imaging (MRI) over CT ensures better tissue characterization in the evaluation of mediastinal masses, chest wall, and diaphragm. In these areas, MRI already has an established role in diagnosis. However, most often, it is performed subsequent to a CT examination not only due to the latter's faster image acquisition but also greater acceptance and familiarity among clinicians. The challenges to MRI of the chest are due to its relatively longer acquisition times, motion artifacts related to respiratory motion, and cardiac pulsations.

Magnetic resonance imaging of the lung especially is a very challenging field. This is because about 70% of the lung consists of air-filled spaces. Protons are localized within the tissues of the lung or blood vessels accounting for only 30% of the volume. The healthy lung, thus, has a tissue proton density, which is about 10 times lower than other tissues producing a signal that is 10 times weaker than other tissues even under perfect conditions.[21] The generation of MR signal from even these protons is hampered by two factors: (1) the lung has countless air–tissue interfaces, which have very different magnetic properties, leading to susceptibility artifacts with resultant loss of signal in structures such as alveolar septae, and (2) the pulsatile nature of blood flow. These problems are further compounded by artifacts due to respiratory and cardiac motion, making lung one of the most difficult organs to image on MR. The susceptibility differences result in rapid dephasing of spins in gradient echo (GRE) imaging; hence, pulse sequences with very short echo times (TE < 1–2 ms) are required.[21]

There have been several advances in hardware and pulse design helping to overcome several of these limitations—such as multichannel MR systems, powerful gradients, parallel imaging, very short TE, and ultrafast turbo spin echo acquisitions. These along with improved technology for k-space sampling and development of contrast agents for perfusion and ventilation studies have put MR on the threshold of a radiation-free alternative to CT in some clinical situations.[22-24]

TECHNICAL CONSIDERATIONS

Magnet Strength and Coils

For MRI of the thorax, scanners with *a field strength* of 1.5 or 3 T and full parallel imaging capability are recommended.[21] Along with the *spine coil* integrated into the table, receive only, *phased array body coils* are used over the chest. These increase SNR and allow parallel imaging, reducing acquisition time. The coverage must be adequate in the craniocaudal and anteroposterior directions.[25]

Respiratory Motion

The availability of fast imaging sequences on modern scanners has ensured that most sequences can be acquired in <20 seconds. Thus, it is advisable to acquire images during a single breath hold or as a multibreath hold sequence. This minimizes blur associated with respiratory motion and is better than triggered or navigator sequences. The success of breath-hold imaging can be significantly increased, provided breath holding is rehearsed with the patient before lying down and the patient is informed about the frequency and duration of breath hold.[26] In patients who are unable to hold breath and for longer sequences, synchronization of the image acquisition to the respiratory cycle is done. This can be done using respiratory or spirometric triggering or gating using external hardware such as pneumatic bellows or the signal of lung itself. Another method is to use navigator echoes to detect the motion of the diaphragm directly via MRI, which can be used for retrospective gating of scans during free breathing.[21]

Cardiac Gating

Cardiac gating is useful to freeze cardiac motion for the evaluation of cardiac and paracardiac lesions. ECG gating is preferred to peripheral gating because it freezes cardiac motion more reliably, eliminating pulsatility artifacts.[26]

PROTOCOL AND SEQUENCES

A basic protocol consists of noncontrast breath hold T1- and T2-weighted sequences without fat saturation. Gadolinium-based contrast agents are required for a number of indications such as evaluation of mediastinal and lung masses or pulmonary nodules, chest wall masses, pleural pathology, lung perfusion, and evaluation of vasculature. A set of precontrast TIW images is acquired without fat saturation to facilitate the detection of mediastinal nodes or masses surrounded by fat, while postcontrast images are acquired with fat saturation. This may be done using the Dixon technique for a more homogeneous fat saturation near the neck. Identical parameters should be used for pre- and postcontrast images when evaluating enhancement.[21,25] The postcontrast images can be acquired as a single postcontrast T1W fat-saturated sequence or as a dynamic contrast-enhanced (DCE) examination where multiple fast 3D-T1W-GRE acquisitions are done after intravenous contrast.

Advantages of the dynamic technique include the ability to show the rate of enhancement over time, eliminating guesswork about when maximal vascular or lesion enhancement will occur. The pattern of enhancement may help to increase the specificity of diagnosis. In addition, because exactly the same imaging parameters are used in the pre- and postcontrast acquisition, it is possible to measure relative ROI assessment of lesion hyperintensity and to subtract postcontrast images from precontrast images, which are very useful to assess enhancement in T1W hyperintense lesions.

The sequences are obtained in the standard axial, coronal, and sagittal planes. Additional planes may be used to optimize lesion characterization, e.g., to better characterize mediastinal or chest wall invasion acquisition can be planned to get images perpendicular or parallel to the site of invasion.[21,25-27]

MAGNETIC RESONANCE PULMONARY ANGIOGRAPHY

Heavily T1W-3D-GRE (FLASH/SPGR/FFE) sequences are used to obtain high-resolution breath-hold pulmonary angiograms. The shortest possible TR and TE are used with modest parallel imaging. Contrast is usually given via a pressure injector in a dose of 0.2 mL/kg body weight at 2–3 mL/second, followed by a saline flush of 20 mL at 5 mL/second. The acquisition is optimized to peak vascular enhancement using a test bolus or care bolus technique.

Alternatively, a time-resolved 3D sequence with echo sharing such as TRICKS/TREAT/TWIST can be used after intravenous injection of gadolinium, the so-called "4D magnetic resonance angiography (MRA)" (3D over time). Acquisition times of 1.5 seconds or less are possible, so that multiple datasets in arterial and venous phases can be acquired **(Figs. 10A to D)**. The postcontrast images are subtracted from the precontrast images to enhance visualization of vasculature.[21]

MAGNETIC RESONANCE PERFUSION IMAGING

Magnetic resonance perfusion of the lung or mediastinum is feasible using a version of the time-resolved pulmonary angiography sequence. At a temporal resolution of <1 second per 3D dataset, this allows generation of passage kinetics curves and parametric maps of regional blood flow and blood volume. The contrast dose needed for a perfusion study is lower than that needed for a pulmonary angiography at 0.05 mL/kg, followed by a 20-mL saline flush at 5 mL/second. Generation of fully quantitative map of pulmonary blood volume (PBV), pulmonary blood flow (PBF), and mean transit time (MTT) requires a deconvolution with arterial input function (AIF) measured in the larger arteries **(Figs. 11A and B)**. This may be challenging due to lack of linearity between local tissue contrast agent concentration and MR signal intensity. MR perfusion can provide information not just on presence or absence of perfusion but also on the time course of perfusion or capillary filling time. Delayed filling presumably via collaterals can be identified. Pulmonary hemodynamics and blood flow can also be analyzed using techniques developed for cardiac MRI.[21,25,28]

Noncontrast methods proposed for assessing pulmonary perfusion include arterial spin labeling (ASL) techniques. Several different variants of this have been proposed and used. In addition, unenhanced perfusion and ventilation MRI can be done using Fourier decomposition MRI.

OTHER ADVANCED/NEWER IMAGING TECHNIQUES

Ultrashort Echo Time and Zero Echo Time Imaging

Ultrashort echo time sequences that use radial K-space sampling are now become available. These shorten echo times to below 1 ms. At these very short TE (<200 ms), the

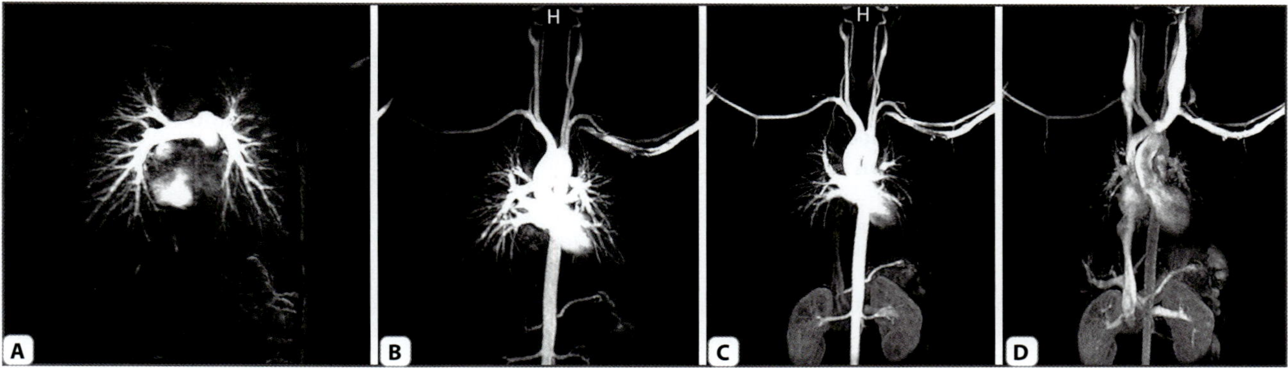

FIGS. 10A TO D: Multiphasic pulmonary angiogram using TWIST on a 3T magnet. Note all the phases from the pulmonary opacification in the first image (A) to venous in the last image (D).

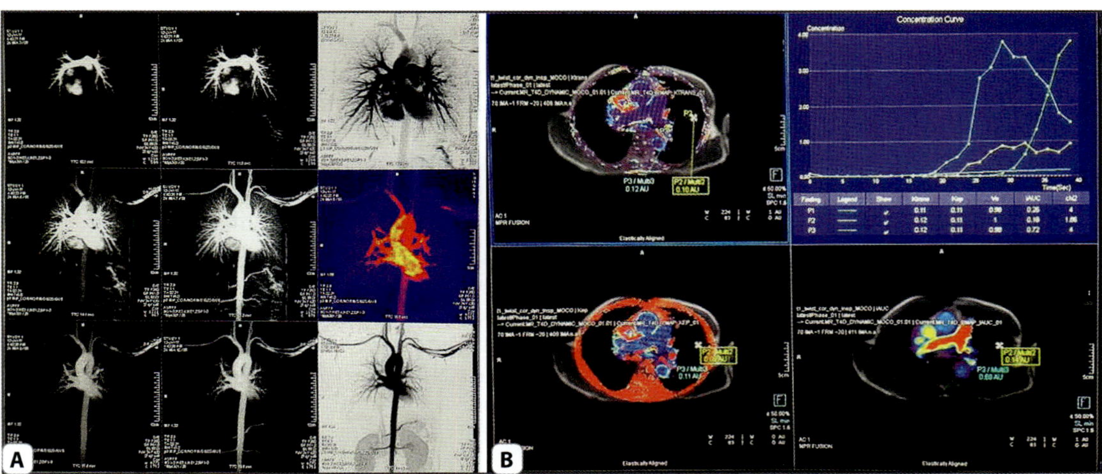

FIGS. 11A AND B: (A) Multiphasic magnetic resonance (MR) acquisition with generation of qualitative perfusion maps and quantitative perfusion curves. (B) The yellow curve represents the pulmonary perfusion.

short T2 of the lung is less problematic, and images with parenchymal sensitivity are possible. Further developments have led to zero echo-time (ZTE) MRI where the signal is sampled directly after the radiofrequency (RF) pulse, resulting in a nominal TE of zero. The resolution of these images is below the routine images; however, they allow visualization of parenchymal lung disease hitherto impossible with MRI. Another application is quantitative regional T2* measurement of the lung by direct T2* decay on 3D-GRE with UTEs, allowing evaluation of lung microstructure and emphysema.

In recent years, high-resolution *synthetic CT* images have been generated from UTE MRI using AI tools such as generative adversarial network (GAN). These images have demonstrated a good SNR, contrast-to-noise ratio, and excellent concordance between real CT and synthetic CT images in patients of cystic fibrosis. They had better image quality than UTE MR.[29]

Novel Contrast Methods and Ventilation Magnetic Resonance Imaging

Ventilation is the second important aspect of gas exchange in the lungs. 4D-MRI can visualize breathing motion and analyze lung volumes, which have demonstrated excellent agreement with spirometric studies.

Direct visualization of lung ventilation can be done using hyperpolarized noble gases, sulfur hexafluoride, or oxygen inhalation. Oxygen is paramagnetic; when the patient breathes in pure oxygen instead of air, it shortens the T1 of blood, plasma, and tissue in the lungs, resulting in an increase in signal. This can be used to generate parametric maps with ventilation and perfusion weighting. Hyperpolarized noble gases such as Xe-129 and He-3 can also be used to give high signal-to-noise images of lung ventilation.

CLINICAL APPLICATIONS OF MAGNETIC RESONANCE OF THORAX

There are a number of accepted and emerging areas of thoracic imaging (besides cardiac applications) where MRI can play a significant role depending on the availability of expertise.

Mediastinum

Magnetic resonance can help to better characterize mediastinal abnormalities and masses. It is superior to CT in distinguishing solid from cystic masses, presence of hemorrhage, and can help to detect both microscopic and macroscopic fat within the lesion. The detection of microscopic fat by chemical shift MR can help to distinguish between thymic hyperplasia (which has microscopic fat) from tumor (which lacks microscopic fat). Dynamic contrast enhancement patterns and low apparent diffusion coefficient (ADC) values have been used to distinguish between benign and malignant lesions. Due to superior demonstration of fat planes and cine imaging capability, MR can help to more accurately demonstrate lesion invasiveness, its relationship to critical vascular structures, and discernment of mediastinal from paramediastinal lesions. Mediastinal and hilar nodes can be easily detected without the use of contrast; however, calcified nodes are difficult to detect.

Pulmonary Embolism and Pulmonary Hypertension

In a meta-analysis, gadolinium-enhanced MRA has reported sensitivity varying from 77 to 100% and specificity of 95–98%.[30] The sensitivity is reported to be 100% for central and lobar arteries, while it falls to 40% for subsegmental branches. MRA with MR perfusion has been shown to be highly accurate (98%) for the detection of embolism with the perfusion sequence, having a sensitivity of 100% and specificity of 91%.[31] MRI using a combination of MRA and perfusion sequence allows differentiation between idiopathic pulmonary artery hypertension and secondary pulmonary artery hypertension due to thromboembolic disease with sensitivity and specificity similar to planar scintigraphy and single-photon emission computed tomography (SPECT). The latter shows features of segmental perfusion defects besides vascular change, while the idiopathic variety shows a more diffuse and patchy perfusion pattern.[24,32] Even more importantly, MR allows assessment of right ventricular dilatation, hypertrophy, and estimation of cardiac strain and pulmonary artery pressures.[23] It has been reported that septal flattening, elevated right ventricular end-diastolic volume index, and delayed contrast enhancement of the septal insertions have prognostic implications in pulmonary hypertension. Quantitative CE-MRA can be used to assess the severity of pulmonary hypertension and therapy effect.[28]

Lung Cancer

In lung cancer MRI has a role in the evaluation of Pancoast tumors where it is reported to be more accurate than CT in demonstrating blood vessel and brachial plexus involvement. It is superior to CT for demonstrating pericardial, heart, mediastinal, vessel, and chest wall involvement and may be indicated in specific situations as a problem-solving tool. MR may also be useful to distinguish between a central mass and postobstructive atelectasis, and the latter shows higher signal intensity on T2W images; the central mass also shows lower ADC values than atelectasis **(Figs. 12A to D)**. Whole-body MRI also provides acceptable accuracy for non-small cell lung cancer (NSCLC) staging compared to positron emission tomography (PET)/CT.[23,24,28]

Detection and Characterization of Pulmonary Nodule

Magnetic resonance imaging and CT have been reported to be equally accurate in distinguishing between benign and malignant pulmonary nodules in a meta-analysis.[32] 3D-GRE sequences with UTE allowed a detection rate of over 90% for nodules between 4 and 29 mm in diameter (nonsolid, part-solid, and solid nodules) compared to thin-section CT **(Figs. 13A and B)**. Nodules < 5 mm are difficult to detect on MR. Malignant nodules have been reported to show lower ADC values than benign nodules.[28,33] Enhancement characteristics can also be assessed using contrast-enhanced dynamic MR sequence. In- and opposed-phase imaging have been used to demonstrate microscopic fat in pulmonary hamartoma.[34]

Cystic Fibrosis

Since patients with cystic fibrosis are young at presentation and require multiple examinations for follow-up, MR has been suggested as a tool for follow-up imaging. MR has been reported to be comparable to CT in detecting morphological lung changes, while it is superior to CT in the assessment of functional alterations. It is possible to visualize bronchiectasis, bronchial wall thickening, mucus plugging, air-fluid levels, and consolidation on MR. Functional assessment includes the evaluation of respiratory mechanics using inspiratory and expiratory 3D-GRE MRI, lung perfusion, blood flow, and pulmonary ventilation using hyperpolarized gases for MRI. MRI perfusion defects may help to reveal even a small airway (<1 mm) obstruction, which is, otherwise, difficult to detect.[22,24,27,28]

Pneumonitis

In children with suspected pneumonitis, MR can detect thoracic abnormalities such as consolidation, ill-defined nodules, and effusions.[23,27] In pediatric patients with suspected pulmonary infection.[35] MR may be used in the follow-up of pulmonary infections in order to reduce radiation exposure associated with CT.[23,27,36]

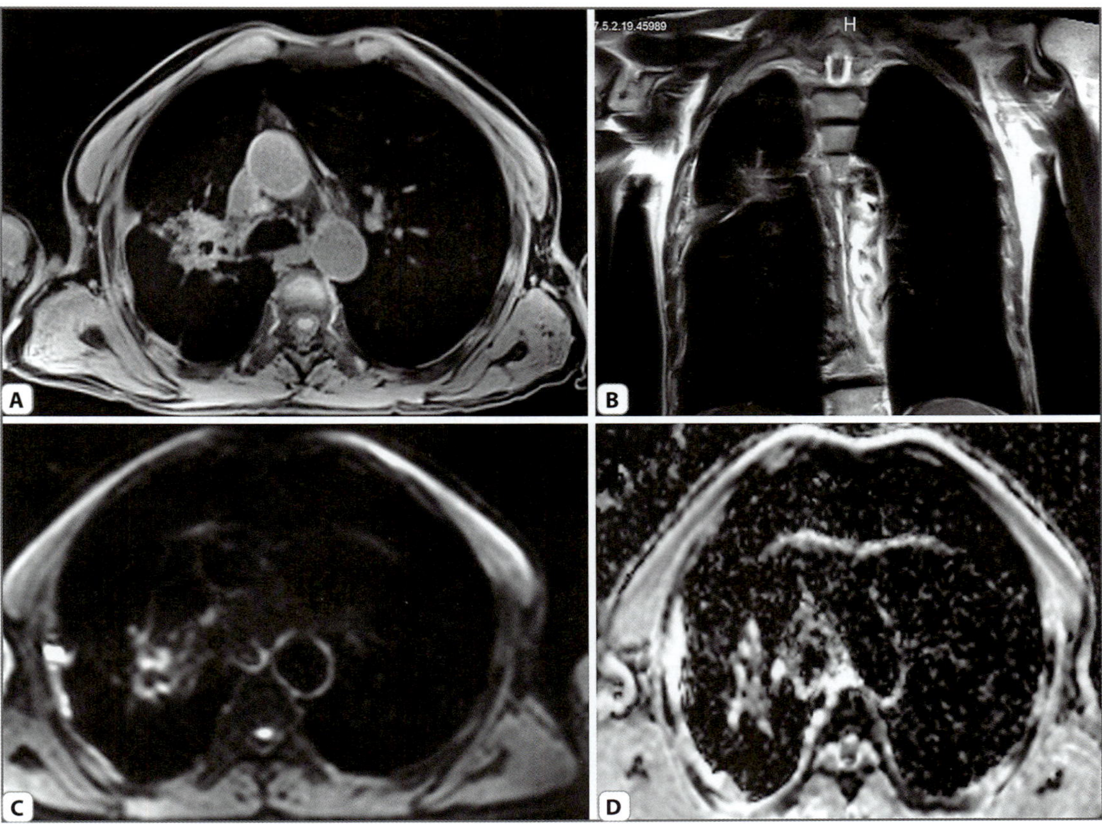

FIGS. 12A TO D: Axial T1W (A) and coronal T2W images (B) in a case of lung cancer. (C and D) Figures show a spiculated mass obstructing the right upper lobe bronchus with a pleural tail, DWI, and ADC map. Note the areas of diffusion restriction within the mass and in the pleura, suggesting pleural spread.

(ADC: apparent diffusion coefficient; DWI: diffusion-weighted imaging)

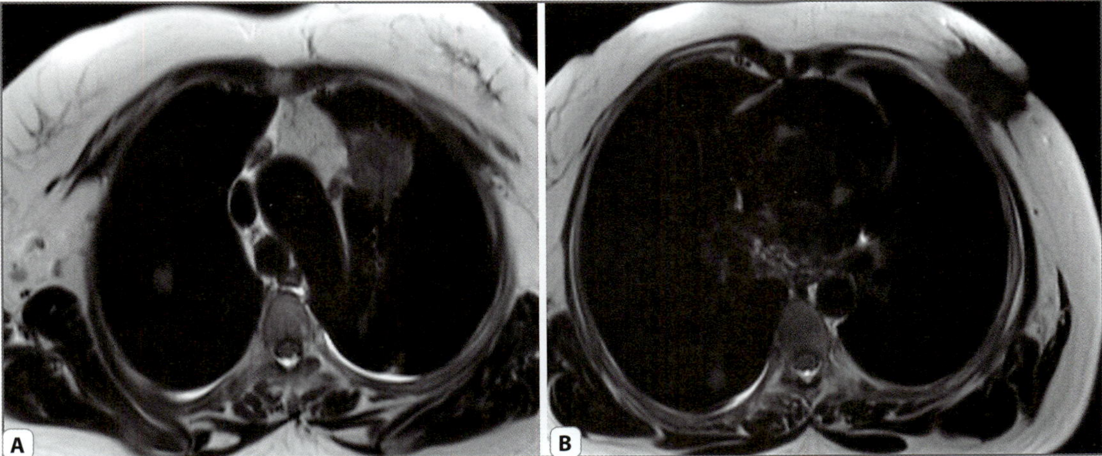

FIGS. 13A AND B: Axial T2W (HASTE) magnetic resonance (MR) images show multiple lung metastases that appear hyperintense to skeletal muscle in a patient with carcinoma of the breast. Note the mass lesion in the right breast.

Emphysema and Chronic Obstructive Pulmonary Disease

Researchers have attempted to use ventilation MR using He-3 to grade and characterize chronic obstructive pulmonary disease (COPD) with large wedge-shaped or lobar defects being typical of advanced COPD. Alveolar filling time can be calculated using dynamic imaging of ventilation kinetics, and alveolar size estimation may be done using ADC. The ADC of hyperpolarized helium MRI correlates with carbon monoxide diffusing capacity of the lung. MR perfusion can show perfusion defects correlating with severity due to hypoxic vasoconstriction.

It can also evaluate diaphragmatic motion and dynamic lung volumes, which are often altered in these patients.[23,27]

Interstitial Lung Disease

Three essential applications of MR have been suggested in literature—(1) assessment of morphological changes and patterns, (2) evaluation of inflammatory disease activity, and (3) effect of morphological changes on functional parameters. Consolidation, fibrotic changes, nodules, reticulation, etc., can be detected due to the increased T2W signal, although subtle changes in the subpleural region are difficult to detect. Postcontrast T1W images, which increase the signal of the lung, have been used to assess honeycombing. Dynamic MR and differences in T2W signal have been used to distinguish between active inflammation from fibrosis **(Figs. 14A and B)**.[27] Recently, UTE-MRI has been shown to have diagnostic accuracy similar to CT in ILD. T1 values and T2 relaxation times have been used to evaluate changes in ILD, while MR elastography has revealed increased lung stiffness.

The Fleischner Society Position Paper in 2020 categorized clinical MR applications of lung into three main categories, which are summarized in **Box 1**.

Pleura, Chest Wall, and Diaphragm

Magnetic resonance can easily demonstrate pleural effusion, deposits, and plaques of asbestosis. It is superior to CT in distinguishing pleural effusion from thickening and discernment of pleural invasion by tumors. Calcifications, a sign of benignity are, however, not well seen. MR is routinely used for evaluating chest wall masses to demonstrate the exact extent and invasion by the mass. MR can also be used to evaluate diaphragmatic pathologies such as eventration, hernia, and paralysis **(Figs. 15A to D)**.[25,27]

NORMAL ANATOMY

MEDIASTINUM

Normal mediastinal anatomy can be evaluated by analyzing CT or MR images at certain predefined anatomical levels due to their characteristic appearance and landmarks.

Axial Sections (Cranial to Caudal)

Thoracic Inlet (Junction of Neck and Thorax)

Most mediastinal structures are vascular at this level. The internal jugular veins join the subclavian veins to form the brachiocephalic veins posterior to the clavicular heads. These veins are the most anterior and lateral vessels at this level. Medially lie the two common carotid arteries, while just posteriorly are the two subclavian arteries (SCAs). The SCA crosses over the first rib to exit the mediastinum

BOX 1: Clinical indications for lung MRI.

Applications currently supported by data:
- Staging of cancer lung
- Characterization of lung nodule
- Pulmonary hypertension
- Cystic fibrosis

Data good but requires either additional validation or regulatory approval:
- Pulmonary parenchymal abnormalities
- Lung nodule detection
- Pulmonary embolism

Investigative applications:
- ILD
- COPD and asthma

(COPD: chronic obstructive pulmonary disease; ILD: interstitial lung disease; MRI: magnetic resonance imaging)

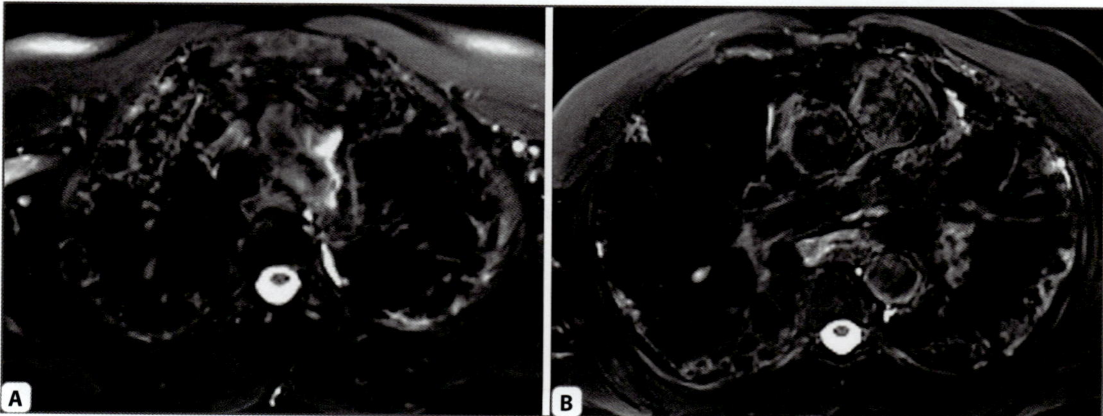

FIGS. 14A AND B: T2W images (FSE-BLADE with fat saturation) show honeycombing in the subpleural regions of both lungs. Note some areas show a higher signal than the rest on the T2W images, suggesting active inflammation according to some researchers.

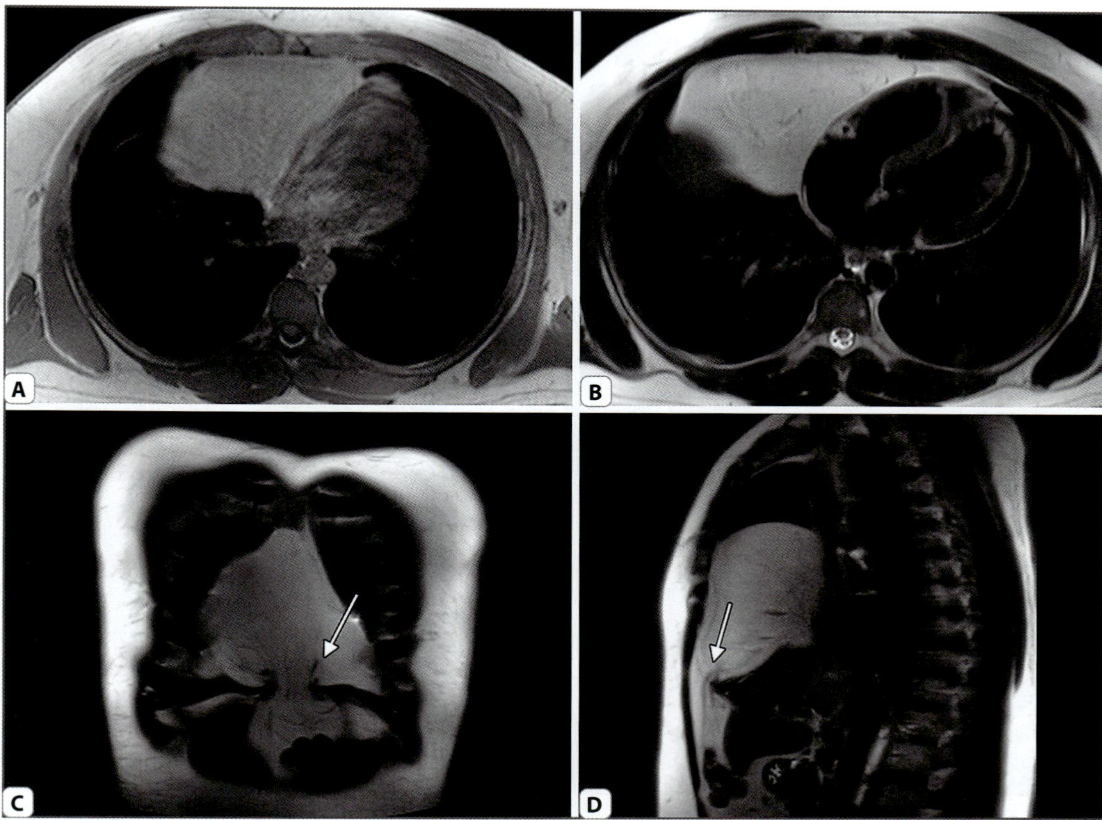

FIGS. 15A TO D: Axial T1W FLASH (A) and T2W HASTE (B) in a case of Morgagni hernia shows a paracardiac mass with a signal identical to subcutaneous fat. (C and D) The diaphragmatic discontinuity (white arrows) through which the omentum is herniating into the thorax is well seen on the coronal and sagittal HASTE images.

and enters the axilla. The esophagus lies posterior or posterolateral to the trachea **(Fig. 16A)**.

Left Brachiocephalic Vein Level

The left brachiocephalic vein crosses the midline just beneath the manubrium to join the vertically oriented right brachiocephalic vein to form the SVC. Between the brachiocephalic vein and trachea are the three major branches of the arch of aorta—(1) the innominate artery, which is nearly midline; (2) the left common carotid artery, which is slightly to the left and posterior; and (3) the left SCA, which is the most posterior and lateral vessel in close contact with the left upper lobe **(Fig. 16B)**.

Aortic Arch Level

The aortic arch traverses obliquely from right-to-left and anterior-to-posterior to left side just anterior to the trachea. The SVC is seen in cross-section adjacent to the anterior portion of the arch to the right side of trachea. The space posterior to the SVC, anterior to the trachea, and lateral to the transverse aorta is the pretracheal space or anterior paratracheal space. Anterior to the great vessels and brachiocephalic vein is prevascular space. Both these spaces contain fat and small lymph nodes. Posterior or posterolateral to the trachea and anterior to the spine is esophagus **(Fig. 16C)**.

Azygos Arch-aortopulmonary Window Level

The azygos vein arches anteriorly from its location just anterior and slightly to the right of the spine to join the SVC. The entire arch may not be visible in a single section and, occasionally, this is poorly opacified, leading to confusion with lymphadenopathy. The ascending aorta lies anterior to the trachea, and the descending aorta lies on the left posterolateral aspect of trachea. The ascending aorta is larger than the descending aorta measuring about 3.5 cm in mean diameter, while the descending aorta measures about 2.5 cm (this varies with age and sex). The aortopulmonary window is also seen at this level as a fat-filled space. It is located between the inferior aspect of aortic arch superiorly and the superior aspect of left pulmonary artery (LPA) inferiorly. The contents of this important space include lymph nodes, left recurrent laryngeal nerve, and the ligamentum arteriosum. The esophagus is seen anterior to the spine and posterior to trachea **(Fig. 16D)**.

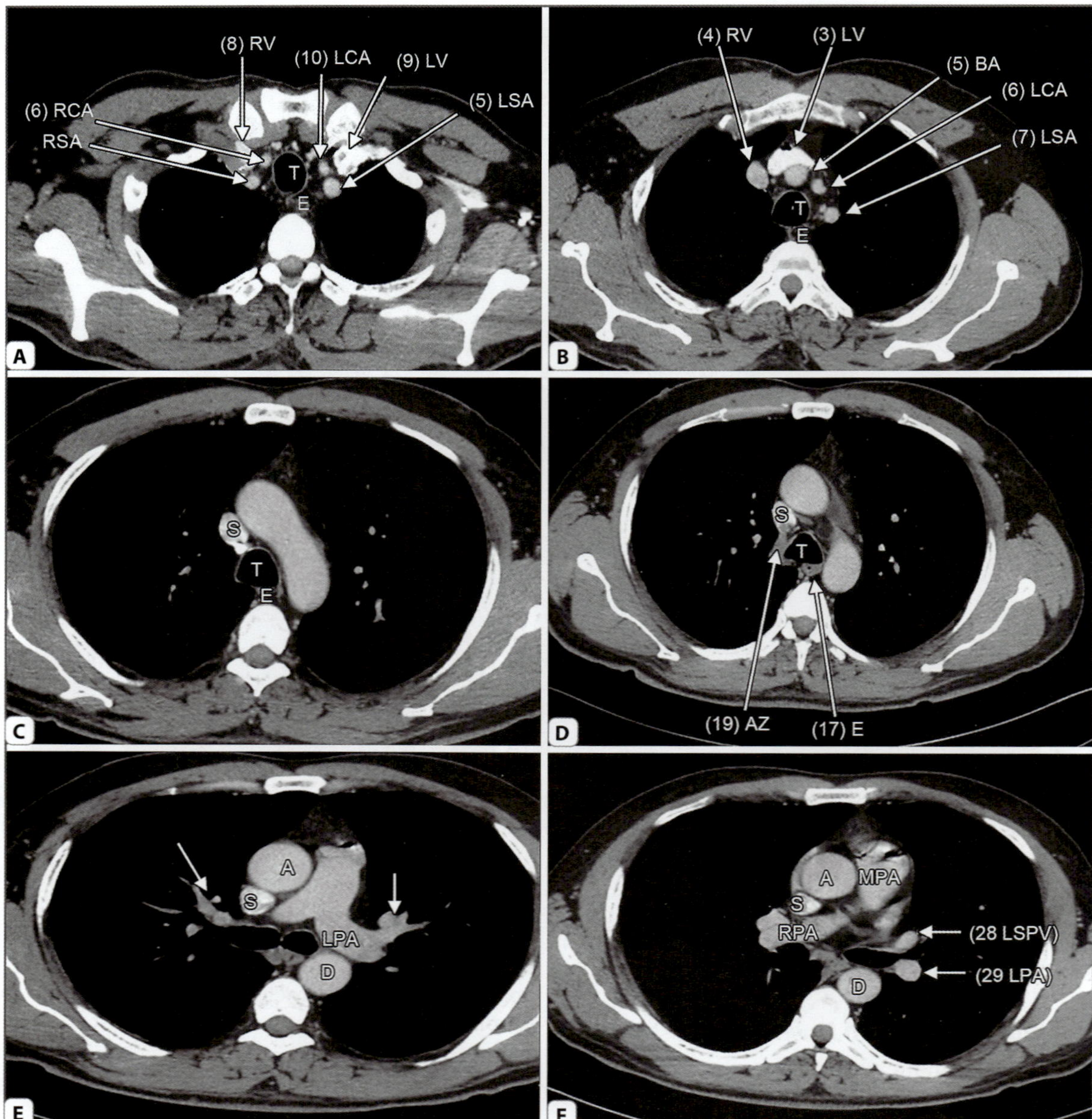

FIGS. 16A TO F: (A) Thoracic inlet level. Trachea (t) and esophagus (E) in midline. (B) Left brachiocephalic vein level. Trachea (t) and esophagus (E). (C) Aortic arch level. The superior vena cava (S) and aortic arch lie anterior to the trachea (t) and esophagus (E). Anterior to the arch is the thymus, which has undergone fatty replacement. (D) Azygos arch aortopulmonary window level. The azygos (AZ) vein arches from a posterior position beside the esophagus to join the superior vena cava (S) crossing over the right upper lobe bronchus. The aortopulmonary window is between the ascending and descending aorta. (E) Left pulmonary artery level. To the left of the left pulmonary artery (LPA) lies the left superior pulmonary vein (arrow). The ascending (A) and descending (D) aorta and superior vena cava maintain their relative positions from the level above. The truncus anterior (tA) or right upper lobe pulmonary artery is anterior to the right upper lobe bronchus (white arrows). (F) Right pulmonary artery level. The left superior pulmonary vein (LSPV) is anterior to the left main bronchus, and left pulmonary artery is posterior. The main pulmonary artery (MPA) divides into right pulmonary artery (rPA) and left pulmonary artery, which is more superior and not visible.

(A: ascending aorta; d: descending aorta; E: esophagus; LCA: left common carotid artery; LCC: left common carotid artery; LSA: left subclavian artery; LV: left brachiocephalic vein; RCA: right common carotid artery; RSA: right subclavian artery; RV: right brachiocephalic vein; S: superior vena cava; T: trachea)

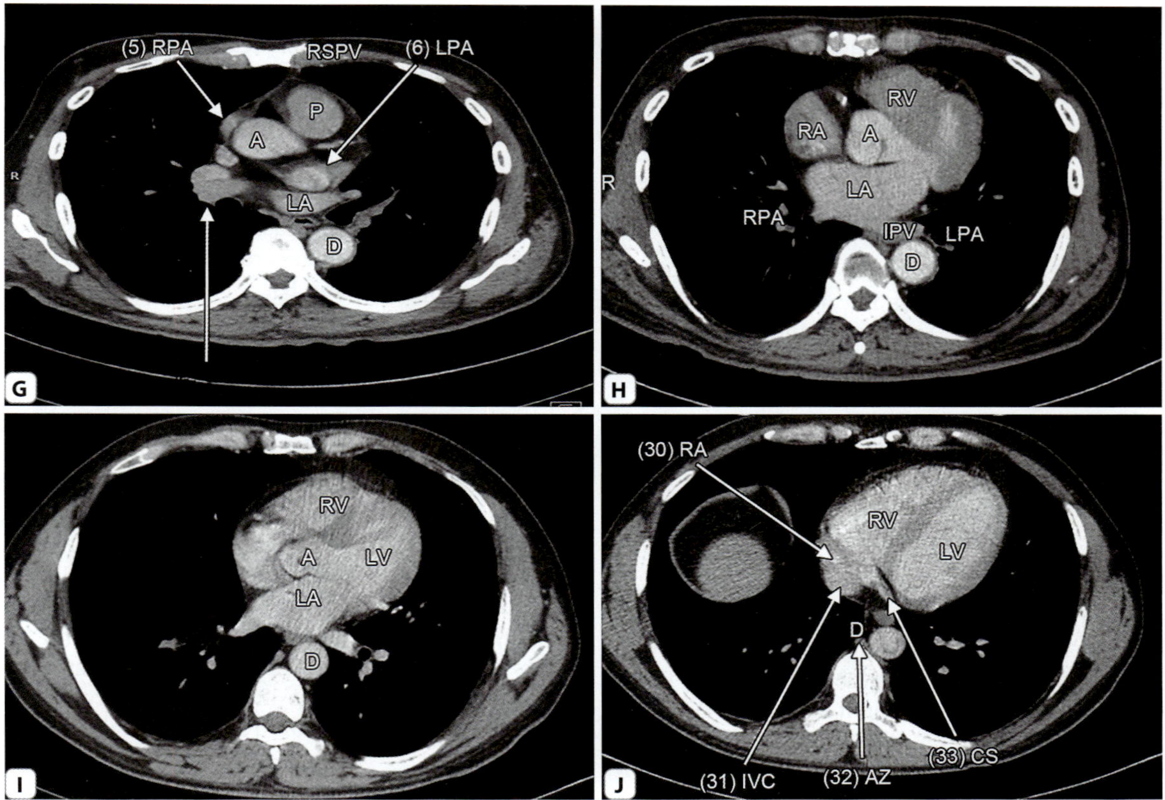

FIGS. 16G TO J: (G) Left atrial level. The right atrial appendage is anterior to the superior vena cava (S) and adjacent to the ascending aorta (A). The left atrial appendage is situated anterior and to the left of the left atrium, adjacent to the main pulmonary artery (P). The left atrium (LA) is the most superior and posterior chamber of the heart. Superior pulmonary veins enter the anterosuperior portion of the left atrium. (H) Left atrial level (at a caudal level). (I) Four-chamber level. (J) Three-chamber level. The left atrium is more cranial to this level and is not visible. The three visualized chambers are the right atrium (RA) with the IVC draining into it, right ventricle (RV), and left ventricle (LV). The coronary sinus (CS) is between the inferior vena cava (i) and the left ventricle.

(A: aortic root; AZ: azygos vein; D: descending aorta; IPV: inferior pulmonary vein; LA: left atrium; LPA: left pulmonary artery; LV: left ventricle; RA: right atrium; RPA: right pulmonary artery; RV: right ventricle)

Left Pulmonary Artery Level

The LPA is seen at a superior level compared to the MPA and is located anterolateral to the left main bronchus at the level of carina. The left superior pulmonary veins are located just lateral to the posterior LPA. The right upper lobe bronchus can be seen arising from the right main bronchus at the level of carina. The right upper lobe pulmonary artery also called truncus anterior lies anterior to the right upper lobe bronchus. To the right of the esophagus lies the azygos vein. The hemiazygos vein lies to the left of the spine and parallels the course of the azygos vein. Along the posterior aspect of ascending aorta and anterior to the carina is a crescentic extension of the pericardium—the superior pericardial recess. It may contain a small amount of fluid or extend to more cephalad location and must not be confused with a lymph node or mass. Demonstrating continuity with the superior pericardial recess on contiguous sections can help to establish the true nature of a high-riding pericardial recess **(Fig. 16E)**.

Right Pulmonary Artery Level

The MPA is situated anterior and to the left of ascending aorta. The right pulmonary artery (RPA) courses posteriorly from the MPA between the SVC anteriorly and bronchus intermedius posteriorly. The right superior pulmonary vein lies to the right of the intrapulmonary portion of RPA. Anterior to the left main and upper lobe bronchus lies the left superior pulmonary vein, while posteriorly is the left lower lobe pulmonary artery **(Fig. 16F)**.

Left Atrial Level

In the upper sections, the right atrial appendage is situated anterior to the SVC. It curves around the ascending aorta, which is situated almost in the center of the mediastinum. The pulmonary artery outflow tract is located anterior and to the left of aorta. Posterior and to the left of the pulmonary artery outflow tract is the left atrial appendage (LAA)—roughly triangular in shape. The left main coronary artery courses in the fat between the LAA and aortic root. The right superior pulmonary veins drain into the LA just posterior to the SVC **(Figs. 16G and H)**.

Four-chamber Level

All four cardiac chambers can be identified at this level. The LA is located posteriorly and is most cranial of the chambers. On the posterolateral aspect, inferior pulmonary veins can be seen entering the LA. The RA is situated anterior and to the right of the LA, which communicates with the right ventricle (RV) situated anteriorly and slightly to the left of RA. Just posterior and to the left of the RV lies the left ventricle (LV). The right coronary artery may be seen in the right atrioventricular groove, the left circumflex artery in the left atrioventricular groove, and the left anterior descending coronary artery in the interventricular groove between the RV and LV **(Fig. 16I)**.

Three-chamber Level

At this level, the LA, which has a more cephalad position, is not visible. The RV is seen just beneath the sternum, and the LV is lying to the left posterolateral aspect. The RA is located posterior and to the right of RV. The IVC opens into the inferior aspect of RA. Between the IVC and LV, the coronary sinus can be seen opening into the RA **(Fig. 16J)**.

The normal axial anatomy on MRI can be seen in **Figures 17 and 18**.

Coronal and Sagittal Planes

These planes can be extremely useful for assessing the relationship between the mediastinal structures and their relationship with pathology. The anatomy is depicted in **Figures 19 and 20**.

THYMUS

The thymus is situated anterior to the aorta and pulmonary artery or right ventricular outflow tract in the prevascular space. It is usually best seen on a section through the aortic arch or great vessels. In children before puberty, most of the mediastinum anterior to the great vessels is filled by the thymus. The size of the gland varies so much in this age group that it is not possible to decide if the gland is normal based on measurements alone; approximate symmetry is the norm. In addition, the normal gland appears to be molded by the anterior chest wall and great vessels **(Fig. 21)**. The size of the gland decreases with age. The average thickness of each lobe on CT decreases from 8–9 mm at 20 years to 5–6 mm at 50 years, with the maximum thickness of each lobe being up to 15 mm.[1] The measurements are slightly greater on MRI probably because MR demonstrates thymic tissue replaced by fat as well. The craniocaudal measurements are 5–7 cm as measured on sagittal MR images. The density of the gland also changes from soft-tissue attenuation prior to puberty to gradual fatty replacement so that above 40 years, the attenuation is near fat, making the gland indistinguishable from surrounding fat. Some streaky or modular densities may be seen, representing residual thymic parenchyma. On T1W MR images, the thymus has a signal similar to that of muscle and lower than that of mediastinal fat; with increasing age, the signal of the gland increases, approaching that of mediastinal fat. On T2W images, the signal intensity differences are minimal and do not change with age **(Figs. 22A and B)**.

LYMPH NODES

Lymph nodes are distributed throughout the mediastinum. Normal lymph nodes are <10 mm in diameter in 95% of cases. Retrocrural nodes (behind diaphragmatic crura), paraspinal nodes, and those in the region of brachiocephalic veins are usually 6 mm or less. On the other hand, nodes in the aortopulmonary window, pretracheal, lower paratracheal, and subcarinal compartment are often 6–10 mm in diameter. The nomenclature of mediastinal nodes should be in accordance with the international lymph node map in the TNM classification of lung cancer given by the International Association for the Study of Lung Cancer (IASLC).

MEDIASTINAL DIVISIONS ON CROSS-SECTIONAL IMAGING[36,37]

Recently, the International Thymic Malignancy Interest Group (ITMIG) has introduced a new definition of mediastinal compartments to be adopted as a new standard with cross-sectional imaging. The three compartments as per this system are: (1) prevascular or anterior, (2) visceral or middle, and (3) paravertebral or posterior **(Figs. 23A to D)**. The boundaries and contents of these are listed in **Table 1**.

TRACHEOBRONCHIAL TREE[38,39]

The trachea is seen as a thin-walled air-containing structure on axial CT scans lying anterior to the dorsal spine and esophagus. It is round or oval in shape with a slightly flattened posterior margin in about 25% of patients. On expiratory scans, the posterior margin of the intrathoracic becomes more concave.

The normal dimensions of the trachea vary with the sex of the patient. In males, it ranges from 13 to 27 mm in transverse dimension and 13–27 mm in sagittal plane, while in females, the corresponding measurements are 10–21 and 10–23 mm. The tracheal index [coronal diameter (in mm)/sagittal diameter (in mm)] is approximately 1. Due to the angled course of the trachea, a true perpendicular cross-section of its lumen is not obtained on axial CT images. The tracheal wall measures 3 mm in thickness.

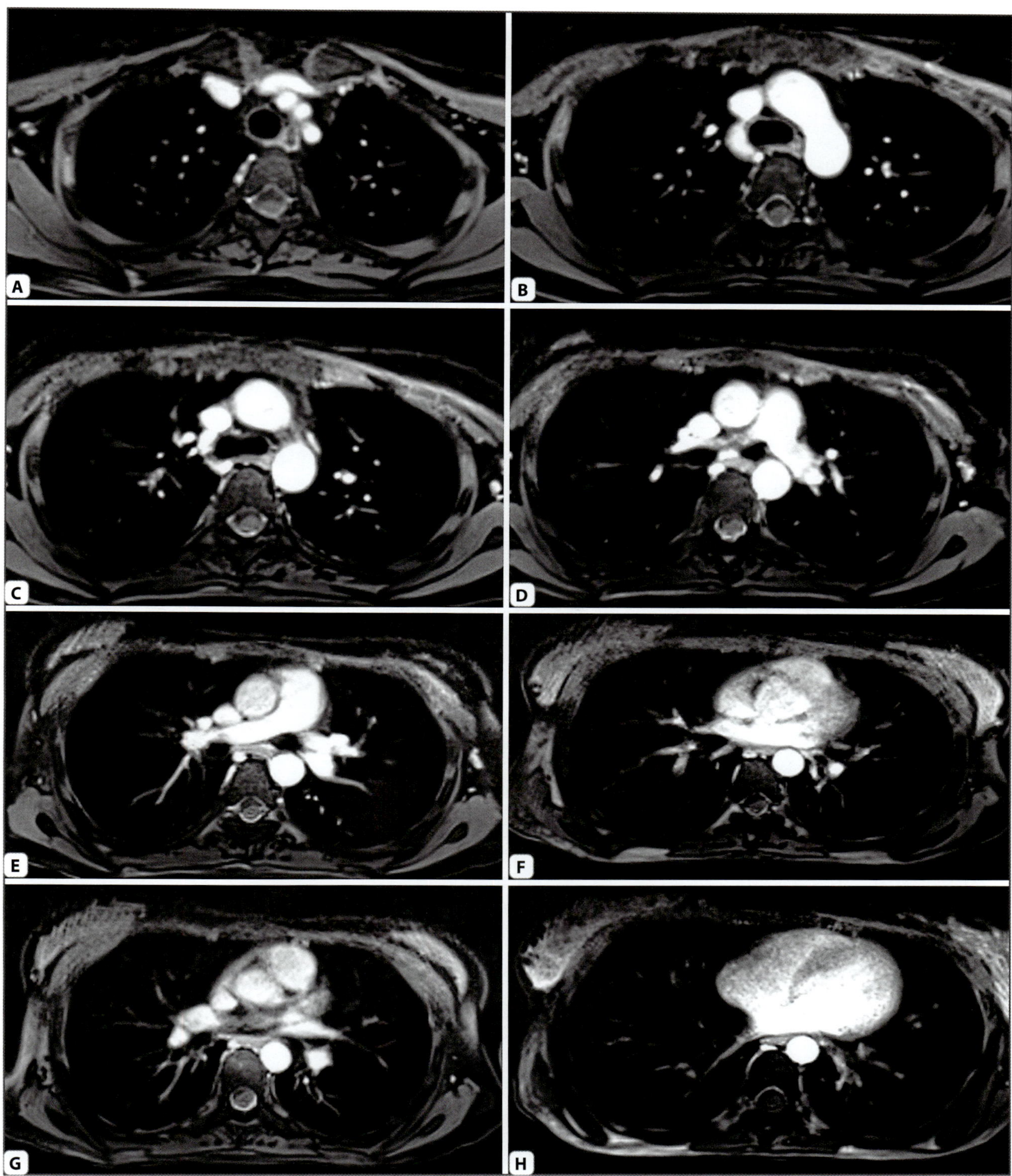

FIGS. 17A TO H: Postcontrast T1W (VIBE) images: Normal mediastinal anatomy on magnetic resonance (MR).

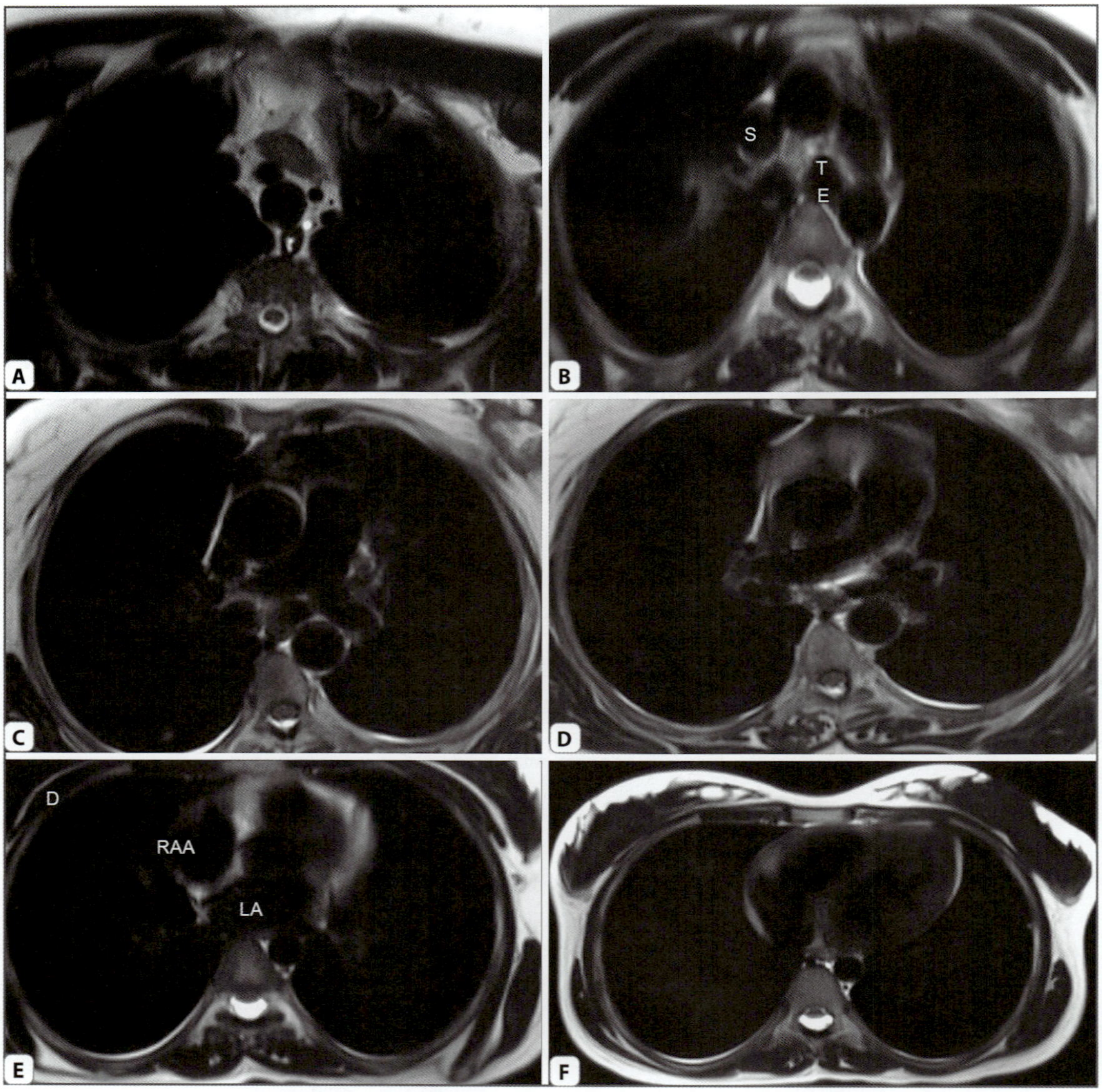

FIGS. 18A TO F: Representative HASTE axial images showing the normal mediastinal anatomy.

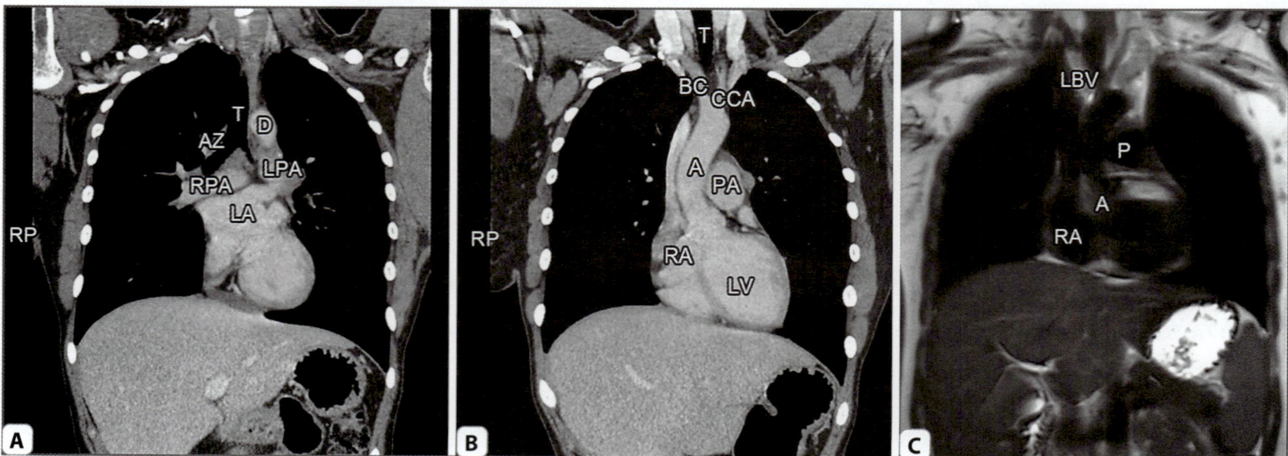

FIGS. 19A TO C: Coronal plane—CT at the level of carina (A) and at aortic outflow tract level (B) and corresponding MR (C).

(A: aorta; CT: computed tomography; D: descending aorta; LB: left brachiocephalic vein; LV: left ventricle; LPA: left pulmonary artery; MR: magnetic resonance; PA: pulmonary artery; RA: right atrium; RPA: right pulmonary artery)

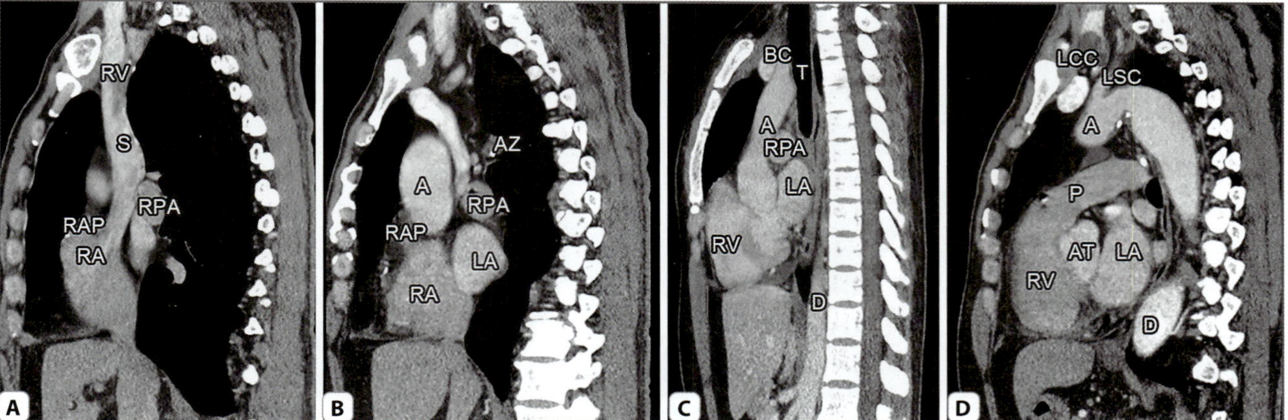

FIGS. 20A TO D: CT images. (A) Sagittal plane—superior vena cava level. (B) Sagittal plane—right atrial level. (C) Sagittal plane—aortic outflow tract level. (D) Sagittal plane—pulmonary artery outflow tract level.

[A: ascending aorta; AT: aortic outflow tract; AZ: azygos vein; BC: brachiocephalic artery; D: descending aorta; LA: left atrium; LCC: left common carotid artery; LSC: left subclavian artery; P: pulmonary artery (outflow tract); RA: right atrium; RAP: right atrial appendage; RPA: right pulmonary artery; RV: right brachiocephalic vein; RV: right ventricle; S: superior vena cava; T: trachea]

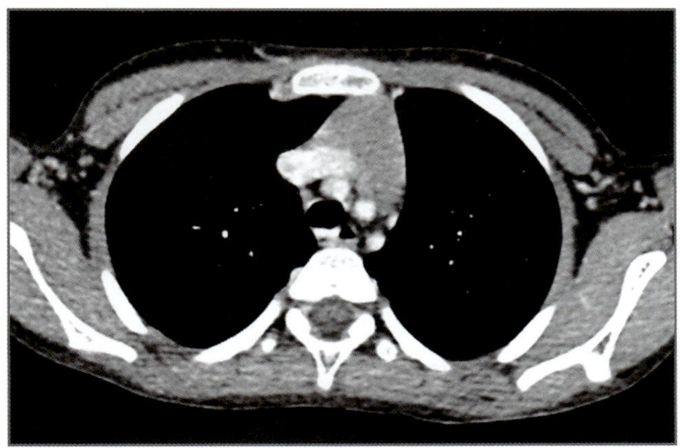

FIG. 21: Axial computed tomography (CT): Normal thymus in a 7-year-old boy seen as a triangular homogeneous soft-tissue density anterior to the great vessels.

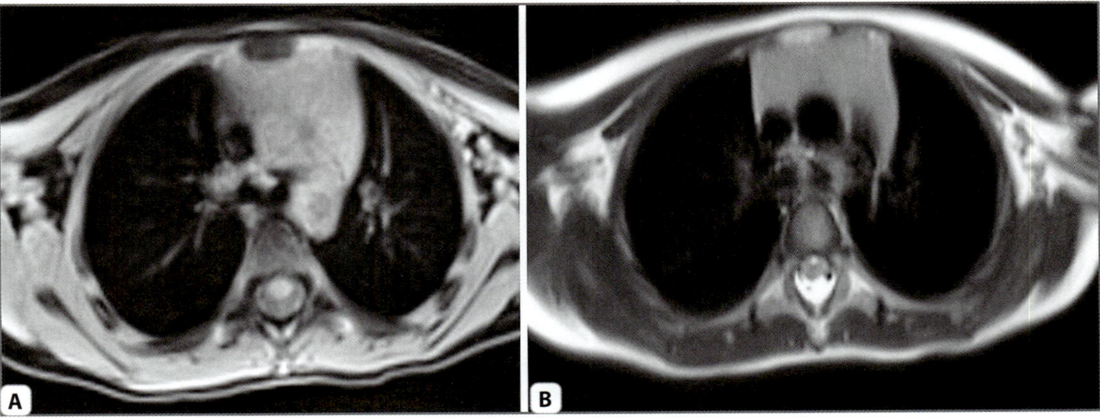

FIGS. 22A AND B: T1W FS (A) and T2W MR (B) images in a 5-year-old demonstrate the thymus in the prevascular space appearing homogeneously isointense to skeletal muscle on T1 and hyperintense to skeletal muscle on T2.

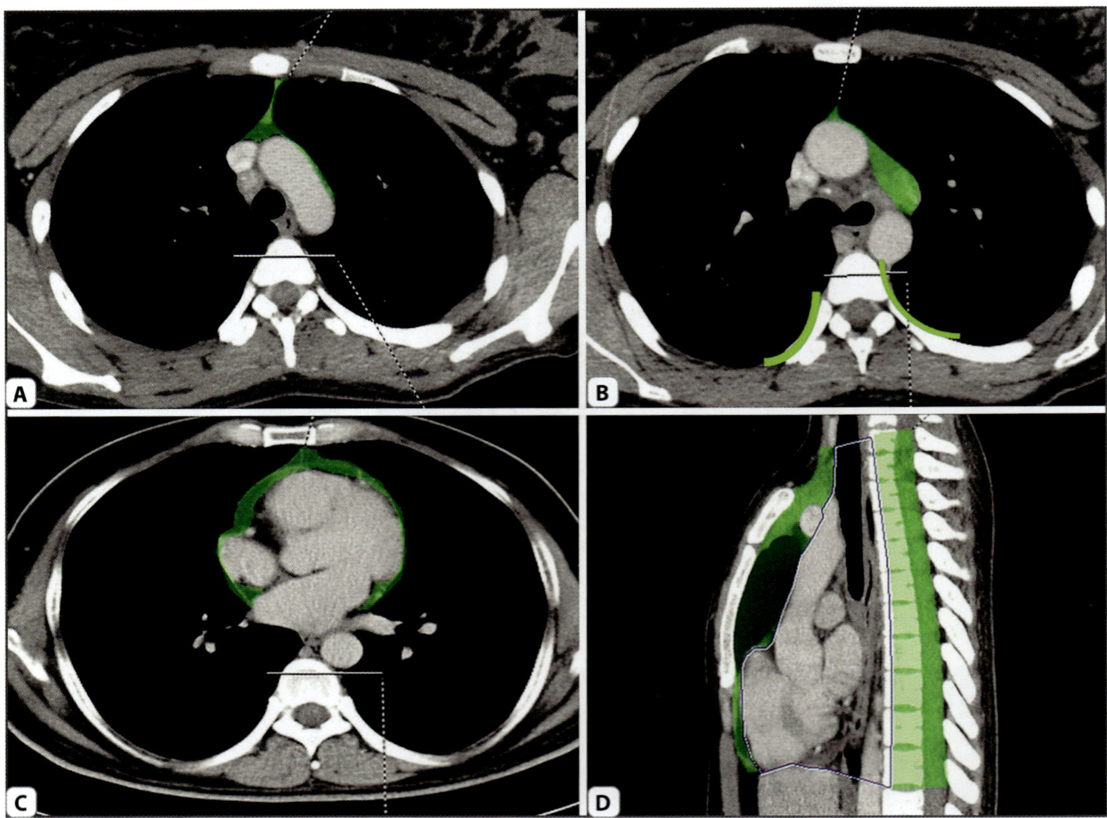

FIGS. 23A TO D: Axial and sagittal CT sections showing the mediastinal divisions according to the ITMIG classification. The prevascular space is depicted in green anteriorly. The horizontal line 1 cm behind the anterior vertebral imaging is the demarcation between the visceral and posterior mediastinal or paravertebral region, which is again shaded in green.

(CT: computed tomography; ITMIG: International Thymic Malignancy Interest Group)

TABLE 1: International Thymic Malignancy Interest Group (ITMIG) classification of mediastinal compartments on cross-sectional imaging.

Compartment	Boundaries	Major contents
Prevascular	• Anteriorly: Sternum • Posteriorly: Anterior aspect of the pericardium as it wraps around the heart in a curvilinear manner Superiorly: Thoracic inlet* • Inferiorly: Diaphragm • Laterally: Parietal mediastinal pleura	• Thymus and lymph nodes • Left brachiocephalic vein and fat
Visceral	• Anteriorly: Posterior boundary of the prevascular compartment • Posteriorly: Vertical line connecting a point on each thoracic vertebral body 1 cm posterior to its anterior margin** • Superiorly: Thoracic inlet inferiorly: Diaphragm	• Trachea, carina, esophagus, and lymph nodes • Heart, ascending aorta, aortic arch, descending thoracic aorta, superior vena cava (SVC), intrapericardial pulmonary arteries, and thoracic duct
Paravertebral	• Anteriorly: Posterior boundary of the visceral compartment • Posteriorly: Vertical line against the posterior margin of the chest wall at the lateral margin of the tran sverse process of the thoracic spine	Thoracic spine and paravertebral soft tissues

*The thoracic inlet is a thin plane demarcated by superior border of manubrium anteriorly, body of 1st thoracic vertebra posterosuperiorly, and 1st ribs and their costal cartilages on each side.

**This line was chosen as the posterior boundary of the visceral compartment and the anterior boundary of the paravertebral compartment, as most abnormalities in the posterior compartment are neurogenic masses that arise from the dorsal root ganglia/neurons adjacent to the intervertebral foramina.

The posterior wall is thinner than the anterior wall. The cartilage within the anterior and lateral walls may appear slightly hyperdense compared to surrounding soft tissue and fat. The cartilage may calcify in the elderly. The trachea divides into the right and left main bronchi at carina. The right and left main bronchi course obliquely in the axial plane and are well seen on multiplanar reconstructions. On axial CT sections, bronchi are seen as ring structures in cross-section, while they appear as tubular structures when horizontally oriented.

The right upper lobe bronchus has a horizontal course and is seen just at or below the carina arising from the lateral aspect of right main bronchus. The anterior and posterior divisions of this, being horizontal in their proximal part, are seen as tubular structures. The middle lobe bronchus arises from the anterior aspect of right main bronchus and is seen as a tubular structure due to its horizontal course. It divides into the medial and lateral segmental bronchi. At nearly the same level, the apical segmental bronchus of the lower lobe can be seen coursing posteriorly in the horizontal plane. The rest of the lower lobe bronchi is seen in cross-section below this level as they have a vertical course. The lung closely abuts the posterior aspect of the right main bronchus and the bronchus intermedius, so that their posterior walls are clearly delineated as a thin stripe on axial CT images.

On the left side, the left upper lobe bronchus arises at a lower level than the right upper lobe bronchus with a horizontal course. The lingular bronchus courses anteriorly in the horizontal plane after arising from the upper lobe bronchus. The lower lobe bronchi have a roughly similar course, as shown in **Figures 24A to F**.

LUNG SEGMENTS, FISSURES, AND PLEURA[1,38,39]

Fissures are poorly seen on routine axial CT sections as avascular areas or broad bands, as they represent subpleural regions with relative paucity of vessels. On HRCT sections, they are well seen as thin white lines and may be better appreciated on MPRs **(Figs. 25A and B)**. The individual lung lobes and segments can be identified by their position within the hemithorax and their relationship to the segmental bronchi and fissures. Segmental anatomy on CT is shown in **Figures 26A to D**. The normal pleura and extrapleural spaces are not visible.

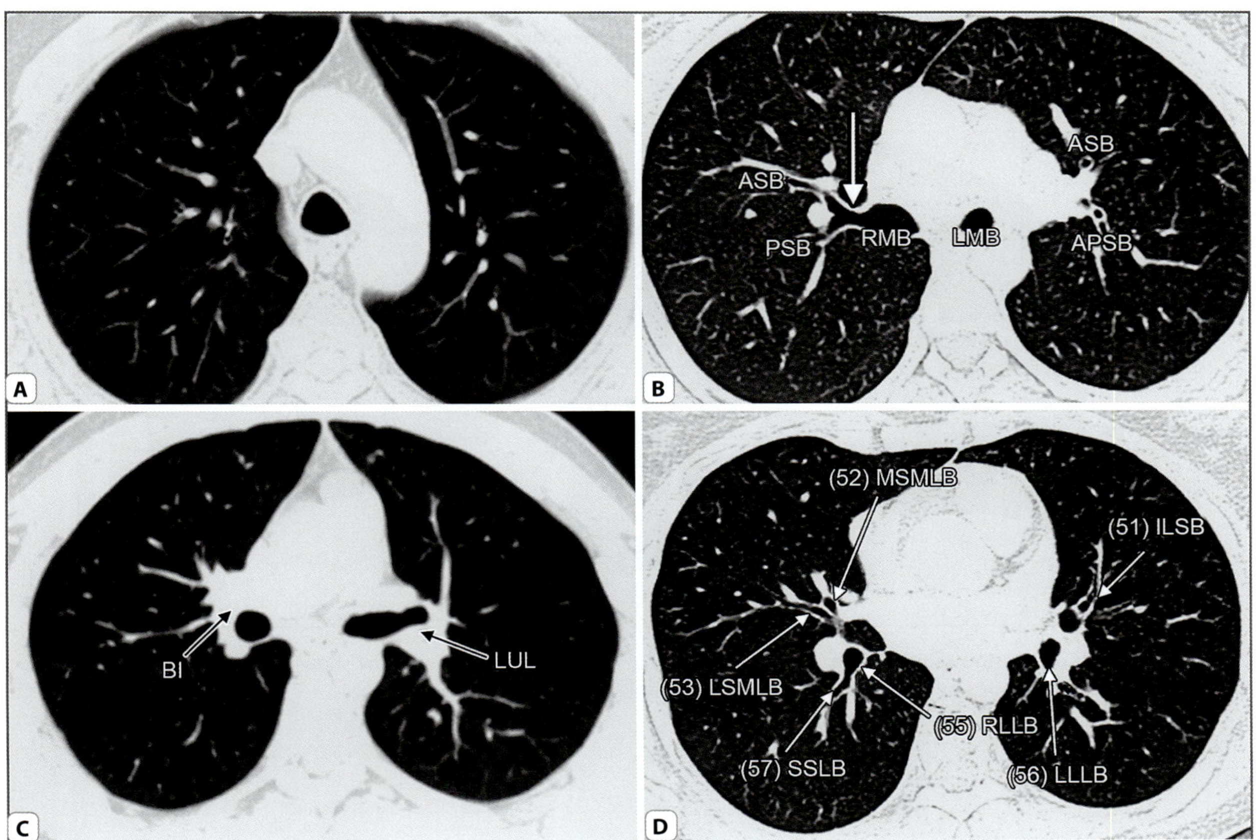

FIGS. 24A TO F: *Continued*

Continued

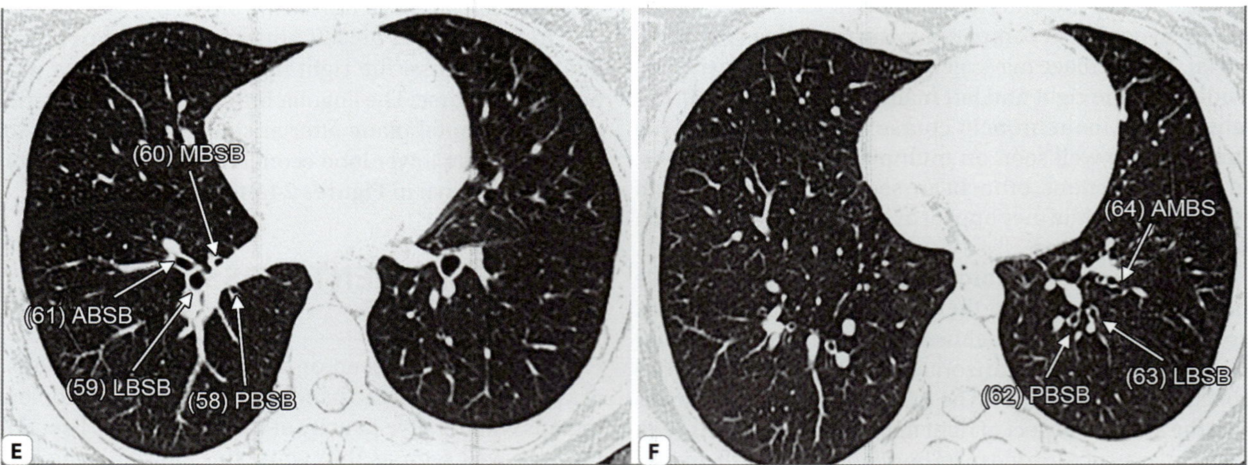

FIGS. 24A TO F: Bronchial anatomy as seen on computed tomography (CT). (A) Section just above the carina shows apical and apicoposterior segmental bronchi in cross-sections on the right and left side, respectively. (B) Section at the level of carina shows right and left main bronchi, right upper lobe bronchus (white arrow), and its division into anterior and posterior segmental bronchi. (C) Section just below carina shows bronchus intermedius on right side and left upper lobe bronchus arising from left main bronchus. (D) On the left side, lingular branch of upper lobe bronchus is seen. On the right side, middle lobe bronchus and its divisions into medial and lateral segmental bronchi. The superior segmental bronchi of both lower lobes are also seen coursing posteriorly. (E and F) Section at further caudal level shows major lower lobe segmental bronchi on both sides.

(RMB: rights main bronchus; LMB: left main bronchus; ASB: anterior segmental bronchus; PSB: posterior segmental bronchus; APSB: apicoposterior segmental bronchus; BI: bronchus intermedius; LUL: left upper lobe bronchus; MSMB: medial segmental middle lobe bronchus; LSMB: lateral segmental middle lobe bronchus; SSLB: superior segmental lower lobe bronchus; RLLB right lower lobe bronchus; LLLB left lower lobe branches; MBSB: medial basal segmental bronchus; ABSB: anterior basal segmental bronchus; PBSB posterior basal segmental bronchus)

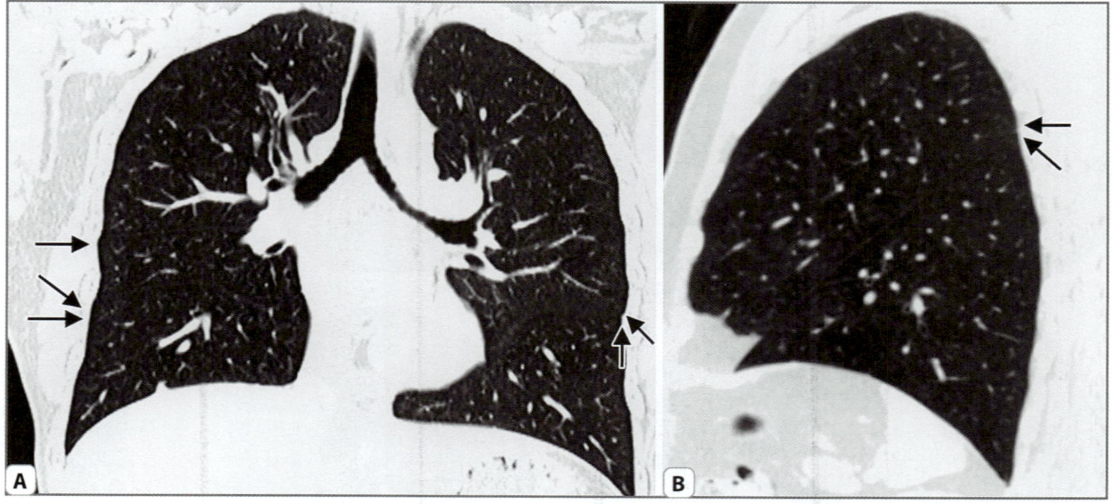

FIGS. 25A AND B: Coronal and sagittal computed tomography (CT) sections in lung window showing the oblique fissures on both sides and the horizontal fissures on the right side (double and single black arrows, respectively).

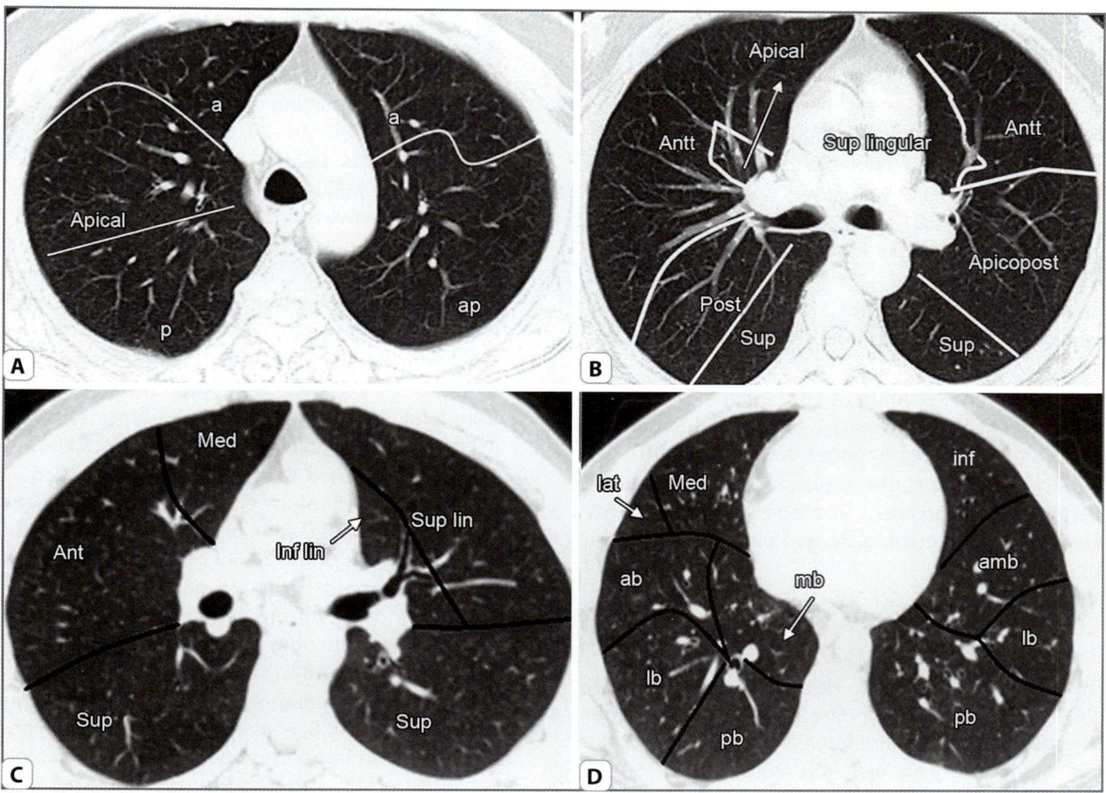

FIGS. 26A TO D: Normal segmental lung anatomy. (A) Section at the level of aortic arch. (B) Left pulmonary artery level. (C) Right pulmonary artery level. (D) Cardiac ventricular level.

[Apical: apical segment of right upper lobe (S1); P: posterior segment of right upper lobe (S2); Apicopost: apicoposterior segment of left upper lobe (S1 + S2); a: anterior segment of right upper lobe (S3); Lat: lateral segment of right middle lobe (S4). Superior lingular segment (S4). Medial: medial segment of right middle lobe (S5); Inferior: inferior lingular segment of left upper lobe (S5); Superior: superior segment of right or left lower lobe (S6); Mb: medial segment of right lower lobe (S7); Ab: anterior segment of right lower lobe (S8); Amb: anteromedial segment of left lower lobe (S7 + S8); Lb: lateral segment of right or left lower lobe (S9); Pb: posterior segment of right or left lower lobe (S10)].

CONCLUSION

The increasing, almost universal, use of CT for thoracic imaging and emerging applications of MRI make it imperative that one is aware of the advancements, strengths, and limitations of these techniques, so that they can be tailored to answer the clinical question at hand while minimizing radiation exposure.

REFERENCES

1. Nair A, Aziz ZA, Hansell DM. Techniques in thoracic imaging. In: Adam A, Dixon AK, Gillard JH, Prokol S (Eds). Grainger and Allison's Diagnostic Radiology, 6th edition. United Kingdom: Elsevier; 2015. pp. 149-83.
2. Thomas FG, Bernhard. CT technology for imaging the thorax: state of the art. In: Schoepf UJ, Meinel FG (Eds). Medical Radiology, 2nd edition. Berlin-Heidelberg: Springer; 2016. pp. 3-28.
3. Hutt A, Tacelli N, Faivre JB, Flohr T, Duhamel A, Remy J, et al. Is bronchial wall imaging affected by temporal resolution? Comparative evaluation at 140 and 75 ms in 90 patients. Eur Radiol. 2016;26(2):469-77.
4. Schulz B, Jacobi V, Beeres M, Bodelle B, Gruber T, Lee C, et al. Quantitative analysis of motion artifacts in high-pitch dual-source computed tomography of the thorax. J Thorac Imaging. 2012;27(6):382-6.
5. McLoud TC, Little BP. Thoracic radiology: recent developments and future trends. Radiology. 2023;306(2):e223121.
6. Nishino M, Schiebler ML. Advances in thoracic imaging: key developments in the past decade and future directions. Radiology. 2023;306(2):e222536.
7. Tack D, Appiah V. Acquisition protocol for thoracic CT. In: Schoepf UJ, Meinel FG (Eds). Medical Radiology, 2nd edition. Berlin-Heidelberg: Springer; 2016. pp. 59-68.
8. Dominik F, Richard HL. Contrast medium injection technique. In: Schoepf UJ, Meinel FG (Eds). Medical Radiology, 2nd edition. Berlin-Heidelberg: Springer; 2016. pp. 37-57.

9. Mayo JR, Webb WR, Gould R, Stein MG, Bass I, Gamsu G, et al. High-resolution CT of the lungs: an optimal approach. Radiology. 1987;163(2):507-10.
10. Murata K, Khan A, Herman PG. Pulmonary parenchymal disease: evaluation with high-resolution CT. In: Nishino M, Boiselle PM, Copeland JF (Eds). Radiology. 2004;170:629-35.
11. Beigelman-Aubry C, Hill C, Guibal A, Savatovsky J, Grenier PA. Multi-detector row CT and postprocessing techniques in the assessment of diffuse lung disease. Radiographics. 2005;25(6):1639-52.
12. Litmanovich DE, Tack D, Lee KS, Shahrzad M, Bankier AA. Cardiothoracic imaging in the pregnant patient. J Thorac Imaging. 2014;29:38-49.
13. Harald B, Heuschmid M, Andreas FK. Vascular: pulmonary veins. In: Medizin S, Heidelberg V (Eds). Dual-Source CT Imaging. Berlin-Heidelberg: Springer; 2008. pp. 140-50.
14. Thorsten RCJ, Konstantin N, Christopher BR, Becker R. Vascular: extended chest pain protocol. In: Medizin S, Heidelberg V (Eds). Dual-Source CT Imaging. Berlin-Heidelberg: Springer; 2008. pp. 130-9.
15. Eibel R, Türk T, Kulinna C, Schöpf UJ, Brüning R, Reiser MF. Value of multiplanar reformations (MPR) in multi-slice spiral CT of the lung. Rofo. 2001;173(1):57-64.
16. Eibel R, Türk TR, Kulinna C, Herrmann K, Reiser MF. Multidetector row CT of the lungs: multiplanar reconstructions and maximum intensity projections for the detection of pulmonary nodules. Rofo. 2001;173(9):815-21.
17. Kuettner A, Anders K, Lell M, Nuremberg E. Dual energy: virtual noncontrast. In: Medizin S, Heidelberg V (Eds). Dual-Source CT Imaging. Berlin-Heidelberg: Springer; 2008. pp. 242-51.
18. Dinkel J, Hintze C, Rochet N, Thieke C, Biederer J. Computed tomography of the lungs: a step into the fourth dimension. Radiology. 2009;49(8):698-704.
19. Wielputz MO, Bardarova D, Weinheimer O, Kauczor HU, Eichinger M, Jobst BJ, et al. Variation of densitometry on computed tomography in COPD–influence of different software tools. PLoS One. 2014;9(11):e112898.
20. Paul NS. Strategies for dose reduction and improvement of image quality in chest CT. In: Schoepf UJ, Meinel FG (Eds). Medical Radiology, 2nd edition. Berlin-Heidelberg: Springer; 2016, pp. 29-36.
21. Wild JM, Marshal H, Bock M, Schad LR, Jakob PM, Molinary MPF, et al. MRI of the lung (1/3): methods. Insights Imaging. 2012;3:345-53.
22. Kauczor HU, Zaporozhan JL, Ley S. Imaging of pulmonary pathologies. Focus on magnetic resonance imaging. Proc Am Thorac Soc. 2009;6:458-63.
23. Hochhegger B, de Souza VVS, Marchiori E, Irion KL, Souza AS, Junor JE, et al. Chest magnetic resonance imaging: a protocol suggestion. Radiol Bras. 2015;48(6):373-80.
24. Henzler T, Bindert GS, Schoenberg SO, Fink C. Diffusion and perfusion MRI of the lung and mediastinum. Eur J Radiol. 2010;76:329-36.
25. Christine UL, White DB, Sykes AMG. Establishing a chest MRI practice and its clinical application: our insight and protocols. J Clin Imaging Sci. 2014;4:17.
26. Ackman JB. MR imaging of mediastinal masses. Magn Reson Imaging Clin North Am. 2015;23:141-64.
27. Mirasadraee JBS, Beer M, Molinary F, Hintze C, Bauman G, Both M, et al. MRI of the lung (3/3)-current application and future perspectives. Insights Imaging. 2012;3:373-86.
28. Hatabu H, Ohno Y, Gefter WB, Parraga G, Madore B, Lee KS, et al. Expanding applications of pulmonary MRI in the clinical evaluation of lung disorders: Fleischner Society Position Paper. Radiology. 2020;297(2):286-301.
29. Longuefosse A, Raoult J, Benlala I, de Senneville BD, Benkert T, Macey J, et al. Generating high-resolution synthetic CT from lung MRI with ultrashort echo times: initial evaluation in cystic fibrosis. Radiology. 2023;308(1):e230052.
30. Stein PD, Woodard PK, Hull RD, Kayali F, Weg JG, Olson RE, et al. Gadolinium-enhanced magnetic resonance angiography for detection of acute pulmonary embolism: an in-depth review. Chest. 2003;124:2324-8.
31. Kluge A, Loboldt W, Bachmann G. Acute pulmonary embolism to the subsegmental level: diagnostic accuracy of three MRI techniques compared with 16-MDCT. AJR Am J Roentgenol. 2006;187(1):W7-14.
32. Nikolaou K, Schoenberg SO, Attenberger U, Scheidhler J, Dietrich O, Kuehn B, et al. Pulmonary arterial hypertension: diagnosis with fast perfusion MR imaging and high-spatial-resolution MR angiography-preliminary experience. Radiology. 2005;236:694-703.
33. Koyama H, Ohno Y, Kono A, Takenaka D, Maniwa Y, Nishimura Y, et al. Quantitative and qualitative assessment of non-contrast-enhanced pulmonary MR imaging for management of pulmonary nodules in 161 subjects. Eur Radiol. 2008;18:2120-31.
34. Hochhegger B, Marchiori E, dos Reis DQ, Souza AS, Souza LS, Brum T, et al. Chemical-shift MRI of pulmonary hamartoma: initial experience using a modified technique to assess nodules fat. AJR Am J Roentgenol. 2012;199:W331-4.
35. Sodhi KS, Khandelwal N, Saxena AK, Singh M, Aggarwal R, Bhatia A, et al. Rapid lung MRI in children with pulmonary infections: time to change our diagnostic algorithms. J Magn Reson Imaging. 2016;43:1196-206.
36. Carter BW, Benveniste MF, Madan R, Godoy MC, de Groot PM, Truong MT, et al. ITMIG classification of mediastinal compartments and multidisciplinary approach to mediastinal masses. Radiographics. 2017;37(2):413-36.
37. Carter BW, Tomiyama N, Bhora FY, de Christenson MLR, Nakajima J, Boiselle PM, et al. A modern definition of mediastinal compartments. J Thorac Oncol. 2014;9(9 Suppl 2):S97-101.
38. Mukherjee S, Gupta R. Imaging in chest disease. In: Pande JN (Ed). Respiratory Medicine in the Tropics, 1st edition. New Delhi: Oxford University Press; 1988. p. 90.
39. Amstrong P. The normal chest. In: Grainger RG, Allison D (Eds). Diagnostic Radiology, 3rd edition. New York: Churchill Livingstone; 1997. p. 207.

Alpana Manchanda, Satyam, Gaurav Shanker Pradhan

CHAPTER 4

Patterns of Lung Diseases on Computed Tomography

INTRODUCTION

High-resolution computed tomography (HRCT) has transformed the evaluation of lung diseases, offering unparalleled visualization of pulmonary structure and pathology. It is the most sensitive imaging modality for detecting focal and diffuse lung abnormalities, surpassing conventional chest radiography, which lacks the resolution to distinguish subtle variations in lung density. This capability makes HRCT indispensable in modern thoracic imaging.

In HRCT, a "pattern" represents a constellation of imaging findings that may suggest specific disease processes.[1] These patterns, when combined with anatomical distribution and clinical context, guide the diagnostic process.[2] These patterns often narrow the differential diagnosis of diffuse lung disease and, in many cases, point directly to a specific diagnosis.

High-resolution computed tomography has revolutionized the evaluation of diffuse lung diseases by enabling superior detection, histospecific diagnosis, and assessment of disease progression or reversibility. It has provided critical insights into interstitial lung diseases, airway abnormalities, and obstructive lung diseases. Furthermore, it aids in evaluating disease progression and reversibility, making it an essential tool in patient management. Although HRCT is not a nascent technique, advancements such as volumetric image acquisition continue to refine its utility, cementing its role as a cornerstone of diagnostic chest imaging.

Diffuse abnormalities of the lung parenchyma on HRCT can be broadly categorized into four primary patterns: (1) reticular and short linear opacities, (2) nodular opacities, (3) increased lung opacity [ground-glass opacity (GGO) or consolidation], and (4) cystic airspaces or areas of decreased lung density.[3] While these patterns often correspond to findings on chest radiographs, HRCT provides superior clarity, enabling precise visualization of the disease's distribution and extent.

HIGH-RESOLUTION COMPUTED TOMOGRAPHY PATTERNS OF LUNG DISEASE

Effective interpretation of HRCT findings requires a systematic approach and an understanding of the pathological basis of various imaging patterns.[4] These findings can generally be classified into two major groups given as follows:

1. Increased lung opacity
2. Decreased lung opacity

Further, subclassification of these patterns simplifies the diagnostic process and aids in forming a differential diagnosis. In some cases, both increased and decreased lung opacity may coexist in the same scan, indicating either multiple concurrent diseases or a single pathological process with both infiltrative and obstructive components.

Increased Lung Opacity

High-resolution computed tomography scan findings manifesting as increased lung opacity can be further subclassified into the following abnormalities or patterns:

- Nodular pattern
- Linear and reticular pattern
- Ground-glass opacity
- Consolidation

Nodular Pattern: Nodules and Nodular Opacities

A variety of lung diseases are characterized by multiple nodules as the primary abnormality. A nodule is defined as a pulmonary opacity that is nearly circular, discrete, and either sharply defined or ill-defined, measuring ≤30 mm in average diameter.[4] A small nodule measures <1 cm, whereas nodules 1 cm or larger are classified as large nodules.[5] Lesions > 30 mm are referred to as masses.[5,6]

The term micronodule has been used to describe very small, discrete, and round opacities. Historically, definitions of micronodules have varied, with thresholds of <7, 5, or 3 mm in diameter.[5] However, the Nomenclature Committee of the Fleischner Society 2024 recommends reserving the term for nodules ≤30 mm. More recent guidelines suggest broadening the definition of micronodules to include opacities <6 mm, particularly for distinguishing incidental findings from larger, potentially actionable nodules.[6,7] This classification is particularly relevant for patients at high risk for malignancy or with a history of cancer, as newly appearing micronodules may warrant further evaluation. While micronodules share characteristics such as shape, margin, and location, as with larger nodules, their small size makes precise characterization more challenging. Importantly, the concept of individual micronodules differs from that of a micronodular pattern, which refers to numerous such opacities. In patients with multinodular lung disease, nodules are typically of varying sizes. The disease characterized solely by micronodules is rare, except in conditions such as miliary disease.

Nodules are typically further described based on their size (uniform or variable), margin (sharply or poorly defined), density (solid and subsolid), number, and location.

On chest radiographs, a nodular pattern is identified by innumerable, small, and rounded opacities, typically ranging from 2 to 10 mm in diameter.[6] These nodules are widespread but not necessarily uniformly distributed. HRCT offers a clearer depiction of these patterns and enables further classification based on three anatomical distributions: (1) centrilobular, (2) perilymphatic, and (3) random. Such categorization, combined with clinical context, aids in narrowing the differential diagnosis of nodular lung disease.

In addition to size and distribution, nodules are also described by their shape (round, ovoid, or polygonal) and as spherical, flat, or elongated in configuration based on their appearance in various imaging planes.[6] Margins may be sharply defined or ill-defined, depending on the clarity of their interface with surrounding lung tissue. A smooth outline is without any indentation or protrusion; however, an irregular margin of nodule may show lobulations or spiculations.[6] Specific features such as pleural tags or linear extensions from the nodule to the pleural surface may further refine diagnostic considerations.[6]

The localization of nodules—whether within the interstitium or air spaces—is another important factor. Interstitial nodules are generally well defined and of soft-tissue attenuation, whereas airspace nodules tend to be ill-defined, with densities ranging from solid to GGO. However, many diffuse lung diseases involve both compartments, making this distinction less reliable for differential diagnosis in certain cases.

The detection and characterization of nodules on CT depend significantly on technical factors. Narrow collimation is superior to thick-section acquisition, as it minimizes partial volume effects that may obscure small nodules.[8] Additionally, advanced imaging techniques such as maximum intensity projection (MIP) reconstructions of contiguous thin sections improve the visualization of minute nodules **(Figs. 1A and B)**. Although not yet routinely performed, these techniques enhance diagnostic accuracy, particularly for small or subtle nodular patterns.[9]

The systematic analysis of nodular patterns on HRCT, combined with an understanding of their size, shape, margin, density, and distribution, is critical for diagnosing underlying lung pathologies and formulating accurate differentials.

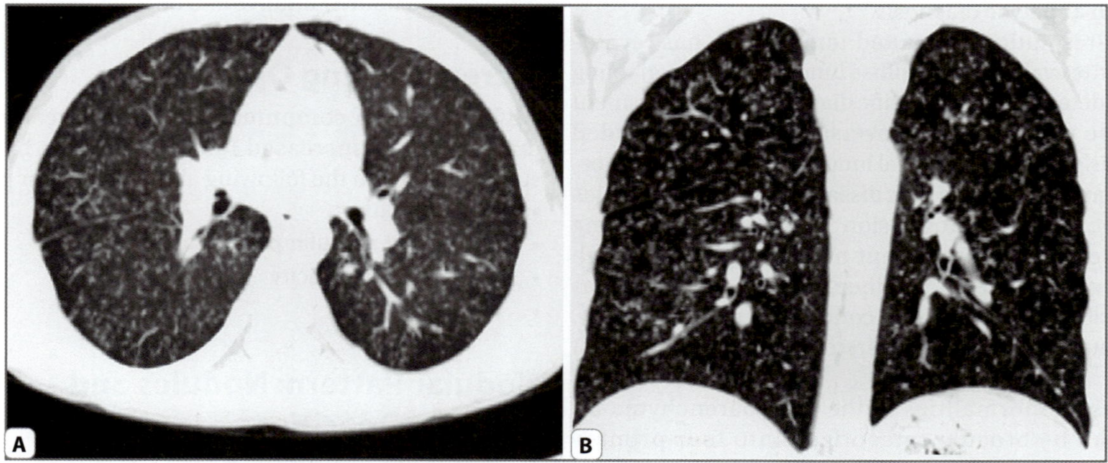

FIGS. 1A AND B: Miliary nodules. (A) Axial CT shows multiple, small, sharply defined nodules uniformly distributed in bilateral lung parenchyma. (B) Coronal reformatted CT MIP reconstruction delineates the miliary nodules better in bilateral lung fields.

(CT: computed tomography; MIP: maximum intensity projection)

The HRCT evaluation of nodular lung disease is based on several key findings and patterns,[10] including:

- Craniocaudal distribution of nodules
- Appearance and attenuation of nodules
- Specific distribution of the nodules relative to lung structures

The above features are essential for narrowing the differential diagnosis and identifying the underlying pathology.

The craniocaudal distribution of nodules helps in the differential diagnosis of nodular lung disease, as certain diseases such as sarcoidosis, pneumoconiosis, Langerhans cell histiocytosis, respiratory bronchiolitis, miliary tuberculosis, and other granulomatous diseases are seen predominantly in the upper lobes, while others such as hematogenous metastases tend to be lower lobe predominant **(Figs. 2A and B)**.

However, this information should not be interpreted in isolation, as overlap in distribution patterns is common, and variability exists even among patients with the same disease.

The appearance and attenuation of nodules provide insights into their origin, whether interstitial or airspace (alveolar).

- *Interstitial nodules* are usually well defined, with soft-tissue (solid) attenuation, and obscure adjacent structures such as vessels.
- *Alveolar nodules* are typically ill-defined and may exhibit homogeneous soft-tissue attenuation or GGO.

The following tables enumerate the differential diagnosis of multinodular lung disease based on sharpness of nodule margin **(Table 1)** and nodule attenuation **(Table 2)**.

Differentiating lung nodules into interstitial and airspace nodules on HRCT scan is not always accurate,

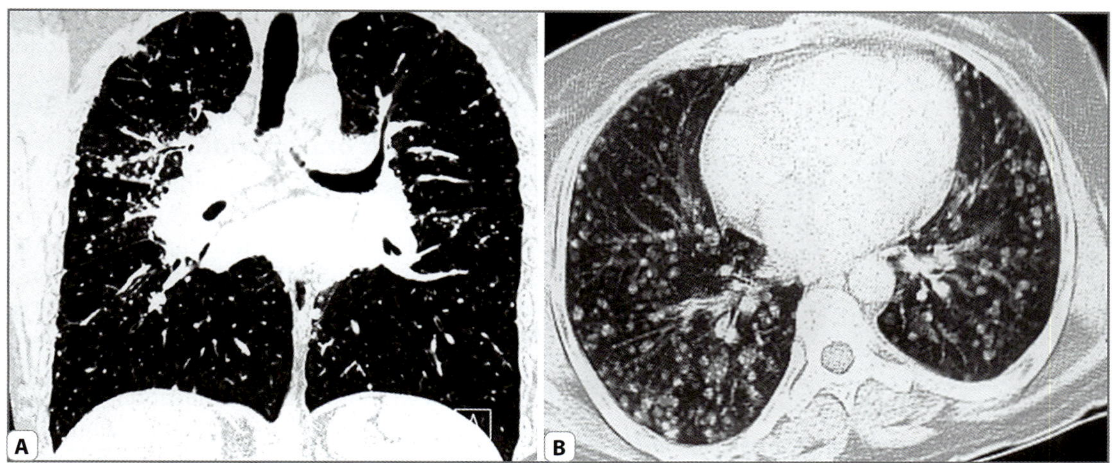

FIGS. 2A AND B: Micronodules and random nodules. (A) Coronal MPR shows typical micronodules of sarcoidosis predominantly in bilateral upper lobes in perilymphatic distribution. (B) Axial CT shows multiple sharply defined random nodular opacities due to hematogenous metastasis.

(CT: computed tomography; MPR: multiplanar reconstruction)

TABLE 1: Differential diagnosis of nodular lung disease based on the sharpness of nodule margin.

Usually well-defined margins	Usually ill-defined margins	Either well- or ill-defined margins
• Sarcoidosis • Metastases • Miliary infection (tubercular, fungal/viral)	• Hypersensitivity pneumonitis • Respiratory bronchiolitis • Follicular bronchiolitis	• Langerhans cell histiocytosis • Lymphoid interstitial pneumonia • Pneumoconioses
Amyloidosis	Infection (bacterial, fungal, or viral)	
	Organizing pneumonia	
	Invasive mucinous adenocarcinoma (previously bronchioloalveolar carcinoma)	
	Aspiration	
	Pulmonary edema	
	Pulmonary hemorrhage	
	Metastatic calcification	

TABLE 2: Differential diagnosis of lung nodules based on nodule attenuation.

Usually solid	Usually ground-glass opacity (GGO)	Either solid or GGO
Sarcoidosis	Hypersensitivity pneumonitis	Lymphoid interstitial pneumonia
Metastases	Respiratory bronchiolitis	Pneumoconioses
Miliary infections	Follicular bronchiolitis	Bronchopneumonia
Amyloidosis	Pulmonary edema	Invasive mucinous adenocarcinoma
Langerhans cell histiocytosis	Pulmonary hemorrhage	Organizing pneumonia
	Metastatic calcification	Aspiration

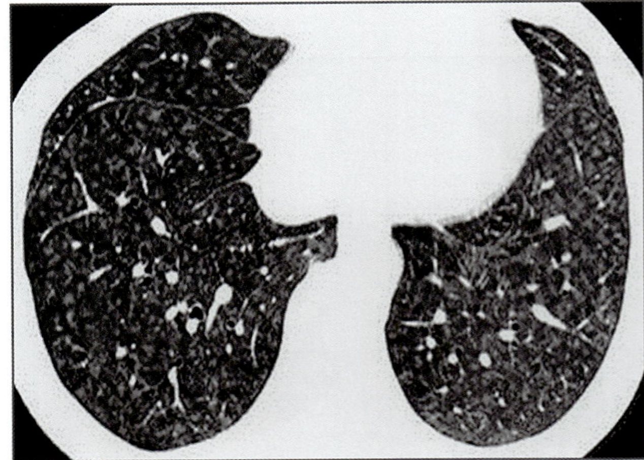

FIG. 3: Ground-glass nodular opacities. Axial high-resolution computed tomography (HRCT) shows poorly defined ground-glass nodular opacities scattered in bilateral lower lobes in hypersensitivity pneumonitis.

as many diffuse lung diseases involve both the interstitial and airspace compartments histologically. Also, there are many exceptions to the rule. For example, hypersensitivity pneumonitis (HP), which is an interstitial lung disease, is characterized by very indistinct nodules **(Fig. 3)**.

Recent updates emphasize the importance of nodule attenuation and structure in characterizing nodular patterns. Nodules may be classified as simple (a single structural component such as soft tissue, ground glass, or fat) or complex (containing multiple components such as soft tissue and ground glass).[11-13] Subtypes include solid and subsolid, and subsolid is further divided into pure ground-glass and part-solid nodules, with specific morphologies correlating to disease progression in entities such as lung adenocarcinoma.[13,14]

In the assessment of diffuse nodular disease, *the anatomic distribution of nodules* relative to the secondary pulmonary lobule has diagnostic value on HRCT scans as it provides a focused differential diagnosis and is reflective of the pathophysiology of the underlying disease.

There are three specific distributions of small nodules in the secondary pulmonary lobule, which can be distinguished on HRCT given as follows:

1. Perilymphatic or lymphatic distribution
2. Random
3. Centrilobular distribution

Recognition of these three distributions is fundamental to the HRCT interpretation of nodular lung disease with an accuracy of 90–95%, as it can aid in formulating differential diagnoses by reflecting the pathophysiology of underlying diseases.[8] Location-specific terms, *such as perifissural or juxtafissural*, improve anatomical precision in describing nodule distribution.[6]

The representative schematic diagrams **(Figs. 4A to D)** depict the normal anatomy of the secondary pulmonary lobule and various distribution patterns of nodules at the level of secondary pulmonary lobule.

Perilymphatic or Lymphatic Nodules

Nodules in a perilymphatic distribution are seen in relation to the pulmonary lymphatics, which are located within the visceral pleura, interlobular septa, and along the bronchovascular bundles. The most common diseases, which show a perilymphatic distribution, are given in **Box 1**.

On HRCT and histologically, perilymphatic nodules are seen in one or more of the four locations given as follows:

1. *Peribronchovascular nodules* are seen individually or in clusters adjacent to large bronchi and vessels in the central lung regions, giving a nodular appearance to the walls of bronchi and arteries. They are most typically seen in sarcoidosis **(Fig. 5)**.
2. *Subpleural nodules* are easily recognized beneath the pleural surfaces and adjacent to the interlobular fissures. Confluent subpleural nodules can result in the appearance of pseudoplaques. Subpleural nodules have been seen in around 80% of patients with silicosis or coal workers' pneumoconiosis (CWP) and at least 50% of patients with sarcoidosis and also common with lymphangitic spread of carcinoma **(Fig. 6)**.[5]
3. *Interlobular septal nodules* give the appearance of "beaded" septa or nodular septal thickening. These are most frequent in patients of lymphangitic spread of carcinoma **(Figs. 7A and B)**.
4. *Centrilobular peribronchovascular nodules* are also seen in relation to small airways and vessels in the centrilobular location (center of pulmonary lobules), giving a beaded appearance to the centrilobular artery.

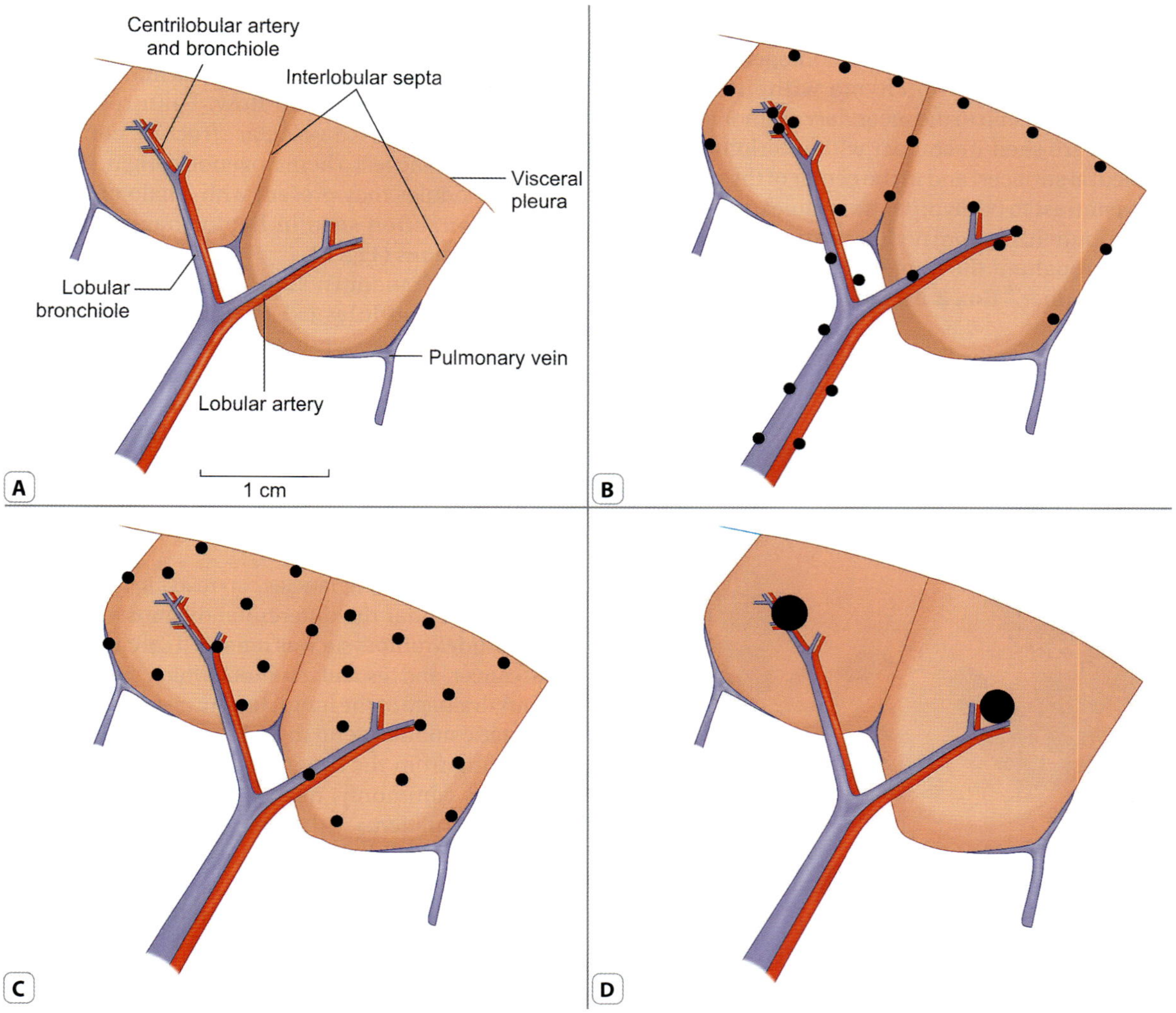

FIGS. 4A TO D: Schematic representations of distribution of nodules at the level of the secondary pulmonary lobule. (A) Normal anatomy of the secondary pulmonary lobule. (B) Perilymphatic distribution of nodules. (C) Random distribution of nodules. (D) Centrilobular distribution of nodules.

BOX 1: Differential diagnosis of perilymphatic nodules.[10]

- Sarcoidosis (common)
- Lymphangitic carcinomatosis
- Pneumoconioses—silicosis, coal workers' pneumoconiosis (CWP), beryllosis, talc, and rare earth
- Lymphoid interstitial pneumonia (rare)
- Amyloidosis (rare)

A combination of two of the above four possible sites has been described to be usually sufficient for perilymphatic nodules for diagnosis.[5] As perilymphatic nodules occur only in relation to these specific locations, the distribution of the nodules is patchy, with both normal and abnormal areas of lung regions seen on HRCT **(Table 3)**.[10]

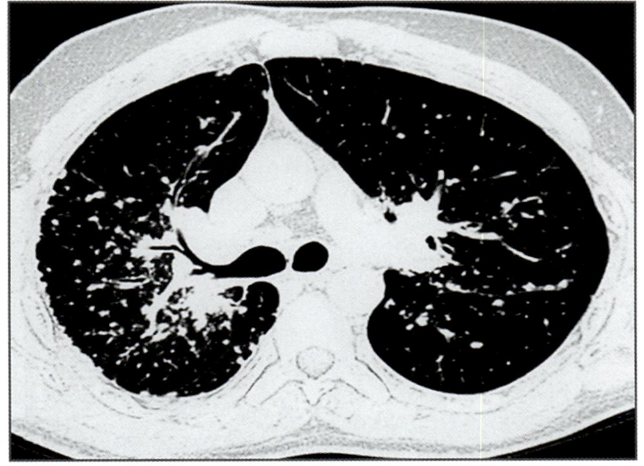

FIG. 5: Nodular interlobular septal thickening: Multiple granulomas in sarcoidosis in peribronchovascular, subpleural, and centrilobular interstitium more marked in the right upper lobe.

Random Nodules

Random nodules show diffuse and homogeneous spread throughout the lung parenchyma without a specific anatomical relationship to the secondary pulmonary lobule. The nodules are seen in contact with interlobular septa, visceral pleural surfaces, and in the center of the pulmonary lobule. In contrast to perilymphatic nodules, which show a patchy distribution, random nodules are usually distributed uniformly throughout the lung parenchyma in a bilateral symmetric manner.[4] **Box 2** lists the differential diagnosis of random nodules.

These nodules, typically well defined and smooth, are most commonly associated with hematogenous spread, as in metastatic disease or miliary infections such as tuberculosis. Random nodules are uniformly distributed in bilateral lungs but may exhibit basilar predominance due to preferential blood flow. Features such as the feeding vessel sign—a vascular structure connecting to a nodule—can suggest a hematogenous origin. Occasionally, random nodules may present with a halo of ground-glass attenuation, often seen in hemorrhagic metastases or fungal infections **(Fig. 8)**.

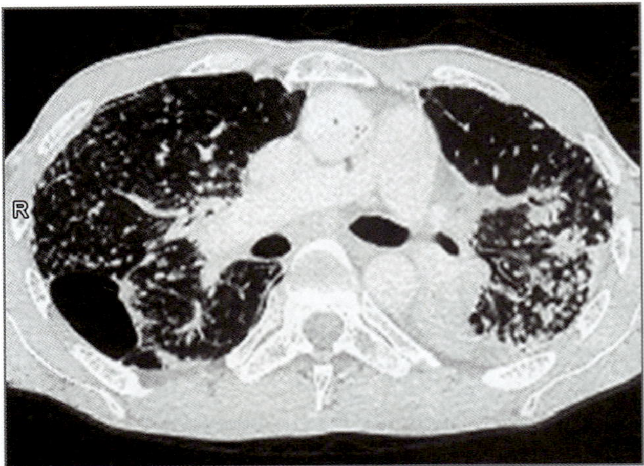

FIG. 6: Perilymphatic distribution of nodules in silicosis: Axial high-resolution computed tomography (HRCT) shows multiple small discrete and confluent micronodules in centrilobular and subpleural regions without tree-in-bud morphology. These are bilateral, symmetrical with upper lobe predominance. Subpleural bulla is noted on the right side.

The size of random nodules provides further diagnostic clues. Larger nodules (>1 cm) are more suggestive of metastatic disease, while tiny nodules (2–5 mm) often indicate miliary tuberculosis or other granulomatous disease. Miliary tuberculosis may show an upper lobe predominance as the organism grows best there due to high oxygen tension, which is in the upper lobes. However, considerable overlap may be seen in the size of nodules that each disease produces. Miliary tuberculosis can result in nodules >5 mm in size.[10]

A number of malignancies can result in a miliary pattern, which can render the differential diagnosis to be difficult. This includes tumors such as renal cell carcinoma, head and neck cancer, and testicular tumors, which have their primary venous drainage in the lungs. In contrast, larger, less profuse metastatic nodules tend to be adenocarcinomas, typically originating from the lung, breast, or the gastrointestinal tract. Less commonly, multiple cavitary nodules may be identified in patients with septic emboli, metastasis usually of squamous cell histology, Wegener's granulomatosis, rheumatoid lung disease, invasive fungal infections, and pulmonary vasculitis **(Fig. 9)**.[1,15] Multiple irregular nodules in a bronchovascular distribution are characteristic of lymphoproliferative disorders, lymphoma, leukemia, and Kaposi sarcoma. When associated with thin-walled cysts, randomly distributed nodules are suggestive of Langerhans cell histiocytosis.

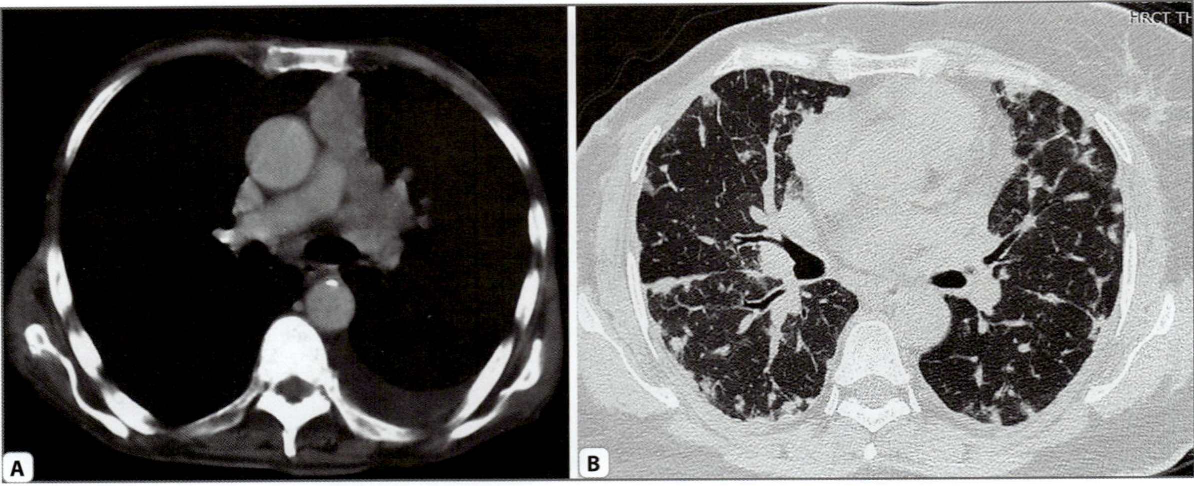

FIGS. 7A AND B: Lymphangitis carcinomatosis. (A) Axial computed tomography (CT) mediastinal window shows a left suprahilar mass involving the left main bronchus, encasing the left main pulmonary artery with left pleural effusion. (B) Lung window depicts nodular interlobular septal thickening and nodular fissural thickening in bilateral lung parenchyma.

TABLE 3: Typical pattern of involvement of the perilymphatic interstitium of some common diseases showing perilymphatic nodules.

	Sarcoidosis	Silicosis	Lymphangitic spread of carcinoma
Site	• Upper lobe predominance • Diffuse distribution/lower lobe involvement is also seen	May be diffuse but in mild disease may be seen in upper lobes	Upper or lower lobes or diffuse
Perilymphatic interstitium is most commonly involved by nodules on high-resolution computed tomography (HRCT)	• Along central bronchi and vessels • In relation to major fissures	Centrilobular and subpleural in location	• Within thickened peribronchovascular interstitium and interlobular septa • Subpleural nodules less profuse
Size of nodules	Few mm to 1 cm	2–5 mm	Seen as beaded appearance of septum
Appearance of nodules	Usually well defined	Well defined	Septal thickening smooth/nodular
Lung involvement	Patchy and asymmetric distribution of nodules	• More evenly distributed • Typical bilateral and symmetrical nodules	Variable-unilateral, patchy, bilateral, or symmetric

BOX 2: Differential diagnosis of random nodules.

- Hematogenous metastases
- Miliary tuberculosis
- Miliary fungal infections (coccidioidomycosis, histoplasmosis)
- Disseminated viral infection
- Silicosis or coal workers' pneumoconiosis (may occasionally appear random)
- Langerhans cell histiocytosis

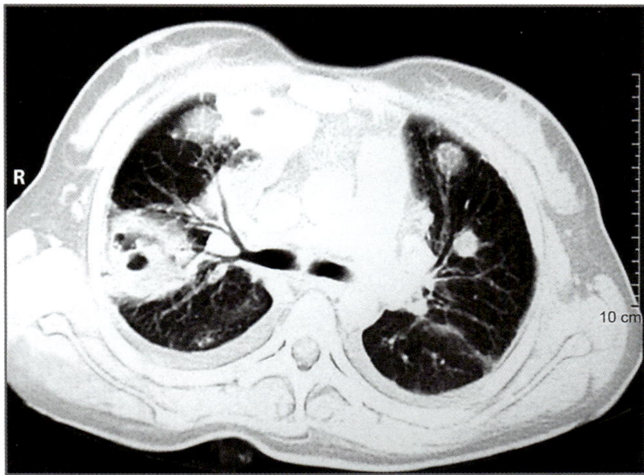

FIG. 8: Feeding vessel sign: Axial computed tomography (CT) shows multiple variable-sized nodules in angiocentric distribution scattered in bilateral lung fields.

When numerous, nodules in patients with sarcoidosis, Langerhans cell histiocytosis, or silicosis may appear to be randomly and diffusely distributed and may be difficult to distinguish from the nodules of miliary infection or metastasis.[5]

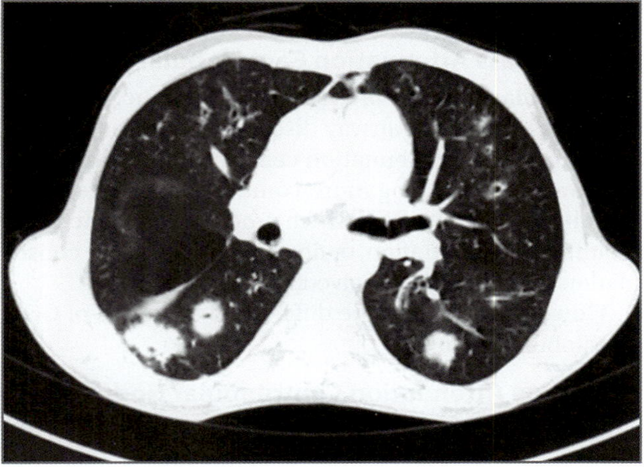

FIG. 9: Cavitating nodules: Axial computed tomography (CT) in a patient of rheumatic heart disease reveals multiple nodules in bilateral lower lobes with central hypodensity consistent with septic emboli.

Correlation with clinical history is important in the differential diagnosis of the nodular pattern. If the patient has a known malignancy, the nodular pattern is diagnostic of hematogenous spread. If signs of infection such as fever or elevated counts are present, miliary tuberculosis or fungal infection is likely. However, it should be remembered that in the elderly or debilitated patients, miliary tuberculosis may be associated with very few symptoms.[10]

Centrilobular Nodules

Centrilobular nodules are located within the center of the secondary pulmonary lobule along the terminal bronchioles and their associated pulmonary arteries and supporting connective tissue with lymph vessels. Centrilobular nodules may result from airway, vascular, or perivascular diseases.[2] They can be due to either interstitial or airspace abnormalities and range in attenuation from ground-glass to soft-tissue density and in size from a few millimeters to about a centimeter.

On HRCT, centrilobular nodular opacities show characteristic distributions, which distinguish them from other patterns. These are given as follows:

- The most peripheral centrilobular nodules show sparing of the visceral pleural surface as the most peripheral pulmonary lobules are 5–10 mm from the pleural surfaces.
- The nodules appear evenly spaced due to uniformity of size of the pulmonary lobules.[5,10]

Differential Diagnosis of Centrilobular Nodules

The differential diagnosis of centrilobular nodules depends on many findings given as follows:

- *Attenuation of centrilobular nodules*: (i) GGO or (ii) homogeneous soft-tissue attenuation
- *Overall distribution of nodules* (whether diffuse/symmetrical/patchy)
- Association with tree-in-bud (TIB) pattern

Ground-glass Attenuation Centrilobular Nodules

Centrilobular nodules of ground-glass attenuation may be seen as a result of airway disease or vascular disease, with ground-glass attenuation centrilobular nodules due to airway disease being more common of the two. They typically reflect processes, which produce peribronchiolar inflammation, infiltration, or fibrosis without dense consolidation or obliteration of alveoli **(Fig. 10)**.

Flowchart 1 depicts the differential diagnosis of GGO centrilobular nodules.

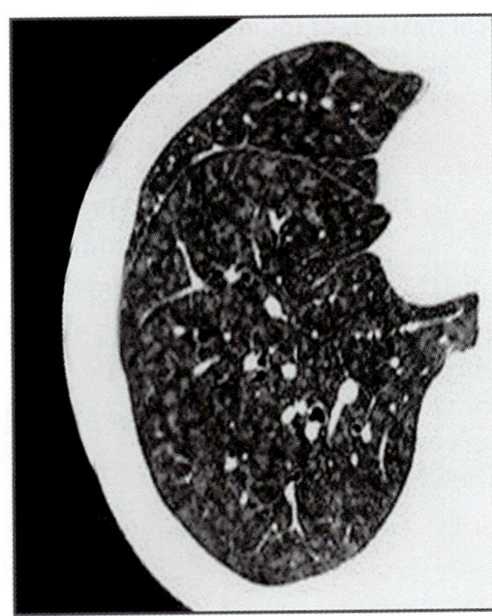

FIG. 10: Ill-defined GGO nodules: Magnified axial HRCT image of right lung depicting diffuse ill-defined GGO nodules in subacute hypersensitivity pneumonitis.

(GGO: ground-glass opacity; HRCT: high-resolution computed tomography)

Differential diagnosis of GGO centrilobular nodules

Airway disease:	*Vascular disease (diffuse, symmetrical GGO):*
• Subacute HP **(Fig. 10)**	• Pulmonary edema
• RB-ILD	• Pulmonary arterial HTN
• Follicular bronchiolitis	• Metastatic calcification
• Pneumoconiosis	

FLOWCHART 1: Differential diagnosis of ground-glass opacity (GGO) centrilobular nodules.[10]

(HP: hypersensitivity pneumonitis; HTN: hypertension; RB-ILD: respiratory bronchiolitis-interstitial lung disease)

Soft-tissue Attenuation Centrilobular Nodules

Centrilobular nodules of homogeneous soft-tissue attenuation are characterized by inflammation or infiltration with consolidation of peribronchiolar alveoli or dense peribronchiolar fibrosis. There may be bronchiolar filling or impaction **(Fig. 11)**, and the entire lobule may be involved with disease progression.[10] The differential diagnosis includes disease processes such as bronchopneumonia **(Fig. 12)**, aspiration **(Fig. 13)**, tumor, and invasive adenocarcinoma (previously known as bronchioalveolar carcinoma).

Table 4 enumerates the differential diagnosis of soft-tissue attenuation centrilobular nodules with their salient features.

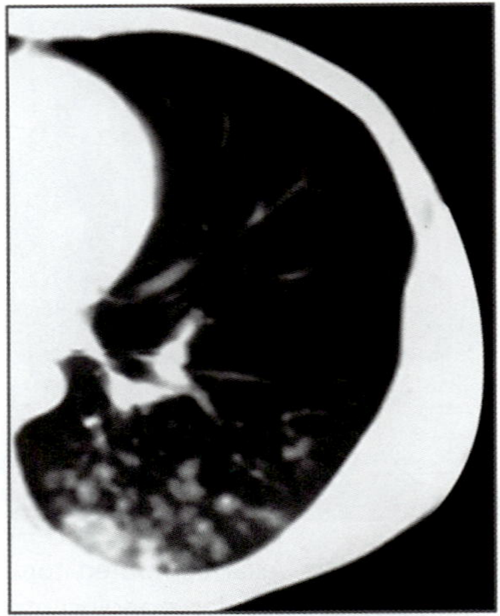

FIG. 11: Soft-tissue centrilobular nodules: Axial computed tomography (CT) image of left lung shows peripheral branching nodular opacities consistent with bronchiolar impaction.

Distribution of Centrilobular Nodules in Differential Diagnosis

When formulating a differential diagnosis of centrilobular nodules, the overall distribution of centrilobular nodules, whether diffuse, symmetrical, or patchy, should be taken

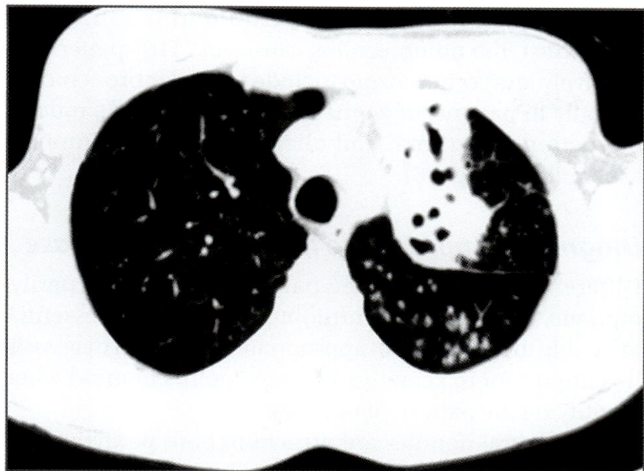

FIG. 12: Airspace nodules in bronchopneumonia: Axial computed tomography (CT) reveals ill-defined soft-tissue nodules in left lower lobe with collapse consolidation of left upper lobe.

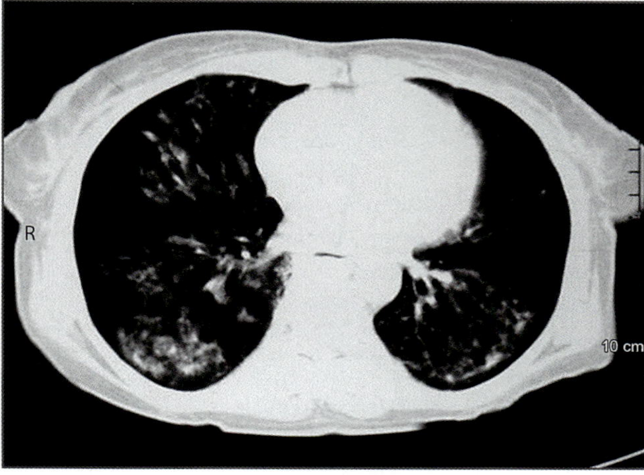

FIG. 13: Centrilobular nodules: Axial computed tomography (CT) shows multiple discrete and confluent centrilobular nodules predominantly in bilateral lower lobes in aspiration pneumonitis.

in conjunction with nodule attenuation (ground-glass or soft-tissue attenuation). **Table 5** enumerates the differential diagnoses of centrilobular nodules based on overall distribution.[10]

Tree-in-bud Pattern

Once nodules are characterized as being primarily centrilobular in distribution, further assessment is required to determine whether they have a "TIB" configuration or not.

"Tree-in-bud" opacities are nearly always the result of inspissated secretions lodged within centrilobular bronchioles, which account for a branching configuration when coursing parallel to the CT scan plane. Normal bronchioles have a diameter of <1 mm and a wall thickness <0.1 mm, which are below the limit of the spatial resolution of HRCT scan. The presence of inspissated secretions results in bronchiolar distension and increased density, allowing their direct visualization.[15]

TABLE 4: Differential diagnosis of soft-tissue attenuation centrilobular nodules.

Soft-tissue attenuation centrilobular nodules	Salient features
Bronchopneumonia results from endobronchial spread of infection—bacterial, mycobacterial, fungal, and viral	• Most common cause • *Acute symptoms*: Nodules are focal, multifocal, or patchy
Endobronchial spread of tumor invasive mucinous adenocarcinoma (formerly BAC)	• Multifocal or patchy nodules ± larger areas of consolidation or GGO • Multiple lobes and both lungs may be involved
Langerhans cell histiocytosis	Early disease and centrilobular nodules in peribronchovascular distribution
Vascular diseases (pulmonary edema and pulmonary hemorrhage)	±GGO or soft-tissue attenuation nodules

(BAC: bronchioloalveolar carcinoma; GGO: ground-glass opacity)

TABLE 5: Differential diagnosis of centrilobular nodules based on distribution.

Distribution of centrilobular nodules	Differential diagnosis
Diffuse distribution	• Hypersensitivity pneumonitis (HP) • Respiratory bronchiolitis (RB) or respiratory bronchiolitis-interstitial lung disease (RB-ILD) • Follicular bronchiolitis • Atypical/viral infection • Pneumoconiosis • Pulmonary edema • Pulmonary hemorrhage • Pulmonary arterial hypertension
Upper or mid-lung predominance	• HP • RB or RB-ILD • Langerhans cell histiocytosis • Pneumoconiosis
Lower lobe distribution	• Aspiration • Endobronchial spread
Patchy distribution	• Endobronchial infection (bacterial, mycobacterial, fungal) • Invasive mucinous adenocarcinoma • Aspiration

The common radiological manifestation of the TIB pattern consists of centrilobular nodules of soft-tissue attenuation connected to multiple branching linear structures of similar caliber, originating from a single stalk, which resembles the branches of a budding tree. **Figure 14** depicts the "TIB" pattern.

On HRCT, the TIB pattern is well recognized by the presence of multiple V- or Y-shaped branching linear opacities 1–2 mm in thickness and 1–2 cm in length, often associated with small nodules at the tips of their branches. The HRCT finding of TIB is due to dilatation and impaction of centrilobular bronchioles by pus or mucus (branches) associated with a small region of peribronchiolar inflammation (buds) and has a characteristic appearance **(Figs. 15A and B)**.[10]

The TIB pattern originally described in cases of endobronchial spread of *Mycobacterium tuberculosis* is highly suggestive of active tuberculosis. However, this pattern is now recognized as a CT manifestation of many diverse entities. **Box 3** enumerates the differential diagnosis of "TIB" pattern.[16]

The "TIB" pattern is most common due to infection with involvement of the small peripheral airways. It is not specific with regard to the type of infection, though bacterial and mycobacterial infections are seen most frequently. Bronchiectasis or bronchial wall thickening may be present depending on the cause or duration of the infection. In contrast, the noninfectious causes of "TIB" pattern are relatively less common and include follicular bronchiolitis (usually in patients of connective tissue disease), mucoid impaction in asthma, and allergic bronchopulmonary aspergillosis **(Fig. 16)**.[10]

Diagnostic Approach to Nodular Lung Disease

Differentiation of the three patterns of nodules (perilymphatic, random, and centrilobular) on HRCT is essential to be able to formulate an appropriate differential diagnosis. It is important to keep the following points in mind when identifying the pattern of nodules:

- Subpleural nodules are present in both perilymphatic and random patterns but should not be present in patients with centrilobular nodules. If the distribution is not clear, then one should pay attenuation to the fissures and peripheral subpleural interstitium to determine if the nodules are present there.

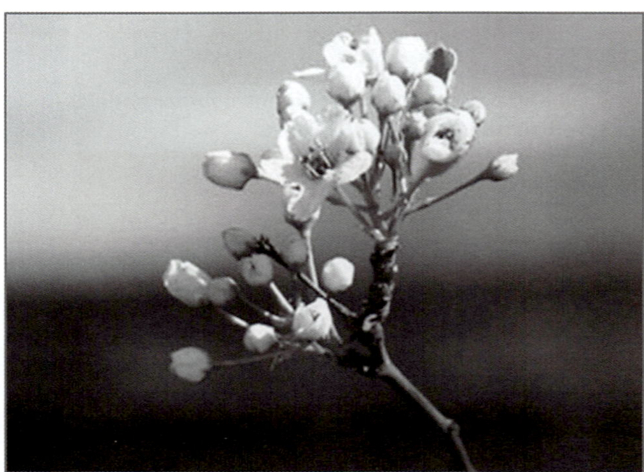

FIG. 14: Photographic representation of "tree-in-bud" pattern.

BOX 3: Differential diagnosis of "tree-in-bud" pattern.

Infections:
- Bacterial infections (*Staphylococcus aureus, Haemophilus influenzae*)
- Mycobacterial infections (*Mycobacterium tuberculosis*, MAIC)
- Fungal infections (airway invasive aspergillosis)
- Viral infections (CMV, RSV)

Infectious variants (congenital/immunological/idiopathic):
- Cystic fibrosis
- Kartagener syndrome
- Allergic bronchopulmonary aspergillosis (ABPA)
- Obliterative bronchiolitis
- Panbronchiolitis, aspiration, and inhalation

(CMV: cytomegalovirus; MAIC: *Mycobacterium avium* intracellulare complex; RSV: respiratory syncytial virus)

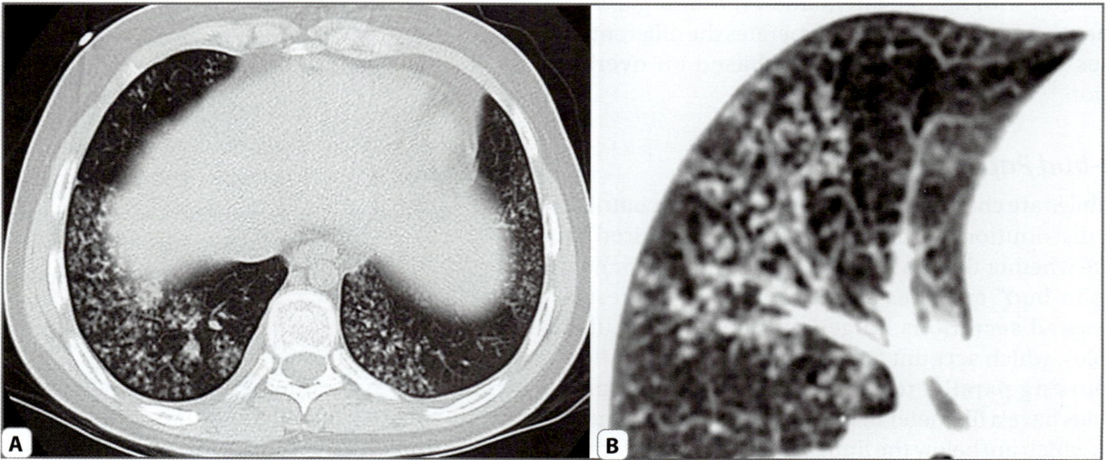

FIGS. 15A AND B: Tree-in-bud (TIB) pattern. (A) Axial computed tomography (CT) showing peripheral poorly defined small (2–4 mm) centrilobular nodules and branching linear opacities of similar caliber originating from a single stalk (TIB) pattern in bilateral lower lobes. (B) Magnified image depicting TIB pattern.

- A diffuse distribution is typical of a random pattern, while a patchy distribution is typical of perilymphatic nodules. Centrilobular nodules may be either diffuse or patchy in distribution, depending on the underlying cause. For example, HP is often diffuse, while endobronchial spread of infection is typically patchy.
- When centrilobular nodules are present, one must ascertain the presence of "TIB" pattern. Infection is very likely when a "TIB" pattern is present, and when not present, the differential diagnosis depends on the attenuation and distribution of nodules.

Flowchart 2 depicts the algorithmic approach for distribution of small nodules on HRCT and their differential diagnosis.[10]

Linear and Reticular Pattern Opacities

Thickening of interstitial fiber network of lung due to fluid, infiltration, or fibrous tissue results in increased linear or reticular opacities in HRCT.

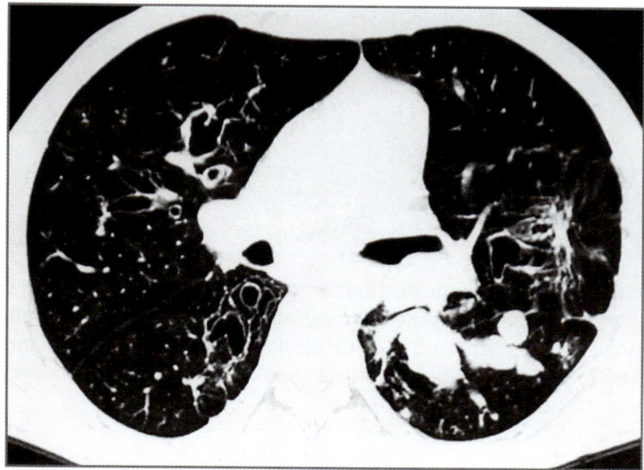

FIG. 16: Allergic bronchopulmonary aspergillosis: Axial computed tomography (CT) shows central bronchiectasis in bilateral lung fields with mucus-filled bronchi in left lower lobe with centrilobular nodules in the adjacent lung.

A reticular pattern consists of intersecting linear opacities forming a mesh or netlike pattern.[3] This pattern almost invariably suggests interstitial injury and represents interstitial lung disease on HRCT. The term "reticular" is purely descriptive (reticulum = network) and encompasses a spectrum of abnormalities, from thickening of the interlobular septa to honeycomb destruction of the lung parenchyma.[8] It is usually associated with features of fibrosis such as architectural distortion and bronchiectasis. These abnormalities are characterized into three recognizable patterns on HRCT given as follows:[17]

1. Interlobular septal thickening
2. Honeycombing
3. Intralobular interstitial thickening

Interlobular Septal Thickening

Interlobular septa form the borders of the secondary pulmonary lobule. They comprise connective tissue and contain pulmonary veins and lymphatics. These septa are around 0.1 mm in thickness and 1–2 cm in length. It is normal to find interlobular septae anteriorly or along mediastinal pleural surfaces.[4] The septae are seen when abnormally thickened, leading to the visualization of numerous septae. In the peripheral lung, the thickened septa of 1–2 cm in length are seen perpendicular to the pleural surface and may outline part or all of the secondary pulmonary lobule. On HRCT, the thickened interlobular septae are the counterpart of Kerley B lines seen on chest radiographs.[18] The thickened interlobular septae outlining the pulmonary lobules appear polygonal in shape and are identified by the presence of a dot-like branching centrilobular artery in the center. This characteristic relationship is valuable in identifying these structures in HRCT.

The terms septal lines or septal thickening may be used to describe interlobular septal thickening. Apart from interstitial lung disease, thickened interlobular septa may be seen in normal elderly patients and smokers.[17]

It should be kept in mind that the differential diagnosis of septal thickening is limited when it is seen as an

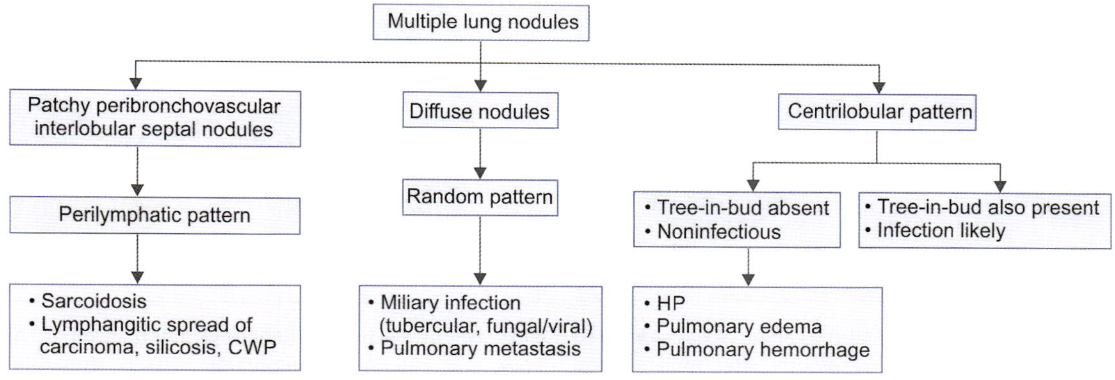

FLOWCHART 2: Algorithm of distribution and differentials of multiple small nodules on HRCT.

(CWP: coal workers' pneumoconiosis; HP: hypersensitivity pneumonitis; HRCT: high-resolution computed tomography)

isolated or predominant abnormality. Septal thickening can be characterized as smooth, nodular, or irregular in morphology in different pathologic processes, and recognizing this morphologic pattern is useful in differential diagnosis.[10,17]

Thickened interlobular septa may be categorized by their morphology.

Smooth septal thickening is present when the septae are thicker than normal and, otherwise, appear normal and are well visualized on HRCT. It is usually a manifestation of pulmonary edema or lymphangitic spread of tumor with fluid or tumor infiltrating the lymphatics located within the septa. Irrespective of the cause, smooth interlobular septal thickening is often associated with smooth peribronchovascular and subpleural interstitial thickening, which is most easily seen as thickening of fissures.[17]

In *pulmonary edema*, the smooth interlobular septal thickening may be diffuse and bilaterally symmetrical with basal predominance. Often, the thickened septa are more defined in the apical and upper lobes, as the interlobular septae are best developed in this region **(Fig. 17)**.[17]

Septal thickening in *lymphangitic spread of tumor* may be either smooth or nodular, with smooth thickening being more common. The abnormality may be unilateral or bilateral, asymmetric, and patchy, having upper or lower lobe involvement. Both pulmonary and extrapulmonary tumors (from breast, stomach, pancreas, and prostate) can result in lymphangitic spread of tumor.[2,10]

Nodular septal thickening is most commonly seen in patients with sarcoidosis or lymphangitic spread of tumor **(Fig. 18)**. It reflects the lymphatic involvement within the septa, with the nodules representing clusters of granulomas or tumor nodules. In both conditions, the nodules are seen in perilymphatic distribution.[19] Sarcoidosis is often associated with architectural distortion, which reflects the underlying pulmonary fibrosis. Lymphangitic spread of carcinoma is a nonfibrosing process, which does not produce any architectural distortion.

Irregular interlobular septal thickening is usually seen in fibrotic lung disease with architectural distortion associated with fibrosis, resulting in the septa to become jagged in appearance. On HRCT, other findings such as honeycombing and traction bronchiectasis are of importance in reaching a differential diagnosis **(Fig. 19)**.[19]

Flowchart 3 illustrates the algorithmic approach to the differential diagnosis of interlobular septal thickening when it is a predominant abnormality.[4,17]

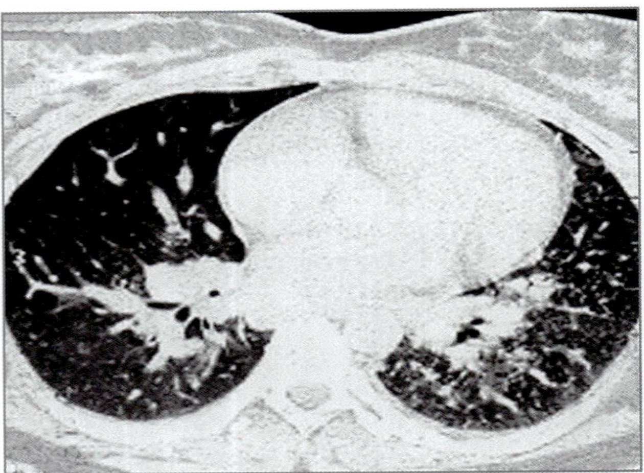

FIG. 18: Perilymphatic distribution of nodules in sarcoidosis: Axial high-resolution computed tomography (HRCT) shows multiple small nodules scattered in centrilobular, peribronchovascular, and perilymphatic distribution. Micronodular beading is seen along major fissures.

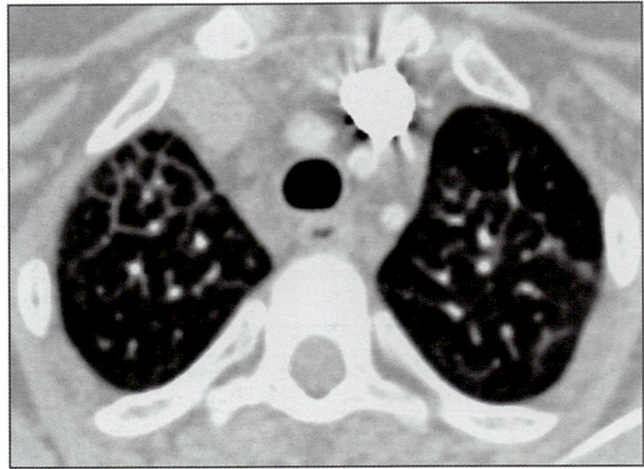

FIG. 17: Smooth interlobular septal thickening: Axial computed tomography (CT) shows diffuse smooth interlobular septal thickening outlining pulmonary lobules with ground-glass opacity in bilateral upper lobes in a patient with pulmonary edema.

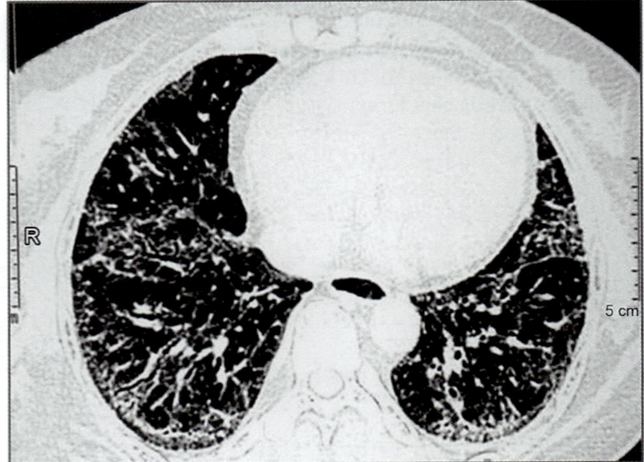

FIG. 19: Irregular interlobular septal thickening: Axial high-resolution computed tomography (HRCT) shows intralobular, interlobular, and subpleural interstitial thickening involving bilateral lower lobes with traction bronchiectasis.

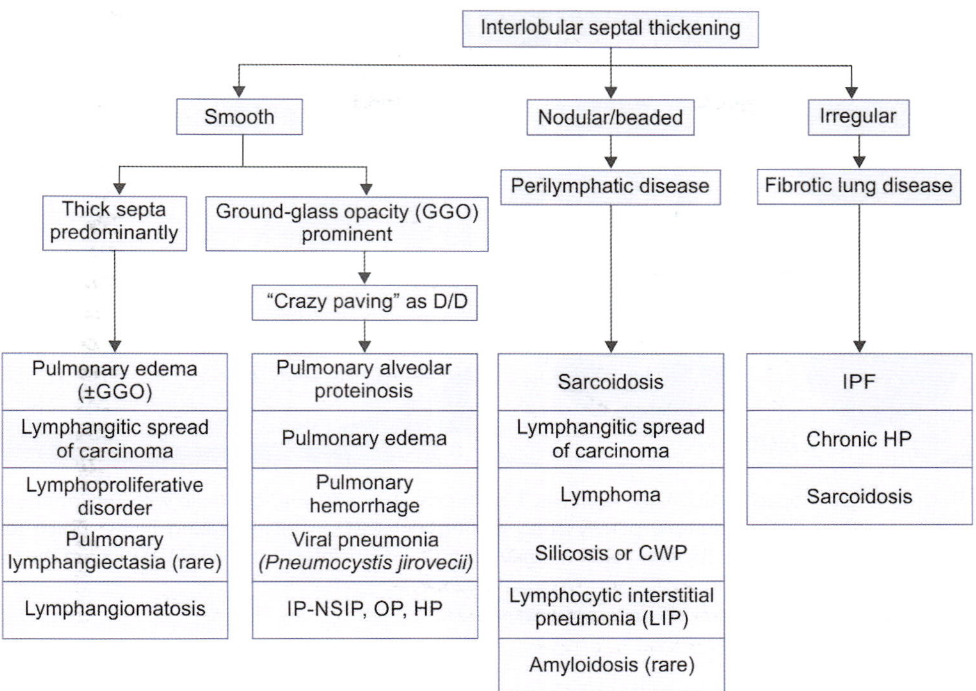

FLOWCHART 3: Algorithmic approach to the differential diagnosis of interlobular septal thickening.
(CWP: coal workers' pneumoconiosis; D/D: differential diagnosis; HP: hypersensitivity pneumonitis; IPF: idiopathic pulmonary fibrosis; NSIP: nonspecific interstitial pneumonia; OP: organizing pneumonia)

Honeycombing

Presence of honeycombing is the most specific HRCT sign of fibrosis, appearing as air-filled cystic spaces. This will be discussed later under the HRCT findings manifesting as decreased lung opacity.

Intralobular Interstitial Thickening

The intralobular interstitium, distinct from the interlobular septa, supports pulmonary lobular structures and is normally invisible on HRCT. It comprises mainly of the fine network of very thin connective tissue fibers within the alveolar walls or the parenchymal interstitium.[1]

Intralobular interstitial thickening is an early sign of fibrosis. It is a nonspecific finding and may be associated with interstitial infiltration or inflammation in the absence of fibrosis. The term "intralobular lines" is used to describe the presence of intralobular interstitial thickening. These lines are <5 mm long, form a fine lace-like network, and usually do not conform to the lobular anatomy. Intralobular interstitial thickening is usually associated with other features of lung fibrosis such as architectural distortion or traction bronchiectasis. The term traction bronchiectasis refers to the bronchial dilatation occurring as a result of interstitial fibrosis, whereby the bronchi appear irregular, but are not associated with any radiological evidence of bronchial inflammation, i.e., bronchial wall thickening or mucus impactions.

They are seen in all types of fibrotic lung disease, especially idiopathic pulmonary fibrosis (IPF), usual interstitial pneumonia (UIP), nonspecific interstitial pneumonia (NSIP), and pulmonary disease, associated with collagen vascular diseases. Intralobular interstitial thickening may also be seen in other idiopathic interstitial pneumonia, pulmonary infections (viral pneumonia), pulmonary edema, pulmonary hemorrhage, and lymphangitic carcinomatosis.

Irregular Reticulation

Irregular reticulation is a nonspecific finding and is said to be present when normal reticular opacities do not represent any of the other two patterns, i.e., interlobular septal thickening and honeycombing. They are known by various names such as parenchymal bands and subpleural lesions. The presence of irregular reticulation is moderately specific for fibrosis.

Ground-glass Opacity

Ground-glass opacity refers to the hazy increase in lung attenuation that does not obscure the underlying vessels or bronchial margins. GGO is a nonspecific but significant finding on HRCT, reflecting a variety of pathological processes, including airspace disease, interstitial disease, or a combination of both. It may represent lung infiltration, active inflammation, fibrosis, or even atelectasis. GGO results from volume averaging of

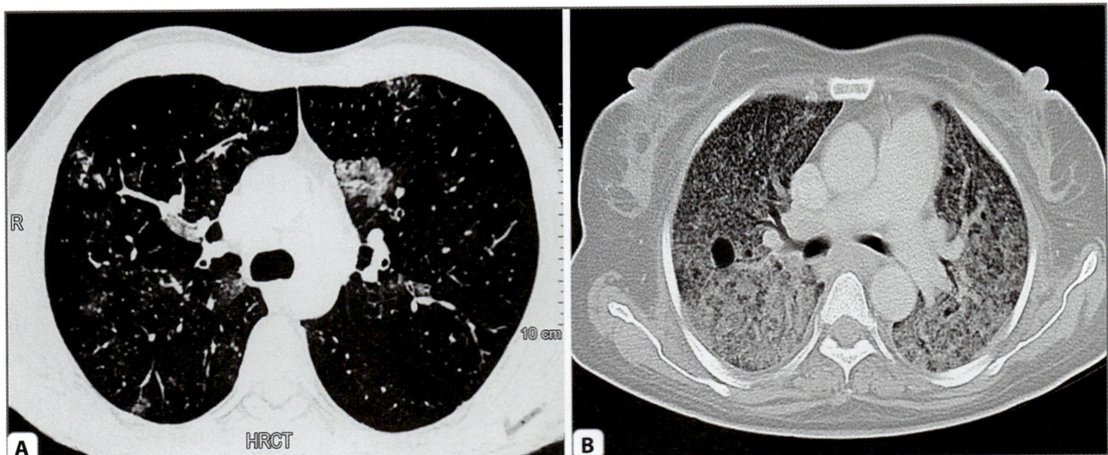

FIGS. 20A AND B: Ground-glass opacity (GGO). (A) Axial HRCT of the chest in a 40-year-old male with recurrent episodes of cough, wheeze, and blood eosinophilia reveal multiple patchy areas of transient GGO in bilateral lung fields, which resolved following antihelminthic therapy—Löffler syndrome. (B) Axial HRCT of *Pneumocystis jirovecii* infection in an HIV patient in the form of symmetric diffuse GGO associated with cyst in right lung.

(HIV: human immunodeficiency virus; HRCT: high-resolution computed tomography)

morphological abnormalities that are too small to be clearly resolved by HRCT.

Ground-glass opacity can be challenging to recognize, especially when minimal or diffuse. However, it is mostly patchy or geographic in distribution, affecting some areas of lung and sparing other regions, thereby making it easier to recognize **(Figs. 20A and B)**. In cases where the presence of GGO is equivocal, comparing the attenuation of the lung parenchyma with air in the bronchi may be helpful. In normal individuals, the density difference is marginal, while with GGO, the airways appear "too black" within an area of lung (the "black bronchus" sign).

Ground-glass opacity is a significant finding on HRCT, as it often indicates an active and potentially treatable or reversible disease process if it is not associated with signs of fibrosis. Its clinical significance depends on the patient's symptomatology (acute vs. chronic), distribution of GGO on HRCT, and presence or absence of other findings on HRCT **(Fig. 21)**.

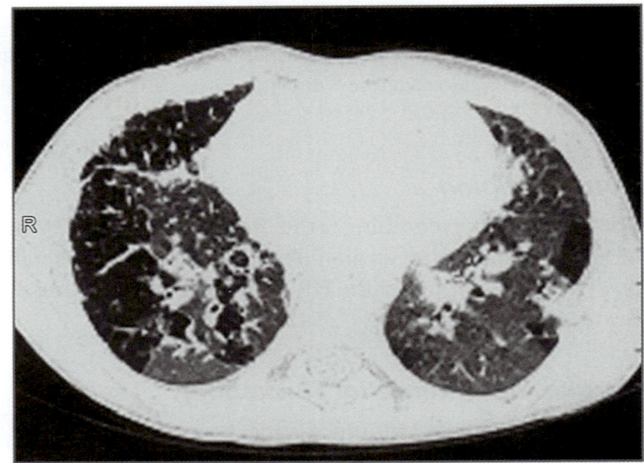

FIG. 21: Ground-glass attenuation: Axial high-resolution computed tomography (HRCT) shows extensive areas of ground-glass attenuation in bilateral lung fields in acute hypersensitivity pneumonitis.

Differential Diagnosis of Ground-glass Opacity

A wide variety of conditions can manifest as GGO, making it crucial to correlate with clinical context, especially the duration of symptoms (acute, subacute, or chronic). **Box 4 and Table 6** depict the differential diagnosis of GGO according to the clinical presentation and distribution.[20]

Pitfalls in Diagnosis of Ground-glass Opacity

There are several potential pitfalls in the recognition and diagnosis of GGO which a radiologist must be aware to avoid misdiagnosis of the same. GGO may be spuriously diagnosed on HRCT in the following circumstances:

- In pediatric patients where immature lung architecture may mimic GGO.
- High-resolution computed tomography performed with thick collimation, where volume averaging may create spurious GGO.
- "Dependent density" in the posterior lung during supine scanning may clear on prone scan.
- Expiratory scans, where reduced alveolar air during expiration can mimic GGO.
- In scans showing patchy emphysema or other causes of hyperlucency such as airway obstruction and air trapping, normal lung regions can mimic the appearance of GGO by appearing relatively dense, which can be distinguished on expiratory scan.

Additional factors, such as inappropriate window settings, contrast and brightness adjustments, or differences

BOX 4: Differential diagnosis of GGO on the basis of clinical presentation.

Acute presentation:
- Pulmonary edema
- Pulmonary hemorrhage
- All types of pneumonia (especially atypical pneumonia):
  - *Pneumocystis jirovecii*
  - Viral—cytomegalovirus (CMV)
  - Mycoplasma
  - Acute interstitial pneumonitis
  - Acute eosinophilic pneumonia
- Hypersensitivity pneumonitis
- Aspiration

Subacute or chronic presentation:
- Nonspecific interstitial pneumonia (NSIP)
- Pneumonia associated with collagen vascular disease
- Desquamative interstitial pneumonia (DIP)
- Respiratory bronchiolitis-interstitial lung disease (RB-ILD)
- Hypersensitivity pneumonitis (HP)
- Organizing pneumonia (OP)
- Chronic eosinophilic pneumonia
- Chronic/recurrent aspiration
- Adenocarcinoma in situ (formerly BAC)
- Pulmonary alveolar proteinosis (PAP)

(BAC: bronchioloalveolar carcinoma; GGO: ground-glass opacity)

TABLE 6: Differential diagnosis of GGO on the basis of distribution.

Distribution of GGO	Causes
Peripheral and subpleural	NSIP, DIP, OP
Patchy and geographic	HP, OP, eosinophilic pneumonia
Peribronchovascular	Sarcoid, OP, eosinophilic pneumonia
Diffuse and extensive	HP

(DIP: desquamative interstitial pneumonia; GGO: ground-glass opacity; HP: hypersensitivity pneumonitis; NSIP: nonspecific interstitial pneumonia; OP: organizing pneumonia)

between CT scanner models, can also contribute to misinterpretation.

Consolidation

Consolidation is characterized by abnormal dense opacification of the lung parenchyma with obscuration of the underlying vessels. It may be alveolar or interstitial in origin; though most commonly, the alveolar air is replaced by fluid, cells, tissue, or pus. Consolidation is detected both on plain radiography and CT and may be visualized earlier on CT than plain radiographs.[8] HRCT provides useful diagnostic information regarding the distribution and characteristics of consolidated lung, but the rate of change of consolidation should always be sought from serial chest radiographs. For example, rapid radiographic resolution in hours rather than days of diffuse lung opacification of acute onset is highly suggestive of pulmonary edema or hemorrhage.

The CT appearances of airspace consolidation differ depending on the degree of involvement. The earliest findings consist of poorly marginated small nodules called acinar nodules approximately 7 mm in diameter, which occur when single acini are replaced by fluid or tissue **(Figs. 22A and B)**. These are not true nodules and represent clusters of single acini filled with fluid, inflammatory cells, or blood, depending on the disease process. With involvement of adjacent acini, the acinar nodules coalesce and may progress to lobular, subsegmental, segmental, lobar, or multilobar areas of consolidation **(Figs. 23 A and B)**. Unlike GGO, on HRCT, consolidation results in an increase in lung opacity, with underlying vessels being obscured. Air bronchogram is usually seen if the bronchi are patent.[21]

Differential Diagnosis

The differential diagnosis of consolidation overlaps considerably with GGO. **Table 7** enumerates the differential diagnosis of consolidation with their salient features.[20]

The differential diagnosis of consolidation depends mainly on:
- Duration of symptoms
- Distribution of consolidation

Consolidation presenting in an acute condition is mostly seen in pneumonia and aspiration. The various causative organisms of pneumonia result in different patterns of parenchymal opacification on HRCT. Aspiration may be focal or patchy and typically involves the lower lobes and posterior upper lobes.

Perihilar "batwing" consolidation with sparing of the periphery of the lung is typical of pulmonary edema **(Fig. 23C)**. This pattern may also be seen with pulmonary hemorrhage, pneumonia such as *Pneumocystis jirovecii* pneumonia, and inhalational lung injury. In patients with pulmonary edema, a perihilar distribution is most often seen when a rapid accumulation of fluid has occurred. Relative sparing of the lung periphery has been attributed to better lymphatic clearance of fluid in this region.[22]

Differential diagnosis of consolidation of chronic symptomatology includes organizing pneumonia **(Fig. 24)**, chronic eosinophilic pneumonia, invasive adenocarcinoma, sarcoidosis, lymphoma, lipoid pneumonia, hypersensitivity pneumonitis, and pulmonary infarction.[20,23]

Presence of focal consolidation within single or cluster of acini or a TIB pattern may help in reducing the differential diagnosis, but the differentiation of adenocarcinoma and organizing pneumonia may rarely be made with certainly on HRCT appearance alone, and a tissue diagnosis is usually required.

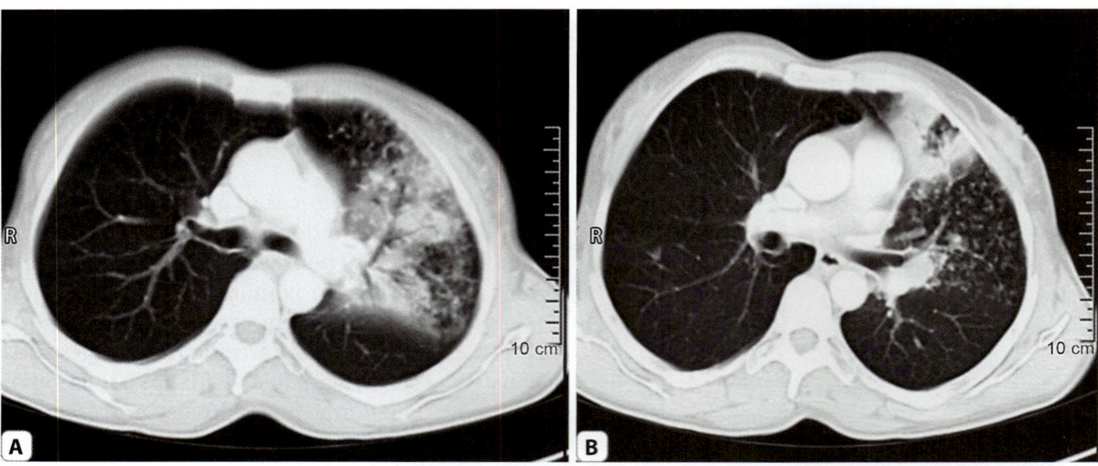

FIGS. 22A AND B: Airspace consolidation: Axial computed tomography (CT) shows consolidation with air bronchogram and adjacent airspace nodules in left upper lobe.

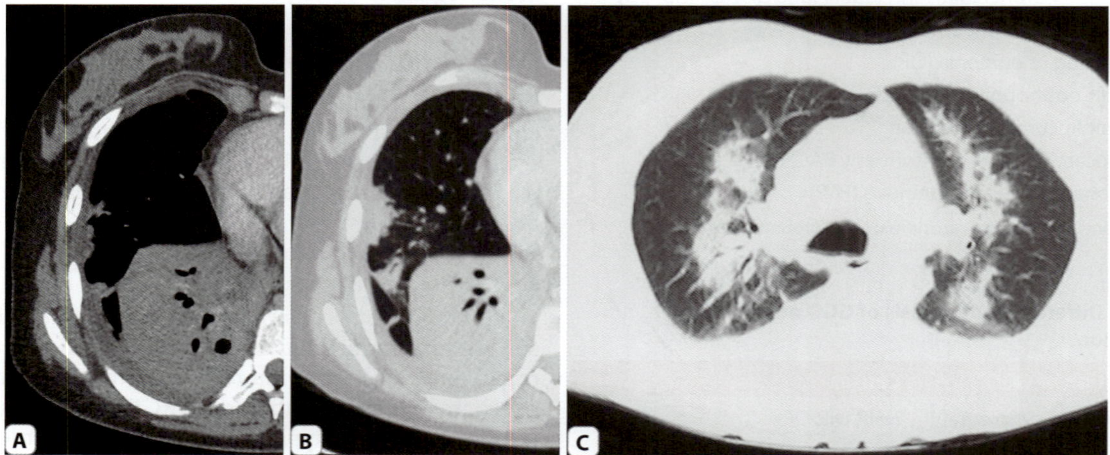

FIGS. 23A TO C: Consolidation. (A and B) Axial computed tomography (CT) shows consolidation with air bronchogram in right lower lobe with subpleural smaller areas of consolidation and mild pleural effusion. (C) CT shows perihilar "batwing" consolidation in pulmonary edema, with peripheral sparing.

TABLE 7: Differential diagnosis of consolidation.

Differential diagnosis	Salient features
Acute consolidation	
Pneumonia (bacterial, mycobacterial, fungal, viral)	Patchy, nodular, lobular, or diffuse, depending on the organism
AIP and ARDS	Patchy or diffuse
Pulmonary edema	Diffuse, GGO more common
Pulmonary hemorrhage	Patchy or diffuse, GGO more common
Acute eosinophilic pneumonia	Diffuse, GGO more common
Radiation pneumonitis	Extent usually corresponds to radiation site
Subacute/chronic consolidation	
Organizing pneumonia (OP)	Mostly peripheral, may be mass like or reverse halo in some
Chronic eosinophilic pneumonia	Patchy or nodular, peripheral, resembles OP
Invasive mucinous adenocarcinoma	Diffuse, patchy, or nodular

Continued

Continued

Differential diagnosis	Salient features
Nonspecific interstitial pneumonia (NSIP)	Patchy, subpleural GGO more common
Hypersensitivity pneumonitis (HP)	Patchy, GGO more common
Lipoid pneumonia	Patchy or lobular, low attenuation consolidation
Lymphoma	Focal, patchy, or mass like in peribronchovascular distribution
Sarcoidosis	Patchy or mass-like confluence of very small granulomas
Alveolar proteinosis	GGO more common, patchy or diffuse
Pulmonary infarction	Wedge shaped, pleural based

(AIP: acute interstitial pneumonia; ARDS: acute respiratory distress syndrome; GGO: ground-glass opacity)

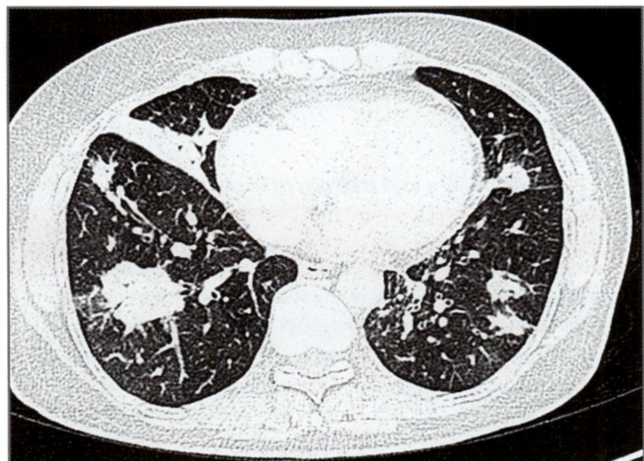

FIG. 24: Organizing pneumonia: Axial HRCT shows multiple focal consolidations with air bronchogram in peribronchial regions with surrounding GGO.

(GGO: ground-glass opacity; HRCT: high-resolution computed tomography)

Decreased Lung Opacity

Area of Decreased Attenuation with Walls

Various abnormalities associated with reduced attenuation in this subgroup include bronchiectasis, honeycombing, lung cysts, cystic lung disease, and pneumatocele.

Bronchiectasis

Bronchiectasis is a chronic condition characterized by irreversible dilatation of the bronchi, usually associated with inflammation, which occurs secondary to bronchial obstruction, bronchial wall damage, or parenchymal fibrosis.[24] In all acute and subacute conditions, the term bronchial dilatation is used.

High-resolution computed tomography findings of bronchiectasis

HRCT is the gold standard for diagnosing and characterizing bronchiectasis. The key findings include:

- *Bronchial dilatation* is the most specific finding of bronchiectasis and is considered when the bronchoarterial ratio exceeds one. However, this may normally be seen in the elderly, people living in high attitude, or in asthmatics. When bronchial dilatation is marked, the cross-section appearance of the bronchus and artery together appears as a ring and is termed as the "signet ring" sign.
- *Lack of bronchial tapering*: This is the earliest sign of bronchiectasis and is easiest to detect when the bronchus is seen in longitudinal section.
- *Visualization of peripheral airway*: Normally, bronchi are not visible within 1 cm of the costal pleura. Their presence in these regions, or abutting the mediastinal pleura, is abnormal and indicative of bronchiectasis (tram-tracking sign).[4]
- *Mucoid impaction*: Dilated bronchi when filled with fluid or mucous are easily appreciated on HRCT. They appear as gloved finger, V- or Y-shaped branching densities. When viewed perpendicular to the imaging plane, impacted bronchi appear as nodular opacities. HRCT also identifies associated findings such as atelectasis or distal hyperinflation.
- *Traction bronchiectasis and bronchiolectasis*: These refer to bronchial or bronchiolar dilatation caused by fibrosis and are typically associated with thickened, irregular bronchial walls, often seen alongside honeycombing or scarring in fibrotic lung disease.[25,26]

Types of bronchiectasis

On the basis of morphological appearance on HRCT or pathology, bronchiectasis is classified into three types in increasing order of severity given as follows:

1. *Cylindrical or tubular bronchiectasis* is the mildest form, which consists of uniformly dilated bronchi with smooth wall thickening **(Fig. 25A)**. They are often associated with chronic airway infections.[27,28]
2. *Varicose bronchiectasis*: In varicose bronchiectasis, the bronchial lumen is characterized by alternating areas of luminal dilatation and narrowing, giving a beaded appearance with irregular or nodular wall thickening **(Fig. 25B)**. This is commonly seen in cystic fibrosis and allergic bronchopulmonary aspergillosis.[27,28]

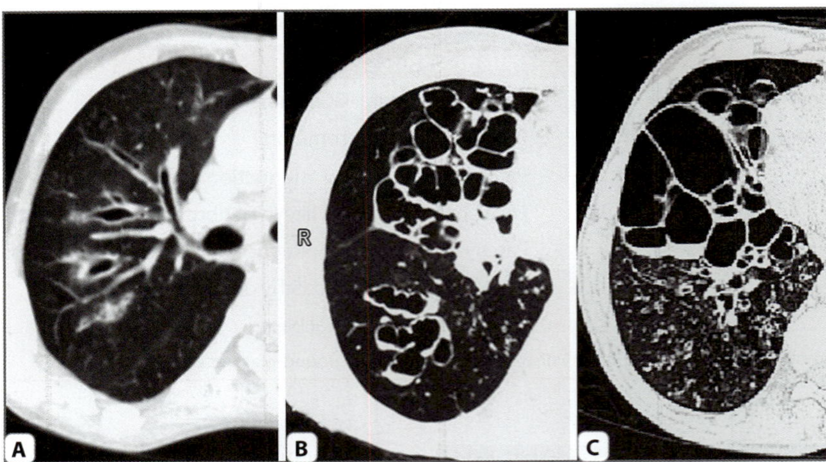

FIGS. 25A TO C: Bronchiectasis. (A) Axial computed tomography (CT) shows cylindrical bronchiectasis with bronchial wall thickening in right upper lobe with mucoid impaction in terminal bronchioles. (B) Varicose bronchiectasis with air-fluid levels in right lung. (C) Cystic bronchiectasis with air-fluid levels and mucoid impaction in right lung.

3. *Cystic bronchiectasis*: Cystic or saccular bronchiectasis is the most severe form of bronchiectasis where the dilated bronchi terminate as a cluster of thin-walled air-filled cysts **(Fig. 25C)**.[27] Air-fluid levels may be present in the dependent portion of the dilated cystic bronchi. Cystic bronchiectasis often reflects an early childhood infection, is often patchy in distribution, and may be lobar.

More than one type of bronchiectasis may be seen in the same patient. The radiologist has an important role in the detection and characterization of bronchiectasis and should be able to differentiate bronchiectasis from motion artifact (most commonly from cardiac pulsation in the middle and lingular lobes) and bronchial dilatation in acute lung disease.[27] CT has limited ability to determine the cause of bronchiectasis, but the distribution and pattern of disease can help suggest the most likely cause, as given in **Table 8**.[21,29]

TABLE 8: Distribution and pattern of bronchiectasis.

Distribution and pattern of bronchiectasis	Likely etiology
Bilateral upper lobe bronchiectasis: • Cystic fibrosis • Allergic bronchopulmonary aspergillosis	• Bilateral symmetrical, central, upper lobe predominance • Bilateral asymmetrical, central bronchiectasis, cylindrical or varicose type with mucoid impaction
Unilateral upper lobe distribution	Most common with tuberculosis
Lower lobe distribution	Most common secondary to childhood viral infection
Right middle lobe and lingular distribution	Bronchiectatic form of atypical mycobacterial infection, immotile cilia syndrome, and hypogammaglobulinemia

Honeycomb Cysts

Honeycomb cysts are characterized by air-containing space having thick walls that are lined by bronchiolar epithelium and fibrous walls. Pathologically, honeycombing represents interstitial fibrosis with lung destruction and dilatation of peripheral air spaces and is the most specific HRCT sign of fibrosis. In patients with extensive disease (fibrosis), the stacked appearance of cysts resembles a "honeycomb," hence, the term honeycomb cysts **(Fig. 26)**.

Honeycombing produces a characteristic appearance on HRCT. A confident diagnosis of honeycombing on HRCT requires the following characteristic findings:

- *Peripheral subpleural location*: Honeycomb cysts are typically distributed in the lower lobes and along the subpleural regions.
- *Clustered or layered cystic structures*: These cysts share walls, forming a honeycomb-like pattern.
- *Cyst size*: They are small in size ranging from 3 to 10 mm in diameter, although larger sizes may be observed in some cases.

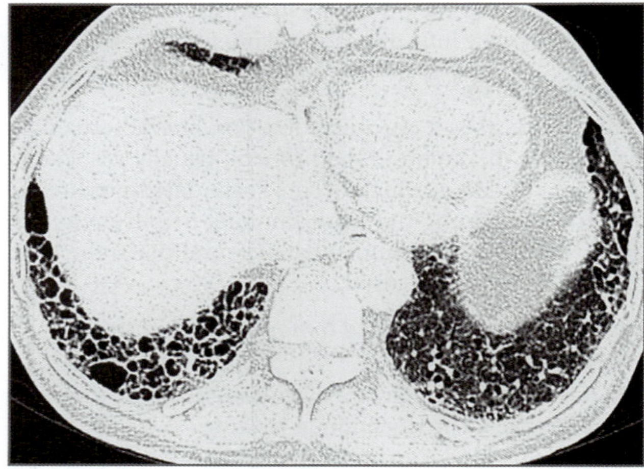

FIG. 26: Honeycomb cysts: High-resolution computed tomography (HRCT) image shows honeycomb cysts with predominance in right basal and subpleural region. The cysts are variable sized, show well-defined thick walls, and occur in several layers.

- *Thick, clearly defined fibrous walls*: These measure 1–3 mm in thickness and help differentiate honeycombing from other cystic lung diseases, such as paraseptal emphysema or subpleural air trapping.
- *Lucent cysts*: Honeycomb cysts are of air attenuation and appear empty or black, without any internal vascular, bronchial, or septal structures.
- *Absence of branching*: Branching cystic structures are indicative of traction bronchiectasis rather than honeycombing.
- *Association with other signs of fibrosis*: Honeycombing is often accompanied by architectural distortion, traction bronchiectasis, irregular reticulation, and volume loss in the affected regions.

Significance of honeycombing

Honeycombing on HRCT usually represents UIP with the most common cause being IPF. The presence of lower lobe subpleural honeycombing in such patients strongly suggests UIP—IPF and obviates the need for surgical lung biopsy **(Figs. 27A to C)**.[4] However, a number of other diseases also show honeycombing on HRCT. **Box 5** enumerates the differential diagnosis of honeycombing on HRCT. The honeycombing in these conditions may be indistinguishable on HRCT and require correlation with clinical exposure or drug history to suggest the appropriate diagnosis.

Pitfalls in diagnosis of honeycombing

Distinguishing honeycombing from mimics is critical to avoid misdiagnosis given as follows:

- *Paraseptal emphysema*: This condition can mimic honeycombing due to its subpleural location; however, the cysts in emphysema lack shared fibrous walls and other features of fibrosis. There are several differentiating features between the two, which are tabulated in **Table 9**.
- *Subpleural air trapping*: It may also appear as cystic spaces but can be differentiated by the absence of fibrotic changes.
- *Single-layer cysts*: While traditionally multiple layers of cysts were required for a confident diagnosis of honeycombing, current practice accepts a single layer of subpleural cysts as honeycombing if other signs of

BOX 5: Differential diagnosis of honeycombing.

- Idiopathic pulmonary fibrosis
- Connective tissue disease (rheumatoid arthritis most common)
- Drug-related fibrosis
- Cyclophosphamide (common) and nitrofurantoin
- Asbestosis

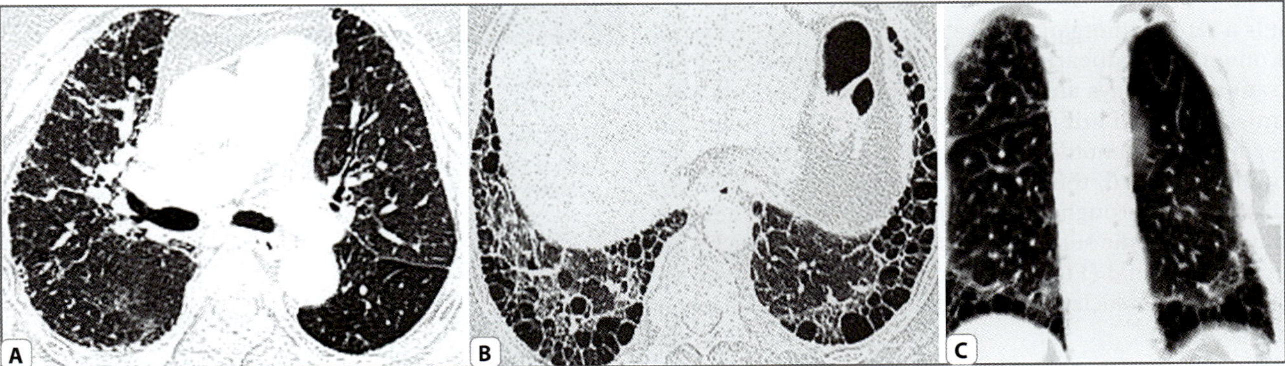

FIGS. 27A TO C: Usual interstitial pneumonia pattern. (A) Axial HRCT at the level of upper lobe bronchus shows mild septal thickening in bilateral lung parenchyma. (B) Axial HRCT through lung bases reveals extensive reticulation and honeycombing with lower lobe and posterior, peripheral predominance. (C) Coronal MPR image reveals an apicobasal gradient of abnormalities typical of UIP pattern.
(HRCT: high-resolution computed tomography; MPR: multiplanar reconstruction; UIP: usual interstitial pneumonia)

TABLE 9: Differentiating features of honeycombing and paraseptal emphysema.

Features	Honeycombing	Paraseptal emphysema
Layers	Cysts of one or more layers	Single layer only
Wall thickness	Thick walled	Very thin wall
Size	Small (few millimeters to 1 cm)	Large (up to several centimeters)
Distribution	Lower lobes	Upper lobes
Associated features	Traction bronchiectasis, irregular reticulation	±Centrilobular emphysema
Overall lung volume	Volume loss	Increased
Reticulation or traction bronchiectasis	Present	Absent

fibrosis, such as traction bronchiectasis or architectural distortion, are present.

Cystic Lung Disease

Lung disease may be characterized by cystic air spaces or lung cysts. Lung cysts are used to describe clearly defined air-containing spaces that are 1 cm or more with a definable epithelial or fibrous usually <3 mm thick wall. Although the precise mechanism of cystic change is not understood, a check-valve mechanism has been advocated in the pathologies of some cysts.[21] On chest radiography, the walls of multiple cysts may superimpose, producing a delicate reticular pattern, making them difficult to identify individually. **Box 6** shows the differential diagnosis of conditions characterized by lung cysts.[8] HRCT is often helpful in suggesting a diagnosis on the basis of their size, wall characteristics, and distribution of the cysts.

Langerhans cell histiocytosis

It is a multiorgan disease with pulmonary involvement seen mostly in ages between 20 and 40 years in cigarette smokers. The predominant HRCT findings consist of cysts and nodules. The cysts are of irregular or bizarre shape, thin or thick walled, may be of unequal sizes, and show a predominant upper lung zone distribution with relative sparing of costophrenic sulci **(Fig. 28)**. Serial CT scan shows the natural history of the disease with nodules which cavitate, become cystic airspaces, and finally coalesce.[30]

Lymphangioleiomyomatosis

It is a rare multiorgan disease that is almost exclusive to women of childbearing age and characterized by infiltration of airways and lymphatics by immature smooth muscle cells. Patients may present with dyspnea or recurrent pneumothorax. The typical HRCT pattern is of multiple, round, thin-walled cysts, which are diffusely distributed throughout the lungs, with involvement of the costophrenic sulci; the intervening lung parenchyma appears normal **(Fig. 29)**. Lymphangioleiomyomatosis (LAM) is not associated with nodules, but pleural effusions are common.[30]

Lymphoid interstitial pneumonia

Lymphoid interstitial pneumonia (LIP) is a part of spectrum of pulmonary lymphoproliferative disorders characterized by HRCT by diffuse GGOs and ill-defined centrilobular nodules. Multiple thin-walled cysts may be seen in patients with LIP **(Fig. 30)**. They are usually associated with a history of connective tissue disease, especially Sjögren's syndrome and immunosuppression. The cysts are less numerous in number than the cysts occurring in patients with histiocytosis or LAM. In patients with LIP, the cysts are seen mainly in the lower lobes with vessels often associated with wall of cysts.[28]

Incidental Lung Cysts

Randomly scattered thin-walled cysts have been seen as a normal finding in 25% of elderly patients older than 75 years

BOX 6: Differential diagnosis of lung cysts.

- Langerhans cell histiocytosis (LCH)
- Lymphangioleiomyomatosis (LAM)
- Lymphoid interstitial pneumonia (LIP)
- *Pneumocystis jirovecii* pneumonia
- Cavitating form of bronchoalveolar carcinoma
- Tracheobronchial papillomatosis
- Birt–Hogg–Dubé syndrome
- Sarcoidosis
- Hypersensitivity pneumonitis (subacute)
- Elderly healthy individuals (>75 years)

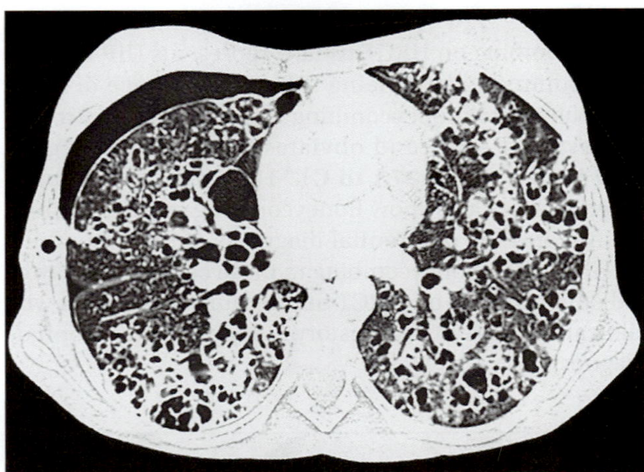

FIG. 28: Thick-walled cysts: Axial high-resolution computed tomography (HRCT) shows multiple thick-walled cysts of varying sizes in bilateral lung parenchyma. A large thin-walled cyst suggestive of bulla is seen along the right mediastinal pleura with associated pneumothorax: Langerhans cells histiocytosis.

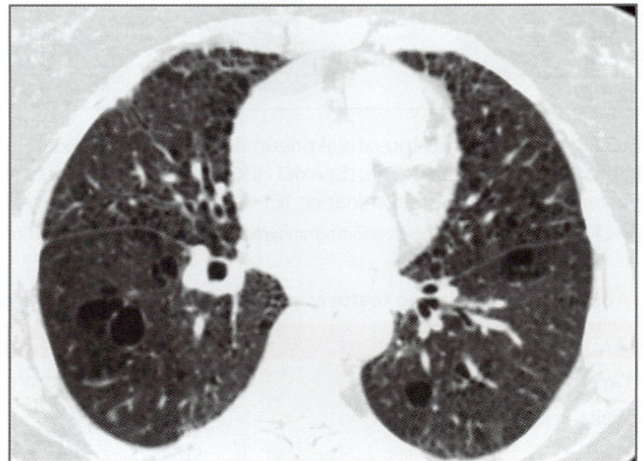

FIG. 29: Thin-walled cysts: Axial high-resolution computed tomography (HRCT) in early lymphangioleiomyomatosis shows subtle thin-walled cysts interspersed with normal lung parenchyma predominantly in lower lobes.

on HRCT. The cysts ranging from 5 to 22 mm have been seen in all lobes in asymptomatic nonsmoking individuals; these are likely to represent part of the aging process.[30]

DECREASED LUNG OPACITY WITHOUT DISCERNIBLE WALL

Emphysema

Emphysema is defined as the permanent and abnormal enlargement of air spaces distal to the terminal bronchiole and is accompanied by destruction of the walls of the involved air spaces. It is the end result of several different processes such as cigarette smoking, enzyme deficiency, and drug abuse. While traditionally the absence of fibrosis was considered a criterion, it is now recognized that localized fibrosis can coexist with emphysema, both histologically and on imaging. Emphysema results in focal areas of very low attenuation without well-defined walls, which can be accurately diagnosed on HRCT.[31] These findings allow for early and accurate diagnosis, often surpassing pulmonary function tests in sensitivity for detecting early-stage emphysema. Emphysema is pathologically and radiologically categorized based on the predominant involvement of the secondary pulmonary lobule into the following types:

- Centrilobular emphysema (CLE)
- Panlobular emphysema (PLE)
- Paraseptal emphysema (PSE)

Table 10 depicts the differences between the three types of emphysema.

Centrilobular emphysema primarily affects the center of the secondary pulmonary lobule and is the most common form in smokers. It predominantly involves the upper lobes, presenting as multiple small areas of low attenuation without perceptible walls, producing a "punched-out" appearance surrounded by normal lung. A centrilobular artery may be visible within the center of these lucencies **(Fig. 31)**. This appearance is diagnostic of CLE, and biopsy is not required for diagnosis if the patient has a smoking history. HRCT is often more sensitive than pulmonary function tests and is able to detect very early stage of CLE.[32] With progression, CLE can involve larger areas spanning multiple lobules but generally respects lobular borders.

Panlobular emphysema is histopathologically characterized by complete destruction of the secondary pulmonary lobule and shows either diffuse or lobar distribution. On HRCT, it is seen as generalized lung lucency with

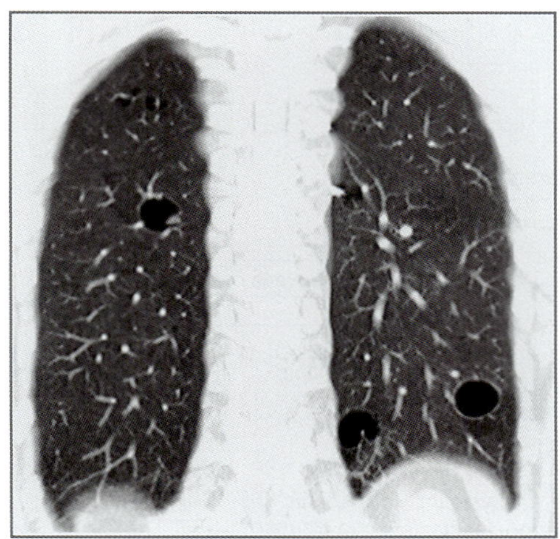

FIG. 30: Coronal MPR showing multiple bilateral thin-walled cysts (LIP) in a 40-year-old female of Sjögren's syndrome having dyspnea on exertion.

(MPR: multiplanar reconstruction; LIP: lymphoid interstitial pneumonia)

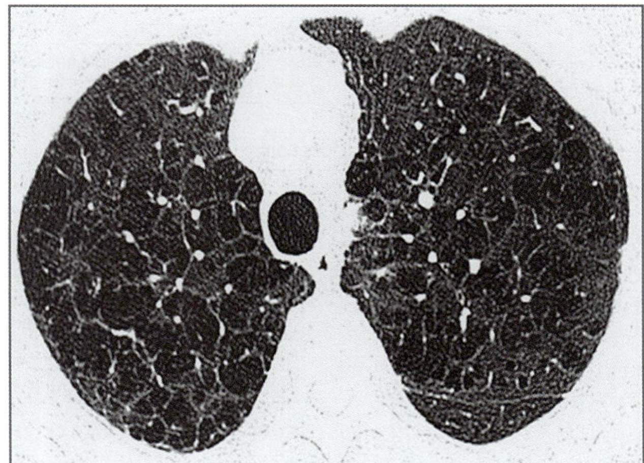

FIG. 31: Centrilobular emphysema: Axial high-resolution computed tomography (HRCT) shows numerous small low attenuation areas with ill-defined borders evenly distributed in bilateral upper lobes in centrilobular emphysema.

TABLE 10: Comparison of different types of emphysema.

Types of emphysema	Causes	Distribution	High-resolution computed tomography (HRCT) appearance
Centrilobular	Cigarette smoking	Upper lobes, central	Focal lucencies without visible walls
Panlobular	Alpha-1 antitrypsin deficiency, cigarette smoking	Lower lobes, diffuse	Generalized increase in lung lucency
Paraseptal	Cigarette smoking or idiopathic	Subpleural	Focal round, well-defined lucencies in a single layer with thin walls

attenuated small vessels with increased lung volume and reduced parenchymal density.[30] The architecture of secondary pulmonary lobules is no longer visualized. Severe PLE may coexist with CLE, resulting in overlapping radiological features.

Paraseptal emphysema preferentially destroys the distal portion of the pulmonary acinus, often near pleural surfaces, the mediastinum, or interlobar fissures. Hence, findings on HRCT are characteristically peripheral in distribution. On HRCT, it typically appears as subpleural air-attenuation cysts arranged in a single layer **(Fig. 32)** and outlined by a thin, discrete wall, which may correspond to interlobular septa. There is no architectural distortion. It is commonly associated with smoking and often coexist with CLE.

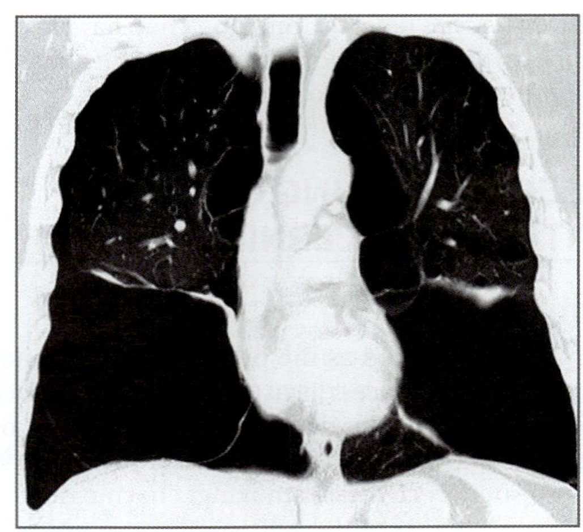

FIG. 32: Emphysema with bullae and pneumothorax: Coronal MPR CT of the chest shows single layer of subpleural areas of low attenuation marginated by interlobular septa in bilateral upper zones along mediastinal pleural surface consistent with paraseptal emphysema. Large subpleural bullae in bilateral lower zones and small centriacinar emphysematous spaces are seen in bilateral upper and mid zones. A small pneumothorax is seen along the right lateral chest wall.

(CT: computed tomography; MPR: multiplanar reconstruction)

Bullous Emphysema

The term is used to refer to emphysema that is associated with large bullae. They occur most commonly in patients of PSE and CLE. A bulla is defined as a sharply demarcated area of emphysema >1 cm in diameter, with thin, hair-like walls on HRCT. These bullae can cause significant lung volume changes and are often a sequela of advanced emphysema. **Flowchart 4** shows the algorithmic approach to cystic air spaces.

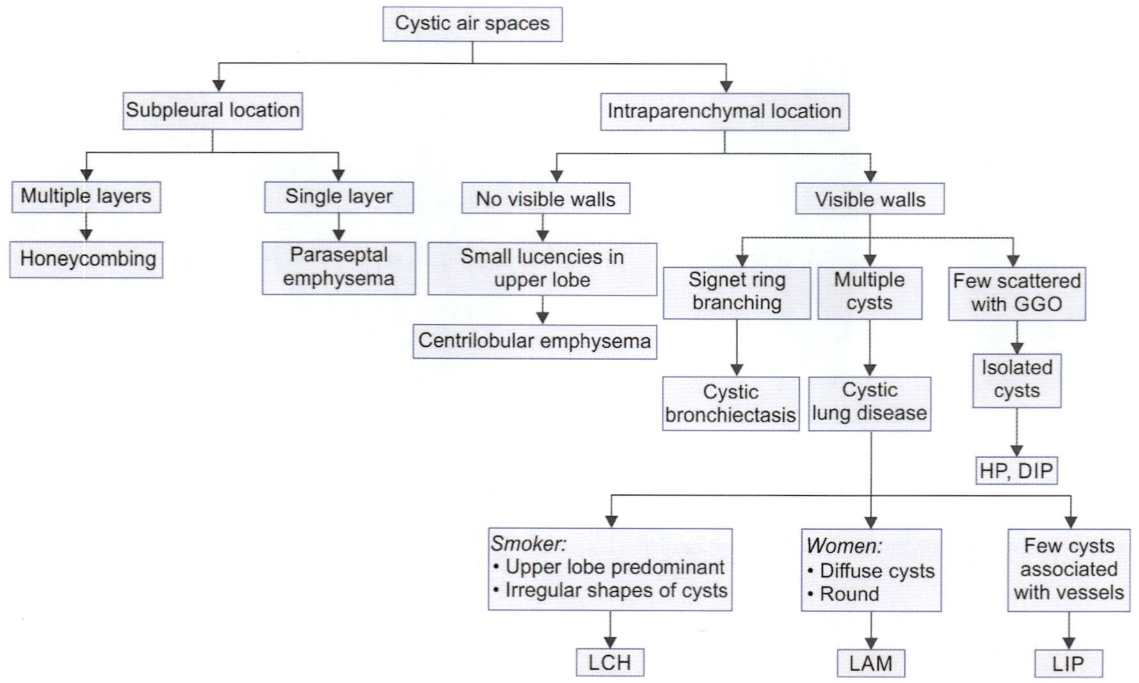

FLOWCHART 4: Algorithmic approach to the diagnosis of cystic air spaces.[34]

(DIP: desquamative interstitial pneumonia; GGO: ground-glass opacity; HP: hypersensitivity pneumonitis; LAM: lymphangioleiomyomatosis; LCH: Langerhans cell histiocytosis; LIP: lymphoid interstitial pneumonia)

HIGH-RESOLUTION COMPUTED TOMOGRAPHY FINDINGS MANIFESTING AS INHOMOGENEOUS LUNG OPACITY

Mosaic Attenuation Pattern

Mosaic attenuation pattern refers to inhomogeneous lung attenuation on HRCT caused by a range of conditions involving the airways, pulmonary vasculature, alveoli, or interstitium, either independently or in combination.[33] This pattern is defined by the Fleischner Society Glossary as a "patchwork of regions of differing attenuation seen on CT of the lung" and is characterized by heterogeneous areas of differing attenuation with well-defined borders **(Fig. 33)**.[6] The nonuniform distribution of disease results in a mosaic appearance on imaging.

The mosaic attenuation pattern poses a diagnostic challenge, as the radiologist must discern whether the low attenuation areas, high attenuation areas, or both represent abnormal lung regions. Mosaic pattern of lung attenuation is now the preferred terminology due to its broader applicability and has replaced the older terms of mosaic oligemia and perfusion.

The mosaic attenuation pattern can result from three categories of disease given as follows:[35]

- Small airway disease
- Pulmonary vascular disease
- Infiltrative lung disease (parenchymal disease)

Small Airway Disease

Small airways are noncartilaginous airways <2 mm in diameter, located from the eighth generation of airways down to the terminal and respiratory bronchioles. These airways are not typically visible in normal individuals on imaging but may become discernible due to underlying disease processes.

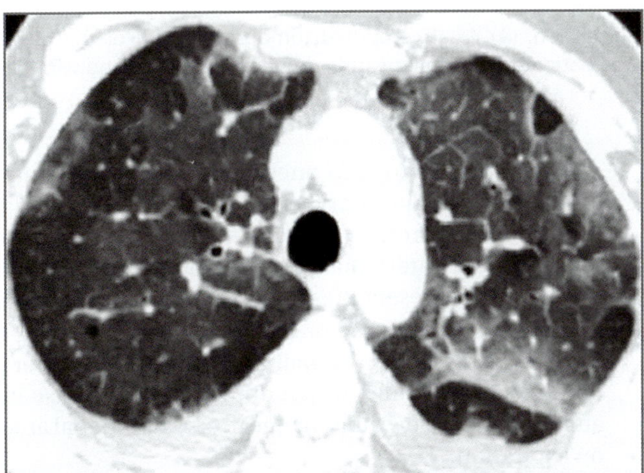

FIG. 33: Mosaic attenuation pattern: Axial HRCT of the chest shows multiple geographic areas of GGO with low attenuation areas showing reduced caliber of vessels within.

(GGO: ground-glass opacity; HRCT: high-resolution computed tomography)

- Small airway disease can be classified given as follows:
  - Primary bronchiolar disorders, which include:
    - Constrictive bronchiolitis
    - Cellular bronchiolitis
    - Diffuse panbronchiolitis
    - Respiratory bronchiolitis
    - Follicular bronchiolitis
  - Bronchiolar involvement in diffuse interstitial lung disease, such as HP.
  - Bronchiolar involvement in large airway disease, such as bronchiectasis or asthma.

Obstruction of small airways due to small airways inflammation is a common pathologic process and is usually reversible. In contrast, in constrictive bronchiolitis, the submucosal and peribronchiolar fibrosis leads to irreversible obstruction of the small airways **(Figs. 34A and B)**.

Pathophysiology of Mosaic Attenuation in Small Airway Disease

Airway obstruction in small airway disease leads to hypoxia of underventilated lung, resulting in reflux vasoconstriction and air trapping. This manifests in HRCT as areas of decreased attenuation with reduced caliber of vessels in affected regions. Conversely, redistribution of blood flow to normally ventilated areas results in higher attenuation and reduced volume in those regions.

On CT scan, there are certain direct signs and indirect signs of small airway disease given as follows:

- Direct signs—thickened peripheral airways and dilatation of peripheral airways
- Indirect signs—air trapping, subsegmental atelectasis, mosaic lung attenuation, centrilobular nodules, and TIB opacities

The radiologist needs to look at the following structures on HRCT of the chest to ascertain the underlying cause of mosaic attenuation pattern:

- *Peripheral vessels*: If these are smaller in the areas of decreased lung attenuation, then it is either a vascular cause or small airway disease and not parenchymal disease (appearing on HRCT as GGO, reticular, or reticulonodular opacities).
- *Heart and pulmonary vasculature*: Among the pulmonary vascular causes, mosaic attenuation is most commonly seen in pulmonary hypertension and pulmonary thromboembolism. In pulmonary hypertension, enlargement of the pulmonary trunk is suggestive of vascular cause of mosaic attenuation and right ventricular enlargement and hypertrophy seen on CT. In patients with left ventricular and/or left atrial dilatation, pulmonary edema may be the cause of mosaic appearance, especially if interlobular septal thickening is present.

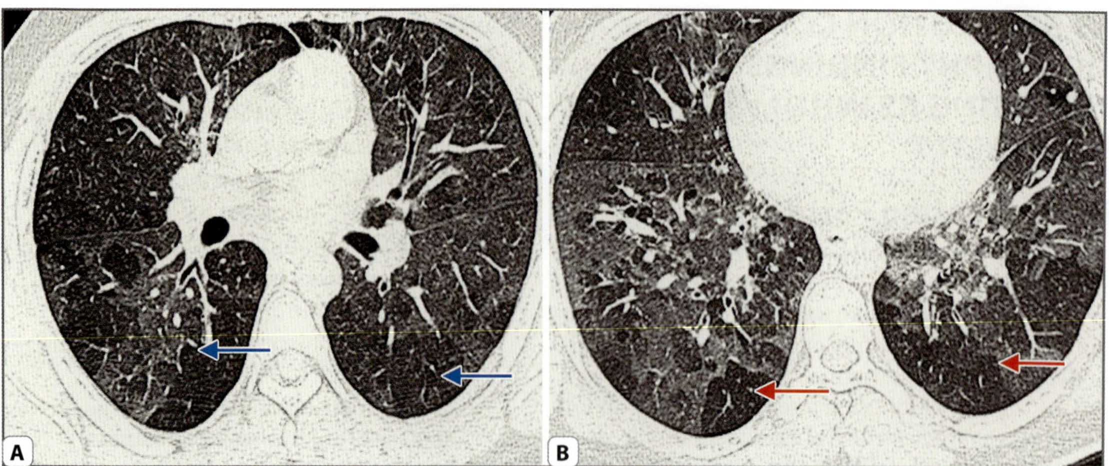

FIGS. 34A AND B: Mosaic attenuation. (A) Axial high-resolution computed tomography (HRCT) inspiratory scan showing patchy areas of mosaic attenuation seen as focal areas of reduced lung density with decreased vessel size within (arrows) along with normal appearing denser lung regions. (B) Corresponding expiratory scan shows persistent lucency in same areas (arrows) confirming air trapping: Constrictive bronchiolitis in a patient of rheumatoid arthritis.

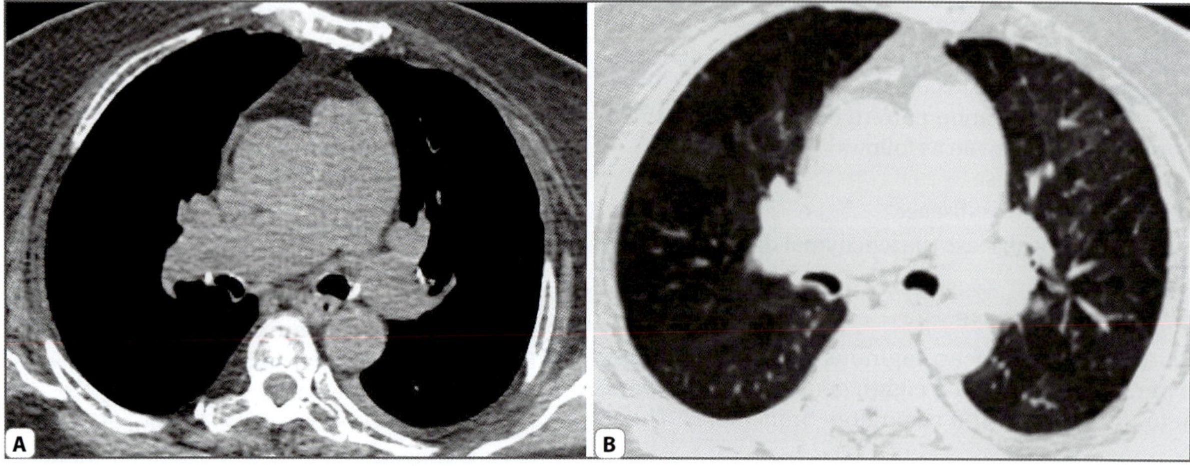

FIGS. 35A AND B: Mosaic attenuation with pulmonary artery hypertension. (A) Axial computed tomography (CT) of the chest mediastinal window image reveals dilated main pulmonary artery in the patient of pulmonary artery hypertension. (B) Lung window image reveals areas of mosaic attenuation in bilateral lung fields.

In pulmonary hypertension, the mosaic attenuation often manifests as scattered areas of low attenuation confined to the secondary pulmonary lobules **(Figs. 35A and B)**. While in pulmonary thromboembolism, the mosaicism is confined to segmental or subsegmental distribution in the vascular distribution of thrombi.

- *Small airways*: Abnormally dilated or thick-walled airways in the lucent areas confirm small airway disease. In addition, presence of centrilobular nodules along with mosaicism on CT is the clue to injury to small airways.
- *Parenchymal changes*: Mosaic attenuation pattern can be produced by interstitial lung disease (parenchymal disease) characterized by GGO and interlobular septal thickening. It may be seen in conditions, such as *Pneumocystis jirovecii* pneumonia, diffuse alveolar hemorrhage, pulmonary edema, HP, or organizing pneumonia, wherein areas of higher attenuation represent the interstitial process and areas of lower attenuation represent the normal lung.
- *Air trapping*: Air trapping on expiratory HRCT is the best clue to the diagnosis of small airway disease. It refers to the regions of lung, which do not show increase in attenuation or show little change in cross-sectional area on expiration.

Pitfalls in Classification[36]

- Areas of air trapping can be seen in normal patients, and some degree of heterogeneity in lung parenchyma is seen on expiratory scan. One should inspect the

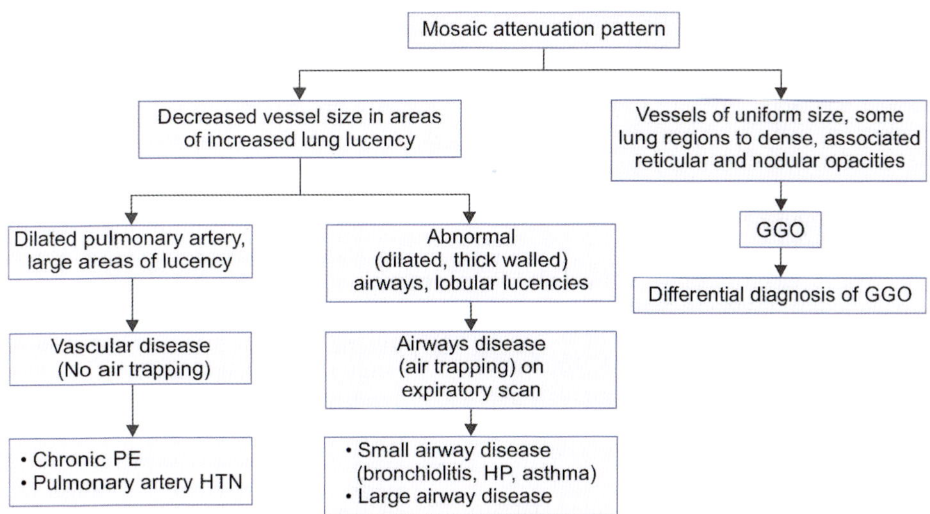

FLOWCHART 5: Algorithmic approach to inhomogeneous lung opacity mosaic attenuation pattern.[35]
(GGO: ground-glass opacity; HP: hypersensitivity pneumonitis; HTN: hypertension; PE: pulmonary embolism)

posterior wall of trachea on CT scan. In case of acquisition during expiratory scan, the posterior wall of trachea shows bowing.

- Presence of air trapping excludes primary parenchymal disease unless there is suspicion of HP, which has mixed features of both parenchymal and small airway disease.
- Rarely, air trapping can occur in pulmonary vascular disease.

Flowchart 5 shows the algorithmic approach to mosaic attenuation pattern.

CONCLUSION

Lung disease can produce recognizable alterations in parenchymal anatomy on HRCT, resulting in various patterns and distributions of abnormalities. However, the various patterns described are not always isolated findings on CT. They commonly occur in combination with other patterns and findings. The use of an organized algorithmic approach in conjunction with clinical data is essential in the evaluation of CT patterns of lung disease, so as to formulate a differential diagnosis or reach a specific diagnosis.

REFERENCES

1. Collins J. CT signs and pattern of lung disease. RCNA. 2001;39(6):1115-35.
2. Elicker B, Pereira CA, Webb R, Leslie KO. High-resolution computed tomography pattern of diffuse interstitial lung disease with clinical and pathological correlation. J Bras Pneumol. 2008;34(9):715-44
3. David MH, David AL, McAdams HP, Alexander AB. Imaging of Diseases of the Chest, 5th edition. USA: Elsevier Limited; 2010. pp. 171-96.
4. Gotway MB, Reddy GP, Webb WR, Elicker BM, Leung JW. High-resolution CT of the lung: patterns of disease and differential diagnosis. Radiol Clin North Am. 2005;43:513-42.
5. Webb RW, Muller NL, Naidich DP. HRCT findings: nodules and nodular opacities. In: Webb RW, Muller NL, Naidich DP (Eds). High-Resolution CT of the Lung, 5th edition. United States: Wolters Kluwer; 2015. pp. 106-39.
6. Bankier AA, MacMahon H, Colby T, Gevenois PA, Goo JM, Leung AN, et al. Fleischner Society: glossary of terms for thoracic imaging. Radiology. 2024;310(2):e232558.
7. MacMahon H, Naidich DP, Goo JM, Lee KS, Leung ANC, Mayo JR, et al. Guidelines for management of incidental pulmonary nodules detected on CT images: from the Fleischner Society 2017. Radiology. 2017;284(1):228-43.
8. Hansell DM, Lynch DA, McAdams HP. Basic HRCT Pattern of Lung Disease in Imaging of Diseases of the Chest. Mosby: Elsevier; 2010. pp. 153-204.
9. Remy JH, Remy J, Artaud D, Deschildre F, Duhamel A. Diffuse infiltrative lung disease: clinical value of sliding-thin-slab maximum intensity projection CT scans in the detection of mild micronodular pattern. Radiology. 1996;200:333-9.
10. Elicker BM, Webb RW. Nodular lung disease. In: Elicker BM, Webb RW (Eds). Fundamentals of High-Resolution Lung CT: Common Findings, Common Patterns, Common Diseases, and Differential Diagnosis, 1st edition. United States: Wolters Kluwer; 2013. pp. 37-54.
11. Azour L, Ko JP, Naidich DP, Moore WH. Shades of gray: subsolid nodule considerations and management. Chest. 2021;159(5):2072-89.
12. de Margerie-Mellon C, Bankier AA. To be or not to be ... a pulmonary nodule. Radiol Cardiothorac Imaging. 2019;1(5):190201

13. van Riel SJ, Sánchez CI, Bankier AA, Naidich DP, Verschakelen J, Scholten ET, et al. Observer variability for classification of pulmonary nodules on low-dose CT images and its effect on nodule management. Radiology. 2015;277(3):863-71.
14. Ridge CA, Yildirim A, Boiselle PM, Franquet T, Schaefer-Prokop CM, Tack D, et al. Differentiating between subsolid and solid pulmonary nodules at CT: inter- and intraobserver agreement between experienced thoracic radiologists. Radiology. 2016;278(3):888-96.
15. Raoof S, Amchentsev A, Vlahos I, Goud A, Naidich DP. Pictorial essay: multinodular disease: a high-resolution CT scan diagnostic algorithm. Chest. 2006;129(3):805-15.
16. Rossi SE, Franquet T, Volpacchio M, Giménez A, Aguilar G. Tree-in-bud pattern at thin-section CT of the lungs: radiologic-pathologic overview. Radiographics. 2005;25:789-801.
17. Webb RW, Muller NL, Naidich DP. HRCT findings: linear and reticular opacities. In: Webb RW, Muller NL, Naidich DP (Eds). High-Resolution CT of the Lung, 5th edition. United States: Wolters Kluwer; 2015. pp. 74-105.
18. Collins J, Stern EJ. Signs and Patterns of Lung Disease in Chest Radiology: The Essentials, 3rd edition. United States: Wolters Kluwer; 2015. pp. 17-37.
19. Elicker BM, Webb RW. Reticular opacities. In: Elicker BM, Webb RW (Eds). Fundamentals of High-Resolution Lung CT: Common Findings, Common Patterns, Common Diseases, and Differential Diagnosis, 1st edition. United States: Wolters Kluwer; 2013. pp. 17-36.
20. Webb RW, Muller NL, Naidich DP. HRCT findings: parenchymal opacification. In: Webb RW, Muller NL, Naidich DP (Eds). High-Resolution CT of the Lung, 5th edition. United States: Wolters Kluwer; 2015. pp. 140-65.
21. Frauquet T. Non-neoplastic parenchymal lung disease. In: Hagga JR, Dogra VS, Forsting M, Gilkeson RC, Ha HK, Sundaram M (Eds). CT and MRI of the Whole Body, 5th edition. Mosby: Elsevier; 2009. pp. 863-926.
22. Pawa S. Basic patterns of lung disease. In: Chowdhury V, Gupta AK, Khandelwal N (Eds). Diagnostic Radiology: Chest and Cardiovascular Imaging, 3rd edition. New Delhi: Jaypee Brothers Medical Publishers Pvt. Ltd.; 2010. pp. 28-59.
23. Elicker BM, Webb RW. Increased lung attenuation: ground-glass opacity and consolidation. In: Elicker BM, Webb RW (Eds). Fundamentals of High-Resolution Lung CT: Common Findings, Common Patterns, Common Diseases and Differential Diagnosis, 1st edition. United States: Wolters Kluwer; 2013. pp. 59-70.
24. Grenier PA, Aubry CB. Airway disease and chronic airway obstruction. In: Adam A, Dixon AK, Gillard JH, Schaefer-Prokop C, Grainger RG (Eds). Grainger and Allison's Diagnostic Radiology: A Textbook of Medical Imaging, 6th edition. United Kingdom: Churchill Livingstone, Elsevier; 2014. pp. 267-97.
25. Aliberti S, Goeminne PC, O'Donnell AE, Aksamit TR, Al-Jahdali H, Barke AF, et al. Criteria and definitions for the radiological and clinical diagnosis of bronchiectasis in adults for use in clinical trials: international consensus recommendations. Lancet Respir Med. 2022;10(3):298-306.
26. Polverino E, Goeminne PC, McDonnell MJ, Aliberti S, Marshall SE, Loebinger MR, et al. European Respiratory Society guidelines for the management of adult bronchiectasis. Eur Respir J. 2017;50(3):1700629.
27. Javidan NC, Bhalla S. Bronchiectasis. Radiol Clin North Am. 2009;47:289-306.
28. Webb RW, Muller NL, Naidich DP. HRCT findings: air-filled cystic lesions. In: Webb RW, Muller NL, Naidich DP (Eds). High-Resolution CT of the Lung, 5th edition. United States: Wolters Kluwer; 2015. pp. 65-86.
29. Cartier Y, Kavanagh PV, Johkoh T, Mason AC, MüllerNL. Bronchiectasis: accuracy of high resolution CT in the differentiation of specific diseases. AJR Am J Roentgenol. 1999;173:47-52.
30. Beddy P, Babar J, Devraj A. A practical approach to cystic lung disease on HRCT insights Imaging. 2011;2(1):17.
31. Webb RW, Muller NL, Naidich DP. HRCT findings: decreased lung attenuation. In: Webb RW, Muller NL, Naidich DP (Eds). High-Resolution CT of the Lung, 5th edition. United States: Wolters Kluwer; 2015. pp. 187-205.
32. Elicker BM, Webb RW. Decreased lung attenuation: emphysema, mosaic perfusion and cystic lung disease. In: Elicker BM, Webb RW (Eds). Fundamentals of High-Resolution Lung CT: Common Findings, Common Patterns, Common Diseases and Differential Diagnosis, 1st edition. United States: Wolters Kluwer; 2013. pp. 71-82.
33. Kligerman SJ, Henry T, Lin CT, Franks TJ, Galvin JR. Mosaic attenuation: etiology, methods of differentiation, and pitfalls. Radiographics. 2015;35:1360-80.
34. Raoof S, Bondalapati P, Vydyula R, Ryu JH, Gupta N, Raoof S, et al. Cystic lung diseases: algorithmic approach. Chest. 2016;150(4):945-65.
35. Stern EJ, Swensen SJ, Hartman TE, Frank MS. CT mosaic pattern of lung attenuation: distinguishing different causes. AJR Am J Roentgenol. 1995;165:813-6.
36. Ridge CA, Bankier AA, Eisenberg RL. Mosaic attenuation. AJR Am J Roentgenol. 2011;197:W970-7.

Mandeep Garg, Anmol Bhatia, Naveen Kalra

CHAPTER

5

Imaging of Pulmonary Tuberculosis

INTRODUCTION

Tuberculosis (TB) is caused by *Mycobacterium tuberculosis* and is responsible for significant morbidity and mortality, particularly in the countries of the developing world. As per the World Health Organization (WHO) Global TB Report 2024, 8.2 million people were globally reported to be newly diagnosed with TB in 2023, compared to 7.5 million in 2022, 6.4 million in 2021, and 5.8 million diagnosed in 2020. The newly diagnosed cases in 2022 and 2023 probably included a sizeable backlog of people who had developed TB in previous years when diagnosis and treatment were delayed by COVID-related disruptions during the pandemic. Among the 30 high TB-burden countries, which accounted for 87% of the global total in 2023, India contributed the highest number (26%) of cases. Further, 80% of the number of deaths caused by TB globally among human immunodeficiency virus (HIV)-negative people were seen in the WHO African and Southeast Asian regions, and India alone accounted for 29% of such deaths.[1]

The disease course and clinical-radiological presentation are dependent upon and altered by the nature of the interaction between the mycobacteria and the response by the host body. Notably, immunocompromised and elderly patients often exhibit atypical presentations due to their altered immune responses. Consequently, radiologists must be familiar with the evolving clinical-radiological spectrum of pulmonary TB to ensure accurate diagnosis and management.

Tuberculosis can affect any organ system, with the lungs being the most common and often the initial ones involved. After lung parenchyma, pulmonary TB commonly affects the lymph nodes, followed by the pleura. The lymph node and pleural involvement are included under extrapulmonary tuberculosis (EPTB).[2]

ROLE OF IMAGING IN PULMONARY TUBERCULOSIS

- Making a diagnosis
- Evaluating treatment response and residual disease activity
- Detecting complications and sequelae

RADIOLOGICAL PATTERNS OF PULMONARY TUBERCULOSIS

Tuberculosis is classified as primary and postprimary TB. Primary TB is the initial infection with *M. tuberculosis* in a previously uninfected individual. It is more common in younger patients, often asymptomatic, and may involve both lungs and lymph nodes. Postprimary TB is the reactivation of a latent *M. tuberculosis* infection or a new infection in an individual with prior exposure to the bacteria. It is more common in adults and typically affects the upper lobes of the lungs.[2]

Radiological patterns of pulmonary TB may be considered under the following groups:

- Typical radiological patterns of primary TB
- Postprimary TB or phthisis
- Patterns encountered in both primary and/or postprimary forms
- Complications and sequelae of TB
- Atypical patterns

Typical Radiological Patterns of Primary Tuberculosis

Four entities are known to occur in primary pulmonary TB: Gangliopulmonary pattern, miliary pattern, tuberculous pleuritis, and involvement of the tracheobronchial airway. Gangliopulmonary TB is seen only in primary TB, while others are seen in both primary and postprimary TB.

Gangliopulmonary form is characterized by the presence of enlarged lymph nodes in the mediastinum and/or hila, with relatively less involvement of parenchyma (Ghon focus). This form preferentially occurs in children and hence is known as "childhood-type TB."

Right paratracheal and hilar lymph nodes are the most commonly enlarged nodes seen in primary TB **(Fig. 1)**, although various other nodal stations can be involved in different combinations. The prevalence of lymph node enlargement decreases with increasing age.[3] On contrast-enhanced computed tomography (CECT), tuberculous nodes >2 cm show central areas of low attenuation, suggestive of caseous necrosis, and peripheral rim enhancement **(Fig. 2)**. In approximately two-thirds of cases of primary TB in the pediatric population, parenchymal lesions are encountered on the ipsilateral side of enlarged lymph nodes.[3] Lesions in parenchyma are typically located in the peripheral lung fields involving the subpleural locations.

The gangliopulmonary form of TB is usually self-limiting, with immunocompetent individuals usually remaining asymptomatic. Sometimes, the only radiological finding is Ranke complex, which includes both the parenchymal lesion (Ghon focus) and affected lymph nodes **(Fig. 3)**. However, the course in gangliopulmonary form may be complicated in the form of lymph node perforating in the bronchus, retro-obstructive pneumonia, and/or atelectasis (known as epituberculosis). Retro-obstructive pneumonia may evolve into a fibrotic lesion, which may get calcified. Destruction of the lung parenchyma results in fibrosis associated with traction bronchiectasis. However, in adults, the primary infection mostly causes parenchymal consolidation without lymphadenopathy **(Fig. 4)**. Cavitatory form is rarely encountered in children.

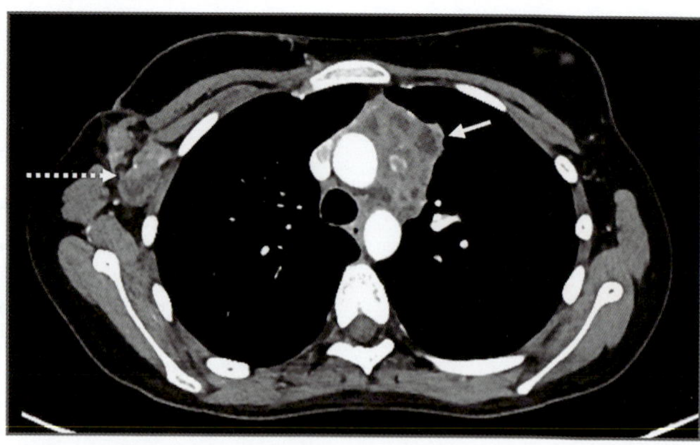

FIG. 2: Contrast-enhanced computed tomography axial image shows multiple enlarged conglomerated necrotic lymph nodes in station 3A (solid white arrow). Necrotic lymph nodes are also seen in the right axilla (dotted white arrow).

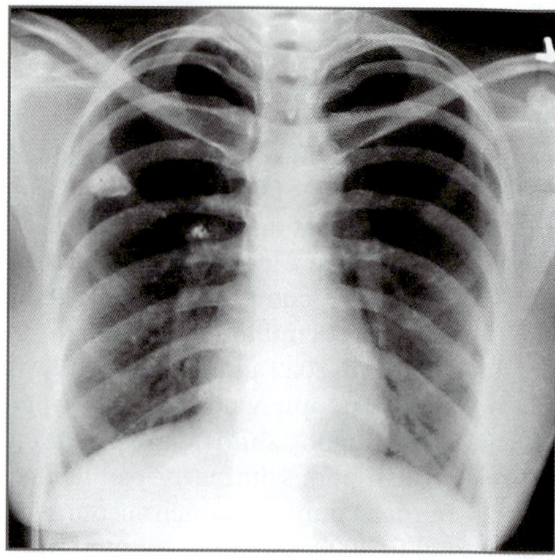

FIG. 3: Ranke complex. Chest radiograph shows a calcified lesion in the right upper zone along with calcification of the right hilar node and the intervening lymphatic channel.

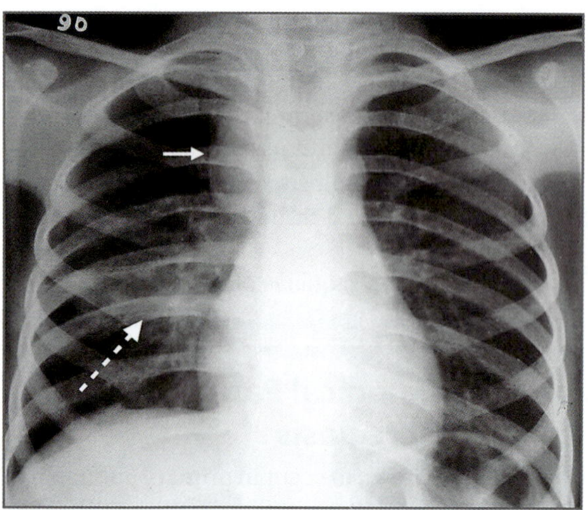

FIG. 1: Chest radiograph showing widening of the right paratracheal stripe (dotted white arrow), suggestive of right paratracheal lymph adenopathy. A patch of consolidation is also seen (solid white arrow).

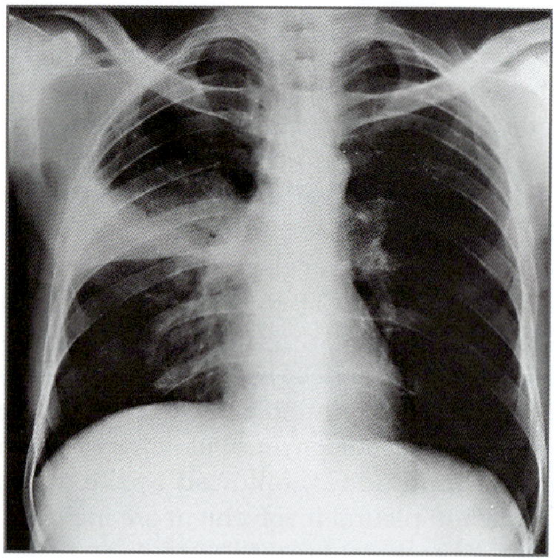

FIG. 4: Primary tuberculosis in a 40-year-old male. Chest radiograph shows multilobar consolidation in the right lung affecting the upper and lower lobes without lymphadenopathy.

Postprimary Tuberculosis or Phthisis

This form is due to the reactivation of residual dormant infective focus and evolves and progresses depending upon the status of acquired immunity. It is mostly, but not always, a disease affecting the adult population.[4] In the pediatric population, it mostly occurs in adolescent children, particularly in girls with menarche.[3] This form of TB is characterized by caseous necrosis undergoing liquefaction, progressive lung destruction associated with fibrosis, and the formation of cavities. The lesions are typically located in the upper lobes (apicoposterior segments) and have a relatively lower degree of involvement in the lower lobes (superior segments). The areas of caseous necrosis undergoing liquefaction later communicate with the adjacent airways, forming cavities **(Figs. 5A and B)**. The findings include parenchymal infiltrates in apicoposterior locations, cavities, pleural effusion, fibrotic areas causing lung parenchyma destruction, pulling up of hila/fissures, traction bronchiectasis, and pleural adhesions.[5] Cavitation may be seen radiographically in 40% of cases in postprimary form. The cavity wall can be thin and smooth, or thick and nodular. Air-fluid levels can be seen in 10% of cases with cavities,[6] which may be due to superimposed infection by bacteria or fungi.

Bronchogenic spread is characterized by multiple, ill-defined nodules, having a lobar/segmental distribution, typically involving lower lung zones.[7] Computed tomography (CT) typically shows 2- to 4-mm sized nodules that are centrilobular in distribution presenting as sharply marginated branching structures within and around terminal and respiratory bronchioles, giving a "tree-in-bud" appearance **(Fig. 6)**.[8] The "tree-in-bud" pattern or sign on CT should be used when both the "tree" and the "bud" are visible. The term "centrilobular branching opacity" is preferable in case only the "tree" is seen, and the "bud" is absent. However, the term "*clusters of micronodules*" may be used on CT in adults with active pulmonary TB, representing aggregated tree-in-bud lesions.[9]

Cicatrization atelectasis is a common finding following postprimary TB, which presents as atelectatic changes in the upper lobe, retracted hilum, lower lobe compensatory hyperinflation, and ipsilateral tracheomediastinal shift. This may also be associated with pleural thickening in the apices along with fibrosis, proliferation of extrapleural soft tissue, and subpleural atelectatic changes on CT.[10]

Galaxy sign (GS) and cluster sign (CS), initially defined in sarcoidosis, have also been described in immunocompetent patients with postprimary TB on CT. They are associated with perilymphatic-predominant nodularity rather than centrilobular-predominant nodularity. The GS is a large parenchymal nodule formed due to the coalescence of small nodules and has multiple tiny surrounding satellite nodules. Clusters of multiple small nodules also characterize the CS, but these nodules do not tend to coalesce as in GS.[11]

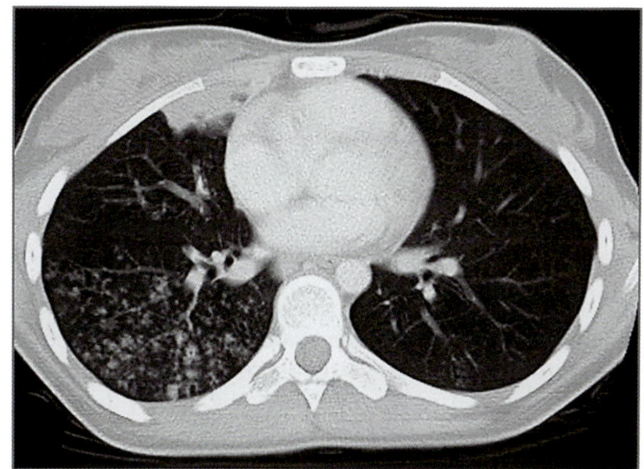

FIG. 6: Coalescing centrilobular nodules with "tree-in-bud" appearance are seen in the right lower lobe.

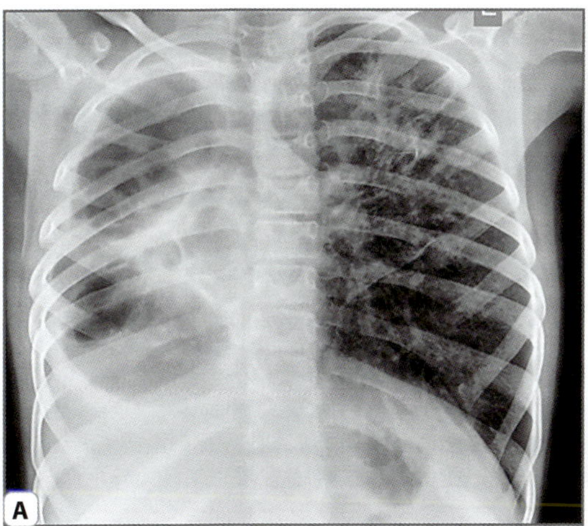

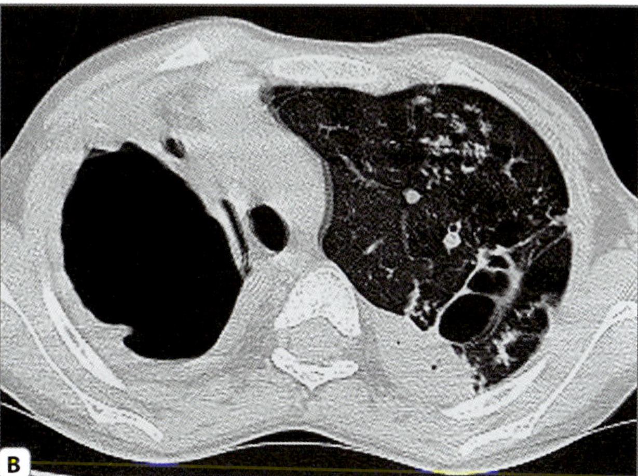

FIGS. 5A AND B: Large areas of cavitation are seen in the right lung on chest radiograph (A) and axial section of computed tomography scan (B). Bronchiectatic changes are also noted in the left lung.

Radiological Patterns Seen in Both Primary and/or Postprimary Tuberculosis

Miliary TB

Miliary TB results from the hematogenous spread of the infection in the lungs and other organs, resulting in innumerable tiny granulomas. A chest radiograph is usually unremarkable at the onset of symptoms, and the nodules only become discernible after 4 weeks **(Fig. 7)**.[11] CT helps to demonstrate the miliary nodules before they become perceptible on radiographs **(Fig. 8)**. It shows a combination of sharply and poorly defined, diffusely distributed 1–4 mm nodules in a random fashion, commonly associated with thickening of the interstitium (both interlobular and intralobular septa).[12] A typical "*snowstorm*" appearance on chest X-ray suggesting an evolution to adult respiratory distress syndrome has also been reported.[13] The second most common finding on high-resolution computed tomography (HRCT) in cases of miliary TB includes ground-glass opacities, which represent small granulomas below the resolution of HRCT superimposed on exudative lung changes.[14] Maximum intensity projection (MIP) reconstructed images in such cases can help delineate tiny lung nodules.

Exudative Pleuritis

The pleural cavity may be involved by a caseating granuloma in the parenchyma adjacent to the pleura or through a hematogenous route. It is usually seen along with parenchymal and/or lymphadenopathy. It may, however, be seen sometimes as the only radiologic finding in 5% of adult patients, suggesting primary TB.[15] CECT shows smooth thickening with the enhancement of parietal and visceral pleura, resulting in split-pleura sign **(Fig. 9)**. Tuberculous pleurisy when localized results in tuberculous empyema, which sometimes ruptures outside forming a subcutaneous abscess, called empyema necessitans. Diffuse pleural thickening without any effusion suggests fibrothorax and indicates disease inactivity. Pleural collection communicating with the bronchial tree results in the development of a bronchopleural fistula and an air-fluid level within **(Fig. 10)**. Diagnosis of the bronchopleural fistula is suggested clinically by a copious amount of sputum production by the patient and radiologically by the appearance of hydropneumothorax with changing air-fluid level. CT may demonstrate the communication between the collection in the pleural cavity and bronchi or lung parenchyma.[16]

Tracheobronchial TB

Tracheobronchial TB is known to occur in 2–4% of patients with pulmonary TB.[17] It usually results from a perforation of

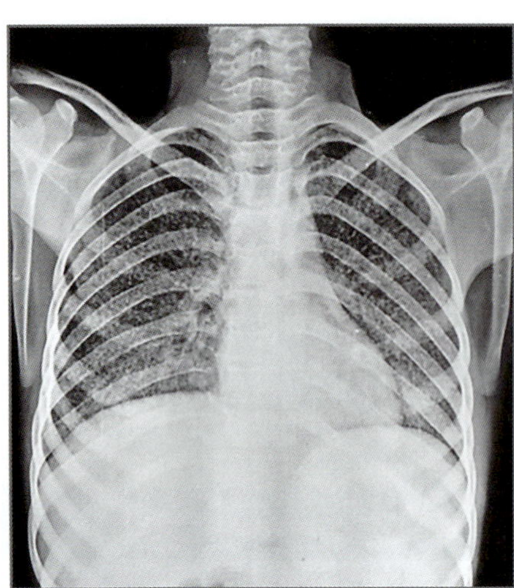

FIG. 7: Chest radiograph showing miliary nodules in bilateral lungs.

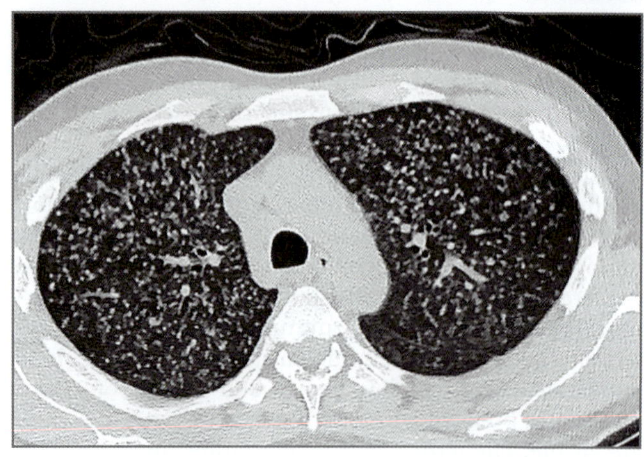

FIG. 8: Axial computed tomography scan section showing miliary nodules in bilateral lungs.

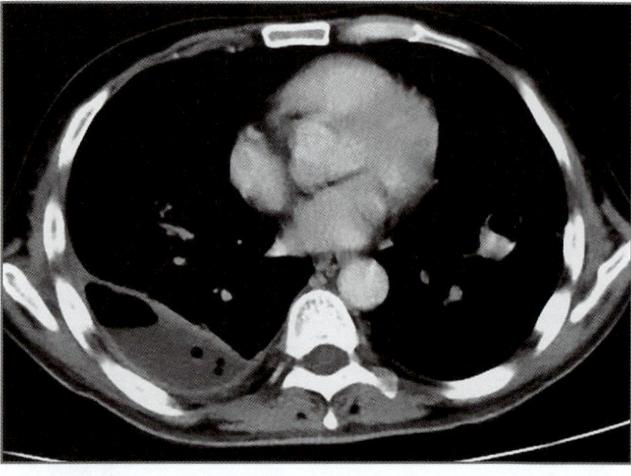

FIG. 9: Tubercular empyema. Axial computed tomography scan section showing loculated empyema in the right lung with thickened and enhancing visceral and parietal pleura. Few air foci are also seen in the collection.

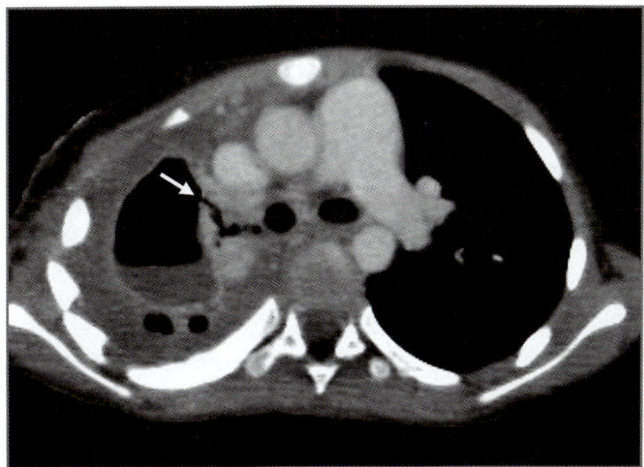

FIG. 10: Bronchopleural fistula in tubercular empyema. Axial computed tomography scan section showing loculated empyema in the right lung with thickened and enhancing visceral and parietal pleura. Air-fluid level is seen in the collection. A bronchus is seen to communicate with the pleural collection (arrow), suggestive of a bronchopleural fistula. Volume loss of the right hemithorax with thickened ribs due to chronic empyema is noted.

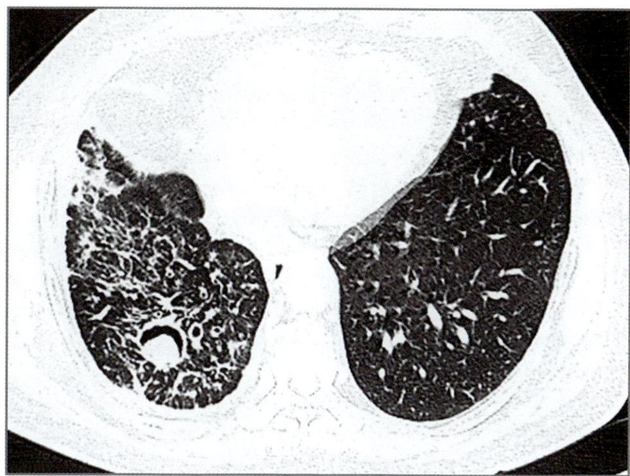

FIG. 11: Fungal ball. Axial section of computed tomography scan showing a cavity in the right lower lobe with soft tissue in its dependent portion. Fibrobronchiectatic changes are seen in the surrounding parenchyma.

enlarged lymph nodes into a bronchus,[18] or may also result from lymphatic and hematogenous dissemination.[19] The ulcerogranulomatous lesions or granulomatous polypoidal growths can be seen involving the bronchi, which result in fibrotic stenoses after healing and lead to postobstructive bronchiectasis. The acute form of tracheobronchial TB manifests as smooth or irregular thickening of the walls, resulting in circumferential bronchial narrowing.[20] Encasement by the enlarged enhancing mediastinal nodes is also commonly seen in the active stage. Cicatricial bronchostenosis may occur lately following the healing of the focal infection involving the walls of the bronchi. The chronic fibrotic stage shows circumferential symmetric thickening of the wall, resulting in concentric narrowing of the bronchus.[21]

Tuberculoma

Tuberculomas are usually sequelae of the healed form of primary TB but can be seen in 3–6% of patients with postprimary TB as the only or the main finding.[22] These can be multiple or solitary, varying in size from 0.4 to 5 cm. The possible pathogenesis resulting in tuberculoma formation includes the rounding of a contracted healing tubercular lesion or a healed filled-in cavity.[22] Most of the tuberculomas remain static in size. Calcification is seen to occur in 20–30% of cases, which can be diffuse or nodular.[23]

Complications and Sequelae of Pulmonary Tuberculosis

A tuberculous cavity can be colonized by *Aspergillus* species, resulting in an "*aspergilloma*," which consists of a bunch of entangled hyphae knotted together with cellular fragments and mucus. It can be associated with thickening of the walls of the cavity or the adjacent pleural lining. CT shows soft tissue in a cavity that is separated from the adjacent wall by a crescent-shaped area of air **(Fig. 11)**.[24] This soft tissue may sometimes be mobile and change position on prone imaging.

Tuberculosis may predispose to malignancy by a local mechanism known as scar cancer, or there may be a coexistence of TB and carcinoma. Malignancy may also cause tubercular reactivation, both by compromising the patient's immunity and by erosion into an encapsulated focus. Hence, any predominant or enlarging nodule on follow-up imaging should raise suspicion for coexisting carcinoma in TB patients.[25]

In the areas of active foci, pulmonary arteries and veins may demonstrate findings of vasculitis and/or thrombosis. There may be increased tortuosity of the bronchial arteries, which commonly are hypertrophied in patients with bronchiectasis associated with TB or in parenchymal TB only **(Figs. 12A and B)**. Rasmussen aneurysm results when a tubercular cavity erodes the branch of the pulmonary artery in the surrounding parenchyma **(Fig. 13)**.[26]

Broncholithiasis is an uncommon complication resulting from the erosion of a calcified node in the peribronchial location into the adjacent bronchus. CT shows a lymph node in an endobronchial or peribronchial location, which causes bronchial obstruction, resulting in focal hyperinflation, atelectasis, obstructive pneumonitis, bronchiectasis, and branching opacities (obstructive bronchoceles).[27]

Esophageal involvement by TB from adjacent lymph nodes results in the formation of strictures, fistulae between the esophagus and mediastinum or airway, and traction diverticulae.[28]

Tuberculous pericarditis is seen to occur in 1% of cases of TB. It may result from the direct invasion of enlarged

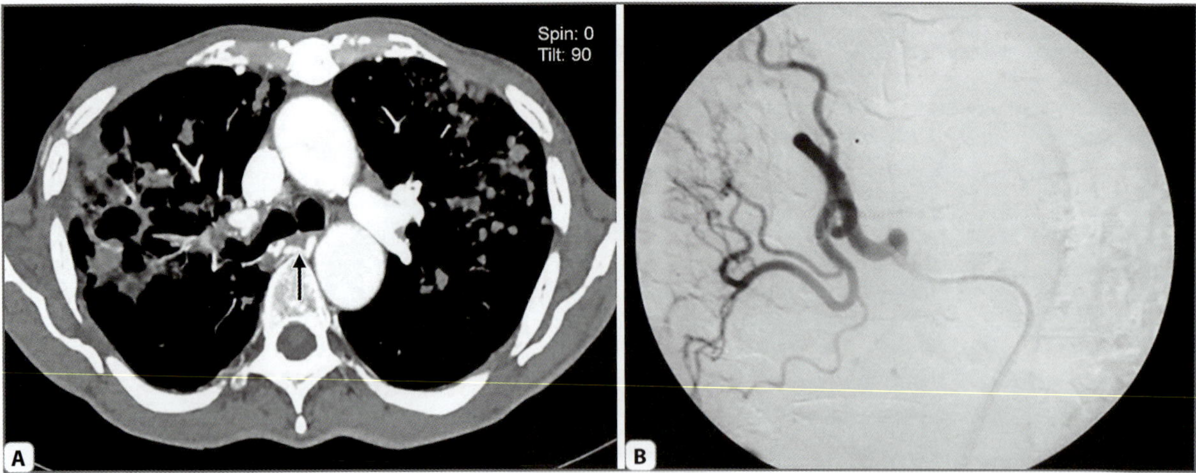

FIGS. 12A AND B: A 62-year-old man with pulmonary TB having massive hemoptysis. (A) Axial bronchial angiography image shows the ostium of the enlarged right bronchial artery (arrow). Bilateral consolidation and multiple nodules are seen. (B) Selective right bronchial angiogram shows an enlarged and tortuous right bronchial artery.

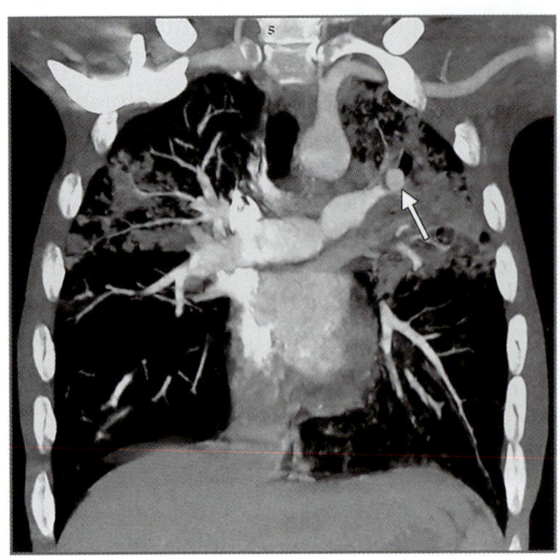

FIG. 13: Rasmussen aneurysm. Coronal section of computed tomography angiography showing a contrast-filled outpouching (arrow) arising from a branch of a pulmonary artery within the consolidation in the left upper lobe. Areas of consolidation and nodules are seen in bilateral upper lobes.

lymph nodes into the pericardium or from the miliary spread of the infection. Pericardial thickening (with or without effusion) along with enlarged lymph nodes is seen on CT. Constrictive pericarditis, characterized by fibrous or calcified pericardial thickening measuring >3 mm, is seen as a delayed complication in 10% of patients with tuberculous pericarditis **(Figs. 14A and B)**.[22]

Pneumothorax is seen in around 5% of cases of the postprimary form, usually in the severe cavitatory form of the disease. It indicates severe and widespread lung involvement, and the inception of empyema and bronchopleural fistula.

Fibrosing mediastinitis in TB is an unusual complication that progresses slowly without obvious clinical symptoms. The findings on CT in fibrosing mediastinitis include a hilar or mediastinal mass showing coarse calcification, narrowing of the tracheobronchial tree, and encasement of pulmonary and other mediastinal vasculature, sometimes presenting as superior vena cava syndrome.[29]

Atypical Patterns

These are usually encountered in elderly and immunocompromised patients. Various factors which may alter the pathogenesis of the atypical patterns include:

- Deficient cellular immunity resulting in reactivation of TB (typical pattern)
- Reinfection or second primary infection can happen[30]
- Elderly subjects contracting the disease for the first time.

A shift from the usual trail (reactivation) to an unusual trail is seen in cases where there is an exogenic reinfection or a second primary infection, thereby the presentation similar to what occurs in the pediatric population.[31,32] These atypical radiographic findings such as infiltrates confined to lower lung fields, hilar/mediastinal lymphadenopathy, and exudative pleuritis can result in the wrong initial diagnosis and thus delayed treatment.

Magnetic Resonance Imaging in Pulmonary Tuberculosis

Magnetic resonance imaging (MRI) is a problem-solving modality, and conventional sequences (T1W and T2W) should be combined with diffusion-weighted imaging (DWI) and contrast-enhanced (CE) imaging for optimal evaluation. It can be used to evaluate mediastinal nodes better and assess disease activity in case of mediastinal

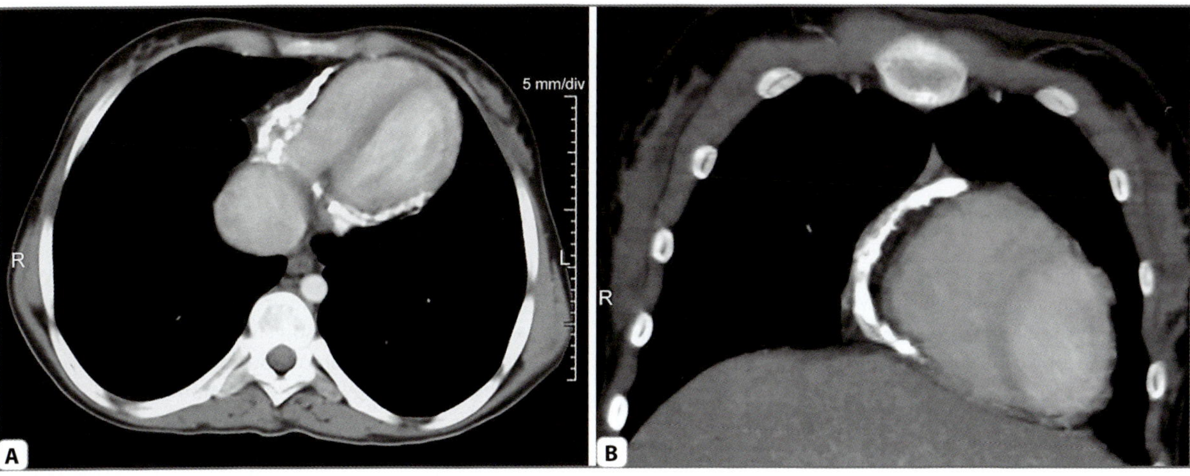

FIGS. 14A AND B: Tubercular calcific pericarditis. Axial (A) and coronal (B) sections of computed tomography scan show a thick sheet of calcification along the right and left ventricles.

nodes/fibrosis. Since MRI is a radiation-free modality, it can be used for follow-up of already known lesions, especially in young patients to reduce radiation exposure.[33-35] MRI is equivalent to CT for detection of lymph nodes, lung cavitation, and pleural effusion, having a sensitivity and specificity of 100%. Sodhi et al. found the sensitivity and specificity of MRI for the detection of nodules in pulmonary TB to be 88.2 and 95.7%, respectively, while for the detection of consolidation, it was 92.9 and 100%.[36] However, high cost and limited availability are its main limitations.

Artificial Intelligence in Pulmonary Tuberculosis

Artificial intelligence (AI) is becoming popular and providing research opportunities and technical underpinnings in pulmonary TB. It has enabled the development of unique, precise, fast, and automated implements for pulmonary TB care. State-of-the-art AI models are being developed using images and genetic data to detect pulmonary TB, distinguish it from other pulmonary disorders, and identify resistance to drugs to assist clinicians in deciding the appropriate treatment schedule in the early stage of the infection.[37] Autoencoder (AE) and convolutional neural network (CNN) were combined, and a new model called autoencoder convolutional neural network (AECNN) was proposed by Li et al. for the analysis of pulmonary TB.[38] A lightweight classification network was proposed by Tian et al. based on a combination of CNN and transformer, which may be used to classify TB cases on chest CT.[39] Studies have also used deep learning models to identify drug-resistant and nondrug-resistant tubercular infections to detect tubercular and nontubercular mycobacterial infections. Studies on AI have also been conducted to detect infectivity in pulmonary TB patients, which is important for preventing and controlling the infection.[40-44]

CONCLUSION

In conclusion, imaging remains indispensable in the diagnosis and management of pulmonary TB, offering crucial insights into disease activity, extent, and complications. Radiologists play a pivotal role in guiding clinical decision-making and optimizing patient outcomes. Future research should focus on refining imaging techniques, and exploring the potential of artificial intelligence to enhance the accuracy and efficiency of radiological interpretation.

REFERENCES

1. WHO Global tuberculosis report 2024. Geneva: World Health Organization; 2024. [online] Available from https://www.who.int/teams/global-tuberculosis-programme/tb-reports/global-tuberculosis-report-2024 [Last accessed February, 2025].
2. Bhalla AS, Goyal A, Guleria R, Gupta AK. Chest tuberculosis: radiological review and imaging recommendations. Indian J Radiol Imaging. 2015;25:213-25.
3. Leung AN, Müller NL, Pineda PR, FitzGerald JM. Primary tuberculosis in childhood: radiographic manifestations. Radiology. 1992;182(1):87-91.
4. Lamont AC, Cremin BJ, Pelteret RM. Radiologic patterns of pulmonary tuberculosis in the paediatric age group. Paediatr Radiol. 1986;16(1):2-7.
5. Palmer PE. Pulmonary tuberculosis: usual and unusual radiographic presentations. Semin Roentgenol. 1979;14:204-42.
6. Woodring JH, Vandiviere HM, Fried AM, Dillon ML, Williams TD, Melvin IG. Update: radiographic features of pulmonary tuberculosis. Am J Roentgenol. 1986;146:497-506.
7. Hadlock FP, Park SK, Awe RJ, Rivera M. Unusual radiographic findings in adult pulmonary tuberculosis. Am J Roentgenol. 1980:134:1015-8.

8. Im JG, Itoh H, Shim YS, Lee JH, Ahn J, Han MC, et al. Pulmonary tuberculosis: CT findings—early active disease and sequential change with antituberculous therapy. Radiology. 1993;186:653-60.
9. Im JG, Itoh H. Tree-in-bud pattern of pulmonary tuberculosis on thin-section CT: pathological implications. Korean J Radiol. 2018;19:859-65.
10. Im JG, Webb WR, Han MC, Park JH. Apical opacity associated with pulmonary tuberculosis: high-resolution CT findings. Radiology. 1991;178:727-31.
11. Wetscherek MTA, Sadler TJ, Lee JYJ, Karia S, Babar JL. Active pulmonary tuberculosis: something old, something new, something borrowed, something blue. Insights Imaging. 2022;13:3.
12. Leung AN. Pulmonary tuberculosis: the essentials. Radiology. 1999;210:307-22.
13. Piqueras AR, Marruecos L, Artigas A, Rodriguez C. Miliary tuberculosis and adult respiratory distress syndrome. Intensive Care Med. 1987;13:175-82.
14. Hong SH, Im JG, Lee JS, Song JW, Lee HJ, Yeon KM. High-resolution CT findings of miliary tuberculosis. J Comput Assist Tomogr. 1998;22:220-4.
15. Choyke PL, Sostman HD, Curtis AM, Ravin CE, Chen JT, Godwin JD, et al. Adult-onset pulmonary tuberculosis. Radiology. 1983;148:357-62.
16. Westcott JL, Volpe JP. Peripheral bronchopleural fistula: CT evaluation in 20 patients with pneumonia, empyema or postoperative air leak. Radiology. 196:175-81.
17. Lee KS, Kim YH, Kim WS, Hwang SH, Kim PN, Lee BH. Endobronchial tuberculosis: CT features. J Comput Assist Tomogr. 1991;15:424-8.
18. Auerbach O. Tuberculosis of the trachea and the major bronchi. Am Rev Tuberc. 1949;60:604-20.
19. Smith L, Schillaci R, Sarlin R. Endobronchial tuberculosis. Serial fiberoptic bronchoscopy and natural history. Chest. 1987;91:644-7.
20. Moon WK, Im JG, Yeon KM, Han MC. Tuberculosis of central airways: CT findings of active and fibrotic disease. Am J Roentgenol. 1997;169:649-53.
21. Kim HY, Song KS, Goo JM, Lee JS, Lee KS, Lim TH. Thoracic sequelae and complications of tuberculosis. Radiographics. 2001;21:839-58.
22. Sochocky S. Tuberculoma of the lung. Am Rev Tuberc. 1958;78:403-10.
23. Lee KS, Song KS, Lim TH, Kim PN, Kim IY, Lee BH. Adult-onset pulmonary tuberculosis: findings on chest radiographs and CT scans. Am J Roentgenol. 1993;160:753-8.
24. Fraser RS. Pulmonary aspergillosis: pathologic and pathogenetic features. Pathol Annu. 1993;28:231-77.
25. Snider GL, Placi B. The relationship between pulmonary tuberculosis and bronchogenic carcinoma: a topographic study. Am Rev Respir Dis. 1969;99:229-36.
26. Santelli ED, Katz DS, Goldschmidt AM, Thomas HA. Embolization of multiple Rasmussen aneurysms as a treatment of hemoptysis. Radiology. 1994;193:396-8.
27. Adler O, Peleg H. Computed tomography in diagnosis of broncholithiasis. Eur J Radiol. 1987;7:211-2.
28. Fraser RS, Muller NL, Colman N, Paré PD. Diagnosis of Diseases of the Chest. Philadelphia: Saunders; 1999. pp. 798-873.
29. Lee JY, Kim Y, Lee KS, Chung MP. Tuberculous fibrosing mediastinitis: radiological findings. Am J Roentgenol. 1996;167:1598-9.
30. Stead WW, Lofgren JP, Warren E, Thomas C. Tuberculosis as an endemic and nosocomial infection among the elderly in nursing homes. N Engl J Med. 1985;312:1483-7.
31. Korzeniewska-Kosela M, Krysl J, Müller N, Black W, Allen E, FitzGerald JM. Tuberculosis in young adults and the elderly: a prospective comparison study. Chest. 1994;106:28-32.
32. Umeki S. Comparison of younger and elderly patients with pulmonary tuberculosis. Respiration. 1989;55:75-83.
33. Sodhi KS, Khandelwal N, Saxena AK, Bhatia A, Bansal D, Trehan A, et al. Rapid lung MRI: paradigm shift in evaluation of febrile neutropenia in children with leukemia: a pilot study. Leuk Lymphoma. 2016;57:70-5.
34. Sodhi KS, Khandelwal N, Saxena AK, Singh M, Agarwal R, Bhatia A, et al. Rapid lung MRI in children with pulmonary infections: time to change our diagnostic algorithms. J Magn Reson Imaging. 2016;43:1196-206.
35. Sodhi KS, Bhatia A, Khandelwal N. Rapid lung magnetic resonance imaging in children with pulmonary infection. Pediatr Radiol. 2017;47:764-5.
36. Sodhi KS, Sharma M, Saxena AK, Mathew JL, Singh M, Khandelwal N. MRI in thoracic tuberculosis of children. Indian J Pediatr. 2017;84(9):670-6.
37. Liang S, Ma J, Wang G, Shao J, Li J, Deng H, et al. The application of artificial intelligence in the diagnosis and drug resistance prediction of pulmonary tuberculosis. Front Med (Lausanne). 2022;9:935080.
38. Li L, Huang H, Jin X. AE-CNN classification of pulmonary tuberculosis based on CT images. In: 9th International Conference on Information Technology in Medicine and Education (ITME) (Piscataway, NJ); 2018. pp. 39-42.
39. Tian J, Zhang Y, Lei J, Sun C, Hu G. Lightweight classification network for pulmonary tuberculosis based on CT images. J Artif Intell Technol. 2023;3:25-31.
40. Gao XW, Qian Y. Prediction of multidrug-resistant TB from CT pulmonary images based on deep learning techniques. Mol Pharm. 2018;15:4326-35.
41. Wang L, Ding W, Mo Y, Shi D, Zhang S, Zhong L, et al. Distinguishing nontuberculous mycobacteria from *Mycobacterium tuberculosis* lung disease from CT images using a deep learning framework. Eur J Nucl Med Mol Imaging. 2021;48:4293-306.
42. Hwang EJ, Park S, Jin KN, Kim JI, Choi SY, Lee JH, et al. Development and validation of a deep learning-based automatic detection algorithm for active pulmonary tuberculosis on chest radiographs. Clin Infect Dis. 2019;69(5):739-47.
43. Vajda S, Karargyris A, Jaeger S, Santosh KC, Candemir S, Xue Z, et al. Feature selection for automatic tuberculosis screening in frontal chest radiographs. J Med Syst. 2018;42:146.
44. Lee S, Yim JJ, Kwak N, Lee YJ, Lee JK, Lee JY, et al. Deep learning to determine the activity of pulmonary tuberculosis on chest radiographs. Radiology. 2021;301:435-42.

Anju Garg, Swati Gupta, Jyoti Kumar, Satyam

CHAPTER

6

Nontubercular Pulmonary Infections

INTRODUCTION

Pulmonary infections or pneumonia are an important cause of morbidity and mortality, especially in our country. Inflammatory diseases of the lung may be referred to as either pneumonia or pneumonitis. Although these terms are used interchangeably, pneumonia usually implies an infection by pathogenic organisms, whereas pneumonitis refers to a noninfective inflammatory process involving the alveolar wall.[1]

Patients with pneumonia commonly present with cough (with or without sputum), and fever—often with chills, dyspnea, and pleuritic chest pain. On physical examination, there may be tachypnea, with bronchial breath sounds and crepts on auscultation. In addition to these clinical features, an infiltrate on the chest radiograph or other imaging modality, with or without supporting microbiological data, is usually considered as an appropriate investigation for the diagnosis of pneumonia. The specific organism causing the infection can be established with certainty only in approximately 50% of patients, despite intensive laboratory investigation.

Although the specific diagnosis requires a microbiological evaluation, the radiologist plays a very important role in the evaluation of a suspected case of pulmonary infection. The radiologist can establish the presence of disease, localize and define the extent of disease, suggest an etiological diagnosis, recognize any underlying pathology, assess the response to treatment, and establish the presence of complications.

IMAGING MODALITIES

Chest radiography and computed tomography (CT) are the most useful imaging modalities available for the evaluation of a patient with a known or suspected pulmonary infection.

A *chest radiograph* (posteroanterior view) is the basic and most useful imaging tool to establish the presence of pneumonia, determine its location and extent, and monitor its response to therapy. Further, the chest radiograph can suggest an etiological agent, prognosis, associated conditions, complications (cavitation, abscess formation, pneumothorax, and pleural effusion), alternative diagnoses, and sometimes even guide invasive diagnostic procedures. Patients who are hospitalized for suspected pulmonary infection but have negative chest radiography findings should be presumptively treated with antibiotics and imaging repeated in 24–48 hours, as chest radiographs can be negative early in the course of the disease.

Computed tomography is not recommended for the initial evaluation of patients with pneumonia but is recommended when there is a strong clinical suspicion of pneumonia that is accompanied by normal, ambiguous, or nonspecific radiography. It is a useful adjunct to conventional radiography in complicated cases or in patients in whom the response to treatment is unexpectedly slow. In these cases, the role of CT is to further characterize the complex types of pneumonia, look for complications, and detect underlying disease within the lung or mediastinum. It also plays an important role in differentiating lung abscess from empyema.

Ultrasonography (US): In recent years, ultrasound has been used as an additional modality both in the diagnosis and follow-up of patients with pneumonia.[2] Multiple studies have compared the findings in pneumonia on lung ultrasound (LUS) with chest radiography and have shown that LUS is at least equivalent, if not superior, to chest radiography.[3] Its use is especially recommended in the emergency setting, among bedridden patients, and in pregnant women and children because of its lack of ionizing radiation, portability (it can be done at the bedside), and repeatability.[4] It can also give quantitative and qualitative information about pleural fluid collections and serve as a guide for aspiration in cases of pulmonary infections. It is however operator dependent with a lack of reproducibility.

Magnetic resonance imaging (MRI): With the recent advances in MRI, resulting in faster and shorter protocols, it has become possible to use MRI to diagnose pulmonary infection and its complications. MRI has been found to have a sensitivity and specificity equal to that of CT in the detection of pneumonia, with better accuracy than chest radiographs. The major advantage of MRI is the lack of ionizing radiation, and therefore, it can be used as a nonradiation alternative in children and pregnant patients. Challenges that remain are the need for sedation/anesthesia in pediatric patients, cost, and motion artifacts.[5,6]

Artificial intelligence (AI) is revolutionizing chest radiology by enhancing the efficiency and accuracy of diagnosing chest pathologies. As the technology continues to evolve, it promises to play an even greater role in improving patient care and streamlining healthcare systems. AI algorithms, particularly those based on deep learning, can process chest X-rays and CT scans with high accuracy. Its role spans various aspects including detection, characterization, and follow-up, offering numerous advantages for clinicians and patients. Efforts are needed to ensure that data represent various populations and infection patterns. Standardization and validation of AI systems are crucial for widespread clinical adoption.[7]

RADIOGRAPHIC PATTERN

Pneumonias can be categorized according to their radiographic appearances. Although widely used, this categorization may have limited value because the same organism may produce several patterns and because patterns often overlap in an individual patient **(Table 1)**.

In *lobar/airspace pneumonia*, the infective organism reaches the acini leading to a rapid production of abundant edema fluid with minimal cellular reaction. There is an initial peripheral localization but as the fluid increases in amount, it flows from alveolus to alveolus limited only by pleural boundaries, leading to a confluent involvement of the lung parenchyma.[8] Airspace disease is typically due to bacterial infection; however, some viruses can also cause this pattern.

On chest radiographs, the classical appearance is a homogeneous nonsegmental consolidation. Eventually, the pneumonia may involve the whole lobe, but usually, symptoms develop before the entire lobe is consolidated and antibiotic therapy, if started, halts the process. The consolidation is usually confined to one lobe, although multilobar involvement is not uncommon. Because the airways are not primarily affected, there is little or no volume loss, and patent airways leading to visible air bronchograms are common **(Fig. 1A)**.

On ultrasound, the consolidated lung appears similar in echogenicity to the liver or spleen ("hepatization" of the lung). Multiple bright dot-like structures and branching linear structures can be seen within the consolidated lung, which represents scattered residual air in alveoli and bronchi—the "sonographic air bronchogram" **(Fig. 1B)**. These air bronchograms may show centrifugal movement with breathing.[9] Consolidation can be differentiated from atelectasis based on this movement—the "dynamic air bronchogram." According to a study, dynamic air bronchograms have a 97% positive predictive value for pneumonia.[10]

On CT, airspace consolidation localizes in the middle and outer zones of the lungs and is seen as dense opacification with air bronchograms or air bronchiolograms. Areas of ground-glass attenuation may be seen around this denser airspace consolidation **(Figs. 1C and D)**.[11]

Lobar pneumonia must be distinguished from atelectasis and pleural involvement. Secondary causes such

TABLE 1: Categorization of pneumonia based on radiographic pattern and the commonly associated organisms.

Chest radiograph pattern	Common findings	Possible pathogen classification	Possible pathogens
Lobar	Homogenous consolidation, air bronchogram	Bacterial	*Streptococcus pneumoniae*, *Klebsiella pneumoniae*, *Haemophilus influenzae*, gram-negative bacilli
Bronchopneumonia	Peribronchial thickening, patchy air space opacities	Bacterial, viral	• *Bacterial*: *Streptococcus pneumoniae*, *Staphylococcus aureus*, *Haemophilus influenzae*, *Klebsiella pneumoniae*, *Pseudomonas aeruginosa*, *Escherichia coli*, *Proteus* species • *Viral*: Adenovirus, HSV, CMV, coronaviruses, influenza, Bocavirus
Interstitial	Diffuse pattern, peribronchial thickening, reticular opacities with para hilar dominance	Viral, atypical pathogens	Viral (RSV, influenza A, adenovirus, SARS-CoV-2, CMV), PCP, *Chlamydia pneumoniae*, *Mycoplasma pneumoniae*, *Legionella pneumophila*, *Chlamydophila psittaci*, *Coxiella burnetii*
Nodular pattern	Nonhomogenous, nodules with branching opacities, spares subpleural space	Tubercular, fungal, viral	*Mycobacterium tuberculosis*, septic emboli, *Aspergillus* species, *Histoplasma capsulatum*, *Cryptococcus neoformans*, *Mycoplasma pneumoniae*, varicella zoster virus

(CMV: cytomegalovirus; HSV: herpes simplex virus; PCP: *Pneumocystis* pneumonia; RSV: respiratory syncytial virus; SARS-CoV-2: severe acute respiratory syndrome coronavirus 2)

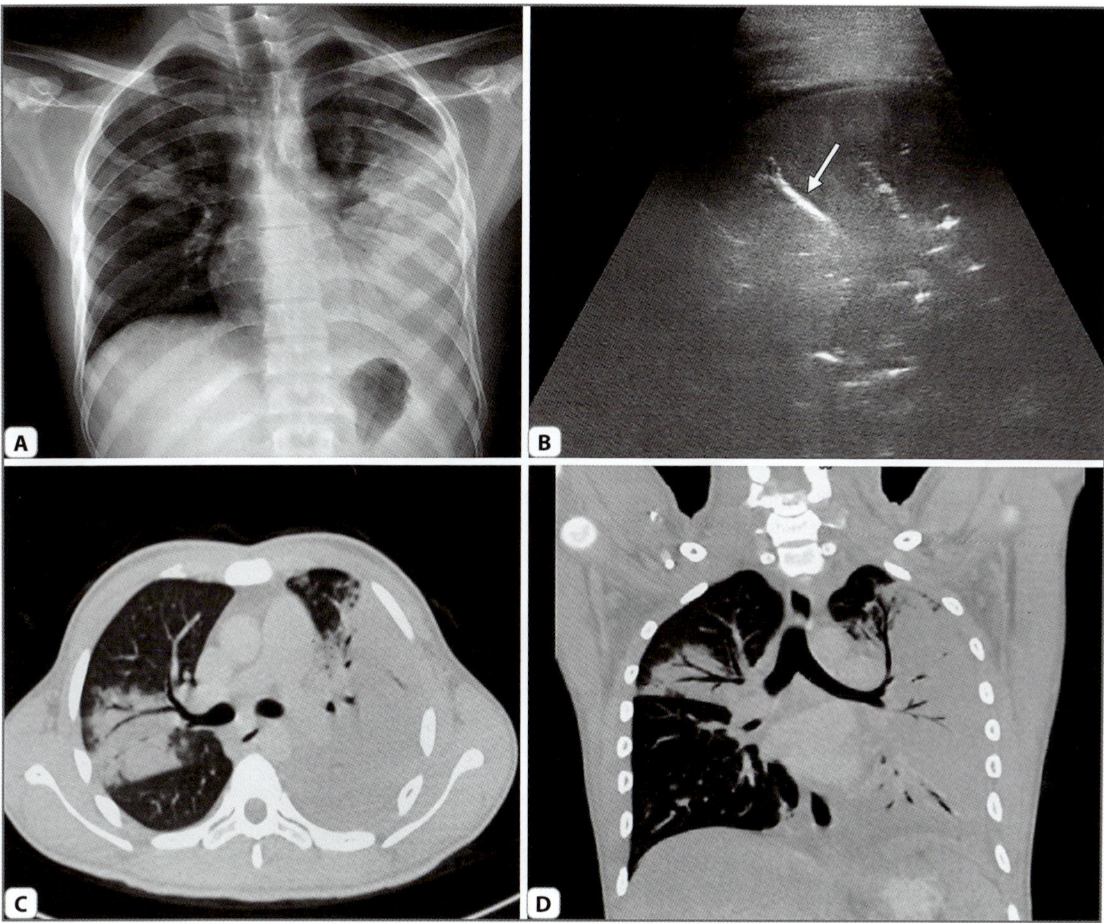

FIGS. 1A TO D: Airspace pneumonia. Chest radiograph (A) shows a homogeneous opacity in the right mid zone, left mid, and lower zone with air bronchogram within. Ultrasound image (B) shows lung parenchyma resembling liver (hepatization) with linear echogenic structure within representing air in bronchi—the sonographic air bronchogram (arrow). CT scan at lung window settings axial (C) and coronal reformat (D) shows airspace consolidation in the left lower lobe and right upper lobe with air bronchogram. Consolidation in the right upper lobe is limited by a major fissure.

(CT: computed tomography)

as pulmonary edema, hemorrhage, or obstructed bronchi should be looked for. In lower lobes involvement, aspiration pneumonia should be considered in an appropriate clinical context. Noninfective causes of lobar pattern include radiation pneumonitis, pulmonary alveolar proteinosis, organizing pneumonia, adenocarcinoma in situ (formerly bronchoalveolar carcinoma), and lymphoma.[12]

In *bronchopneumonia*, it is the mucosal surfaces of the bronchi and bronchioles that are affected, rather than the terminal airspace. There is development of a peribronchiolar focus of infection, which subsequently spreads along the intralobular airway to the alveolus, and then from one alveolus to another, until the pulmonary lobule is partially or completely involved. A bronchopneumonia pattern is most commonly due to infection by staphylococcal or gram-negative organisms; anaerobic organisms may also cause this pattern of involvement.[13]

On chest radiographs, mild bronchopneumonia results in peribronchial thickening and poorly defined airspace opacities. More severe disease results in inhomogeneous, patchy, poorly defined opacities with the absence of air bronchograms. The process is diffuse, as several foci of disease are often seeded at the same time, and frequently both lungs are involved **(Fig. 2)**. It is often difficult to make a radiographic distinction between lobar pneumonia and confluent bronchopneumonia.[13] On CT, consolidation which involves the terminal and respiratory bronchioles and adjacent alveoli results in poorly defined centrilobular nodular opacities measuring between 4 and 10 mm in diameter. When the infection extends to involve the entire secondary lobule, lobular distribution of airspace consolidation is seen **(Fig. 3)**.[11] This pattern can also be seen in adenocarcinoma in situ (formerly bronchoalveolar carcinoma), hypereosinophilic syndrome, and lymphoma, which can present as multifocal alveolar consolidation. In chronic cases, differential diagnoses include lipoid pneumonia, pulmonary alveolar proteinosis, or radiation pneumonitis.[12]

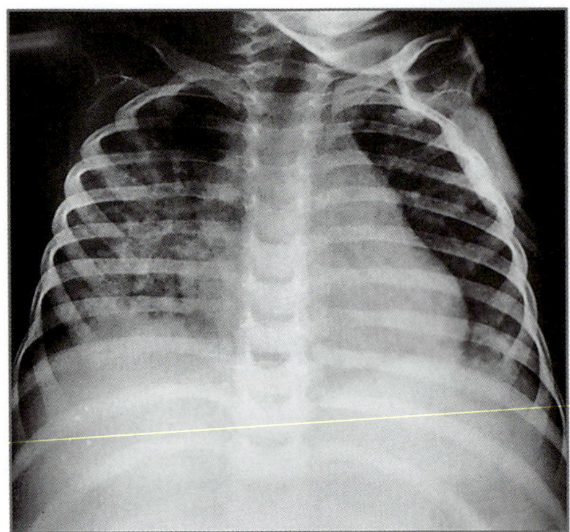

FIG. 2: Bronchopneumonia. Chest radiograph shows patchy opacities in the right mid zone and bilateral lower zones.

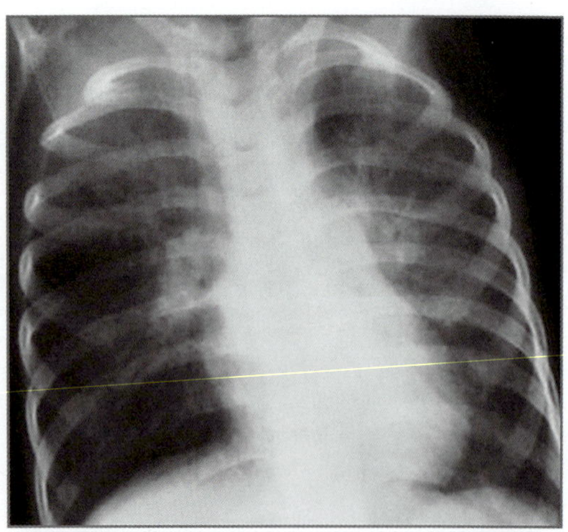

FIG. 4: Interstitial viral pneumonia. Chest radiograph showing bilateral poorly defined linear and nodular shadowing radiating from the hila with hyperinflated lung fields.

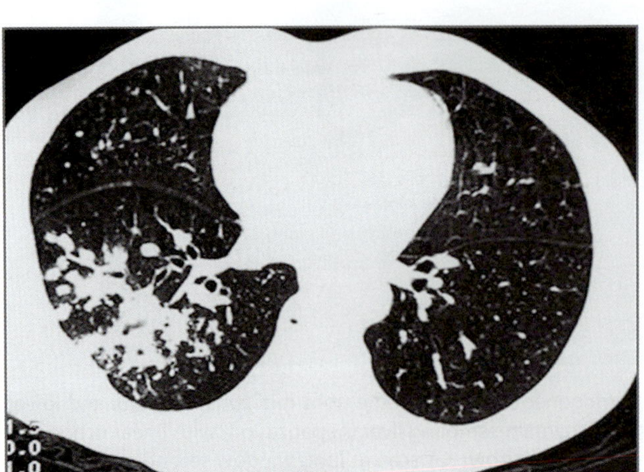

FIG. 3: Bronchopneumonia. CT scan shows acinar and centrilobular nodules along with lobular consolidation in the right lower lobe.
(CT: computed tomography)

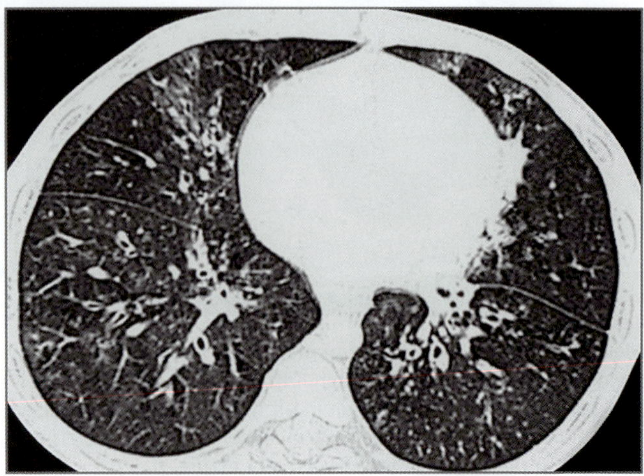

FIG. 5: Interstitial pattern of pneumonia. CT scan in a case of viral pneumonia shows focal areas of ground-glass attenuation with peribronchial thickening and centrilobular nodules.
(CT: computed tomography)

In *interstitial pneumonia*, the infection results in diffuse edema of the airway walls along with inflammatory cellular infiltration, which extends from the peribronchial tissues into the interlobular septa. The usual causes of acute interstitial pneumonia are viral or *Chlamydia pneumoniae* and *Mycoplasma pneumoniae* infection.

The chest radiographs show generalized hyperaeration, widespread peribronchial thickening, increased reticular markings, or small ill-defined nodules **(Fig. 4)**. On CT, the lesions are seen to be distributed in the central zone of the lung as well as middle and outer zones. There is a thickening of bronchial walls, centrilobular shadows, acinar, and lobular shadows **(Fig. 5)**. A predominantly ground-glass pattern and linear, reticular shadows or patchy consolidation may be seen.[11]

A *nodular pattern* may sometimes be seen as presence of random nodules in the lung parenchyma, which can occur due to hematogenous spread of disease or granulomatous infection **(Figs. 6A and B)**. Miliary TB, septic emboli, varicella zoster, and some fungal infections can show a nodular pattern of lung infection.

In practice, these patterns may be of limited use as the radiological appearance may be indeterminate, the pathological and radiological classification can be varied, and the pattern produced by various organisms often may not be constant.[14]

A *spherical or round pneumonia* is a well-circumscribed rounded consolidation, often streptococcal in origin, which mimics a mass lesion.[15] It is seen more commonly in children and involves the posterior segment of the lower lobes. It is thought to represent an early manifestation of the infectious focus that has spread centrifugally. An alternative theory is that round pneumonia occurs in children because of the underdeveloped pores of Kohn and the absence of

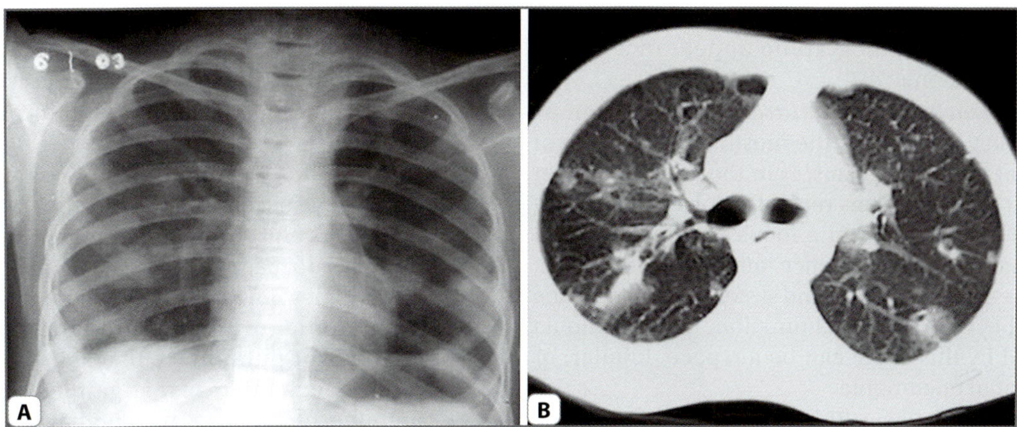

FIGS. 6A AND B: (A) Septic emboli seen as multiple nodular opacities scattered in both lung fields on a chest radiograph. (B) CT scan shows multiple nodular densities scattered in both lung fields, showing the "feeding vessel" sign. Few of the nodules show evidence of cavitation.

(CT: computed tomography)

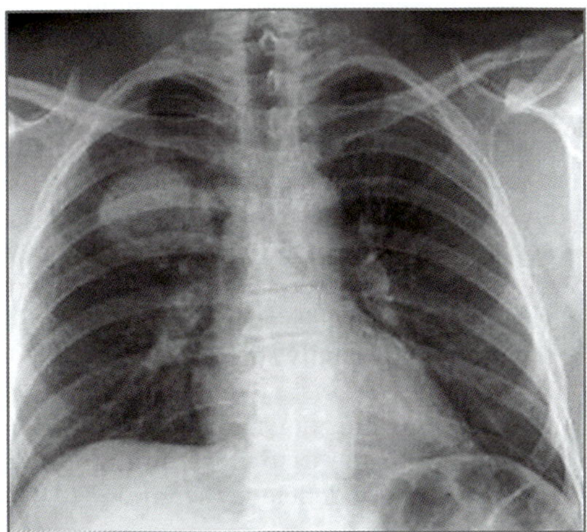

FIG. 7: Round pneumonia. Chest radiograph shows a rounded opacity in the right upper lobe containing an air bronchogram.

TABLE 2: Factors affecting the pathogenesis of pneumonia.

Inherent properties of the organism	• Virulence • Site of invasion • Mode of invasion
Route of entry	• Tracheobronchial route • Bloodstream • Direct spread from adjoining structures
Host factors	• Age • Immune status • Underlying lung disease • Systemic conditions • Aspiration pneumonia
Environmental factors	• Community-acquired pneumonia • Nosocomial pneumonia • Infections in returning travelers

canals of Lambert, which limits the spread of the organism and results in a focal, round mass seen on radiographs and CT scans. As adults have fully developed canals of Lambert, this theory can also explain why round pneumonia is seen less often in adults.[16]

On chest radiographs, the appearance of round pneumonia can vary from a small dense mass to a large ill-defined rounded opacity **(Fig. 7)**. Margins may be smooth, irregular, lobulated, or even occasionally spiculated.[17] Air bronchograms can be seen in some cases but they are not specific for an infective process.

On CT scans, round pneumonia is seen as a heterogeneous mass of soft tissue attenuation that can have spicules, air bronchograms, pleural thickening, and satellite lesions. The last two findings are found to be the most useful for diagnosis, while the presence or absence of air bronchograms does not help in distinguishing between malignancy and round pneumonia. Comparison with prior recent radiographs and short-term (3–7 days) interval follow-up are very useful in establishing the correct diagnosis.[15,17]

ETIOPATHOGENESIS OF PULMONARY INFECTIONS

The radiological manifestations of pneumonia are based on the etiopathological factors **(Table 2)**.[18] The type of pneumonic pattern and the consequent radiographic pattern are dependent on:

- The specific inherent properties of the organism, i.e., its virulence, its site of action, and its mode of action, e.g., the staphylococcal bacteria cause marked destruction and abscess formation; *Klebsiella* leads to a more productive type of inflammation; a fungal or tubercular infection evokes a granulomatous response, etc.

- The route of entry of the organism has a significant influence on the radiographic appearance of the resulting pneumonia:
  - *Via the tracheobronchial tree*: By inhalation or aspiration. Inhalation, the most common route of entry of microorganisms, is in the form of droplet nuclei. The organisms reach the lower respiratory tract where they form a focus of infection, and depending on the virulence, amount of inoculum, and the state of the local and systemic defense of the host, they can cause inflammation. The pneumonia caused by this route can be airspace, lobular, or interstitial pneumonia.
  - *Via the bloodstream*: This kind of spread normally occurs in conjunction with an extrapulmonary source of infection that causes septicemia, which in turn localizes in the lung. Radiographically, this is a random, patchy distribution with increased involvement of the basal segments due to preferential gravity-related blood flow.
  - *Via direct spread* from infective lesions in the chest wall, across the diaphragm, and from the mediastinum. The disease is usually localized to an area contiguous to the source and generally leads to the formation of an abscess.
- Certain host factors also alter the classical appearance of a given pneumonia due to specific organisms and should be evaluated to help narrow the radiographic differential diagnosis:
  - *Age*: In newborns, infection can be congenital or acquired.[19] Congenital infection is generally viral if due to transplacental spread. The acquired type is more often bacterial. Children are prone to respiratory infections with bronchiolitis and pneumonia as the common manifestations and are usually caused by viruses. In adults, streptococcal pneumonia is the leading cause. In young adults, other common causes are viral or mycoplasma-related.
  - *Immune status*: Immunosuppressed patients are unusually susceptible to infection with common pathogens and several microorganisms, which are normally not pathogenic, e.g., *Pneumocystis jirovecii* and cytomegalovirus (CMV). Differentiation between pneumonia, drug reaction, and parenchymal changes of pulmonary disease is difficult and often needs other investigations. Infections in immunocompromised patients have been discussed in detail in the next chapter.
  - *Underlying lung disease*: A decrease in local resistance or a local obstruction leads to increased incidence of infection, e.g., bronchiectasis, sequestrated lung, or chronic obstructive diseases.

    In emphysematous lungs, the pulmonary infection can often assume bizarre radiographic patterns due to the distorted emphysematous pulmonary parenchyma.[20] The consolidation appears to have multiple cavities due to the underlying low attenuation emphysematous areas giving rise to a "Swiss cheese appearance" **(Figs. 8A to C)**. These pseudocavities and pseudohoneycombing should be differentiated from true cavities and honeycombing. Resolution is often delayed in pneumonia associated with pulmonary emphysema.[21]
  - *Systemic conditions*: Diseases associated with increased lung infections are diabetes, alcoholism, connective tissue disorders, malignancy, and acquired immunodeficiency syndrome (AIDS).

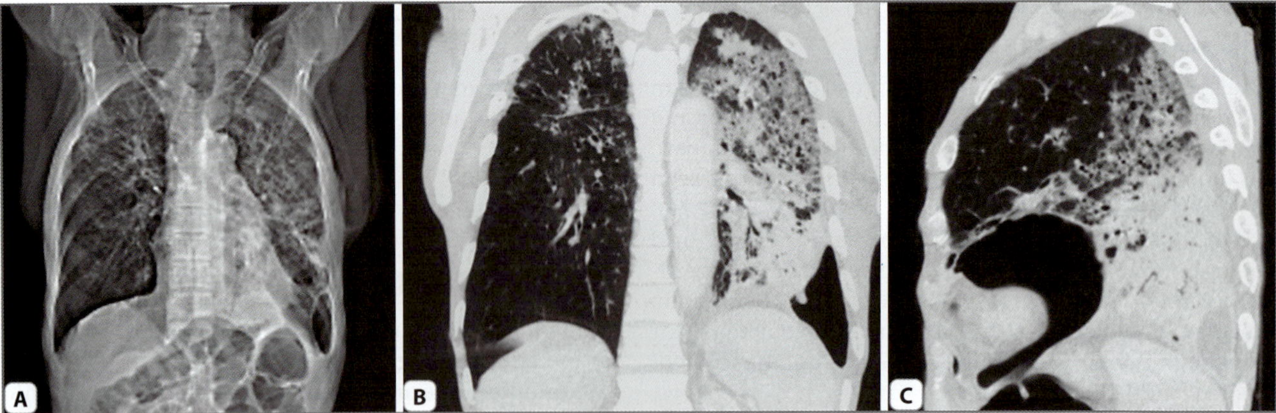

FIGS. 8A TO C: Topogram (A) shows bilateral patchy opacities with a loculated left pneumothorax in a 60-year-old patient with emphysematous lungs. Coronal (B) and sagittal (C) CECT images show dense consolidation with air bronchogram in the left lower lobe, segmental consolidation in the left upper lobe showing multiple small cysts within (Swiss cheese appearance), due to underlying centriacinar emphysematous changes with an associated small left pneumothorax. Few ground-glass opacities and apical nodular opacities were seen in the right lung.

(CECT: contrast-enhanced computed tomography)

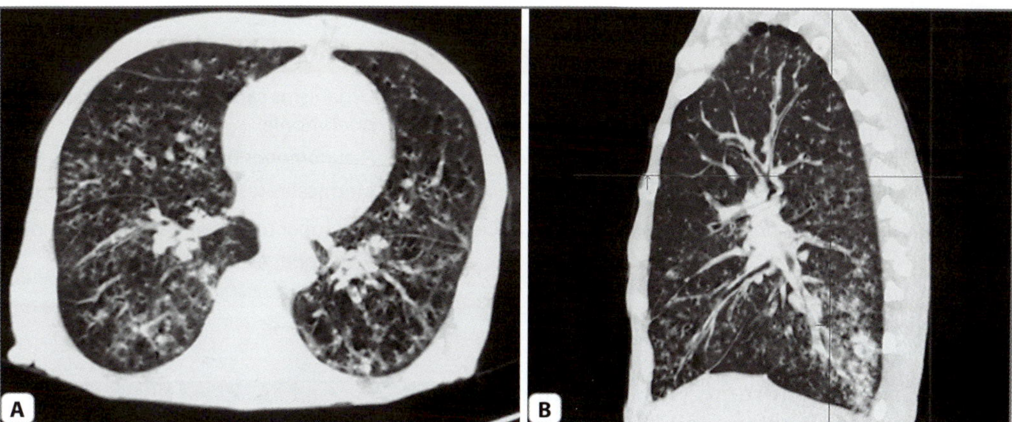

FIGS. 9A AND B: Axial (A) and sagittal CT images, (B) Aspiration pneumonia—In a patient with carcinoma tongue, multiple confluent centriacinar opacities were seen in the posterior aspect of bilateral lower lobes and posterior segment of upper lobes, consequent to aspiration.

- *Aspiration pneumonia* occurs in patients with impaired consciousness, chronic debilitating diseases, structural abnormalities of the pharynx and esophagus, neuromuscular disorders, impaired swallowing mechanisms, indwelling tracheal or esophageal/gastric tubes, and in postoperative patients, due to inhalation of bacteria, food, gastric contents, etc., leading to parenchymal inflammation or edema. It has several different pathophysiological aspects—bacterial pneumonia caused by the oral flora, chemical pneumonitis by gastric acid or exogenous lipids such as paraffin liquid, and granulomatous reaction to foreign bodies. It occurs in the gravity-dependent portions of the lung, so in recumbent patients, it involves the posterior segment of the upper lobes and the superior segment of the lower lobes, whereas in an erect patient, aspiration is more likely to involve bilateral basal segments, middle lobe, and lingular lobe. On imaging, it is often seen as a bronchopneumonia or bronchiolitis pattern **(Figs. 9A and B)**. Aspirated material may sometimes be seen in the bronchial lumen. A lung abscess may also be seen in bacterial aspiration.[22]

- Environmental factors:
  - *Community-acquired pneumonia (CAP)* is defined as a lower respiratory tract infection acquired by a patient in a nonhospitalized setting, which is associated with clinical symptoms of acute infection and new opacities depicted on a chest radiograph, if one is obtained. It can be typical or atypical. The etiological causes of CAP are listed in **Table 3**.[23]
  - *Nosocomial infections (HAP and VAP)*: Hospital-acquired pneumonia (HAP) is defined as pneumonia that develops in patients during their hospital stay, typically 48 hours or more after admission. It is not present or incubating at the time of hospital admission.

TABLE 3: Common causative organisms of community-acquired pneumonia.[23]

Bacteria	*Streptococcus pneumoniae, Staphylococcus aureus, Chlamydia pneumoniae, Mycoplasma pneumoniae, Haemophilus influenzae, Klebsiella pneumoniae, Streptococcus pyogenes, Legionella pneumophila, Mycobacterium tuberculosis*, etc.
Viruses	Influenza virus, parainfluenza virus, respiratory syncytial virus, varicella-zoster virus, adenovirus coronavirus, etc.

Ventilator-acquired pneumonia (VAP) is defined as pneumonia occurring >48 hours after endotracheal intubation.

It is paradoxical but true that pneumonia is more likely to occur in patients who are admitted to a hospital. This is because of the ease with which hospital strains of staphylococci and gram-negative bacilli can be acquired from other patients, hospital staff, or inhalation therapy machines. Also, the frequent use of antibiotics in hospitalized patients suppresses the growth of normal respiratory flora, greatly increasing the susceptibility of treated patients to infection.[19] Causal organisms depend on the onset of disease and host conditions **(Table 4)**.[24] A variety of radiographic patterns are seen, including airspace, interstitial, and mixed compounding the problem. It is often difficult to distinguish atelectasis from HAP, and the two may coexist, although atelectasis often develops rapidly and may resolve rapidly.[25] The incidence of pneumonia in ventilated patients (VAP) can be as high as 20% with a high mortality rate.

Diagnosing pneumonia in ventilated or postoperative patients can be difficult. Portable chest radiography may not show basal consolidation in approximately one-fourth of patients following abdominal surgery.[26] Pneumonia, edema, acute

TABLE 4: Causative organisms of nosocomial pneumonia.[24]

	Early onset (within 48–72 hours)	Late onset (>72 hours)
Hospital-acquired pneumonia (HAP)	• *Haemophilus influenzae, Streptococcus pneumoniae,* • Methicillin-sensitive *Staphylococcus aureus* (MSSA), Enterobacteriaceae (*Klebsiella, Escherichia coli, Serratia*), anaerobes, *Legionella*	• Organisms same as in early-onset hospital-acquired pneumonia, • *Pseudomonas aeruginosa,* • Methicillin-resistant *Staphylococcus aureus* (MRSA)
Ventilator-acquired pneumonia (VAP)	• *Streptococcus pneumoniae, Haemophilus influenzae,* MSSA, • Enterobacteriaceae	• Enterobacteriaceae, *Pseudomonas aeruginosa*, MRSA • *Acinetobacter* species

respiratory distress syndrome (ARDS), drug toxicity, atelectasis, infarction, and hemorrhage have overlapping signs, so a confident diagnosis based on radiographic features alone is often impossible.[25,27] In patients with ARDS, CT may reveal areas of cavitation or empyema, not seen on chest radiographs and are suggestive of coexisting infection.[28] The use of ultrasound in correlation with clinical findings makes it an ideal tool for rapid diagnosis, especially in situations with unstable patients.

- *Infections in returning international travelers*: Some pathogens are related to specific geographic regions and locations. Travel to these regions may result in contracting travel-related pulmonary diseases. Risk depends upon travel destination, activities undertaken, and length of stay. A high degree of clinical suspicion is of paramount importance in early diagnosis.[29]

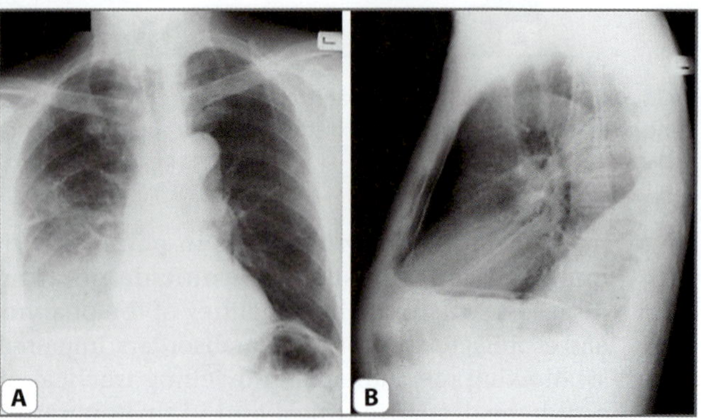

FIGS. 10A AND B: Chest radiographs PA view (A) and lateral view, (B) Streptococcal pneumonia involving the entire right lower lobe.

SPECIFIC PNEUMONIA

Bacterial Infections

Streptococcal Pneumonia

Streptococcal pneumonia is caused by *Streptococcus pneumoniae* and is the most common CAP, affecting individuals of all ages. It typically presents with a sudden onset of fever, chills, cough, and chest pain, often associated with bloody or rusty sputum. The infection initially affects the terminal airways before spreading to the surrounding segments, giving rise to the classical pattern of unilateral airspace pneumonia **(Figs. 1 and 10)**. An air bronchogram is frequently observed, which is a characteristic feature **(Fig. 11)**. The volume of the lobe usually remains unchanged.

Classically, it causes a lobar pattern of consolidation but may sometimes even have a bronchopneumonic or interstitial pattern.[30] Occasionally, early during the disease, a spherical or round pneumonia may be seen, particularly in children. One study that investigated the radiographic appearance in 81 admitted patients with culture-documented pneumococcal pneumonia demonstrated a lobar pattern of consolidation in 81% of patients. Lobar consolidation was focal in 48% and multifocal in 33%. A bronchopneumonic pattern was seen in 19% of cases.[31]

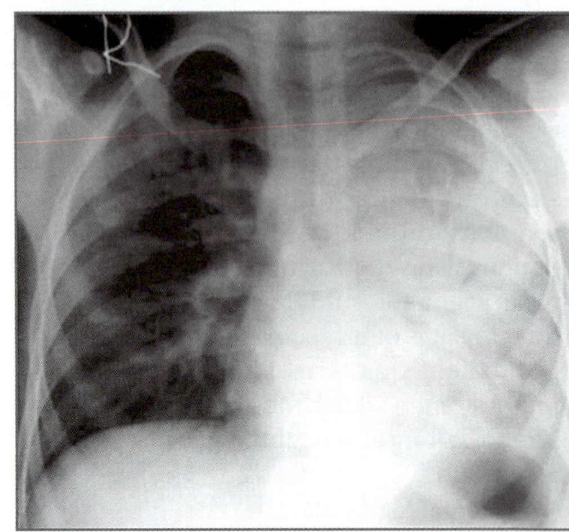

FIG. 11: Pneumococcal pneumonia involving almost the entire left lung with air bronchogram seen within.

Associated small pleural effusions may sometimes be seen, but empyema and cavitation are distinctly unusual. A very rare complication is pulmonary gangrene. Uncomplicated infection usually shows complete radiographic clearance within 10–14 days of appropriate treatment. The presence of multilobar disease is associated with increased morbidity and mortality.

Staphylococcal Pneumonia

It is caused by *Staphylococcus aureus*. The infection follows the aspiration of organisms from the upper respiratory tract, occurring particularly in hospitalized patients. Staphylococcal pneumonia may be community-acquired, particularly in infants and elderly individuals, often complicating influenza. Infection can also occur because of staphylococcal bacteremia.

The chest radiograph typically shows a bronchopneumonic pattern, initially involving the lower zones **(Figs. 2 and 12)**. The consolidation can spread rapidly and become confluent, resembling lobar pneumonia. Volume loss, early and large effusions, empyema, and abscess formation are common **(Figs. 13A to D)**. Resolution is generally slower than streptococcal infections, and residual fibrosis can occur. Pneumatoceles, seen as thin-walled air-filled cysts **(Figs. 14A to C)**, can appear during the first week of infection, mostly seen in children, and may lead to pneumothorax.[32]

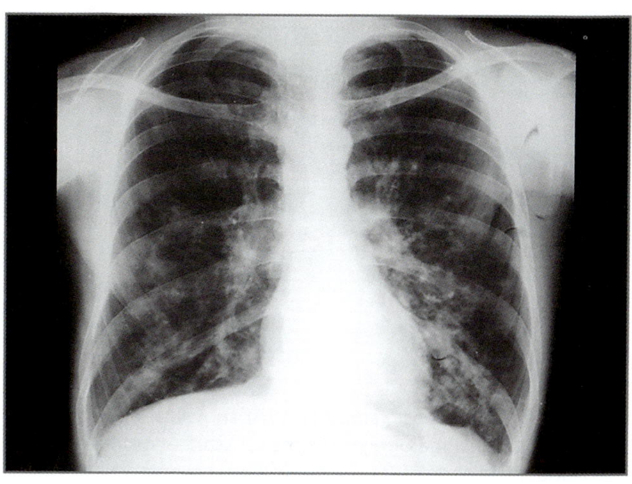

FIG. 12: Staphylococcal pneumonia showing patchy opacities in bilateral lung fields on background of emphysema.

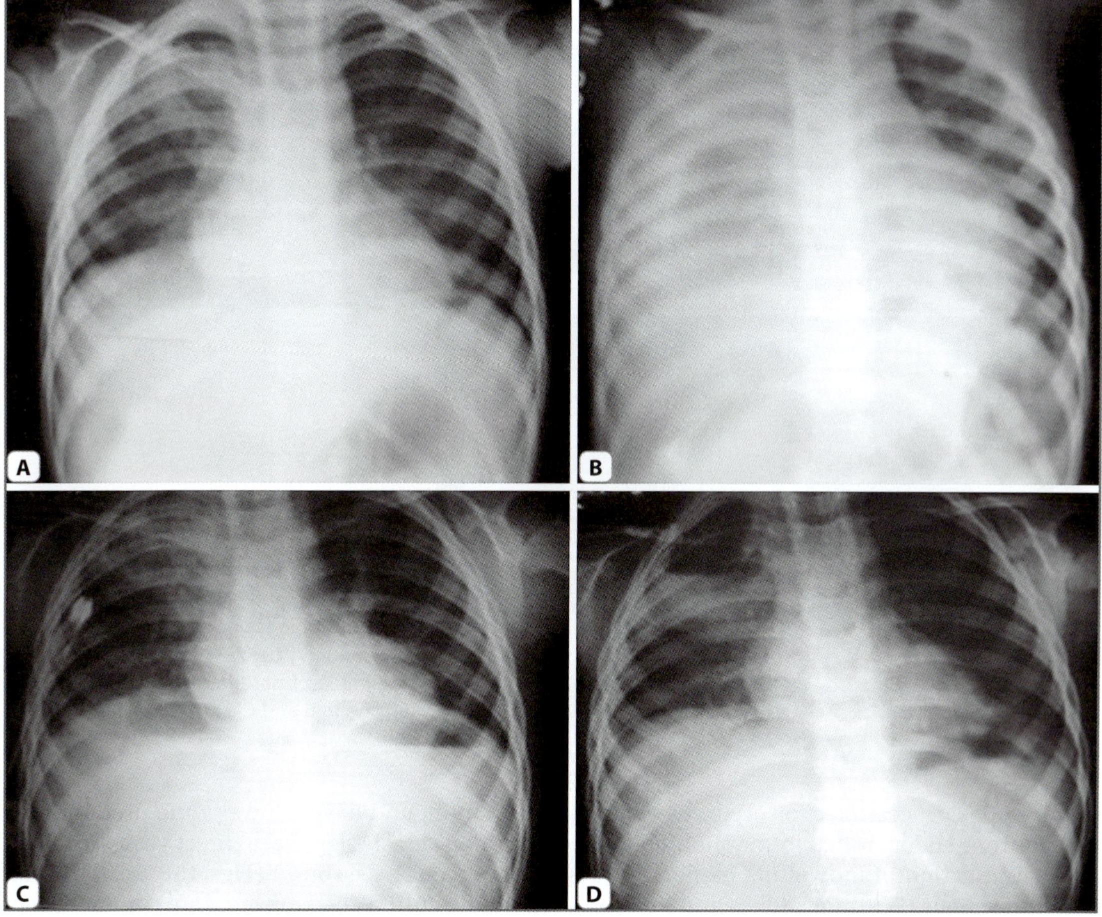

FIGS. 13A TO D: Serial chest radiographs of a 5-year-old child with complicated staphylococcal pneumonia. (A) Areas of patchy consolidation in the right lung with evidence of volume loss. (B) Three days later—complete opacification of right hemithorax was seen. A chest tube was inserted, which drained pus. (C) Chest radiograph taken 2 days after chest tube insertion shows almost complete clearing of the empyema; however, there is an increase in the underlying patchy consolidation in the right upper zone. (D) An abscess has developed in the right upper lobe.

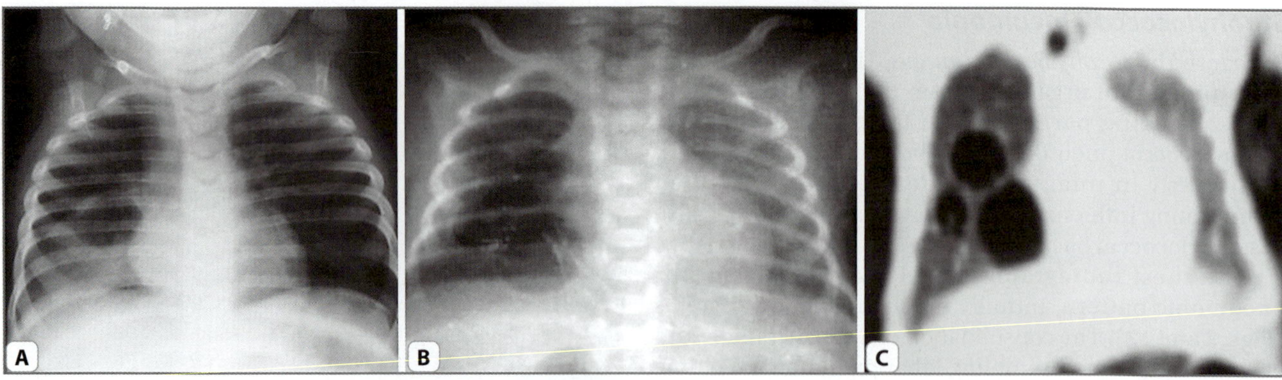

FIGS. 14A TO C: Chest radiograph (A) shows pneumatocele formation in a right lower lobe consolidation due to staphylococcal pneumonia. Chest radiograph, (B) and CT scan—coronal reconstruction, (C) in another infant showing multiple residual pneumatoceles following an episode of staphylococcal pneumonia.

(CT: computed tomography)

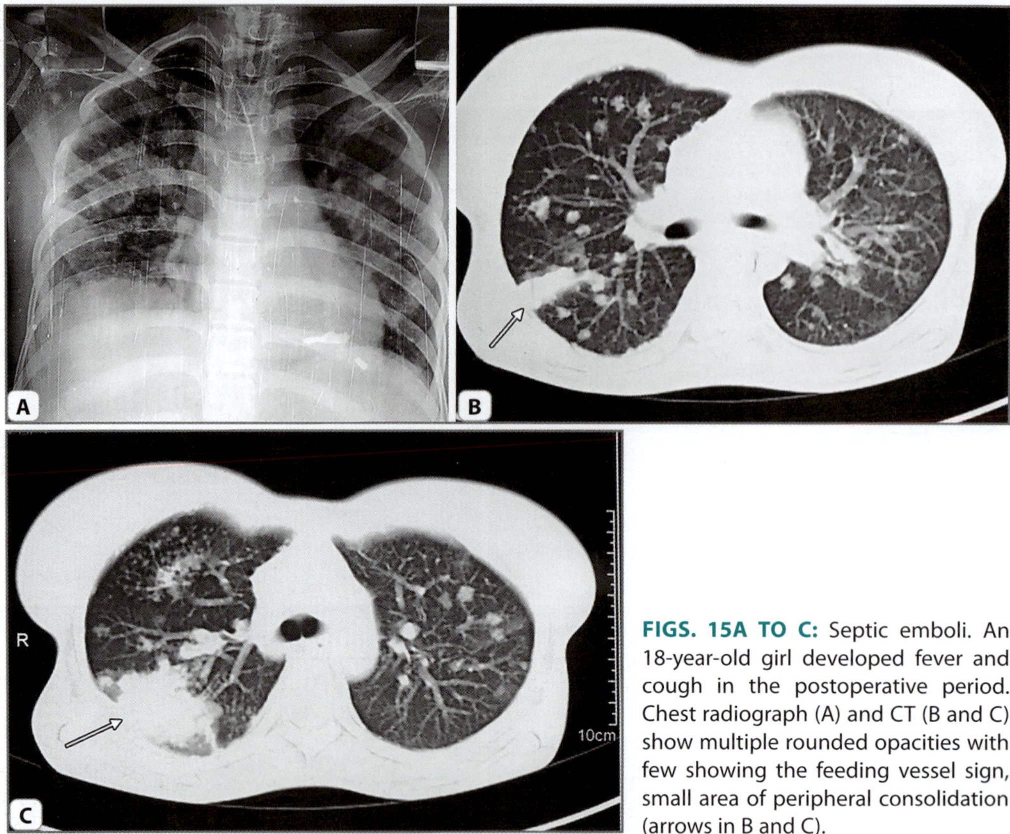

FIGS. 15A TO C: Septic emboli. An 18-year-old girl developed fever and cough in the postoperative period. Chest radiograph (A) and CT (B and C) show multiple rounded opacities with few showing the feeding vessel sign, small area of peripheral consolidation (arrows in B and C).

Septicemic staphylococcal infection occurs by hematogenous spread from endocarditis, thrombophlebitis, or staphylococcal infection of indwelling catheters. It is also seen in intravenous (IV) drug addicts and immunocompromised patients. The usual radiographic and CT appearance is that of multiple pulmonary opacities **(Figs. 7 and 15)**. CT often shows more lesions than plain radiographs. The opacities may be of varying sizes, generally round (sometimes wedge-shaped or irregular), often show cavitation, and have a lower zone predominance.[33] The "feeding vessel" sign, i.e. a direct vessel leading up to the opacity can be seen on CT **(Figs. 15B and C)**. Accompanying pleural effusion and empyema are common features.

Gram-negative Pneumonias

These are caused by a great variety of organisms, the most important being the Enterobacteriaceae (notably

Klebsiella, *Enterobacter*, *Escherichia coli*, and *Proteus mirabilis*), *Pseudomonas aeruginosa*, *Acinetobacter*, and *Haemophilus influenzae*. They are the most important cause of nosocomial infections and a major cause of morbidity and mortality in the hospital setup. Very often, the affected patients have a known predisposing factor such as chronic obstructive pulmonary disease, a major medical condition like diabetes, or history of recent surgery.

The organisms most commonly enter the lungs by aspiration, but pneumonia following inhalation of bacteria or spread by bloodstream can also be seen. Aspiration is particularly important because the carriage of gram-negative organisms in the upper respiratory tract is greatly increased in debilitated patients in hospital.[14] The radiographic pattern is entirely nonspecific and ranges from small ill-defined nodules to patchy consolidation, which may become confluent and resemble lobar pneumonia. Lower lobes tend to be predominantly affected; upper and middle lobe involvement may be seen in 50% of cases. Cavitation, pleural effusions, and empyema are quite commonly associated **(Figs. 16 and 17)**.

The pneumonia caused by *Klebsiella pneumoniae* (also known as Friedlander's pneumonia) differs from other gram-negative pneumonias in that it is not uncommonly acquired outside the hospital and usually affects people with chronic debilitating illnesses or alcoholism. The symptoms include high fever, toxemia, and resemble those of severe pneumococcal pneumonia. On chest radiography, the consolidations are also like those seen with *S. pneumoniae* pneumonia, i.e., a lobar pneumonia pattern. Klebsiella pneumonia has a tendency for the formation of voluminous inflammatory exudates leading to lobar expansion with resulting bulging of interlobar fissures **(Fig. 18)**, a greater tendency for abscess and cavity formation which are frequently multiple and large, and also a greater frequency of pleural effusion and empyema.[34]

Anaerobic Pneumonias

Anaerobic cases of pneumonia are caused by a variety of organisms that are normally found in the oropharynx but which are abnormally aspirated into the lung, including species of *Bacteroides*, *Clostridium*, *Fusobacterium*, *Peptococcus*, etc.[35] Most of these infections are polymicrobial. Predisposing factors such as a recent episode of altered consciousness, dysphagia, or alcoholism are frequent. The disease may be acute but is commonly subacute or chronic with prominent systemic symptoms and an indolent course.

Following aspiration, the chest radiograph is frequently normal initially. The appearance of abnormality is delayed for 24–72 hours. Three types of radiographic appearances may be seen—pulmonary parenchymal infection (bronchopulmonary pattern), pneumonia with cavitation or a discrete lung abscess, each of which may be

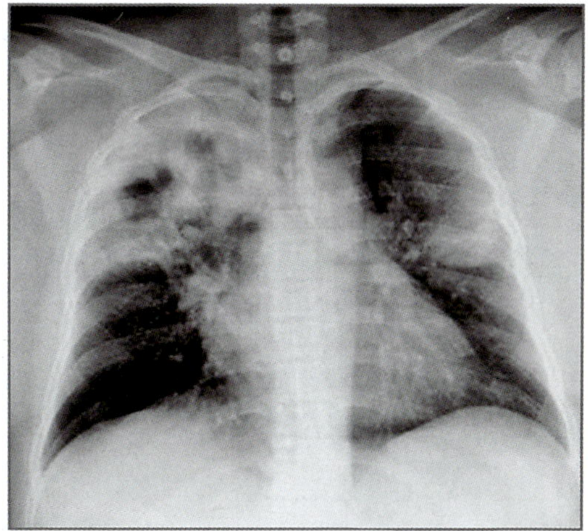

FIG. 16: Bilateral consolidation with extensive cavitation in the right upper lobe caused by gram-negative bacteria in a hospital setting.

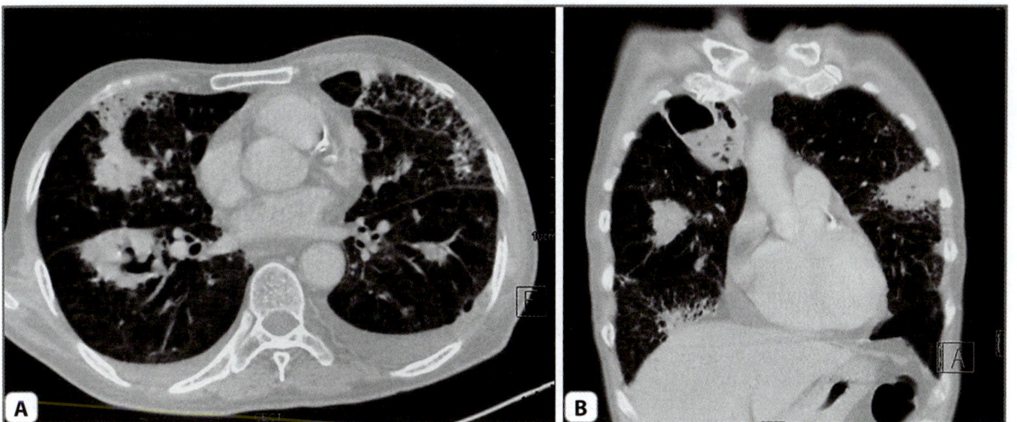

FIGS. 17A AND B: Axial (A) and coronal (B) CT showing multifocal areas of consolidation, bilateral ground-glass opacities, and bilateral pleural effusions in a 65-year-old patient with *Pseudomonas* pneumonia in a hospital setting. Cavitation is seen in some of the consolidated areas.

(CT: computed tomography)

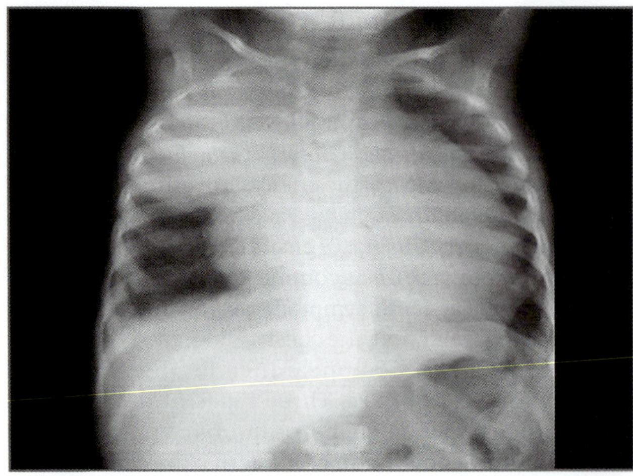

FIG. 18: Bulging fissure seen as downward convexity of the horizontal fissure in a case of consolidation of the right upper lobe with associated pleural effusion.

associated with empyema. These pneumonias commonly involve the superior and posterobasal segments of the lower lobe and/or posterior segment of the upper lobe due to drainage of infected material from the mouth into these segments as the patient lies on their back (gravitational pneumonia). Involvement may be unilateral or bilateral. Heterogeneous opacities may be seen in the involved lobes. Multiple cavities may be seen within the area of consolidation due to severe lung necrosis or the formation of lung abscesses.

The other manifestation of an anaerobic lung infection is a focal cavitary mass with very little surrounding consolidation—the so-called "primary lung abscess." The abscess may vary in size from 2 to 12 cm and characteristically has a thick, irregular wall **(Figs. 19 and 20)**. Hilar or mediastinal lymphadenopathy may accompany the lung abscess, and such cases may closely resemble lung carcinoma.[36] Empyema is a common complication; it

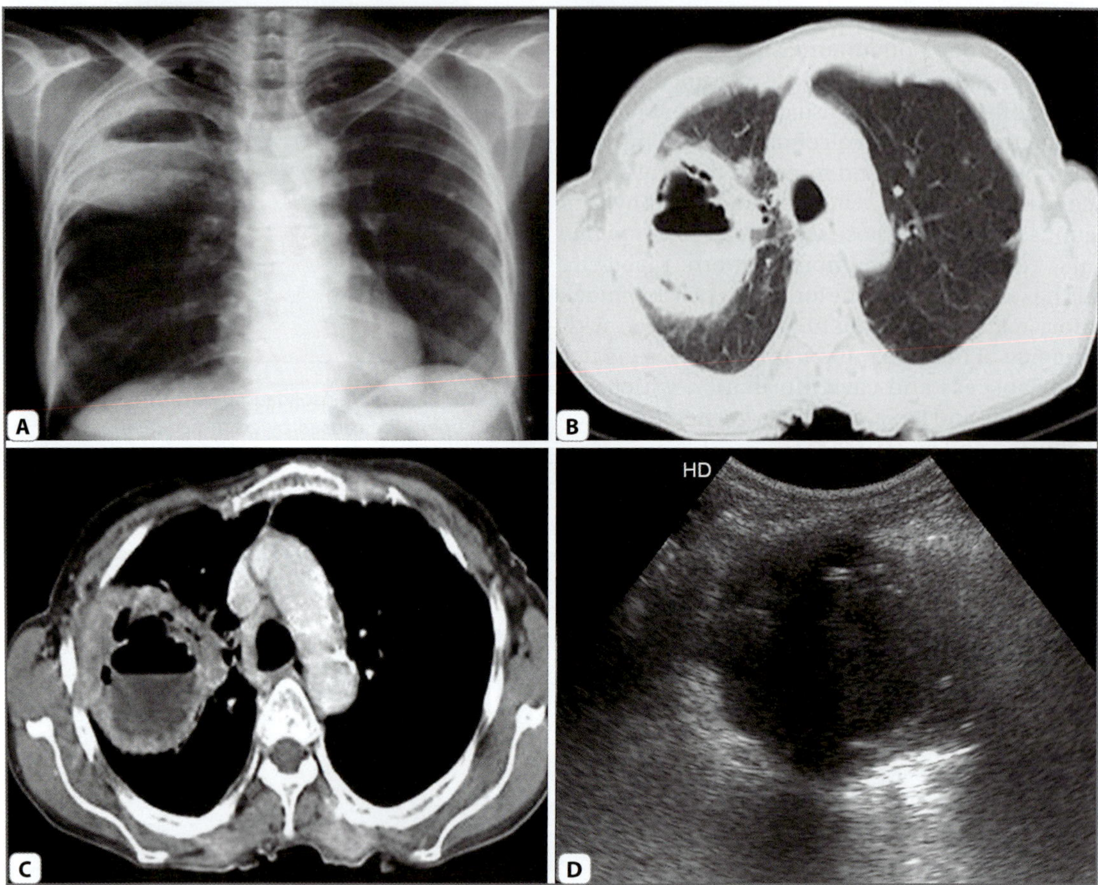

FIGS. 19A TO D: Anaerobic lung abscess in an alcoholic patient with poor orodental hygiene—Chest radiograph (A), CT scan at lung window settings (B), and mediastinal window settings (C). Lung abscess is seen in the posterior segment of the right upper lobe with thick irregular walls. Ultrasound image (D) shows the abscess as an irregularly walled lesion with anechoic contents. This abscess was aspirated under US guidance.

(CT: computed tomography; US: ultrasound)

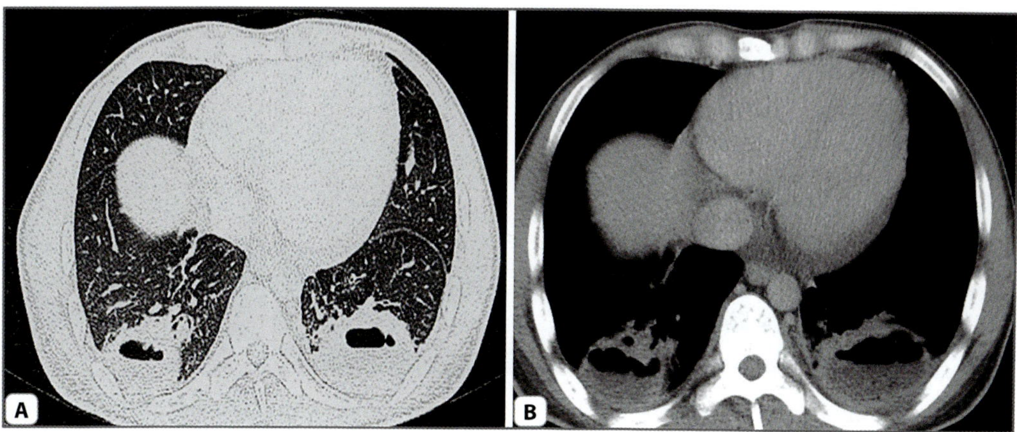

FIGS. 20A AND B: In a patient on ventilator, CT scan with lung window (A) and mediastinal window (B) settings shows bilateral thick-walled abscesses seen in the posterior aspects of both lower lobes.
(CT: computed tomography)

may be large and may occur with or without radiographic evidence of pneumonia.[37]

Actinomycosis

Although previously grouped with mycosis, *Actinomyces israelii* is now regarded as a branching bacterium. It causes infection of the lung by aspiration or direct extension from the abdomen or cervicofacial disease. The organism produces proteolytic enzymes that allow the infection to cross fascial planes. Therefore, pneumonia readily spreads to the pleura, producing empyema, and may spread extrapleurally to give rise to abscesses and sinus tracks in the chest wall, bones of the thorax, pericardium, and mediastinum.[38] The chest radiograph usually shows an area of nonsegmental airspace consolidation, commonly in the periphery of the lung and with a predilection for the lower lobes. If therapy is not instituted, an abscess may develop and infection may extend into the pleura. Pleural involvement manifests as pleural effusion, pleural thickening, or empyema formation but is seldom associated with large accumulations of fluid. Rib involvement causes lytic destruction with periostitis. Actinomycosis may also present as a mass, which can cavitate.[39] On CT, the typical findings are those of chronic low attenuation areas (representing actinomycotic or sulfur granules) with peripheral enhancement (representing granulation tissue in wall of abscess) and adjacent pleural thickening. CT can demonstrate chest wall, pleural, mediastinal, and spinal invasion to advantage.[40] Associated mediastinal lymphadenopathy may be present.

Atypical Pneumonia

Atypical pneumonia is caused by atypical bacteria such as *Mycoplasma pneumoniae*, *Chlamydophila pneumoniae*, and *Legionella pneumophila*. Some viral and fungal pathogens may also give rise to atypical pneumonia. Atypical CAP is characterized by prodromal upper airway symptoms, low-grade fever, myalgias, dry cough, and headache. There may also be associated extrapulmonary manifestations such as diarrhea, abdominal pain, arthritis, and facial rash. As the symptoms differ from those of typical pneumonia and are generally milder, they have been termed atypical pneumonias. The importance of the atypical pneumonias is not related to their frequency (~15% of CAPs) but to difficulties in their diagnosis and their nonresponse to beta-lactam therapy.

Mycoplasma Pneumonia

Mycoplasma pneumonia is caused by *Mycoplasma pneumoniae*, which is the smallest free-living organism, sharing some similarities with bacteria. It is a major nonbacterial cause of CAP in the 20–40 year age group. Spread is via droplets, and the symptoms resemble a viral rather than a bacterial infection. The definitive diagnosis is serological and therefore, delayed and often retrospective. The radiological findings are very variable; the most common pattern is unilateral lower lobe involvement, beginning as a patchy/nodular, peribronchial consolidation that progresses to become sublobar or lobar and homogeneous **(Figs. 21A to C)**.[18] Sometimes the initial features are those of an interstitial process with small, irregular nodules and linear shadows.[41] Slow progression of this pattern to that of a typical consolidation is very suggestive of a mycoplasmal infection. Pleural effusion generally does not occur, and cavitation is rare. Nodal enlargement is common in children and is an unusual, but recognized, finding in adults. The CT findings consist of centrilobular nodules and branching linear opacities in a patchy distribution, thickening of the bronchovascular bundles, and areas of lobular or segmental consolidation.[42]

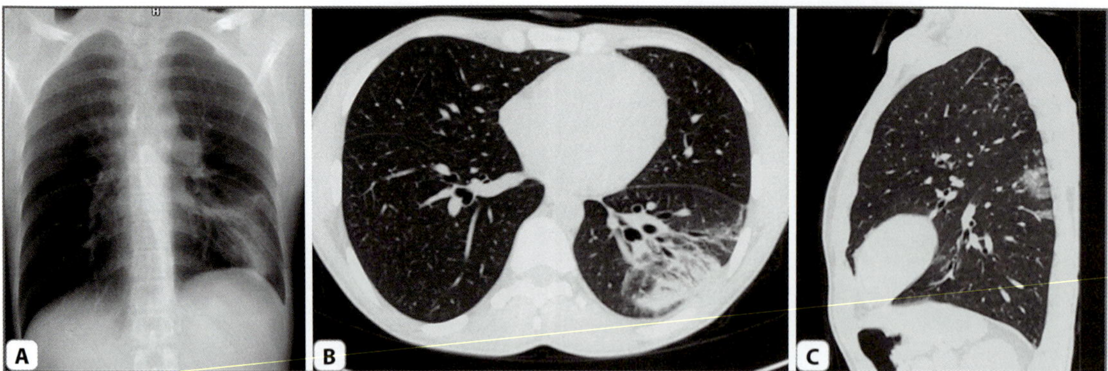

FIGS. 21A TO C: *Mycoplasma pneumoniae*. Chest radiograph (A) shows a homogeneous opacity in the left lower zone. CT scan at lung window settings axial (B) and sagittal reformat (C) shows a peripherally based airspace consolidation in the left lower lobe with air bronchogram.

(CT: computed tomography)

Chlamydia Pneumonia

Chlamydia pneumonia is caused by *Chlamydophila pneumoniae* and is a common cause of CAP. It often affects children and young adults. The radiographic findings are nonspecific with overlap of features with pneumonia from other organisms. The most common radiographic finding is airspace consolidation with interstitial infiltrates, combined interstitial and airspace infiltrates, and pleural effusion.[43] Lymphadenopathy and cavitation are not generally seen.

Legionella Pneumonia

Legionella pneumonia is also known as Legionnaires' disease. It is caused by infection with any *Legionella* species, most commonly by *Legionella pneumophila*. It is seen more often in middle-aged and older adults, smokers, and those with chronic illnesses or a weak immune system. Infection occurs due to inhalation of airborne microscopic sources of contaminated water. It can be more severe than the other atypical pneumonias. The radiographic appearances may often lag behind the clinical picture, and deterioration can be seen on imaging despite clinical improvement. The early radiographic and CT manifestations are nonspecific and similar to those found in CAP from other bacterial origin. The chest radiograph shows asymmetric airspace consolidation, more in the middle and lower zones. Pleural effusion and mediastinal lymphadenopathy may be seen in a few cases. On CT, there is lobar or multilobar consolidation with adjacent ground-glass haze.[44,45]

Viral Infections

Viruses are a major cause of respiratory tract infection in the community, particularly in children. The usual mode of spread is by transmission by droplets. In infants and young children who are immunocompetent, respiratory syncytial virus (RSV), parainfluenza virus, adenovirus, and influenza virus are the most common offenders, whereas in adults, influenza type A and B and adenovirus are more common.[46] Immunocompromised patients are susceptible to CMV and other herpes viruses.[47]

Viruses result in several forms of lower respiratory infections, which include tracheobronchitis, bronchiolitis, and pneumonia. Pneumonia usually begins in the distal bronchi and bronchioles, giving rise to the interstitial pattern of involvement. Parenchymal involvement initially involves the lung adjacent to the terminal and respiratory bronchioles but spread throughout the lobule can occur. In elderly patients, rapidly progressive pneumonia may occur, with diffuse alveolar damage leading to hemorrhagic pulmonary edema. Viral infections commonly predispose to secondary bacterial infection.

The imaging findings of viral pneumonias do not usually allow the diagnosis of a specific viral infection. Clinical features such as patient age, immune status, time of year, illness in other family members, community outbreaks, onset, severity and duration of symptoms, and the presence of a rash remain important aids in diagnosing viral pneumonia.

Chest radiograph shows reticular opacities that are often bilateral and diffuse in distribution. The associated bronchiolitis leads to hyperinflation of the lung fields **(Figs. 4 and 22)**. Presence of hilar lymphadenopathy is variable; it is common in measles pneumonia and infectious mononucleosis but rare with other viral pneumonias. Pleural effusions are not a prominent feature, although small ones do not negate the diagnosis. CT scan may show poorly defined airspace nodules (4–10 mm diameter), patchy areas of peribronchial ground-glass opacity, and consolidation along with hyperinflation **(Figs. 5 and 22C)**. The combination of CT findings varies somewhat between the individual viral pneumonias and has been summarized in **Table 5**.

The progressive form of pneumonia shows large areas of homogeneous or patchy, unilateral or bilateral airspace consolidation or poorly defined centrilobular nodules.[48]

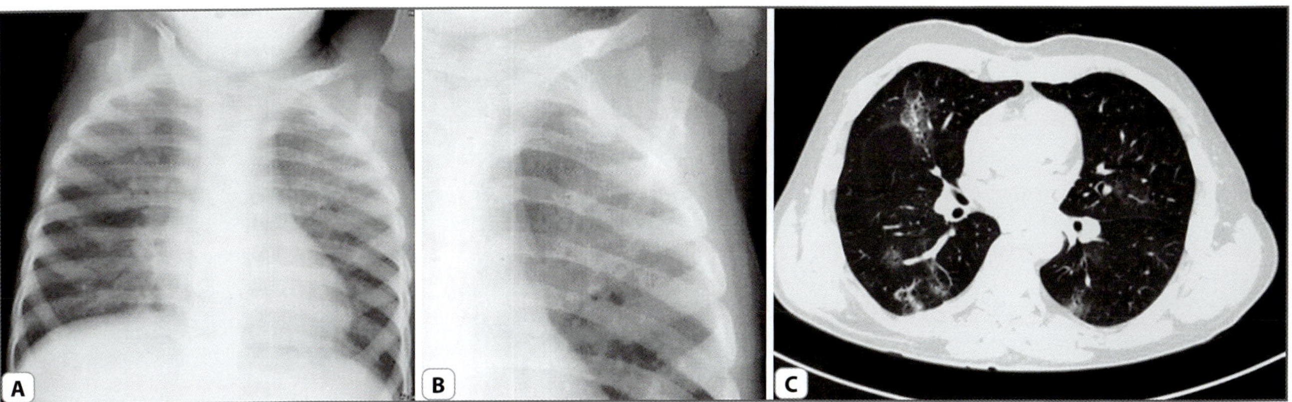

FIGS. 22A TO C: Viral pneumonia. Chest radiograph (A) with a magnified view of the left upper zone (B) shows hyperinflated lung fields with linear streaky opacities representing peribronchial thickening and nodular opacities. (C) Axial CT shows bilateral multifocal peripheral regions of ground-glass opacities in a case of nonspecific viral pneumonia.

(CT: computed tomography)

TABLE 5: Summary of CT findings in viral pneumonias.[46]

Cause of pneumonia	Lobar consolidation	Ground-glass opacity	Reticulo nodular opacities	Peribronchial cuffing	Pleural effusion
Influenza virus	++	+++	++	–	–
Parainfluenza virus	++	++	++	–	–
SARS-CoV-1	++	+++	++	–	–
SARS-CoV-2	++	+++	++	–	–
RSV	++	++	+++	+	+
Varicella-zoster virus	–	+	+++	+	–
Adenovirus	++	+	+	+	–

(SARS: severe acute respiratory syndrome; RSV: respiratory syncytial virus)

Influenza and Parainfluenza Virus

Infections with influenza virus occur in epidemics, pandemics, or sporadically. Influenza subtypes A and B are most commonly responsible for the severe outbreaks associated with pneumonia.

Swine flu is caused by a strain of human influenza A (H1N1) virus, which originated in Mexico in 2009 and spread to more than 190 countries, including India. In June 2009, the World Health Organization had declared it a level 6 (highest level) pandemic. The virus causes a wide spectrum of respiratory illnesses, which range from mild febrile illness to severe respiratory distress.[49] Symptoms include fever, dry cough, myalgia, and headache. The predominant radiological pattern in H1N1 pneumonia is bilateral ground-glass opacities and alveolar consolidation. The opacities are usually in the mid zones and bases in the chest radiograph, while on the CT they are mainly peripheral and peribronchovascular in distribution, with diffuse zonal involvement.[50] Pneumonia is more common in the very young, those over 65 years of age, in late pregnancy, and in those with underlying disease. Pleural effusion is rare.[48]

An acute form of pneumonia with rapid progression shows fast confluence of the consolidation caused by the diffuse alveolar damage, which may be homogeneous or irregular, unilateral or bilateral, giving rise to an ARDS type of picture **(Figs. 23 and 24)**.

Avian influenza or "bird flu" is caused by the H5N1 subtype of the influenza A virus. Human infection occurs because of close contact with infected birds, usually poultry or their products. Chest radiograph commonly shows multifocal consolidations. On CT, the most common findings consist of focal, multifocal, diffuse ground-glass opacities (GGOs), or areas of consolidation. Centrilobular nodules can be seen. There may be associated pseudocavitation, pneumatocele formation, and lymphadenopathy.[51]

Coronavirus

SARS-CoV-1

Severe acute respiratory syndrome (SARS) is caused by a coronavirus, the SARS-associated coronavirus (SARS-CoV-1). It was recognized as a global threat in March 2003, after first appearing in Southern China in November 2002. It leads to a systemic infection clinically manifesting as a progressive pneumonia. Chest radiograph and CT show focal unilateral or bilateral areas of GGO and/or consolidation.

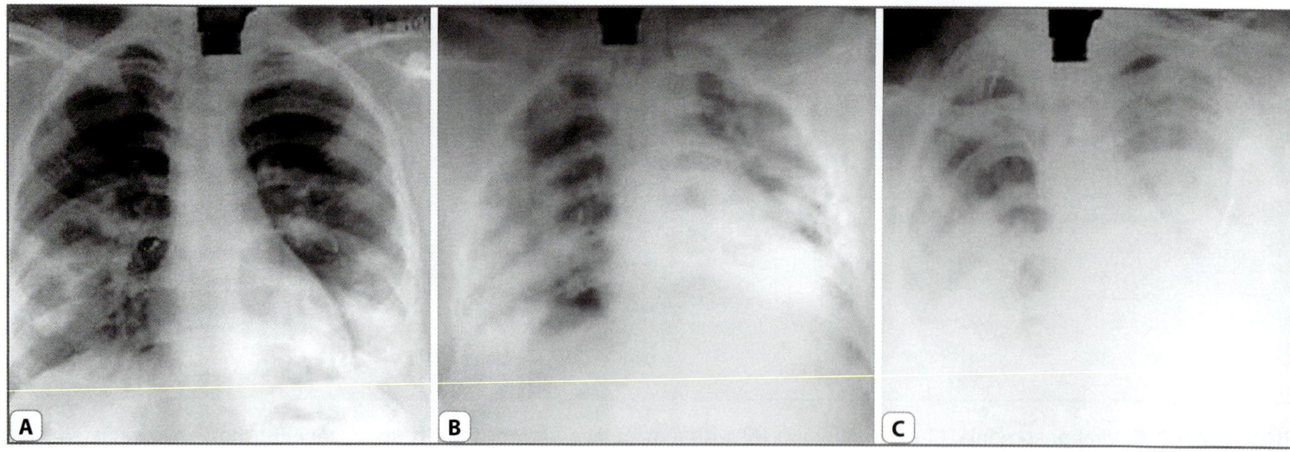

FIGS. 23A TO C: Serial radiographs of a 22-year-old female with swine flu. (A) At presentation areas of ill-defined consolidation are seen in the lower zones. (B) Three days later, there is an increase in the consolidation. (C) A further 3 days later there is extensive bilateral airspace consolidation like that seen in acute respiratory distress syndrome (ARDS).

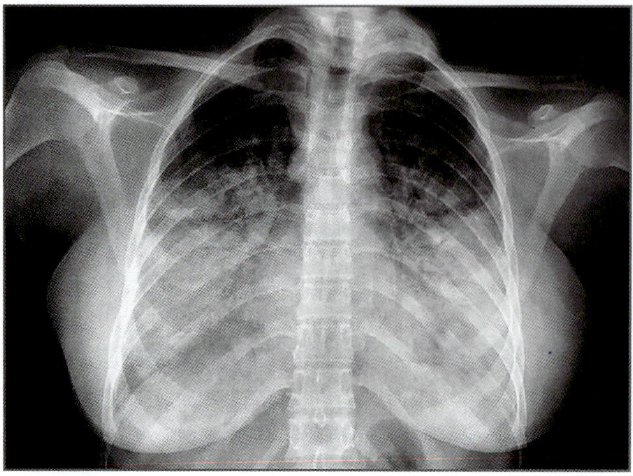

FIG. 24: Swine flu. Confluent fluffy opacities due to alveolar consolidation in bilateral mid and lower zones in a young girl with swine flu.

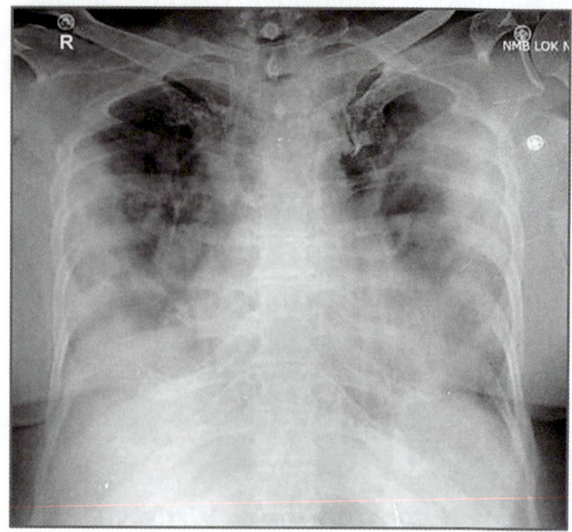

FIG. 25: Frontal chest radiograph in a 58-year-old COVID-19-positive patient shows multifocal peripheral areas of consolidation in bilateral lung fields with middle and lower zone predominance. These are typical features of COVID-19 pneumonia.

The areas of ground-glass opacity may be associated with thickening of the intralobular and interlobular septae.[14]

SARS-CoV-2

COVID-19 (coronavirus disease 2019) is a prime example of a global pandemic, starting from China in 2019 with worldwide spread. As of 2024, ~776 million people have been infected globally with over 7 million deaths.[52] COVID-19, caused by the SARS-CoV-2 virus, predominantly affects the lungs, although nonpulmonary manifestations are also common. While the diagnosis is definitively made through reverse transcription polymerase chain reaction (RT-PCR) testing, imaging provides essential insights, particularly in evaluating disease severity and ruling out other lung pathologies.

Chest radiology plays a pivotal role in the management of COVID-19, primarily in assessing the extent of pulmonary involvement, monitoring disease progression, identifying complications, and facilitating follow-up. Portable chest radiography is crucial in the care of critically ill, debilitated, and intensive care unit (ICU) patients, enabling rapid evaluation without requiring patient transport.

In the early or mild stages of COVID-19, radiographs may appear normal in up to 60% of cases, which means a normal radiograph does not rule out the infection. Chest radiographic findings typically become more apparent around 10–12 days after symptom onset, when the characteristic features of COVID-19 pneumonia emerge. These include bilateral, peripheral, and lower zone predominant airspace opacities, which appear as GGOs and/or consolidation **(Figs. 25 and 26)**. Multifocal bilateral consolidation in the lower lung zones is the most common and easily detectable finding, while subtle GGOs can be difficult to identify. Other possible radiographic findings include ill-defined nodular and linear opacities.[53] However, these features can overlap with other conditions, such as viral pneumonia, atypical bacterial pneumonia, noncardiogenic pulmonary edema, small vessel vasculitis causing alveolar hemorrhage, and drug-induced pneumonitis, necessitating careful differentiation.

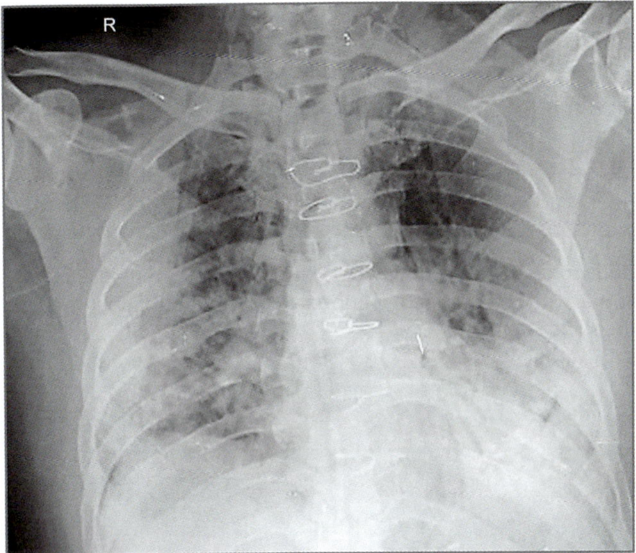

FIG. 26: Frontal chest radiograph in an adult COVID-19-positive patient shows typical pattern of multifocal peripherally distributed airspace consolidation in bilateral mid and lower lung zones.

Computed tomography imaging offers greater sensitivity than chest radiographs in detecting COVID-19-related abnormalities, and it is especially useful in cases where the diagnosis is uncertain or in advanced stages of disease **(Figs. 27A to E)**. It plays a critical role in predicting prognosis, assessing disease progression, and detecting complications such as secondary infections, fibrosis, or thromboembolic events. The typical CT findings in COVID-19 pneumonia include multifocal GGOs, often with a peripheral and subpleural distribution in the bilateral lung parenchyma **(Figs. 28A and B)**. As the disease progresses, patients may develop linear consolidations, and signs of organizing pneumonia, such as the characteristic "reverse halo" sign, particularly in the later stages of the disease **(Figs. 29A to L)**. Pleural effusion and lymphadenopathy are not usually seen.

The COVID-19 reporting and data system (CO-RADS) assessment scheme was developed by the Dutch Radiological Society in patients with moderate to severe symptoms of COVID-19.[54] It provides a level of suspicion for pulmonary involvement in patients suspected of having COVID-19 disease based on the features observed at noncontrast chest CT **(Table 6)**.

Computed tomography severity score was another algorithm that was proposed by Li et al. to standardize and quantify the radiological examinations for evaluating the severity of lung involvement.[55] The severity score is

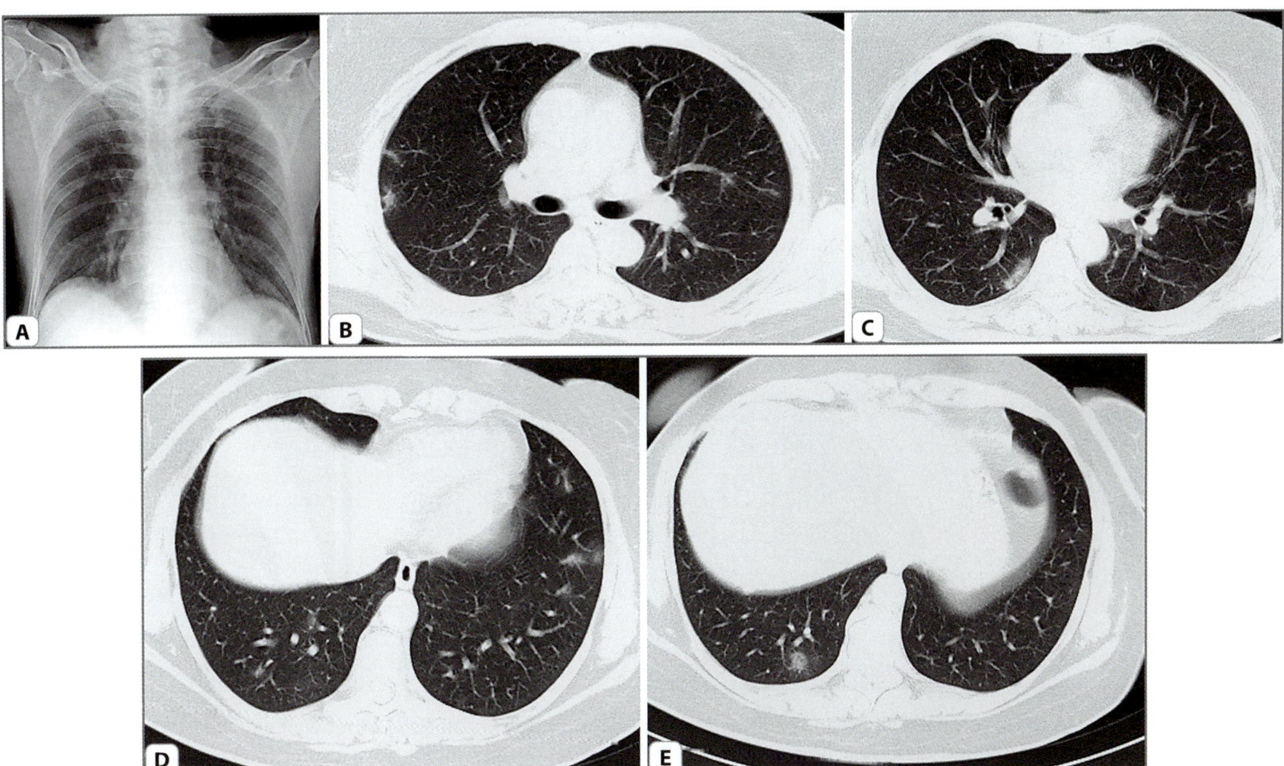

FIGS. 27A TO E: Frontal chest radiograph (A) in a 35-year-old COVID-19-positive patient appears unremarkable. Axial noncontrast CT chest images in lung window (B to E) of the same patient reveal few multifocal ground-glass opacities (arrows) in bilateral upper and lower lobes (CT severity score—4/25).

(CT: computed tomography)

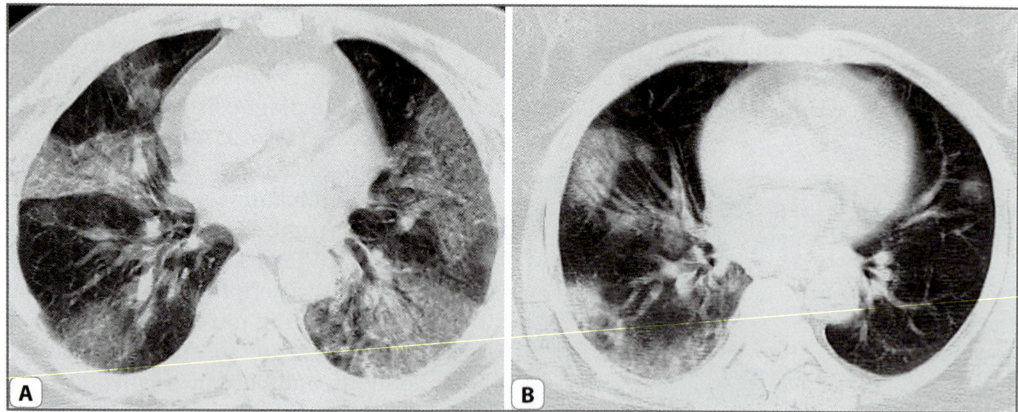

FIGS. 28A AND B: Axial noncontrast CT chest image in the lung window of a 70-year-old COVID-19 suspect shows multiple sharply marginated areas of ground-glass opacity in bilateral lung parenchyma with predominant peripheral distribution. Superimposed consolidation is also noted in some of the ground-glass opacities on the right side.

(CT: severity score)

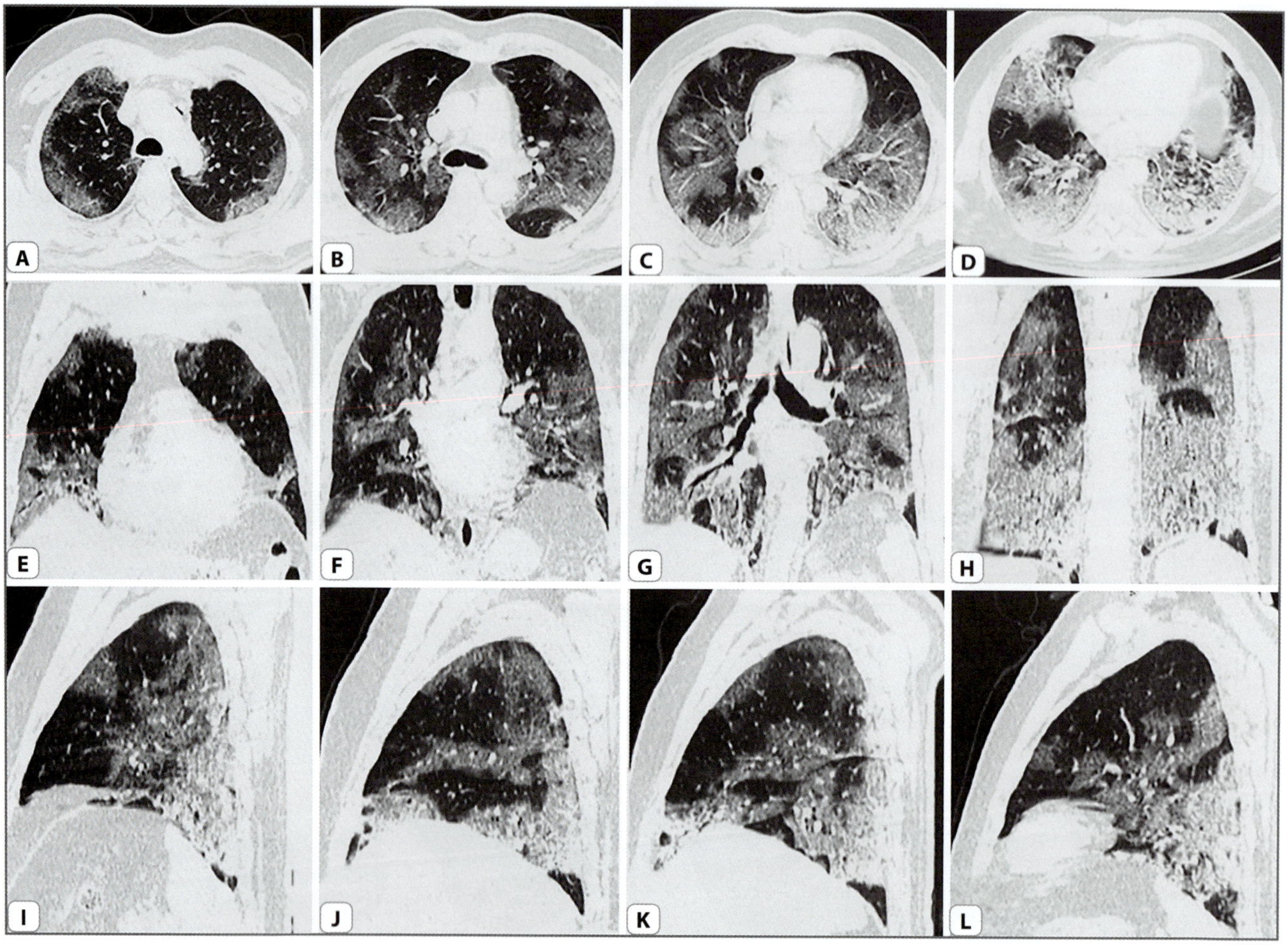

FIGS. 29A TO L: Axial (A to D), coronal (E to H), and sagittal (I to L) CT chest images in the lung window of a COVID-19-positive patient reveal multifocal peripheral ground-glass opacities with areas of consolidation and interlobular septal thickening in bilateral lung parenchyma, predominantly in bilateral lower lobes. The extent of lung involvement in each lobe was assessed subjectively and a CT score of 20/25 was assigned [right upper lobe-3 (25–50%), right middle lobe-4 (50–75%), right lower lobe-5 (>75%), left upper lobe-3 (25–50%), and left lower lobe-5 (>75%)].

(CT: computed tomography)

TABLE 6: CO-RADS categories with the corresponding level of suspicion for pulmonary involvement in COVID-19.

	Level of suspicion for pulmonary involvement of COVID-19	Summary
CO-RADS 0	Not interpretable	Scan technically insufficient for assigning a score
CO-RADS 1	Very low	Normal or noninfectious findings
CO-RADS 2	Low	Typical for other infections but not COVID-19
CO-RADS 3	Equivocal/unsure	Features compatible with COVID-19 that can also be found in other viral pneumonia or noninfectious diseases
CO-RADS 4	High	Typical for COVID-19 but have some overlap with other viral pneumonias. Findings are similar to CO-RADS 5 but with an atypical distribution
CO-RADS 5	High suspicion	Findings are typical for COVID-19 and can be divided into two groups, i.e., mandatory features and confirmatory patterns. *Mandatory features*: • Ground-glass opacities, with or without consolidation, near visceral pleural surfaces • Multifocal bilateral distribution *Confirmatory patterns*: • Ground-glass areas with sharp/unsharp demarcation outlining multiple adjacent secondary pulmonary lobules • Intralobular interstitial thickening with ground-glass opacities giving a "crazy paving" pattern • The pattern can evolve to resemble organizing pneumonia, giving the "reverse halo" sign with the presence of curvilinear subpleural bands
CO-RADS 6	Proven	RT-PCR positive for SARS-CoV-2

(CO-RADS: COVID-19 reporting and data system; RT-PCR: reverse transcription polymerase chain reaction; SARS-CoV-2: severe acute respiratory syndrome coronavirus 2)

calculated based on the assessment of the percentage of lung involvement for each patient and giving each lobe a score from 1 to 5. The final score is the sum of individual lobar scores and ranges from 0 to 25 points; a score of 0 corresponds to no parenchymal involvement, whereas a score of 25 corresponds to involvement of almost the entire lung parenchyma **(Table 7)**. This score was intended to find another objective method to identify significant radiological differences between severe and milder cases of COVID-19. This score has shown positive correlation with age, inflammatory biomarkers, severity of clinical categories, and disease phases. CT score ≥18 had shown to be highly predictive of patient mortality in short-term follow-up. The cutoff value for identifying severe cases of COVID-19 of CT score was 7, with the sensitivity and specificity of 80.0% and 82.8%, respectively **(Figs. 29A to L)**.

In the postrecovery phase of COVID-19, it is not uncommon to have patients presenting with long-term respiratory consequences such as breathlessness and/or hypoxia and deranged pulmonary function test (PFT) results due to fibrotic lung disease. CT imaging features such as bronchovascular bundle distortion, fibrotic stripes, traction bronchiectasis, architectural distortion, and interlobular septal thickening are suggestive of pulmonary fibrosis as seen in post-COVID condition (PCC) or long COVID **(Figs. 30A to C)**.[56]

TABLE 7: CT score based on the extent of lung involvement and severity of the disease.

Score	Percentage of lung involvement
1	<5% involvement
2	5–25% involvement
3	26–50% involvement
4	51–75% involvement
5	>75% involvement

(CT: computed tomography)

Middle East Respiratory Syndrome

Middle East respiratory syndrome (MERS) is a disease caused by the Middle East respiratory syndrome coronavirus (MERS-CoV). It was first detected in Saudi Arabia in September 2012 and spread to other countries by 2015. The spectrum of manifestations ranges from asymptomatic to involvement of upper respiratory tract, to pneumonia, respiratory failure, and multiple organ failure (MOF) resulting in death.[56] On chest radiograph, ground-glass opacity followed by consolidation can be seen. On CT, the lesions are primarily subpleural and involve lower lobes, with extensive consolidation and pleural effusion.[57]

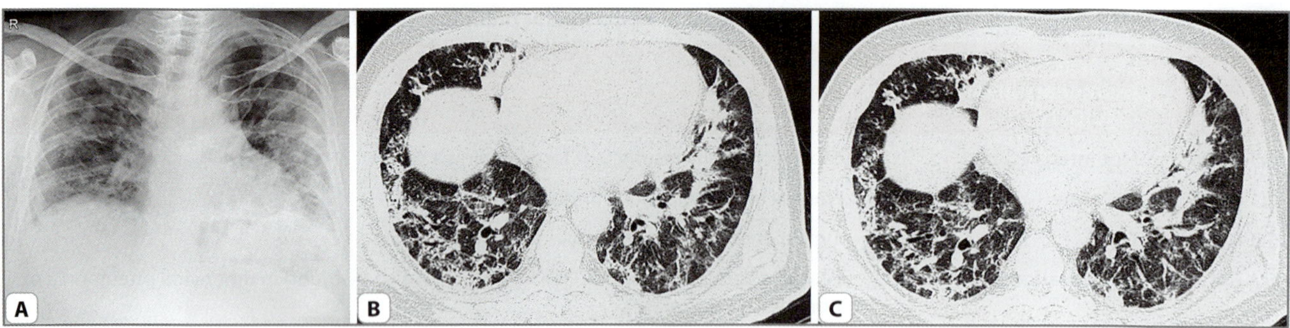

FIGS. 30A TO C: Frontal chest radiograph (A) performed after 3 weeks in a COVID-19 recovered patient reveals prominent interstitial markings with fibrotic opacities predominantly in bilateral middle and lower zones. Axial noncontrast CT images in lung window (B and C) of the same patient reveal fibrotic parenchymal bands predominantly in bilateral lower lobes with associated mild cylindrical tractional bronchiectasis and interlobular septal thickening.

(CT: computed tomography)

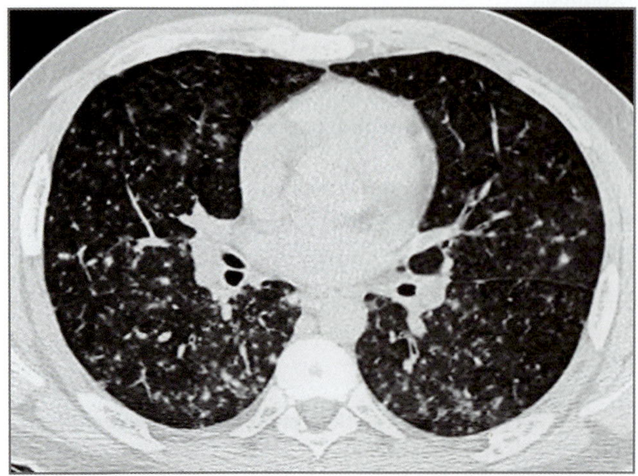

FIG. 31: Varicella pneumonia. Axial CT scan showing multiple nodular opacities scattered in bilateral lung parenchyma.

(CT: computed tomography)

Respiratory Syncytial Virus

Respiratory syncytial virus is a major cause of bronchiolitis and bronchopneumonia in infants and young children. In adults, it can cause prolonged fever, but it rarely causes serious complications, unless the patient is immunocompromised. Chest radiographs show streaky peribronchial infiltrates with associated hyperinflation. Lobar collapse or consolidation is occasionally seen. Hilar lymphadenopathy may be seen.

Varicella

Varicella pneumonia occurs more commonly in adults than in children. It has a specific radiographic appearance of multiple small, discrete acinar nodules scattered throughout both lung fields **(Fig. 31)**. Hilar lymph node enlargement may be present. High-resolution computed tomography (HRCT) findings mirror the radiographic abnormalities, but smaller nodules (1–10 mm) can be identified, and few of them have a halo of ground-glass opacification representing hemorrhage. The nodules usually resolve in a week but may persist for months and in 2% of patients they may calcify.[14]

Adenovirus

The common cold virus may sometimes cause pneumonia in epidemics. Radiographically, widespread scattered patchy/confluent opacities occur, which are peribronchial in distribution. Hilar lymphadenopathy may occur. The infection can be highly damaging particularly if acute infection occurs before 2 years of age, causing bronchiectasis, obliterative bronchiolitis, and in some cases Swyer–James/McLeod's syndrome.[58]

FUNGAL INFECTIONS

Fungi can be divided into two major groups according to the pathogenesis of infection:

1. Primary pathogens
2. Opportunistic pathogens

Primary Pathogens

Fungi that frequently infect healthy individuals constitute the primary pathogens. These include species such as *Histoplasma*, *Coccidioides*, *Blastomyces*, and *Paracoccidioides*. They are natural inhabitants of North and South America and are not commonly found in the Indian subcontinent.[59]

Histoplasmosis

It is caused by the fungus *Histoplasma capsulatum*, which is found in moist soil and in bird excreta in many parts of the world, but human infection is only seen with more frequency in parts of North America.[14] The radiographic picture closely resembles tuberculosis. In both, there is necrosis of pulmonary tissue followed by fibrosis and contraction. Parenchymal and/or nodal calcification is commonly seen. Other manifestations can be pulmonary granulomas or small nodules scattered in both lung fields resembling miliary tuberculosis. An uncommon late manifestation of histoplasmosis is a fibrosing mediastinitis, which can be well evaluated by CT.[14]

Coccidioidomycosis

It is caused by the fungus *Coccidioides immitis* and is found principally in endemic areas in the southwestern United States and northern Mexico. The most common radiological manifestation of primary coccidioidomycosis is a single or multiple foci of airspace consolidation. Thin-walled cavities, pleural effusion, and mediastinal lymphadenopathy may rarely be seen. Most patients with primary coccidioidomycosis recover within 3 weeks. Patients with persisting radiographic abnormalities after 6–8 weeks are considered to have chronic pulmonary coccidioidomycosis. The radiologic manifestations include lung nodules, cavities, and rarely bronchiectasis and scarring. Apical fibrocavitary disease with lobar contraction, bronchiectasis, and rarely calcification may resemble reactivation tuberculosis.[34]

Opportunistic Pathogens

These fungi invade debilitated or immunocompromised individuals and those with a preexisting, diseased, and scarred lung parenchyma. These include species such as *Aspergillus*, *Candida*, and *Cryptococcus*.[13] In contrast to the primary pathogens, these organisms can be found globally and usually are ubiquitous in the environment. In addition to saprophytic and invasive infection, some fungi (particularly *Aspergillus* species) can cause disease by inducing an exaggerated hypersensitivity reaction without invading tissue.

Aspergillosis

Aspergillus infections of the lung are caused by *Aspergillus fumigatus*, which are ubiquitous fungi found throughout nature and may result in disease in susceptible hosts when inhaled. The pathogenesis of *Aspergillus* infection varies with the quality and virulence of the inhaled organism and the status of the host defense mechanisms. Four varieties of pulmonary aspergillosis have traditionally been described.[60]

1. Aspergilloma—a saprophytic noninvasive infection of a preexisting cavity
2. Allergic aspergillosis—including allergic broncho-pulmonary aspergillosis (ABPA) and hypersensitivity pneumonitis caused by hypersensitivity to fungus
3. Semi-invasive aspergillosis or chronic necrotizing aspergillosis, a form of infection seen in patients with mild immunological suppression
4. Invasive aspergillosis—an infection in immuno-compromised hosts, which is invariably fatal without treatment

Aspergilloma: Aspergilloma, also known as mycetoma, is a ball of coalescent mycelial hyphae that typically colonize preexisting chronic cavities. The predisposing causes can range from tuberculosis, sarcoidosis, cavities in rheumatoid lung, or ankylosing spondylitis, etc. In most of the cases reported from India, there was a history of tuberculosis in the past or during detection.[61] Common clinical manifestations include cough and expectoration. Hemoptysis is frequent and has been reported in at least half of the cases. The mechanism of the bleeding is unknown; it has been attributed to friction between the fungus ball and the hypervascular wall, to endotoxins liberated from the fungus, and to a type 3 reaction in the cavity wall.[62]

On chest radiograph, an aspergilloma is seen as a round to oval mass of soft tissue density lying within a preexisting cavity. As most of the preexisting cavities colonized by the fungus are due to tuberculosis, mycetoma is most often found in the upper lobes or in the superior segment of the lower lobes. Typically, there is an airspace separating the fungus ball from the wall of the cavity, resulting in a distinctive "air crescent sign" **(Fig. 32A)**. The air crescent sign is not specific to mycetoma formation, as it can also be seen in patients with blood clots within a preexisting cavity, necrotic carcinoma, ruptured hydatid cyst, and lung abscess with necrosis. If the mycetoma fills the cavity completely, it may obliterate the air crescent. The fungus ball is usually mobile within the cavity and this mobility can be demonstrated on a decubitus chest radiograph **(Fig. 32B)**. Thickening of a cavity wall may be an early sign of *Aspergillus* infection.

Computed tomography demonstrates the finding of a mobile intracavitary mass characteristic of aspergilloma. The fungus ball is a sponge-like mass that contains irregular airspaces. The air crescent sign and the wall of the preexisting cavity are well seen and fungal strands bridging the fungus ball and cavity wall may be seen **(Fig. 33)**. Mobility can be readily demonstrated by supine or prone scan, although it is rarely necessary as the diagnosis is obvious in most cases. Occasionally, flecks of calcification may be seen within the mycetoma.[63]

Allergic aspergillosis is a result of a hypersensitivity reaction that produces ABPA or less commonly an extrinsic allergic pneumonitis, a Loeffler-like syndrome. The common symptoms of ABPA are cough, wheezing, and associated allergic symptoms and radiographic findings include central bronchiectasis and mucoid impaction seen typically as branching opacities, usually central and in an upper lobe distribution—the "gloved finger sign." These opacities are commonly transient and recurrent but may occasionally remain unchanged or even grow over time. CT shows the bronchiectasis and mucoid impaction very well **(Figs. 34 and 35)**.[64] The central distribution of bronchiectasis suggests the diagnosis of ABPA, even though it is not specific for the diagnosis. The findings of ABPA overlap with other entities such as cystic fibrosis or postinfectious bronchiectasis.

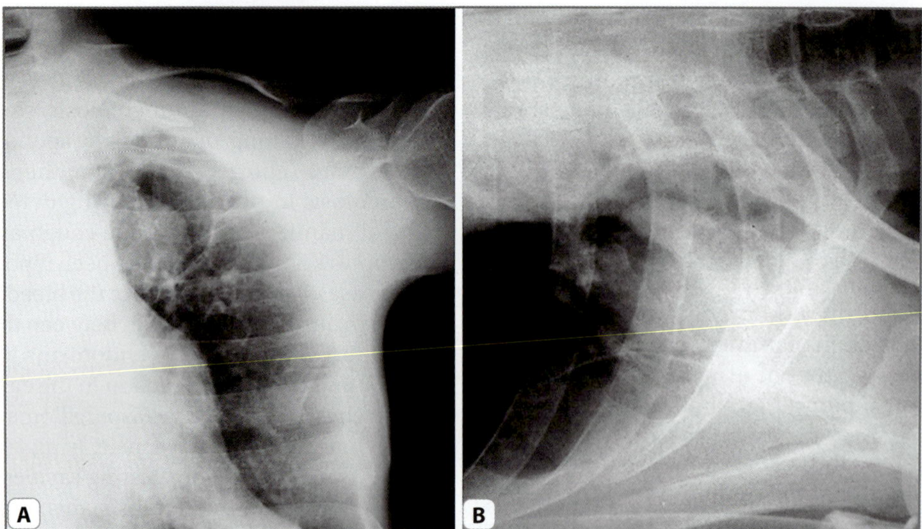

FIGS. 32A AND B: Frontal chest radiograph (A) shows a cavity containing an intracavitary fungus ball with a crescent of air above the mycetoma. Lateral decubitus view (B) shows the fungus ball lying in the dependent part of the cavity suggesting movement of the mycetoma within the cavity.

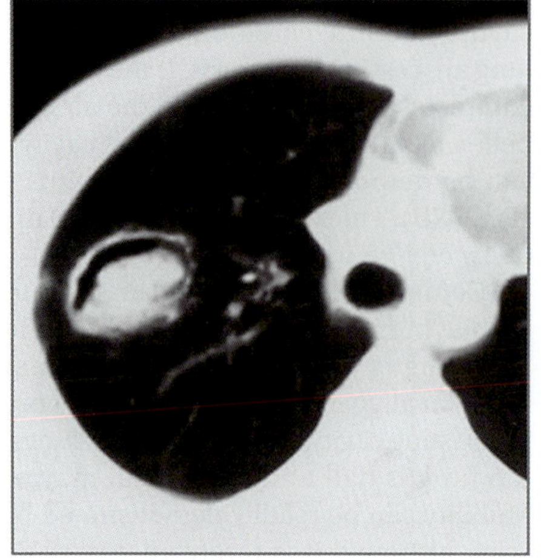

FIG. 33: Aspergilloma: CT shows the fungus ball lying in the dependent portion of the cavity with a characteristic air crescent sign.

(CT: computed tomography)

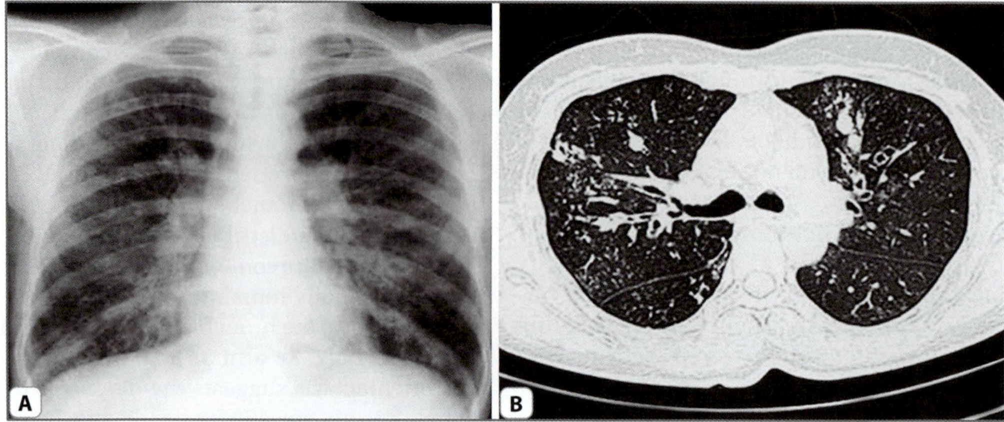

FIGS. 34A AND B: Allergic bronchopulmonary aspergillosis (ABPA). Chest radiograph (A) and HRCT (high-resolution computed tomography) scan (B) showing bronchial thickening, central bronchiectasis, and mucoid impaction within dilated bronchi and bronchioles in bilateral lung fields.

Hypersensitivity pneumonitis can occur with *Aspergillus* inhalation. It is seen on chest radiographs as a ground-glass opacity and/or diffuse small nodules. Sometimes, recurrent transient opacities superimposed on a fine micronodular pattern may be seen.[65] Diffuse, small centrilobular nodules of ground-glass attenuation are seen on CT, which are characteristic of subacute hypersensitivity pneumonitis. Chronic hypersensitivity pneumonitis demonstrates traction bronchiectasis and interstitial thickening often associated with areas of ground-glass opacity and mosaic perfusion. The major differential diagnosis is idiopathic pulmonary fibrosis.[65]

Semi-invasive and invasive aspergillosis occur in immunocompromised patients and will be dealt in detail in another chapter.

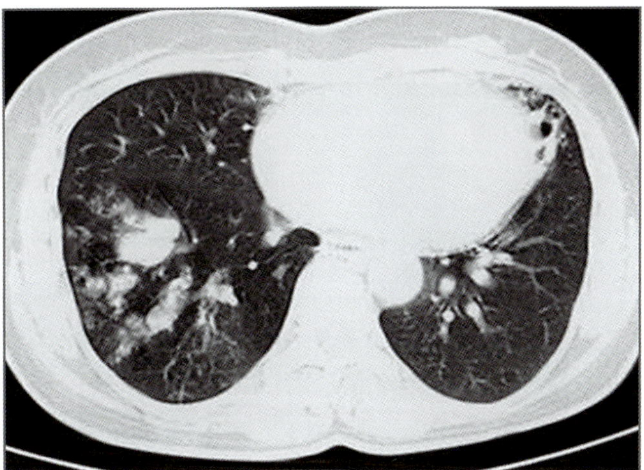

FIG. 35: CT scan in ABPA showing the characteristic "gloved finger" sign of mucoid-filled dilated bronchi in the right lower lobe.
(ABPA: allergic bronchopulmonary aspergillosis; CT: computed tomography)

Cryptococcosis

Cryptococcosis is caused by the fungus *Cryptococcus neoformans*. Although it can occur as a pulmonary or disseminated disease in otherwise normal individuals, cryptococcosis is more frequently seen to affect immunocompromised patients. In immunocompetent individuals, the radiographic findings can be single or multiple pulmonary nodules or areas of segmental or lobar consolidation. Cavitation and pleural effusion are rare. Hilar and mediastinal lymphadenopathy may be seen. Rarely a disseminated pattern of bronchopneumonia may be seen. Many patients with cryptococcal pneumonia have no symptoms and the pulmonary lesions seen radiographically heal spontaneously.[34]

Pulmonary Mucormycosis

Mucormycosis is a group of fungal infections caused by members of the order Mucorales. It can involve multiple organs including skin, paranasal sinus, orbit, brain lungs and gastrointestinal tract. Risk factors include uncontrolled diabetes mellitus and immunocompromised state such as post stem cell transplant, solid organ transplant, neutropenia and corticosteroid use. However, an outbreak of mucormycosis occurred during COVID-19 pandemic, rhino-orbital mucormycosis was the most common manifestation followed by pulmonary mucormycosis **(Figs. 36A to C)**.

In the early stage of pulmonary mucormycosis, peribronchial ground glass opacities are seen. As the disease progresses, consolidation, nodules and masses may be seen. Few features on imaging such as reversed halo sign, bird's nest sign and presence of multiple nodules with pleural effusion help in differentiating pulmonary mucormycosis from invasive pulmonary aspergillosis. Reversed halo sign

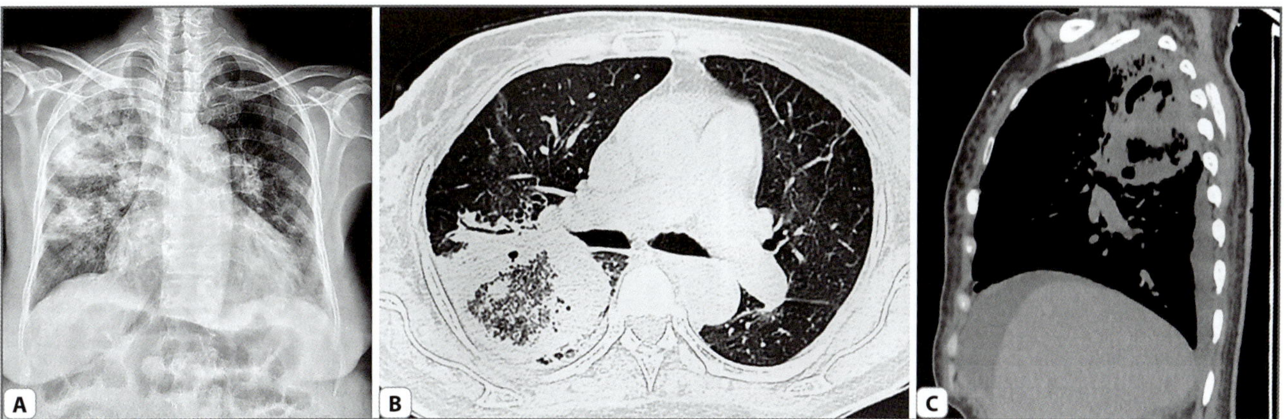

FIGS. 36A TO C: Frontal chest radiograph (A) in a COVID-19 patient with pulmonary mucormycosis reveals an area of consolidation with central necrosis in right upper and mid zone. Axial CT lung window (B) and sagittal reformat soft tissue window (C) reveal bird nest sign in right upper lobe with pleural effusion.

is a term used when ground glass lesion is surrounded by a peripheral rim of consolidation. This peripheral rim tends to be thicker in mucormycosis than cryptogenic organizing pneumonia (COP). Diagnosis is confirmed by identification of hyphae obtained on endobronchial or percutaneous sampling.

PARASITIC INFECTIONS

Protozoal Infections

Pleuropulmonary amebiasis is usually secondary to liver involvement.[66,67] Pleural effusion and lower lobe consolidation may be present contiguous to an amebic abscess in the liver or subdiaphragmatic space, just as they may accompany any other suppurative process in these sites. Changes can occur at the base of either lung but are much more frequent on the right because of the relationship of the liver to the diaphragm. An amebic liver abscess may extend through the diaphragm into the pleural cavity, giving rise to an empyema. If it extends into the lung, it can cause pneumonia or a lung abscess.[68]

Chest radiographs may show an elevated hemidiaphragm, pleural effusion and/or thickening, and basal atelectasis **(Fig. 37)**. If the abscess ruptures through the diaphragm, basal consolidation with cavitation may be seen. Fistulas may develop to airways, pericardium, or rarely skin. The diagnosis can be established by ultrasound, CT or MRI, and serological tests **(Figs. 38A to C)**.

Metazoal Infestations

Roundworm, Hookworm, and Strongyloides Infections

Many parasitic worms including *Ascaris*, *Taenia*, *Ancylostoma*, and *Strongyloides* pass through the lungs as part of their life cycle. In most instances, no pulmonary complications occur with any of these worms, but in a few patients, an allergic reaction takes place in the lung parenchyma, which manifests itself radiographically as dense migratory pulmonary consolidations without recognizable segmental distribution **(Fig. 39)**.[34,69] Blood and sputum eosinophilia are often present, and the entity is therefore included as one of the causes of Loeffler's syndrome.[70]

Filariasis

The most common filarial worm to cause pulmonary manifestations is *Wuchereria bancrofti*, which is responsible for elephantiasis. *W. bancrofti* can cause tropical eosinophilia, a syndrome consisting of cough, wheezing, and severe blood eosinophilia. It is believed to occur due to an immunologic response to microfilariae

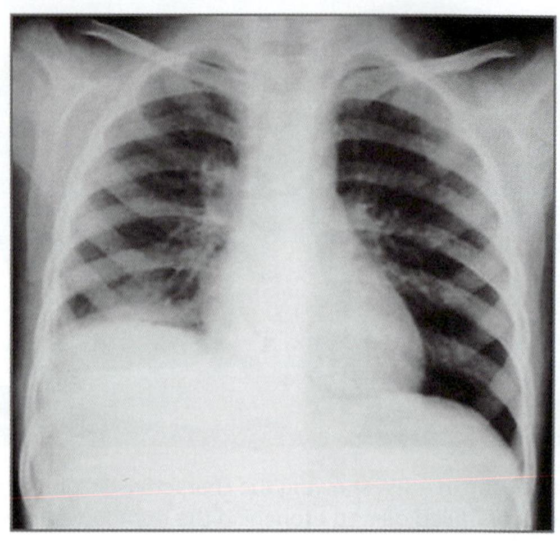

FIG. 37: Chest radiograph shows elevation of the right dome of the diaphragm with associated pleural effusion and basal consolidation. Ultrasound showed a subdiaphragmatic liver abscess.

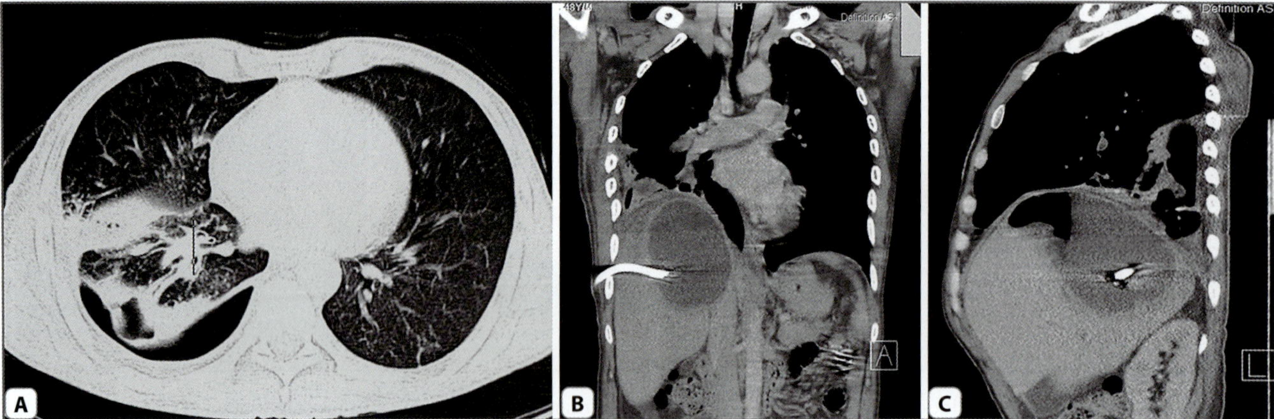

FIGS. 38A TO C: Pleuropulmonary amebiasis. CECT axial-lung window (A), coronal (B), and sagittal (C), mediastinal window: A large abscess in the liver with a drain in situ, with a loculated pyopneumothorax and focal basal consolidation suggestive of an amebic liver abscess, which has ruptured through the diaphragm.

(CECT: contrast-enhanced computed tomography)

rather than a direct infection. The chest radiograph may either be normal or show widespread fine nodular or reticulonodular shadowing, closely resembling miliary tuberculosis. Occasionally, localized consolidation may be seen.[71]

Echinococcus Infection/Hydatid Disease

Echinococcus infection is caused by a tapeworm *Echinococcus granulosus*. Humans are accidental hosts and acquire the infection by ingesting ova from fomites or contaminated water and by direct contact with dogs. Larvae develop in the host's duodenum, enter the bloodstream and travel to the end organs. The liver is the most common organ involved, followed by the lung. Cysts develop around this parasite in the end organs. The cyst wall consists of three layers: An outermost layer or the "pericyst" is a fibrotic capsule formed by the compression of the adjacent lung tissue. The cyst itself has a thin wall composed of two adherent layers, an outer ectocyst and an inner delicate lining—the endocyst. Multiple cysts are seen in approximately one-third of patients and are bilateral in 20%.[72]

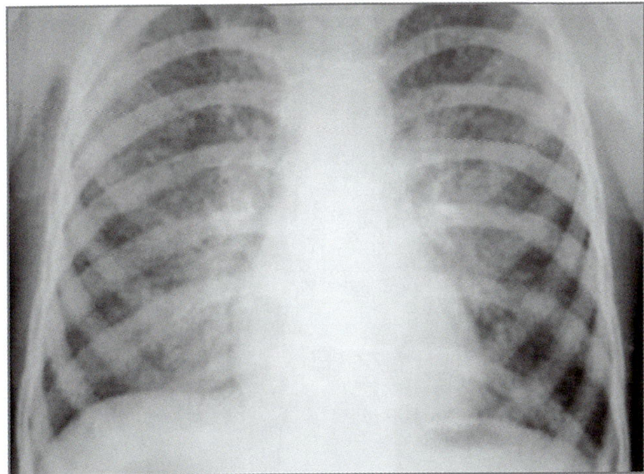

FIG. 39: Tropical eosinophilia. Chest radiograph shows diffuse nodular opacities in a child presenting with cough with a TLC of 40,000 cells/cc with 75% eosinophils.
(TLC: total leukocyte count)

Unruptured pulmonary cysts are generally asymptomatic and may be discovered incidentally on a routine chest film. They are homogeneous, roughly spherical or oval, sharply demarcated mass lesions, ranging in size from 1 to 10 cm and occur more commonly in mid and lower zones **(Fig. 40A)**. CT scan shows the masses to be cystic with a well-defined enhancing wall **(Fig. 40B)**. The internal contents are of water density and daughter cysts, when present, are seen as curved septations within the main cyst. The cysts are relatively pliant and mold to adjacent structures, resulting in indentation, lobulation, and flattening. Calcification, which is a common feature of hydatid cysts in the liver, is very rare in lung cysts. Approximately two-thirds of the cysts rupture. Cyst rupture may occur in the surrounding lung, airways, or pleural space. If the pericyst ruptures, with the two inner layers remaining intact, air dissects between the pericyst and ectocyst, giving rise to a crescent or meniscus sign. If there is disruption of the inner layers, a complex cavitary lesion results, which may show any of the following features such as air-fluid level, a floating membrane—water-lily sign **(Figs. 41A to C)**, a double wall, an essentially dry cyst with crumpled membranes lying at its bottom **(Fig. 42)**, or an empty cyst.[73] All these signs are particularly well seen on CT.[74] CT may also show air bubbles or blebs in the wall of a hydatid cyst, which are specific for detection of rupture.[75] Secondary infection of a hydatid cyst may produce a lung abscess with or without surrounding consolidation. Rupture into the pleural space causes an effusion or if there is an additional airway communication, a hydropneumothorax.

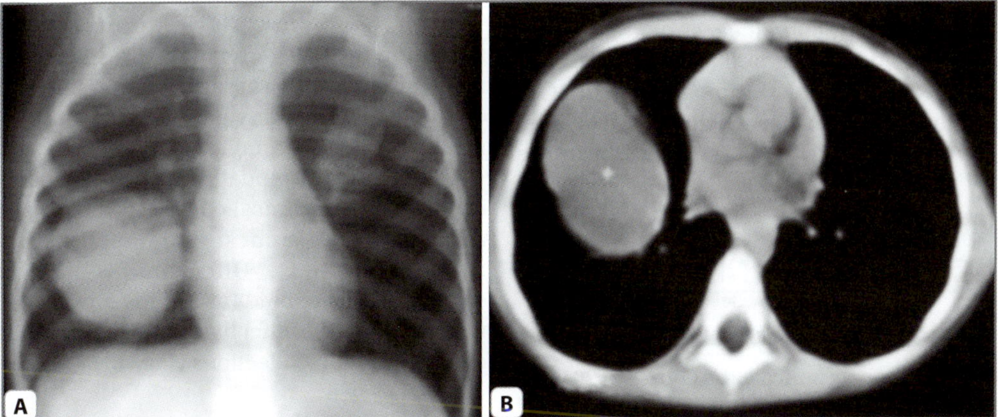

FIGS. 40A AND B: Hydatid cyst. Chest radiograph (A) shows a well-defined slightly lobulated mass in the right lower zone and another oval-shaped mass in the left upper zone. CT scan (B) through the lower mass shows a homogeneous fluid density cyst.
(CT: computed tomography)

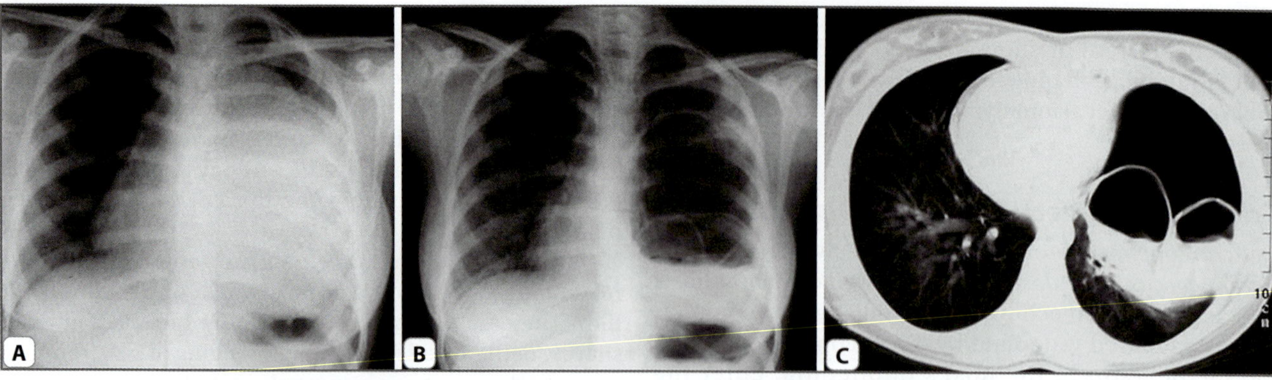

FIGS. 41A TO C: Chest radiograph (A) shows an unusually large unruptured hydatid cyst in the left lung field, displacing the mediastinum to the right. After rupture, chest radiograph (B) and CT scan (C) show air-fluid level within the cyst with floating membranes—water-lily sign.

(CT: computed tomography)

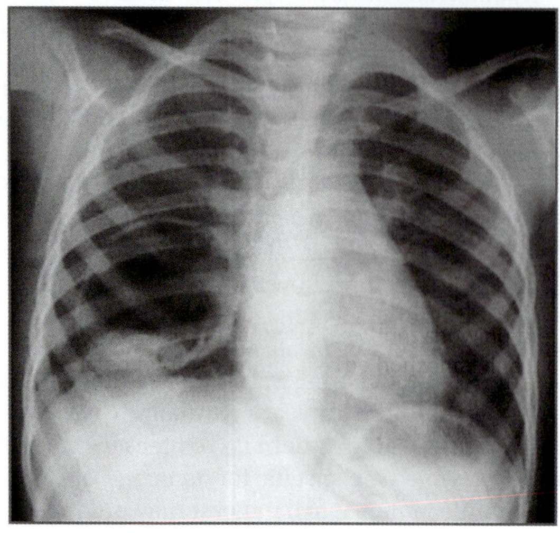

FIG. 42: Chest radiograph shows a ruptured hydatid cyst with crumpled membranes lying at the bottom of the cyst.

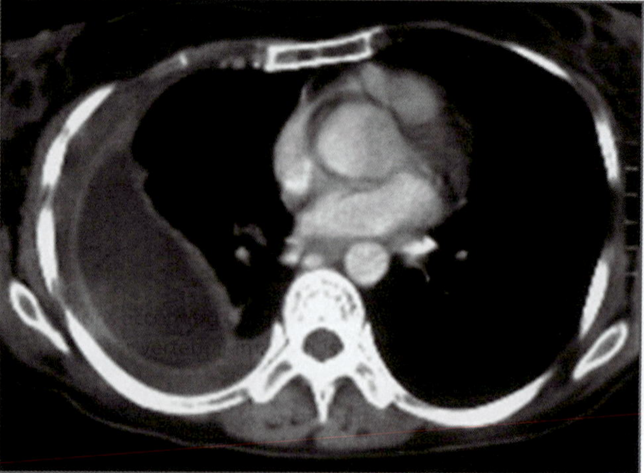

FIG. 43: CT scan in a case of empyema showing a homogeneous lenticular-shaped fluid collection based on the chest wall enclosed within thick enhancing pleura—split pleura sign.

(CT: computed tomography)

Magnetic resonance imaging can display complex cysts contents well, and the cyst membrane, whether collapsed or not, is seen as a low-intensity curvilinear structure on both T1-weighted (T1W) and T2-weighted (T2W) sequences. MRI and multidetector computed tomography (MDCT) reconstructions may be particularly helpful in revealing the exact location of a hydatid cyst in relation to the diaphragm.[76,77]

COMPLICATIONS OF PNEUMONIA

Pleural Effusion and Empyema

Parapneumonic effusions complicate the course of 20–60% of patients hospitalized with bacterial pneumonia.[78] Effusions are quite common in staphylococcal and gram-negative pneumonia, much less common in pneumococcal pneumonias, and distinctly unusual in viral and mycoplasmal infections.

Parapneumonic effusion progresses to empyema formation in 5–10% of patients; resolution occurs in the rest with antibiotic therapy. Progression to empyema in debilitated and elderly patients increases morbidity and the likelihood of mortality.

The choice of modality for the evaluation of effusion depends on the clinical context. Blunting of costophrenic angle occurs in a chest radiograph with pleural fluid up to 200–500 mL.[79] Ultrasound is useful for detecting small amounts of fluid (as little as 5 mL), loculations, and viscosity.[80] On the other hand, CT allows detailed evaluation of complex fluid collections **(Fig. 43)**.

Hydropneumothorax

The appearance of gas in the pleural space together with fluid is usually iatrogenic in origin. It may be associated with a bronchopleural fistula caused by rupture of a pneumatocele or abscess, and is seen particularly with *S. aureus*, gram-negative and anaerobic infections.

Pneumatoceles

Pneumatoceles commonly follow staphylococcal infections in children (not so common in adults). They are thin-walled cavities of variable sizes **(Fig. 14)**. They are formed due to check valve obstruction between the lumen of a small bronchus and adjacent interstitium. They can resolve completely or persist for months in which case they are of no clinical significance unless they cause pressure on adjacent structures.

Bronchiectasis

Bronchiectasis commonly occurs during the acute phase of pneumonia but resolves as the inflammation subsides.[81] Occasionally this can persist and act as a source of hemoptysis or recurrent infections.

Pulmonary Abscess, Necrotizing Pneumonia, and Pulmonary Gangrene

These conditions present a continuum caused by microbial infections, predominantly anaerobic microbes.[82] *Abscess* occurs due to cavitation secondary to necrosis in a variety of bacterial cases of pneumonia, particularly those caused by *S. aureus*, gram-negative bacteria, and anaerobes. Cavitation is also seen in amebic, fungal, and metazoal infections, but it is rare with viral and mycoplasmal pneumonia. Abscesses that fail to establish airway communication do not cavitate and are undetected on chest radiographs, being isodense with surrounding consolidated lungs. However, they can be seen on CT because of the low attenuation center within the abscess **(Figs. 44A and B)**.

Necrotizing pneumonia is characterized by consolidation combined with peripheral necrosis and formation of multiple small cavities. In the continuum, necrotizing pneumonia lies between lung abscess and pulmonary gangrene **(Figs. 45A to C)**.[83,84]

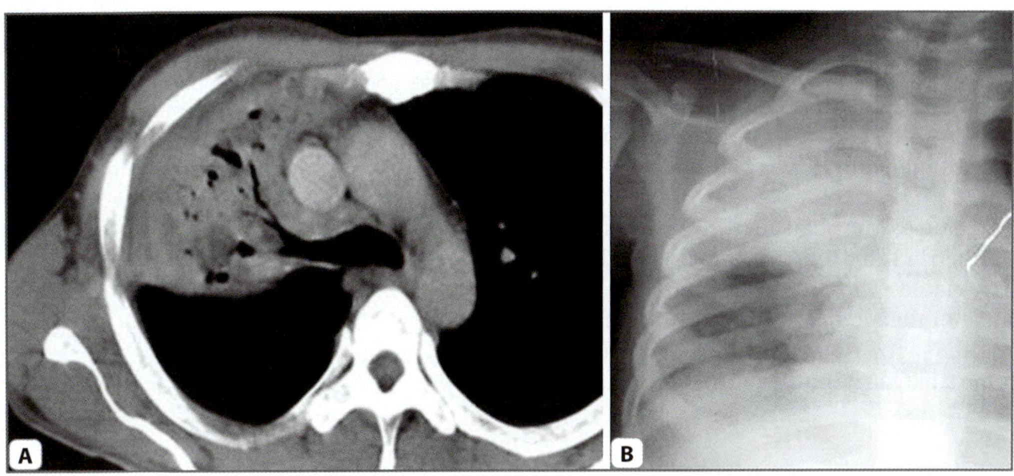

FIGS. 44A AND B: CT scan (A) demonstrates dense consolidation in the right upper lobe containing a focal region of low attenuation and gas consistent with necrosis and abscess formation not appreciated on chest radiograph (B).

(CT: computed tomography)

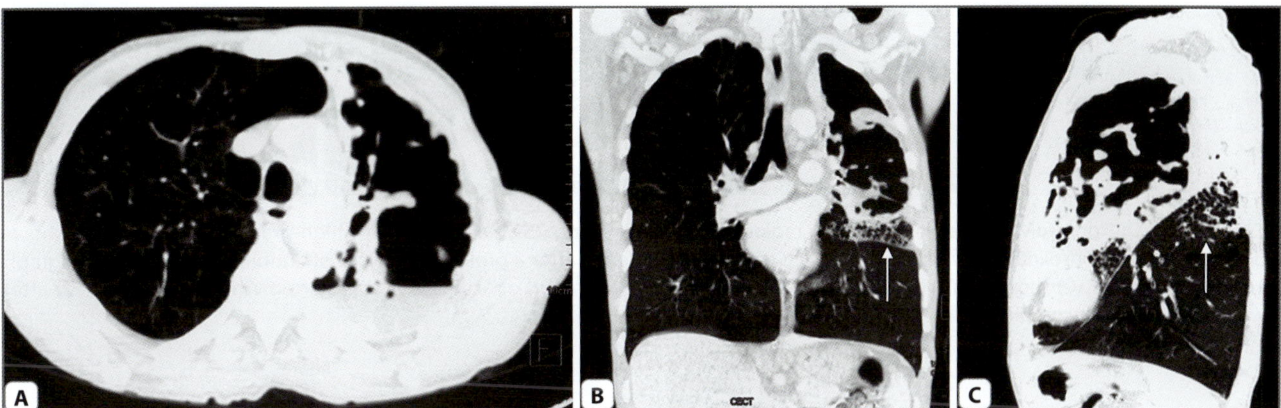

FIGS. 45A TO C: Necrotizing pneumonia. Axial (A), coronal (B), and sagittal (C) CECT in a 65-year-old patient with emphysema shows consolidation of the left upper lobe with marked destruction of the lung parenchyma with an air-fluid level. Adjacent areas of consolidation show small cysts within due to centriacinar emphysema (arrows in B and C).

(CECT: contrast-enhanced computed tomography)

Pulmonary gangrene occurs due to progressive devitalization of pulmonary parenchyma. It is characterized by the sloughing of a pulmonary segment or lobe as a consequence of thrombosis in branches of pulmonary and bronchial arteries supplying the necrotic area.[85] Contrast-enhanced computed tomography (CECT) shows obliteration of the pulmonary artery supply to the segment or lobe, which has large cavities and necrotic parenchyma.[83]

Differential diagnosis of necrotizing pulmonary infections includes infected bullae, pleural empyema, and lung tumors.[82]

Miscellaneous Complications

Miscellaneous complications such as osteomyelitis, obliterative bronchiolitis, and ARDS can occur.

DELAYED RESOLUTION OF PNEUMONIA

Nonresolving or slowly resolving pneumonia (NRP) refers to the persistence of radiographic abnormalities beyond the expected time course and affects 10–20% of patients hospitalized with CAP.[86] It has been defined as either <50% clearing at 2 weeks or less than complete clearing after 4 weeks despite antibiotic therapy for a minimum period of 10 days.[87]

The various causes that can lead to nonresolving pneumonia are listed in **Table 8.**[88] Causes may be pathogen-related or host-related. The presence of complications is another cause of delayed resolution of pneumonia. Noninfectious diseases or "pneumonia mimics" as enumerated in the table can be misdiagnosed as pneumonia and thus be another reason for apparent delayed resolution. In our country, tuberculosis is one of the most common causes of nonresolving pneumonia **(Figs. 46A to D)**.[89]

Further evaluation in the form of CT chest, microbiological tests for etiological agents, bronchoscopy, biopsy, and other tests specific to the suspected organisms/disease are required for these patients.

TABLE 8: Causes of nonresolving pneumonia.

Factors	Causes
Pathogen related	Atypical organism, resistant organism, uncommon organism, nosocomial infection
Host related	Severity of initial illness, presence of comorbidities, immunosuppressed state, metastatic infection
Presence of complications	Parapneumonic effusion/empyema, abscess, gangrene
Noninfectious disease	Neoplastic disorders (adenocarcinoma in situ, lymphoma, lymphangitis carcinomatosis, etc.), pulmonary embolism, systemic vasculitis (Wegener's granulomatosis), connective tissue disorders, drug-induced disorders (amiodarone, nitrofurantoin, methotrexate, etc.), cryptogenic organizing pneumonia, eosinophilic pneumonia, congestive cardiac failure

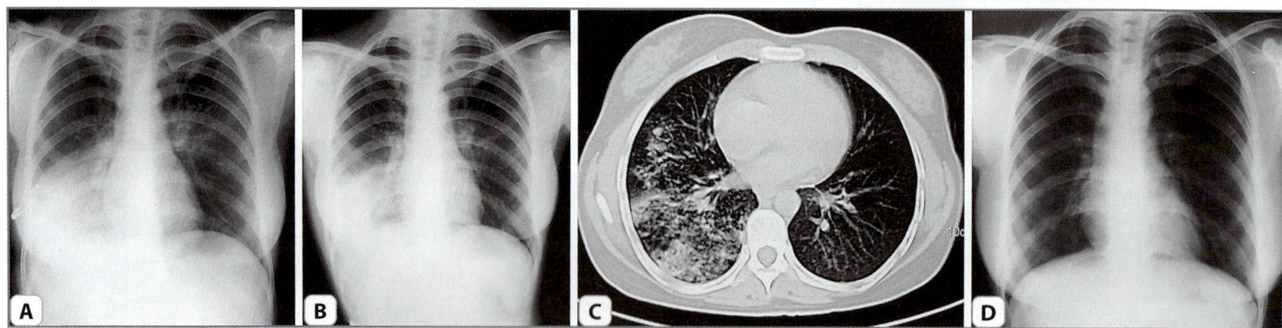

FIGS. 46A TO D: Nonresolving pneumonia. Chest radiograph (A) in a young 25-year-old girl with high-grade fever and cough shows a right lower zone consolidation, which shows only partial clearance even after a prolonged course of antibiotics on chest radiograph (B) after 5 weeks. CT (C) showed multiple focal lobular alveolar and tree-in-bud opacities. ATT was started. Chest radiograph (D) after 4 weeks of ATT shows complete resolution.

(ATT: antitubercular therapy)

DIAGNOSTIC ALGORITHM IN PATIENTS SUSPECTED OF PNEUMONIA

An imaging algorithm for the diagnosis of pneumonia has been suggested in **Flowchart 1**. In patients with mild disease, empirical treatment usually suffices, whereas in patients with severe disease, an aggressive approach is sometimes needed for the identification of specific causative organisms. Demonstration of the pathogen can be done by examination of stained smears of sputum, pleural fluid, culture of respiratory secretions, blood, or other biological material. Interventional procedures such as transthoracic needle biopsy done under ultrasound or CT guidance are a reliable and cost-effective means to obtain material for culture.[90]

In cases with underlying comorbidities or the immunosuppressed state of the host, specific treatment may be initiated accordingly. In cases of complicated pneumonia, CT can assist in the identification of the complication and, hence, aid management. If the disease is suspected to be a "pneumonia mimic," specific and ancillary tests may be needed to reach a conclusive diagnosis.

CONCLUSION

Chest radiography is the imaging technique of choice in evaluating patients with suspected pneumonia because of its low radiation dose, low cost, and wide accessibility. In daily practice, radiographs are used to confirm the clinical diagnosis of pneumonia, characterize the extent and severity of the disease, search for complications, monitor the response to therapy, and examine for possible alternative or additional diagnoses. The radiographic pattern needs to be correlated with the clinical background to suggest an etiological diagnosis as summarized in **Table 9**. CT scan has the advantage of superior contrast resolution and cross-sectional display, which that is helpful in the analysis of complex or slowly resolving cases, particularly when radiographic evidence of associated conditions and complications is equivocal.

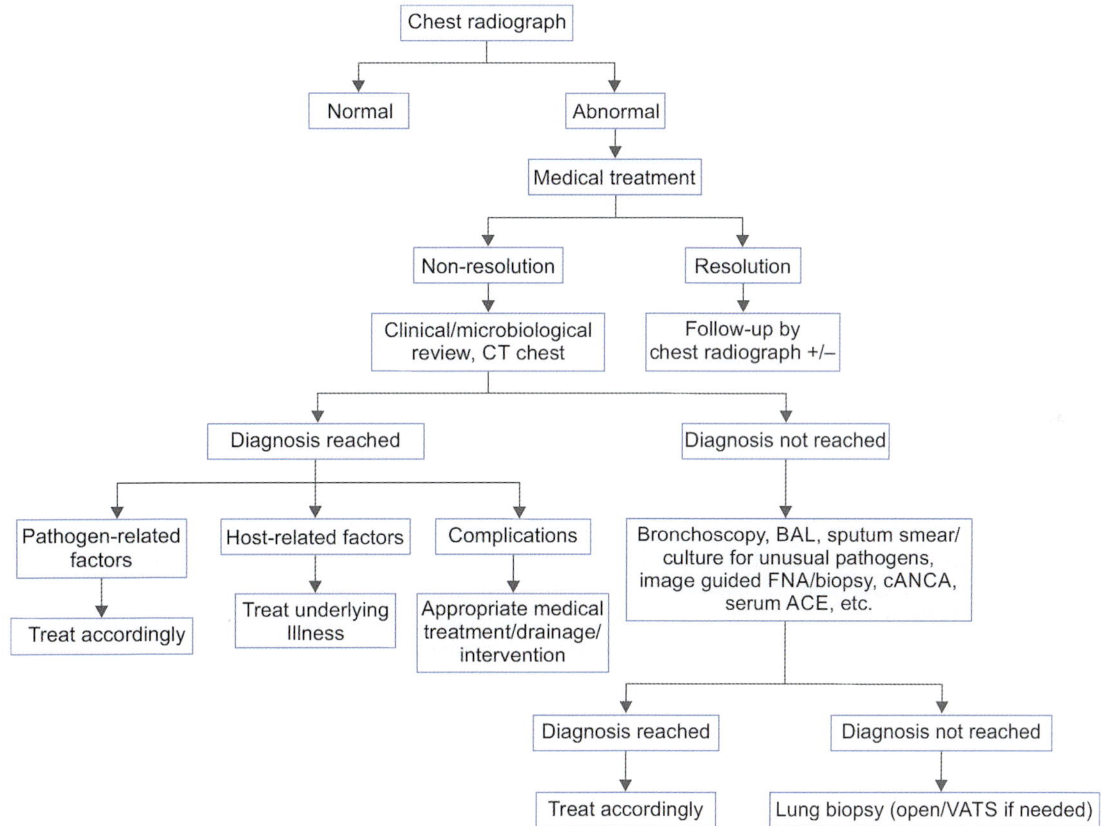

FLOWCHART 1: Clinicoradiological algorithm for diagnosis of pneumonia.

(ACE: angiotensin-converting enzyme; BAL: bronchoalveolar lavage; cANCA: cytoplasmic antineutrophil cytoplasmic antibodies; CT: computed tomography; FNA: fine needle aspiration; VATS: video-assisted thoracoscopic surgery)

TABLE 9: Summary of clinical and radiographic clues to the etiological diagnosis of pneumonia.[90]

Radiographic findings	Clinical circumstance	Organism
Segmental consolidation	Community-acquired	*S. pneumoniae, M. pneumoniae*
Lobar consolidation	Community-acquired, diabetes	*S. pneumoniae* (two-thirds of community-acquired pneumonias), *K. pneumoniae*, gram-negative bacilli
Round pneumonia	Community-acquired	S. pneumoniae
Bronchopneumonia	Hospital-acquired, aspiration	*P. aeruginosa, S. aureus*, streptococci, gram-negative bacilli, anaerobes, *M. pneumoniae*
Interstitial pneumonia	Community-acquired	Virus, *M. pneumoniae*
Cavitation/necrosis	Aspiration, COPD	*S. aureus*, gram-negative bacilli, anaerobes, *Actinomycosis, M. tuberculosis, Aspergillus*
Multiple cavitary nodules	Drug addict, septicemia	*S. aureus*
Pneumatoceles	Postviral, complication	*S. aureus*
Empyema	Complication of pneumonia	*S. pneumoniae, S. aureus*, gram-negative bacilli, *M. tuberculosis*
Chest wall invasion	Alcoholic	Actinomycosis, *M. tuberculosis*, fungi
Lymphadenopathy		*M. pneumoniae, M. tuberculosis*

(COPD: chronic obstructive pulmonary disease)

REFERENCES

1. Padley SPG, Rubens MB. Pulmonary infections. In: David Sutton (Ed). Textbook of Radiology and Imaging, vol. 1. Edinburgh: Churchill Livingstone; 2003. pp. 131-60.
2. Alkhayat KF, Hasan M, Alam-Eldeen. Value of chest ultrasound in diagnosis of community acquired pneumonia. Egypt J Chest Dis Tuberc. 2014;63(4):1047-51.
3. Schenck EJ, Rajwani K. Ultrasound in the diagnosis and management of pneumonia. Curr Opin Infect Dis. 2016;29(2):223-8.
4. Pereda MA, Chavez MA, Hooper-Miele CA, Gilman RH, Steinhoff MC, Ellington LE, et al. Lung ultrasound for the diagnosis of pneumonia in children: a meta-analysis. Pediatrics. 2015;135(4):714-22.
5. Sodhi KS, Khandelwal N, Saxena AK, Singh M, Agarwal R, Bhatia A, et al. Rapid lung MRI in children with pulmonary infections: time to change our diagnostic algorithms. J Magn Reson Imaging 2016;43:1196-206.
6. Liszewski M, Görkem S, Sodhi K, Lee E. Lung magnetic resonance imaging for pneumonia in children. Pediatric Radiol. 2017;47(11):1420-30.
7. Ginsburg AS, McCollum ED. Artificial intelligence and pneumonia: a rapidly evolving frontier. Lancet Glob Health. 2023;11:e1849-50.
8. Spencer H. The bacterial pneumonias. Pathology of the Lung, 4th edition. Oxford: Pergamon Press; 1985. pp. 167-212.
9. Blaivas M. Lung ultrasound in evaluation of pneumonia. J Ultrasound Med. 2012;31(6):823-6.
10. Liechtenstein D, Meziere G, Seitz J. The dynamic air bronchogram: a lung ultrasound sign of alveolar consolidation ruling out atelectasis. Chest. 2009;135(6):1421-5.
11. Tanaka N, Matsumoto T, Kuramitsu T, Nakaki H, Ito K, Uchisako H, et al. High-resolution CT findings in community-acquired pneumonia. J Comput Assist Tomogr. 1996;20(4):600-8.
12. Beigelman-Aubry C, Godet C, Caumes E. Lung infections: the radiologist's perspective. Diagn Intervent Imaging. 2012;93:431-40.
13. Heitzman ER. The radiological diagnosis of pneumonia in the adult: a commentary. Semin Roentgenol. 1989;24(4):212-7.
14. Goodman PC, Wilson AG, Armstrong P, Müller NL, Grainger RG, Allison D, et al. Pulmonary infections in adults. In: Grainger RG, Allison D, et al. (Eds). Diagnostic Radiology. Edinburgh: Churchill Livingstone; 2001. pp. 377-417.
15. Rose RW, Ward BH. Spherical pneumonias in children simulating pulmonary and mediastinal masses. Radiology. 1973;106:179-82.
16. Wang N. Anatomy. In: Dial DH, Hammar SP (Eds). Pulmonary Pathology. New York: Springer Verlag; 1988. pp. 17-40.
17. Wagner AL, Szabunio M, Hazlett KS, Wagner SG. Radiologic manifestations of round pneumonia in adults. AJR Am J Roentgenol. 1998;170:723-6.
18. Scanlon GT, Unger JD. The radiology of bacterial and viral pneumonias. Radiol Clin North Am. 1973;11(2):317-38.
19. Smith CB, Overall JC. Clinical and epidemiologic clues to the diagnosis of respiratory infections. Radiol Clin North Am. 1973;11(2):261-78.
20. Fein AM, Feinsilver SH, Niederman MS. Atypical manifestations of pneumonia in the elderly. Clin Chest Med. 1991;12:319.
21. Nambu A, Ozawa K, Kobayashi N, Tago M. Imaging of community-acquired pneumonia: roles of imaging examinations, imaging diagnosis of specific pathogens and discrimination from noninfectious diseases. World J Radiol. 2014;6(10):779-93.
22. Franquet T, Giménez A, Rosón N, Torrubia S, Sabaté JM, Pérez C. Aspiration diseases: findings, pitfalls, and differential diagnosis. Radiographics. 2000;20:673-85.

23. Gupta D, Agarwal R, Aggarwal AN, Singh N, Mishra N, Khilnani GC, et al. Guidelines for diagnosis and management of community- and hospital-acquired pneumonia in adults: Joint ICS/NCCP(I) recommendations. Lung India. 2012;29(Suppl. 2):S27-62.
24. Kieninger AN, Lipsett PA. Hospital-acquired pneumonia: pathophysiology, diagnosis, and treatment. Surg Clin North Am. 2009;89(2):439-61.
25. Rubin SA, Winer-Muram HT, Ellis JV. Diagnostic imaging of pneumonia and its complications in the critically ill patients. Clin Chest Med. 1995;16(1):45-59.
26. Beydon L, Saada M, Liu N, Becquemin JP, Harf A, Bonnet F, et al. Can portable chest X-ray examination accurately diagnose basal consolidation after abdominal surgery? A comparison with computed tomography scan. Chest. 1992;102(6):1697-703.
27. Winer-Muram HT, Rubin SA, Ellis JV, Jennings SG, Arheart KL, Wunderink RG, et al. Pneumonia and ARDS patients receiving mechanical ventilation: diagnostic accuracy of chest radiography. Radiology. 1993;188(2):479-85.
28. Winer-Muram HT, Steiner RM, Gurney JW, Shah R, Jennings SG, Arheart KL, et al. Ventilator-associated pneumonia in patients with adult respiratory distress syndrome: CT evaluation. Radiology. 1998;208(1):193-9.
29. Trimble A, Moffat V, Collins AM. Pulmonary infections in the returned traveller. Pneumonia. 2017;9:1
30. Kantor HG. The many radiologic faces of pneumococcal pneumonia. AJR Am J Roentgenol. 1981;137(6):1213-20.
31. Shah RM, Gupta S, Angeid-Backman E, O'Donnell J. Pneumococcal pneumonia in patients requiring hospitalization: effects of bacteremia and HIV seropositivity on radiographic appearance. AJR Am J Roentgenol. 2000;175(6):1533-6.
32. Macfarlane J, Rose D. Radiographic features of staphylococcal pneumonia in adults and children. Thorax. 1996;51(5):539-40.
33. Naraqi S, McDonnel G. Haematogenous staphylococcal pneumonia secondary to soft tissue infection. Chest. 1981;79:173-7.
34. Armstrong P. Bacterial pneumonia. In: Hansell DM, Armstrong P, Lynch DA, et al. (Eds). Imaging of Diseases of Chest. Philadelphia: Mosby; 2005. pp. 183-276.
35. Bartlett JG, Finegold SM. Anaerobic infections of the lung and pleural space. Am Rev Respir Dis. 1974;110:56-77.
36. Groskin SA, Panicek DM, Ewing DK, Rivera F, Math K, Teixeira J, et al. Bacterial lung abscess: a review of the radiographic and clinical features of 50 cases. J Thoracic Imaging. 1991;6:62-7.
37. Landay MJ, Christensen EE, Bynum LJ, Goodman C. Anaerobic pleural and pulmonary infections. AJR Am J Roentgenol. 1980;134(2);233-4.
38. Mabeza GF, Macfarlane J. Pulmonary actinomycosis. Eur Respir J. 2003;21:545-51.
39. Frank P, Strickland B. Pulmonary actinomycosis. Br J Radiol. 1974;47:373-8.
40. Cheon JE, Im JG, Kim MY, Lee JS, Choi GM, Yeon KM. Thoracic actinomycosis: CT findings. Radiology. 1998;209(1):229-33.
41. Putnam CE, Curtis AM, Aimeone JF, Jensen P. Mycoplasma pneumonia. Clinical and roentgenographic patterns. AJR Am J Roentgenol Radium Ther Nucl Med. 1975;124(3):417-22.
42. Reittner P, Muller NL, Heyneman L, Johkoh T, Park JS, Lee KS, et al. Mycoplasma pneumoniae pneumonia: radiographic and high-resolution CT features in 28 patients. AJR Am J Roentgenol. 2000;174:37-41.
43. Tarver RD, Teague SD, Heitkamp DE, Conces DJ Jr. Radiology of community-acquired pneumonia. Radiol Clin North Am. 2005;43(3):497-512.
44. Poirier R, Rodrigue J, Villeneuve J, Lacasse Y. Early radiographic and tomographic manifestations of Legionnaire's disease. Can Assoc Radiol J. 2017;68(3):328-33.
45. Kim KW, Goo JM, Lee HJ, Lee HY, Park CM, Lee CH, et al. Chest computed tomographic findings and clinical features of legionella pneumonia. J Comput Assist Tomogr. 2007;31(6):950-5.
46. Greenberg SB. Viral pneumonia. Infect Dis Clin North Am. 1991;5:603-21.
47. Waite S, Jeudy J, White CS. Acute lung infections in normal and immunocompromised hosts. Radiol Clin North Am. 2006;44(2):295-315.
48. Kim EA, Lee KS, Primack SL, Yoon HK, Byun HS, Kim TS, et al. Viral pneumonias in adults: radiologic and pathologic findings. Radiographics. 2002;22:S137-49.
49. Chowell G, Bertozzi SM, Colchero MA, Lopez-Gatell H, Alpuche-Aranda C, Hernandez M, et al. Severe respiratory disease concurrent with the circulation of H1N1 influenza. N Engl J Med. 2009;361(7):674-9.
50. Abdelsalam M, Diab HS, Ragab Y. Radiological findings in patients with H1N1 influenza pneumonia. Egypt J Chest Dis Tuberc. 2016;65(1):135-42.
51. Qureshi NR, Hien TT, Farrar J, Gleeson FV. The radiologic manifestations of H5N1 avian influenza. J Thorac Imaging. 2006;21(4):259-64.
52. COVID-19 Epidemiological Update – 6 November 2024. [online] Available from https://www.who.int/publications/m/item/covid-19-epidemiological-update-edition-173. [Last accessed February, 2025].
53. Jeong YJ, Wi YM, Park H, Lee JE, Kim SH, Lee KS. Current and emerging knowledge in COVID-19. Radiology. 2023;306(2):e222462.
54. Prokop M, van Everdingen W, van Rees Vellinga T, Quarles van Ufford H, Stöger L, Beenen L, et al. CO-RADS: a categorical CT assessment scheme for patients suspected of having COVID-19—definition and evaluation. Radiology. 2020;296(2):E97-104.
55. Li K, Wu J, Wu F, et al. The clinical and chest CT features associated with severe and critical COVID-19 pneumonia. Invest Radiol. 2020;55(6):327-31.
56. Han X, Chen L, Fan Y, Alwalid O, Jia X, Zheng Y, et al. Longitudinal assessment of chest CT findings and pulmonary function after COVID-19 infection. Radiology. 2023;307(2):e222888.
57. Kayali G, Peiris M. A more detailed picture of the epidemiology of Middle East respiratory syndrome coronavirus. Lancet Infect Dis. 2015;15(5):495-7.
58. Teper AM, Kofman CD, Maffey AF, Vidaurreta SM. Lung function in infants with chronic pulmonary disease after severe adenoviral illness. J Pediatr. 1999;134(6):730-3.
59. Fraser RS, Pare JAP, Eraser RG, Pare PD. Infectious diseases of lungs. In: Fraser RG, Pare PD (Eds). Synopsis of Diseases of the

Chest, 2nd edition. Philadelphia: WB Saunders and Co.; 1994. pp. 332-54.

60. Gotway MB, Dawn SK, Caoili EM, Reddy GP, Araoz PA, Webb WR. The radiologic spectrum of pulmonary Aspergillus infections. J Comput Assist Tomogr. 2002;26(2):159-73.
61. Panda BN. Fungal infections of lungs: the emerging scenario. Indian J Tuberculosis. 2004;51:63-9.
62. Johnson J. Pulmonary aspergillosis. Semin Respir Med. 1987;9:87-199.
63. Roberts CM, Citron KM, Strickland B. Intrathoracic aspergilloma. Role of CT in diagnosis and treatment. Radiology. 1987;165:123-8.
64. Neeld DA, Goodman LR, Gurney JW, Greenberger PA, Fink JN. Computerized tomography in the evaluation of allergic bronchopulmonary aspergillosis. Am Rev Respir Dis. 1990;142:1200-5.
65. Patel RA, Sellami D, Gotway MB, Golden JA, Webb WR. Hypersensitivity pneumonitis: spectrum of imaging findings. J Comput Assist Tomogr. 2000; 24:965-70.
66. Wilson ES. Pleuropulmonary amebiasis. AJR Am J Roentgenol Radium Ther Nucl Med. 1971;111:518-24.
67. Kinura K, Stoopen M, Reeder MM, Moncada R. Amebiasis: modern diagnostic imaging with pathological and clinical correlation. Semin Roentgenol. 1997;32(4 Pt 1):250-75.
68. Shamsuzzaman SM, haschiguchi Y. Thoracic amebiasis. Clin Chest Med. 2002;23:479-92.
69. Bean W. Recognition of ascariasis by routine chest or abdomen roentgenograms. AJR Am J Roentgenol. 1965;94:379-84.
70. Gelpi AP, Mustafa A. Ascaris pneumonia. Am J Med. 1968;44:377-89.
71. Udwadia FE. Tropical eosinophilia. In: Herzog H (Ed). Pulmonary Eosinophilia: Progress in Pulmonary Research, vol. 7. Basel: S Karger; 1975. pp. 35-155.
72. Beggs I. The radiology of hydatid disease. AJR Am J Roentgenol. 1985;145:639-48.
73. Von Sinner WN. Radiographic, CT and MRI spectrum of hydatid disease of chest: a pictorial essay. Eur Radiol. 1993;3:62-70.
74. Kervancioglu R, Bayram M, Elbeyli L. CT and MRI spectrum of hydatid disease. Acta Radiol. 1999;40:510-14.
75. Kokturk O, Ozturk C, Diren B, Unsal M, Ayla K. Air bubble: a new diagnostic CT sign of perforated pulmonary hydatid cyst. Eur Radiol. 1999;9(7):1321-3.
76. Von Sinner WN. New diagnostic signs in hydatid disease; radiography, ultrasound, CT and MRI correlated to pathology. Em J Radiol. 1991;12:150-9.
77. Prieto A, Diaz A, Calvo J, López-Negrete L. MR imaging of pulmonary hydatid disease. Eur J Radiol. 1996;23:85-7.
78. Heffner JE. Infection of the pleural space. Clin Chest Med. 1999;20(3):607-20.
79. Blackmore CC Black WC, Dallas RV, Crow HC. Pleural fluid volume estimation: a chest radiograph prediction rule. Acta Radiol. 1996;3(2):103-9.
80. Hirsh JH, Rogers JV, Mack LA. Real-time sonography of pleural opacities. AJR Am J Roentgenol. 1981;136(2):297-301.
81. Nelson SW, Christoforidis AJ. Reversible bronchiectasis. Radiology. 1958;71:375.
82. Poole PS, Stark HE, Stark P. Necrotizing pneumonia, pulmonary abscess, and lung gangrene: multiple pathways to lung parenchymal destruction. Contemp Diagn Radiol. 2011;34(13):1-6.
83. Reimel BA, Krishnadasen B, Cuschieri J, Klein MB, Gross J, Karmy-Jones R. Surgical management of acute necrotizing lung infections. Can Respir J. 2006;13:369-73.
84. Penner C, Maycher B, Long R. Pulmonary gangrene. A complication of bacterial pneumonia. Chest. 1994;105:567-73.
85. Curry CA, Fish EK, Buckley JA. Pulmonary gangrene: radiological and pathologic correlation. South Med J. 1998;91:957-60.
86. Finich S, Chalmers JD. Brief clinical review: non-responding pneumonia. EMJ Respir. 2014;2:104-11.
87. Kirtland SH, Winterbauer RH. Slowly resolving chronic and recurrent pneumonia. Clin Chest Med. 1991;12:303-18.
88. Kuru T, Lynch JP. Nonresolving or slowly resolving pneumonia. Clin Chest Med. 1999;20:623-51.
89. Jayaprakash B, Varkey V, Anithakumari K. Etiology and clinical outcome of non-resolving pneumonia in a tertiary care centre. J Assoc Physicians India. 2012;60:98-101.
90. Franquet T. Imaging of pneumonia: trends and algorithms. Eur Respir J. 2001;18:196-208.

Mandeep Kang, Pankaj Gupta, Mandeep Garg

CHAPTER 7

Pulmonary Manifestations in Immunocompromised Host

INTRODUCTION

Immunocompromised hosts constitute a special group of patients who are predisposed to infections by both opportunistic and nonopportunistic organisms.[1] The number of individuals who are immunocompromised is growing steadily, not only because of the continuing human immunodeficiency virus/acquired immunodeficiency syndrome (HIV/AIDS) epidemic, but also due to the growing incidence of various kinds of malignancies and increasing number of patients undergoing solid organ or bone marrow transplants. Pulmonary infections are a major cause of mortality and morbidity in this group of patients.[2-4] Diagnostic possibilities include infections (opportunistic or routine), hemorrhage, spread of underlying malignancy, chemotherapy- or radiotherapy-induced lung changes, and conditions not directly related to the underlying disease process such as congestive heart failure or pulmonary embolism. Therefore, the development of a pulmonary infiltrate on the chest radiograph is an ominous sign, which poses a considerable diagnostic challenge.[5]

This chapter will separately address two groups of patients, which are HIV/AIDS patients and non-HIV immunocompromised patients who have hematological malignancy or have received solid organ or hematopoietic stem cell transplantation (HSCT).

HUMAN IMMUNODEFICIENCY VIRUS/ACQUIRED IMMUNODEFICIENCY SYNDROME

The pandemic of HIV and AIDS has affected the entire world. According to the World Health Organization (WHO) and Joint United Nations Program on HIV/AIDS, it was estimated in 2007 that there were around 33 million people living with HIV infection throughout the world. Around 25 million deaths have occurred due to AIDS with opportunistic pulmonary infections, accounting for a majority of these.[6] Pulmonary infections will occur in nearly all patients with HIV infection during the course of their illness at some time. HIV infection is associated with an increased risk for lung complications due to alterations in the host defenses in the lung, such as mucociliary functional abnormalities and impairment in the immune response to pathogens.[7] In the past several years, there have been various trends noted in the demographics as well as treatment of HIV patients, which have had an important impact on the incidence of various pulmonary complications.[3,8] A change in the epidemiology with higher rates of infection in women and children and lower rates of infection in intravenous drug abusers (IVDAs) and homosexual or bisexual men has been reported. IVDAs are far more likely to suffer recurrent *Staphylococcus aureus* infections, aspiration pneumonia, lung abscess, septic emboli, and tuberculosis (TB). In IVDAs, the rates of bacterial pneumonia are more than twice of any other risk group, regardless of the CD4+ lymphocyte count. TB is much more common in Africa and Southeast Asia and, globally, is the major cause of mortality (13% according to estimates by the WHO).[9] Kaposi sarcoma (KS) is seen almost exclusively in homosexual males. In the subset of the patient population who have acquired the HIV infection through sexual contact, *cytomegalovirus* (CMV) infection is seen more commonly.

With the introduction of trimethoprim-sulfamethoxazole (TMP-SMX) prophylaxis in 1989, there has been a marked reduction in the frequency of *Pneumocystis jirovecii pneumonia* (PCP); however, opportunistic infections by atypical mycobacteria and CMV have increased in incidence.[8]

The introduction of highly active antiretroviral therapy (HAART), which effectively suppresses viral replication, has resulted in decreased viral loads and increased CD4+ lymphocyte counts, thereby dramatically reducing the HIV-associated morbidity and mortality and improving the prognosis; however, pulmonary infection continues to be the most common complication. With HAART becoming increasingly available, changes have been seen in the clinical presentation, epidemiology, and also the radiographic patterns of lung infections in this group of patients. Conversely, immune restoration, which occurs with the initiation of HAART, has been associated with new clinical syndromes known variously as reversal syndrome, immune reconstitution inflammatory syndrome (IRIS), or paradoxical response.[9-11]

SYSTEMATIC APPROACH TO IMAGING DIAGNOSIS

A systematic approach should be employed for the radiological evaluation of HIV/AIDS patients. The chest radiograph should be carefully analyzed for the pattern of abnormality.[12] This should be integrated with the available demographic, clinical, and laboratory information for interpretation. The clinical presentation of the patient is of vital importance as diseases, which present acutely or in a more insidious fashion, may demonstrate an identical pattern on the chest radiograph. Awareness of the CD4+ lymphocyte count is of critical importance, as it predicts the vulnerability of the patient to specific opportunistic infections and malignancies.

CD4+ count <200 cells/mm^3 marks clinical AIDS in an HIV-positive patient. If CD4+ counts are >500 cells/mm^3, there is an increased risk of infection with virulent pathogens, leading to recurrent community-acquired bacterial pneumonia and reactivation of TB. When the CD4+ counts are between 200 and 499 cells/mm^3, lymphoproliferative disorders and primary lung carcinoma are seen in addition to the above infections. PCP and disseminated TB occur with increasing frequency, with a count <200 cells/mm^3; however, the greatest risk of PCP is seen below a count of 100 cells/mm^3. At profound levels of immune depression with CD4+ counts below 50 cells/mm^3, viral pneumonia (commonly CMV), atypical mycobacterial infection, and disseminated fungal infections have a markedly increased frequency.[7,13]

IMAGING METHODS

After a thorough history and complete physical examination, the next steps in the evaluation of a symptomatic patient are a chest radiograph, sputum, and various blood examinations. If the radiographic and clinical findings are nonspecific or unrevealing, computed tomography (CT) of the chest and fiberoptic bronchoscopy (FOB) with bronchoalveolar lavage (BAL) are the usual next steps. The indications for CT include: (i) evaluation of symptomatic patients with normal chest radiographs, (ii) characterization of abnormalities detected on the chest radiograph, (iii) assessment for complications of pneumonia such as development of empyema or lung abscess, (iv) staging AIDS-related malignancies, and (v) planning and guiding biopsy procedures. CT has been shown to be highly sensitive for the detection of disease and fairly specific in its characterization. Most importantly, a normal CT of the chest virtually rules out pneumonia as the site of infection.[14,15] BAL and transbronchial lung biopsy (TBLB) have been shown to have a high diagnostic yield for the diagnosis of both PCP and CMV infections.[16]

RADIOLOGICAL PATTERN APPROACH TO DIAGNOSIS

A useful approach in the evaluation of a symptomatic patient is to identify the radiological pattern and correlate the differential diagnosis of the specific pattern with the clinical findings and CD4+ counts.

Normal Chest Radiographs

Chest radiographs may be normal in 10–39% of patients with proven PCP at initial presentation **(Figs. 1A and B)**.[3,4,8] About 6–17% of AIDS patients with pulmonary TB with positive sputum may also have normal radiographs.

Ground-glass Opacities

Ground-glass opacity (GGO) on high-resolution CT (HRCT) in a patient with HIV/AIDS is highly sensitive for the diagnosis of PCP and may be seen in 92% of patients **(Figs. 1A and B)**. Viral infections such as CMV or herpes may also present with GGO and tend to occur with severe degrees of immune depression. Lymphocytic interstitial pneumonia may also give rise to patchy GGO. In children, PCP presents at a much lower age (4–5 months) in comparison to lymphocytic interstitial pneumonitis (LIP). In comparison to children infected with PCP, children suffering from LIP generally tend to be older and less acutely ill.[17]

Consolidation

Focal segmental or lobar air space consolidation most likely represents a community-acquired bacterial pneumonia. Multiple areas of consolidation may be seen in TB or bacterial pneumonia with unusual organisms such as *Nocardia* or *Rhodococcus*.[3,8]

Multiple Pulmonary Nodules

A miliary pattern characterized by 1–3 mm nodules diffusely scattered in the lung parenchyma most commonly represents mycobacterial infection **(Fig. 2)**. In endemic areas, disseminated fungal infections such as *Histoplasma* and *coccidioidomycosis* may be the causative organisms. Larger nodules (<1 cm) associated with a reticular pattern are seen with CMV infections. *Cryptococcus* may also present with a reticulonodular pattern or as discrete

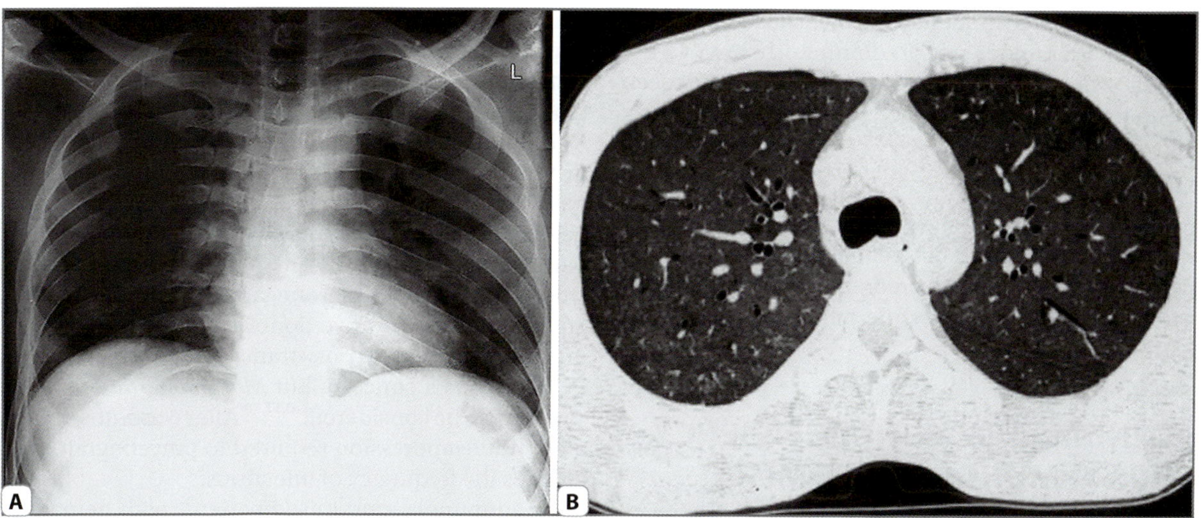

FIGS. 1A AND B: A 30-year-old HIV-positive male with a dry cough. (A) A chest radiograph is normal. (B) HRCT of the chest shows diffuse GGOs. Bronchoalveolar lavage demonstrated pneumocystis.

(GGOs: ground-glass opacities; HIV: human immunodeficiency virus; HRCT: high-resolution computed tomography)

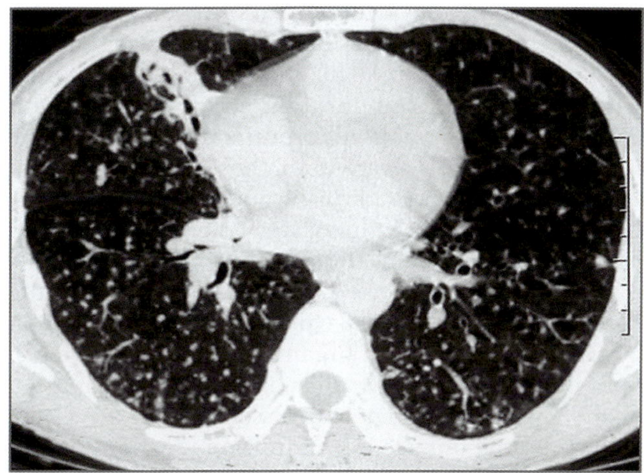

FIG. 2: A 23-year-old HIV-positive male with fever and cough. High-resolution CT of the chest shows multiple, 1–2 mm miliary nodules randomly scattered in the pulmonary parenchyma. Note the subsegmental atelectasis in the RML with bronchiectasis. Sputum was positive for acid-fast bacilli.

(CT: computed tomography; HIV: human immunodeficiency virus)

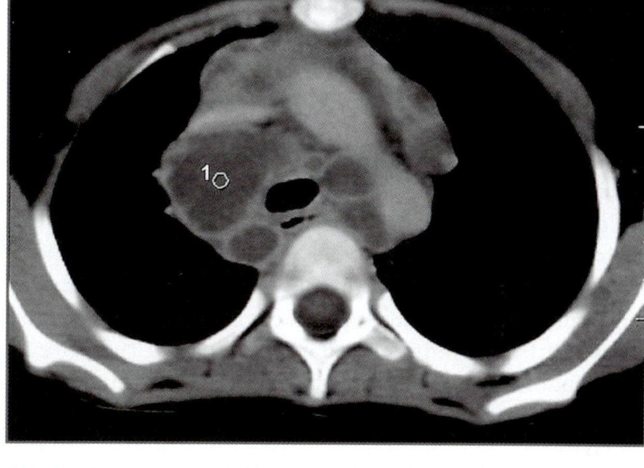

FIG. 3: A 40-year-old HIV-positive female with fever and cough. Contrast enhanced CT of the chest shows conglomerate, hypodense lymph nodes with rim enhancement in the pre- and para-tracheal regions in a case of TB.

(CT: computed tomography; HIV: human immunodeficiency virus; TB: tuberculosis)

nodules. Multiple subpleural nodules of 1–2 cm size with cavitation favor septic emboli. Larger nodules, associated with wedge-shaped, pleural-based opacities, are seen in invasive *aspergillosis*. These nodules may frequently show a "halo" of surrounding GGO. TB or atypical mycobacteria may also present with large nodules, which are typically poorly marginated. Lymphoma may also present with large nodules as may metastases. The nodules in KS are typically clustered along the bronchovascular bundles.[3,7,8,13] A solitary pulmonary nodule with spiculated margins may represent a primary bronchogenic carcinoma.

Lymphadenopathy

The most common cause of hilar and/or mediastinal lymphadenopathy in a patient with AIDS is mycobacterial infections, either TB or atypical mycobacteria.[18] These lymph nodes classically show low-density centers with rim enhancement postcontrast **(Fig. 3)**. Conversely, lymph nodes in KS and bacillary angiomatosis show intense enhancement, reflecting their hypervascular nature. Mediastinal nodes with punctate calcifications are seen in disseminated *Pneumocystis* infection. Calcification may also be seen in the liver, kidneys, and spleen in this situation.

Unlike lymphoma in an immunocompetent host, lymphoma in an AIDS patient does not predominantly involve the lymph nodes; mediastinal or hilar lymphadenopathy is seen in only up to 25% of cases.[19]

Pleural Effusion

The radiographic features of pleural effusion are generally unhelpful in narrowing the differential diagnosis. Large or massive pleural effusions with predominantly lymphocytes on cytology are due to TB, while hemorrhagic fluid is suggestive of KS.

NONHUMAN IMMUNODEFICIENCY VIRUS IMMUNOCOMPROMISED HOSTS

The number of non-HIV immunocompromised patients has significantly increased in the last two decades due to an increase in the number of patients receiving solid organ or hematopoietic stem cell transplants, advances in cytotoxic therapy for various malignancies, and immunosuppressive therapy.[10,11]

Organ transplantation is the most important treatment for end-stage liver, kidney, heart, and lung diseases. The immunosuppression caused by the antirejection medications renders the solid organ transplant recipient vulnerable to a wide variety of infections, causing significant mortality and morbidity. This group of patients is at further risk of pneumonia for several reasons, which are as follows: (i) Prolonged hospitalization, (ii) endotracheal tube injury to the trachea, and (iii) impaired clearance of respiratory secretions due to anesthesia and diminished cough. Lung transplant recipients are also at increased risk due to denervation of the lung and surgically impaired mucociliary transport.[4]

Cytotoxic chemotherapy causes neutropenia. As the granulocyte count declines, the risk of infections increases, and the patient becomes susceptible to infections by pyogenic bacteria and fungi. The common organisms in the setting of neutropenia are bacteria, including *Escherichia coli*, *Klebsiella*, *Pseudomonas aeruginosa*, *S. aureus*, *S. pneumoniae*, and *S. viridans* as well as fungi, including *Aspergillus*, *Candida*, and *Mucor*. Patients are most susceptible to bacterial infections in the early neutropenic phase. As neutropenia persists, fungal infections become more common.[3,10,11] Chemotherapy also causes defects in the humoral immunity, which are associated with infections with encapsulated bacteria such as *S. pneumoniae* and gram-negative organisms such as *Haemophilus influenzae*, *Neisseria meningitidis*, and *P. aeruginosa*.[2]

Cellular immunity mediated by T lymphocytes is affected in patients undergoing chemotherapy and solid organ transplant recipients. Defects in cellular immunity render the patient susceptible to more unusual pathogens, including viruses (CMV, *varicella*, *herpes zoster*), protozoa, fungi (*Pneumocystis jirovecii*, *Aspergillus*, *Cryptococcus*, *Histoplasma*), and bacteria (*Legionella*, *Nocardia asteroides*). Following solid organ transplant, in the first 4 weeks, infections are usually caused by nosocomial bacteria or fungi in patients with prolonged neutropenia. At 1–3 months post-transplant, opportunistic pathogens such as PCP or CMV increase in frequency. One-half to all of the seronegative patients who receive a graft from a seropositive donor suffer from primary CMV infection. In the late post-transplant phase (>3 months), PCP remains a concern, but *Mycobacteria* and *Nocardia* should also be considered.[10,11,20] After 6 months, the degree of immunosuppression required to prevent graft rejection dictates the frequency of infections.

In immunocompromised patients with hematological malignancies, pulmonary involvement occurs in many ways, viz. (i) infection, (ii) recurrence of the underlying hematological disease, (iii) adverse reaction to drugs, (iv) unrelated processes such as pulmonary emboli, and (v) combination of the abovementioned processes. One-third of patients with hematological malignancies suffer a combination of at least two processes such as pneumonia caused by two different pathogens or a drug-related pulmonary complication occurring along with infection. A reasonable differential diagnosis may be considered if one is aware of the host defenses that get compromised. Suppression in the number of granulocytes, B lymphocytes, or T lymphocytes is the most common pattern of impairment, though multiple types of cells may be frequently affected. A critical reduction in the number of each of these cell types predisposes to infection by a particular group of organisms. In these patients, most pulmonary complications, including drug-induced pulmonary disease and pulmonary emboli, are associated with fever that mimics infection. Noninfectious causes comprise one-fourth of the pulmonary complications.[20,21] With improved survival, the late effects of treatment such as second malignancy are becoming more common. Lately, due to better regimens, the incidence of radiation-related complications has decreased.

Hematopoietic stem cell transplantation is now the treatment of choice for malignant diseases such as leukemias, aplastic anemia, and congenital immunodeficiency syndromes. Pulmonary complications in these patients can be divided into two broad categories, i.e., HSCT nonspecific and HSCT-specific complications. HSCT-specific pulmonary complications may develop in approximately half of transplant recipients.[21-23] Stem cells for HSCT may be obtained from the patient's own blood (autologous); related or unrelated donors (allogeneic); or may be obtained from peripheral blood, bone marrow, or cord blood.[24] Complications related to the allogeneic HSCT are due to the toxicity of the conditioning regimen that includes chemotherapy with or without radiation.[23]

Imaging Approach

Chest radiographs remain the basic imaging investigation for the diagnosis of suspected pulmonary infection.[5] However, early in the course of disease, chest radiographs may be normal. CT has a higher sensitivity and allows diagnosis in the setting of a normal chest radiograph in patients with a high clinical suspicion of pneumonia. In a study by Heussel et al., 60% of pulmonary infections in febrile neutropenia were diagnosed by CT scans 5 days before radiographic abnormalities became evident.[25]

BACTERIAL INFECTIONS

Bacterial infections are responsible for most infections in HIV-positive patients, having surpassed PCP. *S. pneumoniae* and *H. influenzae* account for most episodes of community-acquired pneumonia in the general population. Recent hospitalization, antibiotic, or steroid therapy is the predisposing factor for *Pseudomonas* infection. Unusual organisms such as *Rhodococcus* or *Bartonella* can also infect patients with AIDS. The radiological pattern of bacterial pneumonia does not differ from an immune intact host and consists of single or multiple sites of consolidation in a segmental or lobar distribution **(Figs. 4A and B)**.

However, bilateral patchy opacities may be seen with certain organisms such as *Pseudomonas*, *E. coli*, and *S. aureus*. In contrast to immune-intact individuals, there is a higher propensity for bilateral and multilobar diseases in immunocompromised patients with a tendency for rapid progression as well as development of local and systemic complications, including cavitation, abscess formation, and bacteremia. Pleural effusions may also occur.

In IVDAs, *S. aureus* and gram-negative bacteria are common causes of generalized sepsis with secondary pneumonia. Septic embolic appear as multiple, bilateral, 1–2 cm nodules, which frequently cavitate and are more numerous in the lower lobes.

Nocardia infection may be seen in solid organ transplant recipients in the late post-transplant phase (>1 year postheart-lung transplant).[4,11,21] It is also seen in diabetics and patients receiving steroid therapy. It most commonly appears as a solitary nodule or nodular infiltrate with cavitation. Pleural effusion occurs in up to 50% of cases.

Pyogenic airway diseases, viz., infectious bronchitis, bronchiolitis, and bronchiectasis, have increased in frequency in HIV-positive patients. Chest radiographic findings in extensive bronchiolitis present an interstitial pattern with reticulonodular opacities distributed in a symmetrical fashion, which mimics PCP. On CT, small nodular and branching Y- and V-shaped centrilobular opacities (tree-in-bud appearance) are seen, which represent bronchioles impacted with inflammatory secretions **(Fig. 5)**. Similar imaging findings may be noted in viral and mycobacterial infections.

Bronchiectasis is commonly seen in association with HIV infection. It is thought to be a complication of prior lung infections. However, it has also been described in patients without history of previous infections and may represent an accelerated form of lung injury.[7]

Bacterial pneumonia affects 20–50% of HSCT recipients in the neutropenic phase.[25] Gram-negative organisms from the oral mucosa or gastrointestinal tract have been typically associated. However, more recently, gram-positive organisms such as *S. aureus* and coagulase-negative *Staphylococcus* represent 60–70% of infections. The radiographic appearances include consolidation, GGO, centrilobular, acinar, and lobular opacities.

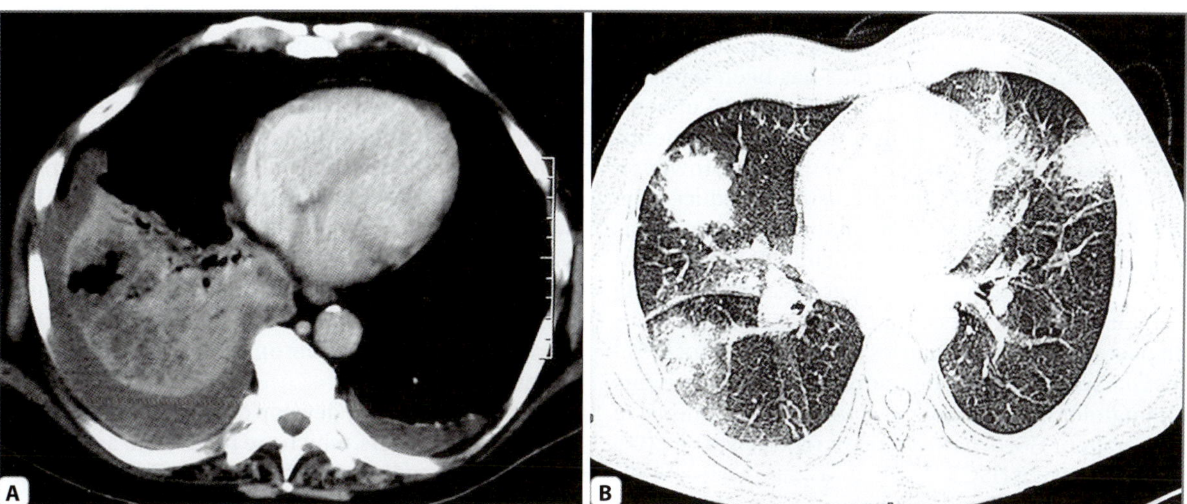

FIGS. 4A AND B: Bacterial pneumonia. (A) Air-space consolidation with air bronchograms and eccentric cavitation with associated pleural effusion. (B) Multifocal, bilateral, patchy air-space consolidation. Sputum culture revealed *Pseudomonas aeruginosa*.

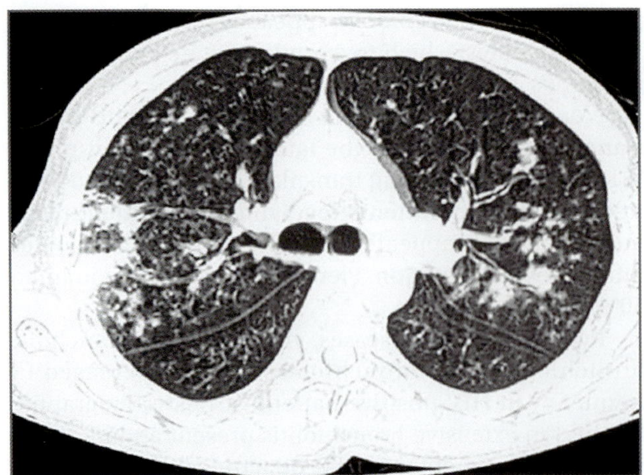

FIG. 5: A 50-year-old male postchemotherapy presented with fever and dyspnea. High-resolution computed tomography (CT) of the chest shows multifocal, patchy consolidation with centrilobular nodules and tree-in-bud appearance. Sputum was positive for *Streptococcus viridans*.

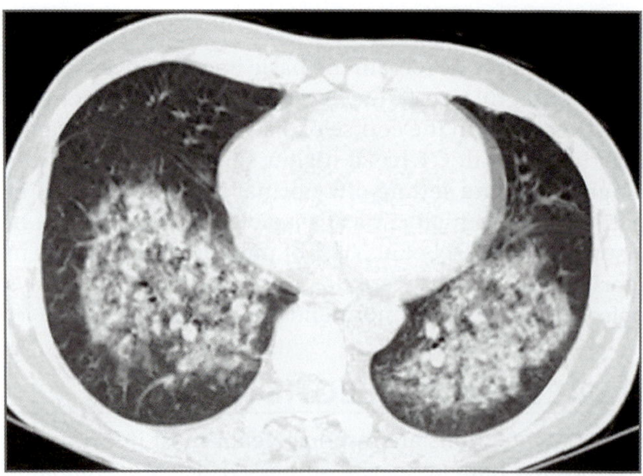

FIG. 6: A 45-year-old HIV-positive lady presented with cough and dyspnea. High-resolution CT of the chest shows typical, diffuse GGOs with subpleural sparing in both lower lobes in a case of *Pneumocystis* pneumonia.

(CT: computed tomography; GGOs: ground-glass opacities; HIV: human immunodeficiency virus)

PNEUMOCYSTIS JIROVECII PNEUMONIA

Pneumocystis jirovecii is classified as a fungus and is an opportunistic eukaryote.[26] The incidence of PCP has decreased secondary to improved prophylaxis regimens and HAART; however, it still remains one of the most common AIDS-defining illnesses as well as the most common cause of serious pulmonary infections in HIV-positive patients.[3,26] In fact, at least one episode of infection with PCP will occur in most (>70%) of the patients with HIV/AIDS during the course of their illness. PCP occurs twice as frequently in homosexual males versus IVDAs. Also, it affects males at twice the frequency of females. Although it can occur at any level of immune depression, it typically occurs at CD4+ counts below 200 cells/mm^3.[27]

Pneumocystis jirovecii pneumonia has been reported in 33% of heart-lung transplant recipients, 3–10% of heart transplant recipients, 0–11% of liver transplant recipients, and 6–14% of kidney transplant recipients. However, prophylaxis with TMP-SMX has dramatically reduced the incidence of PCP. Nebulized pentamidine can be used as the second-line prophylactic agent when TMP-SMX cannot be given.[27] The infection can occur at any time following solid organ transplant but commonly occurs in the 4–6th month post-transplant and carries a mortality rate of 47%.[4]

Pneumocystis jirovecii pneumonia also affects patients with hematological malignancies undergoing intensive chemotherapy or HSCT. Its incidence is reported to be <10% in patients receiving HSCT.[6]

Clinically, affected patients present with a low-grade fever, dry cough, and dyspnea. The initial symptoms may be subtle in HIV-infected patients and be present even up to several weeks before diagnosis. This is in contrast to PCP in non-HIV patients in whom the presentation is more acute.[28] PCP classically presents on a chest radiograph with a bilateral, perihilar, or diffuse, symmetric, interstitial pattern, which may be ground glass, reticular, or granular in appearance. These opacities may progress to air-space consolidation. The typical appearance on HRCT is extensive GGOs, which histopathologically correspond to the presence of intra-alveolar exudates comprising fluid, debris, and organisms **(Fig. 6)**. The ground-glass attenuation shows a patchy or geographical distribution with sparing of the subpleural regions. There may be a mosaic pattern with involved secondary lobules seen adjacent to uninvolved lungs **(Figs. 7A and B)**. The parenchymal opacities have a predilection for the upper lobes, which was earlier thought to be due to prophylaxis with aerosolized pentamidines. However, this upper lobe predominance is still prevalent in the present era of TMP-SMX prophylaxis. Thickening of the interlobular septal lines occurs in the subacute phase of the disease. Thin-walled cystic lesions may develop at any time during the course of the illness with an incidence of 10–34%. Cystic PCP is associated with a 35% risk for spontaneous pneumothoraces, which are often refractory to treatment and may require surgical intervention. Although the radiographic abnormalities may clear within 2 weeks of therapy, it is not uncommon to see residual fibrosis or irregular cystic spaces.

Some patients may develop clinical symptoms and signs over months to years, which are referred to as chronic PCP. This appears radiographically as thickened septal lines with honeycombing and traction bronchiectasis.[3,4,7,8,27] Rare presentations of PCP (5–10%) include focal lobar consolidation, nodules, mediastinal lymphadenopathy, bronchiectasis, or pleural effusion.

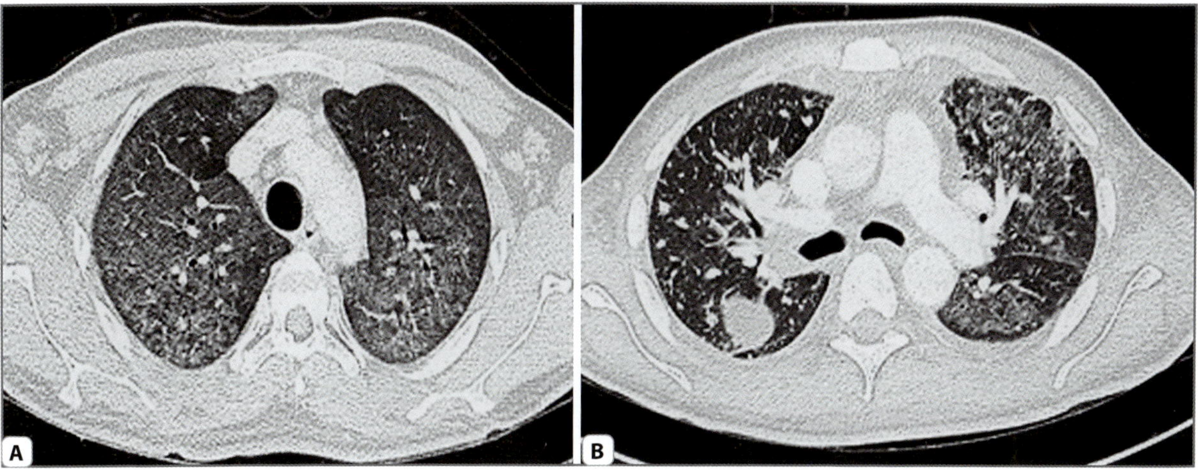

FIGS. 7A AND B: (A) A 30-year-old HIV-positive male with a dry cough of insidious onset. High-resolution CT (HRCT) of the chest reveals diffuse GGOs with interstitial septal thickening, giving a crazy-paving appearance. (B) A 42-year-old HIV-positive male with a dry cough and low-grade fever. HRCT of the chest demonstrates the involvement of the secondary lobules with sparing of adjacent lobules in the left lung. Note the nodules and focal consolidation in the right lung. Bronchoalveolar lavage demonstrated pneumocystis in both patients.

(GGOs: ground-glass opacities; HIV: human immunodeficiency virus)

MYCOBACTERIAL INFECTIONS

Human Immunodeficiency Virus/ Acquired Immunodeficiency Syndrome Patients

It has been estimated that there is a 50–200-fold increased risk of contracting TB by an HIV-positive individual compared to the general population in nonendemic areas. This risk increases for IVDAs and patients in endemic areas such as India and sub-Saharan Africa. TB may accelerate the progression of AIDS. Prompt diagnosis and treatment are, therefore, critical. TB may affect patients with HIV infection at any stage; however, the imaging findings are determined by the level of immune suppression. Early in the course of disease, when the CD4+ counts are >200 cells/mm^3, it usually manifests with the traditional pattern of reactivation TB with upper lobe opacities with cavitation and nodular bronchogenic spread **(Fig. 8)**. Pleural effusions are common. In severely immunocompromised individuals (CD4+ count <200 cells/mm^3), the imaging appearance is reminiscent of primary TB with parenchymal consolidation and mediastinal lymphadenopathy, which typically shows low attenuation centers with peripheral rim enhancement.[10] A miliary pattern is also common.[11] Atypical findings may be seen, including diffuse infiltrates, multiple nodules, frequent middle and lower lobe involvement, or even normal chest radiographs (14–20%). Compared to immunocompetent hosts, AIDS patients infected with TB are more likely to present with extrapulmonary involvement (genitourinary system, bone marrow, central nervous system, and lymph nodes) or systemic dissemination **(Fig. 9)**. These manifestations increase with increasing degrees of immune compromise: 70% of AIDS patients show extrathoracic disease when the CD4+ counts are <100 cells/mm^3 compared to 44% when CD4+ count is >300 cells/mm^3. Almost half of the patients with extrapulmonary involvement will show a miliary pattern in the lungs.[29] TB can involve the central airways with stenosis and wall thickening. Involvement of the lower airways manifests as bronchiectasis or tree-in-bud appearance.

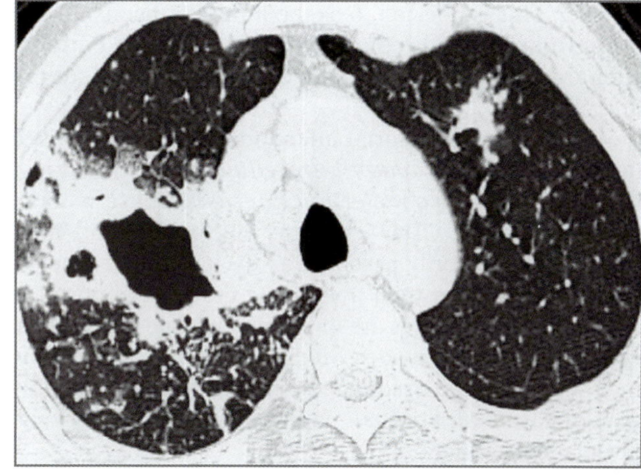

FIG. 8: A 32-year-old HIV-positive lady presented with fever and productive cough. High-resolution CT of the chest shows patchy, multifocal areas of consolidation with cavitation. Sputum was positive for acid-fast bacilli.

(CT: computed tomography; HIV: human immunodeficiency virus)

In patients who are put on HAART, there may be worsening or appearance of new lymphadenopathy, lung parenchymal opacities, or pleural effusion accompanied

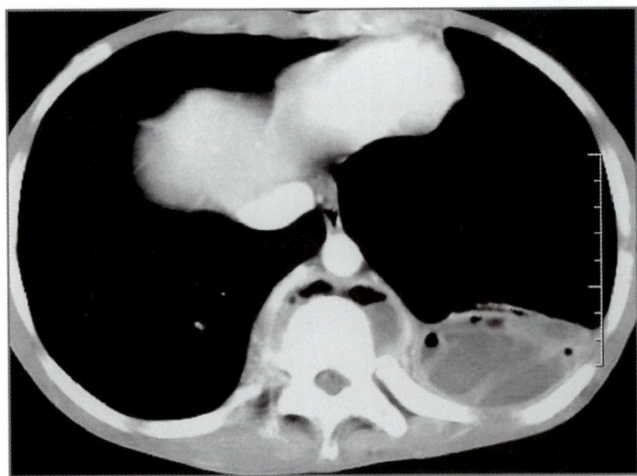

FIG. 9: A 23-year-old HIV-positive male presented with fever, cough, and back pain. Contrast enhanced CT of the chest shows pre- and para-spinal fluid collections with multiple septae and enhancing walls due to spinal TB; miliary nodules were seen in the lungs.

(CT: computed tomography; HIV: human immunodeficiency virus; TB: tuberculosis).

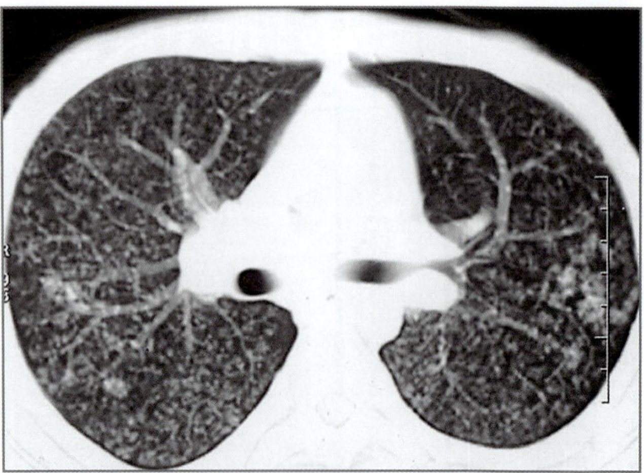

FIG. 10: A 35-year-old renal transplant recipient presented with fever 3 months after transplant surgery. High-resolution computed tomography (CT) of the chest shows multiple, 1–3 mm, randomly distributed nodules in both lungs with tree-in-bud appearance at places. Sputum was positive for acid-fast bacilli.

by fever. This is referred to as the immune reconstitution inflammatory or the paradoxical syndrome. Patients who are severely symptomatic may benefit from steroid therapy.[10]

Atypical mycobacterial infections are usually caused by *Mycobacterium avium intracellulare* (MAI) and less frequently by *Mycobacterium kansasii*. These usually occur when the CD4+ count is <50 cells/mm^3. MAI infection commonly presents as disseminated disease with the gastrointestinal tract being the normal portal of entry. Imaging features are ill-defined nodules, multifocal consolidation, and cavities. Mediastinal lymphadenopathy may occur. The chest radiograph may be normal in roughly 20% of cases. *M. kansasii* commonly presents as focal alveolar consolidation.

Immune reconstitution inflammatory syndrome has also been described in HIV patients with MAI who are started on HAART. This manifests as an acute febrile episode associated with new or enlarging lymphadenopathy.

Human Immunodeficiency Virus-Negative Immunocompromised Patients

Solid organ transplant recipients are at increased risk of contracting TB with 50–100 times the incidence in the general population in the West. However, studies from India have reported a higher incidence, reflecting the endemic nature of the disease.[30] The infection may appear at any time after the surgery ranging from 1 to 96 months following transplant. Steroids and other antirejection medications affect cell-mediated immunity, which are the primary means of controlling and eradicating mycobacterial infections. There is a high (40–64%) incidence of disseminated disease, with pulmonary infection seen in approximately 40% of cases. The rate of progression is also faster than in the general population with higher morbidity and mortality.

The imaging appearance consists of cavitary upper lobe opacities in about one-third of patients. Another one-third of patients demonstrate a miliary pattern **(Fig. 10)**. The rest may show a solitary lower lobe opacity, large nodule, or pleural effusion. Lymphadenopathy is uncommon (3.5%). Nontubercular mycobacterial infection is usually with MAI or *M. kansasii*. These account for a higher fraction of mycobacterial infections in the transplant recipient: 25–43% of mycobacterial infections compared to 5–10% in the general population. These usually present as multiple, moderate-sized pulmonary nodules. Miliary nodules may be seen and are associated with a high mortality.

VIRAL INFECTIONS

Respiratory viral infections are commonly seen in HIV/AIDS patients with CD4+ counts <50 cells/mm^3. CMV is the most common viral pathogen with a reported incidence of up to 90% in advanced HIV disease.

The herpes group of viruses is the predominant viral pathogen in solid organ transplant recipients. Since these are most often reactivation infections of dormant organisms residing in the host or the transplant organ, they occur in the first few months post-transplant.

Although CMV infection affects almost two-thirds of allogeneic HSCT recipients, CMV pneumonia develops in less than one-third of patients.[21] It typically occurs in the early phase and is associated with a high mortality rate of up to 85%. Infection with CMV is associated with increased susceptibility to bacterial, fungal, and protozoal superinfections; increased risk of rejection; and overall mortality.

The imaging appearance of CMV pneumonitis is classically that of diffuse ground glass or patchy interstitial opacities resembling PCP. With severe infection, diffuse alveolar infiltrates may appear, which mimic adult respiratory distress syndrome.[31] Pulmonary nodules may be seen in about two-thirds of cases **(Fig. 11)**. Airway disease, which manifests as bronchiectasis, bronchial wall thickening, and bronchiolitis, may be seen in one-third of cases. *Herpes simplex* (HSV-1, HSV-2) pneumonia is uncommon with a reported incidence of 0.8–10% in solid organ transplant recipients and 0.2% in AIDS patients.[3,4] The chest radiograph will demonstrate multifocal or diffuse consolidation. *Varicella zoster* is also a reactivation infection in the solid organ transplant recipient and usually manifests as a disseminated disease. A 5–15 mm, diffuse, ill-defined, nodular densities with fuzzy outlines are seen on chest radiographs.

Adenovirus and *respiratory syncytial virus* are common causes of viral community-acquired pneumonia. Radiographs may show interstitial opacities, alveolar consolidation, nodules, or pleural effusion.

FUNGAL INFECTIONS

Fungal pneumonias characteristically develop in patients who are neutropenic (from cytotoxic drugs and transplant recipients) or on corticosteroid therapy. The infecting organisms fall into two categories, which are as follows: (1) Those that occur exclusively in immunocompromised hosts such as *Aspergillus*, *Candida*, and *Mucor* species and (2) endemic fungi with increased virulence in immunocompromised hosts such as *Histoplasma*, *Coccidioides*, *Cryptococcus*, and *Blastomyces* species. Invasive aspergillosis and disseminated candidiasis are the most common agents, accounting for 80% of fungal infections in solid organ transplant recipients. Most will occur (80%) within 2 months post-transplant. The incidence varies from 5% in kidney transplants to 40% among liver transplant patients. Fungal pneumonias are relatively uncommon in AIDS occurring in <5% of patients with the most common pathogen being *Cryptococcus*. The incidence of *Aspergillus* infection is increasing and almost exclusively occurs in AIDS patients who are neutropenic due to drugs such as zidovudine or ganciclovir or steroids. Affected individuals are generally in an advanced stage of immune depression with CD4+ counts <50 cells/mm^3. Although meningitis is the most common manifestation of *Cryptococcus* infections, active pulmonary infection is present in 40% of patients with cryptococcosis.

Fungal pneumonia is also common in patients undergoing chemotherapy for hematological malignancies during and following HSCT. Neutropenia is the most important risk factor.[28] Most common pathogen is *Aspergillus*, while *Mucor*, *Candida*, and *Cryptococcus* may also occur. *Aspergillus* infection has the greatest propensity to occur when the peripheral white cell count falls to <1,000 cells/mm^3.

The radiographic abnormalities in angioinvasive aspergillosis consist of nodular or wedge-shaped opacities, frequently abutting the pleural surfaces. These often cavitate reflecting the angioinvasive nature of the fungus and may show central low-density areas or the air crescent sign **(Fig. 12)**. The CT "halo" sign refers to GGOs surrounding

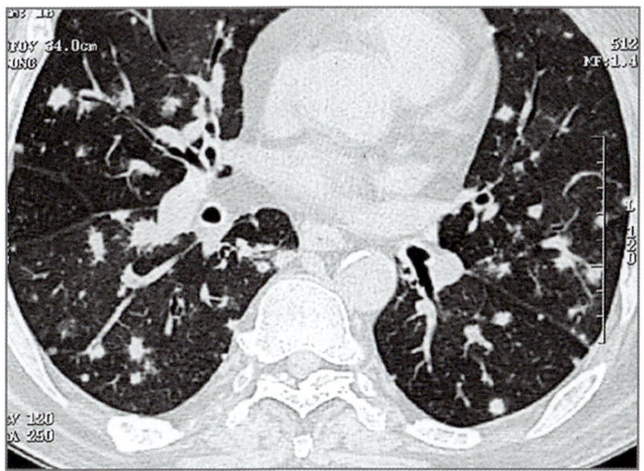

FIG. 11: A 42-year-old HIV-positive male with fever. High-resolution CT of the chest shows multiple, 5–8 mm nodules randomly distributed in both the lungs. Bronchoalveolar lavage showed CMV. Later, autopsy confirmed cytoplasmic inclusion bodies.

(CT: computed tomography; CMV: cytomegalovirus; HIV: human immunodeficiency virus)

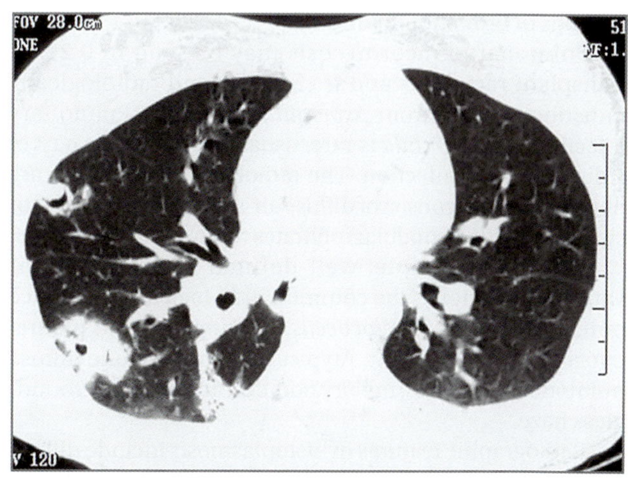

FIG. 12: A 28-year-old male presented with fever and chest pain following chemotherapy. High-resolution computed tomography (CT) of the chest shows multiple nodules with cavitations and air crescent sign with wedge-shaped areas of consolidation. CT-guided fine-needle aspiration cytology revealed *Aspergillus*.

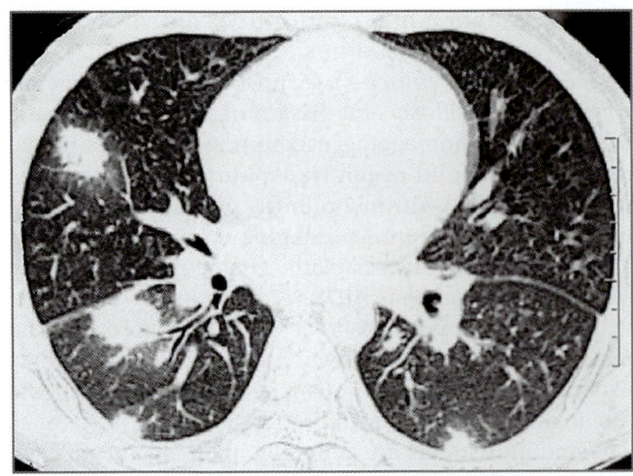

FIG. 13: A 40-year-old male (postrenal transplant) presented with fever and dyspnea. High-resolution computed tomography (CT) of the chest demonstrates multiple, bilateral, large nodules with surrounding ground-glass attenuation—the CT halo sign. Bronchoalveolar lavage revealed *Aspergillus*.

a nodular opacity representing a rim of hemorrhage due to thrombosis within the adjacent vessels caused by the fungus and is an early sign of disease **(Fig. 13)**.[30] Although considered to be characteristic of angioinvasive *Aspergillus*, the "halo" sign may also be seen with *Mucor*, *Candida*, CMV infections, and Wegener's granulomatosis.[31-33] The "air crescent" sign is seen when there is resorption of the necrotic tissue by returning neutrophils and is, therefore, a relatively late sign, representing recovery from the infection.[32] Necrotizing tracheobronchial aspergillosis may be present in 10–30% of patients and may be seen on CT as nodular tracheal or bronchial wall thickening or nonspecific findings of bronchopneumonia.

Pulmonary mucormycosis may be seen in 0.2% of transplant recipients and is clinically and radiologically indistinguishable from *Aspergillus* infection. Pulmonary infection with *Candida* is rare, usually occurring as part of a disseminated infection. The radiologic appearances are nonspecific and consist of diffuse air-space consolidation or single or multiple, nodular infiltrates resembling *Aspergillus*.

Single or multiple, well-defined nodules with or without cavitation is the common radiological appearance of infection with *Cryptococcus*. Adenopathy and pleural effusion may be present. Atypical findings include diffuse pulmonary infiltrates, miliary nodules, and areas of ground-glass haze.[34]

Radiographic features in histoplasmosis include diffuse small nodules (usually <3 mm in size), miliary nodules, or larger nodules around 1 cm in size. Small pleural effusions and mediastinal lymphadenopathy may be seen. Chest radiographs may be normal in 35–50% of patients. In patients with coccidiomycosis, diffuse, small, nodular opacities are the most common radiographic manifestation. Thin-walled cavities, which are characteristically seen in immunocompetent individuals, are uncommon in the immune compromised host. Reports of infection with blastomycosis are rare. Pulmonary findings include focal alveolar infiltrates or bilateral patchy or nodular opacities.[11]

NONINFECTIOUS MANIFESTATIONS OF ACQUIRED IMMUNODEFICIENCY SYNDROME

Kaposi Sarcoma

Kaposi sarcoma is a malignancy, which almost exclusively occurs in bisexual and homosexual males with AIDS. It is also known to affect certain ethnic groups. Its incidence has decreased in recent years due to greater awareness of safe sex habits and the introduction of HAART.[35] The CD4+ counts in patients with KS are generally <100 cells/mm^3.

Kaposi sarcoma is a multisystem disease that affects the skin, lymph nodes, lungs, and gastrointestinal tract. Characteristic findings of pulmonary KS are nodular thickening along the bronchovascular bundles, growing from the perihilar region to the periphery. The nodules may become coalescent, leading to dense air-space consolidation. Pleural effusion occurs in 30–89% of cases and may be unilateral or bilateral. Mediastinal lymphadenopathy is uncommon but when present demonstrates characteristic enhancement following intravenous iodinated contrast.[36]

On MR, KS lesions demonstrate increased signal intensity on T1-weighted images and markedly reduced signal intensity on T2-weighted images with intense enhancement following gadolinium administration. On nuclear scanning, KS lesions are thallium avid; however, in contrast to infectious conditions, they do not take up gallium, thereby allowing differentiation between the two conditions.

Lymphoma

Acquired immunodeficiency syndrome-related lymphoma occurs in AIDS patients at an advanced stage of immune depression when CD4+ counts are <50 cells/mm^3. Most cases consist of non-Hodgkin's lymphoma, usually of high grade with an aggressive nature. Intrathoracic involvement is seen in 10% of cases and is typically extranodal. Pleural effusions are the most common radiographic abnormality. Diffuse, well-defined nodules, focal consolidation, or mediastinal lymphadenopathy may also be seen.

Lymphocytic Interstitial Pneumonitis

Lymphocytic interstitial pneumonitis is a lymphoproliferative disorder characterized by infiltration of the pulmonary interstitium by lymphocytes, histiocytes, and plasma cells. It is much more common in the pediatric population. The radiographic appearance consists of a diffuse, micronodular, interstitial pattern. On HRCT, the most common finding is of GGOs along with poorly defined centrilobular nodules. Cystic air spaces and intestinal thickening may also be seen.[17]

Post-transplant Lymphoproliferative Disorder

Post-transplant lymphoproliferative disorder (PTLD) is a spectrum of lymphoproliferative abnormalities ranging from a benign febrile illness with lymphadenopathy to a rapidly fatal malignant lymphoma. This may develop in 1–10% of transplant patients. The Epstein–Barr virus appears to be causally related to the development of PTLD. With current immunosuppressive regimens, the peak incidence of PTLD is in the third month following transplant.

Radiographically, PTLD manifests as one or multiple, uniform, nonenhancing masses in large organs, including the lung, liver, kidney, bowel, and brain. Lymphadenopathy may be seen in 15–37% of cases, either in isolation or in association with the organ masses. Endobronchial masses resulting in atelectasis have also been reported.[18]

NONINFECTIOUS MANIFESTATIONS IN HEMATOPOIETIC STEM CELL TRANSPLANTATION

Noninfectious lung injury has emerged as a major cause of morbidity and mortality due to a decline in infectious complications due to the widespread use of prophylactic broad-spectrum antibiotics. The frequency of noninfectious complications is similar in allogeneic and autologous HSCT.[37] Definitive diagnosis of noninfectious complications is challenging, as the clinical manifestations overlap with those of the infections and difficulty in obtaining a histological diagnosis. Imaging studies, particularly HRCT, play a major role in the management of these patients. Noninfectious complications usually follow a timeline due to the underlying immunological status of the host. The neutropenic phase following HSCT lasts from 2 to 3 weeks. After allogeneic HSCT, the immunosuppressive phase continues for 1 year. This is divided into an early phase (up to 100 days) and a late phase, which continue for 1 year or more.[38]

PRE-ENGRAFTMENT PERIOD

Noninfectious complications that occur during neutropenic (also known as pre-engraftment period) include idiopathic pulmonary syndrome (IPS), pulmonary edema, diffuse alveolar hemorrhage (DAH), and periengraftment respiratory distress syndrome (PERDS).[39]

Idiopathic Pulmonary Syndrome

It is defined as a diffuse lung injury without an infectious cause. Predisposing factors are pretransplant chemotherapy and total body irradiation. It carries a high mortality. It progresses from an acute exudative to a subacute proliferative to a chronic fibrotic phase. HRCT findings are those of diffuse alveolar damage manifesting as focal or diffuse GGO with a density gradient toward the dependent regions. Consolidation is less common. The chronic phase is characterized by traction bronchiectasis and honeycombing. HRCT findings are, thus, nonspecific, and IPS remains a diagnosis of exclusion.[40,41]

Pulmonary Edema

It is a common complication with a rapid onset, usually occurring in the second or third week after HSCT. Underlying mechanisms include graft-versus-host disease (GVHD), cardiac or renal dysfunction secondary to chemotherapy regimens, pulmonary vasculature hyperpermeability induced by total body irradiation, sepsis, cyclosporine A, or fluid overload.[3,23] Chest X-ray (CXR) suggests a diagnosis when there are diffuse interstitial markings, peribronchial cuffing, perihilar haziness, ground-glass appearance, and vascular prominence. HRCT features include perihilar GGO or consolidation, thickening of interlobular septa, enlargement of pulmonary vessels, and pleural effusions **(Fig. 14)**.

Diffuse Alveolar Hemorrhage

Diffuse alveolar hemorrhage is the most common noninfectious pulmonary complication in leukemia. Around 20% of HSCT patients may develop DAH in the neutropenic phase.[21] The manifestations of DAH are secondary to pulmonary vessel damage by acute GVHD, pretransplantation chemotherapy, or total body irradiation. Clinical presentation is nonspecific; mild hemoptysis occurs in about two-thirds of the patients; frank hemoptysis is rare.[40] It carries a high mortality rate of about 80%. Early diagnosis and prompt steroid therapy improve survival. BAL may aid the diagnosis by demonstrating hemosiderin-laden macrophages. Radiological findings are nonspecific. HRCT findings include widespread GGO or consolidation with interlobular septal thickening (crazy-paving appearance) **(Fig. 15)**. The peripheral lungs are spared.[31]

Periengraftment Respiratory Distress Syndrome

Periengraftment respiratory distress syndrome presents with diffuse capillary leak, cutaneous rash, and fever that occur during the engraftment and neutrophil recovery phases. It is thought to result from proinflammatory cytokines released during engraftment. Autologous HSCT has a greater incidence of this complication. The HRCT findings of interlobular septal thickening with bilateral GGOs and perihilar or peribronchial consolidation and pleural effusions are indistinguishable from those of pulmonary edema and acute respiratory distress syndrome.[39]

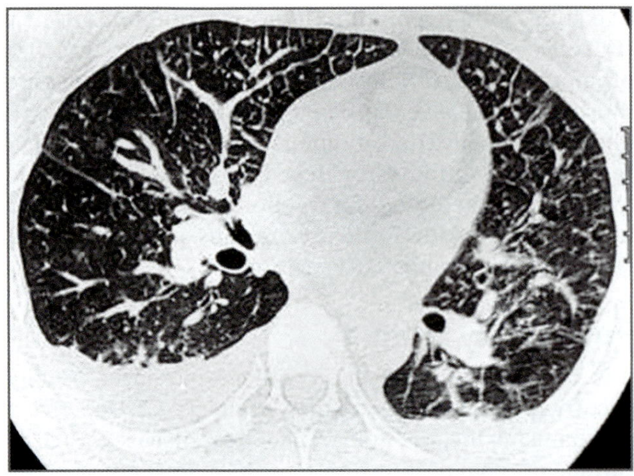

FIG. 14: A 38-year-old female following HSCT developed breathlessness. HRCT shows perihilar ground-glass opacity, thickening of interlobular septa, enlargement of pulmonary vessels, and pleural effusion, suggestive of pulmonary edema.

(HRCT: high-resolution computed tomography; HSCT: hematopoietic stem cell transplantation)

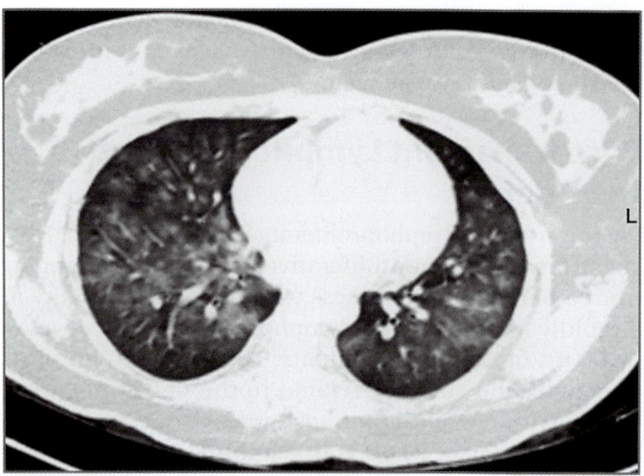

FIG. 15: A 28-year-old female with leukemia following HSCT complained of streaky hemoptysis. HRCT of the chest shows diffuse GGOs due to diffuse alveolar hemorrhage.

(GGOs: ground-glass opacities; HRCT: high-resolution computed tomography; HSCT: hematopoietic stem cell transplantation)

EARLY POST-TRANSPLANT PERIOD

During the early post-transplant period (30–100 days after HSCT), the neutrophil count has recovered. Impaired cellular and humoral immunity, however, persists. Reconstitution of the immune system leads to a reduction in the frequency of infectious complications as well. Noninfectious pulmonary complications during this period include acute GVHD, acute radiation injury, and, rarely, pulmonary cytolytic thrombi.

Drug-induced Lung Injury

Drug-induced lung injury occurs in around 10% of patients with hematopoietic stem cell transplant. There are variable patterns of injury, including nonspecific interstitial pneumonia, hypersensitivity pneumonitis, diffuse alveolar damage, and organizing pneumonia. The HRCT features are nonspecific and include diffuse GGOs, subpleural or peribronchial consolidation, centrilobular nodules, and interlobular septal thickening.[39]

Acute Graft-versus-host Disease

Graft versus host disease is a major cause of morbidity and mortality in patients following allogeneic HSCT and is secondary to the immune reaction of the donor cells to the host tissues. Autologous transplant is not associated with acute GVHD. GVHD occurs in 20–75% of allogeneic HSCT recipients. Skin, liver, and gastrointestinal system are the primary targets. Lung involvement is uncommon, and a broad spectrum of GVHD changes has been described histopathologically—ranging from acute injury to chronic irreversible damage.[42] HRCT demonstrates nonspecific changes, including diffuse interstitial and alveolar opacities that mimic pulmonary edema.

Acute Radiation Pneumonitis

This complication occurs in patients who receive radiation therapy for intrathoracic lymphoma. Most patients are asymptomatic. Moreover, with modern techniques of radiation, the radiation-related acute toxicity has reduced. The early stage changes (8–12 weeks after completion) are characterized by cellular infiltration composed predominantly of macrophages. On imaging, there is patchy consolidation in the radiation field that may coalesce to form a relatively sharp border conforming to the radiation portal. The late stage (6–24 months after completion) is characterized by fibrotic changes, which appear on CT as parenchymal distortion and traction bronchiectasis.[39]

Pulmonary Cytolytic Thrombi

Like GVHD, this is a rare pulmonary complication that occurs exclusively in allogeneic HSCT recipients. In fact, it may be a manifestation of GVHD. Children are primarily affected. A median onset of 72 days after HSCT has been reported.[39] Pathologically, there are intravascular thromboemboli composed of necrotic basophilic debris occluding the small and medium pulmonary vessels, leading to surrounding alveolar hemorrhage or infarct. Multiple bilateral pulmonary nodules with surrounding GGOs are seen on HRCT.

LATE PULMONARY COMPLICATIONS

Late complications occur 3 months after HSCT. During this period, noninfectious causes are more common.[23] The most common complication during this period is chronic GVHD manifesting either as bronchiolitis obliterans, organizing pneumonia, or nonclassifiable interstitial pneumonia. Air-leak syndrome (ALS), PTLD, pulmonary veno-occlusive disease (PVOD), and pleuroparenchymal fibroelastosis are less frequently encountered complications.

Chronic Graft-versus-host Disease

It occurs only in patients with allogeneic HSCT secondary to immune-mediated reaction of the donor T lymphocytes against the host tissues.[42] Lung involvement is common unlike acute GVHD. It manifests either as organizing pneumonia (reversible with favorable prognosis) or bronchiolitis obliterans (irreversible).

Bronchiolitis Obliterans

It occurs most commonly in allogeneic HSCT for leukemia or aplastic anemia. About 10% of patients who develop chronic GVHD develop bronchiolitis obliterans. Factors that increase the risk include immunosuppression with methotrexate, chemotherapy, or irradiation prior to HSCT and low serum immunoglobulin after HSCT. Pathologically, there is constrictive bronchiolitis with submucosal and peribronchiolar fibrosis. HRCT findings are best demonstrated on expiratory CT and include air trapping, mosaic perfusion, and bronchial dilatation.[43]

Bronchiolitis Obliterans Organizing Pneumonia

The pathological hallmark is granulation tissue in the lumen of alveolar ducts and bronchioles followed by fibroblastic proliferation. HRCT findings include patchy, bilateral, multifocal areas of GGO or consolidation in a peribronchial or subpleural distribution. Areas of consolidation tend to be multifocal, bilateral, peripheral, and lower lobe predominant **(Fig. 16)**.[44]

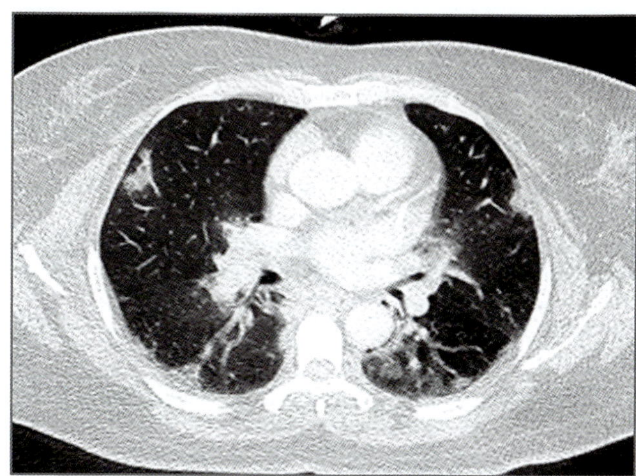

FIG. 16: A 47-year-old female with chronic myeloid leukemia. HRCT shows patchy, bilateral areas of ground glass opacity and consolidation in a subpleural distribution. TBLB confirmed the diagnosis as BOOP.

(BOOP: bronchiolitis obliterans organizing pneumonia; HRCT: high-resolution computed tomography; TBLB: transbronchial lung biopsy)

Air-leak Syndrome

Air-leak syndrome is characterized by spontaneous pneumothorax, pneumomediastinum, pulmonary interstitial emphysema, or subcutaneous emphysema in HSCT recipients. Typically, patients with ALS have chronic GVHD and bronchiolitis obliterans syndrome. On HRCT, the diagnosis of pneumothorax, pneumomediastinum, and subcutaneous emphysema is straightforward; however, changes in interstitial emphysema are subtle and appear as linear lucencies along the bronchovascular bundles. Findings of bronchiolitis obliterans will also usually be evident.[45]

Pulmonary Veno-occlusive Disease

Pulmonary veno-occlusive disease is a rare complication that may be encountered following either autologous or allogeneic HSCT.[46] The diagnosis is based on a triad of pulmonary edema, pulmonary hypertension, and normal pulmonary artery occlusion pressure. HRCT demonstrates main pulmonary artery dilatation, GGOs, and smooth interlobular septal thickening.

Pleuroparenchymal Fibroelastosis

Pleuroparenchymal fibroelastosis is a rare complication with upper lobe involvement characterized by fibrotic thickening of the pleura and fibroelastosis of the subpleural parenchyma.[47]

CONCLUSION

Pulmonary infections are the most common complications in patients with HIV/AIDS and solid organ transplant/HSCT recipients and account for significant morbidity and mortality. It is important for the radiologist to demand and utilize all available clinical information such as signs and symptoms, degree of immunosuppression, risk factor for HIV infection, and time period since solid organ or HSC transplant. In most cases, the clinical and chest radiograph findings are sufficient for a confident diagnosis. However, chest radiographs may be normal or demonstrate subtle or nonspecific findings. Chest CT plays an important role in identifying the presence of disease and may specifically diagnose many conditions. Equally important, a negative HRCT of the chest virtually excludes active infectious disease.

REFERENCES

1. Afessa B, Green B. Bacterial pneumonia in hospitalized patients with HIV infection. Chest. 2000;117(4):1017-22.
2. Aronchick JM. Pulmonary infections in cancer and bone marrow transplant patients. Semin Roentgenol. 2000;35(2):140-51.
3. Daniel DM. Pulmonary infections in HIV/AIDS. Semin Roentgenol. 2000;35(2):124-39.
4. Miller WT. Pulmonary infections in patients who have received solid organ transplants. Semin Roentgenol. 2000;35(2):152-70.
5. Lee C, Colletti PM, Chung JH, Ackman JB, Berry MF, Carter BW, et al. Acute respiratory illness in immunocompromised patients. J Am Coll Radiol. 2019;16(115):5331-9.
6. World Health Organization. (2008). Report on the global AIDS epidemic. [online] Available from https://www.unaids.org/globalreport/Global_report.htm. [Last accessed February, 2025].
7. Beck JM. The immune-compromised host: HIV infection. Proc Am Thorac Soc. 2005;2:423-7.
8. Boiselle PM, Aviram G, Fishman JE. Update on lung disease in AIDS. Semin Roentgenol. 2002;37(1):54-71.
9. Grubb JR, Moorman AC, Baker RK, Masur H. The changing spectrum of pulmonary disease in patients with HIV infection on antiretroviral therapy. AIDS. 2006;20:1095-107.
10. Guillamet CV, Hsu JL, Dhillon G, Guillmet RV. Pulmonary infections in immunocompromised hosts. Clin J Thorac Imaging. 2018;33(5):295-305.
11. Tanaka N, Kunihiro Y, Yanagawa N. Infection in immunocompromised hosts. Imaging J Thorac Imaging. 2018;33(5):306-21.
12. Huang L, Crothers K. HIV associated opportunistic pneumonias. Respirology. 2009;14:474-85.
13. Castaner E, Gallardo X, Mata JM, Esteba L. Radiologic approach to the diagnosis of infectious pulmonary diseases in patients infected with the human immunodeficiency virus. Eur J Radiol. 2004;51:114-29.
14. Allen CM, Al-Jahdali HH, Irion KL, Al-Ghanem S, Gouda A, Khan AN. Imaging lung manifestations of HIV/AIDS. Ann Thorac Med 2010;5(4):201-6.
15. Kang E, Staples CA, McGuinness G, Primack SL, Muller NL. Detection and differential diagnosis of pulmonary infections and tumors in patients with AIDS: value of chest radiography versus CT. Am J Roentgenol. 1996;166:15-9.
16. Hartman TE, Primack SL, Müller NL, Staples CA. Diagnosis of thoracic complications in AIDS: accuracy of CT. Am J Roentgenol. 1994;162:547-53.
17. Calder AD, Perucca G, Johnson SM, Pandey AR, Moshal K, Kusters MA. Lung infections in immunocompromised children. Ped Radiol. 2024;54:530-47.
18. Greenberg SD, Frager D, Suster B, Walker S, Stavropoulos C, Rothpearl A. Active pulmonary tuberculosis in patients with AIDS: spectrum of radiographic findings (including a normal appearance). Radiology. 1994;193:115-9.
19. Carignan S, Staples CA, Muller NL. Intrathoracic lymphoproliferative disorders in the immunocompromised host. J Thorac Imaging. 1995;197:53-8.
20. Franquet T. High resolution computed tomography (HRCT) of lung infections in non-AIDS immunocompromised patients. Eur Radiol. 2006;16:707-18.
21. Mesurolle B, Tanaka N, Kosiuk J, Mignon F, Choquet S. The treated thorax in patients with hematological malignancies. In: Guermazi A (Ed). Radiological Imaging in Hematological Malignancies, 1st edition. Berlin, Germany: Springer-Verlag; 2004. pp. 443-72.
22. Rosenow EC, Wilson WR, Cockerill FR. Pulmonary disease in the immunocompromised host. Mayo Clin Proc. 1985;60(7):473-87.
23. Worthy SA, Flint JD, Muller NL. Pulmonary complications after bone marrow transplantation: high resolution CT and pathological findings. Radiographics. 1997;17:1359-71.
24. Hows JM. Status of umbilical cord blood transplantation in the year 2001. J Clin Pathol. 2001;54:428-34.
25. Heussel CP, Kanczor HU, Heussel GU, Fischer B, Begrich M, Mildenberger P, et al. Pneumonia in febrile neutropenic patients and in bone marrow and blood stem cell transplant recipients: use of high resolution computed tomography. J Clin Oncol. 1999;17:796-805.
26. Huang L, Cattamanchi A, Davis L, den Boon S, Kovacs J, Meshnick S, et al. HIV-associated Pneumocystis pneumonia. Proc Am Thorac Soc. 2010;8:294-300.
27. Cereser L, Dallorto A, Candoni A, Volpetti S, Righi E. Pneumocystis jirovecii pneumonia at chest high resolution computed tomography (HRCT) in non-HIV immunocompromised patients: spectrum of findings and mimickers. Eur J Radiol. 2019;4:116-27.
28. Kramer MR, Marshall SE, Starnes VA, Gamberg P, Amitai Z, Theodore J. Infectious complications in heart lung transplantation: analysis of 200 episodes. Arch Intern Med. 1993;153:2010-6.
29. Spalgais S, Jaiswal A, Puri M, Sarin R, Agarwal U. Clinical profile and diagnosis of extrapulmonary TB in HIV infected patients: routine abdominal ultrasonography increases detection of abdominal tuberculosis. Indian J Tuberc. 2013;60(3):147-53.
30. Gulati M, Kaur R, Jha V, Venkataramu NK, Gupta D, Suri S. High-resolution CT in renal transplant patients with suspected pulmonary infections. Acta Radiol. 2000;41:1-6.
31. Kunihiro Y, Tanaka N, Kawano R, Matsumoto T, Kobayashi T, Yujiri T, et al. Differentiation of pulmonary complications with extensive ground-glass attenuation on high-resolution CT in immunocompromised patients. Jap J Radiol. 2021;39:868-76.
32. Park YS, Seo JB, Lee YK, Do KH, Lee JS, Song JW, et al. Radiological and clinical findings of pulmonary aspergillosis following solid organ transplant. Clin Radiol. 2008;63:673-80.
33. Ray A, Mittal A, Vyas S. CT halo sign: a systematic review. Eur J Radiol. 2020;124:108843.
34. Sui X, Huang Y, Song W, Zheng F, Wang X, Xu X, et al. Clinical features of pulmonary cryptococcosis in thin-section CT in immunocompetent and non-AIDS immunocompromised patients. Radiol Med. 2020;125:31-8.
35. La Ferla L, Pinzone MR, Nunnari G, Martellotta F, Lleshi A, Tirelli U, et al. Kaposi's sarcoma in HIV-positive patients: the

state of art in the HAART era. Eur Rev Med Pharmacol Sci. 2013;17(17):2354-65.

36. Davis SD, Henschke CI, Chamides BK, Westcott JL. Intrathoracic Kaposi sarcoma in AIDS patients: radiographic-pathologic correlation. Radiology. 1987;163(2):495-500.
37. Brodoefel H, Faul C, Salih H, Vogel W, Fenchel M, Horger M. Therapy-related noninfectious complications in patients with hematologic malignancies: high-resolution computed tomography findings. J Thorac Imaging. 2013;28(1):W5-1.
38. Tyndall A. Successes and failures of stem cell transplantation in autoimmune diseases. Am Soc Hematol Educ Program. 2011;(1):280-84.
39. Franquet T, Müller NL, Lee KS, Giménez A, Flint JD. High-resolution CT and pathologic findings of noninfectious pulmonary complications after hematopoietic stem cell transplantation. Am J Roentgenol. 2005;184(2):629-37.
40. Tanaka N, Kunihiro Y, Kawano R, Yujiri T, Ueda K, Gondo T, et al. Chest complications in immunocompromised patients without acquired immunodeficiency syndrome (AIDS): differentiation between infectious and non-infectious diseases using high-resolution CT findings. Clin Radiol. 2021;76:50-9.
41. Panoskaltsis-Mortari A, Griese M, Madtes DK, Belperio JA, Haddad IY, Folz RJ, et al. An official American Thoracic Society research statement: noninfectious lung injury after hematopoietic stem cell transplantation: idiopathic pneumonia syndrome. Am J Respir Crit Care Med. 2011;183(9):1262-79.
42. Yousem SA. The histological spectrum of pulmonary graft-versus-host disease in bone marrow transplant recipients. Hum Pathol. 1995;26(6):668-75.
43. Ooi GC, Peh WC, Ip M. High-resolution computed tomography of bronchiolitis obliterans syndrome after bone marrow transplantation. Respiration. 1998;65(3):187-91.
44. Yoshihara S, Yanik G, Cooke KR, Mineishi S. Bronchiolitis obliterans syndrome (BOS), bronchiolitis obliterans organizing pneumonia (BOOP), and other late-onset noninfectious pulmonary complications following allogeneic hematopoietic stem cell transplantation. Biol Blood Marrow Transplant. 2007;13(7):749-59.
45. Franquet T, Rodríguez S, Hernández JM, Martino R, Giménez A, Hidalgo A, et al. Air-leak syndromes in hematopoietic stem cell transplant recipients with chronic GVHD: high-resolution CT findings. J Thorac Imaging. 2007;22(4):335-40.
46. Mandel J, Mark EJ, Hales CA. Pulmonary veno-occlusive disease. Am J Respir Crit Care Med. 2000;162(5):1964-73.
47. Frankel SK, Cool CD, Lynch DA, Brown KK. Idiopathic pleuroparenchymal fibroelastosis: description of a novel clinicopathologic entity. Chest. 2004;126(6):2007-13.

Uma Debi, Mandeep Garg, Ajay Gulati, Manphool Singhal

CHAPTER 8

Pattern Approach to Interstitial Lung Disease and Imaging of Idiopathic Interstitial Pneumonias

INTRODUCTION

Interstitial lung diseases (ILDs) are defined as a group of diffuse lung parenchymal diseases that result from damage to the lung parenchyma caused by different degrees of inflammation and fibrosis.[1] It refers to variable patterns/diseases characterized histologically by inflammatory infiltrate in the interstitium with variable degrees of fibrosis. Correlation of clinical, radiological, and pathological features is often required to reach a correct diagnosis of ILD. According to the updated American Thoracic Society-European Respiratory Society classification, idiopathic interstitial pneumonias (IIPs) are ILDs of unknown etiology sharing common clinical features and can be categorized into (a) "chronic fibrosing IIPs" [idiopathic pulmonary fibrosis (IPF) and idiopathic nonspecific interstitial pneumonia (NSIP)], (b) "smoking-related IIPs" [respiratory bronchiolitis-associated ILD (RB-ILD) and desquamative interstitial pneumonia (DIP)], (c) "acute or subacute IIPs" [cryptogenic organizing pneumonia (COP) and acute interstitial pneumonia (AIP)], and (d) "rare IIPs" [lymphoid interstitial pneumonia (LIP) and idiopathic pleuroparenchymal fibroelastosis (IPPFE)] **(Table 1)**. In addition, another category "unclassifiable IIPs" has been proposed, which includes IIPs in which final diagnosis is not possible.[2]

IMAGING

Plain Radiography

It is an important part of initial imaging. During imaging interstitial pneumonia, the goals of chest radiograph interpretation are to determine the pattern of lung disease, recognize any change in lung volume, and to determine any other accompanying abnormalities **(Fig. 1)**.

High-resolution Computed Tomography

High-resolution computed tomography (HRCT) is required for evaluating the morphology and density of lung abnormalities and their location in relation to a secondary pulmonary lobule. HRCT is much better than routine CT for this purpose. Previously, sequential HRCT was performed in a supine position with 1–2 cm spacing and 1 mm slice thickness. But, this method is nearly obsolete now except for follow-up imaging as it involves more radiation exposure to the patient. The development of multidetector CT scanners, capable of rapidly imaging the thorax using an isotropic technique, has enabled another way in which HRCT scan may be obtained. HRCT scan can be obtained from thin-section (1–2 mm) reconstruction of volumetric data obtained by using multidetector CT, narrow detector width, and image reconstruction with a high spatial frequency algorithm. Expiratory scans should be performed in patients with obstructive disease at three or more levels. Prone scans may be needed to differentiate dependent densities from early changes of ILD.

ANATOMY OF THE SECONDARY PULMONARY LOBULE (MILLER'S)[3]

The secondary pulmonary lobule is the smallest unit of lung structure, which is demarcated by septae of connective tissue. It is the smallest unit of the lung, which is visible on an HRCT scan **(Fig. 2)**. The secondary pulmonary lobule is a polyhedron that depicts the smallest lung unit, which measures approximately 1–2 cm on one side and contains a few terminal bronchioles, which ultimately supply 5–15 pulmonary acini. Terminal bronchiole and centrilobular artery are present at the center of a secondary pulmonary

TABLE 1: Radiological features and differential diagnosis of the IIPs.[2]

IIP group and clinical, radiological, and pathological diagnosis	HRCT patterns	Typical HRCT distribution	Typical HRCT findings	HRCT differential diagnosis
Chronic fibrosing IIPs				
Idiopathic pulmonary fibrosis	Usual interstitial pneumonia	Peripheral, subpleural, and basal	Reticular opacities, honeycombing, traction bronchiectasis, and architectural distortion	Collagen vascular disease, hypersensitivity pneumonitis, asbestosis, and sarcoidosis
Idiopathic nonspecific interstitial pneumonia	Nonspecific interstitial pneumonia	Peripheral, basal, and symmetric	GGO, irregular lines, traction bronchiectasis, and consolidation	Usual interstitial pneumonia, cryptogenic organizing pneumonia, desquamative interstitial pneumonia, and hypersensitivity pneumonitis
Smoking IIPs				
Desquamative interstitial pneumonia	Desquamative interstitial pneumonia	Lower zone, peripheral predominance in most cases	GGO, reticular lines, and cysts	Respiratory bronchiolitis-associated interstitial lung disease, nonspecific interstitial pneumonia, and hypersensitivity pneumonitis
Respiratory bronchiolitis-associated interstitial lung disease	Respiratory bronchiolitis	Upper lung predominant	Centrilobular nodules, bronchial wall thickening, and patchy GGO	Nonspecific interstitial pneumonia, desquamative interstitial pneumonia, and hypersensitivity pneumonitis
Acute or subacute IIPs				
Cryptogenic organizing pneumonia	Organizing pneumonia	Subpleural or peribronchial	Patchy consolidation or nodules, perilobular pattern, and reverse halo sign	Infection, aspiration pneumonia, eosinophilic pneumonia, nonspecific interstitial pneumonia, vasculitis, sarcoidosis, mucinous adenocarcinoma, and lymphoma
Acute interstitial pneumonia	Diffuse alveolar damage	Bilateral or patchy	Consolidation, GGO, and later traction bronchiectasis	Hydrostatic edema, pulmonary hemorrhage, acute and eosinophilic pneumonia
Rare IIPs				
Lymphoid interstitial pneumonia	Lymphoid interstitial pneumonia	Lower lung predominant	GGO, centrilobular nodules, septal and bronchovascular thickening, and thin-walled cysts	Nonspecific interstitial pneumonia, sarcoidosis, Langerhans cell histiocytosis, and lymphangioleiomyomatosis
Idiopathic pleuroparenchymal fibroelastosis	Idiopathic pleuro-parenchymal fibroelastosis	Peripheral, upper lung predominant	Pleural thickening, subpleural fibrotic changes, or consolidation	Sarcoidosis, pneumoconiosis, postinfective pulmonary fibrosis, connective tissue disease, and hypersensitivity pneumonitis

(GGO: ground-glass opacity; HRCT: high-resolution computed tomography; IIPs: idiopathic interstitial pneumonias)

lobule, and pulmonary veins and lymphatics are present in the periphery. The interlobular septa in the periphery contain connective tissue, venules, and lymphatics. On HRCT, centrilobular artery and intralobular acinar arteries supplying a secondary pulmonary lobule can be discerned, while normal bronchioles supplying it cannot be. Centrilobular arteries measure approximately 1 mm in diameter. Intralobular acinar arteries measure approximately 0.5 mm in diameter. Normal bronchiole supplying a secondary pulmonary lobule measures approximately 1 mm in diameter with wall thickness of approximately 0.15 mm, which is beyond the resolution of HRCT. However, abnormal thickening of the interlobular and intralobular septa, axial interstitium surrounding the bronchovascular bundles, and subpleural peripheral interstitium should always be identified on HRCT.

The correct diagnosis of ILD on HRCT depends on evaluating the morphology and density of the lung abnormalities and their distribution in relationship to the secondary pulmonary lobule. Lung abnormalities are first classified into four categories: (1) Increased lung attenuation, (2) decreased lung attenuation, (3) linear and reticular opacities, and (4) nodules and nodular opacities.

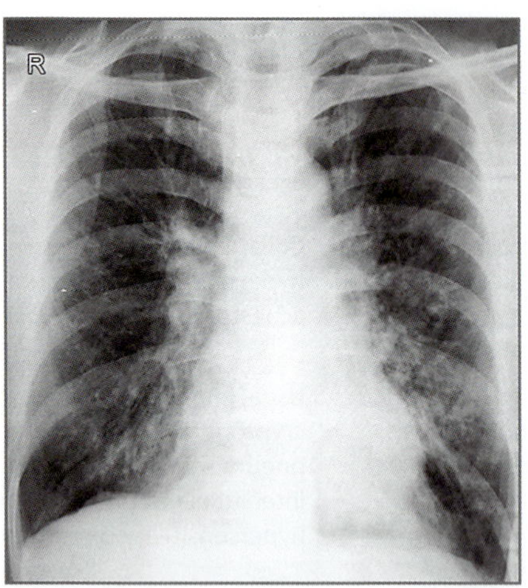

FIG. 1: Frontal chest radiograph posteroanterior (PA) view reveals reticulonodular opacities in bilateral lower lobes.

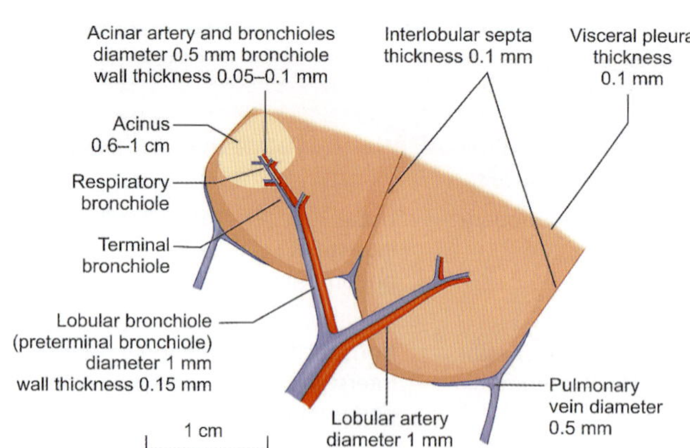

FIG. 2: Anatomy and dimensions of secondary lobule and pulmonary acinus. Two secondary pulmonary lobules in the lung periphery are illustrated along with the dimensions of their components.

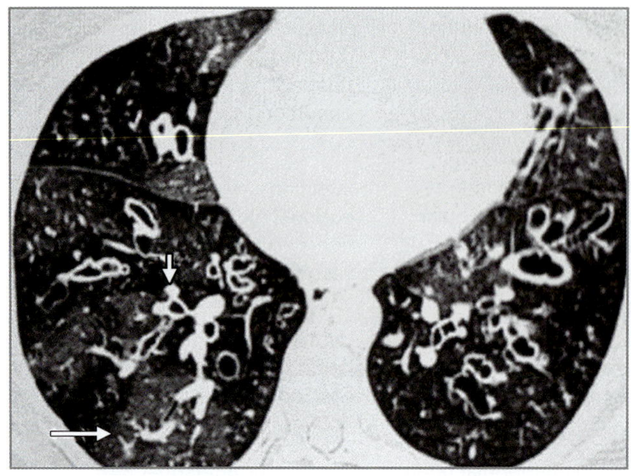

FIG. 3: Axial high-resolution computed tomography (HRCT) of the chest shows patchy areas of ground-glass opacity (long arrow) in bilateral lungs with varicose bronchiectasis, bronchial wall thickening, and signet ring sign (short arrow).

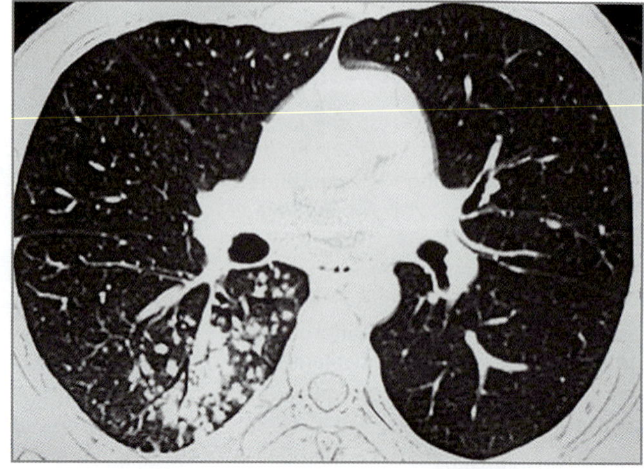

FIG. 4: Axial high-resolution computed tomography (HRCT) of the chest shows patchy areas of consolidation with air bronchogram in right lower lobe surrounded by multiple centrilobular nodules.

Increased Lung Attenuation

It is classified into ground-glass opacity (GGO), consolidation, alveolar microlithiasis, metastatic calcification, and granulomatous diseases (tuberculosis, silicosis, and sarcoidosis). GGO is defined as a mild increase in lung opacity, which does not cause obscuration of the underlying vessel **(Fig. 3)**. It suggests an active or acute disease. Consolidation is defined as increased lung opacity, which causes obscuration of underlying vascular markings **(Fig. 4)**. Air bronchogram is a characteristic finding seen in consolidation.

Decreased Lung Attenuation

It is categorized into mosaic perfusion, honeycombing, bronchiectasis, emphysema, pneumatoceles, and lung cysts. Mosaic perfusion pattern is obtained due to differential attenuation of areas of the lungs, caused due to differences in lung perfusion, either due to pulmonary vascular disease or airway disease. The pulmonary arteries are reduced in size in the lucent lung fields, which help to distinguish mosaic perfusion from GGO **(Fig. 5)**. Honeycombing can be defined as clustered cystic airspaces, which have clearly definable walls and are most commonly seen in peripheral and subpleural lung **(Fig. 6)**. Bronchiectasis is localized, abnormal dilatation of bronchial tree usually segmental and subsegmental bronchi, which occurs as a result of airway inflammation, infections, or impaired mucociliary clearance **(Fig. 3)**. Emphysema is known as irreversible abnormal enlargement and destruction of airspaces distal to terminal bronchiole **(Fig. 7)**. Lung cysts are well-defined,

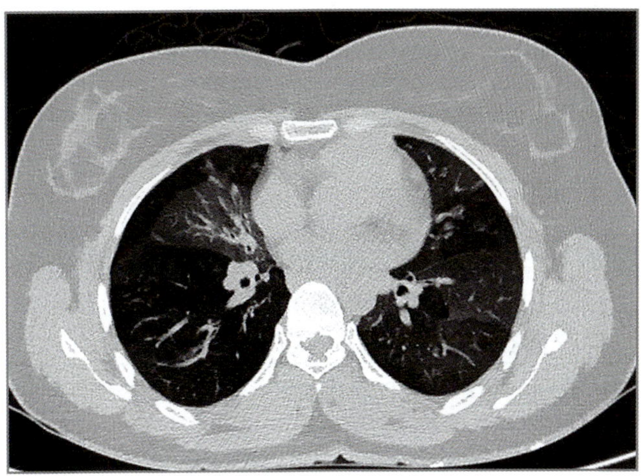

FIG. 5: Axial high-resolution computed tomography (HRCT) of the chest shows areas of mosaic perfusion in bilateral lungs.

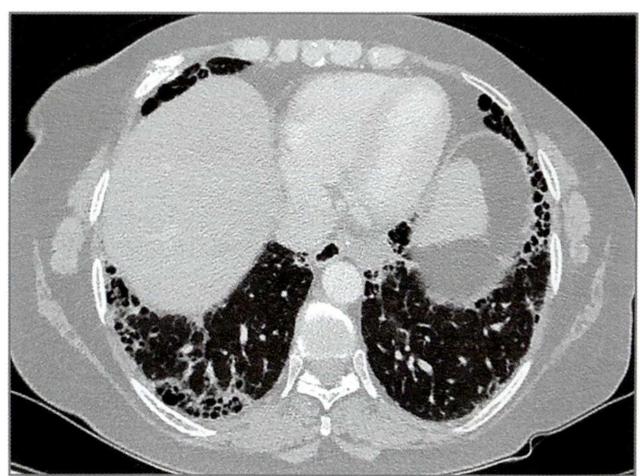

FIG. 6: Axial high-resolution computed tomography (HRCT) of the chest shows honeycombing consisting of multilayered thin-walled cyst.

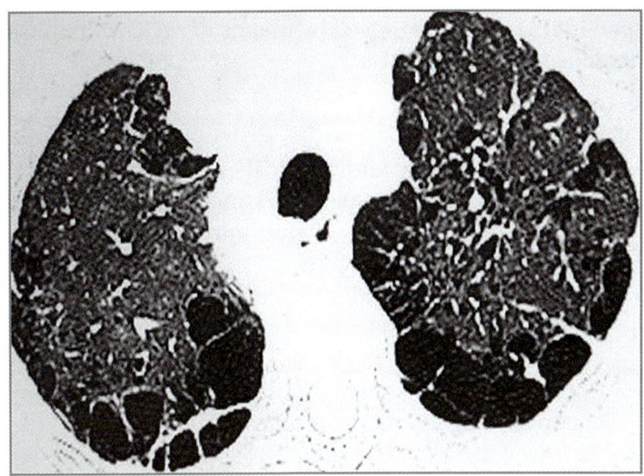

FIG. 7: Axial high-resolution computed tomography (HRCT) of the chest shows centriacinar and paraseptal emphysematous changes in bilateral upper lobes.

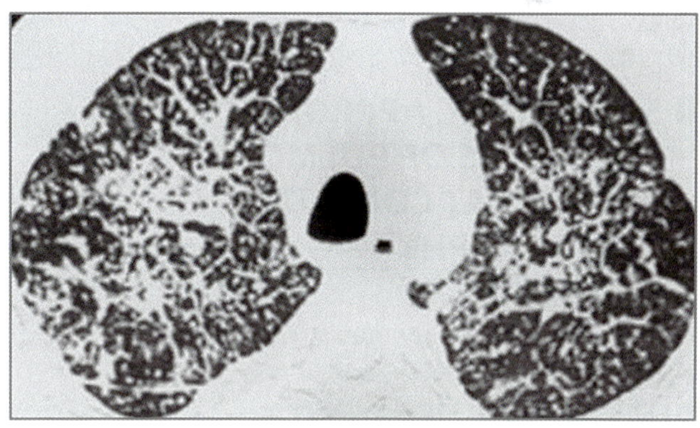

FIG. 8: Axial high-resolution computed tomography (HRCT) of the chest shows intralobular and interlobular septal thickening in bilateral upper lobes.

thin-walled (approximately 1–3 mm) air-containing lesions. Multiple lung cysts are seen in diseases such as lymphangioleiomyomatosis, Langerhans cell histiocytosis, and LIPs.

Nodules and Nodular Opacities

High-resolution computed tomography classifies nodules into three categories depending on location, i.e., which portion of the secondary pulmonary lobule is involved. Centrilobular nodules involve terminal/respiratory bronchioles **(Fig. 4)**. Perilymphatic nodules are seen in subpleural and peribronchovascular regions. Random nodules have no particular anatomic distribution. Common causes of centrilobular nodules are infectious airway diseases, hypersensitivity pneumonitis (HP), and RB. Perilymphatic nodules are seen in sarcoidosis, lymphangitic carcinomatosis, silicosis, and coal workers' pneumoconiosis (CWP). Random nodules are seen in tuberculosis, angioinvasive fungal infections, and hematogenous metastasis.

Linear and Reticular Opacities

These are categorized into intralobular septal thickening, interlobular septal thickening **(Fig. 8)**, parenchymal bands, peribronchovascular interstitial thickening, and subpleural lines. Intralobular septal thickening is seen in IPF, chronic HP, NSIP, and asbestosis. Interlobular septal thickening is seen in lymphangitis carcinomatosis, LIP, IPF, sarcoidosis, pulmonary edema, silicosis, CWP, and pneumocystis pneumonia. Parenchymal bands are linear opacities, which are several millimeters thick and approximately 2–5 cm in length. They are seen in patients with fibrosis. A crazy-paving pattern is formed when there is concurrence of GGO with reticulations **(Table 2)**.

TABLE 2: Factors to check for the history and examination of an individual with suspected idiopathic interstitial lung disease (ILD).[4,5]

ILD of known cause	Factors to check for patient's history and examination
Occupational/environmental lung disease	Occupational exposures (current or previous) known to be a risk factor for lung disease
Systemic disease	• Serological findings, symptoms, or signs of a systemic autoimmune disorder • Extrapulmonary involvement
Hypersensitivity pneumonitis	Exposure to a potential antigen in the home or work environment
Drug-induced lung disease	Use of medicines, over-the-counter supplements, or recreational drugs that may be associated with lung disease
Genetic syndromes	Family history of lung fibrosis, evidence of premature graying, cryptogenic cirrhosis, aplastic anemia, myelodysplasia, macrocytosis, or thrombocytopenia

SYSTEMATIC APPROACH TO DIAGNOSIS OF PULMONARY FIBROSIS AT COMPUTED TOMOGRAPHY[6]

Classify fibrosis patterns:
- Usual interstitial pneumonia (UIP) pattern
- Fibrotic NSIP pattern
- Fibrotic HP pattern
- Other rare patterns (PPFE, sarcoidosis, etc.)

Analyze the distribution of fibrosis:
- Upper lobe, middle lobe, lower lobe, and diffuse
- Central or peripheral
- Subpleural or peribronchovascular

Identify CT features:
- Honeycombing
- Traction bronchiectasis or bronchiolectasis
- Reticulation
- Ground-glass opacity
- Mosaic attenuation and air trapping

Evaluate possible complications:
- Acute exacerbation
- Infection
- Lung cancer
- Pulmonary hypertension

Assess progression with follow-up CT:
- Increased traction bronchiectasis or bronchiolectasis
- New GGO with traction bronchiectasis
- New or increased fine reticulation
- New or increased honeycombing
- Increased lobar volume loss

ROLE OF MULTIDISCIPLINARY DISCUSSION IN PATIENT WITH INTERSTITIAL LUNG DISEASE

The diagnosis of IIP relies on a multidisciplinary discussion (MDD) among pulmonologists, radiologists, and pathologists, often including rheumatologists. Distinguishing between IIPs and known-cause ILDs is crucial for treatment and prognosis. In one-third of cases, MDD can result in a modified diagnosis and in 75% of initially unclassified ILD cases, a consensus unified diagnosis can be achieved. Improved survival rate can be seen in ILD cases diagnosed by means of MDD with those diagnosed without MDDs.[4,6,7]

Key points include:

Diagnostic process:
- A thorough history and physical examination are vital to identify known causes of ILD, including exposure to birds or mold and signs of autoimmune diseases (e.g., lupus, rheumatoid arthritis).
- Serologic testing may be needed, and referrals to rheumatologists can assist in confirming autoimmune conditions.
- Comprehensive histories should cover family, smoking, occupational, and medication exposures.

Imaging:
- High-resolution computed tomography is critical for classifying ILDs and may reduce the need for invasive biopsies if clear patterns are identified.
- Radiologists must be knowledgeable about HRCT patterns associated with IIPs to guide diagnosis effectively.

Surgical biopsy:
- If noninvasive assessments do not provide a diagnosis, surgical lung biopsy may be required, although it carries significant risks.

Treatment implications:
- For HP, drug-induced, and occupational ILDs, removal of exposures is essential.
- Conditions such as connective tissue disease-associated ILD (CTD-ILD) may respond to immunosuppression, while it is contraindicated in IPF, which has a worse prognosis.

IDIOPATHIC INTERSTITIAL PNEUMONIAS

The final diagnosis of an IIPs should always be a consensus diagnosis made after evaluation by the chest physician, radiologist, and pathologist. The diagnosis may be altered, as more details emerge from the patient's history, fine-needle aspiration cytology, biopsy, bronchoalveolar lavage, or postsurgery lung histopathology. Lung damage similar to that seen in IIPs is also seen in diseases such as connective tissue disorders, asbestosis, chronic HP, and drug reaction. The term idiopathic is used when the cause of lung damage is not known and other known etiologies of lung damage have been excluded.

CHRONIC FIBROSING IDIOPATHIC INTERSTITIAL PNEUMONIAS

Idiopathic Pulmonary Fibrosis

Idiopathic pulmonary fibrosis is a chronic fibrosing form of IIP, which is associated with the radiological or histopathological pattern of UIP. It occurs predominantly in older adult population and is associated with median survival of <5 years. The term IPF is used when other recognized causes of ILD have been excluded, and there is UIP pattern seen on HRCT. IPF particularly excludes IIPs such as NSIP and DIP.[8] IPF is the most common ILD accounting for 25–50% of diffuse lung diseases. According to the current guidelines of American Thoracic Society and European Respiratory Society, an algorithm has been devised on the basis of which three levels of certainty can be assigned for UIP on the basis of HRCT findings (UIP, possible UIP, and inconsistent with UIP) **(Table 3)**.[9]

Radiologic Features

Chest Radiograph

Almost all patients of IPF who present with symptoms have abnormal chest radiograph findings. The most common chest radiograph pattern is peripheral reticular opacities, which are predominant in the lower zones and are sometimes associated with honeycombing and volume loss of lower zones. Chest radiographs may sometimes also be normal.

High-resolution Computed Tomography

The diagnosis of UIP is usually made on the basis of clinical and imaging features because of the high diagnostic accuracy of HRCT for cases of UIP.[8] Those cases without a confident HRCT diagnosis may require a biopsy. Characteristic HRCT features of UIP include reticular lines, traction bronchiectasis and bronchiolectasis, and honeycombing, which are predominant in lower lobes and subpleural, peripheral lung. They may be associated with lower lobe volume loss **(Figs. 9A and B)**. GGO is much less common. Architectural distortion due to lung fibrosis is often seen. The HRCT findings of GGOs, which occur in association with reticular opacities and traction bronchiectasis, always indicate lung fibrosis. Patients with preponderant reticular opacities or honeycombing on HRCT usually progress despite being given treatment.[10]

TABLE 3: High-resolution computed tomography imaging patterns in suspected cases of idiopathic pulmonary fibrosis.[11]

	Typical usual interstitial pneumonia (UIP)	Probable UIP	Indeterminate for UIP	Features suggestive of an alternative diagnosis
Degree of confidence for UIP features on histopathology	>90% confidence	High confidence between 70 and 89%	Intermediate confidence between 51 and 69%	Low confidence < 50%
Distribution	Basal predominance subpleural occasionally asymmetric often heterogeneous	Basal subpleural heterogeneous	Diffuse axial or craniocaudal distribution	Subpleural-sparing peribronchovascular distribution and perilymphatic distribution (upper and mild predominance)
CT features	Honeycombing with or without traction bronchiectasis/ bronchiolectasis and irregular septal thickening. Reticulations with minimal to mild superimposed ground-glass ossified nodules may be present	Traction bronchiolectasis or bronchiolectasis reticulations, minimal ground glass, subpleural sparing is absent, and honeycombing is absent	CT features that do not fit into definite, probable, or an alternative diagnosis or non-UIP pattern	Diffuse cysts, mosaic attenuation will extensive, lobular air trapping on expiratory scan predominant or extension pure ground glass (exclude acute exacerbation) predominant consolidation/nodules, mediastinal findings, pleural plaques, dilated esophagus

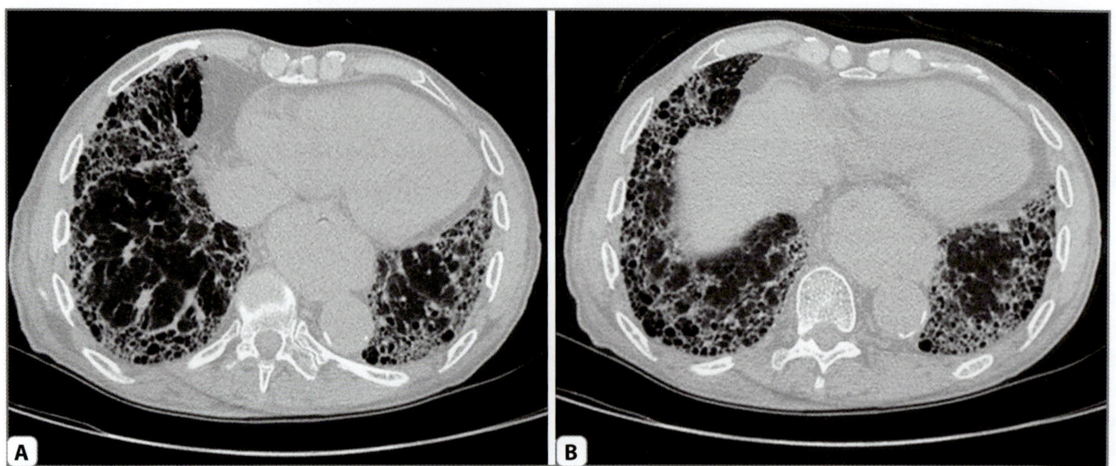

FIGS. 9A AND B: Idiopathic pulmonary fibrosis (IPF)—axial high-resolution computed tomography (HRCT) of the chest shows intralobular and interlobular septal thickening with honeycombing and tractional bronchiectasis more pronounced in bilateral lower lobes.

Acute Exacerbations of Idiopathic Pulmonary Fibrosis[12]

Acute exacerbations of IPF primarily occur in patients with advanced disease and carry a high mortality risk. Patients typically present with a rapid worsening of dyspnea or cough.

Key points include:

- *Diagnosis*: Comparison with clinical history, baseline symptoms, and prior imaging is crucial.
- *Computed tomography findings*:
  - Computed tomography scans may show new bilateral GGOs and/or consolidations over existing fibrosis, often leading to indeterminate patterns for UIP.
  - A diffuse phenotype is linked to higher morbidity and mortality.
- *Exclusion of other conditions*: It is important to rule out acute conditions such as heart failure, pneumothorax, pulmonary embolism, and infections.
- *Histopathology*: Acute exacerbations often show patterns of diffuse alveolar damage (DAD) and/or organizing pneumonia (OP superimposed on UIP).

Nonspecific Interstitial Pneumonia

Nonspecific interstitial pneumonia is less common than UIP. The mean age of patients at onset is about 40–50 years.[13] Onset of NSIP is gradual, but some patients may have subacute onset. Patients usually present with symptoms of breathlessness and cough. Histological and radiological findings of NSIP can be found in patients with drug-induced lung diseases, collagen vascular diseases, and HP. Hence, when HRCT pattern of NSIP is seen, these etiologies should be ruled out. In addition, HRCT features similar to those seen in NSIP may be seen in patients of organizing pneumonia, UIP, and DIP, and surgical biopsy may sometimes be required to differentiate them. NSIP is further classified into two types: (1) fibrotic and (2) cellular subtypes. Fibrotic NSIP is more common than cellular subtype. On histology, interstitial thickening is mainly due to fibrosis with mild inflammation. In cellular NSIP, thickening of interstitium is due to infiltration by plasma cells and lymphocytes. Cellular NSIP has a better prognosis and usually shows response to corticosteroids.[14] It is sometimes difficult to differentiate fibrotic NSIP and UIP on histology. While fibrotic NSIP shows temporal homogeneity, UIP shows heterogeneity with collagen and fibroblastic foci, representing old and active disease together. This may aid in differentiating the two.[15]

Radiologic Features

Chest Radiograph

NSIP shows infiltrates in bilateral lungs, which are more common in lower zones.

High-resolution Computed Tomography Features

The predominant HRCT finding of NSIP is GGO, which is usually bilateral, symmetric, and preponderant in lower lobes and peripheral lung. Pathologically, GGO corresponds to homogeneous interstitial inflammation.[16] Irregular linear or reticular opacities are seen, which may be associated with traction bronchiectasis or bronchiolectasis **(Figs. 10A and B)**. Honeycombing is rarely seen. Other occasional findings include nodules, pleural effusion, and hilar or meditational lymphadenopathy.

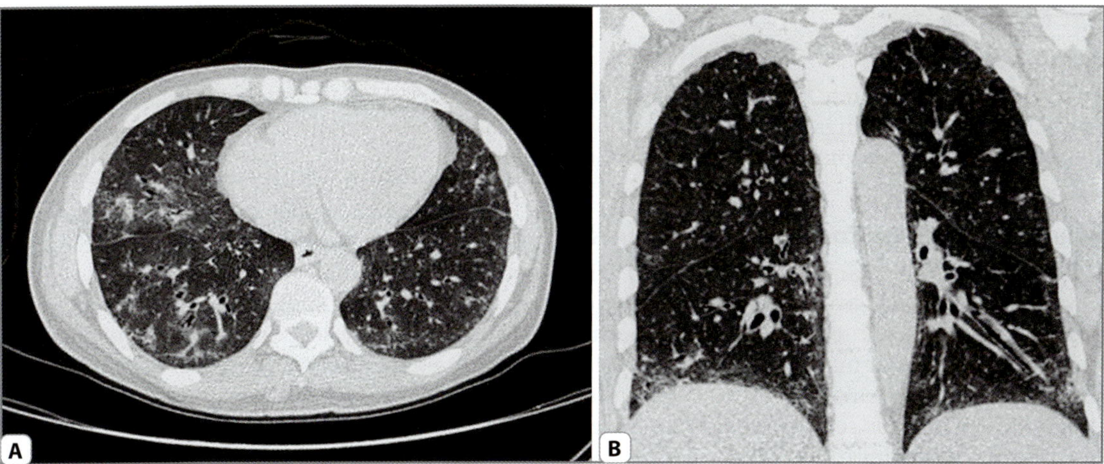

FIGS. 10A AND B: Nonspecific interstitial pneumonia (NSIP)—axial and coronal HRCT of the chest shows bilateral patchy areas of ground-glass opacity and subpleural reticulations with mild traction bronchiectasis in bilateral lower lobes. Fissural nodularity and fibronodular lesions are also seen in bilateral upper lobes and RML.

(HRCT: high-resolution computed tomography; RML: right middle lobe)

SMOKING-RELATED INTERSTITIAL PNEUMONIAS

Respiratory bronchiolitis, RB-ILD, and DIP are currently thought of as a continuum of smoking-related lung diseases. There is similarity in their clinical, radiological, and histological findings.[2] RB is asymptomatic and is detected at autopsy. RB-ILD is the term used when RB is associated with pulmonary symptoms or radiological findings. DIP represents the worst of this spectrum, in which imaging and histological findings are more extensive.

Respiratory Bronchiolitis-associated Interstitial Lung Disease

Both RB and RB-ILD on histology show pigmented macrophages within first- and second-order respiratory bronchioles.[17] In RB-ILD, the degree of abnormality is generally more.[18] The course of this disease following smoking cessation generally improves.[19]

Radiologic Features

Chest Radiograph

The most common abnormality in RB-ILD on chest radiograph is thickening of the central or peripheral airway walls, which is seen in approximately 76% of patients. GGO is seen in 57% of patients.[20]

High-resolution Computed Tomography Features

The common findings of RB-ILD include centrilobular nodules, patchy GGOs, and thickening of the central or peripheral airway walls **(Fig. 11)**. RB-ILD can be usually diagnosed in smokers with these HRCT findings, without the aid of lung biopsy.[9] The HRCT features of HP may overlap with those of RB and RB-ILD. However, the centrilobular nodules, mosaic attenuation, air trapping, and GGO found in HP are usually more extensive. Additionally, almost all patients with HP are nonsmokers.

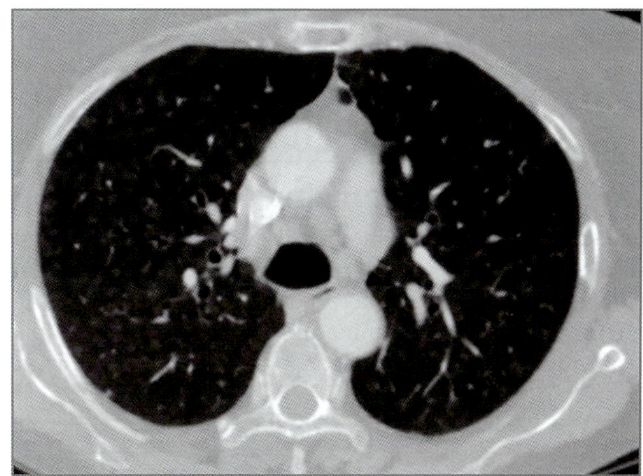

FIG. 11: Respiratory bronchiolitis-associated interstitial lung disease (RB-ILD)—axial high-resolution computed tomography (HRCT) of the chest shows multiple ill-defined ground-glass density nodules in a chronic smoker with RB-ILD.

Desquamative Interstitial Pneumonia

Desquamative interstitial pneumonia is an uncommon interstitial pneumonia. It overlaps with RB-ILD in that the quality of the pigment-laden macrophages is identical, but their distribution and extent differ, with pigment-laden macrophages being more diffuse and extensive in DIP.[2]

Radiologic Features

Chest Radiograph

It may be normal in approximately 3–22% of cases of DIP. On the chest radiograph, findings that can be seen are diffuse patchy GGOs, with predominance in lower zones and in periphery.[21]

High-resolution Computed Tomography Features

The most common and characteristic finding of DIP is GGOs, which are present on HRCT in all cases of DIP **(Fig. 12)**. This occurs due to the homogeneous accumulation of intra-alveolar macrophages and alveolar septal thickening. Mid and lower lobes predominance with peripheral distribution is seen in most of the cases. Reticular opacities are sometimes present. Well-defined and thin-walled cysts may be seen. The GGOs usually resolve with treatment. The main imaging difference between RB-ILD and DIP is the distribution of disease, which is predominantly centrilobular in RB-ILD and diffuse in DIP. Centrilobular nodules are uncommonly seen in patients with DIP. GGOs are usually patchier, less well defined, and less extensive in RB-ILD.

ACUTE AND SUBACUTE INTERSTITIAL PNEUMONIAS

Cryptogenic Organizing Pneumonia

Cryptogenic organizing pneumonia was previously referred to as bronchiolitis obliterans organizing pneumonia. However, COP is the preferred term because organizing pneumonia is the predominant feature and is responsible for the physiologic abnormalities and radiological findings.

Radiologic Features

Chest Radiograph

The most common chest radiograph findings in COP are unilateral or bilateral areas of consolidation.

High-resolution Computed Tomography Features

HRCT typically shows patchy, possibly migratory, unilateral or bilateral areas of consolidation and/or GGOs in a peribronchovascular or subpleural location **(Fig. 13)**. Air bronchograms with mild cylindrical bronchial dilatation may be frequently seen in areas of consolidation. Pleural effusions may uncommonly occur.[22] Nodules are seen in 30% of cases. They are usually small and present predominantly along the bronchovascular bundles. Reticular opacities may be sometimes present and signify histological evidence of fibrosis.

Acute Interstitial Pneumonia

Acute interstitial pneumonia is a type of interstitial pneumonia that progresses rapidly. On histology, there is the presence of DAD. The term AIP is used when there is DAD of unknown origin. Patients with AIP often have a clinical prodrome, suggesting viral upper respiratory tract infection. Patients have hypoxemia, which rapidly progresses to respiratory failure, with a mortality rate of 50% or more. Treatment is generally supportive, and mechanical ventilation is usually required.

Radiologic Features

Chest Radiograph

The chest radiograph shows patchy/diffuse areas of airspace opacities bilaterally **(Fig. 14A)**.

FIG. 12: Desquamative interstitial pneumonia (DIP)—axial high-resolution computed tomography (HRCT) of the chest shows diffuse ill-defined bilateral ground-glass opacification. Centrilobular emphysema with large left-sided bulla is also noted in this 45-year-old heavy smoker.

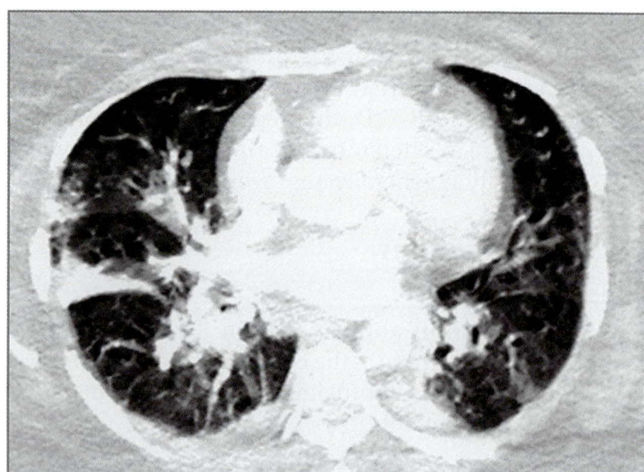

FIG. 13: Cryptogenic organizing pneumonia (COP)—axial high-resolution computed tomography (HRCT) of the chest shows bilateral ill-defined ground-glass opacities with patchy areas of consolidation in bilateral upper lobes.

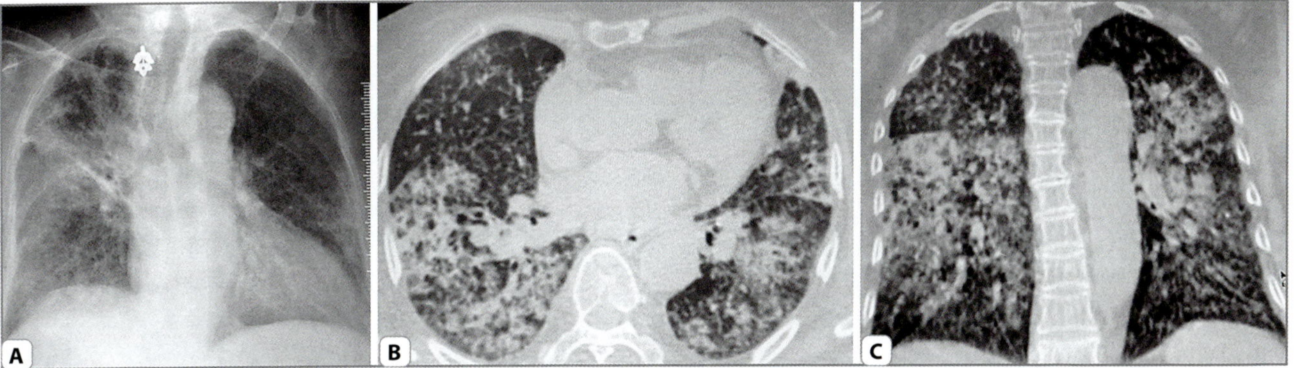

FIGS. 14A TO C: Acute interstitial pneumonia (AIP). (A) Frontal chest radiograph PA view reveals bilateral airspace opacification with air bronchograms, with sparing of the costophrenic angles. (B and C) Axial and coronal HRCT shows bilateral diffuse ground-glass opacity and consolidation of the dependent lung.

(HRCT: high-resolution computed tomography; PA: posteroanterior)

High-resolution Computed Tomography Features

AIP is characterized by three stages: (1) Early exudative phase, (2) subacute proliferative phase, and (3) chronic fibrotic phase. The first exudative phase of AIP shows bilateral patchy GGOs with areas of focal sparing, often with consolidation in the dependent part of lungs **(Figs. 14B and C)**, while the later fibrotic stage of AIP shows distortion of bronchovascular bundles and traction bronchiectasis. AIP can progress to severe fibrosis with areas of honeycombing.[2] Few patients who survive this disease show progressive resolution of the areas of GGO and consolidation. On later HRCT scans, areas of hypoattenuation, reticular pattern, traction bronchiectasis, and associated architectural distortion occurring predominantly in the nondependent part of the lungs can be seen.

RARE INTERSTITIAL PNEUMONIAS

The recently created category of rare IIPs includes idiopathic LIP and IPPFE.[2]

Lymphoid Interstitial Pneumonia

Lymphoid interstitial pneumonia is a lymphoproliferative disorder in which there is infiltration of lung interstitium predominantly by lymphocytes. The incidence of idiopathic LIP is low. LIP is most frequently associated with Sjögren's syndrome, autoimmune thyroid diseases, acquired immunodeficiency syndrome (AIDS), and Castleman syndrome.

Radiologic Features

Chest Radiograph

It is neither sensitive nor specific. Findings include bilateral basal reticular opacities and ill-defined nodules.[23]

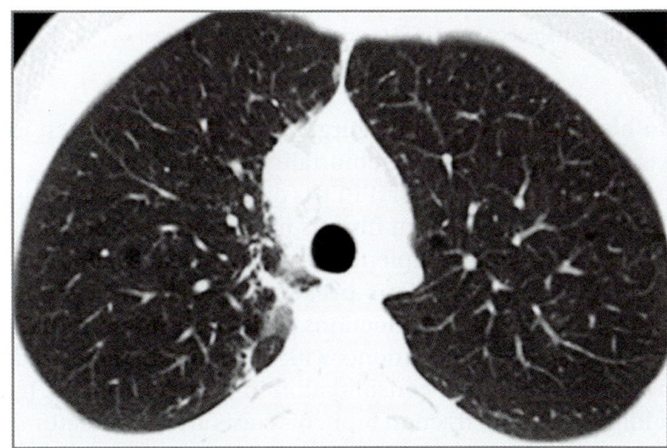

FIG. 15: Lymphoid interstitial pneumonia (LIP)—axial HRCT of the chest shows few thin wall perivascular cysts in bilateral lungs in a patient with AIDS and LIP.

(AIDS: acquired immunodeficiency syndrome; HRCT: high-resolution computed tomography)

High-resolution Computed Tomography Features

The predominant HRCT findings are usually GGO and perivascular cysts **(Fig. 15)**, sometimes leading to misdiagnosis of lymphangioleiomyomatosis. However, cysts related to LIP usually predominate in the lower lungs and around bronchi and vessels, in contrast to the diffuse distribution of cysts in lymphangioleiomyomatosis. Peribronchovascular and interlobular septae thickening are also seen frequently in cases of LIP. Centrilobular nodules may also be seen. Rarely, perivascular honeycombing can be seen.[24,25]

Idiopathic Pulmonary Fibroelastosis

Pleuroparenchymal fibroelastosis is a rare IIP with variable clinical and radiological features. Diagnosis is based

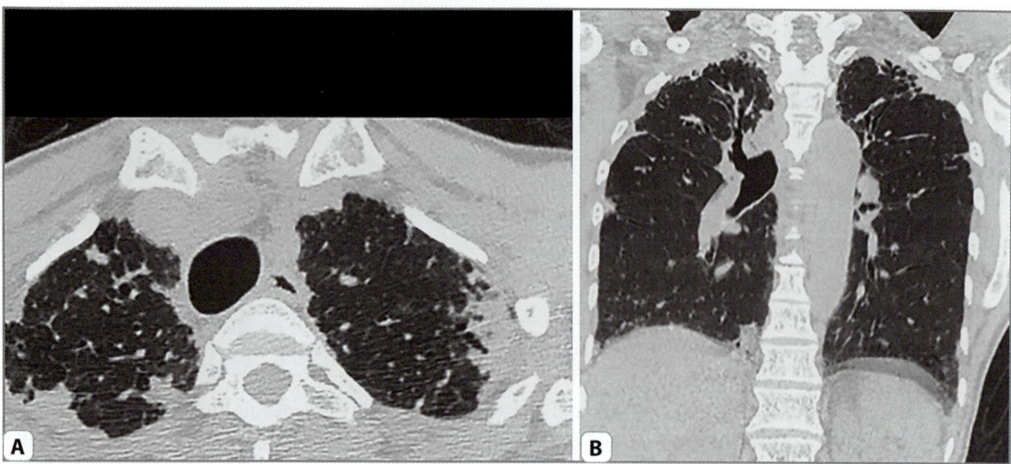

FIGS. 16A AND B: Idiopathic pleuroparenchymal fibroelastosis (IPPFE)—axial and coronal HRCT of the chest shows bilateral apical pleural thickening with patchy areas of consolidation in peripheral region with traction bronchiectasis and architectural distortion in an elderly male patient. No prior history of TB.

(HRCT: high-resolution computed tomography; TB: tuberculosis)

on histology obtained by surgical lung biopsy, which is associated with significant mortality and morbidity.[26]

This rare condition of IPPEE is diagnosed when there is upper lobe predominant fibrosis involving the subpleural lung parenchyma and pleura. On histological evaluation, intra-alveolar fibrosis is present, and the fibrosis is elastotic.[27] Recurrent infections have been noted in half of patients. HRCT in patients with IPPFE is characterized by dense subpleural consolidation in the upper lobes. In addition, areas of traction bronchiectasis and architectural distortion may be seen.[28] The upper lobes were always more severely involved, with involvement of the lower lobes being absent or less marked (apical-caudal distribution) **(Figs. 16A and B)**. Associated features included upper lobe volume loss, architectural distortion, and traction bronchiectasis.[26]

CONCLUSION

The information provided by high resolution computed tomography imaging of the chest has changed the approach to the diagnosis and treatment of interstitial lung diseases. Being able to describe and discern the different radiographic patterns offers providers invaluable information that, when combined with other patient data (subjective history, physical examination, laboratory measurements, etc.), can yield a definitive diagnosis without invasive testing such as tissue biopsy or bronchoscopic evaluation. This in turn, can change the course of a disease as many of the interstitial lung disease have known modifiable risk factors and pharmacologic treatment options. It is therefore imperative for clinicians to be acquainted with accurately identify these radiographic patterns on CT imaging.

REFERENCES

1. American Thoracic Society/European Respiratory Society international multidisciplinary consensus classification of the idiopathic interstitial pneumonias. This joint statement of the American Thoracic Society (ATS), and the European Respiratory Society (ERS) was adopted by the ATS board of directors, June 2001 and by the ERS Executive Committee, June 2001. Am J Respir Crit Care Med. 2002;165(2):277-304.
2. Sverzellati N, Lynch DA, Hansell DM, Johkoh T, King TE, Travis WD. American Thoracic Society–European Respiratory Society Classification of the idiopathic interstitial pneumonias: advances in knowledge since 2002. Radiographics. 2015;35:1849-72.
3. Hobbs S, Lynch D. The idiopathic interstitial pneumonias: an update and review. Radiol Clin North Am. 2014;52:105-20.
4. Lynch DA, Sverzellati N, Travis WD, Brown KK, Colby TV, Galvin JR, et al. Diagnostic criteria for idiopathic pulmonary fibrosis: a Fleischner Society white paper. Lancet Respir Med. 2018;6:138-53.
5. Chung JH, Goldin JG. Interpretation of HRCT scans in the diagnosis of IPF: improving communication between pulmonologists and radiologists. Lung. 2018;196:561-7.
6. Chae KJ, Hwang HJ, Duarte Achcar R, Cooley JC, Humphries SM, Kligerman S, et al. Central role of CT in management of pulmonary fibrosis. Radiographics. 2024;44(6):e230165.
7. Zhan X, Koelsch T, Montner SM, Zhu A, Vij R, Swigris JJ, et al. Differentiating usual interstitial pneumonia from nonspecific interstitial pneumonia using high-resolution computed tomography: the "straight-edge sign". J Thorac Imaging. 2018;33:266-70
8. American Thoracic Society. Idiopathic pulmonary fibrosis: diagnosis and treatment—International Consensus Statement: American Thoracic Society (ATS), and the

European Respiratory Society (ERS). Am J Respir Crit Care Med. 2000;161:646-64.

9. Mueller-Mang C, Grosse C, Schmid K, Stiebellehner L, Bankier AA. What every radiologist should know about idiopathic interstitial pneumonias Radiographics. 2007;27:595-615.
10. Travis WD, Matsui K, Moss J, Ferrans VJ. Idiopathic nonspecific interstitial pneumonia: prognostic significance of cellular and fibrosing patterns-survival comparison with usual interstitial pneumonia and desquamative interstitial pneumonia. Am J Surg Pathol. 2000;24:19-33.
11. Batra K, Adams TN. Imaging features of idiopathic interstitial lung diseases. J Thorac Imaging. 2023;38:S19-29.
12. Collard HR, Ryerson CJ, Corte TJ, Jenkins G, Kondoh Y, Lederer DJ, et al. Acute exacerbation of idiopathic pulmonary fibrosis. An international working group report. Am J Respir Crit Care Med. 2016;194:265-75.
13. Flaherty KR, Thwaite EL, Kazerooni EA, Gross BH, Toews GB, Colby TV, et al. Radiological versus histological diagnosis in UIP and NSIP: survival implications. Thorax. 2003;58:143-8.
14. Ferguson EC, Berkowitz EA. Lung CT: part 2, the interstitial pneumonias–clinical, histologic, and CT manifestations. AJR Am J Roentgenol. 2012;199(4):W464-76.
15. Remy-Jardin M, Remy J, Gosselin B, Becette V, Edme JL. Lung parenchymal changes secondary to cigarette smoking: pathologic-CT correlations. Radiology. 1993;186(3):643-51.
16. Holt RM, Schmidt RA, Godwin JD, Raghu G. High-resolution CT in respiratory bronchiolitis-associated interstitial lung disease. J Comput Assist Tomogr. 1993;17(1):46-50.
17. Vassallo R, Ryu JH. Tobacco smoke-related diffuse lung diseases. Semin Respir Crit Care Med. 2008;29(6):643-50.
18. Portnoy J, Veraldi KL, Schwarz MI, Cool CD, Curran-Everett D, Cherniack RM, et al. Respiratory bronchiolitis-interstitial lung disease: long-term outcome. Chest. 2007;131(3):664-71.
19. Travis WD, Costabel U, Hansell DM, King TE Jr, Lynch DA, Nicholson DG, et al. An official American Thoracic Society/ European Respiratory Society Statement: update of the international multidisciplinary classification of the idiopathic interstitial pneumonias. Am J Respir Crit Care Med. 2013;6(188):733-48.
20. Dalphin JC, Debieuvre D, Pernet D, Maheu MF, Polio JC, Toson B, et al. Prevalence and risk factors for chronic bronchitis and farmer's lung in French dairy farmers. Br J Ind Med. 1993;50(10):941-4.
21. Lynch DA, Travis WD, Müller NL, Galvin JR, Hansell DM, Grenier PA, et al. Idiopathic interstitial pneumonias: CT features. Radiology. 2005;236:10-21.
22. Lee JS, Lynch DA, Sharma S, Brown KK, Müller NL. Organizing pneumonia: prognostic implication of high-resolution computed tomography features. J Comput Assist Tomogr. 2003;27(2):260-5.
23. Johkoh T, Muller NL, Pickford HA, Hartman TE, Ichikado K, Akira M, et al. Lymphocytic interstitial pneumonia: thin-section CT findings in 22 patients. Radiology. 1999;212(2):567-72.
24. Ichikawa Y, Kinoshita M, Koga T, Oizumi K, Fujimoto K, Hayabuchi N. Lung cyst formation in lymphocytic interstitial pneumonia: CT features. J Comput Assist Tomogr. 1994;18(5):745-8.
25. Becker CD, Gil J, Padilla ML. Idiopathic pleura parenchymal fibro elastosis: an unrecognized or misdiagnosed entity? Mod Pathol. 2008;21(6):784-7.
26. Esteves C, Costa FR, Redondo MT, Moura CS, Guimarães S, Morais A, et al. Pleuroparenchymal fibroelastosis: role of high-resolution computed tomography (HRCT) and CT-guided transthoracic core lung biopsy. Insights Imaging. 2015;7(1):155-62.
27. Frankel SK, Cool CD, Lynch DA, Brown KK. Idiopathic pleura parenchymal fibroelastosis: description of a novel clinico-pathologic entity. Chest. 2004;126(6):2007-13.
28. Reddy TL, Tominaga M, Hansell DM, von der Thusen J, Rassl D, Parfrey H, et al. Pleuroparenchymal fibroelastosis: a spectrum of histopathological and imaging phenotypes. Eur Respir J. 2012;40(2):377-85.

Surabhi Vyas, Stanzin Spalkit, Smriti Hari

CHAPTER 9

Imaging of Interstitial Lung Disease of Known Etiology

INTRODUCTION

Interstitial lung diseases (ILDs) are a group of disorders characterized by diffuse parenchymal lung abnormalities and clinically present with dyspnea, restrictive pulmonary function, and impaired gas exchange. The etiological cause is sometimes yet to be discovered. The consensus statement on interstitial pneumonia classifies ILDs into idiopathic interstitial pneumonia (IIP) and those secondary to a known cause, namely:[1,2]

- Systemic autoimmune rheumatic diseases (SARDs)
- Granulomatous diseases
- Exposure-related diseases
- Miscellaneous

Although ILDs more commonly affect adults, some entities such as Langerhans cell histiocytosis (LCH), hypersensitivity pneumonitis (HP), and IIPs are seen in children as well.[3] Diagnosis is based on history, clinical examination, pulmonary function tests, imaging in the form of chest radiographs and computed tomography, and occasionally histopathology from lung biopsy.

In this chapter, we shall discuss the common ILDs with known causes in detail.

SYSTEMIC AUTOIMMUNE RHEUMATIC DISEASES INTERSTITIAL LUNG DISEASE

Systemic autoimmune rheumatic diseases are chronic autoimmune disorders that lead to inflammation and organ damage. This term serves as an umbrella for connective tissue diseases (CTDs) and systemic vasculitis. ILD is a common manifestation of several SARDs and contributes significantly to increased morbidity and mortality. Earlier, conditions such as systemic sclerosis (SSc), Sjögren's syndrome (SS), idiopathic inflammatory myopathies (IIM), mixed connective tissue disease (MCTD), and systemic lupus erythematosus (SLE) were referred to as CTDs or collagen vascular diseases. However, these terms no longer accurately reflect the pathophysiology or the variety of organ systems affected by these diseases. As a result, the term SARD is now preferred. SARD-related ILD also includes ILD associated with conditions such as axial spondyloarthropathy and antineutrophil cytoplasmic antibodies (ANCA)-associated vasculitis, in addition to the ILDs linked to classic CTDs.[4] At histopathologic examination, ILDs associated with collagen vascular disease are diverse and include usual interstitial pneumonia (UIP), nonspecific interstitial pneumonia (NSIP), cryptogenic organizing pneumonia (COP), diffuse alveolar damage, lymphocytic interstitial pneumonia (LIP), and apical fibrosis. The radiologic and pathological manifestations of systemic autoimmune rheumatic diseases-interstitial lung disease (SARDs-ILD) are similar to the idiopathic counterpart, particularly in cases with UIP patterns. However, certain radiologic features are more commonly observed in UIP associated with SARDs-ILD than in UIP associated with idiopathic pulmonary fibrosis (IPF) **(Table 1)**. Identifying these specific signs is clinically significant, as radiologists may be the first to suggest the diagnosis of SARDs-ILD, sometimes even before the underlying SARDs are recognized. The presentation of SARDs-ILD may be the initial manifestation of the underlying disease, making early identification crucial for timely diagnosis and management.[5] High-resolution computed tomography (HRCT) has proved to be very sensitive in detecting and characterizing various histopathologically confirmed ILDs in patients with collagen vascular diseases **(Tables 2 and 3)**.

Systemic Sclerosis

Pulmonary involvement is more common and more severe in SSc than in other collagen vascular diseases.[9]

TABLE 1: Radiological signs associated with SARDs-ILD.[5-8]

Radiological signs suggesting SARDs-ILD versus idiopathic pulmonary fibrosis	
Anterior upper lobe sign **(Figs. 1A and B)**	The concentration of fibrosis within the anterior aspect of the upper lobes (with relative sparing of the other aspects of the upper lobes) and concomitant lower lobe involvement
Exuberant honeycomb sign **(Figs. 1C and D)**	Extensive honeycomb-like cyst formation within the lungs comprising >70% of the fibrotic portions of the lung
Straight edge sign **(Fig. 1E)**	Isolation of fibrosis to the lung bases without substantial extension along the lateral margins of the lungs on coronal images
Four corner signs **(Figs. 1A and B)**	The presence of reticular opacities, ground-glass attenuations, and/or honeycombing distributed in the "4 corners regions of the thorax": The anterolateral regions of mid-upper lobes (from the top of the aortic arch to the carina) and the posterosuperior regions of lower lobes (carina through the inferior pulmonary veins)

(SARDs-ILD: systemic autoimmune rheumatic diseases-interstitial lung disease)

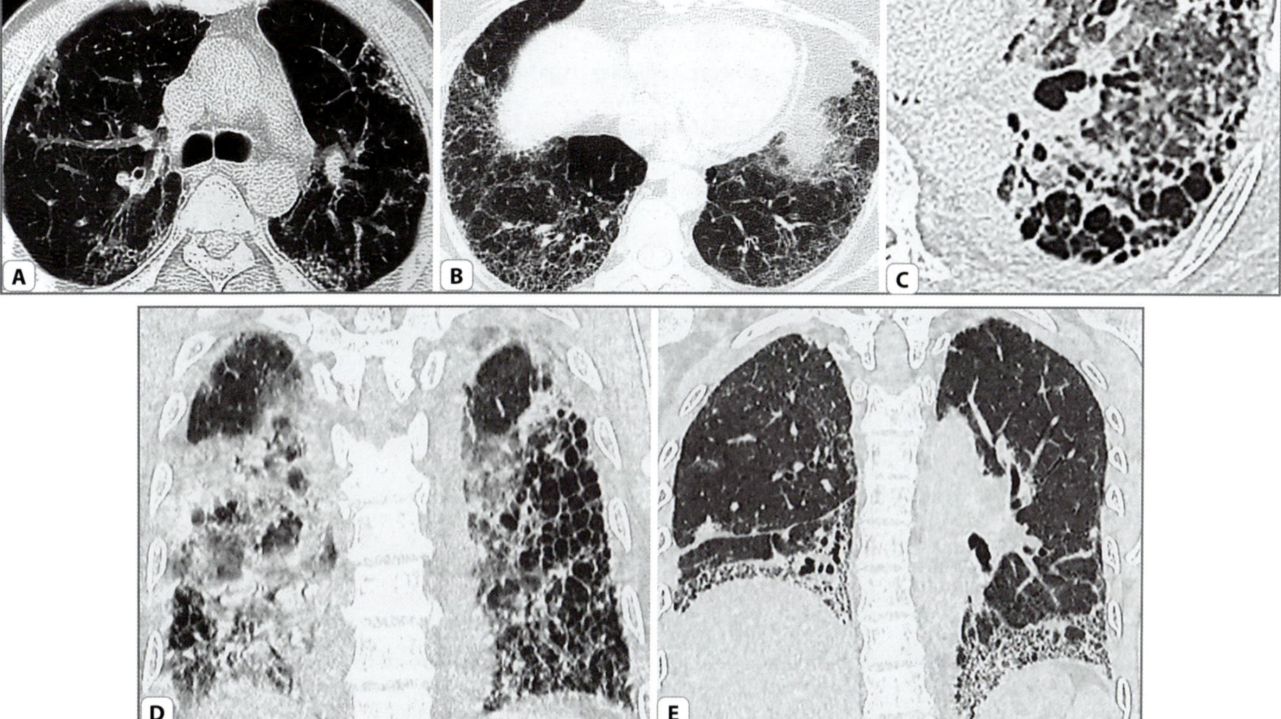

FIGS. 1A TO E: "Anterior upper lobe sign" and "four corner sign" (A and B): Axial section through the upper lobes in a case of progressive systemic sclerosis (PSS) shows the concentration of fibrosis in the anterior segments of upper lobes (in A) and bilateral lower lobes (in B), the anterolateral regions of mid-upper lobes and the posterosuperior regions of lower lobes. "Exuberant honeycomb sign" (C and D): The extensive honeycomb-like cyst formation (in C and D) within the lower lobes of the lung involving >70% of the fibrotic component. Straight edge sign (E): Reveals fibrosis limited to the lung bases with a clear demarcation from the relatively less affected lung in the craniocaudal plane.

Interstitial fibrosis is the most common manifestation (in approximately 80% of patients) followed by pulmonary artery hypertension. The histological features are those of NSIP or UIP, the former being more common and associated with a worse prognosis.[10]

Imaging Features

Pulmonary involvement due to SSc could be classified as:

- *Systemic sclerosis-related ILD* **(Figs. 2A and B)**: Evidence of interstitial fibrosis has been reported in chest radiography in 20–65% of patients. Serial

TABLE 2: Thoracic manifestations of SARDs.[12]

Common and less common manifestations of SARDs					
	Progressive systemic sclerosis	Rheumatoid arthritis	Systemic lupus erythematosus	IIM	Sjögren's syndrome
Common	• NSIP • PAH	• UIP • NSIP	• Edema • Hemorrhage • DAD	• NSIP • OP	LIP
Uncommon	UIP	• Airway disease • OP	Fibrosis	DAD	Airway disease

(DAD: diffuse alveolar damage; IIM: idiopathic inflammatory myopathies; LIP: lymphocytic interstitial pneumonia; NSIP: nonspecific interstitial pneumonia; OP: organizing pneumonia; PAH: pulmonary arterial hypertension; SARDs: systemic autoimmune rheumatic diseases; UIP: usual interstitial pneumonia)

TABLE 3: Compartment-wise imaging findings in SARDs.

SARD	Pulmonary parenchyma	Airway	Pleura	Vascular	Others
Systemic sclerosis	• *ILD*: NSIP, UIP, OP • Aspiration pneumonia			PAH	Dilated esophagus
Rheumatoid arthritis	• *ILD*: UIP, NSIP, AIP, OP • Drug-induced ILD (methotrexate)	• *Small airway disease*: Follicular and constrictive bronchiolitis • *Large airway*: Cricoarytenoid arthritis	Pleural effusion/ thickening	*Vasculitis*: Small and medium vessel vasculitis	Rheumatoid nodules
SLE	• Pulmonary hemorrhage, pulmonary edema, lupus pneumonitis • Infection	Bronchiolitis (rare)	Pleural effusion/ thickening	Pulmonary thrombo-embolism	Diaphragmatic involvement, shrinking lung syndrome
IIM	• Aspiration pneumonia, pulmonary hypo-ventilation, Infection, ILD (NSIP, UIP, OP), DAD (especially in DM) • DAH				
Sjögren's syndrome	*ILD*: NSIP (most common), LIP (less common but more specific), UIP, OP	• Bronchiectasis, bronchiolitis • Air trapping			Increased risk for lymphoma (B-cell NHL)

(AIP: acute interstitial pneumonia; DAD: diffuse alveolar damage; DM: dermatomyositis; DAH: diffuse alveolar hemorrhage; IIM: idiopathic inflammatory myopathies; ILD: interstitial lung disease; LIP: lymphocytic interstitial pneumonia; NHL: non-Hodgkin lymphoma: NSIP: nonspecific interstitial pneumonia; OP: organizing pneumonia; PAH: pulmonary arterial hypertension; RA: rheumatoid arthritis; SARDs: systemic autoimmune rheumatic diseases; SLE: systemic lupus erythematosus; UIP: usual interstitial pneumonia)

radiographs obtained over several years may show progressive loss of lung volume and a worsening of the interstitial disease.

High-resolution computed tomography frequently shows evidence of interstitial pneumonitis and fibrosis in patients with normal or equivocal radiographic findings and may be used to monitor the disease over time. The abnormalities have a predominant peripheral and posterior distribution. The most common abnormalities seen on CT are peripheral and basal ground-glass opacities and fibrosis (often with subpleural sparing)-NSIP pattern **(Figs. 3A to C)**. UIP and organizing pneumonia is a less commonly seen pattern in SSc-ILD.

- *Pulmonary artery hypertension*: A dilated pulmonary trunk, >29 mm in diameter, and enlarged right and left pulmonary arteries are seen. The ratio of the main pulmonary artery to the ascending aorta tends to be >1.
- *Indirect involvement of lung*: Aspiration pneumonia secondary to esophageal dilatation is often noted.
- *Others*: Mediastinal lymphadenopathy and pleural or pericardial effusion are other manifestations.[7]

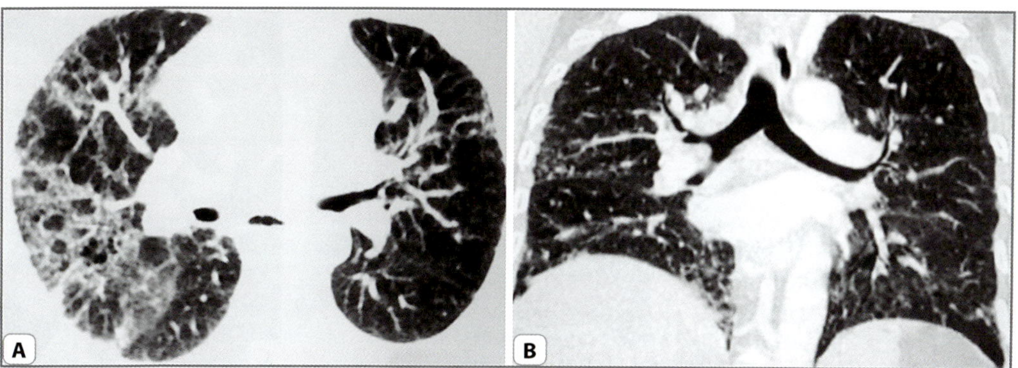

FIGS. 2A AND B: Progressive systemic sclerosis-associated ILD. (A) Axial HRCT shows fine intralobular and interlobular septal thickening and ground-glass opacification in NSIP pattern. (B) Coronal multiplanar reconstruction shows the predominantly basal distribution of the patchy ground-glass opacities.

(HRCT: high-resolution computed tomography; ILD: interstitial lung disease; NSIP: nonspecific interstitial pneumonia)

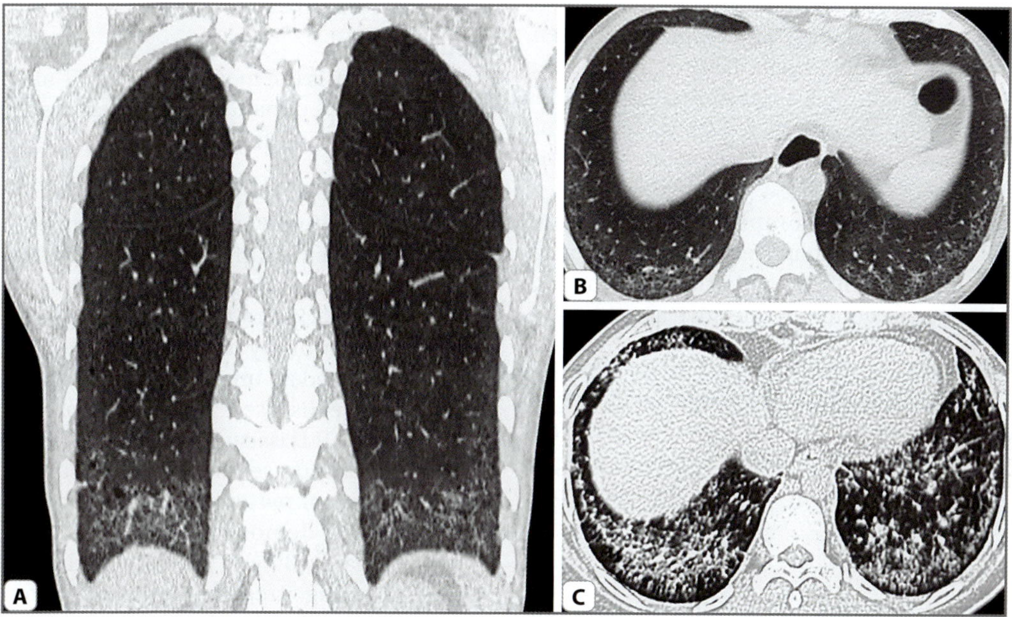

FIGS. 3A TO C: NSIP pattern: Coronal and axial sections (A and B) in a patient with PSS showing subtle reticular opacities with interspersed GGO showing bilateral peripheral and basal predominance. Note the dilated lower esophagus in the axial image (B). Axial image in another patient with PSS showing extensive reticular changes with bronchiolectasis in bilateral lower lobes with peripheral distribution and subpleural sparing (C).

(GGO: ground-glass opacity; NSIP: nonspecific interstitial pneumonia; PSS: progressive systemic sclerosis)

Rheumatoid Arthritis-associated Interstitial Lung Disease

About 5–40% of patients with rheumatoid arthritis (RA) have respiratory system involvement with involvement of the lung parenchyma, airways, and pleura. Various manifestations include interstitial pneumonitis and fibrosis, rheumatoid (necrobiotic) nodules, COP, obliterative bronchiolitis, follicular bronchiolitis, and pleural effusion. Interstitial pneumonitis and fibrosis are the most common pulmonary manifestations of RA, with the latter present in almost 5% of patients on radiography and 30–40% on HRCT.[11]

Imaging Features

Interstitial Lung Disease

Interstitial lung disease is one of the most common pulmonary manifestations of RA and the second leading cause of mortality. UIP is the most common pattern of RA-related ILD, with a fine reticular lower zone predominant pattern in early disease on radiography. With disease progression, these reticulations become coarser and more diffuse in distribution. Honeycombing may also be seen in advanced disease. Similar to the findings in radiography, the predominant abnormality at HRCT consists of irregular

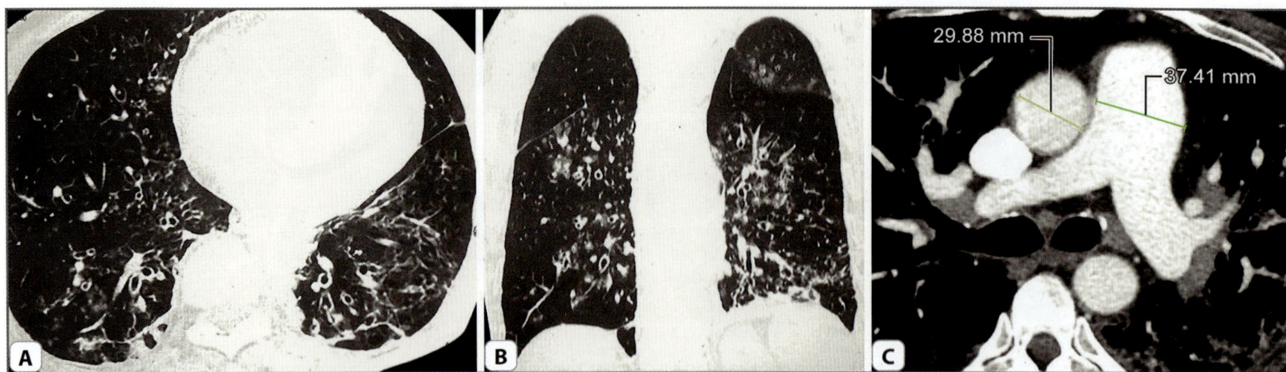

FIGS. 4A TO C: Airway involvement in RA: Axial and coronal lung window CT images (A and B) show bronchial wall thickening and dilatation and small centrilobular nodules suggestive of bronchiolitis. (C) Axial section mediastinal window in the same patient showing dilated pulmonary trunk with main pulmonary artery to the ascending aorta ratio >1 suggestive of PAH.

(CT: computed tomography; PAH: pulmonary artery hypertension; RA: rheumatoid arthritis)

linear opacities caused by a combination of thickening of interlobular and intralobular septa. Honeycombing is seen, most markedly near the diaphragm. NSIP is seen as the second most common pattern, with ground-glass opacities and microcyst formation. Acute interstitial pneumonia and organizing pneumonia are less commonly seen patterns in RA-ILD.

Drug-induced ILD may complicate the imaging appearance of RA-ILD with temporal relation between onset and offending drug helping differentiation between the two. Methotrexate is the most common causative agent.[12]

Airway Involvement

Airway disease in RA can involve the large and small airways from the cricoarytenoid joint (cricoarytenoid arthritis) in the larynx to the smallest bronchioles manifesting as bronchiectasis, bronchiolitis obliterans, and rarely follicular bronchiolitis **(Figs. 4A to C)**.

Pleural Disease

Pleural thickening is seen more commonly than pleural effusion.

Other Parenchymal Lung Disease

Rheumatoid (necrobiotic) nodules: These typically appear as round or lobulated masses, ranging in size from several millimeters to several centimeters. They are often located peripherally in the lungs, with a preference for the mid-upper lung regions. Most patients remain asymptomatic, although symptoms may develop if the nodules cavitate or invade the pleural space.[13]

Systemic Lupus Erythematosus

Thoracic manifestations of SLE involve the parenchyma, pleura, vasculature, and airways. The most common radiologic abnormality is pleural effusion (25–35%). Pericardial effusion is seen in approximately 20% of patients, and pulmonary parenchymal involvement is seen in 20%.[14]

Imaging Features

Pleura

Lupus serositis is the most common CT abnormality seen in up to 50–60% of patients, manifesting as pleuritis and pleural/pericardial effusions.

Parenchyma

Parenchymal involvement can be acute (pulmonary hemorrhage, acute lupus pneumonitis, and pulmonary edema) and chronic (interstitial pneumonitis and fibrosis) manifestation. Unlike the high prevalence of pleuritis and acute pulmonary manifestations (50–60%), fibrotic ILD is considered an unusual finding in SLE than in other collagen tissue diseases. The clinical progression in SLE-related fibrotic ILD is usually slow, often remaining a stable disease. NSIP represents the most frequent radiological and pathological pattern encountered, followed by LIP and OP; HRCT demonstrates interstitial abnormalities in approximately 30% of patients, including interlobular septal thickening, irregular linear hyperattenuating areas, and architectural distortion. Honeycombing is uncommon. Ground-glass attenuation and consolidation on HRCT may be due to acute lupus pneumonitis, hemorrhage, or interstitial pneumonitis/fibrosis.[14]

Vascular

Pulmonary hypertension manifests as enlarged pulmonary vessels and a raised pulmonary/aorta ratio. Pulmonary thromboembolism, seen as filling defects on CT pulmonary angiography, is also a common manifestation of SLE, especially in association with APL (antiphospholipid) antibodies.

Airway

Airway involvement is rare and may manifest as bronchiolitis obliterans.

Others

Diaphragmatic dysfunction, a rare complication of SLE, may result from weakened diaphragm strength, diaphragm

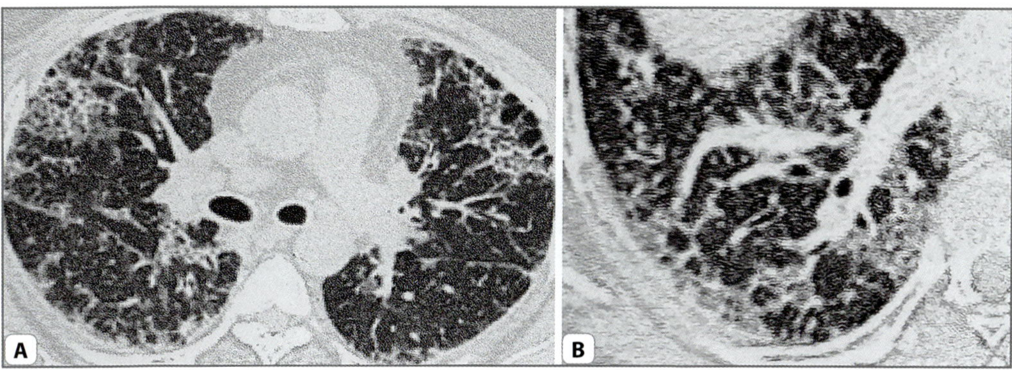

FIGS. 5A AND B: Organizing pneumonia pattern: Axial lung window image (A) and zoomed-in image (B) reveal peripheral subpleural as well as peribronchovascular patchy GGO, areas of consolidation, and interspersed reticular opacities in a patient with IIM (dermatomyositis).

(GGO: ground-glass opacity; IIM: interstitial inflammatory myopathy)

fibrosis, or phrenic nerve damage. This condition leads to decreased lung volume, which is often referred to as "shrinking lung syndrome." Infections may occur secondarily, including community-acquired pneumonia, atypical pneumonia and tuberculosis.[6]

Idiopathic Inflammatory Myopathies

Polymyositis and dermatomyositis are IIMs with pulmonary involvement seen in around 40% of patients in the form of ILD, aspiration pneumonia, and infections.

Pulmonary involvement, particularly ILD, is the most common nonmusculoskeletal manifestation of IIMs. The most common pattern is NSIP, followed by UIP and organizing pneumonia **(Figs. 5A and B)**. A chronic, indolent course is mostly seen in polymyositis, whereas an acute and rapidly progressive course is more common in dermatomyositis. Additionally, respiratory complications can arise from hypoventilation, and respiratory failure may occur due to the weakening of respiratory muscles. Another frequent pulmonary issue is aspiration pneumonia, which results from pharyngeal muscle weakness.[12]

Sjögren's Syndrome

Sjögren's syndrome, also known as *Sicca syndrome*, is a chronic inflammatory autoimmune disease of the exocrine glands, characterized by parenchymal lymphocytic infiltration with resultant xerostomia and xerophthalmia. Pulmonary manifestations usually develop late in the course of the disease and include involvement of airways (as follicular bronchiolitis, common findings), interstitial abnormalities, and lymphoproliferative disorders.

Imaging Features

Parenchymal

Nonspecific interstitial pneumonia is now recognized as the most common pulmonary parenchymal manifestation of SS, followed by LIP. While LIP is specific to SS, it is no longer considered the most common pattern, a shift from earlier perspectives where LIP was considered the predominant finding. This change in the frequency of pulmonary manifestations may be attributed to recent revisions in the diagnostic criteria for LIP, leading to the reclassification of some cases previously diagnosed as LIP as cellular NSIP. Typical HRCT pattern of LIP includes GGO (reflecting the lymphocytic infiltration), thin-walled peribronchovascular cysts, and centrilobular and subpleural nodules **(Figs. 6A to C)**.

Lymphoproliferative Disorders

Lymphoma occurs in ~20% of patients with SS and may manifest as consolidations, large nodules, or pleural effusions.

Airways

Follicular bronchiolitis is a common finding.[15]

GRANULOMATOUS DISEASE

Granulomatous diseases refer to a spectrum of diseases characterized by granuloma formation on histology. Sarcoidosis, granulomatosis with polyangiitis (GPA), and eosinophilic GPA (EGPA) are the important noninfectious conditions in this group.

Sarcoidosis

Sarcoidosis is a chronic, multisystem disease of unknown etiology characterized pathologically by noncaseating granulomas. It commonly affects young and middle-aged patients, females more than males. Patients have nonspecific signs and symptoms, including fatigue, weight loss, and, less commonly, fever. About 50% of patients remain asymptomatic. Pulmonary manifestations occur in 90% of the patients.[16]

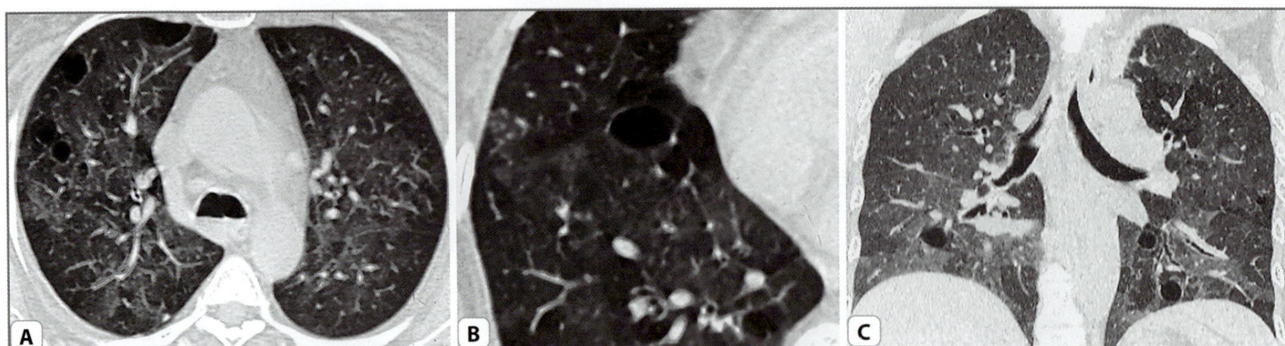

FIGS. 6A TO C: Lymphocytic interstitial pneumonia (LIP): Axial (A), and zoomed axial (B) and coronal (C) lung window images in a patient with Sjögren's syndrome show thin-walled cysts in peribronchovascular distribution, background lung GGO, and few patchy areas of centrilobular nodules (seen in B).

(GGO: ground-glass opacity)

Imaging Features

Chest Radiography

Five stages of intrathoracic abnormalities on radiography are described:

- *Stage 0*: Normal chest radiograph
- *Stage 1*: Mediastinal and hilar lymphadenopathy
- *Stage 2*: Lymphadenopathy with pulmonary parenchymal lesions
- *Stage 3*: Pulmonary parenchymal lesions in the absence of hilar lymphadenopathy
- *Stage 4*: Significant lung fibrosis with architectural distortion or bullae

The staging system is helpful in predicting disease outcomes.

Hilar adenopathy is easily recognized on radiographs **(Fig. 7)**. Garland triad/1-2-3 sign/Pawnbroker's sign is the characteristic nodal involvement at the right paratracheal and bilateral hilar groups, which may be identified on radiography.[17]

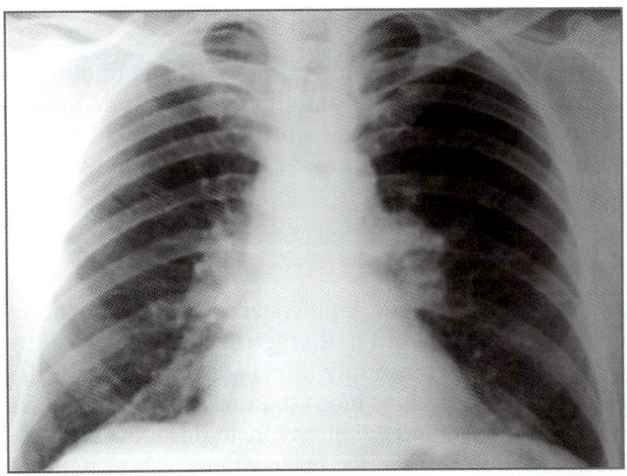

FIG. 7: Sarcoidosis: Frontal chest radiograph shows bulky, bilateral hilar lymphadenopathy.

High-resolution Computed Tomography

Computed tomography is more sensitive for detection of parenchymal abnormalities and thoracic lymphadenopathy. CT also may be helpful in patients for whom there is a high clinical suspicion of complications such as aspergilloma, concurrent infection, or malignancy. It is also beneficial for guiding transbronchial biopsy and endobronchial ultrasound (US)-guided fine-needle aspiration.

Lymphadenopathy: Contrast-enhanced CT is the modality of choice for demonstrating subtle mediastinal lymphadenopathy in the right paratracheal, aortopulmonary window, and subcarinal region. In contrast to tubercular adenopathy, enlarged sarcoidosis lymph nodes tend to remain discrete, maintain their shape, and do not have central necrosis. Sometimes, the nodes are calcified, which may be amorphous, punctate, popcorn-like, or eggshell-like peripheral in nature **(Figs. 8A and B)**.

Parenchymal changes:

- *Nodules*: On HRCT, nodules are seen at initial evaluation in 90–100% of patients with parenchymal abnormalities. They are small (5–10 mm), well-defined nodules **(Figs. 9A and B)** occurring in a perilymphatic distribution in relation to the bronchovascular interstitium, pleural surfaces, interlobular septa, and interlobar fissures, predominantly in the upper and mid lungs. Miliary nodules may also occur. In about 15–25% of the patients, coalescing granulomas form large mass-like nodules (1–4 cm in diameter), the so-called "alveolar sarcoid pattern." When discrete nodules surround these confluent masses, it is termed the "Galaxy sign." Unlike metastasis, these nodules are poorly defined and may contain air bronchogram within. Cavitating nodules are rare in sarcoidosis. Cavitary disease should prompt the exclusion of other conditions, such as vasculitis, tuberculosis, and necrotizing sarcoidosis.
- *Fibrosis*: Roughly 20% of patients develop pulmonary fibrosis (stage 4 disease). Conglomerated parahilar

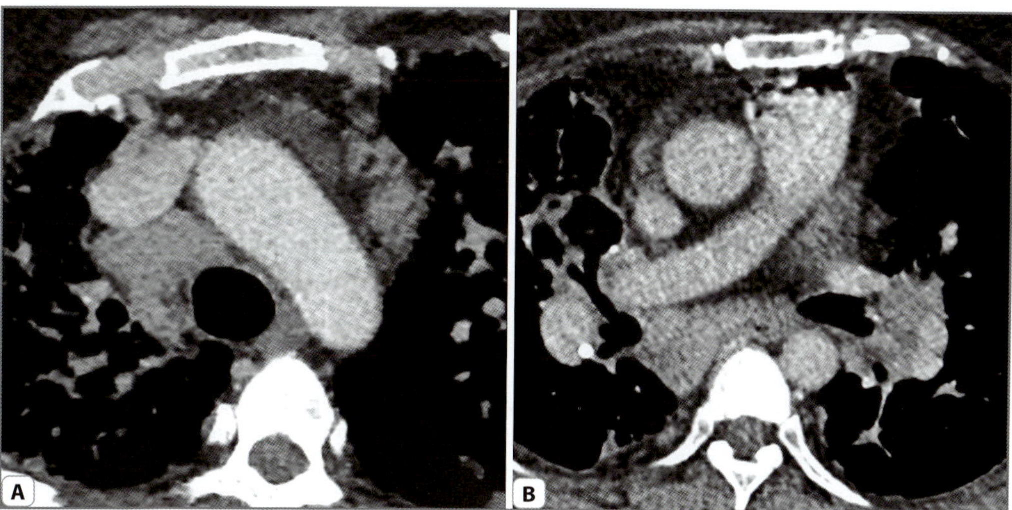

FIGS. 8A AND B: Sarcoidosis: Mediastinal lymphadenopathy—axial contrast-enhanced CT images (A and B) in soft tissue window shows homogeneously enhancing, nonnecrotic right paratracheal, prevascular, subcarinal, and bilateral hilar lymph nodes.
(CT: computed tomography)

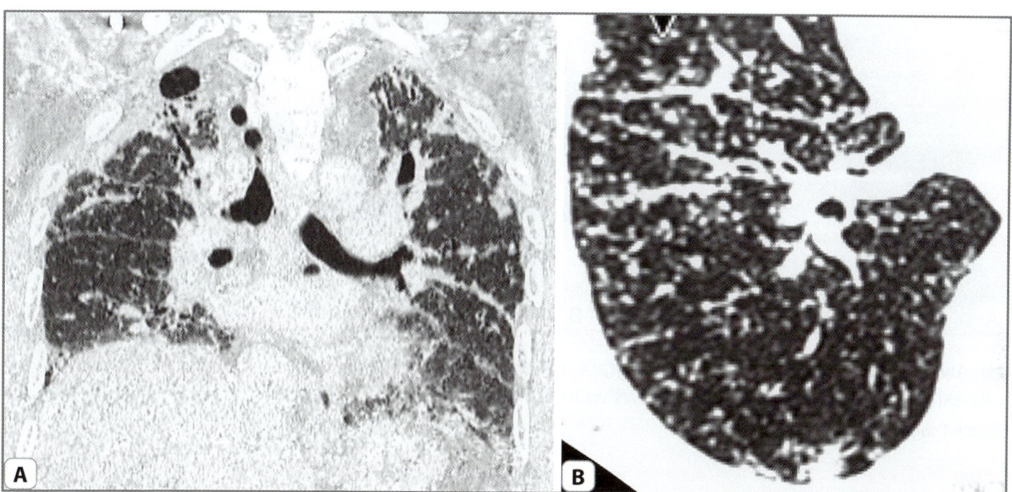

FIGS. 9A AND B: Sarcoidosis: Axial (A) and zoomed axial (B) CT lung window images show numerous micronodules in perilymphatic distribution (subpleural, centrilobular, and peribronchovascular distribution) showing upper lobe predominance. Micronodular beading is seen along the bilateral major fissures.
(CT: computed tomography)

masses distort bronchi and vessels **(Figs. 10A and B)**, resulting in traction bronchiectasis, septal thickening, and honeycombing. The conglomerate masses near the hila, with surrounding cicatricial emphysema, resemble progressive massive fibrosis (PMF) in complicated silicosis. Extensive calcification may be present within fibrotic granulomas.

Airway involvement: It is seen in the form of air trapping, mosaic attenuation, and bronchial stenosis, which are nonspecific findings yet not uncommon.[18]

Alveolar sarcoidosis is an atypical pulmonary manifestation of sarcoidosis **(Figs. 11A and B)** that manifests as opacities ranging in size from 1 to 4 cm, with irregular borders and potential air bronchograms along bronchovascular bundles or adjacent to the pleura.

Radionuclide Scanning

Historically, gallium scanning was performed for activity assessment, with limited specificity. Fluorodeoxyglucose positron emission tomography (FDG-PET) is used for disease activity, identifying occult disease/extrathoracic sites, and prebiopsy planning.[19]

Magnetic Resonance Imaging

Magnetic resonance imaging (MRI) has a role in the evaluation of cardiac involvement of sarcoidosis.[19]

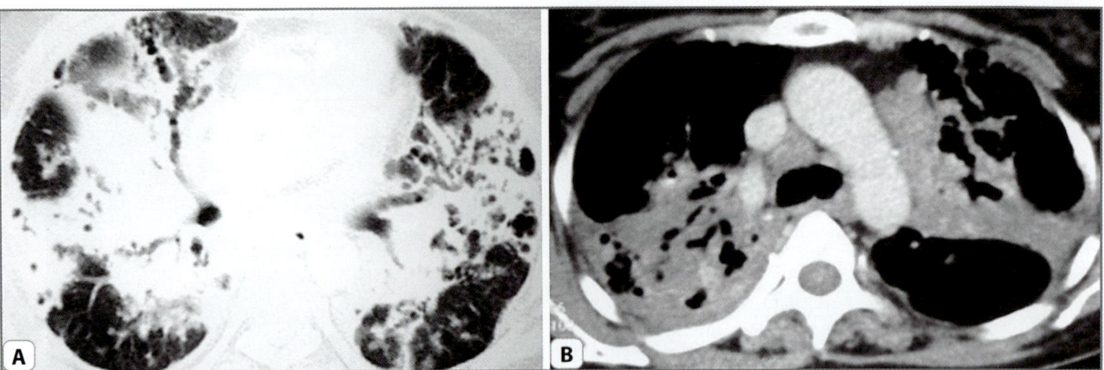

FIGS. 10A AND B: Sarcoidosis: (A) CECT chest (lung window) shows extensive, parahilar fibrotic masses with traction bronchiectasis, findings that indicate stage 4 disease. (B) CECT chest (mediastinal window) shows large fibrotic lesions, mediastinal adenopathy, and irregularly thickened pleura.

(CECT: contrast-enhanced computed tomography)

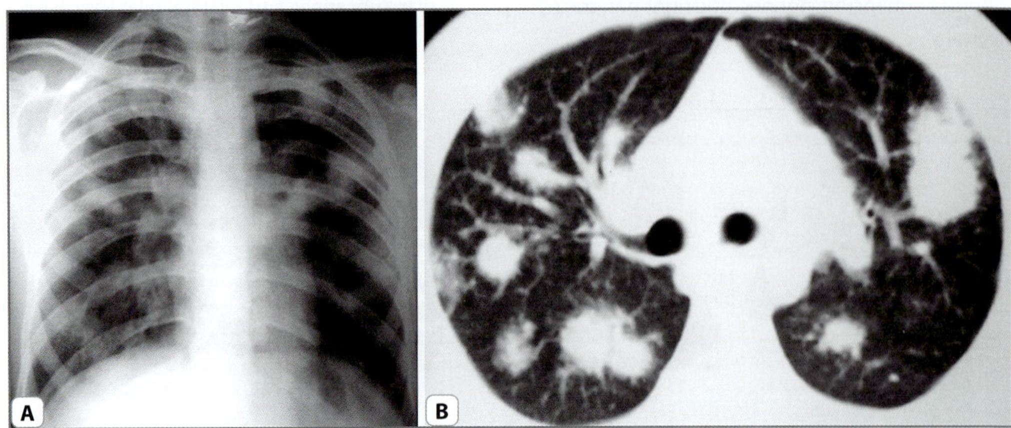

FIGS. 11A AND B: Alveolar sarcoidosis: (A) Frontal radiograph shows bulky hilar adenopathy and multiple lung nodules in bilateral upper and mid zones. (B) Axial CECT in the same patient shows well-defined, irregular parenchymal nodules indicating alveolar sarcoidosis.

(CECT: contrast-enhanced computed tomography)

EXPOSURE-RELATED DISEASES

This group includes diseases associated with environmental antigenic exposures such as HP or occupational exposure to various dusts.

Hypersensitivity Pneumonitis

Hypersensitivity pneumonitis is a diffuse granulomatous ILD caused by an abnormal immune response to various organic dusts. The clinical manifestations and radiologic and histological patterns are nonspecific and may be similar to other interstitial and small airway diseases. A high index of suspicion, detailed exposure, occupational history, bronchoalveolar lavage (BAL) lymphocytosis, and classic HRCT features help make the diagnosis. Still, the causative antigen may remain unidentifiable in up to 40% of histologically proven cases of HP.[20]

Imaging Features

Hypersensitivity pneumonitis is classified into two phenotypic subtypes: Nonfibrotic (purely inflammatory) and fibrotic HP (mixed inflammatory/fibrotic or purely fibrotic). In the past, HP was divided into three categories: Acute, subacute, and chronic forms. However, this classification system is no longer preferred due to the difficulties in clearly distinguishing between these subtypes.[21]

Radiograph

The chest radiographs may be normal early in the course of the disease. Later, bilateral, patchy areas of ground-glass opacity appear, which may be diffuse or show variable zonal distribution. These abnormalities frequently resolve if the antigenic exposure is stopped. If exposure is continued or repeated, the diffuse nodular or ground-glass pattern is

TABLE 4: HRCT chest features of hypersensitivity pneumonitis.[21]

	Nonfibrotic		Fibrotic	
	Parenchymal infiltration	Small airway disease	Parenchymal fibrosis	Small airway disease
Typical	• GGOs • Mosaic attenuation • Diffuse distribution	• Ill-defined, centrilobular nodules • Air trapping • Diffuse distribution	• Irregular linear opacities/coarse reticulation with lung distortion • ±Traction bronchiectasis and honeycombing • *Distribution*: Random, mid-lung zone—predominant or relative lower lobe sparing	• Ill-defined, centrilobular nodules and/or GGOs • Mosaic attenuation, three-density pattern, and/or air trapping
Compatible	• Uniform and subtle GGOs, air-space consolidation, lung cysts • *Distribution*: Diffuse, variant—peribronchovascular, upper lung zones	–	• *UIP pattern*: Extensive GGOs with superimposed subtle features of lung fibrosis • *Distribution*: Variant—peribronchovascular, upper lung zones	Ill-defined centrilobular nodules, or three-density pattern and/or air trapping
Indeterminate	–	–	• UIP pattern • NSIP pattern • Organizing pneumonia pattern (in the absence of other features of HP)	–

(GGO: ground-glass opacities; HP: hypersensitivity pneumonitis; HRCT: high-resolution computed tomography; NSIP: nonspecific interstitial pneumonia; UIP: usual interstitial pneumonia)

replaced by a reticular pattern characteristic of interstitial fibrosis.

High-resolution Computed Tomography

The HRCT features can be categorized into three patterns: Typical for HP, compatible with HP, and indeterminate for HP for both nonfibrotic and fibrotic types **(Table 4)**.

Nonfibrotic HP: The "typical HP" pattern requires at least one HRCT abnormality indicative of parenchymal infiltration and at least one HRCT abnormality indicative of small airway disease, both in a diffuse distribution **(Figs. 12A and B)**. *Compatible-with-HP* patterns are nonspecific patterns that have been described in HP **(Figs. 13A and B)**.

Fibrotic HP: The "typical HP" pattern requires an HRCT pattern of lung fibrosis in one of the distributions and at least one abnormality that is indicative of small airway disease. "compatible-with-HP" patterns are described when the HRCT pattern and/or distribution of lung fibrosis varies from that of the typical HP pattern; signs of small airway disease should accompany the variant fibrosis. The "indeterminate-for-HP" pattern is used when it is neither typical nor compatible **(Figs. 14A to C)**.[22]

Silicosis and Coal Worker's Pneumoconiosis

Silicosis and coal worker's pneumoconiosis (CWP) are ILDs related to exposure to dust-containing crystallized silicon dioxide and coal dust. A positive inhalational history with characteristic findings on imaging is often sufficient to make the diagnosis.

Both silicosis and CWP can be classified as "simple" and "complicated." On imaging, CWP and silicosis show overlapping features.[23]

Imaging Features

Classic Simple Silicosis

- *Radiographs*: It is characterized by multiple well-defined nodular opacities that are uniform in shape and attenuation, ranging from 1 to 10 mm in diameter. These nodules are primarily located in the dorsal lung zones of the upper lobes.
- *HRCT*: On CT, numerous small pulmonary nodules, again predominantly seen in the upper lobes, are often associated with calcifications. The nodules typically follow a perilymphatic distribution and can include

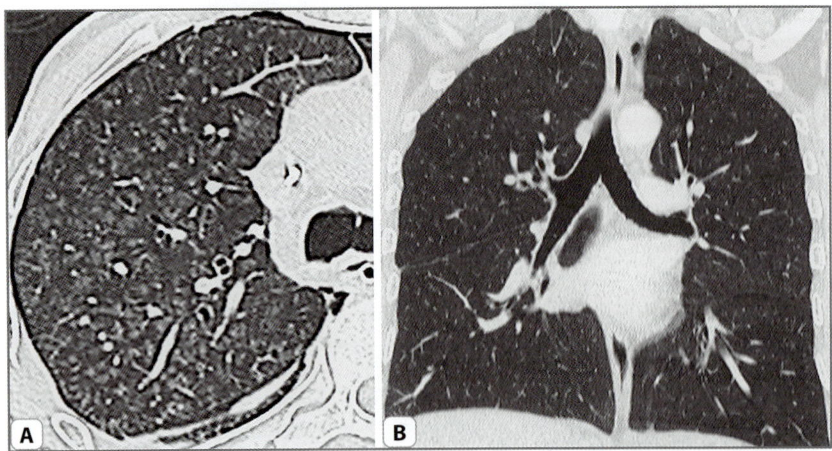

FIGS. 12A AND B: Typical nonfibrotic hypersensitivity pneumonitis: Axial (A) and coronal (B) lung window CT chest images reveal ill-defined centrilobular GGO nodules showing diffuse distribution.

(CT: computed tomography; GGO: ground-glass opacity)

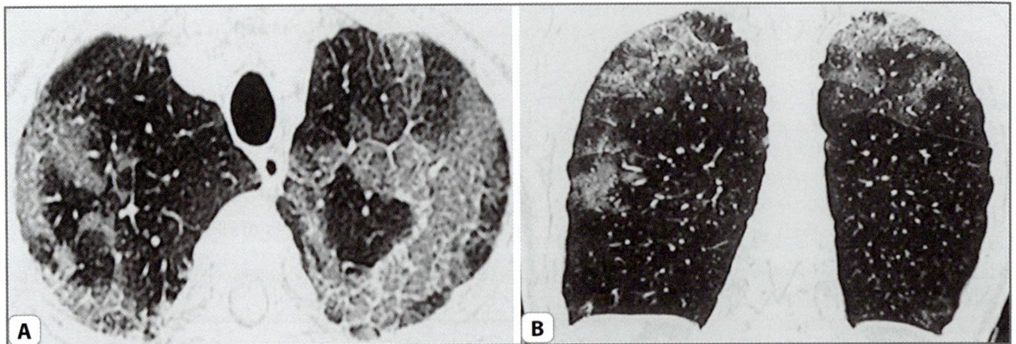

FIGS. 13A AND B: Nonfibrotic hypersensitivity pneumonitis: (A) Axial HRCT shows extensive patchy ground-glass attenuation. (B) Coronal multiplanar reconstruction shows the predominantly upper lobar distribution of the patchy ground-glass opacities.

(HRCT: high-resolution computed tomography)

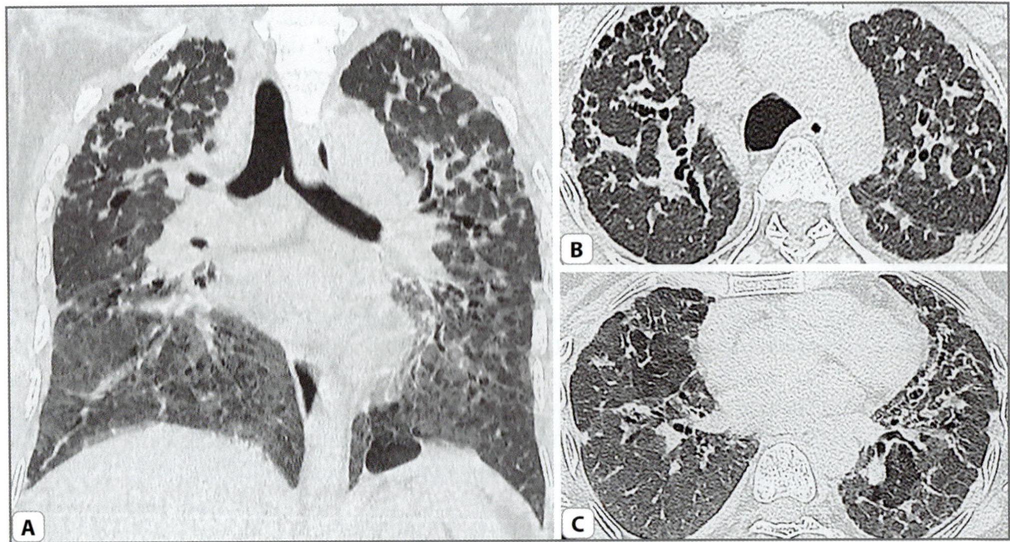

FIGS. 14A TO C: Fibrotic hypersensitivity pneumonitis: Coronal (A), axial lung window images (B and C) show fibrotic changes in the form of traction bronchiectasis and peripheral reticular changes seen in the upper and mid lung sections; note the relative lower lobe sparing and mosaic attenuation with air trapping.

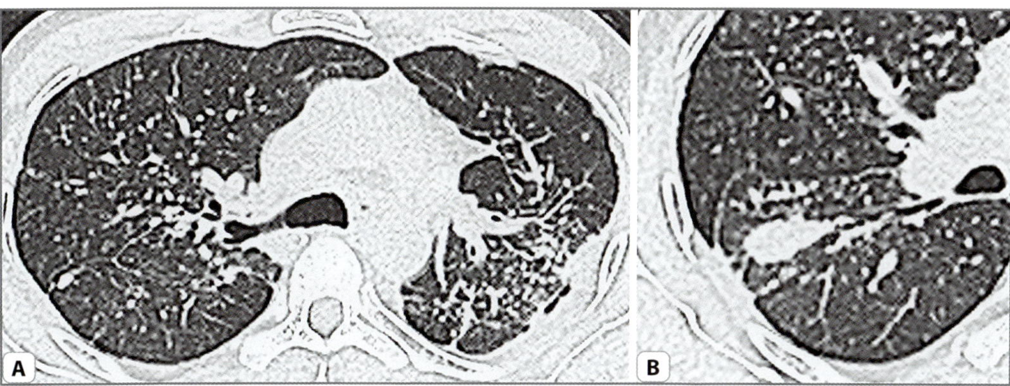

FIGS. 15A AND B: Simple silicosis: Axial HRCT images show clusters of tiny centrilobular and subpleural micronodules in a foundry worker with silicosis. Some of the nodules are seen aggregating into PMF masses.

(HRCT: high-resolution computed tomography; PMF: progressive massive fibrosis)

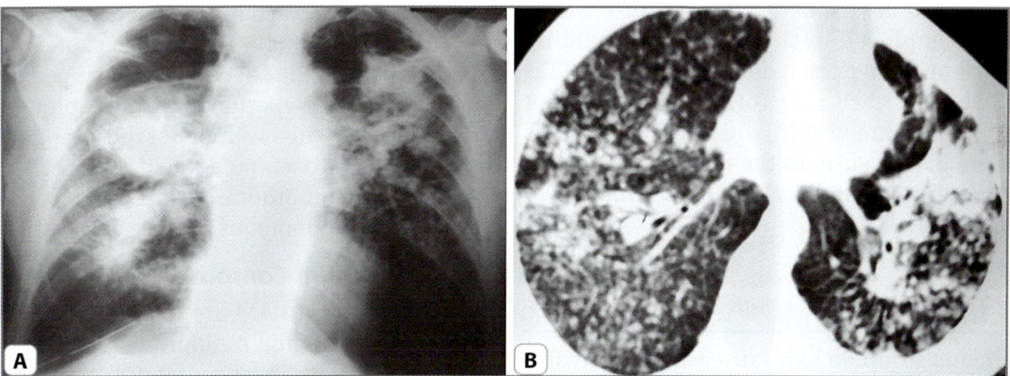

FIGS. 16A AND B: Complicated Silicosis with PMF: Frontal chest radiograph (A) and axial CT lung window in another patient show large, parahilar fibrotic masses with surrounding cicatricial emphysema (in A). (B) Shows clusters of tiny centrilobular and subpleural micronodules, many of them aggregating to form variable-sized PMF lesions. As PMF progresses, the number of nodules decreases because of their aggregation into fibrotic lesions.

(CT: computed tomography; PMF: progressive massive fibrosis)

subpleural nodules that may merge. Additionally, hilar and mediastinal lymphadenopathy may be present and can appear before parenchymal nodules are visible. Lymph node calcification, commonly occurring at the periphery of the nodes, is a frequent finding and is particularly indicative of silicosis when seen as the classic "eggshell" pattern **(Figs. 15A and B)**.

Complicated Silicosis

- *Radiographs*: Radiographs show large, symmetric bilateral opacities (≥1 cm) with irregular margins. These opacities are commonly located in the middle lung zones and may gradually migrate toward the hilum, leaving emphysematous tissue between the fibrotic areas and the pleural surface.
- *HRCT*: On CT scans, the disease appears as focal soft-tissue masses with irregular or ill-defined margins, sometimes containing calcifications, and surrounded by regions of emphysematous change **(Figs. 16A and B)**.[24]

Simple Coal Worker's Pneumoconiosis

- *Radiograph*: Typically, small (1–5 mm) round nodular opacities, sometimes with a reticular or reticulonodular pattern, are seen. These nodules tend to have less well-defined margins and a more granular appearance than silicosis. Few patients may have small central calcifications within the nodules, contrasting with the diffuse calcifications in silicosis. The eggshell calcification pattern of silicosis is rare in CWP cases.
- *HRCT*: Small nodules are seen diffusely distributed, more so in the upper lungs, with about 30% of patients showing nodular calcifications. Hilar or mediastinal lymph node enlargement is also seen.

Complicated Coal Worker's Pneumoconiosis

- *Radiographs*: It may reveal large fibrotic masses indicative of PMF that can have either irregular borders with surrounding emphysema or regular borders without emphysema.

- *HRCT*: The nodules tend to coalesce and initially form clusters and later form large conglomerate masses, i.e., PMF. Conglomerate masses are seen more in apical and posterior segments of the upper lobes. Associated peripheral parenchymal distortion with paracicatricial emphysema is common. PMF is typically bilateral and often symmetric. PMF lesions may uncommonly calcify or show central cavitation.
- *MRI*: Complicated coal workers' pneumoconiosis (CWP) typically appears as a low signal intensity lesion on both T1- and T2-weighted images, in contrast to neoplastic processes, which usually show high signal intensity on T2-weighted images. When contrast is administered, lesions in complicated CWP often display peripheral enhancement.[25]

Asbestosis

Asbestos (inhalational) exposure is seen in miners, millers, persons employed in shipyards, and building trades. Asbestosis on plain chest radiography and HRCT is indistinguishable from other causes of lung fibrosis except when pleural plaques are visible, which then indicates asbestosis as the likely cause. In the absence of pleural plaques, the pattern of fibrosis alone is insufficient to differentiate from UIP.

MISCELLANEOUS

The miscellaneous group includes diseases that involve accumulation of cellular or noncellular material in the alveoli and includes lymphangioleiomyomatosis (LAM), LCH, and pulmonary alveolar proteinosis (PAP).

Lymphangioleiomyomatosis

Lymphangioleiomyomatosis is a rare pulmonary disorder characterized by the abnormal proliferation of perivascular epithelial cells (PECs) or LAM cells. LAM was initially categorized as an ILD because of its diffuse pattern of involvement. However, subsequent genetic studies have revealed that it is more accurately characterized as a destructive, low-grade malignancy. In the latest World Health Organization (WHO) classification of lung tumors, LAM is classified as a low-grade, metastatic PEComatous neoplasm.[26] Proliferation of LAM cells leads to formation of air cysts due to bronchiolar obstruction, which may rupture to cause pneumothorax. Similarly, pulmonary venous obstruction can occur with consequent pulmonary hypertension and hemoptysis. LAM cell proliferation in the lymphatic system can result in enlarged lymph nodes in the hilar, mediastinal, and extrathoracic regions, potentially causing dilation of lymphatic vessels in the lungs and thoracic duct, leading to chylous pleural or abdominal effusion.[27,28] LAM in the lungs manifests with exertional dyspnea and recurrent pneumothorax. Less frequently, patients may experience chest pain, dry cough, hemoptysis, ascites, and chylous effusion, complications such as sepsis, hematuria, pericardial effusion, and lymphedema. These symptoms often worsen during pregnancy. Spontaneous pneumothorax is a hallmark feature of LAM and frequently serves as a diagnostic clue.[27,28]

Lymphangioleiomyomatosis presents in two main forms: The hereditary form associated with tuberous sclerosis complex (TSC)-LAM and the sporadic form (S-LAM), with the latter accounting for approximately 85% of cases. Symptomatic cystic lung disease almost exclusively affects women and is associated with s-LAM; this is explained by the fact that LAM cells express estrogen and progesterone receptors.

Imaging Features

Radiographs

Pleural and parenchymal abnormalities are visualized on chest radiography in around 70% of patients. A bilateral, symmetrical reticular pattern is seen involving all lung zones to a similar degree (80%) or the lower zones predominantly in the remaining 20% of patients. Cysts can be identified in 50–60% of cases. Hyperinflation and expiratory air trapping are often found. Involvement of the lymphatics may cause obstruction and accumulation of chylous pleural effusions. Recurrent pneumothorax is a frequent complication (30–40%) due to spontaneous rupture of the thin-walled cysts.

High-resolution Computed Tomography

HRCT features of LAM are characteristic in the form of uniformly distributed multiple thin-walled cysts of 2 mm to 5 cm size, with intervening normal lung parenchyma **(Fig. 17)**. The wall thickness of the cysts is variable up to a few millimeters. The cysts in LAM typically range from 2 to 5 mm in diameter but can become larger as the disease progresses. Patients with TSC-LAM may exhibit nodular hyperplasia, characterized by small pulmonary nodules (1–8 mm) distributed randomly, a finding not seen in S-LAM patients.

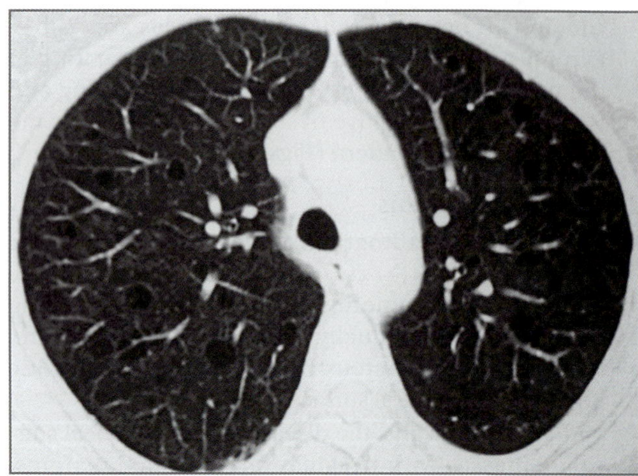

FIG. 17: Axial HRCT shows early LAM with subtle thin-walled cysts interspersed with normal lung parenchyma.
(LAM: lymphangioleiomyomatosis; HRCT: high-resolution computed tomography)

The 2017 guidelines from the American Thoracic Society and the Japanese Respiratory Society endorse a clinical diagnosis of LAM when typical lung CT findings are observed in conjunction with any of the following conditions: TSC, renal angiomyolipoma (AML), cystic lymphangioleiomyoma, or the presence of chylothorax and/or chyloperitoneum.[28] These additional features help to support the diagnosis of LAM in patients presenting with characteristic imaging findings.

Lymphangioleiomyomatosis may stabilize or regress spontaneously over time, which could explain the delayed diagnosis and diagnostic confusion often encountered in primary care settings. Few medications have been shown to benefit patients with LAM, with mTOR (mammalian target of rapamycin) inhibitors, such as sirolimus, among the primary treatment options. Other potential therapies, depending on the specific clinical manifestations, include bronchodilators. For those with recurrent pneumothorax, video-assisted thoracoscopic surgery (VATS), and pleurodesis may be considered. In cases of respiratory failure, lung transplantation is an option. However, it is important to note that recurrent LAM can occur in transplanted lungs, often due to the persistence of the original tuberous sclerosis mutation.[26]

Differential Diagnosis

The primary differential diagnosis on HRCT is LCH. However, the cysts in LCH typically involve the middle and upper lung zones, with sparing of the lung bases. In addition, most patients with LCH also have nodules, a finding rarely seen in LAM. The presence of pleural effusion further helps distinguish cystic lung disease in LAM from LCH.

Langerhans Cell Histiocytosis

Langerhans cell histiocytosis refers to a group of diseases primarily affecting children with unknown etiology, in which Langerhans cells accumulate in one or more body systems such as bone, lung, pituitary gland, mucous membranes, skin, lymph nodes, and liver. On the other hand, pulmonary Langerhans cell histiocytosis (PLCH) is a disease of adults affecting the lungs, usually in isolation or less commonly in other organ systems.[29]

Up to 100% of PLCH patients are current or former smokers, and there is a slight male predominance. The peak is at 20–40 years of age.

Extrapulmonary manifestations of PLCH (bone lesions, diabetes insipidus, and skin lesions) may occur in 5–15% of patients. About 20–25% of patients are asymptomatic.

Dry cough and dyspnea are common presenting complaints, followed by constitutional symptoms, such as weight loss, fever, night sweats, and anorexia. Spontaneous pneumothorax may occasionally be seen.

A key histological feature of LCH is peribronchiolar nodules containing Langerhans and inflammatory cells in the early stages. With time, these nodules become fibrotic, causing stellate peribronchiolar scars.

Cessation of smoking is sufficient for stabilization of symptoms in most patients. Medical therapy includes corticosteroids, which are the mainstay. Chemotherapeutic drugs such as vinblastine, methotrexate, and cyclophosphamide may be used in nonresponders and multi-organ involvement.[30]

Imaging Features

Chest Radiographs

Radiographs show nodular or reticulonodular opacities predominantly in the upper lungs. Costophrenic angles are spared. Lung volumes are preserved. With disease progression, cystic changes and bullae develop in the upper lungs, and lung volume increases.

High-resolution Computed Tomography

It shows characteristic findings of nodules and cysts predominating in the upper and mid lungs, with sparing of the bases. Early in the disease, peribronchiolar centrilobular nodules of 1–5 mm diameter predominate.

With disease evolution, thick- or thin-walled cysts (usually <10 mm in diameter) are identified in 80% of the patients (**Figs. 18A and B**). These cysts may be round, lobulated, irregular, or bizarre in shape, often with normal intervening parenchyma. The rupture of cysts into the pleural space causes episodic pneumothorax. Longitudinal HRCT studies have shown the progression of solid nodules to cavitary nodules to thick-walled cysts and, finally, thin-walled cysts.[29]

In patients showing isolated nodular disease on HRCT, the differential diagnosis includes sarcoidosis, silicosis, metastatic disease, and tuberculosis. The distribution in the upper and mid lungs and the centrilobular nature of the nodules in PLCH may aid in differentiation. Cystic changes may simulate the appearance of LAM; however, the cysts in LAM occur throughout the lung without sparing the lung bases, and nodules are rarely seen. In both conditions, lung volumes are preserved, and pneumothorax can occur.

The natural history of LCH is variable and unpredictable. Approximately, 50% of patients may have partial or complete clearing of radiologic abnormalities with symptom resolution. Follow-up CT scans may show regression of nodules, whereas any cysts that have formed are permanent. In 30–40% of patients, persisting symptoms are of variable severity; scarring supervenes, which results in reticulation, thickening of the cyst walls, and architectural distortion. In 10–20% of patients, recurrent pneumothorax or progressive respiratory failure with cor pulmonale occurs.[30]

Pulmonary Alveolar Proteinosis

Pulmonary alveolar proteinosis is a rare disease characterized by the accumulation of abnormal proteinaceous

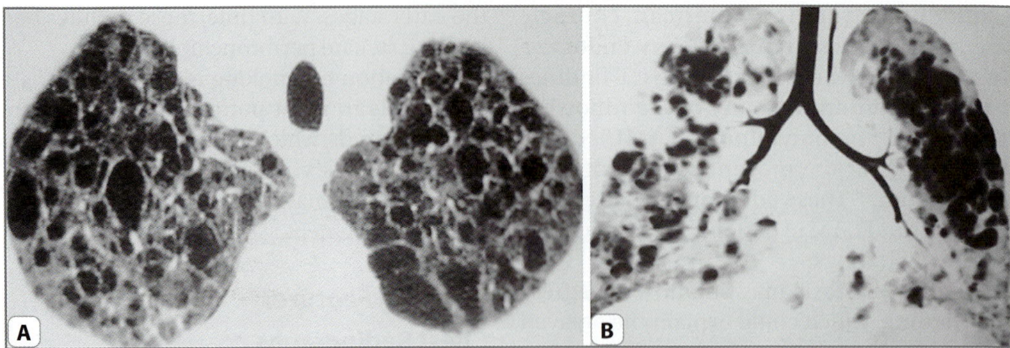

FIGS. 18A AND B: LCH: (A) Axial HRCT shows multiple, varying-sized thick-walled cysts diffusely involving bilateral lungs; (B) Coronal multiplanar reconstruction shows the relative sparing of the bilateral lung bases.
(HRCT: high-resolution computed tomography; LCH: Langerhans cell histiocytosis)

material in the alveoli, causing hypoxemia, restrictive lung disease, and a radiological appearance like pulmonary edema. Idiopathic PAP accounts for up to 90% of cases. Secondary PAP (5–10% of cases) is seen in patients with industrial inhalational exposure to silica particles, cement dust, aluminum dust, titanium dioxide, nitrogen dioxide, and fiberglass; underlying hematologic malignancy; or immunodeficiency disorders such as cytotoxic or immunosuppressive therapy and human immunodeficiency virus infection.

Imaging Features

Chest Radiography

Bilateral central and symmetric lung opacities, with relative sparing of the apices and costophrenic angles. Less commonly, radiographs show multifocal asymmetric opacities or extensive diffuse consolidation without any clear zonal predominance. Opacities may be ground-glass, reticular/reticulonodular, to consolidation with air bronchogram. Although the radiographic appearance of PAP may suggest pulmonary interstitial edema, pleural effusion, and cardiomegaly are absent.

There is often discordance between marked radiographic abnormalities in the presence of more benign clinical symptoms (clinicoradiologic discrepancy).[31]

High-resolution Computed Tomography

Shows bilateral, symmetric alveolar consolidation or ground-glass opacity in a perihilar or hilar distribution. Geographic ground-glass attenuation, sharply demarcated from the surrounding normal parenchyma, with superimposed polygonal shape intra- and interlobular septal thickening **(Fig. 19)**, creates the "crazy paving" appearance.[32] The crazy paving appearance for alveolar proteinosis, although highly sensitive, is not specific.

The radiological differential diagnosis includes diffuse alveolar damage superimposed on UIP, acute interstitial pneumonia, acute respiratory distress syndrome, and bronchoalveolar carcinoma.

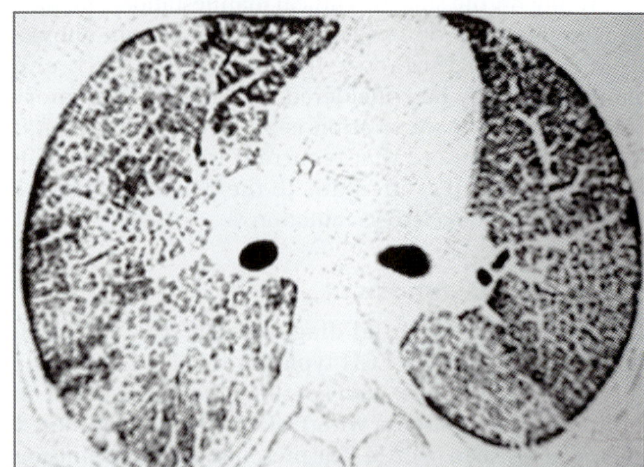

FIG. 19: Pulmonary alveolar proteinosis (PAP): Axial HRCT shows classic findings of "crazy paving"; geographic ground-glass attenuation superimposed with thickening of interstitium producing polygonal opacities.
(HRCT: high-resolution computed tomography)

Sequential therapeutic whole-lung lavage is the primary treatment in idiopathic PAP, which involves using saline solution and chest percussion to remove the lipoproteinaceous material from pulmonary alveoli. Post-therapeutic whole-lung lavage CT may reveal the resolution of ground-glass opacity; however, the septal lines may persist.[31]

CONCLUSION

A whole gamut of conditions in the wide group of ILD due to a known cause has similar clinical presentation. A meticulous history with regards to the underlying disease such as SARD, offending allergens, if any, with thorough biochemical evaluation helps in narrowing down the diagnosis. A multidisciplinary approach with radiologists, pulmonary physicians, and pathologists is desired to achieve optimum care for such patients.

REFERENCES

1. American Thoracic Society, European Respiratory Society. American Thoracic Society/European Respiratory Society International Multidisciplinary Consensus Classification of the Idiopathic Interstitial Pneumonias. This joint statement of the American Thoracic Society (ATS), and the European Respiratory Society (ERS) was adopted by the ATS board of directors, June 2001 and by the ERS Executive Committee, June 2001. Am J Respir Crit Care Med. 2002;165(2):277-304.
2. Travis WD, Costabel U, Hansell DM, King TE, Lynch DA, Nicholson AG, et al. An official American Thoracic Society/European Respiratory Society statement: update of the international multidisciplinary classification of the idiopathic interstitial pneumonias. Am J Respir Crit Care Med. 2013;188(6):733-48.
3. Kuo CS, Young LR. Interstitial lung disease in children. Curr Opin Pediatr. 2014;26(3):320-7.
4. Johnson SR, Bernstein EJ, Bolster MB, Chung JH, Danoff SK, George MD, et al. 2023 American College of Rheumatology (ACR)/American College of Chest Physicians (CHEST) guideline for the treatment of interstitial lung disease in people with systemic autoimmune rheumatic diseases. Arthritis Care Res. 2024;76(8):1051-69.
5. Chung JH, Cox CW, Montner SM, Adegunsoye A, Oldham JM, Husain AN, et al. CT features of the usual interstitial pneumonia pattern: differentiating connective tissue disease-associated interstitial lung disease from idiopathic pulmonary fibrosis. Am J Roentgenol. 2018;210(2):307-13.
6. Brady D, Berkowitz EA, Sharma A, Ackman JB, Bernheim A, Chung M, et al. CT morphologic characteristics and variant patterns of interstitial pulmonary fibrosis in systemic lupus erythematosus. Radiol Cardiothorac Imaging. 2021;3(4):e200625.
7. Richter P, Cardoneanu A, Dima N, Bratoiu I, Rezus C, Burlui AM, et al. Interstitial lung disease in systemic lupus erythematosus and systemic sclerosis: how can we manage the challenge? Int J Mol Sci. 2023;24(11):9388.
8. Walkoff L, White DB, Chung JH, Asante D, Cox CW. The four corners sign: a specific imaging feature in differentiating systemic sclerosis-related interstitial lung disease from idiopathic pulmonary fibrosis. J Thorac Imaging. 2018;33(3):197-203.
9. Goldin JG, Lynch DA, Strollo DC, Suh RD, Schraufnagel DE, Clements PJ, et al. High-resolution CT scan findings in patients with symptomatic scleroderma-related interstitial lung disease. Chest. 2008;134(2):358-67.
10. Chung JH, Walker CM, Hobbs S. Imaging features of systemic sclerosis-associated interstitial lung disease. J Vis Exp. 2020;(160).
11. Bendstrup E, Møller J, Kronborg-White S, Prior TS, Hyldgaard C. Interstitial lung disease in rheumatoid arthritis remains a challenge for clinicians. J Clin Med. 2019;8(12):2038.
12. Palmucci S, Galloto F, Fazio G, Ferlito A, Cancemi G, Di Mari A, et al. Clinical and radiological features of lung disorders related to connective-tissue diseases: a pictorial essay. Insights Imaging. 2022;13(1):108.
13. Kadura S, Raghu G. Rheumatoid arthritis-interstitial lung disease: manifestations and current concepts in pathogenesis and management. Eur Respir Rev. 2021;30(160):210011.
14. Kallianos K. Imaging of pulmonary manifestations of connective tissue disease. Rheum Dis Clin North Am. 2024;50(3):409-22.
15. Lin W, Xin Z, Zhang J, Liu N, Ren X, Liu M, et al. Interstitial lung disease in primary Sjögren's syndrome. BMC Pulm Med. 2022;22(1):73.
16. Ganeshan D, Menias CO, Lubner MG, Pickhardt PJ, Sandrasegaran K, Bhalla S. Sarcoidosis from head to toe: what the radiologist needs to know. RadioGraphics. 2018;38(4):1180-200.
17. Koyama T, Ueda H, Togashi K, Umeoka S, Kataoka M, Nagai S. Radiologic manifestations of sarcoidosis in various organs. RadioGraphics. 2004;24(1):87-104.
18. Dhagat PK, Singh S, Jain M, Singh SN, Sharma RK. Thoracic sarcoidosis: imaging with high-resolution computed tomography. J Clin Diagn Res. 2017;11(2):TC15-8.
19. Silva M, Nunes H, Valeyre D, Sverzellati N. Imaging of sarcoidosis. Clin Rev Allergy Immunol. 2015;49(1):45-53.
20. Hirschmann JV, Pipavath SN, Godwin JD. Hypersensitivity pneumonitis: a historical, clinical, and radiologic review. RadioGraphics. 2009;29(7):1921-38.
21. Raghu G, Remy-Jardin M, Ryerson CJ, Myers JL, Kreuter M, Vasakova M, et al. Diagnosis of hypersensitivity pneumonitis in adults: an official ATS/JRS/ALAT clinical practice guideline. Am J Respir Crit Care Med. 2020;202(3):e36-69.
22. Dabiri M, Jehangir M, Khoshpouri P, Chalian H. Hypersensitivity pneumonitis: a pictorial review based on the new ATS/JRS/ALAT clinical practice guideline for radiologists and pulmonologists. Diagnostics. 2022;12(11):2874.
23. Chong S, Lee KS, Chung MJ, Han J, Kwon OJ, Kim TS. Pneumoconiosis: comparison of imaging and pathologic findings. RadioGraphics. 2006;26(1):59-77.
24. Ozmen CA, Nazaroglu H, Yildiz T, Bayrak AH, Senturk S, Ates G, et al. MDCT findings of denim-sandblasting-induced silicosis: a cross-sectional study. Environ Health. 2010;9:17.
25. Remy-Jardin M, Degreef JM, Beuscart R, Voisin C, Remy J. Coal worker's pneumoconiosis: CT assessment in exposed workers and correlation with radiographic findings. Radiology. 1990;177(2):363-71.
26. Travis WD, Brambilla E, Nicholson AG, Yatabe Y, Austin JHM, Beasley MB, et al. The 2015 World Health Organization classification of lung tumors: impact of genetic, clinical and radiologic advances since the 2004 classification. J Thorac Oncol. 2015;10(9):1243-60.
27. Almoosa KF, Ryu JH, Mendez J, Huggins JT, Young LR, Sullivan EJ, et al. Management of pneumothorax in lymphangioleiomyomatosis: effects on recurrence and lung transplantation complications. Chest. 2006;129(5):1274-81.
28. McCormack FX, Gupta N, Finlay GR, Young LR, Taveira-DaSilva AM, Glasgow CG, et al. Official American Thoracic Society/

Japanese Respiratory Society Clinical Practice Guidelines: lymphangioleiomyomatosis diagnosis and management. Am J Respir Crit Care Med. 2016;194(6):748-61.

29. Tazi A, Soler P, Hance A. Adult pulmonary Langerhans' cell histiocytosis. Thorax. 2000;55(5):405-16.
30. Castoldi MC, Verrioli A, De Juli E, Vanzulli A. Pulmonary Langerhans cell histiocytosis: the many faces of presentation at initial CT scan. Insights Imaging. 2014;5(4):483-92.
31. Da Nam B, Kim TJ, Chung MP, Chung MJ, Kim TS, Lee KS. CT findings in pulmonary alveolar proteinosis: serial changes and prognostic implications. J Thorac Dis. 2018;10(10): 5774-83.
32. Kunal S, Gera K, Pilaniya V, Jain S, Gothi R, Shah A. "Crazy-paving" pattern: a characteristic presentation of pulmonary alveolar proteinosis and a review of the literature from India. Lung India. 2016;33(3):335.

Manisha Jana, Ashu Seith Bhalla, Ekta Dhamija

CHAPTER 10

Miscellaneous Interstitial Lung Diseases

INTRODUCTION

This chapter includes a wide range of diffuse lung diseases (DLDs) not covered in the previous chapters. Some of them are interstitial lung diseases (ILDs), whereas some are diseases mimicking ILD. Since the description of all of these is beyond the scope of this chapter, a pattern approach on high-resolution computed tomography (HRCT) will be followed. Uncommon DLDs presenting with ground-glass opacity (GGO), septal thickening, and nodules are covered. This is followed by a discussion of "cystic lung diseases."

DIFFUSE LUNG DISEASES PRESENTING WITH GROUND-GLASS OPACITY AND CONSOLIDATION

More common DLDs presenting with a predominant GGO and/or consolidation pattern have been discussed in detail in earlier chapters. **Table 1** enlists less frequent etiologies.

Various infections may present with predominant GGO pattern. Interstitial pneumonia[1,2] may appear as ill-defined areas of GGOs. Severity can range from mild forms to those causing respiratory failure. A few more severe specific forms are described here.

Viral Pneumonia

Several viruses can result in an interstitial pattern of pneumonia. Coronavirus disease 2019 (COVID-19) pneumonia and influenza virus are a few of the important causes and are discussed separately here.

TABLE 1: Uncommon DLDs presenting with GGO (with or without consolidation) pattern.

Infections	• *Interstitial pneumonia:* ○ Viral pneumonia ○ Mycoplasma pneumonia ○ Pneumocystis pneumonia
Others	• DAD/ARDS • Pulmonary edema • Diffuse alveolar hemorrhage • Eosinophilic lung diseases • Lipoid pneumonia • PAP

(ARDS: acute respiratory distress syndrome; DAD: diffuse alveolar damage; DLDs: diffuse lung diseases; GGO: ground-glass opacity; PAP: pulmonary alveolar proteinosis)

Coronavirus Disease 2019 Pneumonia

Coronavirus disease 2019 is the pneumonia caused by a novel coronavirus, which was first detected in Wuhan, Hubei Province, China, in early December 2019. During the pandemic, which lasted for nearly 2 years, lung involvement with variable degrees of severity has been reported. Multifocal peripheral GGOs are the most common CT finding described.[3] Multifocal patchy consolidation was the second most common finding, followed by unusual findings such as perilesional ground-glass halo, crazy paving, and reverse halo sign. Features such as pure consolidation, pleural effusion, and septal thickening are more commonly associated with severe disease.[4] Bronchial and vascular dilations in the affected area of the lung are also reported as suggestive imaging features.[4,5] Semiquantitative CT scorings are described, having a good correlation with clinical severity.[6]

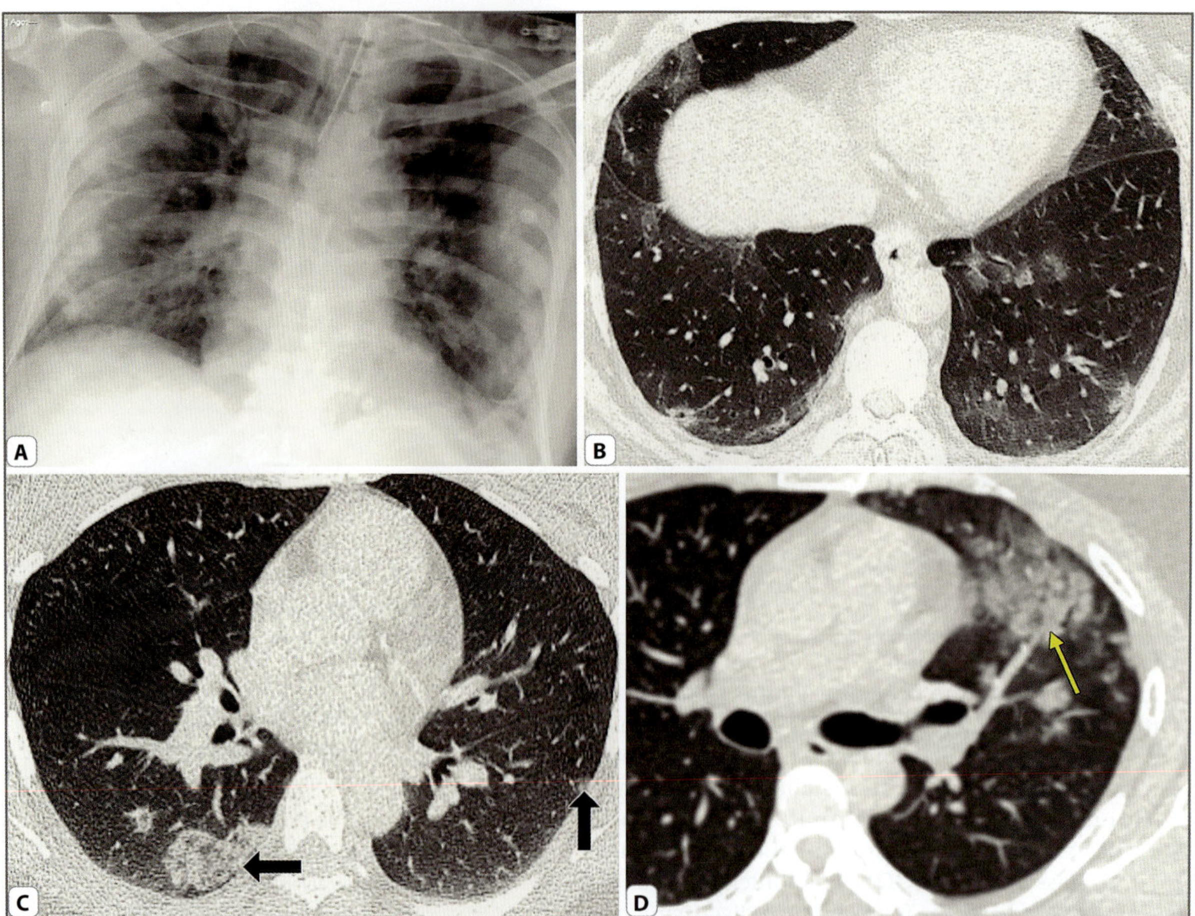

FIGS. 1A TO D: Imaging patterns in COVID-19 in four different patients. (A) Typical radiographic finding of peripheral subpleural consolidations. (B) CT showing subpleural GGOs in another patient. (C) Reverse halo/atoll sign in another patient (black arrows). (D) Focal consolidation with arterial dilation in a different patient (yellow arrow).

(CT: computed tomography; GGOs: ground-glass opacities)

The temporal changes in lung imaging may follow a pattern of GGO to begin with, which might progress to a more extensive GGO/consolidation/crazy-paving pattern **(Figs. 1A to D)**. In some cases, COVID-19 pneumonia may result in variable post-COVID-19 fibrosis with respiratory symptoms **(Figs. 2A to D)**. Other than lung involvement, thromboembolic manifestations involving the cardiovascular system, central nervous system (CNS), and other vessels are also described in active COVID-19 pneumonia or post-COVID-19 complications.

Swine Influenza (H1N1)

It is caused by *Swine-origin influenza A (H1N1)* virus. The pathology is a diffuse alveolar damage (DAD). Patients present with dry cough and dyspnea usually following a prodromal period of 2–7 days. Swine influenza is usually a mild disease but can be complicated by acute respiratory distress syndrome (ARDS) or secondary pneumonia. On HRCT, the predominant findings can be unilateral or bilateral GGO. Consolidations can be peribronchovascular or subpleural consolidations.

Mycoplasma Pneumonia

It is a common cause of community-acquired pneumonia in children and young adults, caused by *Mycoplasma pneumoniae* (walking pneumonia). The usual presenting symptoms are fever and productive cough, nonspecific complaints, fatigue, and myalgia. Chest radiographs can show diffuse reticulonodular opacities, peribronchial thickening, or even frank consolidation. HRCT findings include centrilobular nodules, peribronchovascular and interlobular septal thickening, and lobular or segmental consolidation **(Figs. 3A to D)**.

Pneumocystis Jirovecii Pneumonia

This is the most common cause of opportunistic infection in human immunodeficiency virus (HIV)-infected patients. The causative organism is an atypical fungus *Pneumocystis jirovecii.* The clinical features depend on the immune status of the patient. While it presents as an acute illness with severe hypoxia and respiratory failure in an immunocompetent individual, the symptoms are more gradual in onset in HIV-infected patients. It is common in patients with a CD4 count <100.

A chest radiograph reveals a bilaterally symmetric perihilar reticulonodular pattern that can progress to consolidation subsequently. HRCT reveals bilateral symmetric perihilar GGOs **(Figs. 4A and B)**. In the subacute stage of the disease, consolidation with septal thickening produces a "crazy-paving" pattern. Thin-walled varying-

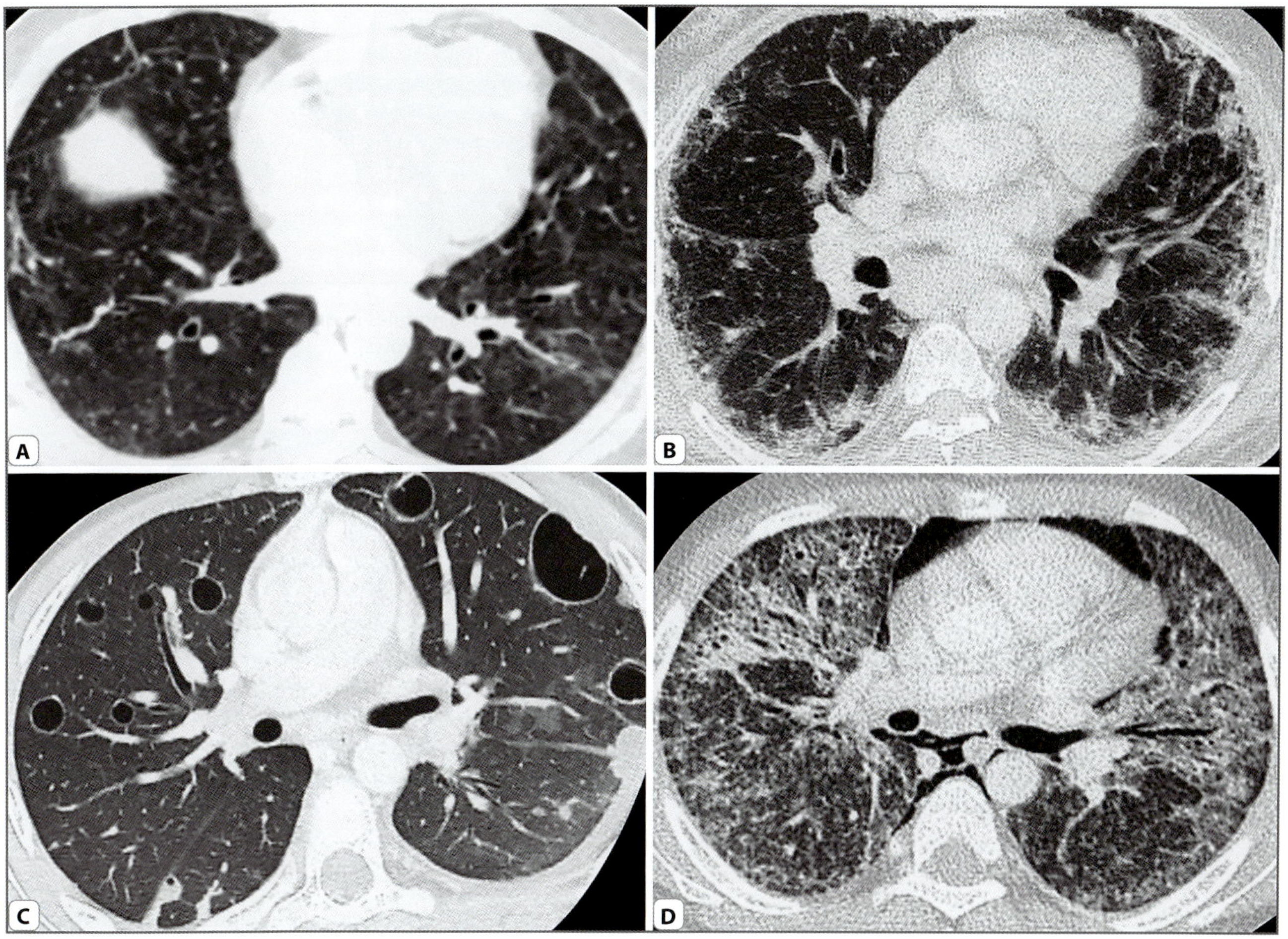

FIGS. 2A TO D: Post-COVID-19 changes in four different patients. (A) Mild post-COVID-19 fibrosis in a patient with mild-COVID-19 pneumonia. (B) Extensive fibrosis affecting the peripheral subpleural parts of the lungs in another patient with severe COVID-19 pneumonia. (C) Superadded staphylococcal pneumonia with pneumatoceles in another patient. (D) Extensive fibrosis with pneumomediastinum in a child with MIS-C.

(COVID-19: coronavirus disease 2019; MIS-C: multisystem inflammatory syndrome in children)

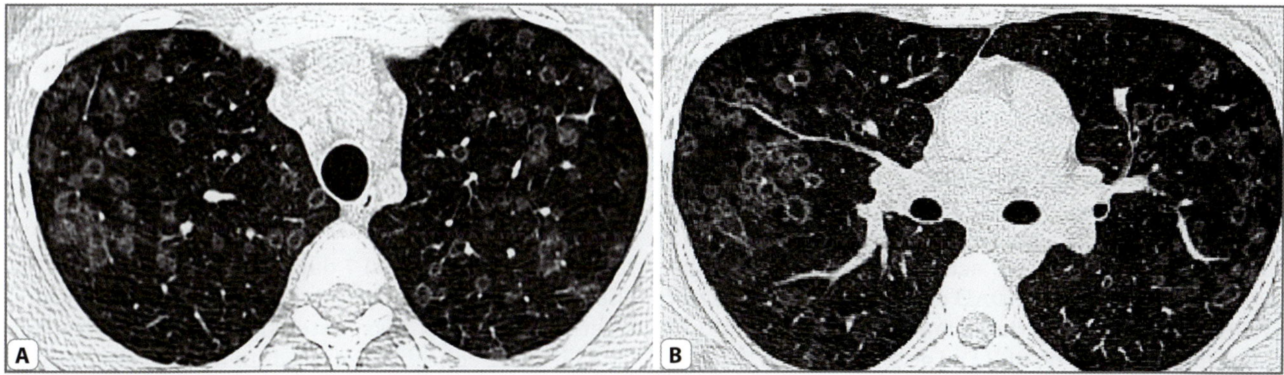

FIGS. 3A TO D: *Continued*

Continued

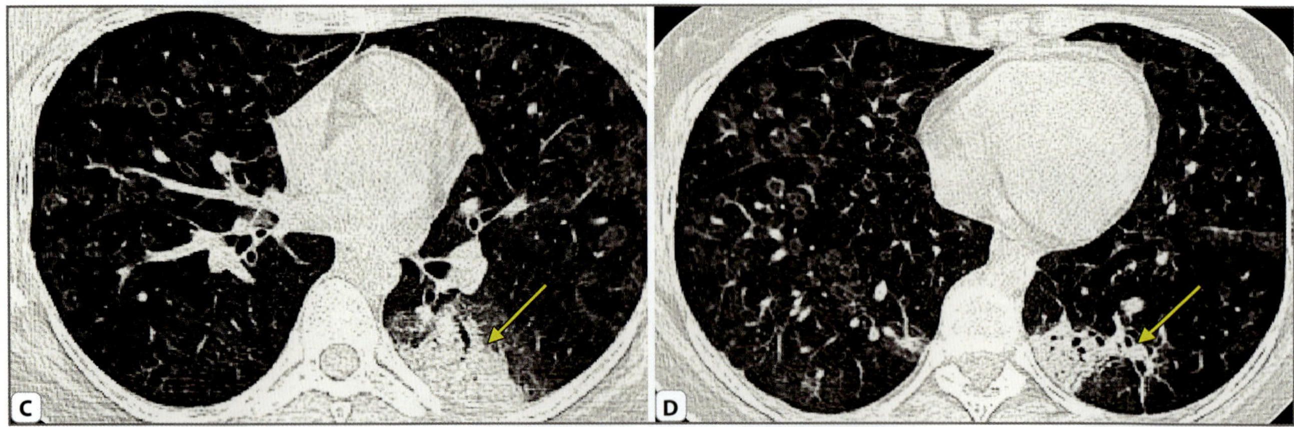

FIGS. 3A TO D: Mycoplasma pneumonia. Extensive areas of ground-glass opacity (GGO) nodules in both lobes, most of them showing central lucency/halo. Left lower lobe shows posterior basal segment consolidation (yellow arrows).

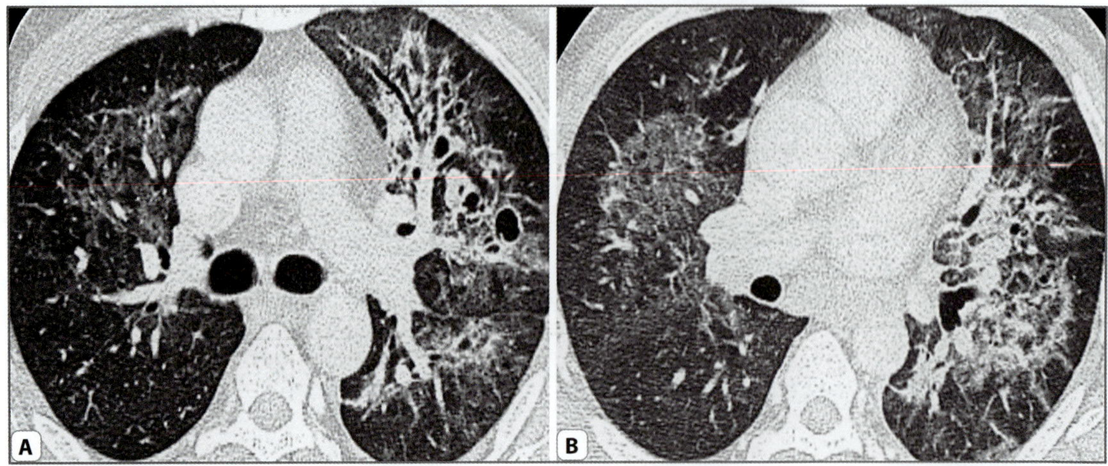

FIGS. 4A AND B: Subacute *Pneumocystis jirovecii* pneumonia. CT reveals central perihilar GGO with superimposed septal thickening and thin-walled cysts.

(CT: computed tomography; GGO: ground-glass opacity)

sized cysts can also develop in subacute stages, which can rupture and lead to spontaneous pneumothorax/pneumomediastinum.

Diffuse Alveolar Damage/Acute Respiratory Distress Syndrome

Diffuse alveolar damage is one of the two common pathological patterns observed in acute lung injury (ALI). ARDS is the clinical syndrome associated with the pathological pattern of DAD. However, it has to be kept in mind that these two are not always synonymous. ARDS can happen without DAD, acute pneumonia being the most common example. DAD can also happen without ARDS, as seen in lung transplant primary graft failure and acute exacerbation of ILD. The term "diffuse alveolar damage" has been excluded from the revised glossary of terminology in Fleischner Society Guidelines 4th edition 2024; however, it is being discussed here for conceptual understanding.

Diffuse alveolar damage can result from a variety of insults and may require mechanical ventilation. The causes of DAD are listed in **Box 1**. The pathology involves damage to all alveolar layers (alveolar epithelium, capillary epithelium, and interstitium), fluid exudation into the alveoli, and subsequent fibrosis and organization.[7,8]

Acute (Exudative) Phase

This is seen in the initial 7 days following the insult. The chest radiograph can be normal in the first 24 hours. Over the next 2–3 days, extensive, bilateral airspace opacification/consolidation ("white lung") can develop. The consolidation can be patchy and multifocal. Radiographic criteria for the diagnosis of ARDS include bilateral opacities (consistent with pulmonary edema), findings not explainable by pleural effusion, lung collapse, or nodules. CT findings can appear in 12 hours. HRCT findings include GGO and consolidation having a diffuse or patchy distribution. Usually, there is an apicobasal gradient, with more opacification of the lung bases.

Increasingly, there is an emphasis on the use of lung ultrasound (US) in critical care settings. The advantages include rapid bedside dynamic evaluation of the lungs, no radiation burden, and ease of following up. Approaches include a combination of intercostal and longitudinal (across intercostal spaces) windows. The lung US findings include bilateral B-lines and/or consolidations.

BOX 1: Causes of diffuse alveolar damage (DAD).

- *Pulmonary causes:*
  - Infection
  - Aspiration
  - Near drowning
  - Acute exacerbation of interstitial lung diseases (ILDs)
  - Noxious fume inhalation
- *Systemic causes:*
  - Sepsis
  - Pancreatitis
  - Burn
  - Trauma
  - Surgery
- *Idiopathic:*
  - Acute interstitial pneumonia (AIP)*
  - Transfusion-associated lung injury (TRALI)

*Have been excluded from 2024 edition of the Fleischner Society Glossary of Terms.

Subacute (Proliferative) Phase

It is between 1 and 2 weeks, when there is a conversion of alveolar exudates into cellular granulation tissue. Imaging in the subacute phase shows an increasing consolidation in the early phase, followed by the appearance of interlobular septal thickening, "crazy-paving pattern," and bronchiectasis and bronchiolectasis **(Figs. 5A and B)**.

Chronic (Fibrotic) Phase

It is seen 2 weeks or more following injury. Diffuse parenchymal fibrosis and architectural distortion ensue. HRCT reveals fibrosis, bronchiectasis, and bronchiolectasis, with distortion of airways and volume loss with bullae formation. Morphological changes may persist in survivors even when imaged months after the acute episode.

Long-term Sequelae

Long-term sequelae can be observed in most ARDS survivors. These can be either because of the DAD or subsequent complications such as nosocomial infections, barotrauma, and ventilator-induced lung injury. It is prudent not to label the injuries in the first year, as they tend to evolve with time. Imaging features may consist of airspace opacities, fibrotic-like changes causing traction bronchiolectasis and bronchiectasis, architectural distortion, pneumatoceles, focal emphysema/mosaic attenuation, or air trapping. The changes are usually more pronounced in the anterior lungs in case of ventilator-induced lung injury.

Pulmonary Edema

The term essentially refers to the accumulation of fluid in the extravascular compartment of the lung, initially in the

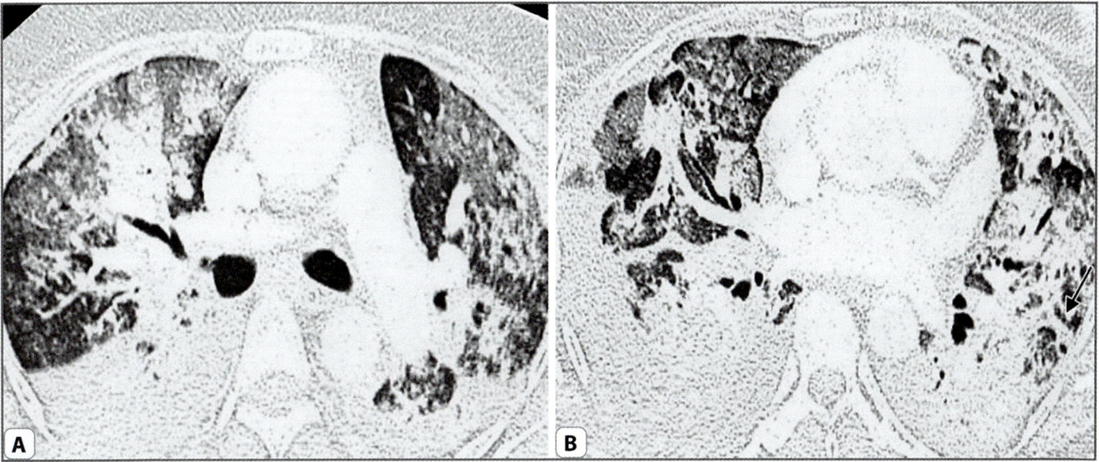

FIGS. 5A AND B: Acute respiratory distress syndrome in subacute phase. HRCT images reveal multifocal nonsegmental patchy consolidation and GGO with superimposed septal thickening (black arrow). Bilateral pleural effusion is also present.

(GGO: ground-glass opacity; HRCT: high-resolution computed tomography)

interstitium, and subsequently in the alveolar filling. Two broad mechanisms in the pathogenesis include hydrostatic (associated with increased capillary pressure resulting in fluid exudation into the alveoli) and permeability edema (exudation of fluid from leaky capillaries, with normal pressure). The latter may or may not be associated with DAD. Hydrostatic edema can be seen in the setting of cardiac failure or volume overload. Permeability edema can be seen in a number of causes, including noxious fume exposure, neurogenic edema, transfusion-associated lung injury (TRALI), high altitude edema, etc. Histopathologically, there is interstitial edema in the initial phase, followed by alveolar filling.

Imaging features may vary depending on the cause of edema. The hydrostatic form shows an enlargement of upper lobe pulmonary veins (due to diversion of blood flow) in an early phase. Later on, airspace opacities with central/parahilar (bat-wing distribution) develop. CT reveals diffuse/patchy, parahilar GGO, and smooth interlobular septal thickening **(Figs. 6A and B)**. Transudative pleural effusion is commonly seen. It has a preponderance toward involvement of the dependent areas that differentiate it from the permeability edema, which has more subpleural and peripheral distribution.

Diffuse Alveolar Hemorrhage

Diffuse alveolar hemorrhage (DAH) can be secondary to various causes, including coagulation disorders, collagen vascular disorders, and vasculitis.[9] The idiopathic form is termed idiopathic pulmonary hemorrhage (IPH). The clinical presentation is variable; hemoptysis and anemia are some of the presenting symptoms. In pathology, three different patterns have been described—(1) associated with pulmonary capillaritis, (2) bland alveolar hemorrhage with no vasculitis, and (3) DAD-related DAH. HRCT reveals bilateral GGO/consolidation having a lobular appearance and more involvement of central parts of the lungs and peripheral sparing **(Figs. 7A and B)**. There is relative sparing of the immediate paraseptal region, causing the septae

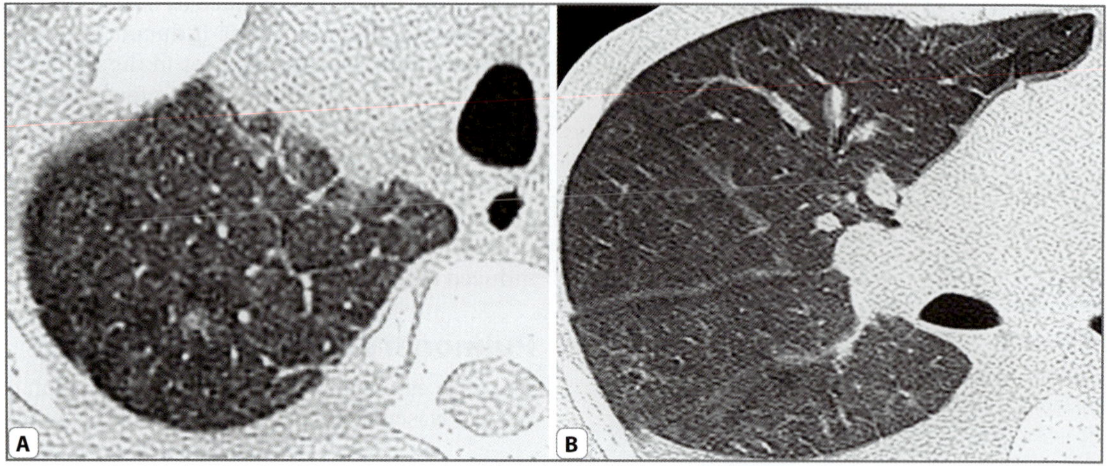

FIGS. 6A AND B: Hydrostatic pulmonary edema. High-resolution computed tomography (HRCT) images reveal smooth septal thickening, fissural thickening, and right pleural effusion.

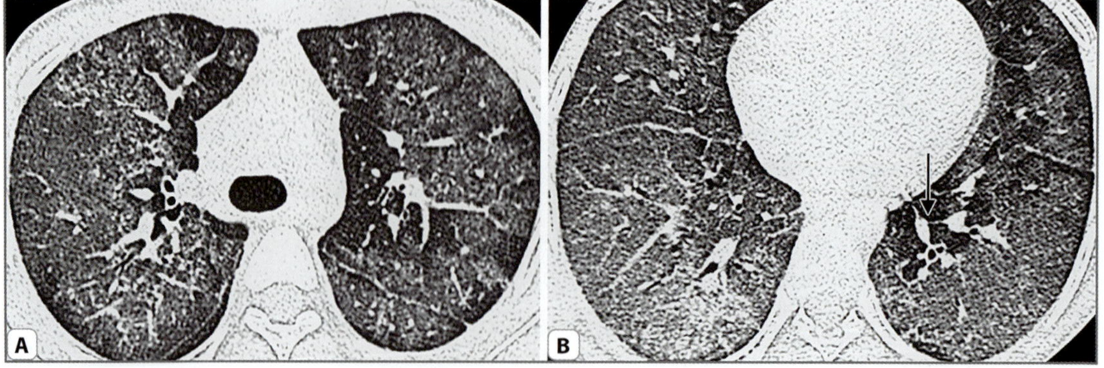

FIGS. 7A AND B: Diffuse alveolar hemorrhage in a 15-year-old male patient with anemia. HRCT images show diffuse GGO and septal thickening with sparing of lung bases and the periphery. Note the lobular sparing (black arrow).

(GGO: ground-glass opacity; HRCT: high-resolution computed tomography)

to appear lucent. In subacute phases, interlobular septal thickening may be superimposed, and fibrosis can be seen in recurrent DAH. In most cases, the pulmonary changes are reversible, except in those with DAD.

Eosinophilic Lung Disease

Eosinophilic lung disease comprises of varied disease entities, which are characterized by pulmonary manifestations and eosinophilia (peripheral or tissue eosinophilia).[10] The diagnostic criteria include eosinophilia in lung parenchyma/airway as seen on histopathology, elevated bronchoalveolar lavage (BAL) eosinophils (>10%) with or without peripheral blood eosinophilia (≥500/μL), and lung parenchymal or airway abnormalities on chest imaging.[11,12] On the basis of etiology, they can be classified as—eosinophilic lung diseases of unknown cause, eosinophilic lung diseases of known cause, and eosinophilic vasculitis. On the basis of clinical presentation, the following subtypes are described.

Acute Eosinophilic Pneumonia (Figs. 8A and B)

It presents with acute onset of fever and respiratory distress that shows immediate response to steroids. Usually, there are >25% eosinophils in BAL fluid. HRCT findings include bilateral patchy GGO and septal thickening. Ill-defined nodules and consolidation are other unusual findings.

Chronic Eosinophilic Pneumonia

The diagnosis of chronic eosinophilic pneumonia should be made after the exclusion of the secondary causes, especially helminthic infestation and drugs. It usually affects middle-aged women, is more common in asthmatics, and has an insidious onset and mild peripheral as well as BAL fluid eosinophilia. HRCT shows GGO and peripheral nonsegmental consolidation with an upper lobe predominance. The radiological distribution appears to be inverse that of pulmonary edema. It usually responds to steroids; however, it may occasionally result in fibrosis.

Idiopathic Hypereosinophilic Syndrome

In contrast, idiopathic hypereosinophilic syndrome usually affects males in their 30s and presents with multiorgan dysfunction. There is persistent eosinophilia without any demonstrable allergic or parasitic cause. HRCT shows a focal or diffuse nonlobar distribution of nodules, perinodular GGO, and patchy GGO.

Other Eosinophilic Lung Diseases

- Tropical pulmonary eosinophilia (TPE) presents with ill-defined nodules, and eosinophilic bronchitis presents with features of small airway disease **(Figs. 9A and B)**.
- Loeffler syndrome presents with transient opacities on imaging, along with peripheral eosinophilia. It is most commonly associated with *Ascaris* infestation; however, it is also seen with *Ancylostoma duodenale* (hookworm) and *Strongyloides stercoralis*.
- In visceral larva migrans, helminthic larvae may get deposited in the lung and other organs through the bloodstream and evoke an eosinophilic response. Imaging features are similar to Loeffler syndrome.
- Eosinophilic bronchitis is a form of airway disorder involving the periphery and small airways associated with BAL/peripheral eosinophilia.
- Various medications namely nonsteroidal anti-inflammatory drugs (NSAIDs), antibiotics (e.g., minocycline, nitrofurantoin), and sulfasalazine can cause eosinophilic lung disease. Inhalation of particulate

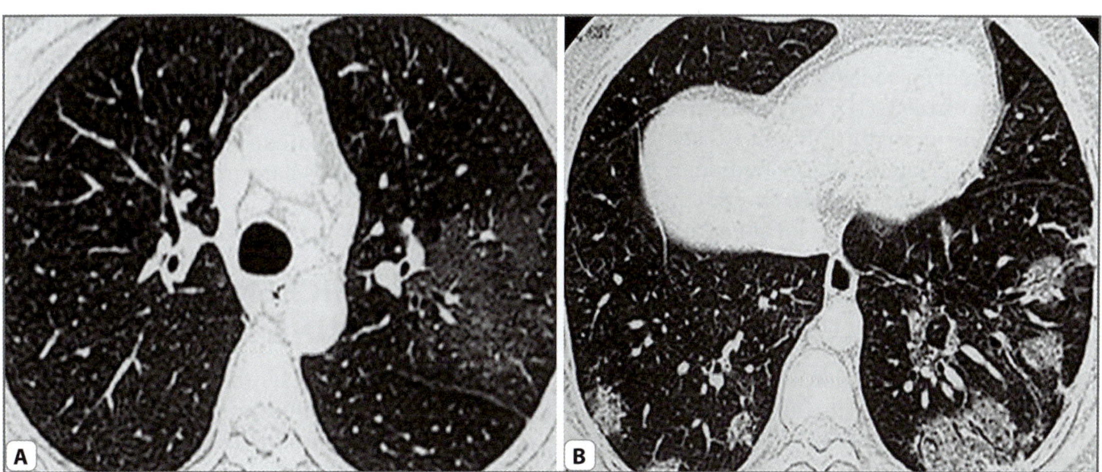

FIGS. 8A AND B: Acute eosinophilic pneumonia in a 30-year-old male with acute onset cough. High-resolution computed tomography (HRCT) images reveal bilateral peripheral ground-glass opacities.

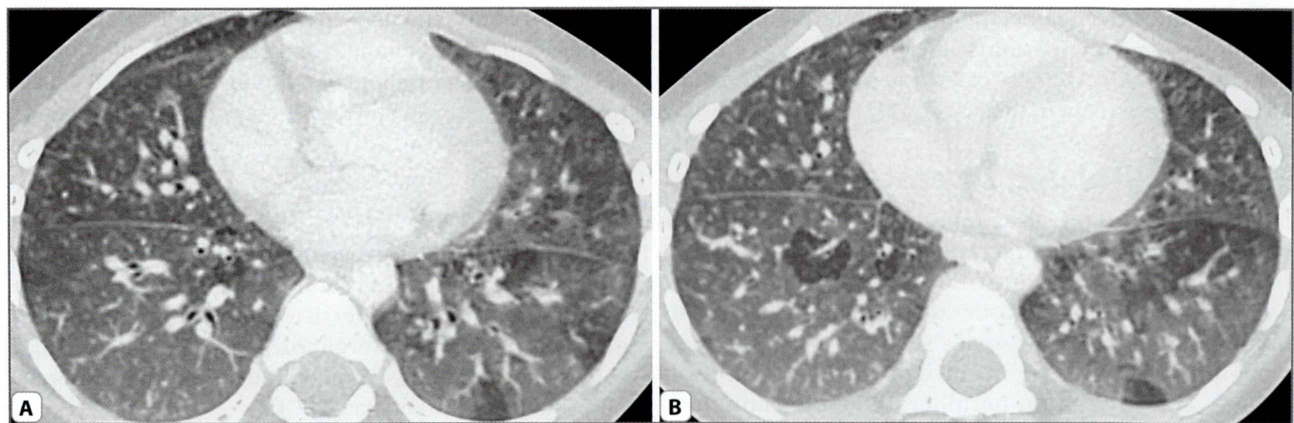

FIGS. 9A AND B: Tropical pulmonary eosinophilia. Axial computed tomography (CT) of the lungs shows multiple ill-defined centrilobular nodules in both lungs without any zonal predominance, accompanied by areas of air trapping in the lower lobes.

metals, recreational inhalational drugs (heroin, cocaine), dust exposure, and several others are also known to cause eosinophilic lung disease.

Lipoid Pneumonia

Lipoid pneumonia is characterized by the alveolar accumulation of lipids.[13,14] It can be of three main types depending on the source and presentation—(1) exogenous acute, (2) exogenous chronic, and (3) endogenous forms.

Acute Exogenous Lipoid Pneumonia

It is caused by inhalation/aspiration of large quantities of animal fats/mineral or vegetable oils. The radiological manifestations develop within 30 minutes to 24 hours. The findings include bilateral segmental or lobar GGO/consolidation, having a middle and lower lobe preponderance. Ill-defined nodules, pneumatoceles, and pleural effusions are uncommon findings.

Chronic Exogenous Lipoid Pneumonia

It is caused by recurrent episodes of aspiration/inhalation. On imaging, segmental GGO/consolidation with a peribronchovascular distribution can be seen in the lower lobes. Other associated imaging findings are septal thickening or fibrosis. Sometimes, the consolidation shows a mass-like appearance with fat attenuation within **(Figs. 10A to D)**.

Endogenous Lipid Pneumonia

It is caused by bronchial obstruction or chronic pulmonary infection causing accumulation of fat within intra-alveolar macrophages. In contrast to the exogenous form, endogenous "cholesterol pneumonia" usually does not show any fat attenuation on CT. It presents as a consolidation distal to a central obstructing lesion. The diagnosis is histopathologic.

Pulmonary Alveolar Proteinosis

Pulmonary alveolar proteinosis (PAP) is characterized by the alveolar accumulation of surfactant-like proteins.[15] It can be of three types—(1) congenital, (2) idiopathic (primary), and (3) secondary. Secondary PAP is seen in patients of hematological malignancies, dust/metal exposure, chemotherapy, or infection and responds well to treatment of the predisposing cause. Congenital form results from inherited disorders of surfactant proteins. A complete discussion of genetic disorders leading to a PAP pattern is beyond the scope of the chapter. Patients with PAP can have variable symptoms. They can either be asymptomatic or can even present with an insidious onset of dyspnea, dry cough, and easy fatigability.

A chest radiograph reveals bilateral symmetric or patchy airspace opacification. HRCT shows the "crazy-paving pattern," caused by GGO and septal thickening **(Figs. 11A and B)**.[15] The involvement of the lungs is usually patchy, with geographic/lobular sparing. Differential diagnoses include—pulmonary hemorrhage, pulmonary edema, radiation exposure, drug-induced, inhalation disorders, mucinous carcinoma, and storage disorders in children.

SEPTAL THICKENING PREDOMINANT DIFFUSE LUNG DISEASES

Uncommon DLDs presenting with septal thickening are listed in **Table 2**. Lymphangitis carcinomatosa, Kaposi sarcoma, and lymphoma are covered elsewhere in this book.

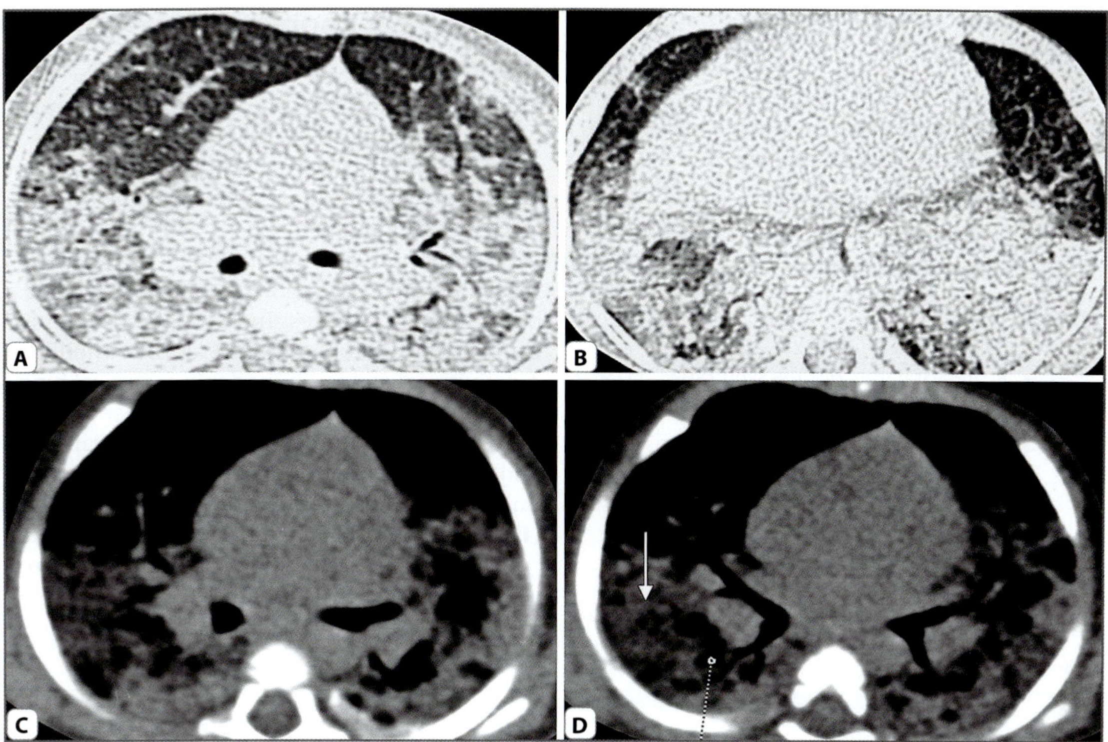

FIGS. 10A TO D: Exogenous lipoid pneumonia in a 7-year-old male child. (A and B) High-resolution computed tomography (HRCT) images reveal bilateral dense consolidation in a dependent location. (C and D) Soft-tissue window images reveal low attenuation areas within the areas of consolidation (white arrow).

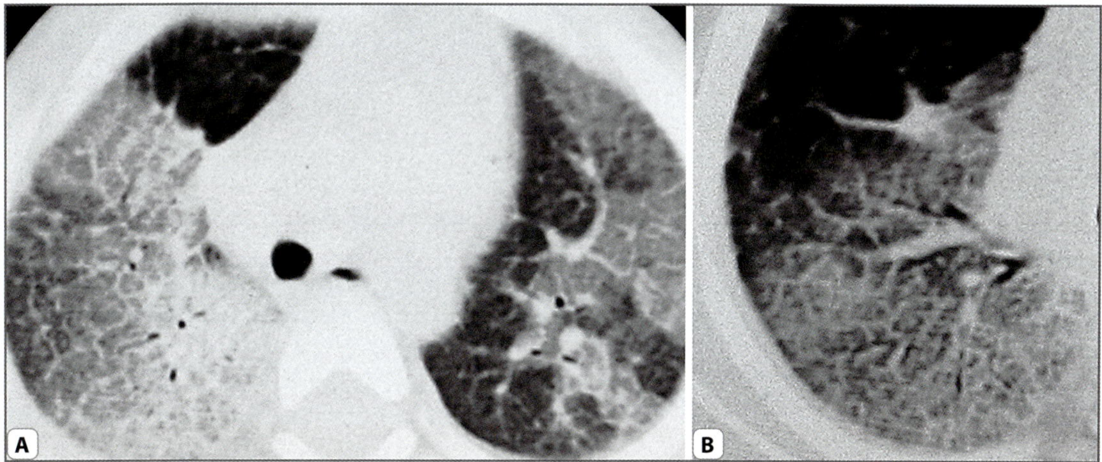

FIGS. 11A AND B: Pulmonary alveolar proteinosis pattern in storage disorder in a 6-year-old girl. Computed tomography (CT) images reveal a diffuse "crazy-paving" pattern.

Pulmonary Leukostasis

Pulmonary leukostasis is a complication observed in acute myeloid leukemia M4 (myelomonocytic type). When white blood cell count exceeds 100,000/μL, leukemic cells start accumulating within the small vessels of lungs, heart, brain, and testis and clog these small vessels. The clinical and radiographic findings are often discordant.[16,17] Chest radiograph can either be normal even in the presence of severe dyspnea or may show alveolar or interstitial opacities. CT may reveal thickened bronchovascular bundles and segmental GGOs **(Figs. 12A and B)**.

TABLE 2: Uncommon diffuse lung diseases (DLDs) with predominant septal thickening.

Infections	• Atypical pneumonia—mycoplasma • *Pneumocystis jirovecii* pneumonia (PCP) • Severe acute respiratory syndrome (SARS)
Neoplastic	• Lymphangitis carcinomatosa • Lymphoma • Pulmonary leukostasis • Kaposi sarcoma
Vascular	• Hydrostatic pulmonary edema • Acute respiratory distress syndrome (ARDS) • Pulmonary veno-occlusive disease (PVOD) • Pulmonary capillary hemangiomatosis (PCH)
Others	• Pulmonary alveolar proteinosis (PAP) • Diffuse alveolar septal amyloidosis • Diffuse alveolar hemorrhage (DAH) • Kaposiform lymphangiomatosis

Pulmonary Veno-occlusive Disease and Pulmonary Capillary Hemangiomatosis

Pulmonary veno-occlusive disease (PVOD) and pulmonary capillary hemangiomatosis (PCH) are rare disorders characterized by severe pulmonary arterial hypertension with normal pulmonary artery occlusion pressure and signs of pulmonary edema.[18-22] Although both are causes of pulmonary arterial hypertension, the pathology in PVOD lies at the postcapillary level. There is fibrous occlusion of pulmonary venules. In PCH, the problem lies at the capillary level [proliferation of alveolar capillaries (PCH)]. A definitive diagnosis is made on a surgical lung biopsy.

The clinical features of both these entities include dyspnea on exertion, chronic cough, cyanosis, syncope, and chest pain. In addition, hemoptysis is seen in PCH. The imaging findings **(Table 3)** are often quite characteristic **(Figs. 13A and B)** in an appropriate clinical setting.

Diagnosing these entities on imaging is crucial, as the administration of vasodilators on a presumptive clinical

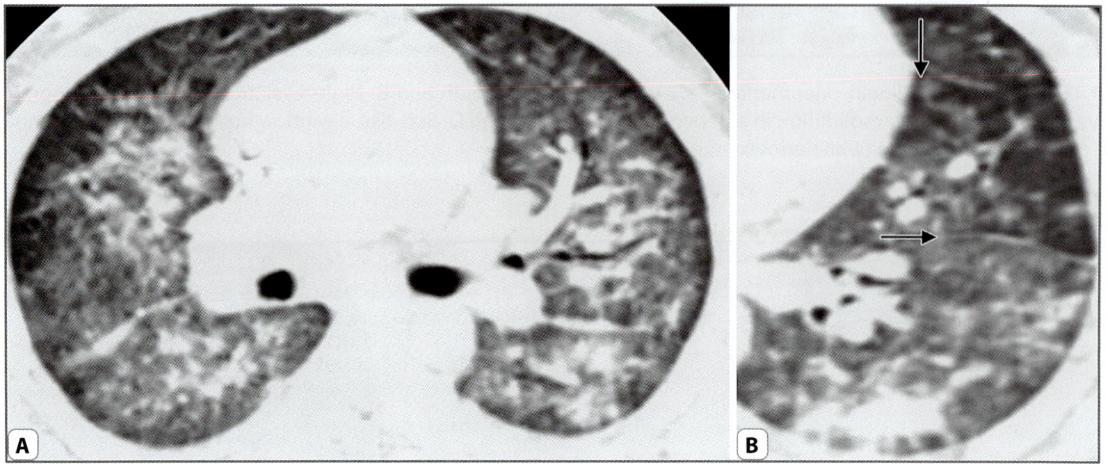

FIGS. 12A AND B: Leukostasis in a 38-year-old male patient with AML. CT reveals diffuse GGO, patchy consolidation, and smooth septal thickening (black arrows).

(AML: acute myeloid leukemia; CT: computed tomography; GGO: ground-glass opacity)

TABLE 3: Clinical and imaging findings of PVOD and PCH.

	PVOD	PCH
Gender predilection	M = F	F > M
Hemoptysis	Uncommon	Common symptom
HRCT	• Dilated main pulmonary artery • Smooth septal thickening • Patchy ground-glass opacities • Uncommon findings—multiple small nodules and consolidation in dependent lungs	• Dilated main pulmonary artery • Bilateral ill-defined ground-glass centrilobular nodules
Hemorrhagic pleural effusion	Uncommon	Common

(PCH: pulmonary capillary hemangiomatosis; PVOD: pulmonary veno-occlusive disease)

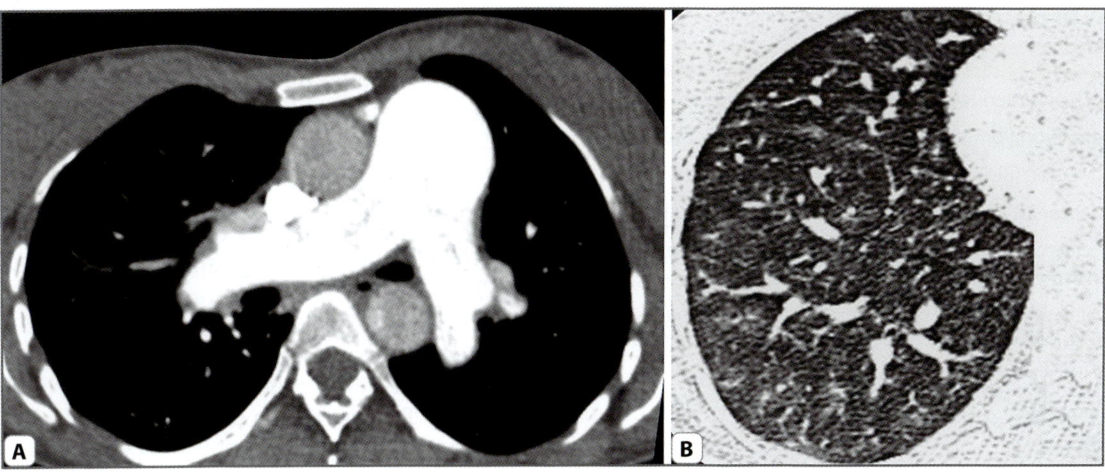

FIGS. 13A AND B: Pulmonary capillary hemangiomatosis in a 33-year-old lady with hemoptysis and PAH. (A) CT reveals a dilated main pulmonary artery. (B) HRCT image reveals diffuse ground-glass nodules in the lungs.
(CT: computed tomography: HRCT: high-resolution computed tomography; PAH: pulmonary arterial hypertension)

diagnosis of primary pulmonary hypertension can cause pulmonary edema in case of PVOD/PCH.

Pulmonary Amyloidosis

Amyloidosis is characterized by the abnormal extracellular deposition of proteins. Thoracic involvement can be localized or a part of systemic disease. Three main patterns of pulmonary involvement are described—(1) nodular parenchymal, (2) diffuse alveolar septal, and (3) airway/tracheobronchial amyloidosis.[23]

Diffuse Alveolar Septal Amyloidosis

It is usually associated with systemic involvement and presents with cough and dyspnea. The prognosis is poor, and progression to pulmonary hypertension and respiratory failure may ensue. A chest radiograph reveals well-defined small nodules and reticular opacities. HRCT findings **(Fig. 14)** include well-defined, small nodules, smooth septal thickening, bilateral basal consolidations, areas of punctate calcifications and occasional cysts, and traction bronchiectasis.

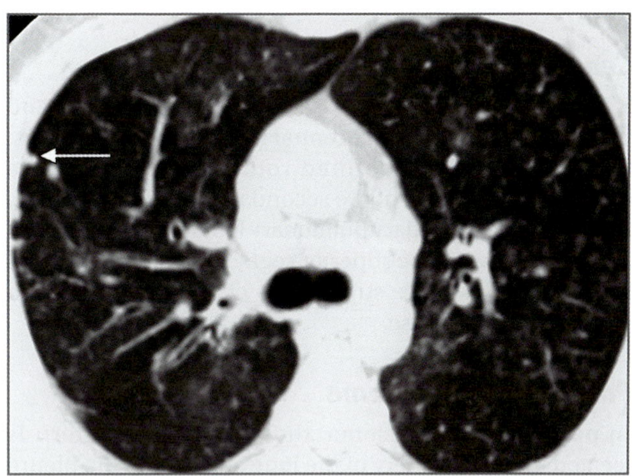

FIG. 14: Pulmonary amyloidosis. CT image reveals multiple small nodules, bronchovascular thickening, patchy GGO, and peripheral bigger and well-defined subpleural nodules (white arrow).
(CT: computed tomography; GGO: ground-glass opacity)

DIFFUSE LUNG DISEASES PRESENTING WITH NODULES

Many DLDs have a predominantly nodular pattern. These disorders have been discussed elsewhere in this book/previously in this chapter **(Table 4)**.

TABLE 4: Uncommon ILDs presenting with nodules.

Centrilobular	Random	Perilymphatic
• Viral pneumonia • *Haemophilus* • *Chlamydia* • *Mycoplasma* • PCH	Pulmonary nodular amyloidosis	• Lymphangitis carcinomatosa • LIP • Amyloidosis

(ILDs: interstitial lung diseases; LIP: lymphoid interstitial pneumonitis; PCH: pulmonary capillary hemangiomatosis)

DIFFUSE LUNG DISEASES PRESENTING WITH CYSTS

Lung cysts are defined as small air-containing lesions in the lungs. Cystic lung diseases **(Table 5)** refer to a pattern where lung cysts are the predominant finding. These need to be differentiated from honeycombing, emphysema, and cystic bronchiectasis.

TABLE 5: DLDs presenting with cysts.

Cystic DLDs	Mimics of lung cysts
Pulmonary Langerhans cell histiocytosis	Emphysema
Lymphangioleiomyomatosis (LAM)	Bronchiectasis
Birt–Hogg–Dubé (BHD) syndrome	Honeycombing
Lymphoid interstitial pneumonia (LIP)	Pneumatoceles
Cysts associated with other DLDs—LIP, DIP, PJP, and any fibrosing ILD	Postinfective cyst/ cavity

(DIP: desquamative interstitial pneumonia; DLDs: diffuse lung diseases; ILD: interstitial lung disease; PJP: *Pneumocystis jirovecii* pneumonia)

Emphysema

Emphysema is caused by permanent dilatation of the airspace distal to the terminal bronchioles with associated destruction of the alveolar wall. Three main types of emphysema are—(1) centrilobular, (2) panlobular, and (3) paraseptal.

Centrilobular Emphysema

It is the most common type, seen usually in smokers, and affects lobules around the central respiratory bronchioles. HRCT reveals well-defined round lucencies in the centrilobular portion of the secondary pulmonary lobule. Borders of the secondary pulmonary lobule are preserved.[24] Apices and lower lobe superior segments are usually more involved. CT is more superior to chest radiography in detecting early disease.

Paraseptal Emphysema

In paraseptal emphysema, the destruction pattern is located in the periphery of the lung adjacent to the pleura or along the interlobular septa. Upper lung zones are more affected. On CT, paraseptal emphysema is seen as small subpleural lucencies arranged as a single tier of "cystic" spaces. Large emphysematous bullae may be seen and can cause pneumothorax.

Panlobular Emphysema

It is associated with α1-antitrypsin deficiency. Panlobular patterns can also be seen in advanced smoking-related emphysema and emphysema related to intravenous drug abuse. It affects the whole secondary lobule and on imaging seen as a generalized diffuse decrease in CT attenuation mainly in the lower lobe.

Combined Pulmonary Fibrosis and Emphysema

Combined pulmonary fibrosis and emphysema (CPFE) is a relatively new entity, which is characterized by upper lobe emphysema and lower lobe fibrosis. On pulmonary function tests, the typical findings include preserved lung volume and severely diminished capacity of gas exchange [diffusing capacity of the lungs for carbon monoxide (DLCO)]. Smoking, connective tissue disorders, and mineral dust exposure are labeled as a few risk factors for this disease. It usually presents with symptoms of exertional dyspnea and is frequently complicated by pulmonary hypertension, ALI, and lung cancer. The prognosis is poor. This entity is defined radiographically by the presence of classic features of emphysema in the upper lobes and pulmonary fibrosis [mainly idiopathic pulmonary fibrosis/ usual interstitial pneumonia (IPF/UIP)] in the lower lobes. HRCT **(Figs. 15A to D)** shows upper lobe centrilobular and/or paraseptal emphysema with multiple bullae and lower lobe honeycombing with subpleural reticular opacities and traction bronchiectasis and sometimes GGOs.[25,26]

Pulmonary Langerhans Cell Histiocytosis

Pulmonary Langerhans cell histiocytosis (LCH)[27,28] is the preferred term for isolated pulmonary involvement; it occurs most commonly in young adult smokers. The clinical features include dyspnea, nonproductive cough, fatigue, chest pain, weight loss, or spontaneous pneumothorax. In children, pulmonary LCH is usually seen as a part of multisystem involvement.

Imaging

A chest radiograph reveals bilateral diffuse symmetrical reticulonodular opacities, which are predominantly distributed in upper zones. The lung volume is usually preserved. Small irregular-shaped nodules are seen in early disease; which later on cavitate and result in pneumothorax.

Computed tomography findings **(Figs. 16A to C)** depend on the stage of the disease. In early disease, multiple small (1–10 mm in size), irregular-shaped nodules are seen. They have distribution in centrilobular, peribronchial, and peribronchiolar locations. The nodules can cavitate. Cystic pattern dominates in the later stage. These cysts are irregular, small (1–3 cm), and sometimes bizarre shaped. Nodules and cysts are usually seen in the upper/mid-lung zone. The cysts can rupture and produce spontaneous pneumothorax (in 10–15%). When LCH is confined to the lungs, the prognosis is good.

Lymphangioleiomyomatosis

Lymphangioleiomyomatosis (LAM) is a disorder caused by abnormal smooth muscle and lymphatic proliferation. It can present either as a sporadic form or a syndromic

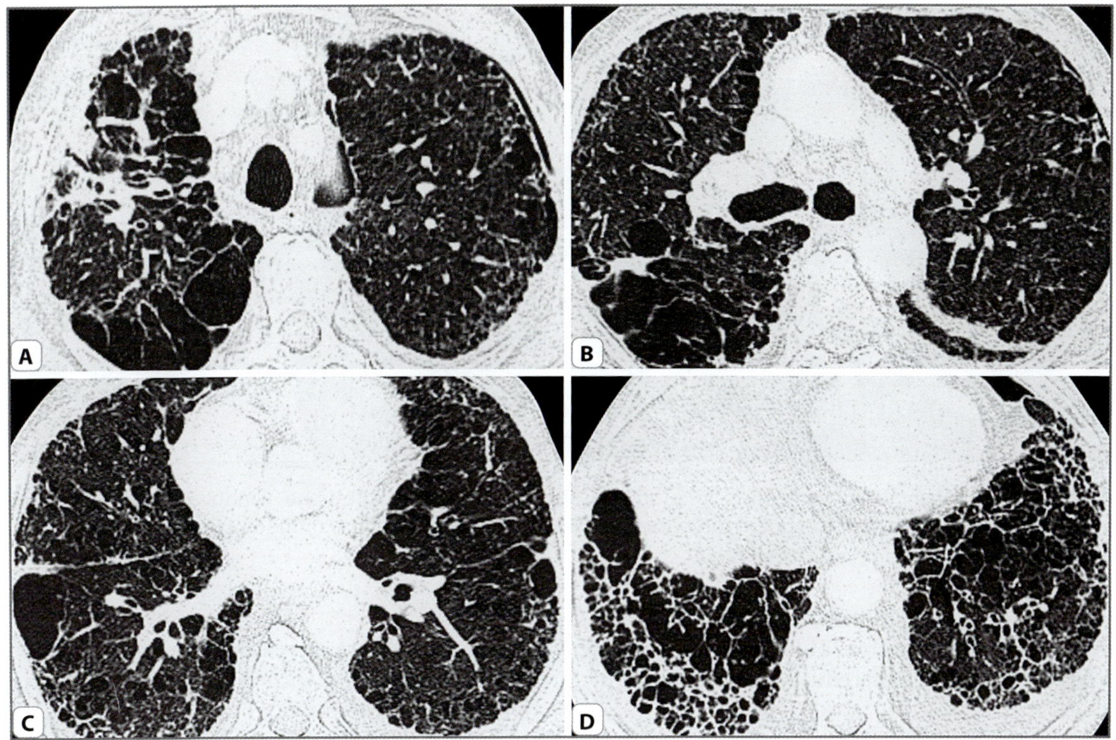

FIGS. 15A TO D: Combined pulmonary fibrosis and emphysema. High-resolution computed tomography (HRCT) images reveal upper lobe centrilobular and/or paraseptal emphysema and lower lobe honeycombing with subpleural reticular opacities.

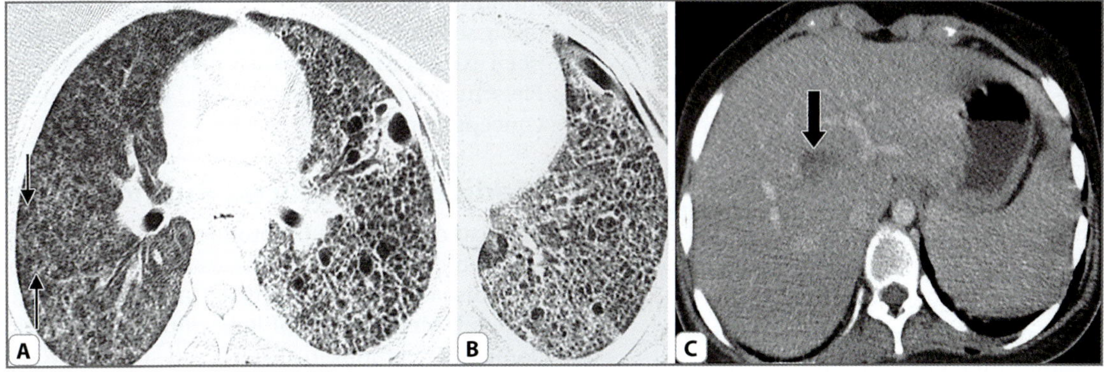

FIGS. 16A TO C: Langerhans cell histiocytosis in a 16-year-old girl. (A and B) High-resolution computed tomography (HRCT) images reveal multiple irregular parenchymal nodules (black arrows) in the right lung and multiple cysts in the left lung. Note the left-sided pneumothorax. (C) Soft-tissue image reveals a focal, small hypodense liver lesion (block arrow).

form (associated with tuberous sclerosis). In proven cases of tuberous sclerosis, about 30–40% of patients can have LAM. Patients of tuberous sclerosis with LAM may not have the classical imaging triad of tuberous sclerosis (epilepsy, mental retardation, and adenoma sebaceum). The sporadic form of LAM is more common than the syndromic form and is seen almost exclusively in women of childbearing age. Syndromic LAM can affect both males and females, although incidence is higher in females.

The pulmonary imaging findings of sporadic and syndromic LAM are similar. Chest radiographs may reveal bilateral reticular shadows with preserved lung volumes. HRCT **(Figs. 17A and B)** shows the presence of thin-walled cysts uniformly distributed in the lungs and chylous pleural effusion. The parenchymal cysts are usually thin-walled (<2 mm in size), uniform in size, and randomly distributed without zonal predominance. The intervening lung parenchyma is usually normal. Rupture of cysts may cause pneumothorax; recurrence of

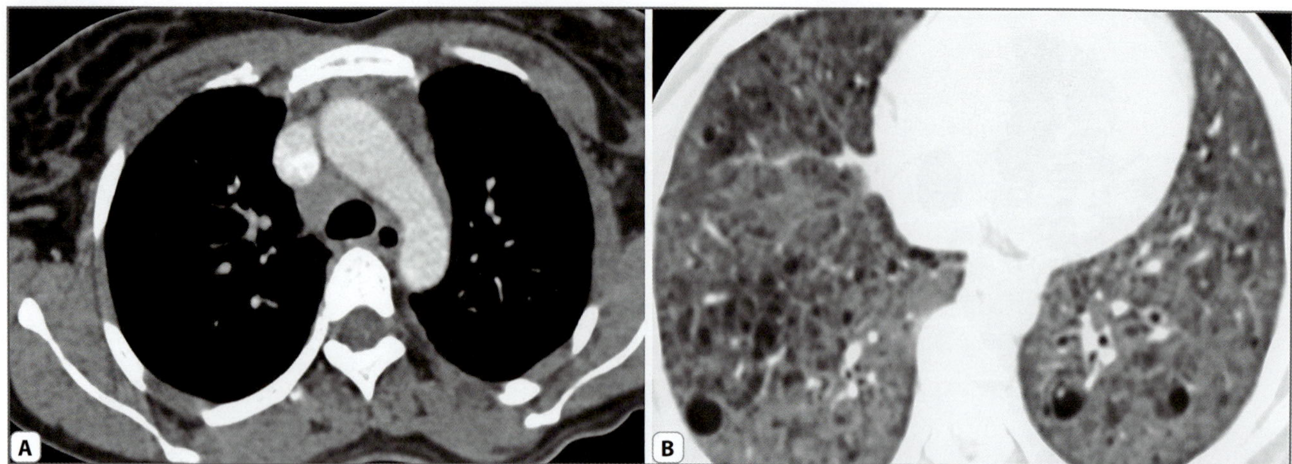

FIGS. 17A AND B: Lymphangioleiomyomatosis in a 30-year-old lady. (A) Axial soft-tissue window image reveals mediastinal lymphadenopathy. (B) High-resolution computed tomography (HRCT) image reveals diffuse ground-glass opacities in both lungs, with scattered thin-walled cysts.

pneumothorax is quite common. Hilar and mediastinal lymphadenopathy and pericardial effusion are other imaging findings.

Langerhans cell histiocytosis cysts are more irregular and bizarre shaped; intervening lungs are often abnormal, and systemic manifestations are commonly associated with pediatric LCH. LAM is a disease, which is characterized by the proliferation of peribronchovascular smooth muscle, causing air trapping and subsequent development of cysts.

Tuberous Sclerosis-associated Lymphangioleiomyomatosis

Tuberous sclerosis is a genetic disorder having an autosomal dominant inheritance. It affects multiple systems, and the classic triad comprises epilepsy, mental retardation, and facial angiofibroma (adenoma sebaceum). While the disease equally affects men and women, pulmonary involvement is more commonly observed in females.

High-resolution computed tomography findings of tuberous sclerosis are similar to those of LAM. Multiple uniformly distributed cysts and a few small nodules (multifocal micronodular pneumocyte hyperplasia) may be seen. Chylous pleural effusions are usually not seen in tuberous sclerosis compared to LAM.

Birt–Hogg–Dubé Syndrome

Birt-Hogg-Dubé (BHD) syndrome is a multisystem disease[29,30] caused by a deletion mutation on the *FLCN* gene (chromosome 17). The disease affects multiple organ systems; abnormalities include cutaneous angiofibromas, perifollicular fibromas, acrochordons, fibrofolliculomas, and renal masses. On imaging, multiple lung cysts are seen, along with multiple bilateral renal tumors (renal cell carcinoma, oncocytoma), multiple lung cysts and secondary spontaneous pneumothorax. CT reveals multiple small cysts **(Figs. 18A to D)** located in lower zones and subpleural location. The cysts may be septated when they become large.

Lymphoid interstitial pneumonia (LIP) and desquamative interstitial pneumonia (DIP) have been discussed in the idiopathic ILD chapter. Although they have been excluded in the glossary of terminology in the revised Fleischner Society Guidelines 2024, they are discussed for conceptual understanding.

Medication-induced Pulmonary Injury

Medication-induced pulmonary injury (MIPI) is a broad terminology that encompasses drug-induced interstitial lung disease (DILD) and drug-induced pulmonary toxic effects.[31] Mechanisms of lung injury include direct DNA damage, alterations in alveolar cell signaling that enhance apoptosis or suppress cell proliferation, and T-cell-mediated immunologic injury.

The diagnostic criteria include newly identified pulmonary parenchymal opacities at imaging, temporal association of presentation with the initiation of a systemic therapeutic agent, and the exclusion of other likely causes.[32,33]

The Pneumotox website (https://www.pneumotox.com) offers a comprehensive overview of respiratory disorders caused by medications. It serves as a guide for understanding and managing drug-related lung conditions. **Table 6** enlists a few common drugs associated with MIPI.

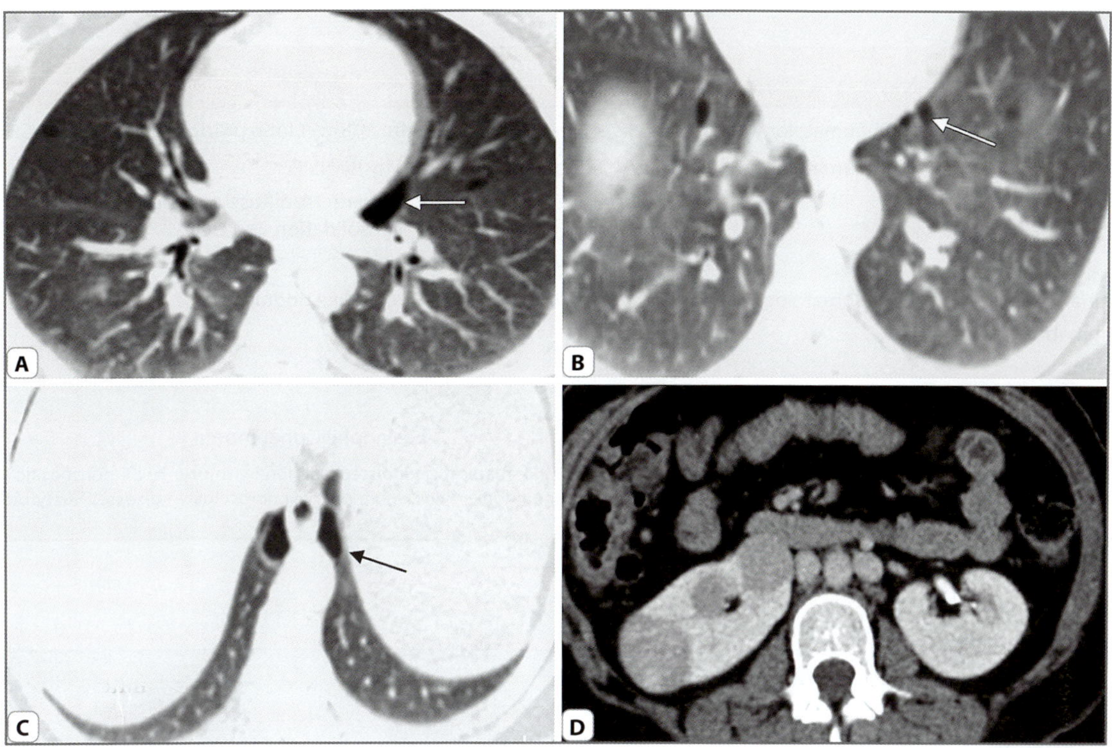

FIGS. 18A TO D: Birt–Hogg–Dubé syndrome in a 39-year-old lady. Note the thin-walled cysts in subpleural locations (black arrow and white arrows) and multiple solid-enhancing right renal masses.

TABLE 6: Common drugs associated with medication induced pulmonary injury (Figs. 19 and 20).

Name of the drugs	Used in	Onset of pulmonary complications	Imaging pattern
Bleomycin	Oncology	10 weeks to 2 years	• Lung base • Acute eosinophilic pneumonia and diffuse alveolar damage **(Figs. 19A to C)** • Chronic fibrotic/OP pattern
Busulfan	Oncology	3–4 years	Lower lobes—OP/NSIP/DAD
Cyclophosphamide	Oncology	1–6 months	Diffuse OP/NSIP
• TKI • Imatinib • Gefitinib • Erlotinib • Afatinib	Oncology	• 4–8 weeks • 10–282 days	• Nonspecific area with ground-glass opacity (GGO) • Multifocal area of airspace consolidations. Patchy distribution of GGO accompanied by interlobular septal thickening
• mTOR inhibitors • Everolimus • Tacrolimus	Oncology	• 12–24 weeks • Median time to onset of 56 days	Cryptogenic organizing pneumonia (COP)—multifocal areas of airspace consolidation—subpleural, peribronchial, or band-like pattern, NSIP
Gemcitabine **(Figs. 20A to D)**	Oncology	3 days to 2 months	Acute capillary leak, pulmonary edema, and PVOD
Amiodarone	Rheumatology	6–12 months	Asymmetric centrilobular nodules and asymmetrical areas of dense GGOs with few consolidations—eosinophilic pneumonia
Hydralazine	Rheumatology	3 months to 1 year	Interstitial lung disease and pulmonary hemorrhage (hydralazine-induced vasculitis)

Continued

Continued

Name of the drugs	Used in	Onset of pulmonary complications	Imaging pattern
Methotrexate	Rheumatology	1–4 weeks	Diffuse/lower lobe predominant GGOs/NSIP
Rituximab	Rheumatology	• Hours < 24 hours to weeks • 0–158 days • Mean—2–4 weeks	• Mostly NSIP • OP pattern/diffuse or patchy bilateral consolidation and GGO
• TNF-alpha • Adalimumab • Etanercept • Infliximab	Rheumatology	1 month to years	Sarcoid-like nodules
NSAID	Rheumatology	1–2 weeks	Eosinophilic pneumonia

(DAD: diffuse alveolar damage; mTOR: mammalian target of rapamycin; MIPI: medication-induced pulmonary injury; NSIP: nonspecific interstitial pneumonia; NSAID: nonsteroidal anti-inflammatory drug; OP: organizing pneumonia; PVOD: pulmonary veno-occlusive disease; TKI: tyrosine kinase inhibitor; TNF-alpha: tumor necrosis factor-alpha)

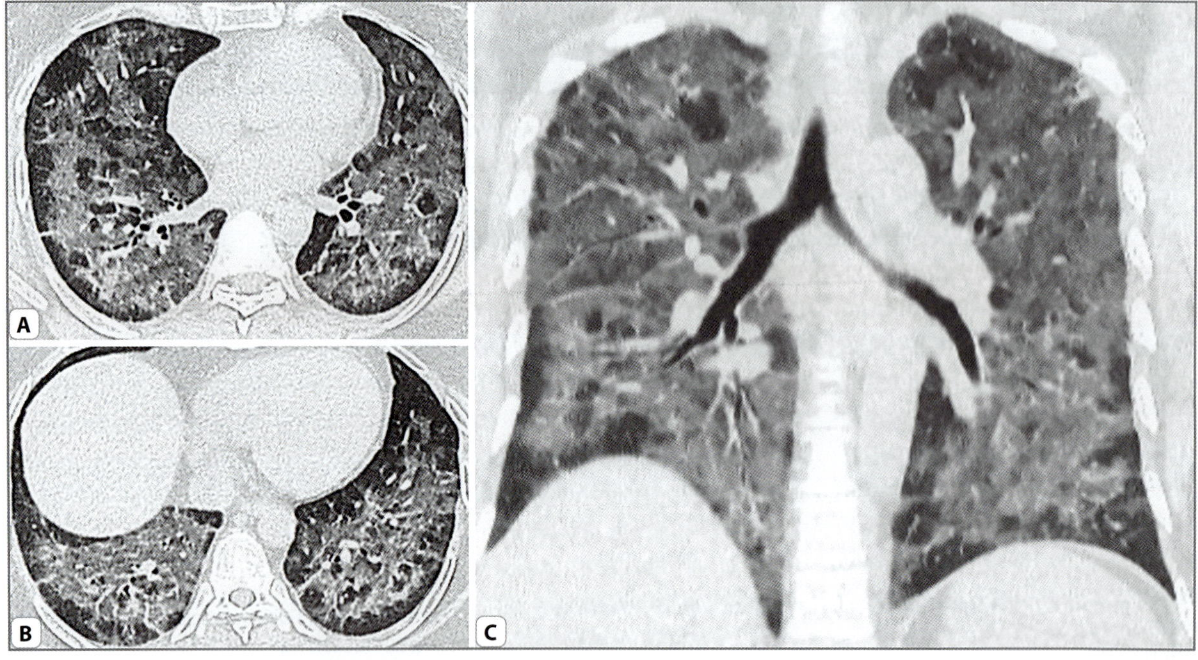

FIGS. 19A TO C: Acute bleomycin-induced lung damage in a patient of Hodgkin lymphoma. (A and B) Axial HRCT lung images show diffuse GGO and occasional septal thickening, sparing extreme lung periphery. (C) Coronal MPR image shows uniform apicobasal distribution.

(GGO: ground-glass opacity; HRCT: high-resolution computed tomography; MPR: multiplanar reconstruction)

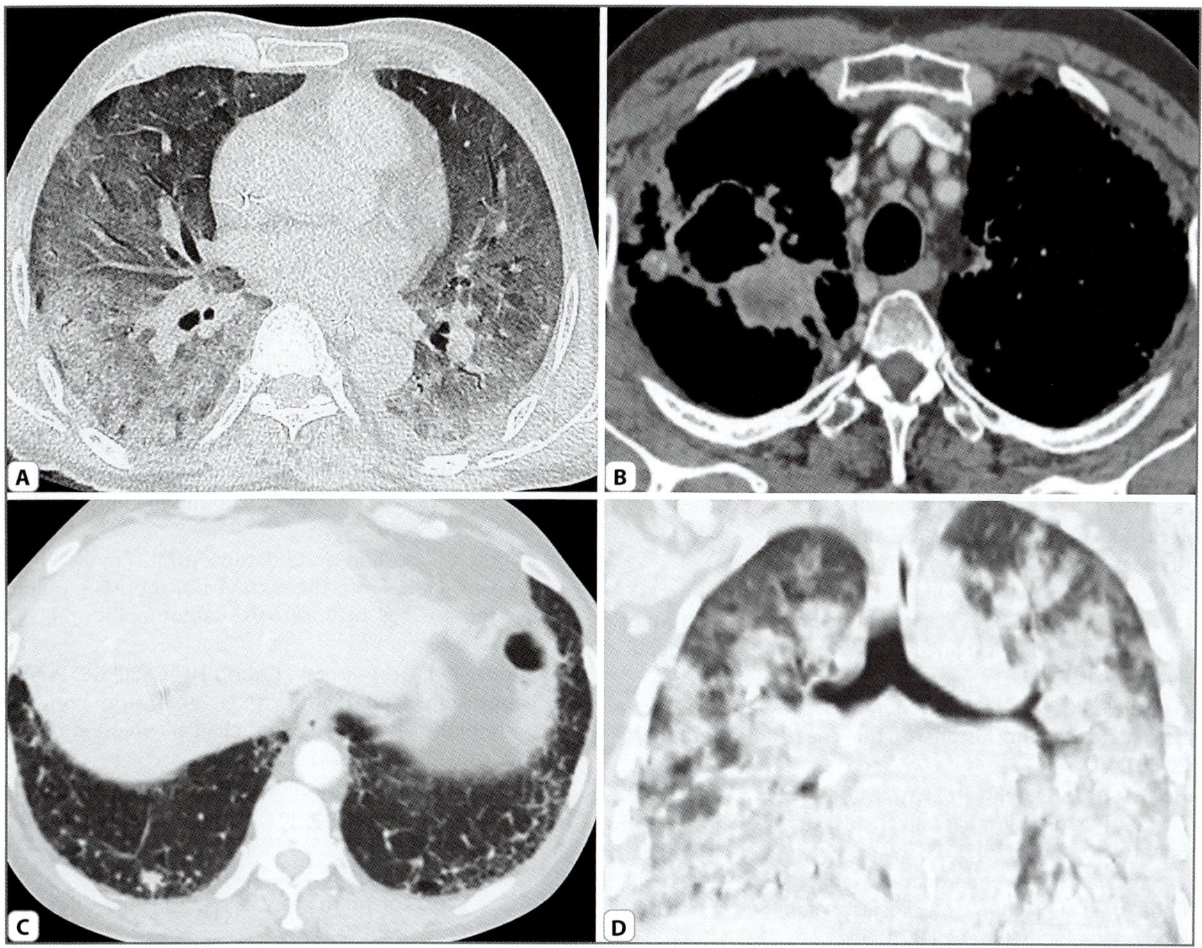

FIGS. 20A TO D: Spectrum of drug-induced lung changes. (A) Gemcitabine-induced acute lung toxicity in a 70-year-old male is seen as nonspecific areas of ground-glass opacities in both lung fields. (B and C) Another patient with carcinoma of lung of the right upper lobe developed chronic ILD changes with NSIP pattern in lung bases sequel to same drug therapy. (D) Differentiation syndrome/all-trans retinoic acid (ATRA) toxicity in a young female with acute promyelocytic leukemia on day 3 of initiation of therapy seen as bilateral confluent airspace opacities predominantly in central lungs.

(ILD: interstitial lung disease; NSIP: nonspecific interstitial pneumonia)

CONCLUSION

Diffuse lung disease is a complex disease with various etiologies, sometimes without any identifiable cause. While reaching a precise diagnosis, it requires a team effort and a combination of clinical, laboratory, and radiological findings; the adoption of a pattern approach on HRCT can help the radiologist to narrow down the differential diagnoses.

REFERENCES

1. Franquet T. Imaging of pulmonary viral pneumonia. Radiology. 2011;260:1.
2. Kim EA, Lee KS, Primack SL, Yoon HK, Byun HS, Kim TS, et al. Viral pneumonias in adults: radiologic and pathologic findings. Radiographics. 2002;22(Spec Issue):S137-49.
3. Koo HJ, Choi SH, Sung H, Choe J, Do KH. Radiographics update: radiographic and CT features of viral pneumonia. Radiographics. 2020;40(4):E8-15.
4. Yu M, Xu D, Lan L, Tu M , Liao R, Cai S, et al. Thin-section chest ct imaging of COVID-19 pneumonia: a comparison between patients with mild and severe disease. Radiol Cardiothorac Imaging. 2020;2(2):e200027.
5. Shirani F, Shayganfar A, Hajiahmadi S. COVID-19 pneumonia: a pictorial review of CT findings and differential diagnosis. Egypt J Radiol Nucl Med. 2021;52(1):38.

6. Prokop M, Everdingen WV, Vellinga TVR, Ufford HQV, Stöger L, Beenen L, et al. CO-RADS: a categorical ct assessment scheme for patients suspected of having COVID-19—definition and evaluation. Radiology. 2020;296(2):E97-104.
7. Chiumello D, Froio S, Bouhemad B, Camporota L, Coppola S. Clinical review: lung imaging in acute respiratory distress syndrome patients—an update. Crit Care. 2013;17(6):R243.
8. Ashbaugh DG, Bigelow DB, Petty TL, Levine BE. Acute respiratory distress in adults. Lancet. 1967;2:319-23.
9. Pnimack SL, Miller RR, Nestor L. Diffuse pulmonary hemorrhage: clinical, pathologic, and imaging features. AJR Am J Roentgenol. 1995;164(2):295-300.
10. Jeong YJ, Kim KI, Seo IJ, Lee CH, Lee KN, Kim KN, et al. Eosinophilic lung diseases: a clinical, radiologic, and pathologic overview. Radiographics. 2007;27(3):617-39.
11. De Giacomi F, Vassallo R, Yi ES, Ryu JH. Acute eosinophilic pneumonia. Causes, diagnosis, and management. Am J Respir Crit Care Med. 2018;197(6):728-36.
12. Fernández-Pérez ER, Olson AL, Frankel SK. Eosinophilic lung diseases. Med Clin North Am. 2011;95(6):1163-87.
13. Betancourt SL, Martinez-Jimenez S, Rossi SE, Truong MT, Carrillo J, Erasmus JJ, et al. Lipoid pneumonia: spectrum of clinical and radiologic manifestations. AJR Am J Roentgenol. 2010;194(1):103-9.
14. Gaerte SC, Meyer CA, Winer-Muram HT, Tarver RD, Conces DJ. Fat-containing lesions of the chest. Radiographics. 2002;22:S61-78.
15. Holbert MJ, Costello P, Li W, Hoffman RM, Rogers RM. CT features of pulmonary alveolar proteinosis. AJR Am J Roentgenol. 2001;176(5):1287-94.
16. Van Buchem MA, Wondergem JH, Kool LJ, Velde J, Kluin PM, Bode PJ, et al. Pulmonary leukostasis: radiologic-pathologic study. Radiology. 1987;165(3):739-41.
17. Tanaka N, Matsumoto T, Miura G, Emoto T, Matsunaga N. HRCT findings of chest complications in patients with leukemia. Eur Radiol. 2002;12(6):1512-22.
18. Frazier AA, Franks TJ, Mohammed TL, Ozbudak IH, Galvin JR. Pulmonary veno-occlusive disease and pulmonary capillary hemangiomatosis. Radiographics. 2007;27(3):867-82.
19. Mandel J, Mark EJ, Hales CA. Pulmonary veno-occlusive disease. Am J Respir Crit Care Med. 2000;162:1964-73.
20. Ito K, Ichiki T, Ohi K, Egashira K, Ohta M, Taguchi K, et al. Pulmonary capillary hemangiomatosis with severe pulmonary hypertension. Circ J. 2003;67(9):793-5.
21. Masur Y, Remberger K, Hoefer M. Pulmonary capillary hemangiomatosis as a rare cause of pulmonary hypertension. Pathol Res Pract. 1996;192:290-5.
22. Dufour B, Maitre S, Humbert M, Capron F, Simonneau G, Musset D. High-resolution CT of the chest in four patients with pulmonary capillary hemangiomatosis or pulmonary veno-occlusive disease. AJR Am J Roentgenol. 1998;171(5):1321-4.
23. Czeyda-Pommersheim F, Hwang M, Chen SS, Strollo D, Fuhrman C, Bhalla S, et al. Amyloidosis: modern cross-sectional imaging. Radiographics. 2015;35(5):1381-92.
24. Washko GR, Hunninghake GM, Fernandez IE, Nishino M, Okajima Y, Yamashiro T, et al. Lung volumes and emphysema in smokers with interstitial lung abnormalities. N Engl J Med. 2011;364(10):897-906.
25. Lin H, Jiang S. Combined pulmonary fibrosis and emphysema (CPFE): an entity different from emphysema or pulmonary fibrosis alone. J Thorac Dis. 2015;7(4):767-79.
26. Cottin V, Nunes H, Brillet PY, Delaval P, Devouassoux G, Tillie-Leblond I, et al. Combined pulmonary fibrosis and emphysema: a distinct underrecognised entity. Eur Respir J. 2005;26(4):586-93.
27. Abbott GF, Rosado-de-Christenson ML, Franks TJ, Frazier AA, Galvin JR. From the archives of the AFIP: pulmonary Langerhans cell histiocytosis. Radiographics. 2004;24(3):821-41.
28. Sundar KM, Gosselin MV, Chung HL, Cahill BC. Pulmonary Langerhans cell histiocytosis: emerging concepts in pathobiology, radiology, and clinical evolution of disease. Chest. 2003;123(5):1673-83.
29. Agarwal PP, Gross BH, Holloway BJ, Seely J, Stark P, Kazerooni EA. Thoracic CT findings in Birt-Higg-Dubé syndrome. Am J Roentgenol. 2011;196(2):349-52.
30. Souza CA, Finley R, Müller NL. Birt-Hogg-Dubé syndrome: a rare cause of pulmonary cysts. AJR Am J Roentgenol. 2005;185:1237-9.
31. Sridhar S, Kanne JP, Henry TS, Revels JW, Gotway MB, Ketai LH. Medication-induced pulmonary injury: a scenario- and pattern-based approach to a perplexing problem. Radiographics. 2022;42(1):38-55.
32. Johkoh T, Lee KS, Nishino M, Travis WD, Ryu JH, Lee HY, et al. Chest CT diagnosis and clinical management of drug-related pneumonitis in patients receiving molecular targeting agents and immune checkpoint inhibitors: a position paper from the Fleischner Society. Radiology. 2021;298(3):550-66.
33. Dhamija E, Meena P, Ramalingam V, Sahoo R, Rastogi S, Thulkar S. Chemotherapy-induced pulmonary complications in cancer: significance of clinicoradiological correlation. Indian J Radiol Imaging. 2020;30(1):20-6.

Ankur Goyal, Ankita Aggarwal, Raju Sharma

CHAPTER

11

Imaging Approach to Mediastinal Pathology

INTRODUCTION

The mediastinum is a complex anatomical space in the central part of the thorax, surrounded by lungs on either side. It extends from the thoracic inlet to the diaphragm and contains all the major vital structures of the chest. Many classification systems divide the mediastinum into various compartments to narrow down the list of differential diagnoses, based on their location and morphology. Chest radiograph is the first screening modality, whereas contrast-enhanced computed tomography (CECT) is the imaging modality of choice for the characterization and extent delineation of mediastinal masses. Ultrasound and magnetic resonance imaging (MRI) are problem-solving tools and prove useful in certain cases. This chapter highlights the salient features of various diseases, which affect the mediastinum.

COMPARTMENTS OF THE MEDIASTINUM

Various classification systems have been described to divide the mediastinum into various compartments, thus aiding in the identification, categorization, and management of the pathologies. In principle, these systems divide the mediastinum into three compartments anteroposteriorly or a separate fourth compartment superiorly. It may be noted that these are not anatomically distinct compartments, since there is no demarcation between them, and, thus, these classifications serve only as a guide for proposing the differential diagnoses.

Shields classification system is the most commonly used system in the clinical practice. This system is more relevant to surgeons and divides the mediastinum into anterior, visceral, and paravertebral sulcus compartments. The traditional systems used in radiology literature are Fraser and Paré, Felson, Heitzman, Zylak, and Whitten models.

Felson's classification is the most commonly used system for mediastinal masses on a lateral chest radiograph. Felson divided the mediastinum into anterior, middle, and posterior compartments **(Fig. 1)**. Two lines are drawn on the lateral radiograph: First line along the anterior wall of trachea extending along the posterior margin of the heart and the second line 1.0 cm posterior to the anterior vertebral margins. Any mass situated between the sternum and the first line is said to be in the anterior mediastinum, between the two lines in the middle mediastinum and posterior to the second line in the posterior mediastinum.

The Japanese Association for Research on the Thymus (JART) model given by Fujimoto et al. in 2014 proposed a

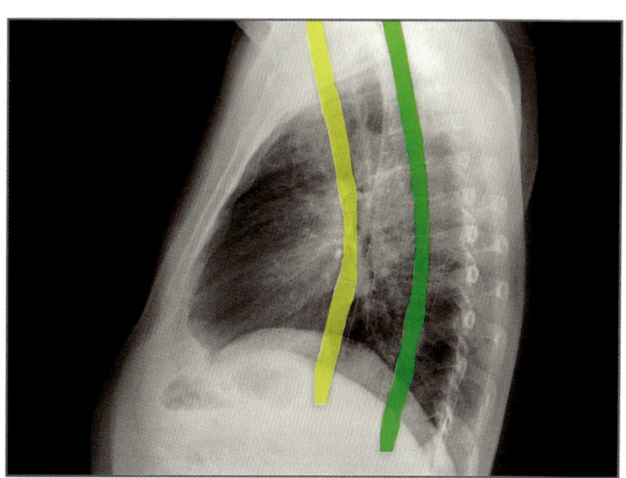

FIG. 1: Mediastinal compartments on lateral chest radiograph. The lateral chest radiograph shows the two lines drawn to divide the mediastinum into compartments, as per Felson classification. The first line is drawn along the anterior border of trachea to back of the heart extending to the diaphragm and a second line joining a point 1.0 cm behind the anterior margin of the dorsal vertebrae. Space anterior to first line is anterior mediastinum, between first and second is middle and posterior to second line is posterior mediastinum.

CT-based classification of the mediastinum and divided it into four compartments: (1) superior, (2) anterior, (3) middle, and (4) posterior. The boundaries are discussed in **Table 1**.[1]

The most commonly used classification system currently used in cross-sectional imaging was given by the International Thymic Malignancy Interest Group (ITMIG) in 2017. This is based on the modification of the JART model and currently the standard of practice. ITMIG classification divides the mediastinum into three compartments: (1) prevascular (anterior), (2) visceral (middle), and (3) paravertebral (posterior) **(Table 2)**.[2]

TABLE 1: JART classification of the mediastinum.

	Superior mediastinum	Anterior mediastinum (prevascular zone)	Middle mediastinum (peritracheoesophageal zone)	Posterior mediastinum (paravertebral zone)
Superiorly	Thoracic inlet	Inferior boundary of the superior portion of the mediastinum	Inferior boundary of the superior portion of the mediastinum	Inferior boundary of the superior portion of the mediastinum
Inferiorly	Horizontal plane at the junction of the inferior margin of the LBCV with the trachea	Diaphragm	Diaphragm	Diaphragm
Anteriorly		Posterior cortex of the sternum	Posterior margin of the LBCV, SVC, ascending aorta, bilateral main pulmonary arteries, and heart	M-PBL
Posteriorly	Anterior margin of the thoracic vertebral body	Pericardium, anterior margins of the LBCV, SVC, RSPV, LSPV, RIPV, LIPV, ascending aorta, and lateral margin of the aortic arch	Anterior margin of the descending aorta and M-PBL	
Laterally	Posterolaterally vertical line against the posterior margin of the chest wall at the lateral margin of the thoracic vertebral process	Parietal (mediastinal) pleural reflections, ITAV, RSPV, LSPV, RIPV, and LIPV		Posterolaterally vertical line against the posterior margin of the chest wall at the lateral rim of the thoracic vertebral process

Note: M-PBL is a vertical line connecting a point 1.0 cm posterior to the anterior vertebral margin.

(ITAV: internal thoracic artery and vein; JART: Japanese Association for Research on the Thymus; LBCV: left brachiocephalic vein; LIPV: left inferior pulmonary vein; LSPV: left superior pulmonary vein; M-PBL: middle-posterior boundary line; RIPV: right inferior pulmonary vein; RSPV: right superior pulmonary vein; SVC: superior vena cava)

TABLE 2: ITMIG classification of the mediastinum.

	Prevascular	Visceral	Paravertebral
Superiorly	Thoracic inlet	Thoracic inlet	Thoracic inlet
Inferiorly	Diaphragm	Diaphragm	Diaphragm
Anteriorly	Posterior cortex of the sternum	Posterior boundaries of the prevascular compartment	Posterior boundaries of the visceral compartment
Posteriorly	Anterior aspect of the pericardium as it wraps around the heart in a curvilinear fashion	Vertical line connecting a point on each thoracic vertebral body 1.0 cm posterior to its anterior margin	Vertical line against the posterior margin of the chest wall at the lateral margin of the transverse process of the thoracic spine
Laterally	The parietal mediastinal pleura	The parietal mediastinal pleura	Parietal mediastinal pleura
Contents	Thymus, fat, lymph nodes, and left brachiocephalic vein	• Nonvascular: Trachea, carina, esophagus, and lymph nodes • Vascular: Heart, ascending aorta, aortic arch, descending thoracic aorta, SVC, intrapericardial pulmonary arteries, and thoracic duct	Thoracic spine and paravertebral soft tissues

(ITMIG: International Thymic Malignancy Interest Group; SVC: superior vena cava)

IMAGING MODALITIES

Radiograph

Chest radiograph is the first imaging modality used for screening any chest pathology. Both frontal posteroanterior (PA) and lateral views are utilized for the assessment of mediastinal pathologies. Various signs have been described on a chest radiograph that help in the localization of mediastinal masses. The majority of these were first described by Benjamin Felson.

Silhouette Sign

As described by Felson, an intrathoracic opacity, which is in anatomical contact with a border of the heart, aorta, or diaphragm, will obscure its margin. The two prerequisites for this sign are that the two masses should be in direct contact with each other, and that they should be of the same density on the radiograph.

Any mass, which obliterates the right heart border or the right border of ascending aorta, is in the anterior mediastinum **(Fig. 2)** or is located in the right middle lobe. In contrast, if the radiopacity overlaps but does not obliterate the right heart border or the right border of the ascending aorta, it is likely to be in the posterior mediastinum. Similarly, an opacity obliterating the left border of the aortic knob is likely to be in the posterior mediastinum. Similarly, obscuration of left heart border suggests the mass to be in the anterior mediastinum or in the lingular segments.

Hilum Overlay Sign

If the hilar vessels are seen through the mass, then mass is placed either anteriorly or posteriorly to the "real" hilum.

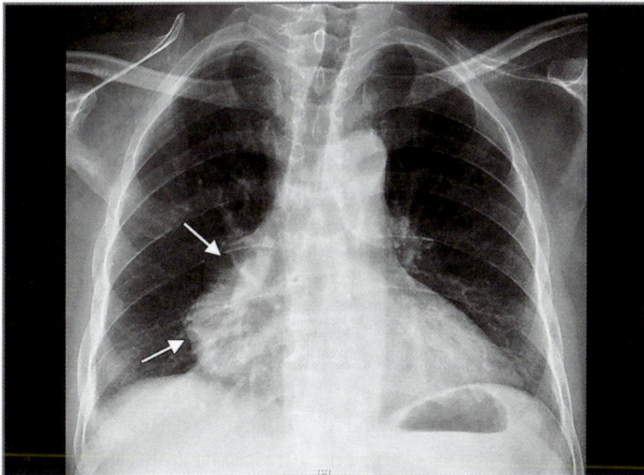

FIG. 2: Silhouette sign. Chest radiograph (PA view) showing a homogeneous mass in the right hemithorax (arrows) with broad base toward the mediastinum and silhouetting the right cardiac margin suggesting anterior mediastinal mass. Hilum can be seen through the mass.

However, if the hilar vessels are not seen separately, then the mass is hilar vessels in location. Originally, this was described as that if the hilar vessels are seen >1 cm within the lateral edge of the mediastinal silhouette, then the lesion is not cardiac; rather, it is anterior or posterior to the hilum.

Hilum Convergence Sign

If the pulmonary vessels are seen to converge the mass, then it signifies that the mass is hilar/pulmonary arterial in origin. However, if the hilar vessels are seen to be converging to the hilum rather than the mass, then it is a perihilar mediastinal mass and not an enlarged pulmonary artery.

Cervicothoracic Sign

If a thoracic mass is in continuity with the soft tissues of the neck, it will lose its contiguous border. The superior border of an anterior mediastinal mass ends at the level of the clavicles, whereas that of the posterior mediastinal mass extends beyond that. Hence, a mass, which is distinctly seen above the clavicle, with clearly defined lateral border, is in the posterior mediastinum and entirely within the thorax. On the other hand, if the superior border of the mass is obscured at the level of the clavicle, it is in the anterior mediastinum extending to neck, and cervicothoracic sign in these cases will be positive.

Thoracoabdominal sign is positive when the inferior border of the mass is not sharp and divergent toward the diaphragm signifying its extension into the abdominal cavity from the intrathoracic location. A completely intrathoracic mass will have a sharp inferior margin and convergent borders.

Sometimes the mediastinal mass may be small and suspected on the basis of thickening of the anterior junctional line. The problem is that the latter may be identified only on about 20% of the normal chest radiographs.[3]

Mediastinal versus Pulmonary Mass

The distinction between mediastinal and pulmonary mass starts from the chest radiograph. A mass, which is sharply marginated, broad-based toward mediastinum (obtuse-angled), extends to both sides of midline is more likely to be mediastinal than pulmonary.

Consolidation in the adjacent lung, poorly-defined margins, and air bronchogram within the mass are pointers toward a pulmonary mass. A mass causing destruction of the spine, sternum, or rib is likely to be extrapulmonary. If a mass is based toward the chest wall (broad-based obtuse-angled), again it is likely to be extrapulmonary.

Mediastinal widening is inferred when the width of the mediastinum is >8 cm or more than a third of the transthoracic width on PA radiograph at the level of carina. Various causes of mediastinal widening are mediastinal hematoma, aortic dissection, aortic aneurysm, or mediastinal tumors. Right paratracheal stripe is the region to the right of trachea, measuring ~4 mm. The most common cause of its widening is lymphadenopathy. Mediastinal mass containing gas can be an esophageal diverticulum, dilated esophagus (e.g., achalasia), hernia, mediastinal abscess, or complicated duplication cyst.

Lateral chest radiograph can add useful information over the frontal radiograph; however, it is underutilized because of increased reliance on computed tomography (CT). Obliteration of retrosternal space and masses overlying the upper dorsal spine are better depicted on lateral radiographs.

Fluoroscopy

In earlier days, fluoroscopy was also utilized for distinguishing the mediastinal from lung mass. A pulmonary mass would move along lung bronchovascular markings with respiration, whereas a mediastinal mass is unlikely to move.

Another utility of fluoroscopy is in the determination of phrenic nerve palsy due to a mediastinal mass. Elevated hemidiaphragm with lack of mobility on respiration on fluoroscopy/ultrasound suggests phrenic nerve palsy. Eventration may also show similar findings but usually shows mild excursion (compared to no excursion in palsy). Presence of paradoxical diaphragmatic movement is more in favor of phrenic nerve palsy. Sniff test may be done to better assess diaphragmatic mobility.

Barium Swallow

Barium swallow is not the primary imaging modality for mediastinal masses. It is done for patients presenting with complaints of dysphagia. Displacement of the esophagus can give indirect evidence of presence of a mediastinal mass. Also, it is useful in the detection of masses arising from the esophagus.

Computed Tomography Scan

According to the American College of Radiology (ACR) appropriateness criteria, CECT scan is the diagnostic imaging modality for mediastinal masses.[4] It is also appropriate as an initial investigation instead of chest radiograph in case of clinically suspected mediastinal mass. The categorization of the mediastinal mass can be aptly done on the CT scan based on various classification systems, ITMIG being the most commonly used system. Lesion characterization, whether cystic or solid, content characterization as fat, calcification, soft tissue, enhancement pattern, etc., can be very aptly done with CT scan. It is a safe, easy, relatively cheaper, and fast modality with easy access. CT is mostly done for presurgical mapping of the lesion, as it can correctly determine the fat planes with various vital vascular structures. Also, multiplanar reformats help in the excellent depiction of the masses in relation to various mediastinal structures, which helps the surgeon in planning the resection. At last, a CT scan can be utilized for guiding biopsies of mediastinal masses.

Magnetic Resonance Imaging

Due to its inherent excellent soft-tissue resolution, the characterization of mediastinal masses can also be done with MRI. It can detect even microscopic (intravoxel) fat and can differentiate hemorrhage from proteinaceous contents. It can confirm the cystic nature of masses, which appear hyperdense on CT and avoid unnecessary biopsies. Diffusion-weighted MRI along with postcontrast sequences can help determine the grade of various tumors, such as thymic masses, and also assist in determining the biopsy site in case of hemorrhage within the mass. According to ACR appropriateness criteria, both CT and MRI with or without contrast are appropriate for definite diagnosis of mediastinal lesions. In a resource-limited nation such as India, it is not possible to offer MRI in all cases; hence, for all practical purposes, MRI is used as a problem-solving tool when there is a diagnostic dilemma on CECT or it is a posterior mediastinal mass to look for spinal/neural foraminal extension. Another use is of "cine MRI" in which multiple sequential acquisitions are done in free breathing to determine the adherence of the mediastinal mass to the adjacent vascular structures[4] **(Box 1)**.

Ultrasonography/Endoscopic Ultrasound/Endobronchial Ultrasound

There is little utility of ultrasound in the detection of mediastinal masses. Only when the mass is in close approximation to the chest wall, it can be visualized with ultrasound. Endoscopic ultrasound (EUS) offers a way to evaluate masses from the esophagus, while endobronchial ultrasound (EBUS) is for lesions abutting the trachea.

Positron Emission Tomography

Fluorine-18-2-fluoro-2-deoxy-D-glucose (FDG)-positron emission tomography (PET)/CT does not offer much utility in the primary diagnosis of mediastinal mass. The only exception is mediastinal lymphoma, where it is always done for primary staging and surveillance. It is often done to rule out distant metastases and response assessment postsurgery/chemotherapy. At times, PET is

BOX 1: Indications of MRI in mediastinal masses.

- Solid versus cystic (in case of hypodense lesions not showing fluid attenuation on CT)
- Detection of intravoxel fat (thymic neoplasm vs. hyperplasia)
- Esophageal leiomyoma versus duplication cyst
- Evaluate neural foraminal and intraspinal extension
- Cine MR to determine adherence to mediastinal vascular structures
- Noncontrast MR is better where contrast administration is not feasible on CT

(CT: computed tomography; MRI: magnetic resonance imaging)

done to determine benign versus malignant masses. If it is negative, the mass has a high likelihood of being benign; however, if positive, it may or may not be malignant. It also shows some promise in determining the aggressiveness in thymic tumors based on the standardized uptake value (SUV) values.[4]

MEDIASTINAL MASSES

Anterior Mediastinum

Thymus

Thymus is a bilobed, encapsulated soft-tissue structure seen in prevascular location in young individuals having prime function of T-cell maturation in childhood. In children, thymus is a homogeneous soft tissue, isodense to muscle on CT, and located anterior to the proximal aortic arch and the superior vena cava (SVC). Up to 5 years of age, it is quadrilateral in shape with convex margins. After that, it gradually becomes smaller, becoming more triangular in shape with straight edges. By 15 years, it should have straight or concave margins, assume triangular configuration, and start having heterogeneous attenuation due to fatty replacement.[5] It is completely replaced by fat after the age of 40 years **(Figs. 3A to C)**.

Normal thymus on pediatric chest radiograph has to be differentiated from a mediastinal mass. Thymic opacity projects from the upper mediastinum, mostly bilateral (can be unilateral on right), produces a triangular sail shadow, has sharp inferior border, and will shrink with deep inspiration.[6] Because of the anterior placement of the thymus, it may have the impressions of the osteocartilaginous junctions, giving a wavy margin, called the thymic wave sign. This sign will not be present in the thymic tumors as they are firm and not soft such as the thymus tissue. Thymus starts to involute by 1–3 years of age and is not appreciated on the radiograph after the age of 5–8 years.

Thymic Hyperplasia

Thymic hyperplasia refers to the enlargement of the thymic tissue that is uniform and maintains the normal bilobed triangular shape. Presence of homogeneous soft tissue in the location of the thymus after the age of 15 years suggests thymic hyperplasia. The presence of convex contours after the age of 15 years is also abnormal; so, it is soft-tissue thickness >13 mm after the age of 20 years.

This can be of two types. True thymic hyperplasia occurs as a response to chemo-/radiotherapy or steroid administration or after a stressful event such as a burn injury. It is also called rebound hyperplasia. There should be an increase in the thymic tissue by >50% from the baseline. Lymphoid thymic hyperplasia is seen in immunological diseases such as myasthenia gravis, human immunodeficiency virus (HIV), hyperthyroidism, and collagen vascular diseases. There is proliferation of lymphoid follicles on histopathology. On imaging, this can be suggested on the basis of increase in the thymic soft tissue with preserved triangular shape. Imaging is unable to make the distinction between the two types of hyperplasia, though few articles say that attenuation >40 Hounsfield unit (HU) suggests lymphoid hyperplasia.

Thymic Neoplasms

Thymoma is the most common tumor of the anterior mediastinum in adults, usually occurring after the age of 40 years. They are most commonly situated in the location of normal thymus; however, they are rarely can be seen in posterior mediastinum or neck.[7,8] They are slow-growing tumors with the potential of local extension into the adjoining serosal surfaces such as the pleura or pericardium. Metastasis, however, is rare. Thymomas are usually seen in patients of myasthenia gravis, pure red cell aplasia, Diamond–Blackfan syndrome, hypogammaglobulinemia, or aplastic anemia. They are usually detected due to the compression or invasion of the adjoining thoracic structures

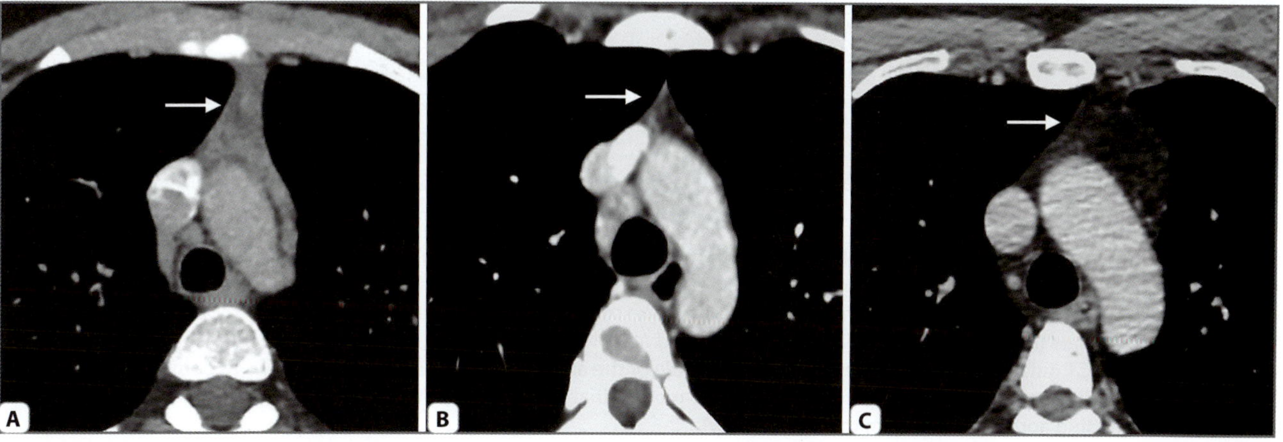

FIGS. 11.3A TO C: Normal appearance of the thymus at different ages. Triangular configuration of normal thymus (arrow) at age 15 years (A), 35 years (B), 50 years (C). There is progressive atrophy and replacement of the soft tissue with fat attenuation.

or incidentally while being scanned for other pathologies or due to the associated systemic paraneoplastic syndromes.

On chest radiograph, thymomas appear as a smooth, well-marginated, ovoid, or lobulated mediastinal mass projecting on one or sometimes both sides of the mediastinum.[9] At times, they are large and extend from the thoracic inlet to the cardiophrenic angle, whereas at times, they are small with very subtle changes on the chest radiograph.

Thymoma appears as a well-defined lobulated anterior mediastinal mass on CT, mostly showing homogeneous enhancement after contrast injection. At times, they can be heterogeneous with presence of necrosis, hemorrhage, and calcification **(Figs. 4A to F)**. Thymoma is said to be cystic when there is a large cystic component in the mass **(Figs. 5A to D)**. The role of CT is mainly in identifying the local invasion and helps in the presurgical mapping of the tumor. Masaoka–Koga (MK) staging system is used for staging the thymoma on surgery and histopathology of the excised specimen[10] **(Table 3)**. This serves as a prognostic indicator as well as a predictor of tumor recurrence.

The updated World Health Organization (WHO) classification for thymic tumors (5th edition) is shown in **Table 4**, in which thymoma has been subdivided based on histopathology.[11] Tumor-node-metastasis (TNM) staging of thymoma is given in **Table 5**.[12]

It is important for the radiologist to differentiate thymoma from thymic hyperplasia. While hyperplasia is characterized by the preservation of triangular shape, thymoma shows convex contours and is usually a well-demarcated soft-tissue lesion. CT-based texture analysis is also useful in making this distinction. Besides, it can also differentiate low from high WHO grade and low from high Masaoka–Koga/ITMIG stage.[13] MRI may prove to be helpful in indeterminate cases on CT scan. Detection of intralesional intravoxel fat is suggestive of thymic hyperplasia over thymoma **(Figs. 6A and B)**. Chemical shift imaging will show drop in signal in opposed phase images in thymic hyperplasia whereas in thymic tumors, no drop in signal is noted. This can be objectively calculated by chemical shift ratio (CSR) as described below:

$$CSR = (\text{thymic } SI_{opp}/\text{muscle } SI_{opp})/(\text{thymic } SI_{in}/\text{muscle } SI_{in})$$

where, CSR: chemical shift ratio; in: in phase; opp: opposed phase; SI: signal intensity.

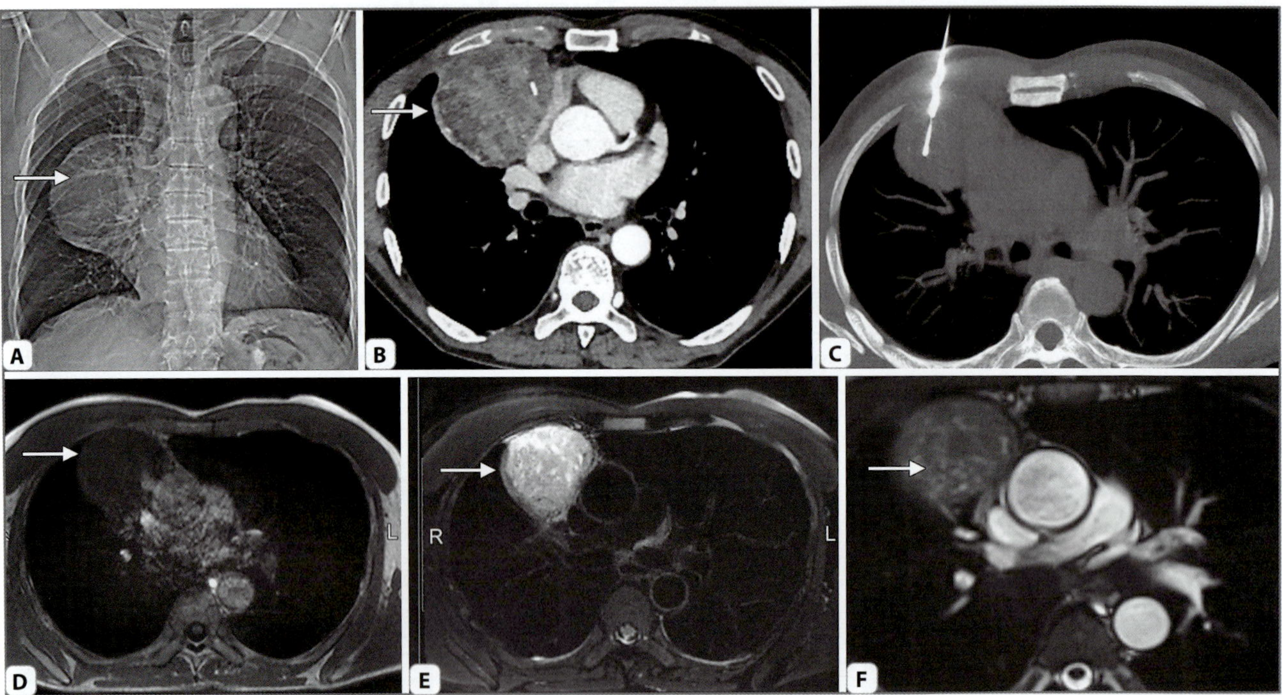

FIGS. 4A TO F: Thymoma in a 45-year-old male patient with myasthenia gravis. Topogram of chest CT (A) showing well circumscribed mediastinum-based mass (arrow) projecting on the right side. Contrast enhanced (CE) CT (B) showing a well defined heterogeneously enhancing mass (arrow) anterior to the heart with focus of calcification suggestive of thymoma. There was >3 cm contact and indentation of the cardiac chambers (suggesting pericardial involvement) and abutment of ascending aorta. Maximum intensity image (MIP) axial CT image (C) shows CT guided biopsy using semiautomatic needle of the anterior mediastinal mass (D) shows hypointense signal while T2W (D) image shows heterogeneously hyperintense anterior mediastinal mass (arrow). Axial BTFE cine image (F) showed preserved pulsations of ascending aorta separate from the mass (arrow).

(BTFE: balanced turbo field echo; CT: computed tomography; MRI: magnetic resonance imaging; T1W: T1-weighted; T2W: T2-weighted)

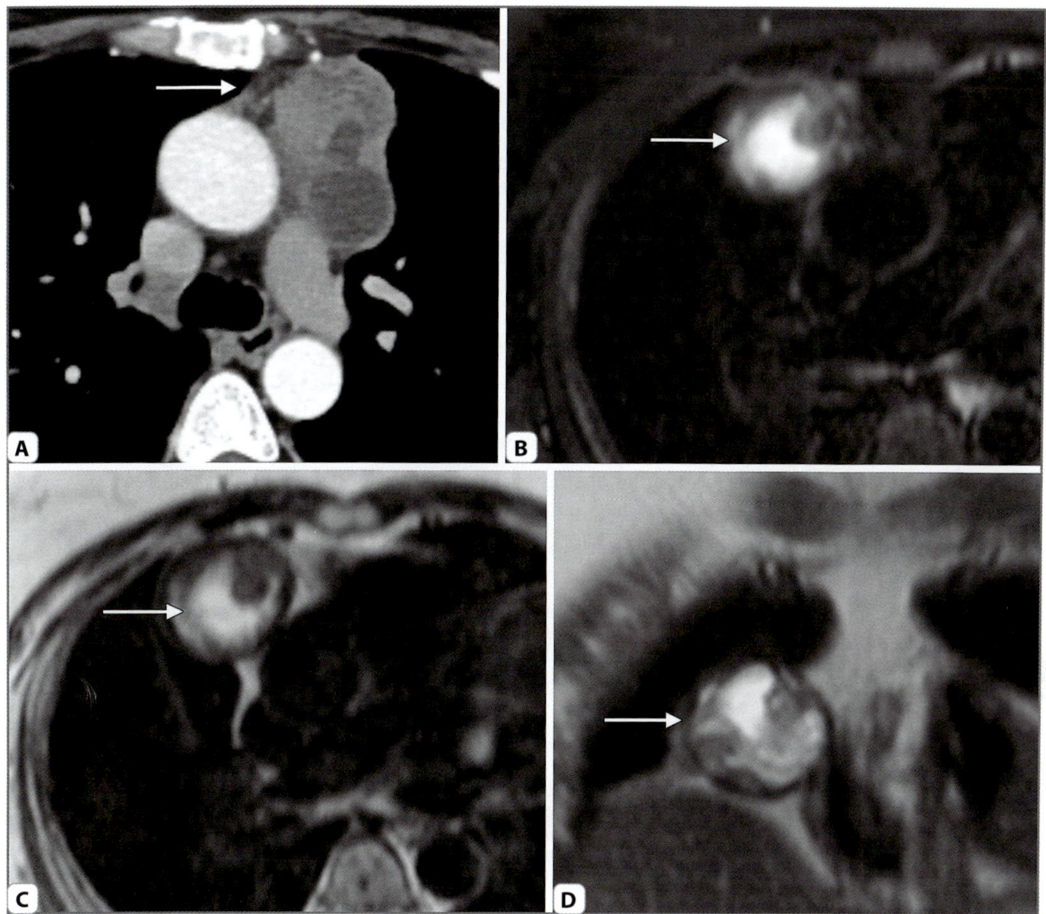

FIGS. 5A TO D: Cystic thymoma. CECT image (A) shows heterogeneous mass (arrow) with low density areas (suggesting necrosis) in anterior mediastinal mass on the left side. MRI of another case: Axial T2 FS (B), axial T2W (C), coronal T2W (D) images show cystic morphology with thick wall and mural nodule in anterior mediastinal mass (arrow) anterior to ascending aorta on the right side, suggesting cystic thymoma.

(CECT: contrast-enhanced computed tomography; MRI: magnetic resonance imaging; T2 FS: T2-weighted fat-saturated; T2W: T2 weighted)

TABLE 3: Masaoka–Koga staging system of thymoma.

Stage I	Encapsulated tumor
Stage IIa	Microscopic invasion into surrounding fatty tissue or mediastinal pleura
Stage IIb	Macroscopic invasion through the capsule into surrounding fatty tissue or mediastinal pleura
Stage III	Macroscopic invasion into a neighboring organ (pericardium, great vessels, or lung)
Stage IVa	Pleural or pericardial dissemination
Stage IVb	Lymphogenous or hematogenous metastatic disease

Stages III and IV patients are given neoadjuvant therapy, whereas stages I and II can directly go for surgical management

The proposed cutoff as per the literature is 0.849, with values lower than this suggesting thymic hyperplasia.[14]

Thymoma is said to be invasive when there is extension beyond the fibrous capsule into adjacent mediastinal structures, pleura or the chest wall **(Figs. 7A to D)**. On imaging, invasive thymoma is suggested when the margins are ill-defined, lobulated, irregular interface with the lung, internal necrosis/multifocal calcification, and presence of pleural nodularity or phrenic nerve palsy.[15]

Thallium 201 nuclear scan can also be used to differentiate normal thymus, hyperplastic thymus, and thymoma in patients with myasthenia gravis.[16] Indium-111 octreotide can also show uptake in thymoma.[17]

TABLE 4: WHO classification of thymoma.[11]

Types	Pathologic classification	Prognosis
Type A thymoma	Spindle and oval epithelial cells showing strong expression of epithelial markers and lack necrosis, have low Ki-67 index and absence of immature TdT-positive T cells	Excellent prognosis
Type AB thymoma	Lobulated growth pattern with mixture of spindle cell, predominant lymphocyte-poor component and lymphocyte-rich component with ≥10% area showing moderate infiltrate of TdT-positive T cells	Moderate prognosis
Type B1 thymoma	Dispersed, nonclustered thymic epithelial cells among densely packed lymphocytes; TdT-positive immature T cells interspersed with TdT-negative nodular (medullary) areas	Moderate prognosis
Type B2 thymoma	Abundance of lymphocytes with clusters of neoplastic epithelial cells stain for keratin and/or p40/p63	Moderate prognosis
Type B3 thymoma	Sheets of mildly/moderately atypical, polygonal tumor cells with interspersed perivascular spaces and paucity of lymphocytes	Poor prognosis
Micronodular thymoma with lymphoid stroma	Multiple small discrete nodules of epithelial cells with abundant epithelial cell-free lymphoid stroma (predominant CD20 positive)	
Metaplastic thymoma	Biphasic thymic tumor; anastomosing islands of polygonal epithelial cells, which may show variable nuclear atypia with background of bland-looking spindly cells	
Lipofibroadenoma	A benign thymic tumor resembling fibroadenoma of the breast with a predominance of fibrous tissue over adipocytes and delicate strands of epithelial cells	

(TdT: terminal deoxynucleotidyl transferase; WHO: World Health Organization)

TABLE 5: TNM staging of thymic tumors.[12]

T component	
T1a	Encapsulated without extension into mediastinal fat
T1b	Extends into mediastinal fat
T2	Direct invasion into pericardium
T3	Direct invasion of lung, chest wall, phrenic nerve, brachiocephalic vein, superior vena cava, and hilar vessels
T4	Direct invasion into trachea, esophagus, myocardium, MPA, aorta, and arch vessels
N component	
N0	No nodal involvement
N1	Involvement of perithymic nodes
N2	Involvement of intrathoracic or cervical nodes
M component	
M0	No metastasis
M1a	Separate pleural or pericardial nodule
M1b	Lung or distant organ metastasis
Stage group	
I	T1N0M0
II	T2N0M0
IIIa	T3N0M0
IIIb	T4N0M0
IVa	Any T, N1, M0 to any T, N0, N1, M1a
IVb	Any T, N2, M0, M1a to any T, any N, M1b

(MPA: main pulmonary artery; TNM: tumor-node-metastasis)

Thymic carcinoma is a rare malignancy with incidence varying between 0.07 and 0.38/100,000 per year.[18] They are suspected when the mass is large, infiltrative, heterogeneous, and locally invasive, with associated lymphadenopathy or has distant metastasis. Common sites of metastases include pleura and mediastinal nodes.

Thymolipomas are benign, fat-containing lesions with an average content of fat ranging from 50 to 95%. They are lobulated, usually large (even up to 20 cm), and seen to extend up to the cardiophrenic angle. They may have variable degrees of soft-tissue attenuation and intervening septations.[19,20] They lack a capsule and do not produce mass effect despite their large size **(Figs. 8A and B)**.

Thymic carcinoids (neuroendocrine tumor) are rare and may be suspected based on the presence of intensely enhancing lesions in the region of thymus **(Figs. 9A to C)**. These may present with endocrine abnormalities such as Cushing syndrome or syndrome of inappropriate secretion of antidiuretic hormone.

Uncommonly, pure cystic lesions may also be seen in the thymic location called thymic cyst. These are benign lesions detected incidentally.[21] On imaging, they are of water attenuation on CT and follow the fluid signal characteristics on MRI [hypointense on T1-weighted (T1W) and hyperintense on T2-weighted (T2W) images] **(Figs. 10A and B)**. They are thin-walled lesions, which can be unilocular or multilocular, with peripheral curvilinear calcification. They may be hyperdense when there is hemorrhage or superadded infection.

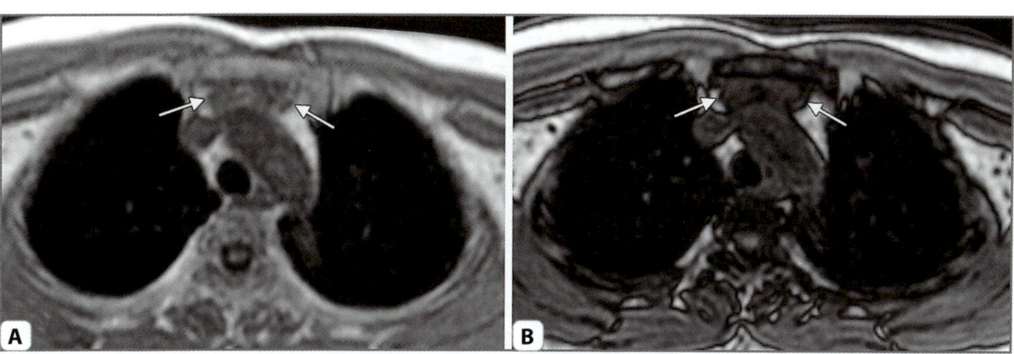

FIGS. 6A AND B: Chemical-shift MRI in thymic hyperplasia. Axial T1-weighted MR images with TE – 4.6 ms (in phase; A) and TE – 2.3 ms (opposed phase; B) showing small lesion in the anterior mediastinum (arrows). The lesion showed a mean signal intensity of 448 in in-phase and 267 in opposed-phase, suggestive of thymic hyperplasia.

(MRI: magnetic resonance imaging; TE: time to echo)

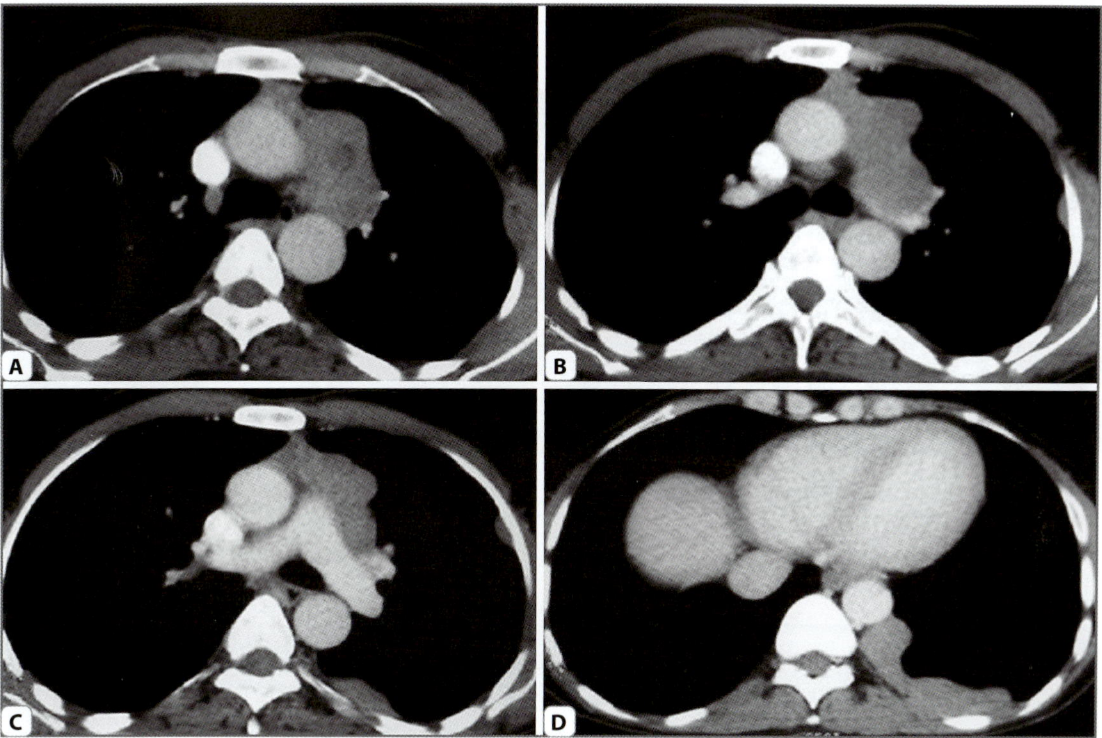

FIGS. 7A TO D: Invasive thymoma. CECT showing lobulated anterior mediastinal mass (A and B) with an ill-defined fat plane with the ascending aorta and pulmonary artery. Nodular pleural metastases are also seen (C and D) suggestive of invasive thymoma with pleural metastases.

Germ Cell Tumor

Anterior mediastinum is the most common site of extragonadal germ cell tumors (GCTs) accounting for 50–70% of all cases.[22] Posterior mediastinal GCTs are rare. They can be teratomas, other nonseminomatous tumors, and seminomas. They are more commonly seen in young men (10–40 years) with mean age of 31 years.[23] They may be detected incidentally or may produce symptoms due to pressure effects on the adjacent mediastinal structures. Various biomarkers may be elevated such as beta-human chorionic gonadotropin (β-hCG), alpha-fetoprotein (AFP), and lactate dehydrogenase (LDH), which should be done in all patients suspected to have mediastinal GCT.[22]

Teratoma

Biochemical markers are not elevated in the benign mature cystic teratoma. A prevascular mass containing visible fat (–40 to –120 HU) in a young adult is highly suggestive

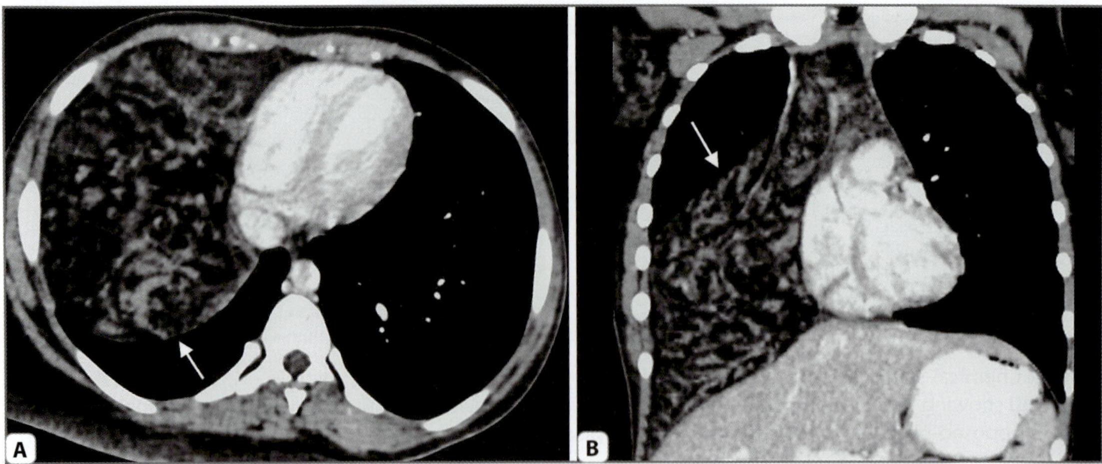

FIGS. 8A AND B: Thymolipoma. Axial (A) and coronal (B) contrast enhanced CT images showing a large right sided anterior and middle mediastinal mass (arrow) containing fat and soft tissue density, suggesting thymolipoma.

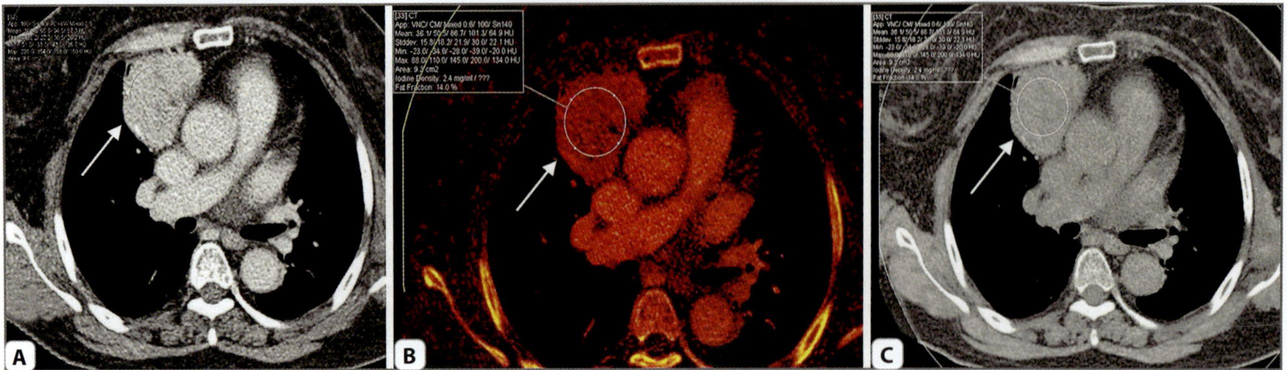

FIGS. 9A TO C: Thymic carcinoid. Monoenergetic (A), iodine (B) and virtual non-contrast (C) axial CT scans performed on dual energy scanner shows a homogeneously intensely enhancing mass in the anterior mediastinum (arrow).

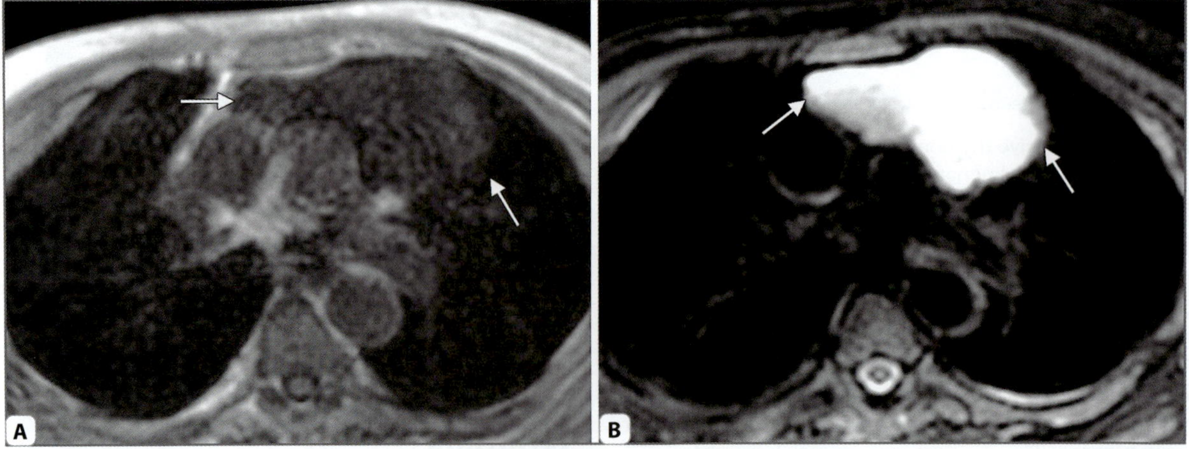

FIGS. 10A AND B: Thymic cyst. Axial T1-weighted (A) and T2-weighted (B) MR images showing a well defined lesion in the anterior mediastinum (arrows) appearing hypointense on T1W and hyperintense on T2W, suggestive of a cyst. No contrast enhancement was seen.

of the diagnosis of mature teratoma **(Figs. 11A to C)**. Fat within the lesion is seen in about 50% of the cases, while calcification is seen in 20–40% of the cases (which may be central, curvilinear, or peripheral). In addition, soft tissue and fluid levels can also in variable amounts, signifying embryological origin from primordial cells of two or three germ layers. On radiograph, they appear as lobulated or rounded anterior mediastinal mass. Presence of tooth-like structures or lucent areas on the radiograph is pathognomonic of the diagnosis[24] **(Figs. 12A to D)**.

These lesions can spontaneously rupture into pleural or pericardial space, lung, and tracheobronchial tree and produce inflammatory changes. Very rarely, they may undergo malignant transformation into sarcoma, adenocarcinoma, squamous cell carcinoma, and carcinoid tumor.[25] Surgical resection is the treatment of choice in benign teratomas.

Immature teratoma shows aggressive behavior with a tendency to infiltrate into surrounding structures. On imaging, they are more solid looking tumors with a tendency

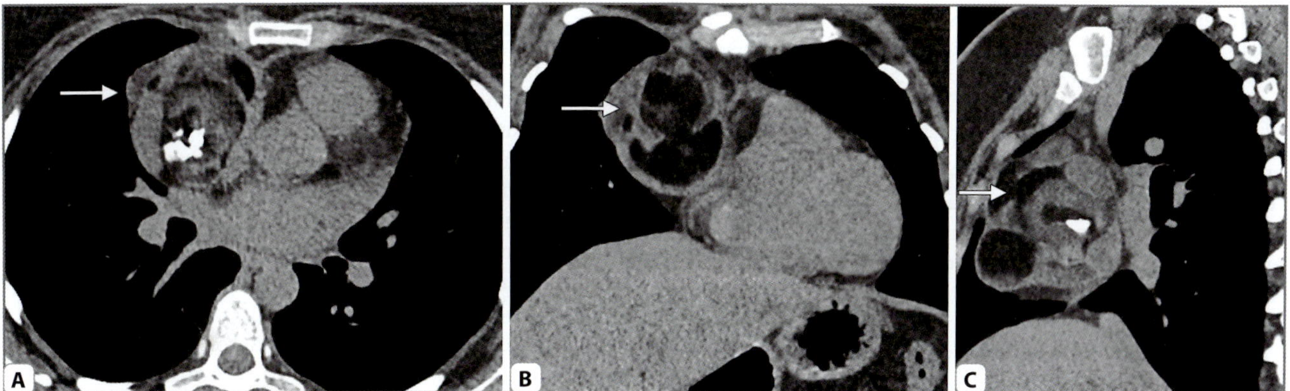

FIGS. 11A TO C: Mature cystic teratoma. NCCT chest axial (A), coronal (B), sagittal (C) images showing a large well encapsulated anterior mediastinal mass in right paracardiac location having low attenuation areas suggestive of fat and hyperdense calcification within, suggestive of teratoma.

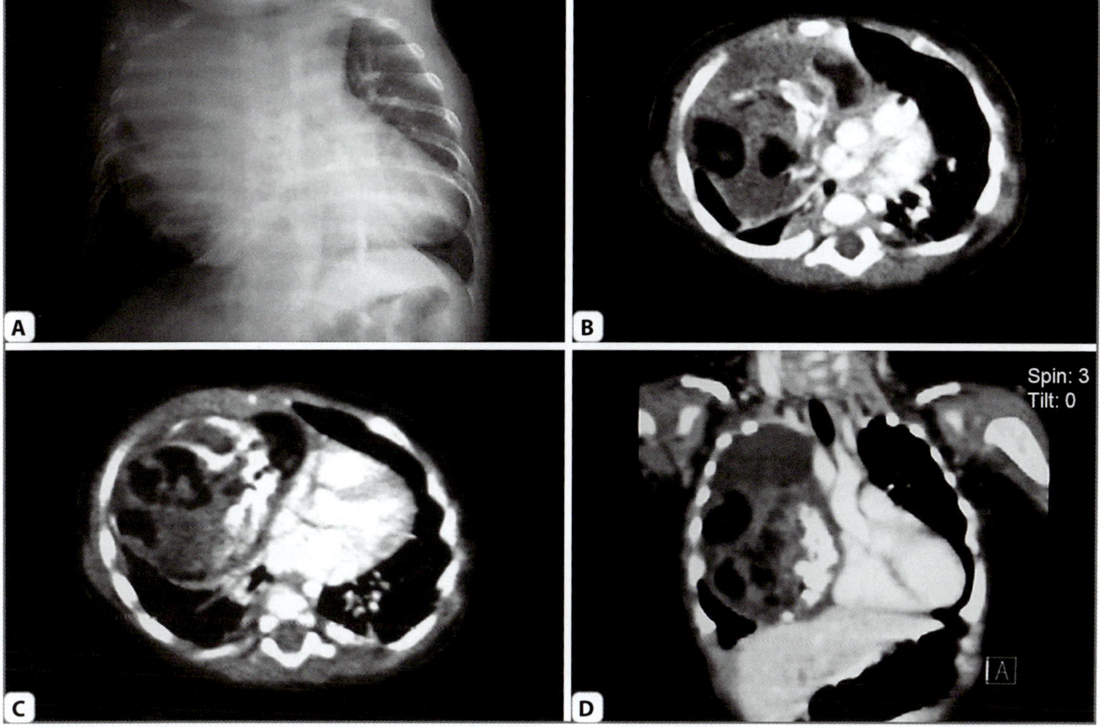

FIGS. 12A TO D: Teratoma in infant. Chest radiograph (A) of a 3-month-old child showing a large mediastinal mass with foci of calcification, and contralateral mediastinal shift. Axial CT (B and C) and coronal reformatted image (D) show a large right-sided low attenuation mass with calcification and fat within it, diagnostic of teratoma.

for local infiltration. Chemotherapy with surgical resection is the preferred treatment in such cases.[26]

Malignant Germ Cell Tumor

Malignant GCTs account for 2–6% of all the mediastinal tumors and 5–13% of malignant mediastinal tumors. These can be of two types: Seminoma and nonseminomatous GCT. Seminoma is the most common malignant GCT.[27,28] They tend to occur in young men (10–39 years). β-hCG will be elevated in ~80% of the advanced cases and helps in the assessment of the tumor burden and tumor growth. They are large, bulky lobulated masses extending to middle or posterior mediastinum. Calcification is usually absent, if seen may be stippled or ring like. Post-treatment they appear as calcified masses, and PET/MRI is required to differentiate fibrotic versus residual mass. They are radiosensitive tumors and respond very well to radiotherapy. When large, surgical resection with radiotherapy is done with a good outcome.

Nonseminomatous malignant GCT includes embryonal, endodermal sinus tumor, choriocarcinoma, or a mix-up of these histological varieties. However, 90% of these cases will be symptomatic.[29] In 80% of the cases, AFP will be elevated. This will usually occur in embryonal or endodermal sinus tumors.[30] β-hCG will be raised in 30% of the cases, especially in choriocarcinoma. LDH will be raised in 60% of the cases and correlates with tumor burden. On radiograph, these are large lobulated masses with indistinct lateral margins with the lungs. There may be associated pleural or pericardial effusion. Multiple rounded lung nodules, signifying lung metastasis, are not uncommon. On CT, they are large heterogeneous masses with invasion into adjacent lung or other parts of the mediastinum. They have a central area of necrosis or hemorrhage in 50% of the cases, showing predominant peripheral enhancement on postcontrast images. Calcification may or may not be there. Associated lymphadenopathy, pleural or pericardial effusion, or metastasis in lungs or liver may be seen. Treatment of choice is cisplatin-based chemotherapy followed by surgical resection. The prognosis, however, is poor.

Differentiation from lymphoma or thymoma is difficult on imaging; however, clinical profile along with the tumor markers and epicenter of the lesion helps to clinch the diagnosis. Lungs are the common site of metastasis, unlike lymphoma.[31]

Other less common fat-containing lesions in the prevascular compartment can be thymolipoma, lipoma, and liposarcoma.

Lipoma

It is a benign mesenchymal soft-tissue tumor composed of fat. They are well encapsulated and seen most commonly near the diaphragm. Malignant degeneration is extremely uncommon, and they are almost always asymptomatic. On CT scan, they will appear as well-defined, homogeneous, fat-containing masses (attenuation of –50 to –100 HU) with no contrast enhancement. MRI shows a uniformly hyperintense signal on T1W images with complete suppression of T1-weighted fat-saturated (T1 FS) images.

Mediastinal Fat Necrosis

This is a close differential of mediastinal lipoma. They present with a classic triad of acute pleuritic chest pain, fat-containing mass, and surrounding fat stranding in the mediastinal fat and the epipericardial fat. There may be thickening of the adjacent pericardium or pleura with mild pleural effusion.[32]

Liposarcoma

This is the malignant counterpart of the fat-containing mesenchymal masses. These are most commonly seen in the extremities and retroperitoneum. Mediastinum is an uncommon site of occurrence. On imaging, they can have variable ratios of fat and enhancing soft tissue depending upon the grade of differentiation and aggressiveness. They can produce symptoms due to the mass effect on the adjacent structures. The presence of thick septations or a discrete soft-tissue component in an adipocytic lesion should raise the suspicion of liposarcoma. However, GCTs with similar morphology are far more common.

Mediastinal Lipomatosis

Mediastinal lipomatosis is said to occur when there is excessive proliferation of mediastinal fat due to exogenous steroid intake, obesity, Cushing syndrome, adrenocorticotropic hormone-producing tumors, or rarely familial disorders. On radiograph, they can appear as smooth mediastinal widening with prominent epicardial fat pads. On CT, they appear as insinuating fat-containing infiltrative masses causing no compression or infiltration of the adjacent structures. The presence of capsule, septa, soft tissue, or enhancement suggests alternative diagnosis.

Omental Hernia

Congenital or post-traumatic defects in the diaphragm can lead to herniation of omental fat with or without other abdominal viscera in the thoracic cavity. In Morgagni hernia, there is defect in the anteromedial part of right hemidiaphragm **(Figs. 13A to D)**, whereas in Bochdalek hernia, the defect is in the left posterior hemidiaphragm **(Figs. 14A to D)**. At times, there may be incarceration of the herniated omental fat, which brings about the symptoms. Surgical repair is done in these cases to avoid complications.[33]

Mediastinal Extension of Thyroid Mass

Large thyroid masses can extend retrosternally into the mediastinum. This usually happens in multinodular goiter but occasionally may be seen in thyroid malignancies. The extension is usually into the superior mediastinum but can be even lower. A heterogeneous mass can be identified

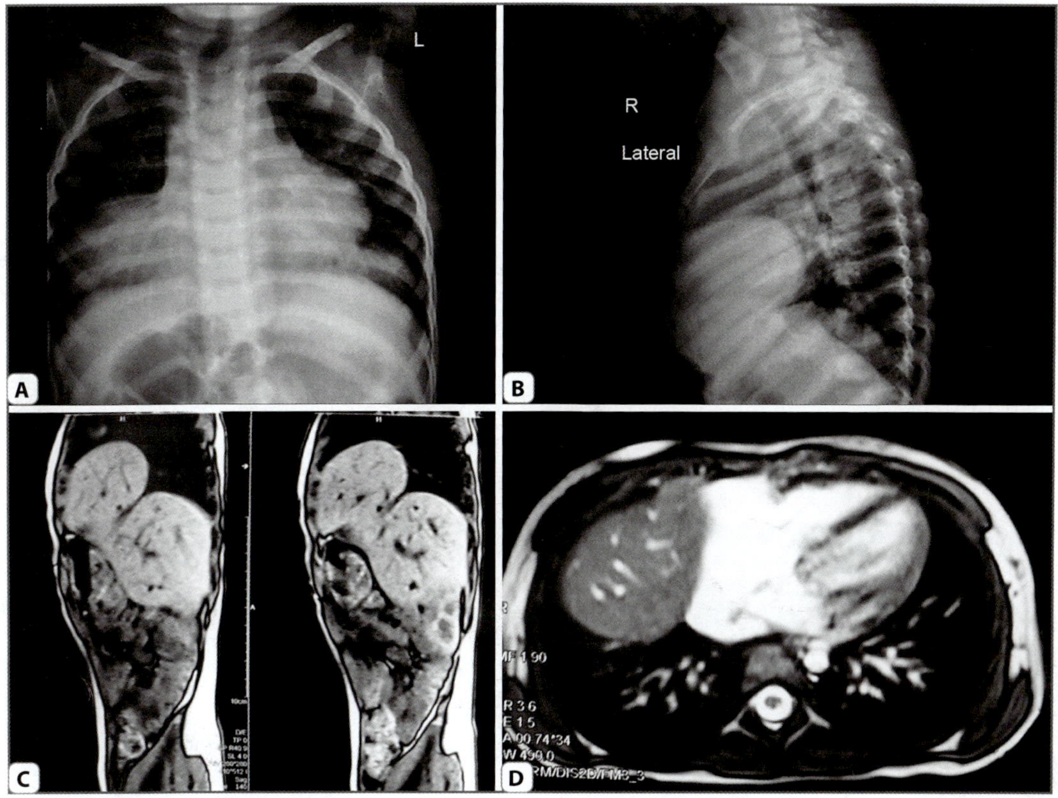

FIGS. 13A TO D: Morgagni hernia. Chest radiograph frontal (A) and lateral (B) projection showing an anteriorly located right cardiophrenic angle mass (C). T1W sagittal and T2W axial (D) MRI scans confirm the herniated liver in a Morgagni hernia.

(MRI: magnetic resonance imaging; T1W: T1-weighted; T2W: T2-weighted)

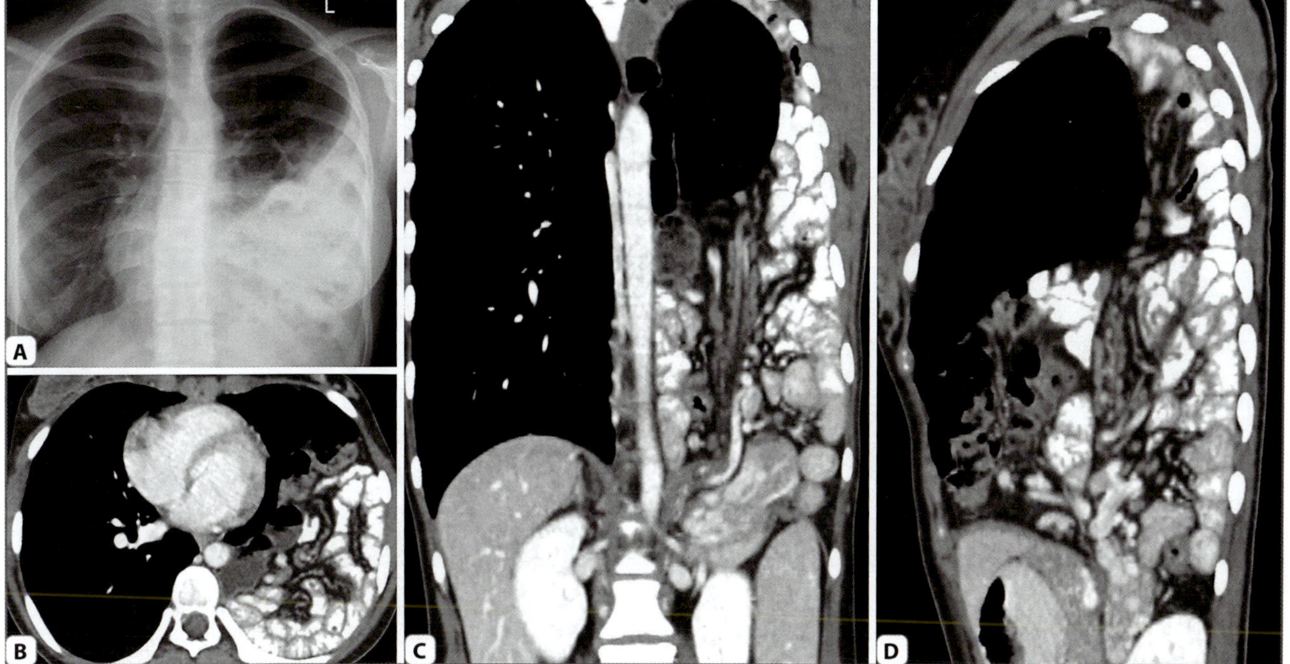

FIGS. 14A TO D: Bochdalek hernia. Chest radiograph (A) shows obscuration of left dome of diaphragm with bubbly lucencies in left lower zone, suggesting left diaphragmatic hernia. Axial CT (B) shows fat and bowel loops in the left hemithorax. Coronal (C) and sagittal (D) T2W MRI scans show herniation of mesenteric fat and bowel loops through a defect in the posterior part of the left dome suggestive of a Bochdalek hernia.

(CT: computed tomography; MRI: magnetic resonance imaging; T2W: T2-weighted)

in the prevascular region showing continuity with the cervical thyroid gland. It is very rare to have an anterior mediastinal mass arising in ectopic thyroid tissue without a demonstrable continuity with the cervical thyroid. On a radiograph, it appears as a lobulated mass in the anterior mediastinum with positive cervicothoracic sign (indicating extension in the neck) with areas of coarse calcification (in ~25% of cases) causing tracheal narrowing at the thoracic inlet. Concomitant anterior neck mass is seen on lateral radiograph of the neck. The mass is hyperdense (70–80HU) on noncontrast computed tomography (NCCT) scan due to presence of iodine in thyroid gland. On administration of contrast, the mass shows marked and sustained contrast enhancement (CE). However, multinodular goiters may not show these features of normal thyroid gland attenuation because the gland is replaced by multiple nodules. Internal cystic changes and calcifications may also be seen. Coarse calcifications are seen in up to 75% of the cases. The mass usually extends anterior to the trachea **(Figs. 15A to F)**.

Surgical removal of the intrathoracic goiter is usually done to avoid complications arising due to inflammation or hemorrhage within the mass. Planes with the surrounding vascular structures, the vertical depth of the thyroid tissue inferior to the upper sternal margin (measured on a sagittal CT image), and associated lymph nodes should be well communicated to the surgeon. Small retrosternal extension of the thyroid mass can be managed by cervical approach; however, large components in the mediastinum or posterior mediastinum may require both cervical and thoracic approaches.

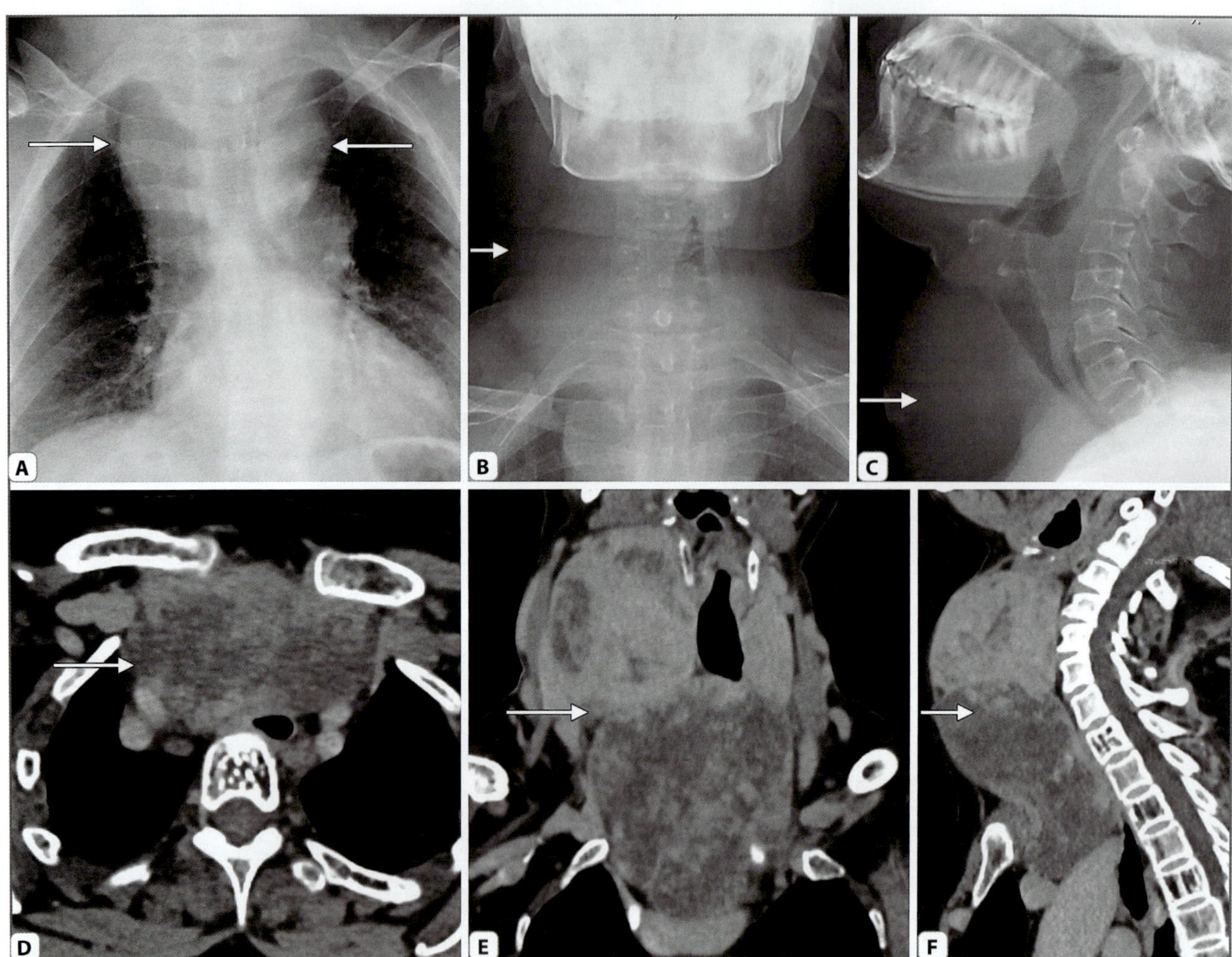

FIGS. 15A TO F: Thyroid mass with superior mediastinal extension. (A) Chest radiograph showing superior mediastinal widening (white arrows), with obscured margins above the clavicles, suggesting positive cervicothoracic sign. Neck radiographs AP(B), lateral (C) show a large neck mass causing compression of the trachea and deviation to the left. Axial (D), sagittal (E), coronal (F) CECT images showing heterogeneously enhancing mass in the anterior mediastinum showing continuity with the thyroid gland in the neck suggesting thyroid origin in a case of multinodular goiter with retrosternal extension.

(AP: anteroposterior; CECT: contrast-enhanced computed tomography)

Lymphoma

Lymphomas are the most common mediastinal malignancy, constituting ~50–60% of all the mediastinal malignancies.[34] Among these, non-Hodgkin lymphoma (NHL) constitutes 65% of the cases. These are homogeneous, mildly enhancing, lobulated masses extending to either side of the mediastinum. These are usually seen in the prevascular compartment or may have transcompartmental extension **(Figs. 16A to C)**. The major feature of differentiation from GCT or thymic tumor is the presence of infiltration. Lymphomas tend to encase or encircle the mediastinal vessels without causing any significant narrowing or infiltration. Nodal masses in other parts of the body further strengthen the diagnosis. Primary mediastinal lymphoma presents as a single confluent mass, whereas secondary lymphoma usually has discrete nodal masses. Necrosis and calcification are unusual in untreated cases. In addition, constitutional symptoms, such as fever, weight loss, and night sweats, may be seen in 50% of the cases.[35]

Lymphoma is the most common mediastinal tumor in the pediatric age group. It can be Hodgkin lymphoma (HL) or NHL. HL is characterized by thymic involvement and contiguous extension. NHL spares the thymus, may involve noncontiguous nodal stations, and is more likely to be homogeneous **(Table 6)**.

MISCELLANEOUS

Parathyroid Adenoma

Parathyroid adenomas are commonly seen in relation to thyroid gland. They may, however, be ectopically present in the mediastinum. Any enhancing prevascular soft tissue in the clinical setting of primary hyperparathyroidism should be suspected to be ectopic parathyroid adenoma. Four-dimensional (4D) CT is a highly sensitive and specific tool to detect these lesions. Parathyroid adenoma classically is hypodense on plain CT scan and shows intense

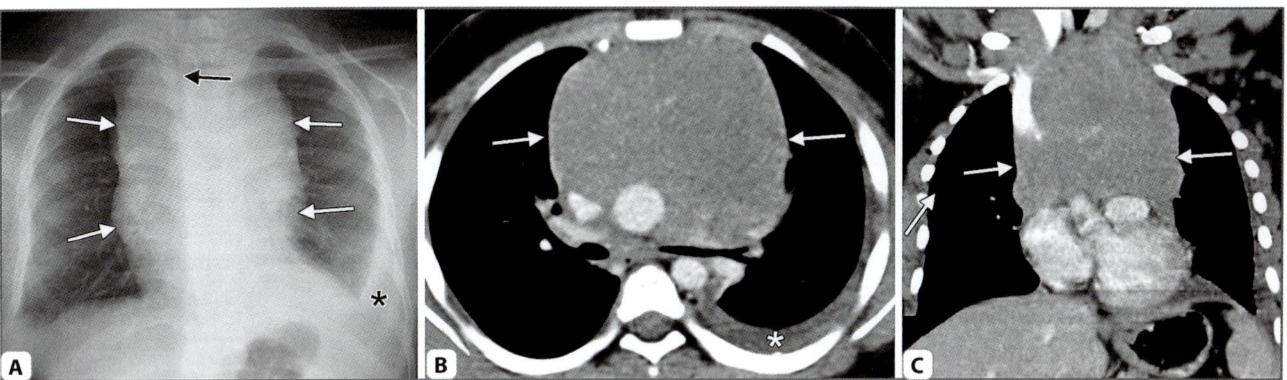

FIGS. 16A TO C: Mediastinal lymphoma. (A) Chest radiograph of a 20-year-old male presenting with respiratory distress showing mediastinal based mass extending on either side of midline (white arrows), compressing and displacing the trachea (black arrow) and silhouetting cardiac margins suggesting anterior location. Left pleural effusion is noted (asterisk). Axial (B) and coronal (C) CT images showing a homogeneous anterior mediastinal mass (arrows) encasing the ascending aorta and left pleural effusion (asterisk in B).

TABLE 6: Differences between Hodgkin lymphoma [HL and non-Hodgkin lymphoma (NHL)].

	HL	NHL
	More common in the second decade	More common in the first decade
Types	Classic HL and nodular lymphocyte predominant HL	Burkitt lymphoma, diffuse large B-cell lymphoma, lymphoblastic lymphoma, and anaplastic large cell lymphoma
	Associated with Epstein–Barr virus and/or an immunocompromised state	
	Night sweats, fever, and weight loss and with painless cervical or supraclavicular adenopathy	
5-year survival rate	90%	70–85%
Histopathology	Reed–Sternberg cells diagnostic positive for CD30 and CD15 and negative for CD20 and CD79a	Large, similar to the Reed–Sternberg cells of HL, lack prominent nucleoli; mitotic figures seen; CD19, CD20, CD22, and CD79a positivity, with results negative for CD5 and CD15
After treatment	Residual benign mediastinal tissue with necrotic and fibrotic components in 88% of cases	Residual tissue is rare in NHL

enhancement on arterial phase, with washout in the venous phase **(Figs. 17A to C)**. Further correlation with sestamibi scan may be done to confirm the diagnosis.[36,37] Castleman disease (CD) is another differential of hypervascular anterior mediastinal mass.

Lymphatic Malformations

These usually present in infancy and are transcompartmental involving neck as well as mediastinum. Neck is the most common site of occurrence in about 75% of the cases followed by axilla. Isolated involvement of the mediastinum is rare (~10%). The mediastinal component is usually asymptomatic, very rarely producing compressive symptoms due to narrowing of vital structures **(Figs. 18A to D)**. It is an insinuating mass lesion and can be of three morphological subtypes depending upon the size of the individual loculations/cysts: Macrocystic (>1 cm), microcystic (<1 cm), or mixed type. They develop due to failure to develop communication between the fetal lymphatic channels and venous system. On imaging, they appear as multiseptated (macrocystic) or solid appearing lesions (microcystic) having internal high density/variable intensity contents due to bleed with the enhancement of only the wall and septae. Mass effect may be seen in macrocystic variety; however, microcystic ones show infiltrative nature without any displacement or symptoms.[38,39] MRI is more definitive of the diagnosis as it demonstrates the cystic nature of the mass. On administration of the contrast, there is no postcontrast enhancement.

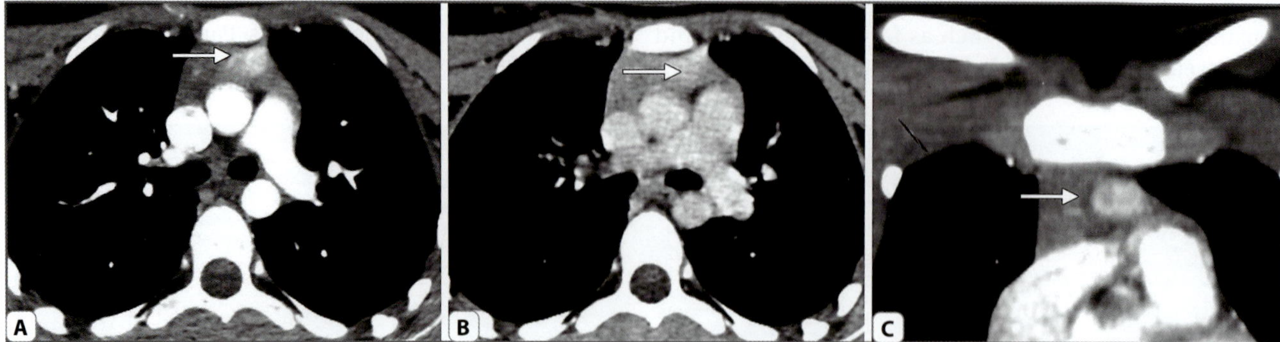

FIGS. 17A TO C: Ectopic parathyroid adenoma. Axial CECT image in arterial phase (A) in a patient with hyperparathyroidism shows a small markedly enhancing anterior mediastinal mass (arrow) just behind the sternum. Axial CECT in venous phase (B) shows mild washout of contrast. Coronal reformat (C) better depicts the mass (arrow). Fluorocholine PET-CT confirmed it to be ectopic parathyroid adenoma.

(CECT: contrast-enhanced computed tomography; PET-CT: positron emission tomography-computed tomography)

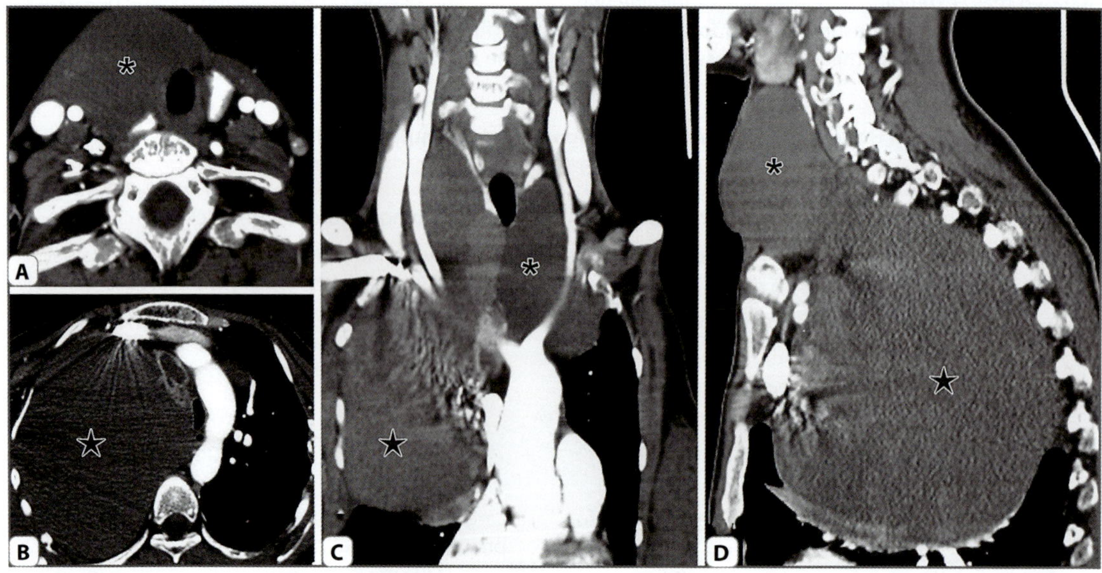

FIGS. 18A TO D: Mediastinal lymphatic malformation. Axial (A and B), coronal (C) and sagittal (D) contrast enhanced CT scans showing a hypodense cystic lesion in the neck region (asterisk) with a large component in the mediastinum (star).

Castleman Disease

This is an uncommon entity in which there is proliferation of the lymphoproliferative tissue. It can be unicentric or multicentric. Unicentric CD appears as avidly enhancing mediastinal mass, which is usually detected incidentally. At times, they become large and lead to compression of adjacent structures leading onto symptoms such as cough, dyspnea, and dysphagia.

Multicentric CD, on the other hand, is always symptomatic and produces systemic constitutional symptoms such as fever, weight loss, and anorexia. Other findings would be lymphadenopathy, organomegaly, renal dysfunction, pleural effusion, pulmonary edema, skin rash, and endocrine dysfunction.[40]

A differential for intensely enhancing mediastinal lesion is solitary fibrous tumor or fibromatosis. T2 hypointensity and absence of necrosis suggest these lesions.

Middle Mediastinum

Benign Cysts

Presence of a well-defined cystic lesion having an attenuation value of 0–20 HU points toward the diagnosis of a benign cystic lesion. This can either be bronchogenic or esophageal duplication cysts. Sometimes, the attenuation on CT appears a little higher because of proteinaceous contents. In such cases, MRI resolves the dilemma.

Bronchogenic duplication cysts arise due to abnormal budding of the foregut and are lined by respiratory epithelium. They are well-circumscribed, homogeneous, and low-density lesions **(Figs. 19A and B)**. They are most often seen at the carina, followed by the paratracheal location, although they may be seen in any part of the mediastinum. They may show sudden increase in size due to internal hemorrhage or infection. They may appear heterogeneous or hyperdense due to the presence of hemorrhage or proteinaceous contents. At times, there may be calcification in the wall or contents. MRI may be done to depict T2-hyperintensity and absence of contrast enhancement, which will confirm the cystic nature of the mass. T1 signal may be variable. Air within the cyst is uncommon unless there is airway/esophageal communication or secondary infection.[41]

Esophageal duplication cysts are less common than bronchogenic cysts. The imaging morphology is similar, except that they may have thicker walls. The major point of differentiation is the location. Esophageal cysts are seen in relation to the esophagus rather than the tracheobronchial tree[41] **(Figs. 20A to D)**. They may have ectopic gastric tissue, which may bleed or rupture, and can be detected on technetium 99m sodium pertechnetate scans. Gut signature (layered pattern of the wall) may be identified on EUS.

Pericardial Cysts

These cysts form as a result of aberrations in the formation of coelomic cavities. They are seen in relation to the pericardium and show typical morphology of cyst on CT and MRI without any solid component. At times, they may have thin peripheral calcification **(Figs. 21A and B)**.

Enhancing Masses

Solid enhancing masses in the visceral compartment can be paraganglioma, CD, or metastasis from vascular primary malignancies.

Paragangliomas are intensely enhancing solid masses and represent extra-adrenal pheochromocytomas **(Figs. 22A and B)**. They may be secreting, when they release catecholamines or nonfunctional. Clinical presentation may be with dysphagia, hoarseness of voice, dyspnea, or chest pain. Metaiodobenzylguanidine (MIBG) and DOTANOC PET scan may help to diagnose these tumors. CD is nonclonal proliferation of plasma cells. Metastasis from highly vascular primary such as renal cell and thyroid neoplasms, melanoma, choriocarcinoma, and some sarcomas also manifests as markedly enhancing nodal masses in the mediastinum.

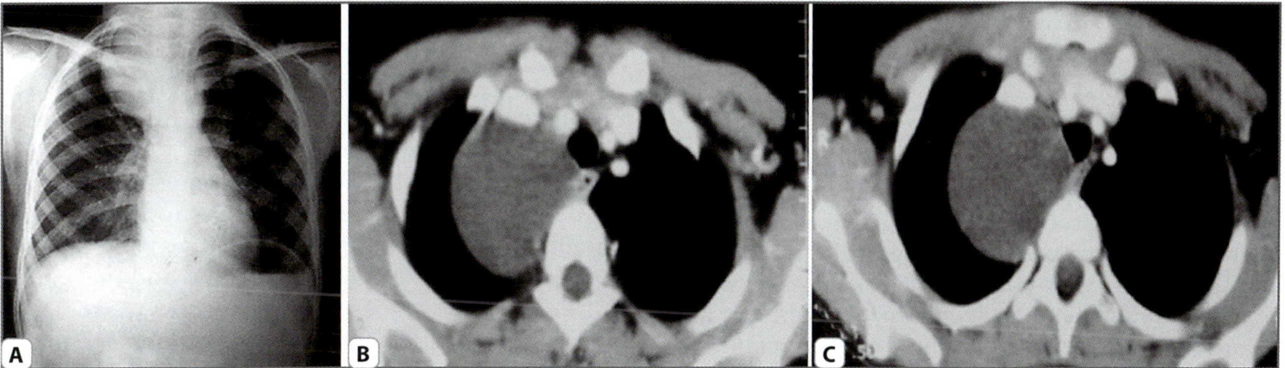

FIGS. 19A TO C: Bronchogenic cyst. Chest radiograph (A) showing a large right paratracheal mediastinal mass. Axial computed tomography (CT) (B and C) shows a fluid attenuation lesion closely related to the trachea, suggesting the diagnosis of a bronchogenic cyst.

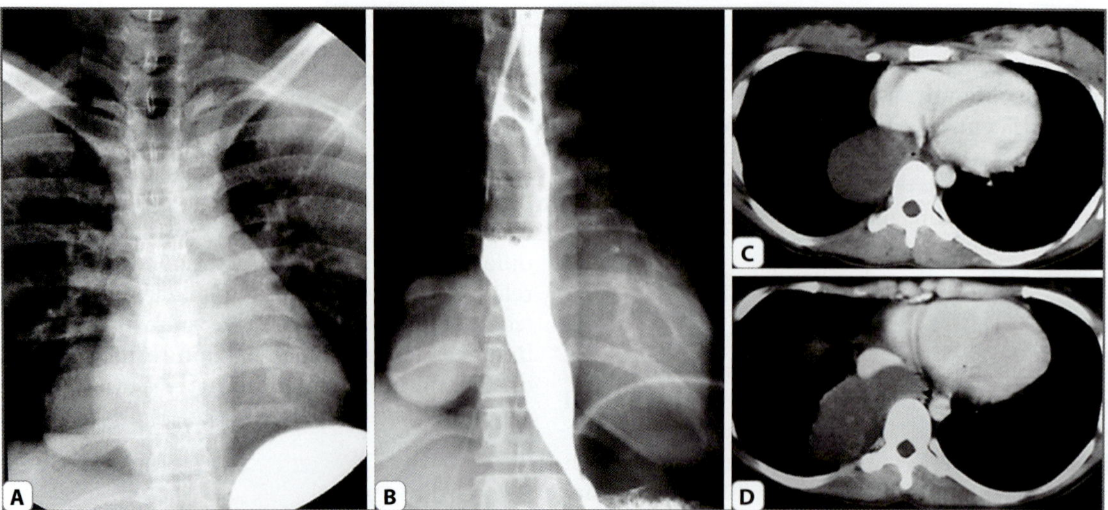

FIGS. 20A TO D: Esophageal duplication cyst. Coned down radiograph (A) showing a right paracardiac mass which is not silhouetting the cardiac border; suggesting posterior mediastinal location. Barium swallow spot (B) shows no communication/impression on the esophagus. Axial CECT scans (C and D) show a fluid density mass intimately related to the esophagus, causing anterior displacement of the inferior vena cava. Diagnosis: Esophageal duplication cyst.

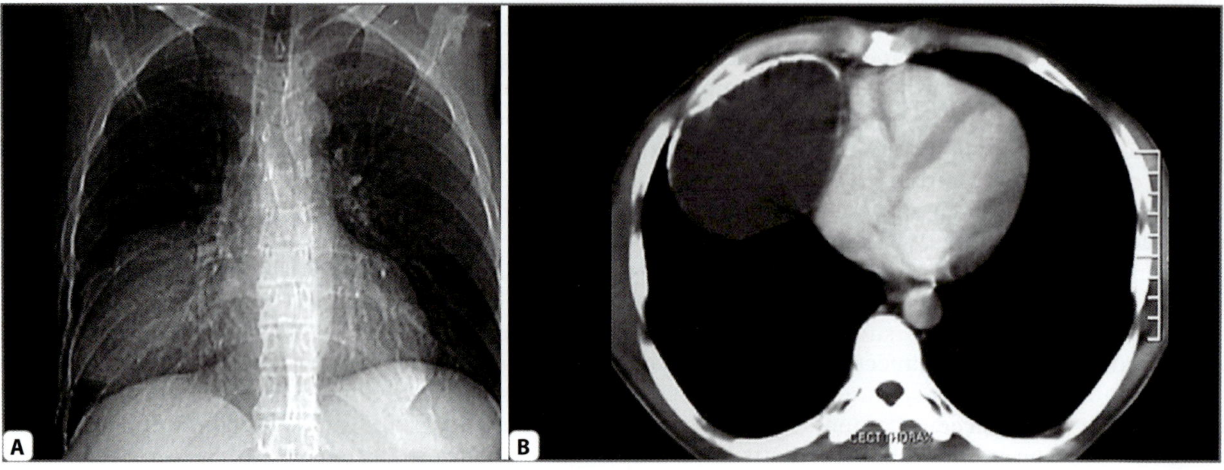

FIGS. 21A AND B: Pericardial cyst. Chest topogram image (A) showing a large right cardiophrenic angle mass; CECT (B) shows a fluid attenuation non-enhancing lesion with peripheral rim calcification in right paracardiac location suggesting a diagnosis of pleuropericardial cyst.

Lymph Nodes

Lymph node enlargement can be seen in all the mediastinal compartments but more commonly in middle and anterior mediastinum. They can be rounded, elliptical, or oval-shaped discrete masses surrounded by mediastinal fat. They can be enlarged due to a wide variety of causes such as infections, granulomatous disorders, neoplasms, and autoimmune disorders. In the mediastinum, the classification for lymph node station has been devised by the International Association for the Study of Lung Cancer in 2009 **(Table 7)**.[42]

Lymph node enlargement is suggested by measuring the short-axis diameter of the node. Any node >1 cm or subcarinal node >1.5 cm is said to be enlarged. The morphology of the nodal enlargement can be variable depending upon particular pathology.

In tuberculosis (TB), the nodes are necrotic (central low density with peripheral rim enhancement), show periadenitis (loss of perinodal fat planes) and matting (conglomeration) **(Figs. 23A and B)**, and may show obliteration of azygoesophageal recess. Associated changes in the lungs in the form of centrilobular nodules in tree-in-bud fashion, consolidation, pleural effusion, or necrotic nodes in other parts of the body may be seen. The nodes may persist in healed TB as small calcified mediastinal nodes. At times, the nodes may become fibrotic and do not shrink much in size. In such cases,

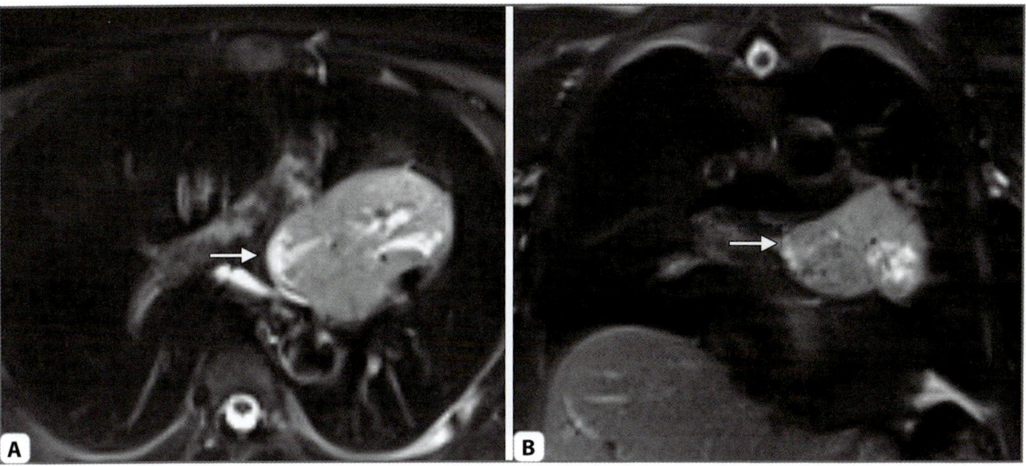

FIGS. 22A AND B: Mediastinal paraganglioma. MRI T2W axial (A), coronal (B) images showing heterogeneously T2 hyperintense mass in visceral compartment, confirmed to be paraganglioma on DOTANOC PET scan.

(MRI: magnetic resonance imaging; PET: positron emission tomography; T2W: T2-weighted)

TABLE 7: Mediastinal lymph nodal stations [International Association for the Study of Lung Cancer (IASLC)].

Nodal zone	Description	Station
Upper zone	Right upper paratracheal	2R
	Left upper paratracheal	2L
	Prevascular	3
	Right lower paratracheal	4R
	Left lower paratracheal	4L
Aortopulmonary zone	Subaortic	5
	Paraaortic	6
Subcarinal zone	Subcarinal	7
Lower zone	Paraesophageal	8
	Pulmonary ligament	9
	Hilar	10
	Interlobar	11
Peripheral zone	Lobar	12
	Segmental	13
	Subsegmental	14

MRI or PET may be helpful to differentiate active versus healed infection.

In sarcoidosis, multiple level nodes are enlarged, especially bilateral hilar and right paratracheal. They are discrete, homogeneous with no necrosis and matting. Intrapulmonary node enlargement is specific for sarcoidosis. Also, specific pulmonary findings such as perilymphatic nodules aid in establishing the diagnosis. In silicosis, multiple mediastinal nodes may be homogeneously enlarged and may show eggshell type of calcification. Mediastinal nodes in lymphoma may present as large mass usually in the anterior mediastinum.

The nodes can also be enlarged in metastases, which do not show any specific pattern or morphology. Presence of a primary neoplasm with enlarged, round, or heterogeneous mediastinal nodes suggests metastatic involvement.

Esophageal Lesions

Esophageal lesions can appear as a focal or a diffuse wall thickening or an irregular mass. The clinical history of dysphagia is supportive of an esophageal lesion. Endoscopy followed by endoscopic biopsy is paramount to establish the diagnosis. Benign masses of the esophagus include fibrovascular polyp and leiomyoma. Fibrovascular polyp is an intraluminal enhancing polypoidal mass, while leiomyomas are smoothly marginated homogeneous intramural masses so that the mucosa is intact. Leiomyoma is the most common benign tumor of the esophagus. It can be detected on barium study as a smoothly marginated mass lined by barium having obtuse angles with the esophageal wall. CT is more confirmatory as it shows well-circumscribed, ovoid, and intramural mass with specks of calcification and homogeneous enhancement with no evidence of infiltration **(Figs. 24A to D)**. Esophageal malignancies appear as irregular circumferential or eccentric wall thickening causing luminal obstruction and may show infiltration into adjacent structures and associated lymphadenopathy. The incidence of lower-end adenocarcinomas is on the rise due to rising incidence of gastroesophageal reflux.

Motility disorders such as achalasia cardia can also present as a mediastinal mass. Achalasia cardia is an idiopathic condition, which arises due to inability of the lower esophageal sphincter to relax with absence of primary peristalsis. This results in marked dilatation of the esophagus with narrowing at the lower end. On chest radiograph, it projects as a large mediastinal mass on the right side, less commonly on the left side, with mottled

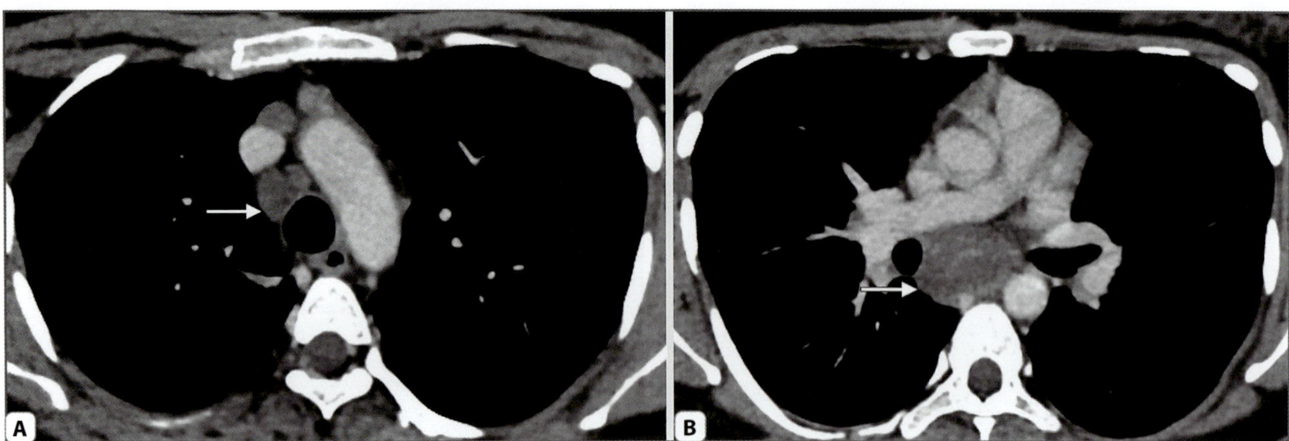

FIGS. 23A AND B: Nodal tuberculosis. Axial CECT scans (A and B) show necrotic conglomerate lymph nodes (arrow) with peripheral enhancement in anterior (A) and visceral compartments (B).

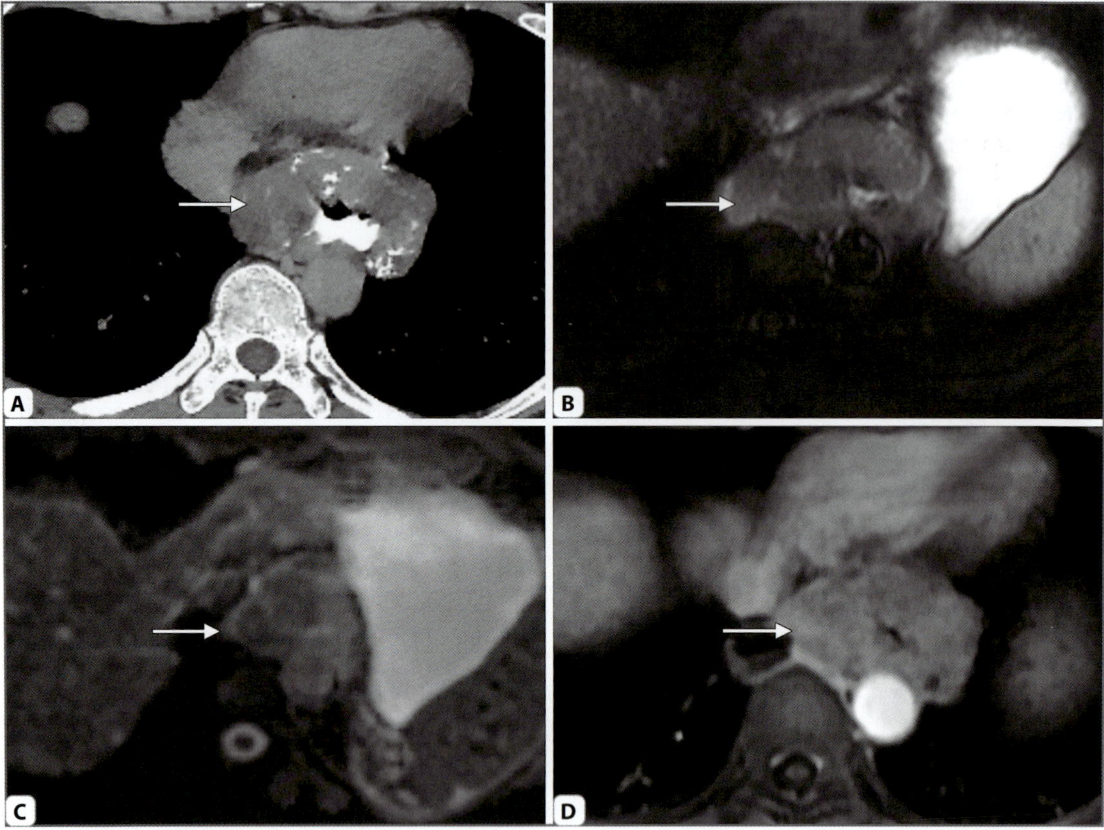

FIGS. 24A TO D: Esophageal leiomyoma. CECT (A) Shows mass like hypodense thickening (arrow) of the lower esophagus with foci of calcification; MRI T2W axial (B) image shows intermediate signal mass (arrow) in lower esophagus which shows diffusion restriction on ADC map (C) with mild contrast enhancement on post-contrast image (D).

(ADC: apparent diffusion coefficient; CECT: contrast-enhanced computed tomography; MRI: magnetic resonance imaging; T2W: T2-weighted)

lucencies or air-fluid level within (suggestive of retained food). Barium swallow is diagnostic of this condition. There is marked dilatation of the esophagus with absent primary contractions and presence of multiple tertiary contractions. There is short segment narrowing of the lower end (<3.5 cm) with delayed clearance of contrast **(Figs. 25A and B)**.

Vascular Origin Lesions

Various vascular lesions can give the appearance of mediastinal mass on a chest radiograph and account for 10% of the radiographically detected mediastinal masses. The distinction can be clearly made on a cross-sectional contrast-enhanced imaging. They can be classified based

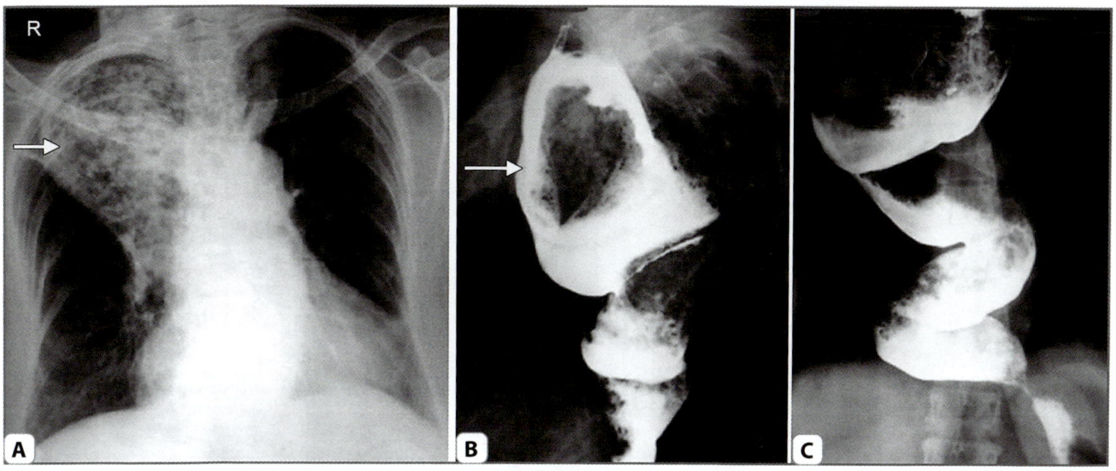

FIGS. 25A TO C: Achalasia cardia. Chest radiograph (A) shows a large right-sided mediastinal mass (arrow) with air lucencies within it. Barium swallow (B and C) shows a grossly dilated sigmoid-type esophagus (arrow) with a smooth narrowing at the lower end suggestive of achalasia cardia.

on the vascular structure from which they take origin such as systemic arterial, systemic venous, pulmonary arterial, pulmonary venous, or lymphatic in nature. Right aortic arch can appear as a rounded homogeneous opacity in the right upper anterior mediastinum between SVC and trachea causing their displacement to the right and left, respectively, with absence of aortic knuckle on the left side.[43] Double aortic arch will have both the opacities on either side.[44] Thoracic aortic aneurysms or pseudoaneurysms are the most common among the vascular anomalies **(Figs. 26A to D)**. They can arise due to atherosclerosis, trauma, infection, inflammation, cystic medial necrosis, etc. On chest radiographs, they cause mediastinal widening. Depending on the site of involvement, segment can appear as a mediastinal mass with a peripheral rim of calcification. Persistent left-sided SVC can also appear as widening of the aorta or mediastinum and may mimic lymphadenopathy.[45] Other causes could be aberrant subclavian artery, dilatation of pulmonary artery, SVC, azygous and hemiazygous system, aortic aneurysm or dissection, SVC syndrome, and mediastinal varix.

Posterior Mediastinum

Neurogenic Tumors

Neurogenic tumors constitute about 60–70% of the posterior mediastinal masses, ~20% of the adult and 35% of pediatric mediastinal masses.[46] Depending upon the cell of origin, they can be peripheral nerve sheath tumors (PNSTs) from peripheral nerves (most common), neuroblastoma group from sympathetic ganglia, and paragangliomas from paraganglion cells.

Peripheral nerve sheath tumors can be schwannoma, neurofibroma, or malignant PNST. They can arise from spinal nerves, proximal intercostal nerves, and rarely from vagus or phrenic nerve. They are well-circumscribed, round, or ovoid masses in the paravertebral location **(Figs. 27A and B)**. They may have an intraspinal extension through the neural foramina when they form a dumbbell shape, which is quite specific for these tumors. Majority of the neurogenic tumors are benign masses, which cause mass effect over the surrounding structures such as pressure erosion of adjoining ribs or the vertebra. MRI is the modality of choice for posterior mediastinal masses as it best demonstrates the intraspinal extension **(Figs. 28A to F)**. Neurofibromas are more homogeneous, whereas cystic changes and hemorrhage are more commonly seen in schwannomas. Fascicular sign represents multiple, small T2 hypointense rings and is usually seen in schwannomas, whereas target sign, which represents central T2 hypointensity with surrounding T2 hyperintensity, is more commonly a feature of neurofibroma. Malignant transformation is suspected when there is a sudden increase in the size of mass, heterogeneity, or invasion of the adjacent structures.

Other paravertebral neurogenic masses include sympathetic ganglion cell tumors such as ganglioneuroma, ganglioneuroblastoma, and neuroblastoma. Ganglioneuroma is the benign counterpart, seen in relatively older children (>7 years), whereas ganglioneuroblastoma and neuroblastoma are the malignant tumors seen in children <5 years of age. On imaging, they appear as vertically oriented masses, placed anterolateral to the vertebra. Ganglioneuromas are well-defined masses, which have high signal on T2W sequence with gradual uptake of contrast on postcontrast images. Ganglioneuroblastoma and neuroblastoma may be well- or ill-defined masses (as they lack a true capsule) and are heterogeneous with necrosis and calcification **(Figs. 29A and B)**.

Paragangliomas are tumors arising from the paraganglia cells placed at two sites in the mediastinum. One along the great vessels is termed as aortopulmonary paraganglioma, and the other is along the sympathetic chain in posterior mediastinum. They are highly vascular masses, which on imaging appear as relatively homogeneous masses, showing intense enhancement. There may be internal flow voids due

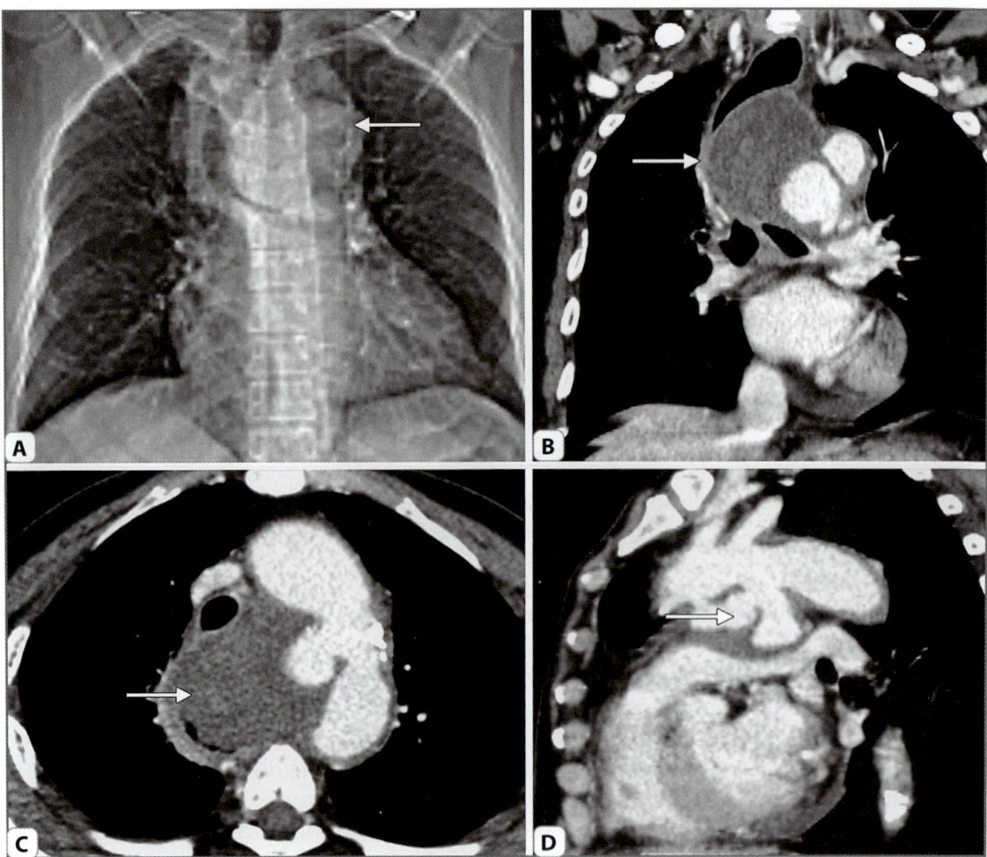

FIGS. 26A TO D: Aortic arch pseudoaneurysm with mediastinal hematoma. Chest topogram (A) depicting mediastinal mass (arrow) on the left side causing compression of the trachea and deviating it to the right side suggestive of middle mediastinum origin. CECT coronal (B), axial (C), sagittal (D) images showing contrast filled outpouching from the arch of aorta surrounded by a large hypodense soft tissue (arrow) consistent with pseudoaneurysm with mediastinal hematoma.

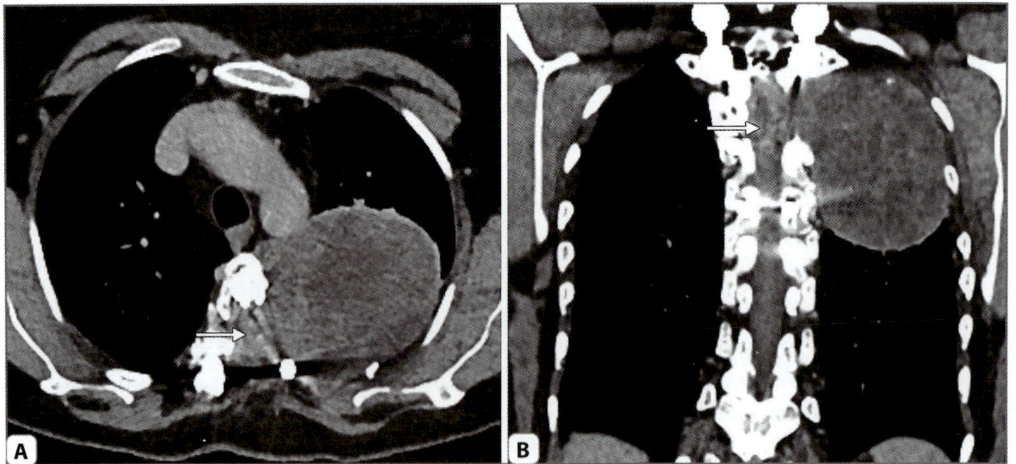

FIGS. 27A AND B: Peripheral nerve sheath tumor. CECT axial (A), coronal (B) images depict a large posterior mediastinal mass having intraspinal extension (arrows) in a case of posterior mediastinal schwannoma. Streak artefacts are due to spine fixation devices.

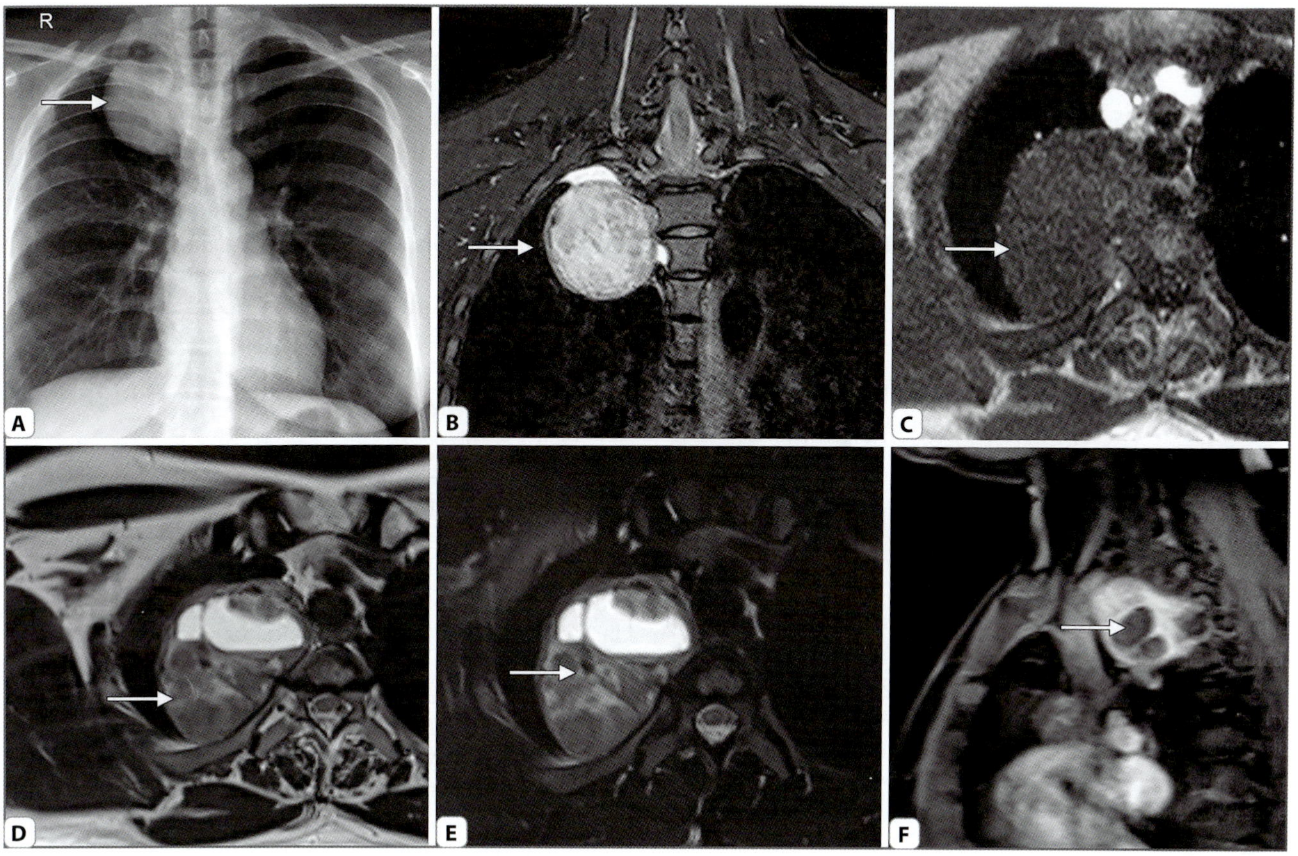

FIGS. 28A TO F: : Posterior mediastinal peripheral nerve sheath tumor. Chest radiograph frontal (A) view showing a posterior mediastinal mass with well demarcated borders above the clavicle, suggesting posterior mediastinal location. T2W fat sat coronal (B), axial T1W (C), axial T2W (D), axial T2W FS (E) and sagittal postcontrast (F) MR images show heterogeneous mass with fluid levels having neural foraminal extension (arrow heads).

(MR: magnetic resonance; T2W: T2-weighted)

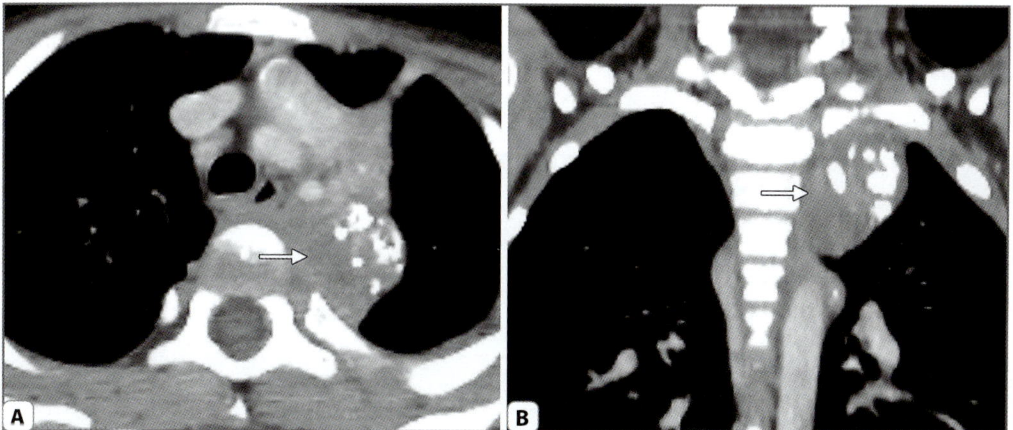

FIGS. 29A AND B: Thoracic Neuroblastoma. CECT axial (A), coronal (B) images showing a posterior mediastinal mass (arrow) in left paravertebral location having coarse calcification within, in a 5-year-old child, findings consistent with neuroblastoma.

to high vascular flow. MIBG scintigraphy and DOTANOC PET scan are helpful in the diagnosis of these tumors.[47]

Meningoceles

Intrathoracic meningocele is the herniation of the meninges through the vertebral defect/cleft or the intervertebral foramina. These are cystic masses in paravertebral location, showing communication with the cerebrospinal fluid (CSF) space.

Neurenteric Cysts

These cysts contain both neural and gastrointestinal components. The diagnosis is suggested when there is a purely cystic lesion in the paravertebral location in association with vertebral anomalies. These do not usually communicate with the CSF space **(Figs. 30A to C)**.

Abscesses

Collections can form in the mediastinum usually as a result of extension of infection from other adjoining sites. They appear as well-defined peripherally enhancing cystic areas with surrounding fat stranding. Tuberculous Spondylodiscitis with bird's nest appearance of paravertebral abscess is very common in our country **(Figs. 31A to G)**. Rarely, pancreatitis-related collections may dissect across the tissue planes and appear as collection in the posterior mediastinum **(Figs. 32A to C)**.

Extramedullary Hematopoiesis

Multiple bilateral enhancing paravertebral masses in the setting of marrow disorders points toward the diagnosis of extramedullary hematopoiesis. They may show variable fat content and enhancement. Multiplicity, bilaterality, intralesional fat, and intense enhancement along with marrow expansion and coarsened trabeculae should suggest this diagnosis.

Multicompartmental Masses

These include lymphatic malformations, lymph nodes, hematoma, fibrosing mediastinitis (FM), and lipomatosis. It is difficult to localize the origin in case of masses involving multiple compartments. Two signs have been described in this scenario.[2] One is to look for the epicenter of the lesion (where the maximum dimension or waist is there). The second is to look at the pattern of displacement of mediastinal vascular structures. Anterior displacement suggests paravertebral origin, while posterior displacement suggests prevascular origin.

Fibrosing Mediastinitis

This is also called sclerosing mediastinitis or mediastinal fibrosis. This is a benign lesion but involves progressive proliferation of fibroinflammatory tissue replacing the mediastinal fat. This can be potentially life-threatening due to encasement and narrowing of the vital vascular structures in the mediastinum and also the hilar structures. It has been classified into the granulomatous or nongranulomatous subtypes.

Granulomatous or focal FM is the predominant subtype (80–90% of FM), which occurs in relatively younger population (35–46 years). This develops due to an abnormal immunological response, which results in the proliferation of the fibroinflammatory tissue. The most common inciting antigens are fungal infections (histoplasmosis) and TB. Other causes include sarcoidosis, blastomycosis, mucormycosis, or cryptococcosis, etc.[48]

Nongranulomatous or diffuse/idiopathic FM is the less common type. It is seen to occur in the mediastinum as well as extrathoracic sites. It is seen to develop as an inflammatory response to autoimmune diseases such as systemic lupus erythematosus (SLE), rheumatoid arthritis (RA), Behçet's disease, and previous radiation.

On chest radiograph, this can appear as mediastinal widening with the presence of mediastinal or hilar

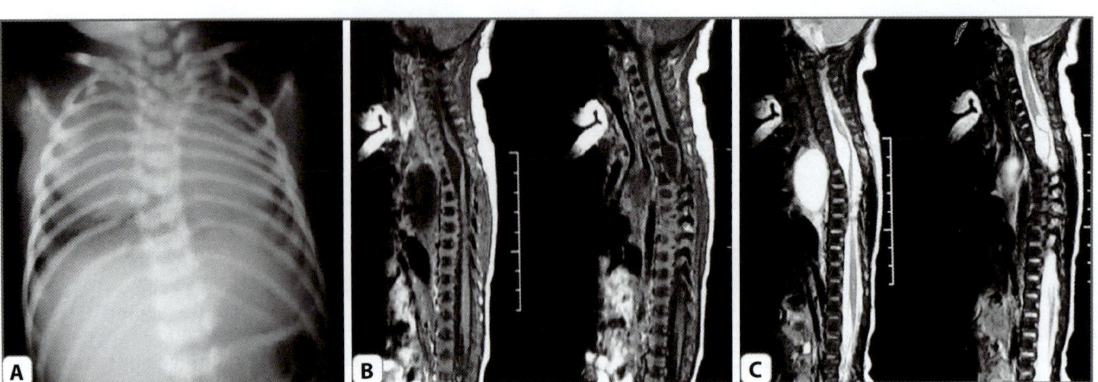

FIGS. 30A TO C: Neurenteric cyst. Chest radiograph (A) shows a large mediastinal mass, with congenital vertebral anomalies and scoliosis of dorsal spine. T1W (B) and T2W (C) sagittal images show a prevertebral mass with intraspinal extension which is hypointense on T1 and bright on the T2W image. Diagnosis: Neurenteric cyst.

(T1W: T1-weighted; T2W: T2-weighted)

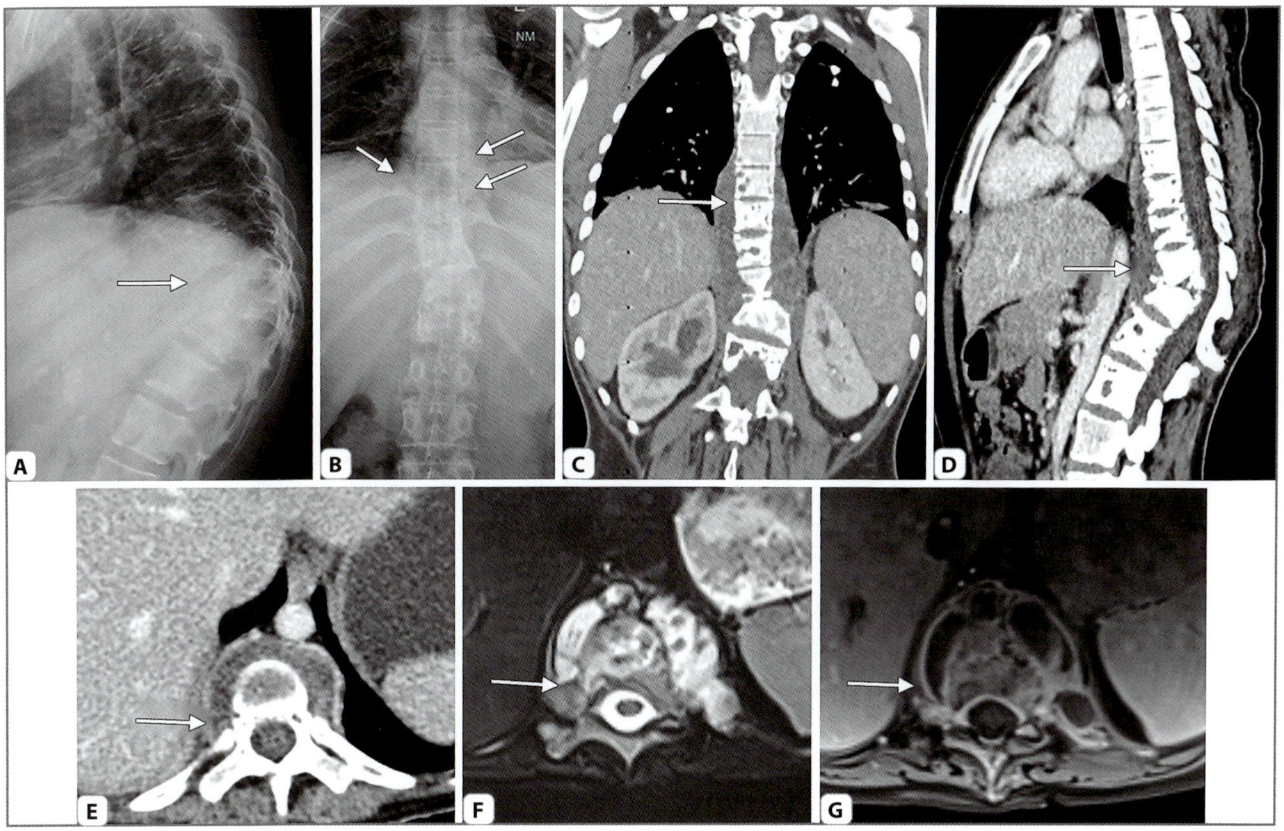

FIGS. 31A TO G: Pott's spine. Dorso-lumbar radiographs, lateral (A), AP view (B) showing destruction of lower dorso-lumbar vertebra (resulting in focal kyphosis) and paravertebral mass (arrows delineating the margins). CECT coronal (C), sagittal (D) axial (E) images showing partial destruction of multiple contiguous dorso-lumbar vertebra with prevertebral and paravertebral collection (arrow); MRI T2W (F), Postcontrast (G) images showing T2 hyperintensity of the vertebrae showing postcontrast enhancement with paravertebral abscess (arrow).

(AP: anteroposterior; CECT: contrast-enhanced computed tomography; MRI: magnetic resonance imaging; T2W: T2-weighted)

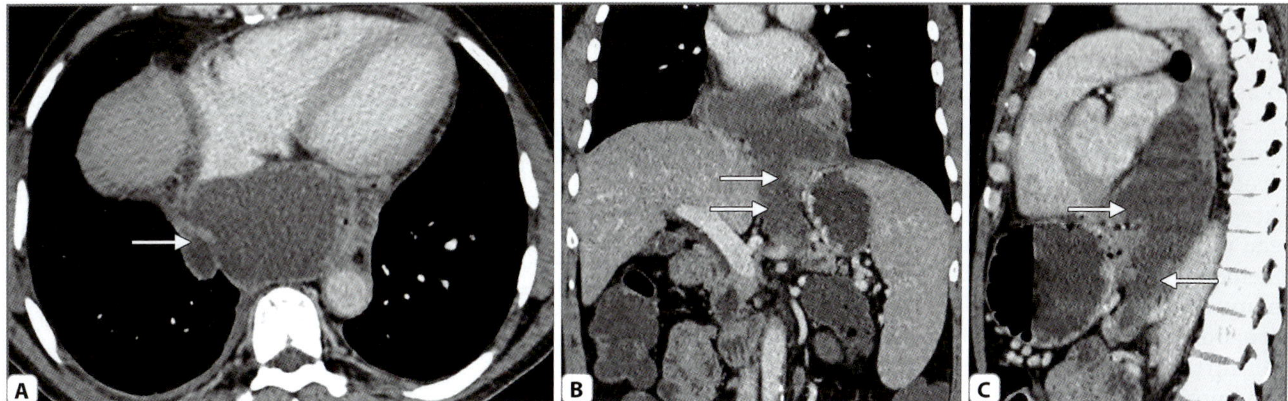

FIGS. 32A TO C: Pancreatitis associated mediastinal collection. CECT axial (A), coronal (B), sagittal (C) showing extension of peripancreatic collection (arrow) into lesser sac and further into the visceral mediastinum across the diaphragm.

calcification (in 85% of cases of focal FM). On CECT, this can appear as a mediastinal mass epicentered in the visceral compartment in the focal type of FM. In the diffuse type, the usual presentation is infiltrating, ill-defined mass **(Figs. 33A and B)**. It encases and causes stenosis of the mediastinal structures, such as tracheobronchial tree, resulting in atelectasis of that segment of the lung, of the pulmonary veins resulting in pulmonary edema, major

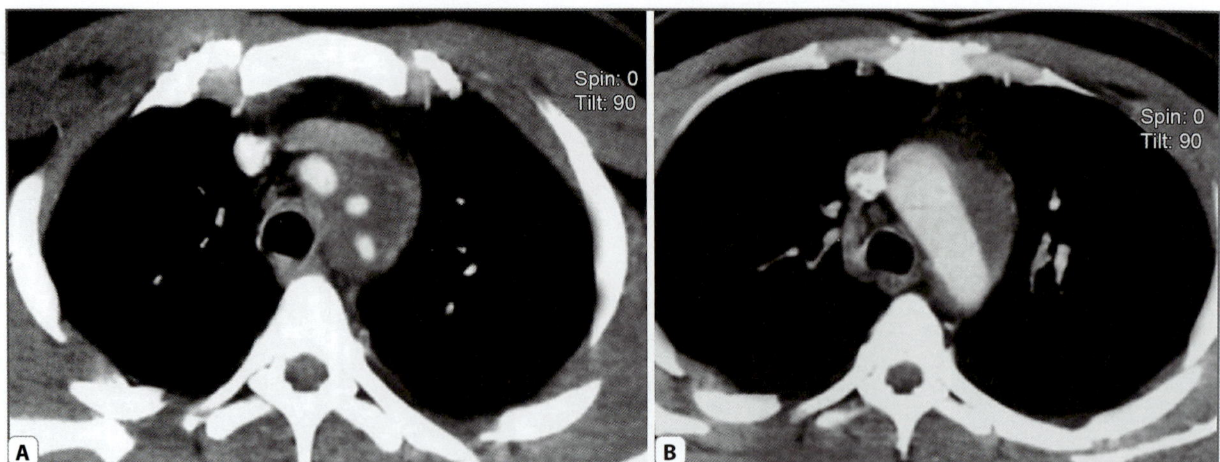

FIGS. 33A AND B: Mediastinal fibrosis. Axial contrast-enhanced computed tomography (CECT) (A and B) showing a plaque-like soft tissue in the mediastinum and encasing brachiocephalic trunk, left common carotid, and left subclavian artery.

branches of the aorta or pulmonary artery, esophagus causing dysphagia, etc. It may even invade the pleura and cause its focal thickening. Calcification may also be seen. They usually respond to corticosteroids, and, at times, may require surgical intervention.

Mediastinitis

This is an acute surgical emergency wherein there is rapid spread of infection resulting in compression of vital structures. It may result from esophageal rupture or spread of infection from the neck or adjoining ribs/ sternum. Patients present with symptoms of sepsis and urgent drainage may be needed to avoid life-threatening complications.

Pneumomediastinum

Any extraluminal air in the mediastinum is referred to as pneumomediastinum, also called by the name of mediastinal emphysema. It can occur due to many causes. The most common cause is rupture of the alveoli as in mucous plugging, mechanical ventilation, excessive coughing or emesis, etc., which can initially lead to pulmonary interstitial emphysema and then to pneumomediastinum. Other causes are tracheobronchial injury, esophageal perforation, tracking of retroperitoneal air or from the neck or chest wall, etc. Pneumomediastinum can further track into various spaces and lead onto pneumothorax, pneumopericardium, pneumorrhachis, pneumoperitoneum, or pneumoretroperitoneum **(Figs. 34A and B)**. On a chest radiograph, pneumomediastinum is marked by lucent streaks or bubbles of gas outlining the mediastinal structures. When it outlines the superior surface of the diaphragm, it seems to separate the heart from the diaphragm, called the "continuous diaphragm sign."[49] When the air outlines the lateral margin of the descending aorta and is seen to extend between parietal pleura and medial left hemidiaphragm, it is called "Naclerio's V sign." Another similar V sign can be seen at the junction of the brachiocephalic veins where the air outlines their superior margins. When this air surrounds the extrapericardial portion of the right pulmonary artery it is called the "ring around the artery sign."

Mediastinal Hematoma

Mediastinal hemorrhage is the collection of blood in the mediastinum as it dissects the fascial planes and extends into the mediastinal fat.[50] can occur due to both traumatic and atraumatic causes. Trauma can lead to vascular injury most commonly involving the aorta or its branches resulting in mediastinal hematoma. Atraumatic causes include underlying coagulopathies or vasculopathies, rupture of aneurysm/pseudoaneurysms, etc. On radiograph, it presents as mediastinal widening.[51] On CT scan, it will appear as a nonenhancing hyperdense mediastinal soft tissue. All the major vessels should be carefully assessed to determine the cause of the hematoma formation. Not only can it lead onto massive blood loss but also produce symptoms due to compression of the vital mediastinal structures. MRI can also be done, which can show mediastinal hematoma of varying signal intensity, depending upon the stage of hematoma. In the early stage, it will be hypointense on T1W and hyperintense on T2W, which in subacute phase will be hyperintense on both T1W and T2W sequences **(Figs. 35A to C)**. In chronic phase, the signal can be variable depending on the degree of conversion from methemoglobin to ferritin and hemosiderin.

APPROACH

A list of commonly encountered differential diagnoses based on the location and imaging features is listed in **Table 8**.

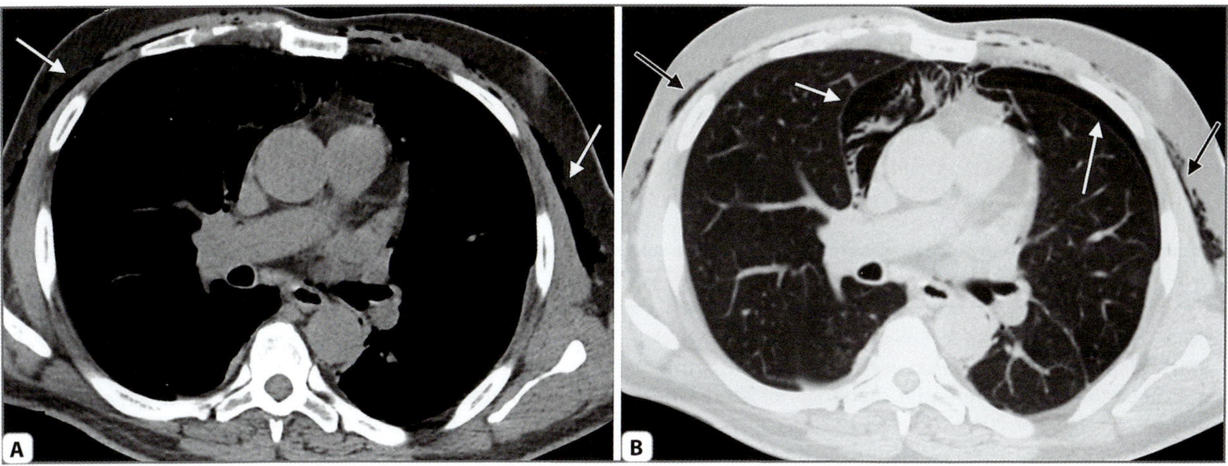

FIGS. 34A AND B: Pneumomediastinum. (A) Axial CT scan in mediastinal window shows air in chest wall (white arrows) suggesting surgical emphysema. Mediastinal air cannot be appreciated; (B) Lung window at the same level shows the pneumomediastinum clearly (white short arrow) along with left pneumothorax (long thin arrow) and surgical emphysema (black arrows).

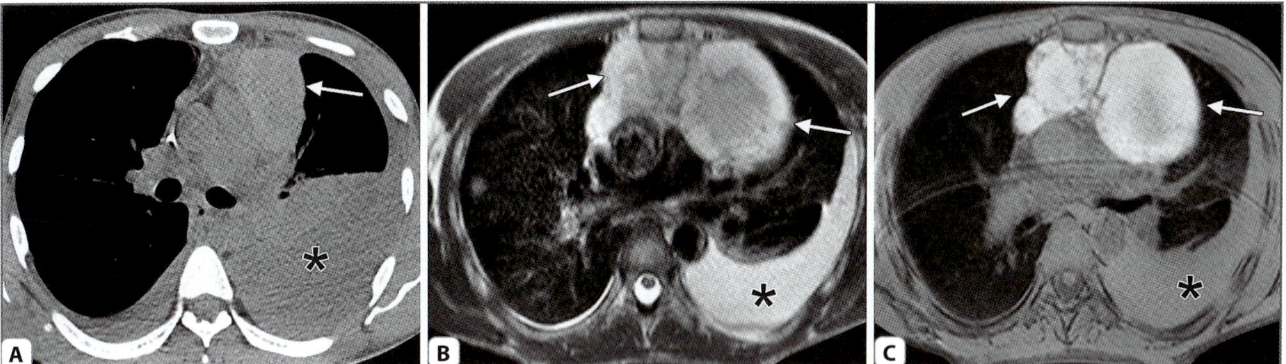

FIGS. 35A TO C: Mediastinal hematoma. (A) Axial noncontrast CT image showing hyperdense hematoma in the anterior mediastinum (arrow) with hyperdense moderate left pleural effusion (asterisk) and mild right effusion; (B and C) Axial T2-weighted (B) and T1-weighted fat saturated (C) MR images showing anterior mediastinal hematoma (arrows) appearing hyperintense on both sequences. Left pleural effusion is noted (asterisk).

(MR: magnetic resonance; T2W: T2-weighted)

TABLE 8: Differential diagnosis of mediastinal lesions based on the location and imaging features.

	Hyperdense/intense CE	Hypodense but enhancing	Hypodense cystic	Fat
Anterior	Thyroid mass extending from neck, thymic carcinoid, CD, ectopic parathyroid adenoma	Thymoma, lymphoma, GCT (Ca)	Thymic and pericardial cysts, cystic thymoma	Thymolipoma, GCT (Ca), fat pads
Middle	Vascular origin (aneurysm/ hematoma)	Lymphadenopathy	Duplication cyst, necrotic nodes	Lipoma
Posterior	Aortic aneurysm, hematoma	Neurogenic tumors (look for foraminal extension)	Neurenteric cyst, meningocele	Extramedullary hematopoiesis (usually bilateral multifocal, may show variable CE)
Multicompart-mental	Hematoma	Lymphoma, venous malformation (phleboliths, progressive CE), infection/ abscess (rim CE)	Lymphatic malformation	Liposarcoma

(Ca: calcification; CD: Castleman disease; CE: contrast enhancement; GCT: germ cell tumor)

CONCLUSION

Imaging plays an important role in the diagnosis and management of mediastinal pathologies. While a chest radiograph is the first investigation, CECT is the workhorse for evaluating these lesions. The three-compartment division proposed by ITMIG should be uniformly followed on CT. Anterior mediastinal masses are much more common than the lesions in other compartments. The radiologist's job is not only to characterize but also stage the lesions, sample them under CT guidance, and assess treatment response.

REFERENCES

1. Nakazono T, Yamaguchi K, Egashira R, Takase Y, Nojiri J, Mizuguchi M, et al. CT-based mediastinal compartment classifications and differential diagnosis of mediastinal tumors. Jpn J Radiol. 2019;37(2):117-34.
2. Carter BW, Benveniste MF, Madan R, Godoy MC, de Groot PM, Truong MT, et al. ITMIG classification of mediastinal compartments and multidisciplinary approach to mediastinal masses. Radiographics. 2017;37(2):413-36.
3. Carter BW, Okumura M, Detterbeck FC, Marom EM. Approaching the patient with an anterior mediastinal mass: a guide for radiologists. J Thorac Oncol. 2014;9(9 Suppl 2):S110-8.
4. Expert Panel on Thoracic Imaging; Ackman JB, Chung JH, Walker CM, Bang TJ, Carter BW, et al. ACR appropriateness criteria® imaging of mediastinal masses. J Am Coll Radiol. 2021;18(5S):S37-51.
5. Ranganath SH, Lee EY, Restrepo R, Eisenberg RL. Mediastinal masses in children. AJR Am J Roentgenol. 2012;198(3): W197-216.
6. Goodman LR. Felson's Principles of Chest Roentgenology: A Programmed Text, 4th edition. Philadelphia: Elsevier Health Sciences; 2014. p. 424.
7. Ko SF, Tsai YH, Huang HY, Ng SH, Fang FM, Tang Y, et al. Retrotracheal thymoma masquerading as esophageal submucosal tumor. World J Gastroenterol. 2005;11(20):3165-6.
8. Orki A, Patlakoglu MS, Tahaoglu C, Kutlu CA. Malignant invasive thymoma in the posterior mediastinum. Ann Thorac Surg. 2009;87(4):1274-5.
9. Restrepo CS, Pandit M, Rojas IC, Villamil MA, Gordillo H, Lemos D, et al. Imaging findings of expansile lesions of the thymus. Curr Probl Diagn Radiol. 2005;34(1):22-34.
10. Detterbeck FC, Nicholson AG, Kondo K, Schil PV, Moran C. The Masaoka–Koga stage classification for thymic malignancies: clarification and definition of terms. J Thorac Oncol. 2011;6(7 Suppl 3):S1710-6.
11. Marx A, Chan JKC, Chalabreysse L, Dacic S, Detterbeck F, French CA, et al. The 2021 WHO classification of tumors of the thymus and mediastinum: what is new in thymic epithelial, germ cell, and mesenchymal tumors? J Thorac Oncol. 2022;17(2):200-13.
12. Ahmad U. The eighth edition TNM stage classification for thymic tumors: what do I need to know? J Thorac Cardiovasc Surg. 2021;161(4):1524-9.
13. Rajamohan N, Goyal A, Kandasamy D, Bhalla AS, Parshad R, Jain D, et al. CT texture analysis in evaluation of thymic tumors and thymic hyperplasia: correlation with the international thymic malignancy interest group (ITMIG) stage and WHO grade. Br J Radiol. 2021;94(1128):20210583.
14. Priola AM, Priola SM, Ciccone G, Evangelista A, Cataldi A, Gned D, et al. Differentiation of rebound and lymphoid thymic hyperplasia from anterior mediastinal tumors with dual-echo chemical-shift MR imaging in adulthood: reliability of the chemical-shift ratio and signal intensity index. Radiology. 2015;274(1):238-49.
15. Rosado-de-Christenson ML, Galobardes J, Moran CA. Thymoma: radiologic-pathologic correlation. Radiographics. 1992;12(1):151-68.
16. Higuchi T, Taki J, Kinuya S, Yamada M, Kawasuji M, Matsui O, et al. Thymic lesions in patients with myasthenia gravis: characterization with thallium 201 scintigraphy. Radiology. 2001;221(1):201-6.
17. Marom EM. Imaging thymoma. J Thorac Oncol. 2010;5(10 Suppl 4):S296-303.
18. Roden AC, Ahmad U, Cardillo G, Girard N, Jain D, Marom EM, et al. Thymic carcinomas–a concise multidisciplinary update on recent developments from the thymic carcinoma working group of the international thymic malignancy interest group. J Thorac Oncol. 2022;17(5):637-50.
19. Gaerte SC, Meyer CA, Winer-Muram HT, Tarver RD, Conces DJ. Fat-containing lesions of the chest. Radiographics. 2002;22 Spec No:S61-78.
20. Molinari F, Bankier AA, Eisenberg RL. Fat-containing lesions in adult thoracic imaging. AJR Am J Roentgenol. 2011;197(5):W795-813.
21. Ackman JB, Verzosa S, Kovach AE, Louissaint A, Lanuti M, Wright CD, et al. High rate of unnecessary thymectomy and its cause. Can computed tomography distinguish thymoma, lymphoma, thymic hyperplasia, and thymic cysts? Eur J Radiol. 2015;84(3):524-33.
22. Albany C, Einhorn LH. Extragonadal germ cell tumors: clinical presentation and management. Curr Opin Oncol. 2013;25(3):261-5.
23. Bokemeyer C, Nichols CR, Droz JP, Schmoll HJ, Horwich A, Gerl A, et al. Extragonadal germ cell tumors of the mediastinum and retroperitoneum: results from an international analysis. J Clin Oncol. 2002;20(7):1864-73.
24. Lewis BD, Hurt RD, Payne WS, Farrow GM, Knapp RH, Muhm JR. Benign teratomas of the mediastinum. J Thorac Cardiovasc Surg. 1983;86(5):727-31.
25. Dhond AP, Agrawal S, Sirmukaddam S, Swapnil V, Srinath S, Roplekar P, et al. Mediastinal teratoma: a case report with review of literature. J Sci Soc. 2016;43(1):57-9.
26. Shameem M, Qaseem SMD, Siddiqui MA, Shah NN, Ahmad A. Mature mediastinal teratoma in adult. Respir Med CME. 2010;3(2):116-7.

27. Knapp RH, Hurt RD, Payne WS, Farrow GM, Lewis BD, Hahn RG, et al. Malignant germ cell tumors of the mediastinum. J Thorac Cardiovasc Surg. 1985;89(1):82-9.
28. Luna MA, Valenzuela-Tamariz J. Germ-cell tumors of the mediastinum, postmortem findings. Am J Clin Pathol. 1976;65(4):450-4.
29. Nichols CR. Mediastinal germ cell tumors. Clinical features and biologic correlates. Chest. 1991;99(2):472-9.
30. Levitt RG, Husband JE, Glazer HS. CT of primary germ-cell tumors of the mediastinum. AJR Am J Roentgenol. 1984;142(1):73-8.
31. Wright CD, Kesler KA, Nichols CR, Mahomed Y, Einhorn LH, Miller ME, et al. Primary mediastinal nonseminomatous germ cell tumors: results of a multimodality approach. J Thoracic Cardiovasc Surg. 1990;99(2):210-7.
32. Pineda V, Cáceres J, Andreu J, Vilar J, Domingo ML. Epipericardial fat necrosis: radiologic diagnosis and follow-up. AJR Am J Roentgenol. 2005;185(5):1234-6.
33. Shahrzad M, Le TSM, Silva M, Bankier AA, Eisenberg RL. Anterior mediastinal masses. AJR Am J Roentgenol. 2014;203(2):W128-38.
34. Zhang ML, Sohani AR. Lymphomas of the mediastinum and their differential diagnosis. Semin Diagn Pathol. 2020;37(4):156-65.
35. Au V, Leung AN. Radiologic manifestations of lymphoma in the thorax. AJR Am J Roentgenol. 1997;168(1):93-8.
36. Kukar M, Platz TA, Schaffner TJ, Elmarzouky R, Groman A, Kumar S, et al. The use of modified four-dimensional computed tomography in patients with primary hyperparathyroidism: an argument for the abandonment of routine sestamibi single-positron emission computed tomography (SPECT). Ann Surg Oncol. 2015;22(1):139-45.
37. Rodgers SE, Hunter GJ, Hamberg LM, Schellingerhout D, Doherty DB, Ayers GD, et al. Improved preoperative planning for directed parathyroidectomy with 4-dimensional computed tomography. Surgery. 2006;140(6):932-40.
38. Ueno S, Fujino A, Morikawa Y, Iwanaka T, Kinoshita Y, Ozeki M, et al. Treatment of mediastinal lymphatic malformation in children: an analysis of a nationwide survey in Japan. Surg Today. 2018;48(7):716-25.
39. White CL, Olivieri B, Restrepo R, McKeon B, Karakas SP, Lee EY. Low-flow vascular malformation pitfalls: from clinical examination to practical imaging evaluation--part 1, lymphatic malformation mimickers. AJR Am J Roentgenol. 2016;206(5):940-51.
40. Kligerman SJ, Auerbach A, Franks TJ, Galvin JR. Castleman disease of the thorax: clinical, radiologic, and pathologic correlation: from the radiologic pathology archives. Radiographics. 2016;36(5):1309-32.
41. Jeung MY, Gasser B, Gangi A, Bogorin A, Charneau D, Wihlm JM, et al. Imaging of cystic masses of the mediastinum. Radiographics. 2002;22 Spec No:S79-93.
42. McCarthy A, Mohan S, Saeed A, Kumaran M. Mediastinal lymphadenopathy, a review of nodal anatomy, pathology and sampling techniques. Imaging. 2014;23(1):20120003.
43. Kelley MJ, Mannes EJ, Ravin CE. Mediastinal masses of vascular origin. A review. J Thorac Cardiovasc Surg. 1978;76(4):559-72.
44. Carter BW, de Groot PM, Godoy MCB, Marom EM, Wu CC. Imaging of the mediastinum: vascular lesions as a potential pitfall. Semin Roentgenol. 2015;50(3):241-50.
45. Wong PS, Goldstraw P. Left superior vena cava: a pitfall in computed tomographic diagnosis with surgical implications. Ann Thorac Surg. 1990;50(4):656-7.
46. Strollo DC, Rosado-de-Christenson ML, Jett JR. Primary mediastinal tumors: part II. Tumors of the middle and posterior mediastinum. Chest. 1997;112(5):1344-57.
47. Nakazono T, White CS, Yamasaki F, Yamaguchi K, Egashira R, Irie H, et al. MRI findings of mediastinal neurogenic tumors. AJR Am J Roentgenol. 2011;197(4):W643-52.
48. Garrana SH, Buckley JR, Rosado-de-Christenson ML, Martínez-Jiménez S, Muñoz P, Borsa JJ. Multimodality imaging of focal and diffuse fibrosing mediastinitis. Radiographics. 2019;39(3):651-67.
49. Bejvan SM, Godwin JD. Pneumomediastinum: old signs and new signs. AJR Am J Roentgenol. 1996;166(5):1041-8.
50. Hammer PM, Schwab CW. Mediastinal hematoma. In: Vincent JL, Hall JB (Eds). Encyclopedia of Intensive Care Medicine. Berlin: Springer; 2012. pp. 1367-71.
51. Li X, Liu L, Cao D, Sun Y. Spontaneous hematoma of posterior mediastinum with an uncommon cause: a case report and review of the literature. Clin Pract. 2016;6(1):838.

Sapna Singh, Anjali Prakash, Jyoti Kumar

CHAPTER

12

Imaging of Solitary Pulmonary Nodule

INTRODUCTION

According to "Fleischner Society Glossary of Terms for Thoracic Imaging 2024", a solitary pulmonary nodule (SPN) is defined as a circumscribed, typically round opacity, ≤30 mm in average diameter **(Figs. 1A and B)**. A rounded lesion > 30 mm is called a mass and a rounded lesion <6 mm in diameter is called a micronodule[1]. SPN is seen in about 0.2% of chest radiographs with a marked increase in its prevalence following the advent of chest CT **(Figs. 2A and B)**.[2]

Differentiation between benign and malignant SPNs forms the goal of imaging. This differentiation is important because lung cancer is the leading cause of cancer-related deaths with an overall mortality rate of 18.7%[3] and about 12.4 %[4] of SPN discovered in routine chest CT are malignant.

SPURIOUS SOLITARY PULMONARY NODULE

Pleural based and chest wall lesions, nipple shadow, skin nodules like neurofibroma, artifacts may be the causes of spurious SPNs, however, oblique views, repeat radiographs or even CT at times may help to differentiate these from a true SPN **(Figs. 3A to C)**.

MORPHOLOGICAL CHARACTERISTICS OF SPN

Of the malignant lesions, adenocarcinoma is the most common carcinoma to give rise to a SPN though all the histological types may present as intrapulmonary nodules.[5,6]

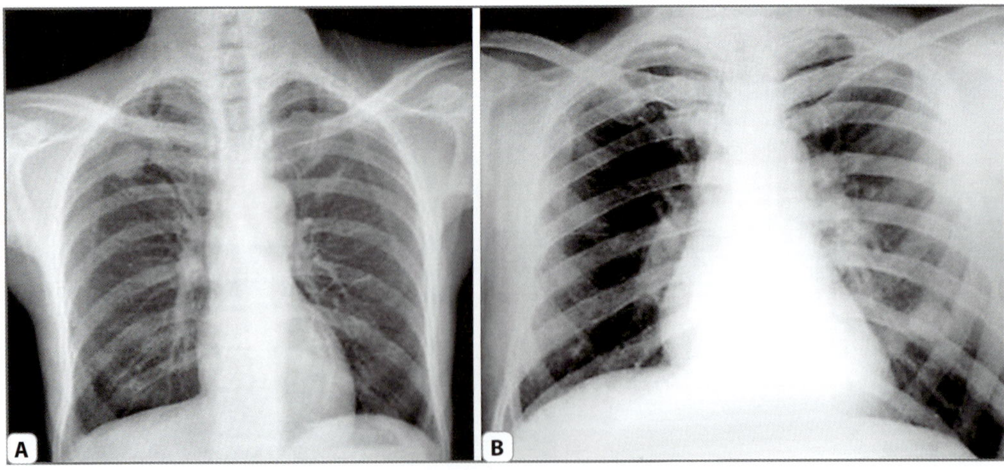

FIGS. 1A AND B: Chest radiographs in two patients showing a circumscribed typically round opacity < 30 mm in average diameter in the right upper zone in one (A) and in the left lower zone in the other; (B) Solitary pulmonary nodules.

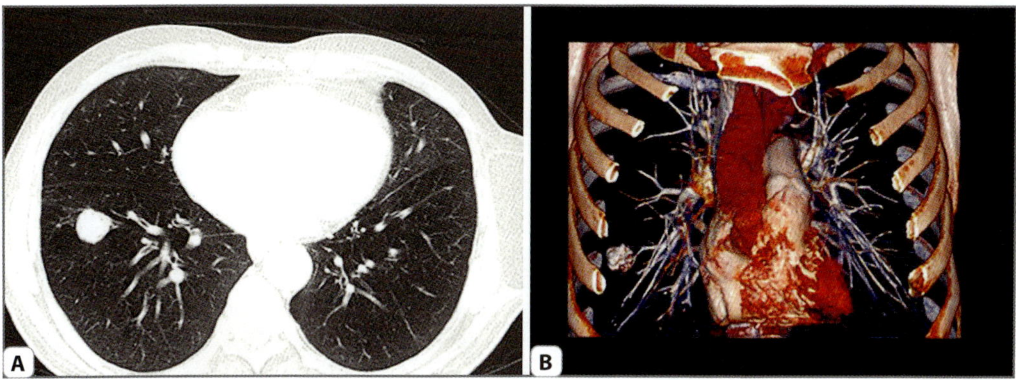

FIGS. 2A AND B: CT scan (A) in patient with suspected pulmonary embolism reveals an incidental solitary pulmonary nodule (SPN) in the right lower lobe. VRT pulmonary angiogram image (B) showing the normal vasculature with the nodule in the lower lobe.

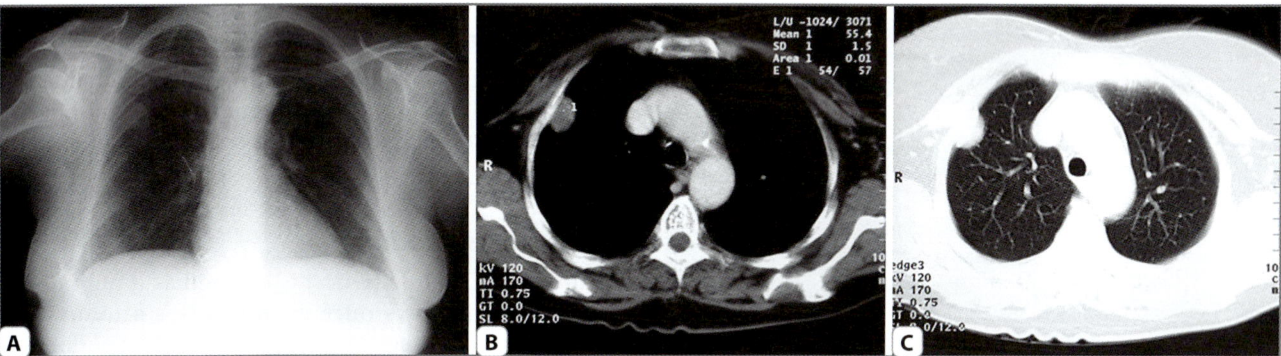

FIGS. 3A TO C: Chest radiograph (A) revealing a solitary nodule in the right lung. CT mediastinal window (B) and lung parenchymal window settings (C) reveal the lesion to be clearly pleural based—a case of pleural fibroma mimicking solitary pulmonary nodule (SPN).

Of the benign nodules, granulomas and intrapulmonary lymph nodes account for 80% while hamartomas account for about 10% of the nodules.[6]

Morphological characteristics of the nodule such as shape, margin, attenuation, structure and location help to describe and characterize pulmonary nodules.

Shape and Margin

A nodule can have a round, ovoid or polygonal shape and can have spherical, flat or elongated configuration, depending upon its appearance in different imaging planes.[1] Owing to its interface with surrounding lung, a nodule can have smooth/well-defined or irregular/ill-defined margin. A smooth nodule margin is even and free of substantial protrusions or indentations **(Figs. 4A and B)**. An irregular nodule margin can be lobulated (showing lobule-like protrusions) and/or spiculated (showing multiple radiating small sharp projections). Malignant lesions often show irregularity, spiculation and lobulation **(Fig. 5)**. The presence of spiculation is a strong predictor of malignancy. A radial extension of malignant cells, along the interlobular septa, lymphatics, small airways or blood vessels is the cause for the spiculation and has been likened to the spokes of a wheel or "corona radiata" or "corona maligna" or the "sunburst appearance" **(Fig. 6)**.[7-9] In patients with adenocarcinoma and adenocarcinoma in situ (bronchioloalveolar carcinoma) it reflects the presence of fibrosis surrounding the tumor.[10] The fibrosis usually reflects a desmoplastic reaction and not a preexisting lung fibrosis. Carcinoma can show the presence of a "pleural tail" or a "pleural tag" in which a thin linear opacity is seen extending from the edge of the lung nodule to the pleural surface. The presence of spiculation is more indicative of the lesion being malignant rather than pleural tail as pleural tail may also be seen with lesions which are benign such as granulomatous disease like tuberculosis.[11,12]

Attenuation and Structure

Nodules have been classified as solid, part-solid and ground-glass based on their attenuation. Use of thick sections precludes accurate nodule characterization due to volume averaging.[1]

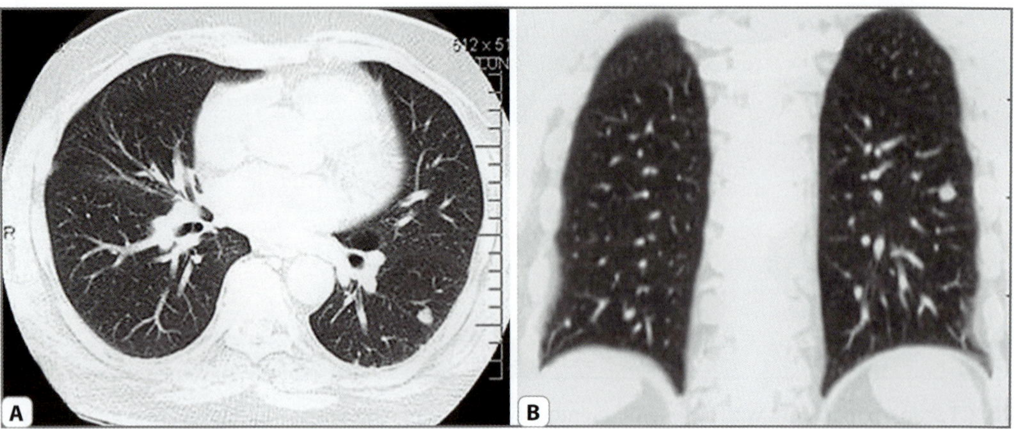

FIGS. 4A AND B: Chest CT scans showing a well-defined smooth marginated, rounded nodule in the left lower lobe with no evidence of calcification/cavitation likely—benign SPN/granuloma.

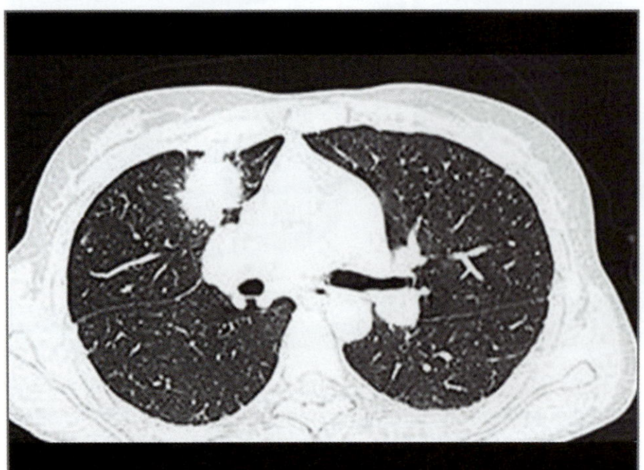

FIG. 5: CT scan showing a nodule in the right upper lobe. The nodule shows lobulations and evidence of notching. Edge irregularity and spiculation is clearly seen.

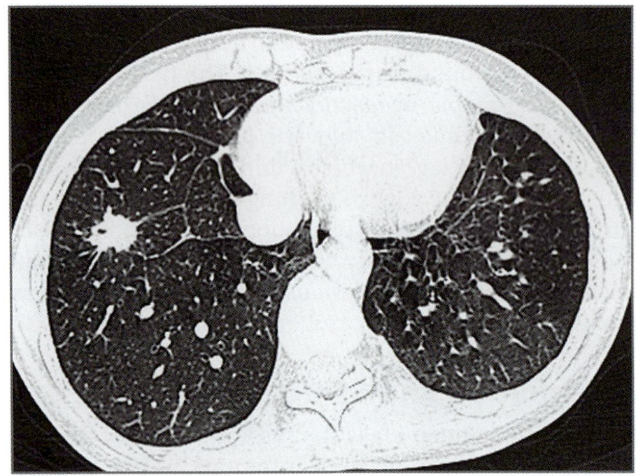

FIG. 6: CT chest showing a nodule in the right upper lobe with irregular, spiculated margins termed the "sunburst appearance" or corona radiata. Multiple pleural tails are seen extending from the mass to the pleural surface. A small eccentric cavitation is noted—bronchogenic carcinoma.

Solid Nodule

Pulmonary nodules which show pure soft tissue attenuation are called solid nodules. This is the commonest type but less malignant as compared to the part-solid and ground-glass nodules.[13,14]

Ground-glass Nodule

Ground-glass nodule (GGN) is defined as a pulmonary nodule which shows pure ground-glass attenuation. Contiguous thin CT sections (1 mm) should be performed to establish lesions as true GGNs whenever possible to avoid the pitfall of interpreting them as solid or part-solid nodules (PSNs).[15]

Part-solid Nodules

This term is used for nodules showing both ground-glass and soft tissue attenuation **(Figs. 7A and B)**. It is important to know the percentage of ground-glass versus solid components of part-solid lesions as ground-glass components conform to lepidic growth pattern and solid component represents an invasive growth pattern.

Based on their structure, nodules can be described as simple or complex. Nodules with a single structural component (soft tissue, ground-glass, fat, calcium) are termed as simple nodules while those with more than one structural components (soft tissue, ground-glass, fat, calcium, air) are termed as complex nodules. Simple nodules can evolve into complex ones and vice versa.

Calcification

Calcification is an important imaging feature that can be used to distinguish between benign and malignant SPNs.

Calcification in a Benign Nodule (Figs. 8A to D)

- Concentric rings of calcification (target calcification)
- Conglomerate foci of calcification involving a large part of the nodule (popcorn calcification)

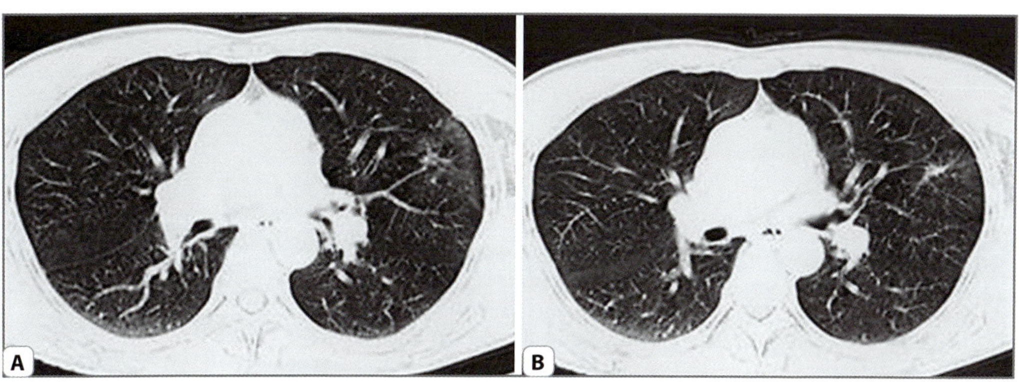

FIGS. 7A AND B: CT scans show an ill-defined central nodule along with ground glass attenuation: part-solid nodule.

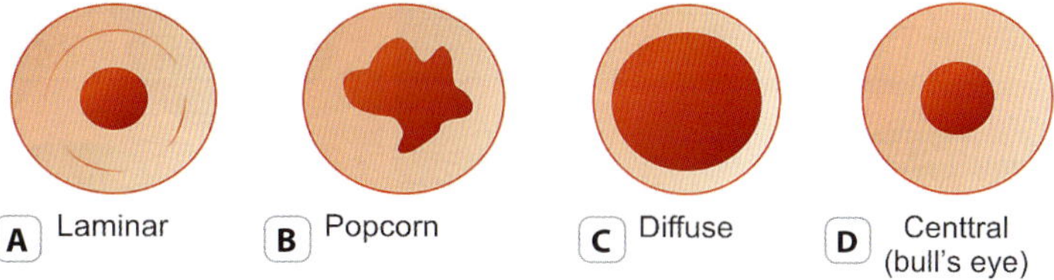

FIGS. 8A TO D: Calcification in benign module.

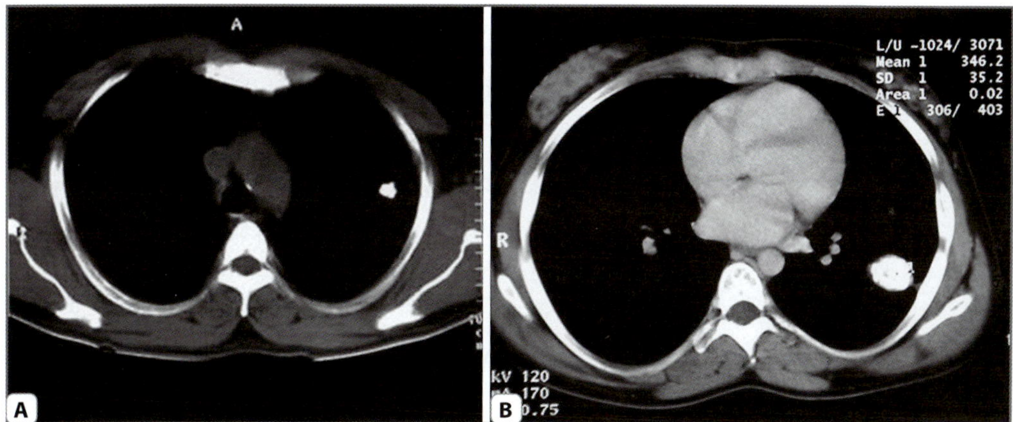

FIGS. 9A AND B: CT scans showing uniform homogeneous calcification in two cases of tuberculomas.

- Homogenous calcification/uniform calcification
- Dense central (bull's eye) calcification.

When any of these patterns is seen, the probability of the lesion being benign is almost 100%[16] **(Figs. 9A and B)**. Popcorn calcification is virtually diagnostic of cartilage containing tumors like hamartomas **(Figs. 10A to C)**. Concentric (laminated) and uniform calcifications are suggestive of a calcified tuberculous or fungal granuloma.

Indeterminate Calcification

Eccentric calcification may be seen in a benign lesion which gets calcified in an eccentric fashion or when a benign calcified lesion is engulfed by a malignant lesion. Stippled/punctate calcification may be seen in both benign and malignant lesions and is thus classified as indeterminate.[17]

Calcification in a Malignant Nodule

A malignant nodule may show calcification which is diffuse and amorphous or psammomatous (in case of metastasis from mucin secreting tumors from the colon or ovary) or dystrophic (in areas of tumor necrosis).[17,18] Centrally located calcification in a spiculated SPN also suggests malignancy.[19]

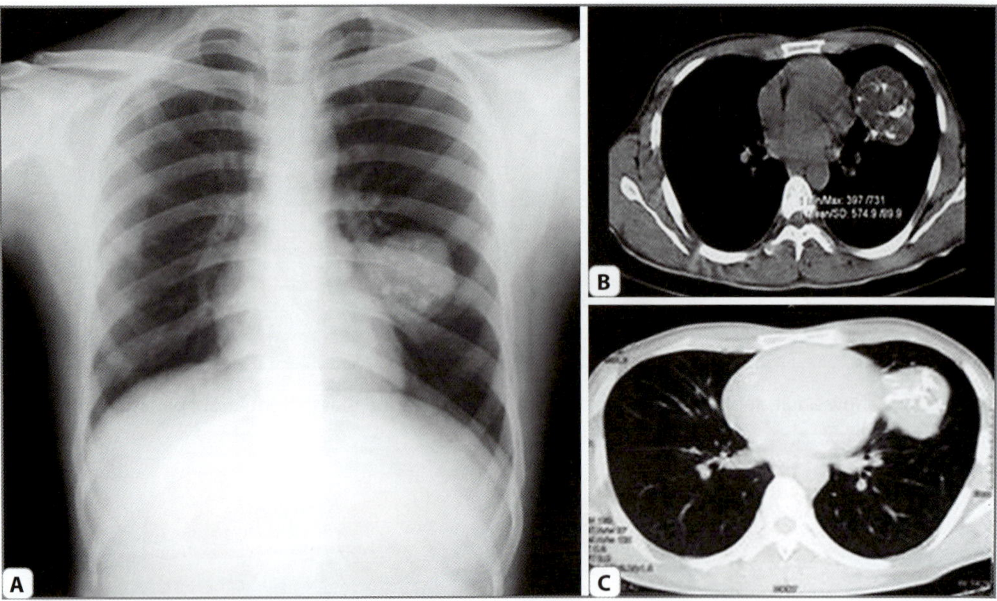

FIGS. 10A TO C: Chest radiograph (A) showing a large solitary nodule in the left lung with dense nodular foci of calcification within suggestive of characteristic popcorn calcification/central cartilage calcification. Non-contrast CT scan mediastinal window; (B) showing a 3 × 3 cm nodule containing overlapping, randomly distributed small rings of calcification or the popcorn calcification and lung parenchymal window settings; (C) reveal the nodule to be round in shape and sharply marginated—pulmonary hamartoma.

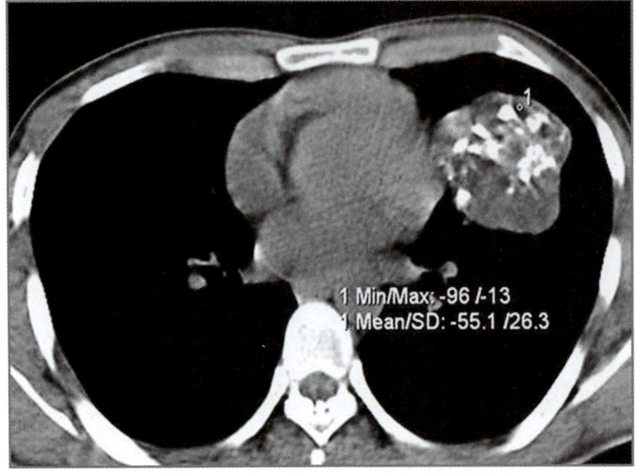

FIG. 11: Non-contrast CT scan showing foci of fat or negative attenuation (–50 to –100 HU) within the nodule in the left lung consistent with pulmonary hamartoma.

Fat

The presence of fat (-40 to -120 HU) within a lesion is virtually diagnostic of a hamartoma **(Fig. 11)**. Other lesions that may show fat include lipoid pneumonia, lipoma and metastatic liposarcoma.[20]

Cavitation

Both benign and malignant SPNs can cavitate. A thick irregular cavity with wall thickness >16 mm is likely to be malignant. About 95% of the nodules with wall thickness < 5 mm are benign.[21] About 75% of the cavities with wall thickness 5-15 mm are benign. Cavitation usually occurs in squamous cell carcinoma, large cell carcinoma and adenocarcinoma while small cell cancers rarely show cavitation.

Association of Nodule Attenuation with Adenocarcinoma

Adenocarcinoma which accounts for about 50% of all lung cancers presents more commonly as a solitary part-solid nodule than the other histologic types of carcinoma. According to the IASLC (International Association for the Study of Lung Cancer), ATS (American Thoracic Society) and European Respiratory Society (ERS), adenocarcinomas can be classified as preinvasive and invasive.[22] Preinvasive lesions comprise atypical adenomatous hyperplasia (AAH) and adenocarcinoma in situ (AIS). These are lesions which typically exhibit growth along the alveolar surface called lepidic growth.[23] Atypical adenomatous hyperplasia (AAH) is a lesion which is purely ground glass in attenuation and usually < 1 cm in size.[24] Adenocarcinoma in situ (AIS) is a lesion with ground glass attenuation and < 3 cm in size. The invasive lesions include minimally invasive carcinoma (MIC) and invasive adenocarcinoma. MIC is defined as a lesion that shows a predominant lepidic growth with no necrosis, no lymphatic, vascular or pleural invasion, is < 3 cm in size with an invasive component not > 5 mm in any location.[22,23] MIA may be seen as ground glass nodule (GGN) or PSN on CT.[25] Classification of invasive adenocarcinoma as having a lepidic, acinar, papillary, micropapillary or solid pattern is based on the histological features. The MIA, AIS and lepidic forms may have both mucinous and non-mucinous forms **(Table 1)**. The term bronchioloalveolar carcinoma is now an obsolete term and should be called adenocarcinoma in situ.[26,27]

The solid component of a PSN is important as it predicts the prognosis of the patient, the solid component representing the invasive foci of adenocarcinoma. A direct correlation has been reported between the presence of a solid component, the size of the solid component and increasing attenuation with the invasiveness or aggressiveness of a PSN.[26,27] The higher the attenuation value of the PSN, the greater the degree of invasion.

Location

According to "Fleischner Society Glossary of Terms for Thoracic Imaging 2024", nodules located in the center of secondary pulmonary lobule are called centrilobular nodules while those distributed along the bronchovascular bundles are termed as peribronchovascular nodules.[1] The nodules arising from the fissure are called "fissural nodules" while those in contact with fissure and not arising from it are called "perifissural nodules". Similarly, nodules arising from the pleura are called "pleural nodules" while those in contact with pleura and not arising from it are called "pleural-based nodules". "Subpleural nodules" are the ones located in close proximity to the pleura but not in contact with the same. Since, the term subpleural is variably used in literature, term "peripheral" is preferred for these nodules. Also, the prefix *juxta-* is inconsistently used to represent nodules around fissure and pleura therefore, its usage should be avoided.

TABLE 1: Correlation of the histological patterns with CT features of part-solid nodules (PSNs).[22,23]

2011 IASLC, ATS and ERS classification	CT features
• Atypical adenomatous hyperplasia (AAH)	• Ground-glass nodule (GGN)
• Adenocarcinoma in situ (AIS)	• GGN with a possible solid component
• Minimally invasive adenocarcinoma (MIA)	• GGN, PSN
• Lepidic predominant adenocarcinoma	• PSN, solid nodule
• Invasive adenocarcinoma	• PSN with a solid component, solid nodule

About 70% of lung cancers are located in the right upper lobe, the right lung being a more common site for malignancy than the left lung.[28-30] While squamous cell carcinoma is more likely to be centrally located, adenocarcinoma is usually peripheral in location **(Figs. 12A to C)**.[31] Metastatic lesions usually involve the outer one third and bases of the lungs. Location, however, cannot be used as an independent predictor of malignancy because benign nodules are equally distributed throughout the upper and lower lobes.[32]

Size of Solitary Pulmonary Nodule

The larger the lesion, the more likely it is to be malignant. For a SPN to be detected on chest radiographs, it should be at least 9 mm in diameter while CT detects smaller lesions.[33] Lung cancer screening trials show mean probability of cancer in nodules 5–10 mm in diameter to be ~1.3%.[34] Though a very small lesion can turn out to be malignant, lesions >3 cm in diameter are more likely to be malignant while those <1 cm are usually benign **(Figs. 13A and B)**.[35,36]

It is essential to measure the nodules accurately for following reasons: (a) determination of risk of malignancy at baseline CT, (b) appropriate allocation of patients to management algorithm, (c) detection of change in follow-up imaging.

To avoid inter-observer or even intra-observer variability in nodule measurement, the Fleischner Society has formulated recommendations for manual measurement of nodule diameter by utilizing contiguously reconstructed sections having thickness <1.5 mm acquired at full inspiration.[37,38]

- The size of small nodules (<10 mm) must be conveyed as the average of both maximal long-axis and perpendicular

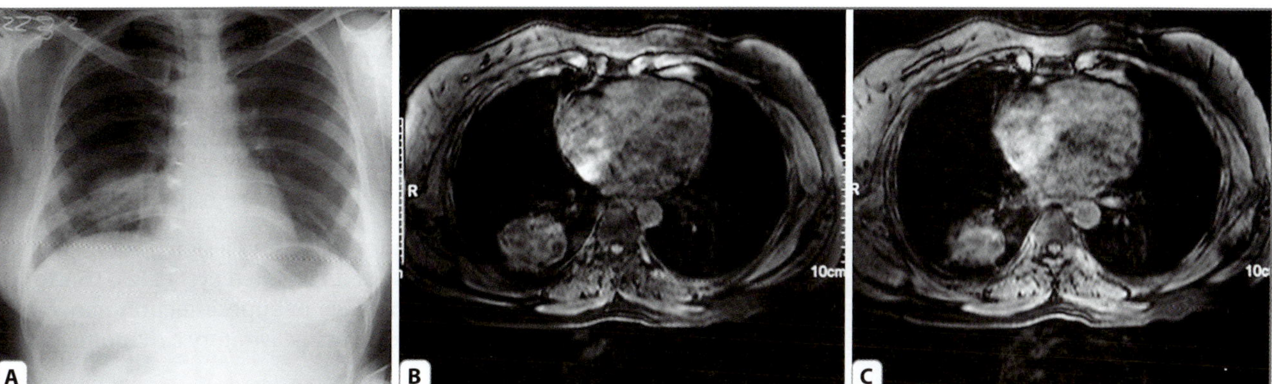

FIGS. 12A TO C: Chest radiograph (A) showing a solitary nodule in the right lower lobe. MR images in the same case (B and C) showing the large nodule in the right lung, it has irregular and spiculated margins—Adenocarcinoma manifesting as a peripheral solitary pulmonary nodule (SPN).

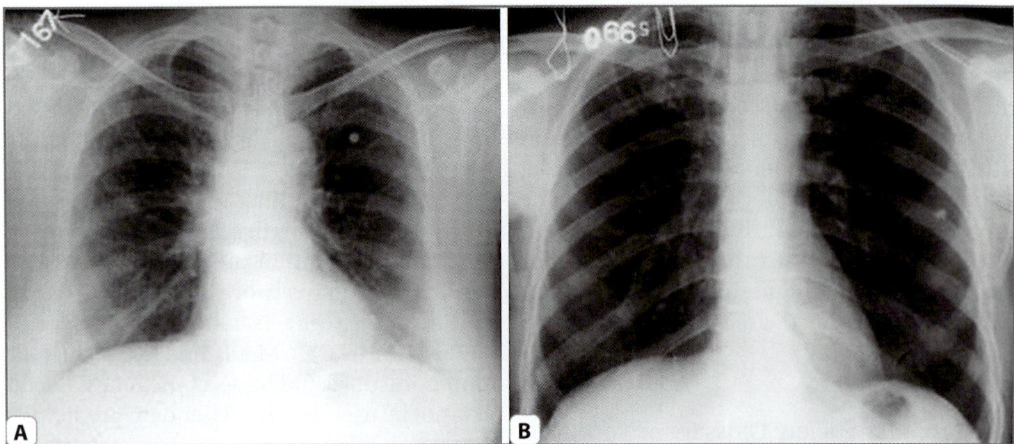

FIGS. 13A AND B: Chest radiographs in two cases showing well-defined nodules < 1 cm clearly seen on plain radiographs due to being calcified—benign SPNs/calcified granulomas.

short-axis measurements in the same plane. For larger nodules (>10 mm) and masses both long- and short-axis measurements should be recorded.

- All the measurements must be given to the nearest whole millimeter.
- For nodules <3 mm in size no measurement to be recorded due to accuracy limitations and they must be reported as micronodules.
- For smaller (<10 mm) PSNs, the average of long- and short-axis dimensions including the ground-glass and any cystic component must be reported and for larger nodules both long and short axis dimensions must be reported.
- If the maximum diameter of solid component measures >3 mm in PSN, the dimensions of both solid and nonsolid components must be reported.
- All measurements must be carried out in axial plane, except for the nodule whose maximal dimension lies in coronal or sagittal plane.
- For small (<10 mm) nodules, the measurements must be performed using high-spatial-frequency (sharp) filter while for larger nodules any reconstruction algorithm will suffice. For evaluation of change in nodule density, soft-tissue window should be utilized.[37]

OTHER CHARACTERISTICS OF SPN

Presence of a Halo

Ground-glass opacity surrounding the nodule gives a "halo sign" to the nodule.[39] This peripheral non-solid component surrounding a nodule should not be confused with corona radiata.

Halo sign is seen in:[40]

- Invasive aspergillosis
- Adenocarcinoma
- Adenocarcinoma in situ (formerly Bronchioloalveolar carcinoma)
- Pulmonary hemorrhage

In lesions such as aspergillosis, the halo sign represents hemorrhage, while in malignancies it represents the lepidic spread of tumor.

Air Bronchiolograms and Pseudocavitation

Air bronchiologram or bubble like lucencies or pseudocavitation may simulate cavities and are more commonly seen in malignant nodules (29%) than in benign nodules (6%).[41-43] Pseudocavitation results from sparing of alveoli and bronchi by tumor infiltration in malignant lesions.

Air Crescent Sign

An "air crescent" or "air meniscus" sign results from a peripheral halo of air between the intracavitatory mass and the cavity wall **(Figs. 14A and B)**. The commonest cause is a fungal ball, i.e., aspergilloma/mycetoma. Other causes include blood clot in a cavity, cavitatory carcinoma, complicated hydatid disease, Rasmussen's aneurysm, mucous plug in bronchiectasis and pulmonary gangrene.

Air-fluid Level

Presence of an air-fluid level within a lesion favors benignity such as a lung abscess or an infected cyst **(Figs. 15A to C)**. Intracavitatory hemorrhage or superinfection may rarely give rise to an air fluid level in cavitatory carcinoma.

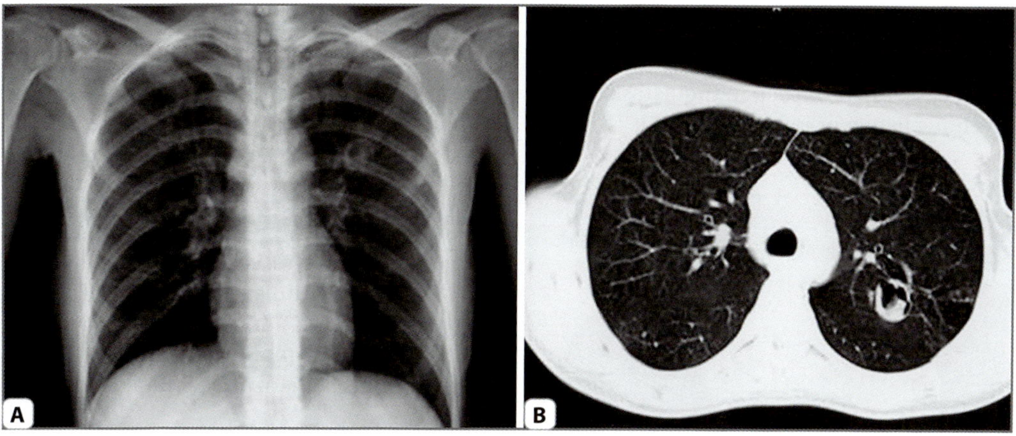

FIGS. 14A AND B: Chest radiograph (A) showing a small solitary lesion in the left upper lobe with a crescent of air between the intracavitatory mass and the cavity wall giving rise to the "air crescent" or air meniscus sign. CT scan (B) showing the same—aspergilloma/ mycetoma.

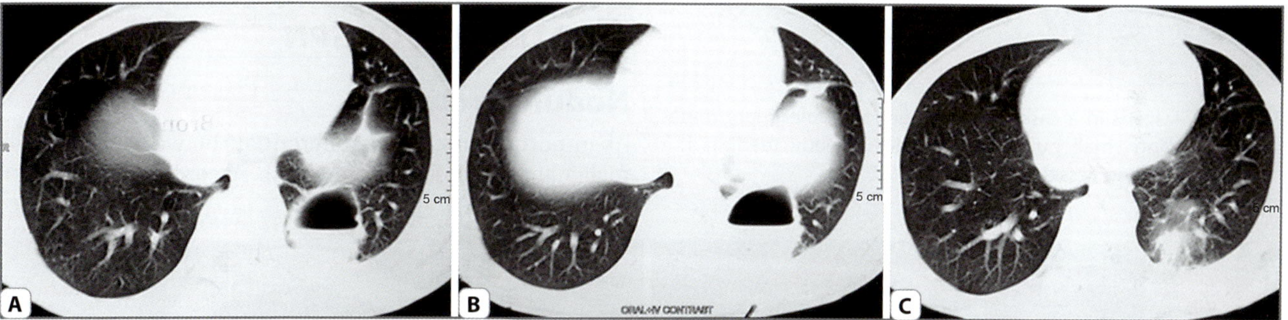

FIGS. 15A TO C: CT scans in a case showing a well-defined cavity with an air-fluid level with wall thickness < 5 mm and surrounding consolidation—lung abscess.

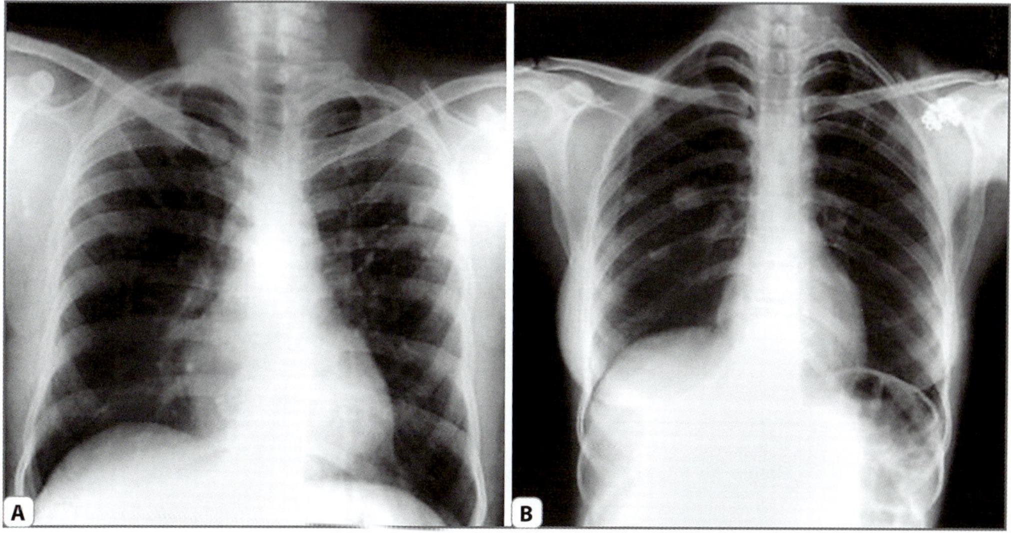

FIGS. 16A AND B: Chest radiograph in two cases showing a calcified tuberculoma with multiple small nodules adjacent to it in the left lung in one case (A) and the right lung in the other; (B) Satellite nodules predicting a benign disease.

Satellite Nodules

The presence of small nodules adjacent to a large nodule or mass favors a benign lesion such as tuberculosis and sarcoidosis. A cluster of small nodules seen within a segment or subsegment of the lung, 3–15 mm in diameter usually indicates a granulomatous process **(Figs. 16A and B)**. In sarcoidosis, the term "galaxy-sign" refers to the presence of multiple satellite nodules.

Feeding Vessel Sign

This refers to a small pulmonary artery directly leading to a nodule. A "feeding vessel sign" is seen in metastasis, septic emboli, arteriovenous fistula or infarct **(Fig. 17)**.[44,45]

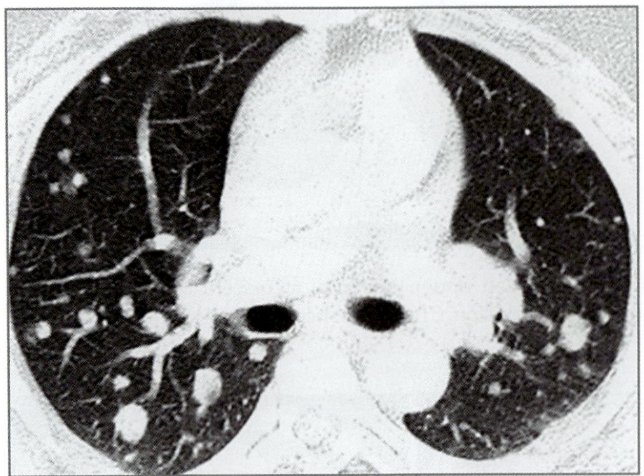

FIG. 17: CT scans in a case of hematogenous pulmonary metastases showing small pulmonary arteries directly feeding the nodules—"feeding vessel sign".

Positive Bronchus Sign

When a bronchial carcinoma infiltrates around but does not occlude an adjacent bronchus it gives rise to a "positive bronchus sign".[46] This is seen as a patent bronchus entering the nodule **(Figs. 18A and B)**.

Vascular Convergence Sign

The convergence of vessels toward the nodule without contacting the nodule margin is termed as "vascular convergence sign" and is seen predominantly in peripheral part-solid malignant lung nodules. Its presence suggests neovascularization which is a feature of malignant nodules.[47]

The morphological characteristics of SPN are summarized in the form of flowchart **(Flowchart 1)**.

ASSESSMENT OF MALIGNANT POTENTIAL OF SPN

Nodule Growth

An important criterion to differentiate between benign and malignant nodules is nodule growth. According to Fleischner

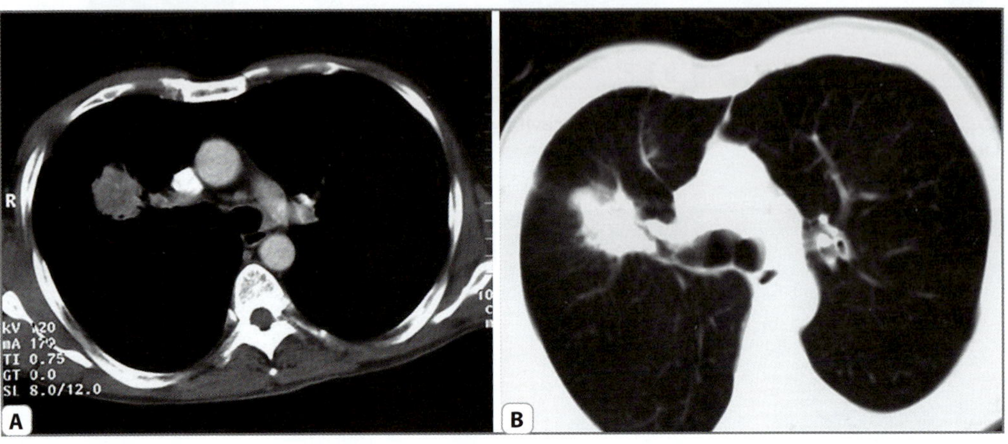

FIGS. 18A AND B: CT scan of the chest showing a pulmonary lesion abutting and narrowing the right upper lobe bronchus without completely occluding it—the positive bronchus sign in bronchogenic carcinoma.

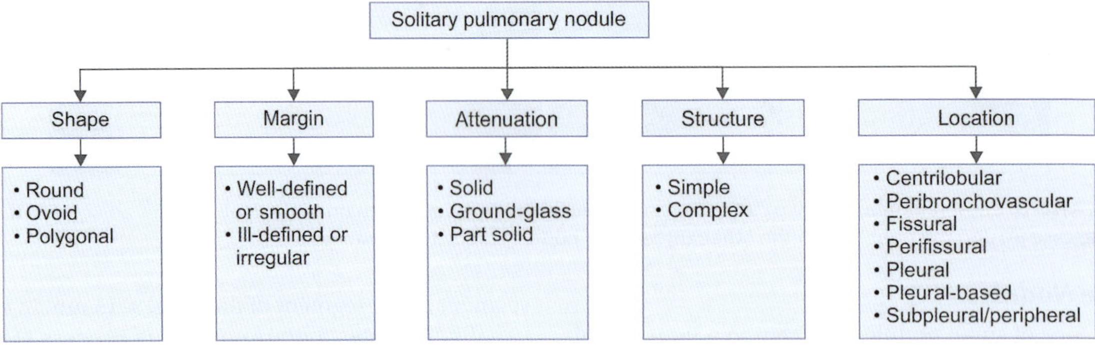

FLOWCHART 1: Flowchart for the evaluation of a solitary pulmonary nodule (SPN).

Society recommendations for nodule measurement, determination of change in size of pulmonary nodule must be ascertained if its average diameter has increased or decreased by at least 2 mm. Change in size smaller than this can reflect spurious measurement especially for ill-defined nodules.[37] Nodule growth is also assessed by volume doubling time (VDT) defined as the time in which the volume of a nodule becomes double. As the most common shape is spherical, the volume is calculated using the equation $4\pi r^3$. A 26% increase in diameter is taken as a doubling in volume based on:

$$VDT = [t \times \log 2]/\log (V_t/ V_o)$$

Where, V_o is the initial volume and V_t is the volume at time t.[48]

This formula is based on an exponential model of nodule growth, i.e, a 5-mm nodule will reach a diameter of 20.3 mm in 12 months if the doubling time (DT) is 60 days but will reach a diameter of only 7.1 mm in 12 months if the doubling time is 240 days. Also, the 26% increase in axial diameter taken as the volume doubling time is difficult to assess in case of nodules ≤ 5 mm in size because 5 mm nodule which doubles its volume increases in diameter by 1.25 mm only.[49] It has been seen that two-dimensional measurements obtained with electronic calipers are unreliable as compared to the three-dimensional measurements.

The volume doubling time (VDT) of a nodule decides the frequency of follow-up imaging and is dependent upon the nodule attenuation and presumed histology.[50] The radiologic pathologic correlation of part-solid and pure ground glass nodule with the histologic spectrum of adenocarcinoma has been described.[51] For solid nodules, volume doubling time has been reported between 100 and 400 days which suggests that detectable growth must be seen between 1 and 2 years of follow-up imaging. Part-solid nodules and ground-glass nodules have a longer volume doubling time ranging from 300 to 450 days and 600 to 900 days respectively, requiring a longer interval between follow-up imaging and longer duration of follow-up imaging. Carcinoids and adenocarcinomas in situ may remain stable for >2 years. Therefore, the dictum that 2-year stability indicates a benign process should be used with caution.[52] NELSON lung cancer screening trial revealed that VDT of 400 days or less, 400–600 days and >600 days corroborates with lung cancer risk of 9.9%, 4.0% and 0.8% respectively.[53]

Three-Dimensional Volume Quantification

Three-dimensional volume quantification utilizes the entire CT data to calculate nodule volume **(Figs. 19A and B)**.[54] Volume quantification method is able to detect smaller differences in nodule size than the two-dimensional method. In order to separate/segment out the nodules from the lung parenchyma, threshold method is used, which takes into account the voxel attenuation above and below a particular threshold as nodule or parenchyma.[54,55] It is important to include the ground glass component of a PSN in volume determination as ground glass component has a high incidence of malignancy.[56] In the case of PSN, growth may occur in the form of an increase in size, an increase in attenuation, appearance of a solid component or increase in the size of the solid component. For optimal CT evaluation of part-solid pulmonary nodules, it is essential to obtain thin section CT.[57] Measurement of attenuation values on serial CT examinations is less variable than measurements of volume and diameter.[58] For these nodules, an increase in mass is calculated which is the product of mean volume and attenuation.

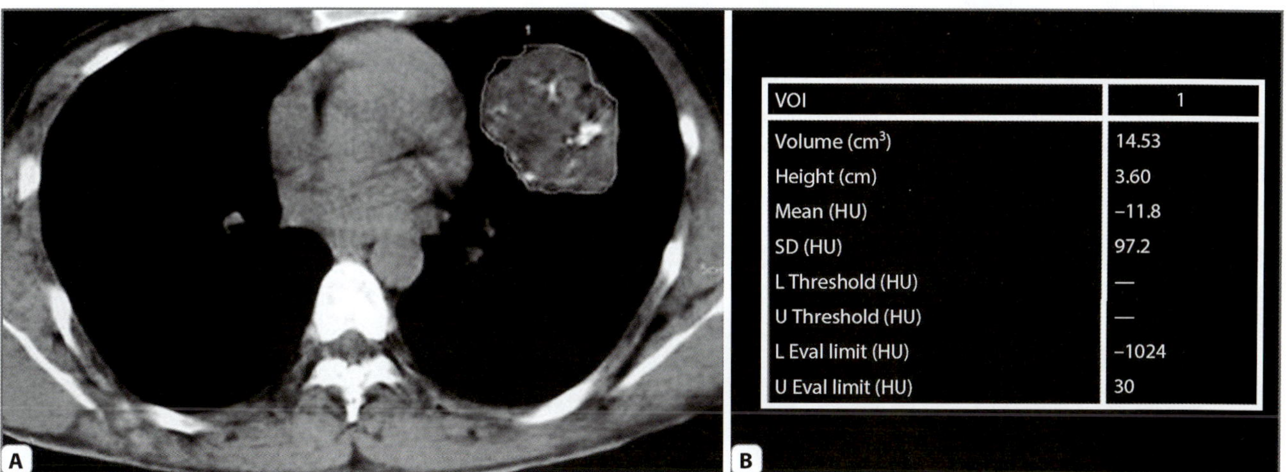

FIGS. 19A AND B: Measurement of volume in a case of pulmonary hamartoma. The volume of the nodule is measured on each axial section and then summed to obtain the total nodule volume (B).

Nodule Enhancement

Dynamic contrast enhanced computed tomography (Dynamic CECT) is a functional imaging technique which reflects the vascularity of pulmonary nodules, which helps in differentiation of benign from malignant pulmonary nodules.[59] The protocol for dynamic contrast enhanced imaging varies widely amongst different studies in terms of contrast concentration used, timing of serial imaging, rate of contrast administration and slice thickness. A standard protocol for acquisition of dynamic CECT dedicated to solitary pulmonary nodules is yet to be formulated. Recent meta-analysis reveal high diagnostic accuracy of dynamic CECT which is comparable to PET/CT in diagnosing solitary pulmonary nodules[60].

Enhancement pattern can be studied by administration of iodinated contrast material intravenously (300 mg/ mL) with a pressure injector. The protocol consists of 3 mm images of the nodule at 1, 2, 3 and 4 minutes after contrast injection.[61,62] Enhancement value is obtained by subtraction of the precontrast value from the peak enhancement. Measurements should be done on mediastinal window and the region of interest (ROI) should be so placed as to cover 70% of the diameter of the nodule **(Figs. 20A to C)**. A cut-off value of 15 HU for enhancement has been found to have a sensitivity of 98% and specificity of 58% for benignity with benign lesions showing enhancement <15 HU.[63] An enhancement of > 20 HU is indicative of tumor neovascularity or malignancy **(Figs. 21A to C)**. The limitation of this technique includes its use in lesions <2 cm as larger lesions would have areas of necrosis and placement of cursor would be a problem. This technique is more applicable for lesions which are relatively spherical in shape and relatively homogenous in attenuation with no large areas of necrosis, fat, calcification or cavitation **(Figs. 22A to C)**. Also, benign vascular tumors and granulomas show enhancement leading to a considerable overlap.[64] An analysis of combined wash-in and wash-out characteristics (studied at 15-minute delay) gives a more precise evaluation of the nodule enhancement.

For benign nodules:

- Wash in <25 HU
- Wash in ≥25 HU with a washout ≥31 HU
- Wash in ≥25 HU and a persistent enhancement without a washout.

For malignant nodules:[65]

- Wash in ≥25 HU
- Washout of 5–31 HU (not >31 HU).

The arterial supply of a nodule is via the bronchial arteries while the washout is via the bronchial veins. In the case of malignancy, a retarded flow in the intravascular and interstitial space accounts for contrast retention.[66] In the case of benign nodules, this washout takes place through relatively straight vessels and active lymphatic flow resulting in a significant washout. A persistent enhancement when seen in a benign nodule occurs due to the presence of fibrosis in the nodule, the fibrotic portion of the nodule retaining contrast for a long-time without washout.

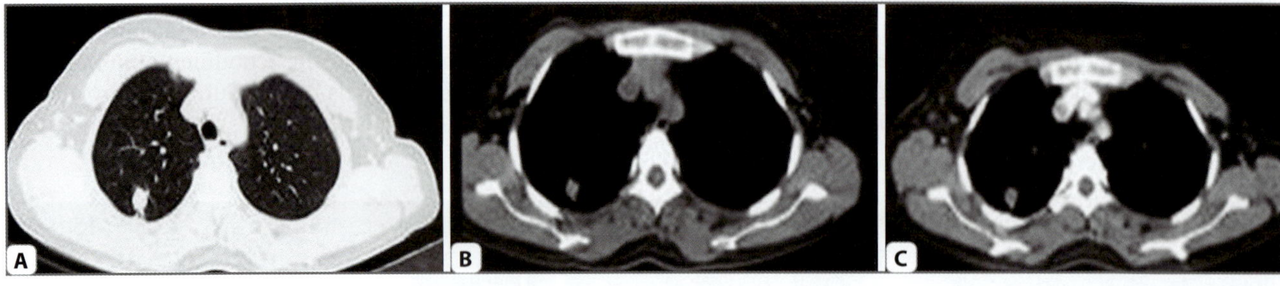

FIGS. 20A TO C: Lung parenchymal window settings on chest CT (A) showing a small (< 1 cm) smooth rounded lesion with a small pleural tail in the right upper lobe. Non-contrast and contrast enhanced scans with mediastinal window settings, (B and C) showing no enhancement of the lesion on the postcontrast scans—benign lesion/tuberculoma.

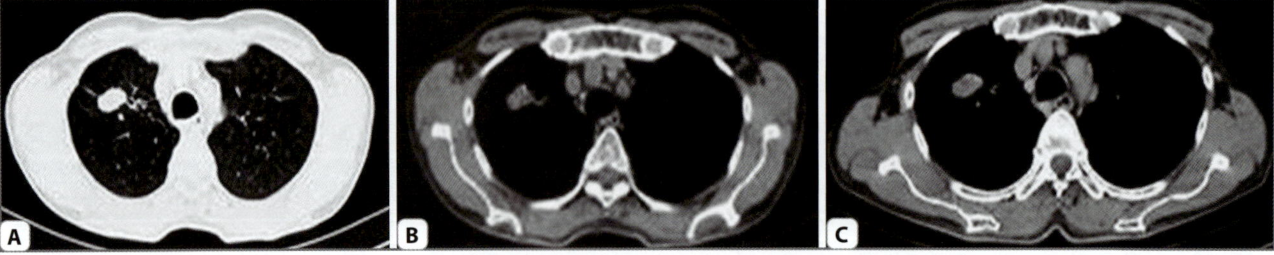

FIGS. 21A TO C: Lung parenchymal window settings (A) showing a small (1 cm) solitary lesion in the right upper lobe. The lesion is irregularly marginated with spiculated contour and multiple pleural tails. Non-contrast and contrast enhanced scans with mediastinal window settings (B and C) reveal significant enhancement > 15 HU on the postcontrast scans—malignant lesion.

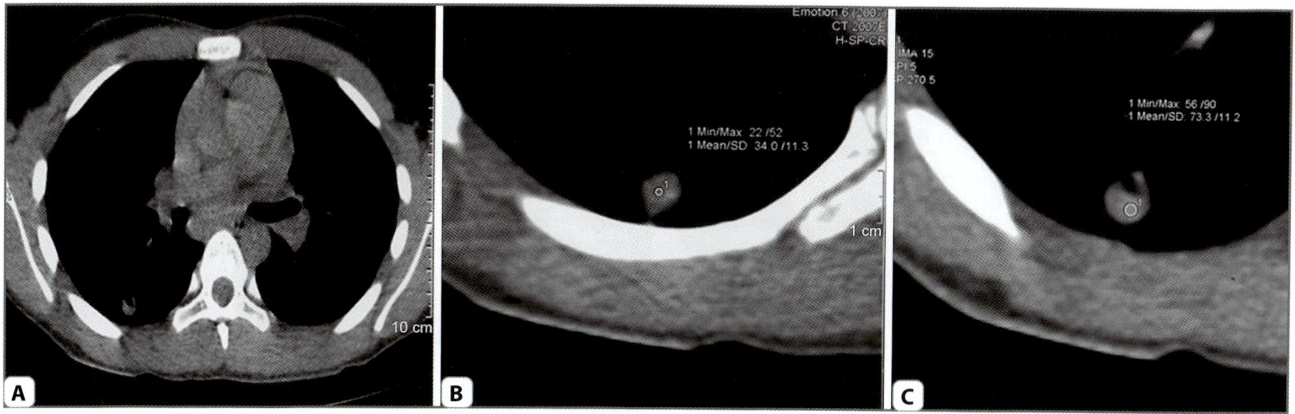

FIGS. 22A TO C: CT scan (A) image showing a lesion <1 cm in size in the right lower lobe with an eccentric cavitation. Pre (B) and post-contrast images (C) reveal an enhancement of 34 HU (56-22 HU) suggestive of a malignant nodule.

Bayesian Analysis

The risk factor of the patients should be evaluated when a SPN is considered to be indeterminate in the initial examination. Age is an important factor in the evaluation with lung cancer being uncommon in patients > 40 years and being rare in those below 35 years of age (<1% of all cases).[67] The risk of developing cancer in male smokers is about 10 times than in non-smokers and the risk is related to the degree and duration of cigarette smoking.[68,69] A history of cancer in first degree relative, occupational exposure, exposure to asbestos, radon and uranium are other risk factors for the development of lung carcinoma.[70]

Bayesian analysis can be useful in the evaluation of these indeterminate solitary pulmonary nodules by allowing more precise determination of the probability of malignancy (pCa). Bayesian analysis uses likelihood ratio (LRs) for numerous radiological findings and clinical features associated with solitary pulmonary nodules to estimate pCa **(Table 2)**.

The likelihood ratios of malignancy in minimally lobulated and deeply lobulated margin were found to be 0.735 and 1.888, respectively.[74] In a new Bayesian model that has been proposed, certain morphological features like edge have been added, criteria such as VDT, minimum HU and CT enhancement have been introduced as predictive features. The new model is an important update on Bayesian analysis and allows for a better differentiation between benign and malignant entities.[74]

TABLE 2: Likelihood ratio (LRs) for selected radiologic features of nodules and patient characteristics.[71-73]

Feature or characteristic	Likelihood ratio
Spiculated margin	5.54
>3 cm	5.23
>70 years of age	4.16
Malignant growth rate	3.40
Smoker	2.27
Upper lobe location	1.22
<1 cm	0.52
Smooth margins	0.30
30–39 years of age	0.24
Never smoked	0.19
20–29 years	0.05
Benign calcification	0.01
Benign growth rate	0.01

Fluorodeoxyglucose Positron Emission Tomography

Nodule metabolism can be evaluated by functional imaging with fluorine 18 (^{18}F)-labelled fluorodeoxyglucose (FDG) positron emission tomography (PET). The technique is a measure of glucose metabolism and aids in the differentiation of benign and malignant nodules[75] **(Figs. 23A to D)**. A standardized uptake value (SUV) of > 2.5 is usually seen in malignancy while a value < 2.5 is seen in benign lesions. PET has a sensitivity and specificity of about 90% for detecting malignant nodules which are larger than 10 mm in diameter, but this high sensitivity and specificity is applicable to solid nodules. In the case of PSN and GGN FDG uptake cannot be used to reliably distinguish between benign and malignant lesions. PET has been found to have a sensitivity as low as 10% and specificity of about 20% for evaluating ground glass opacities.[76] Also, FDG PET can give false negative results in the case of carcinoid tumors, mucinous adenocarcinomas and adenocarcinomas in situ and false positive results in the case of inflammation and infection.[77,78] There may be a respiratory mismatch between CT and PET images leading to an underestimation of the SUV with resultant false negative result. It has been suggested that a respiratory averaged CT, i.e., CT cine images obtained over different portions of the respiratory cycle rather than a mid-expiratory CT improves SUV quantification.

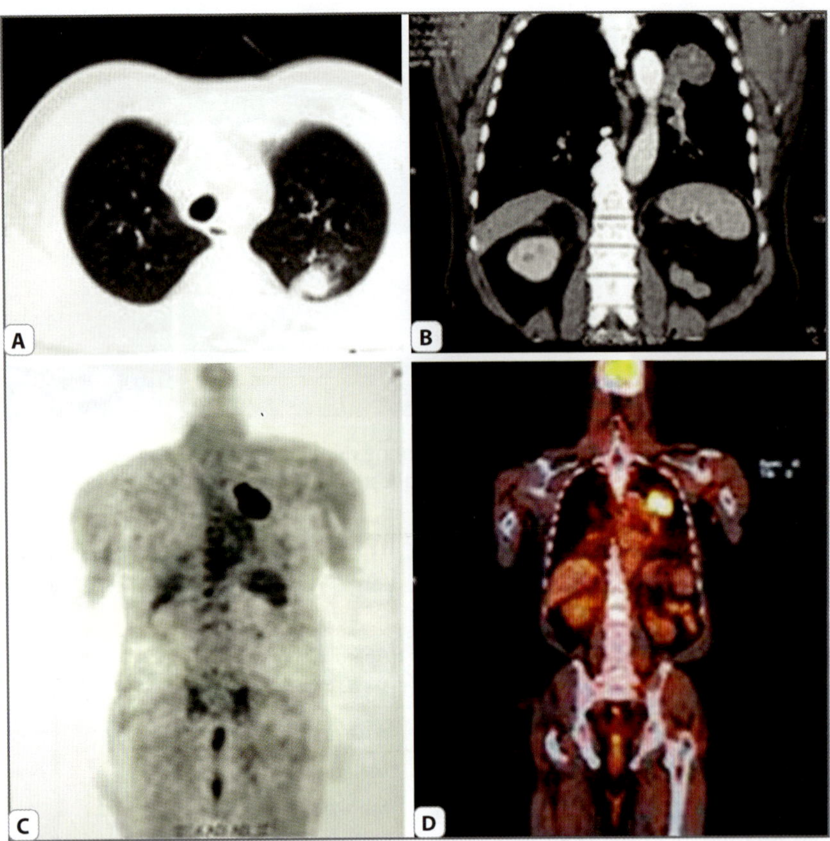

FIGS. 23A TO D: CT chest axial and MPR images (A and B) showing an irregularly marginated lesion with surrounding halo in the left upper lobe. FDG PET scans (C and D) in the patient showing an increased uptake and accumulation of FDG in the nodule—malignant lesion/bronchogenic carcinoma.

Transthoracic Needle Aspiration Biopsy (TNAB)

For a SPN with a high clinical suspicion of malignancy, surgical resection is the best option if the lesion is operable as needle biopsy does not alter management. If the biopsy result is positive, resection has to be done, a negative result does not exclude malignancy and has to be followed by resection if there is a high clinical suspicion of malignancy as the sensitivity of this technique is about 60% for lesions <2 cm in diameter **(Figs. 24A to D)**. The diagnostic yield further falls to 51% for GGO dominant lesions.[79] Thus, needle biopsy is usually indicated for inoperable SPN to confirm the histology. As compared to bronchoscopy, the complication rate of TNAB is high. Complications include pneumothorax and hemorrhage seen in about 5-30% of cases.[80] According to ACR (American College of Radiology) appropriateness criteria given in 2023, tissue sampling may be appropriate next step for solid pulmonary nodules >8 mm detected on chest CT.[81]

Fiberoptic Bronchoscopy

Fiberoptic bronchoscopy (FOB) with transbronchial biopsy and washing has a limited role in evaluating SPN. Although transbronchial biopsy is accurate for assessing endobronchial lesions, the yield for peripheral nodules is less than 60% and is only 25-30% for a SPN <2 cm. The sensitivity of FOB is best when a bronchus leads directly to or is seen within the SPN (the positive bronchus sign).[82]

NEWER IMAGING TECHNIQUES FOR THE EVALUATION OF SPN

Dynamic MR Imaging

Blood patterns and tissue perfusion have been studied by dynamic MR imaging in liver, brain and breast. This technique can be used to characterize SPNs as well.[82] Signal intensity time curves are generated following intravenous injection of gadolinium and maximum relative enhancement ratio and shape of enhancement can be calculated from these. A ratio >0.15 indicates a malignant SPN, a ratio <0.80 indicates benign lesion and ratio between 0.8–0.15 usually indicates active infection. These MR indices are useful for differentiating between benign and malignant SPNs.[83,84] Some recent studies have demonstrated that specificity and accuracy of dynamic MR indices were significantly better than SUVmax.[85]

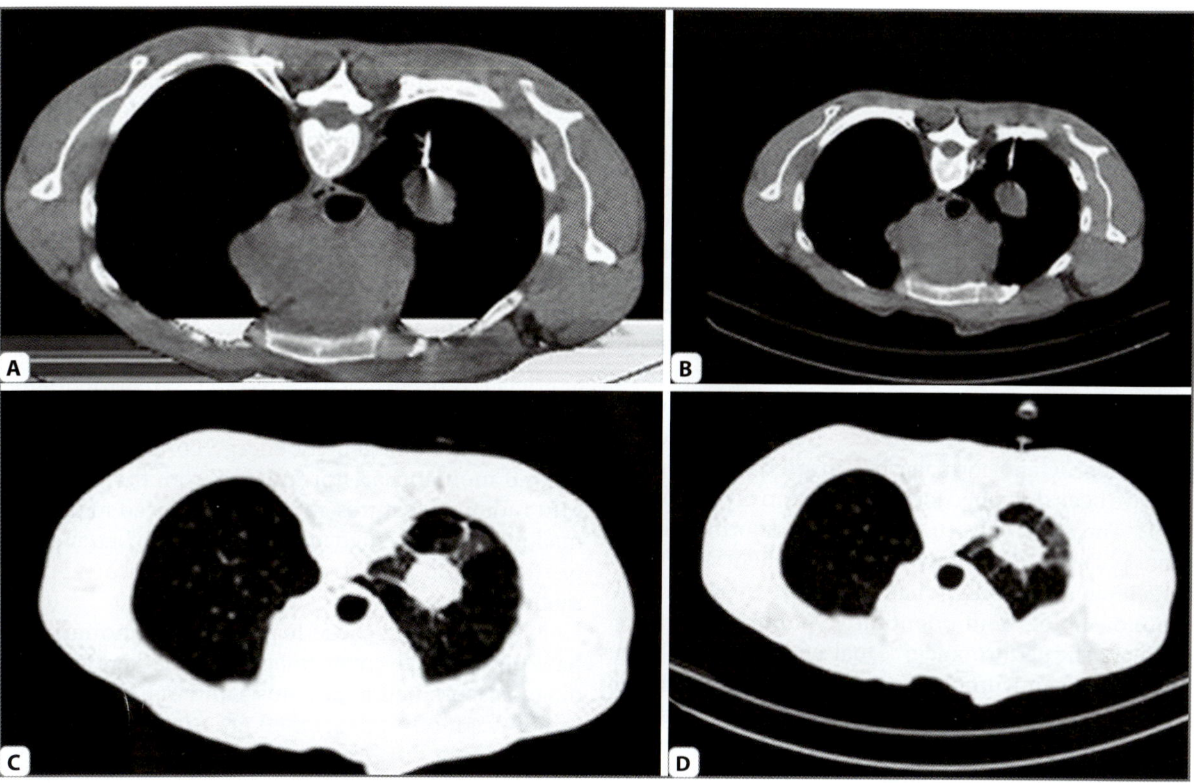

FIGS. 24A TO D: Transthoracic needle aspiration in the case of a nodule in the right lung with needle in situ (A and B) in prone position. The nodule is irregularly marginated with evidence of corona radiata and multiple pleural tails (C and D)—bronchogenic carcinoma.

Diffusion Weighted MRI Imaging

Diffusion weighted imaging (DWI) is a functional imaging technique revealing information regarding the pathological and physiological mechanisms. It offers the following parameters for nodule evaluation:[86]

- Qualitative parameter—visual assessment and grading. Most widely used five point visual assessment grading was described by Satoh et al., to differentiate between benign and malignant nodules.[87] These were: (1) nearly no signal intensity as seen in an almost normal lung; (2) signal intensity between 1 and 3; (3) Signal intensity almost equal to the spinal cord at thoracic spine; (4) higher signal than spinal cord; (5) much higher signal than that of the spinal cord. A score of 3 (a nodule with signal intensity equal to that of the spinal cord) was considered the threshold for differentiation between benign and malignant pulmonary nodules in their study.[87]
- Semiquantitative parameter—lesion to spinal cord signal intensity ratio (LSR). LSR is measured as the ratio of signal intensity of the pulmonary nodule and spinal cord at the same level
- Quantitative parameters—minimum ADC value measurement (ADC min) and lesion to spinal cord ADC ratio (LSAR). LSAR is the ratio of minimum ADC value of pulmonary nodule and spinal cord at the same level

These semiquantitative and quantitative parameters have been evaluated in recent studies showing high sensitivity and accuracy in differentiating benign and malignant lesions. Malignant lesions show lower ADC values, higher LSR and lower LSAR.[86]

Specific threshold for diffusion parameters cannot be universally implemented owing to differences in hardware, protocols for scanning and b-values used, however, ADC value cutoff ranging from 1.1–1.4 × 10^{-3} mm^2/s can be used effectively to distinguish benign from malignant nodules with pooled accuracy of 91% which is comparable to other functional techniques (accuracy of dynamic CECT, FDG PET/CT and dynamic CE-MRI being 92%, 94% and 94% respectively).[88,89]

The disadvantages of DWI include: (a) low ADC value of certain benign lesions like pulmonary abscesses and necrosis, and (b) high ADC value observed in mucinous adenocarcinomas which can be erroneously categorized as benign. However, the use of T2 weighted images in conjunction with DWI helps in differentiating T2 bright abscesses from malignant lesions.[90]

Recently, studies have been conducted to compare turbo-spin echo DWI (TSE-DWI) and echo-planar imaging DWI (EPI-DWI) as the former yield's distortion free images in comparison with latter and may be used as an excellent substitute for EPI-DWI.[91]

Dual-energy CT in the Evaluation of SPN

Angiogenesis of malignant nodules leads to a stronger enhancement of malignant tumors on CT. Iodine is the main ingredient of contrast medium and directly reflects blood flow. Iodine concentration (CI) maps can assess the vasculature and relative vascularity of pulmonary nodule. By single scanning after contrast injection, the degree of enhancement can be obtained without an additional non-enhanced scan. CI in malignant nodules has been found to be significantly higher than benign nodules, thus allowing for the differentiation between benign and malignant nodules.[92] Owing to its material decomposition ability, DECT allows differentiation of calcification from enhanced tissue. Various spectral parameters including effective atomic number, IC and normalized IC in arterial and venous phases have been described for the evaluation of pulmonary nodules.[93] Threshold of IC ~0.95 mg/mL and normalized IC in venous phase ~17.98% have revealed excellent sensitivity and specificity, concluding that composite evaluation of nodule morphology and quantitative parameters yields better diagnostic performance.[93] Dual-energy CT has been found to significantly improve the sensitivity of artificial intelligence (AI) in characterizing pulmonary nodules and showed improved image quality with reduced radiation exposure but its accuracy is poor.[94]

Perfusion CT in the Evaluation of SPN

Perfusion CT is an imaging technique which utilizes multiple consecutive scanning of the lesion after administration of intravenous contrast.[95] The time density curves (TDC), blood volume (BV), blood flow (BF), mean transit time (MTT), time to peak (TTP), pulmonary nodule enhancement peak (PPnod), aorta enhancement peak (PPao) and the ratio of peak enhancement of pulmonary nodule and aorta (PPnod/PPao) are the parameters used to evaluate microvascular structure of pulmonary nodules. Malignant nodules show higher BF, BV, MTT, PPnod, PPao, PPnod/PPao with lower TTP. In a recent study, BV, BF, PPnod and PPnod/PPao revealed significant difference between benign SPN and malignant SPN with cutoff values of 4.13 mL/100 g, 69.32 mL/100 g/min, 44 and 5.48, respectively.[96]

Radiomics in the Evaluation of SPN

Radiomics provides a way to extract large quantity of imaging features from CT, MRI, PET-CT, or other databases via high-through put extraction which is beyond the resolution of human eye and is utilized to analyse the correlation between these features and underlying pathological changes of disease. Therefore, radiomics not only assists in differentiation of malignant from benign tumors, but also plays an important role in metastasis prediction, pathological grading, malignancy staging, and effectiveness of therapy since it reflects the heterogeneity within tumors efficiently and improves the diagnostic accuracy. Extraction of radiomic features from each pulmonary nodule is mostly performed by dedicated software after nodule segmentation. They are divided into first-order features (which includes shape and shape 2D features), texture features and wavelet features. Among these, textural features are most extensively employed in radiomics as they represent the spatial distribution of areas with different intensities and reflect tumor heterogeneity.[97] The DWI-MR images are intensity normalized to have the same 99th percentile grayscale value followed by first-order texture features extraction. Shape-based features are not extracted since air-lung interface affects DWI leading to unreliable lesion edges and shapes. Using each image, four gray level co-occurrence matrix (GLCM) corroborating with four directions are obtained, and six features (contrast, dissimilarity, homogeneity, energy, correlation and angular second moment) are formulated from the GLCMs. DWI-MRI radiomic features could be employed to differentiate malignant from benign lung nodules with better diagnostic performance than traditional quantitative imaging methods.[98]

Insights about these features of pulmonary nodules have been used to create imaging biomarkers for detection, diagnosis, predicting prognosis and monitoring. AI based radiomics models developed after incorporating clinical and imaging data have excellent prediction of risk of malignancy in pulmonary nodules.[99] The advantage of radiomics in discriminating benign from malignant pulmonary nodules lies in its ability to identify characteristic features, which aid in depiction of the detailed imaging differences between them. Radiomics can also be used as an additional critical technique for comprehensively detecting tumor heterogeneity and compensate for the shortcomings of traditional imaging diagnosis. It also serves as a valuable additional tool in cases with overlapping morphological and perfusional analyses of malignant and benign pulmonary nodules.

Role of Artificial Intelligence in the Evaluation of SPN

Artificial intelligence has long been used in the detection of pulmonary nodules with earlier applications involving computer-aided detection (CAD) techniques which revealed variable sensitivity and false-positive rates. Recent applications utilize deep learning algorithms including convolutional neural networks which provide in depth analysis of pulmonary nodules with higher sensitivity and decreased false positive rates.[100,101] Identification of the nodule, size of the nodule, morphology and internal architecture of the nodule can all be evaluated. Association between nodule characteristics and rate of malignancy can be undertaken with the help of these techniques.[102] Multiple FDA approved artificial intelligence solutions are available each focusing on variable degree of lung nodule assessment, including nodule detection, nodule segmentation, nodule characterization, image registration and subtraction.[103] The size and morphology including shape, margin, attenuation, structure and location of nodules can be assessed utilizing artificial intelligence. Low inter-observer and intra-observer variability amongst radiologists in nodule classification especially for PSNs, can be partially overcome using same deep learning algorithm for detection and tracking of nodules. To assess the likelihood of malignancy in pulmonary nodules multiple mathematical models have been developed including the PanCan model, Veterans Affairs model and Mayo Clinic model, but these depend on patient's history which might not be available all the time.[100,104]

The follow-up of the pulmonary nodules emphasizes the need for image registration techniques. Image registration entails superimposing image data or determining the spatial alignment between different images from the same modality at different points in times (intramodality registration) or between different imaging modalities, such as CT, MR PET (intermodality registration). To correlate a nodule accurately on CT study with its matching counterpart on a subsequent CT, global registration of the thorax and the local registration of nodules and smaller structures need to be performed. An interactive system enables easy identification of corresponding structures on initial and subsequent CT studies, recording of nodules and their characteristics including volume and storage of image results for future analysis and documentation.[105]

ACR APPROPRIATENESS CRITERIA FOR INCIDENTALLY DETECTED INDETERMINATE PULMONARY NODULES

The American College of Radiology committee on Appropriateness criteria formulated criteria for determination of appropriate next imaging examination of incidentally detected indeterminate pulmonary nodules to guide radiologists, radiation oncologists and physicians in 2023.[81] These guidelines apply to similar population as Fleischner Society guidelines. Four evidence-based variants were proposed for commonly encountered clinical scenarios: (a) In the evaluation of pulmonary nodules detected on chest radiograph with no prior study to confirm that it has been stable for 2 years, CT chest without contrast is usually appropriate as the next imaging study. For a nodule that is stable for 2 years, no further imaging is required; (b) For pulmonary nodules <6 mm detected on chest CT, follow-up CT chest without contrast may be appropriate when the nodule shows suspicious morphology, upper lobe location, or both in high-risk patients; (c) CT chest without IV contrast is usually appropriate for follow-up of pulmonary nodules >6 mm detected on chest CT irrespective of nodule attenuation. FDG-PET/CT whole body or CT chest without IV contrast is usually appropriate for pulmonary nodules >8 mm detected on chest CT; (d) For pulmonary nodules >6 mm detected on incomplete thoracic CT, CT chest without IV contrast is usually appropriate and the time of next imaging is dependent on nodule size, morphology and clinical risk of malignancy.

GUIDELINES FOR THE MANAGEMENT OF SOLITARY PULMONARY NODULE

Following the Fleischner Society Guidelines of solid nodules in 2005[106] and the subsolid nodules in 2013[107-109] several modifications have taken place leading to the new guidelines of the Fleischner Society in 2017 **(Table 3)**.

The Fleischner Society guidelines are not for:

- Patients with known primary cancer
- Immunocompromised patients who are at risk of infection
- Lung cancer screening population (evaluated using Lung-RADS)
- Children and adults younger than 35 years management in these groups should be based on the specific clinical situation and on a case-by-case basis.

Changes in the revised guidelines include:

- The minimum threshold of the nodule for follow-up has been increased to 6 mm rather than 5 mm.
- Follow up intervals have been given a range rather than a precise time period.
- The guidelines for solid and semisolid nodules are now included in one single table with specific recommendations for multiple nodules.

For multiple nodules, the subsequent management is based on suspicious nodule which may not be the largest nodule. Pure GGNs > 10 mm, part solid GGN with solid component > 5 mm, bubbly appearance of reticulation, atypical subsolid nodules with spiculation should be interpreted with high degree of suspicion.

Low risk (estimated risk of cancer < 5%) category includes patients with young age, less smoking, smaller nodule size, regular margins, and location other than upper lobe. High risk (estimated risk of cancer ≥5%) category comprises of patients with older age, heavy smoking, larger nodule size, irregular or spiculated margins, and upper lobe location.

It has been recommended that thin CT sections of the thorax (≤1 mm) should be performed to enable accurate characterization of the small pulmonary nodules. Sagittal and coronal reconstruction should always be obtained.

A low radiation dose technique is recommended for follow up CT scans with the use of dose modulation and iterative reconstruction techniques to reduce radiation. According to the ACR recommendations for screening CT, the CT dose index volume (CTDI vol) should not be more than 3 mGy.[111]

TABLE 3: Fleischner Society 2017 guidelines for management of incidentally detected pulmonary nodules in adults.*[110]

A: Solid nodules				
Nodule type	**Size**			**Comments**
	<6 mm (<100 mm^3)	6–8 mm (100–250 mm^3)	>8 mm (>250 mm^3)	
Single				
Low risk	No routine follow-up	CT at 6–12 months, then consider CT at 18–24 months	Consider CT, PET/CT, or tissue sampling at 3 months	Nodules <6 mm do not require routine follow-up in low-risk patients
High risk	Optional CT at 12 months	CT at 6–12 months, then CT at 18–24 months	Consider CT, PET/CT, or tissue sampling at 3 months	Certain patients at high risk with suspicious nodule morphology, upper lobe location, or both may warrant 12-month follow-up
Multiple				
Low risk	No routine follow-up	CT at 3–6 months, then consider CT at 18–24 months	CT at 3–6 months, then consider CT at 18–24 months	Use the most suspicious nodule as guide to management. Follow-up intervals may vary according to size and risk
High risk	Optional CT at 12 months	CT at 3–6 months, then at 18–24 months	CT at 3–6 months, then at 18–24 months	Use the most suspicious nodule as guide to management. Follow-up intervals may vary according to size and risk
B: Subsolid nodules				
Nodule type	**Size**			**Comments**
	<6 mm (<100 mm^3)	≥6 mm (>100 mm^3)		
Single				
Ground glass	No routine follow-up	CT at 6–12 months to confirm persistence, then CT every 2 years until 5 years		In certain suspicious nodules <6 mm, consider follow-up at 2 and 4 years. If solid component(s) or growth develops, consider resection.
Part solid	No routine follow-up	CT at 3–6 months to confirm persistence. If unchanged and solid component remains 6 mm, annual CT should be performed for 5 years		In practice, part-solid nodules (PSNs) cannot be defined as such until ≥6 mm, and nodules <6 mm do not usually require follow-up. Persistent PSNs with solid components ≥6 mm should be considered highly suspicious
Multiple	CT at 3–6 months. If stable, consider CT at 2 and 4 years	CT at 3–6 months. Subsequent management based on the most suspicious nodule(s)		Multiple <6 mm pure ground-glass nodules are usually benign, but consider follow-up in selected patients at high risk at 2 and 4 years

*These are the new guidelines given by the Fleischner Society 2017 for incidentally detected pulmonary nodules in adult patients >35 years of age.[110]

It is stated that volumetric measurements can be performed instead of linear measurements with volume of 100 and 250 mm^3 corresponding to the 6- and 8-mm thresholds. Volumetric measurements should be performed with identical software versions.[110]

Lung CT screening Reporting and Data System (Lung RADS) was first formulated in 2014 to standardize lung cancer screening CT reporting, provide management guidelines and outcome monitoring.[112] The latest Lung-RADS version 2022 classifies nodules into four categories according to the risk of malignancy: benign (category 2), probably benign (category 3), suspicious (category 4A) and very suspicious (category 4B or 4X).[113] Category 1 includes either no pulmonary nodules or nodules with specific calcifications and fat containing nodules. The management plan depends upon the nodule category which can be up- or down-graded during surveillance in accordance with interval change. Recommendations for categories 2, 3 and 4A are annual screening, CT at 6 months and CT at 3 months, respectively. Workup for malignancy is recommended for category 4B and 4X[114].

The differential diagnosis of a SPN include neoplasms, infective, non-infectious, congenital and vascular causes which are summarized in **Box 1**.[115]

BOX 1: Differential diagnosis of solitary pulmonary nodule.[115]

Malignant neoplasm:
- Carcinoma (squamous cell, small cell, adenocarcinoma, bronchioloalveolar carcinoma)
- Lymphoma
- Carcinoid
- Pulmonary metastasis (colon, melanoma, renal cell, breast, osteosarcoma)

Benign neoplasm and neoplasm like condition:
- Hamartoma
- Chondroma
- Fibroma

Infective causes:
- Round pneumonia
- Abscess
- Granuloma (fungal, mycobacterial)

Noninfectious inflammatory:
- Sarcoidosis
- Rheumatoid arthritis
- Amyloidosis
- Wegener's granulomatosis

Airway and inhalational disease:
- Mucoid impaction (mucous plug)
- Bronchial atresia
- Cystic fibrosis
- Conglomerate mass or progressive massive fibrosis (e.g., silicosis)
- Lipoid pneumonia

Vascular lesions:
- Pulmonary artery aneurysm
- Hematoma
- Infarct
- Arteriovenous malformation (AVM)

Congenital lesions:
- Sequestration
- Bronchogenic cyst
- Bronchial atresia

Idiopathic/Miscellaneous:
- Amyloidosis
- Fluid filled bulla
- Round atelectasis

MORPHOLOGICAL CHARACTERISTICS IN SPECIFIC LESIONS

Lung Malignancies

About 20% of lung cancers are present as SPNs **(Figs. 25A and B)**. The most common type presenting as a nodule is adenocarcinoma. Bronchogenic carcinoma will show irregular, spiculated margins with absence of calcification. However, presence of calcification does not completely rule out malignancy as cancers may develop in a scar or granuloma which shows pre-existing calcification. The pre-existing calcification is usually of the stippled or eccentric type and occupies < 10% of the nodule.

Metastasis

Though metastatic nodules are usually multiple, rarely these may present as solitary pulmonary nodule. Carcinoma of the colon, melanoma and carcinomas of the kidney and testicle may present with solitary metastasis **(Figs. 26A and B)**.

The metastatic nodules are usually sharply marginated though local invasion, and surrounding hemorrhage may lead to the nodules being poorly defined. Metastatic lesions are predominantly seen in the lung bases because of greater blood flow. "Feeding vessel sign" may be seen in these nodules owing to a hematogenous origin because these nodules are usually seen at the tips of small arteries.[116]

Carcinoid Tumor

These account for 10–20% of SPNs. These are neuroendocrine tumors, and two forms have been described: typical and atypical. Typical carcinoids account for 85–90% of these lesions and occur in the main, lobar or segmental bronchi in a central location. The atypical ones usually have a peripheral location with a worse prognosis than the typical variety.[117] Carcinoids can be intraluminal or extraluminal and are seen as well-defined, lobulated, round or notched with a smooth edge. Spiculation is rarely seen. Curvilinear or multiple nodular calcifications may be seen. Rarely, dense ossification may be seen within the lesion.

A triad of:
- Well defined, lobulated round lesion
- Location adjacent to bronchial bifurcation
- Eccentric calcification:
  - Is highly suggestive of bronchial carcinoid **(Figs. 27A to C)**?[118]

Lymphoma

Both Hodgkin's and non-Hodgkin's lymphoma involves the lung in about 10–15% cases and is characterized by single/multiple nodules, masses or consolidation which may cavitate. Associated hilar and mediastinal adenopathy is usually present.[119]

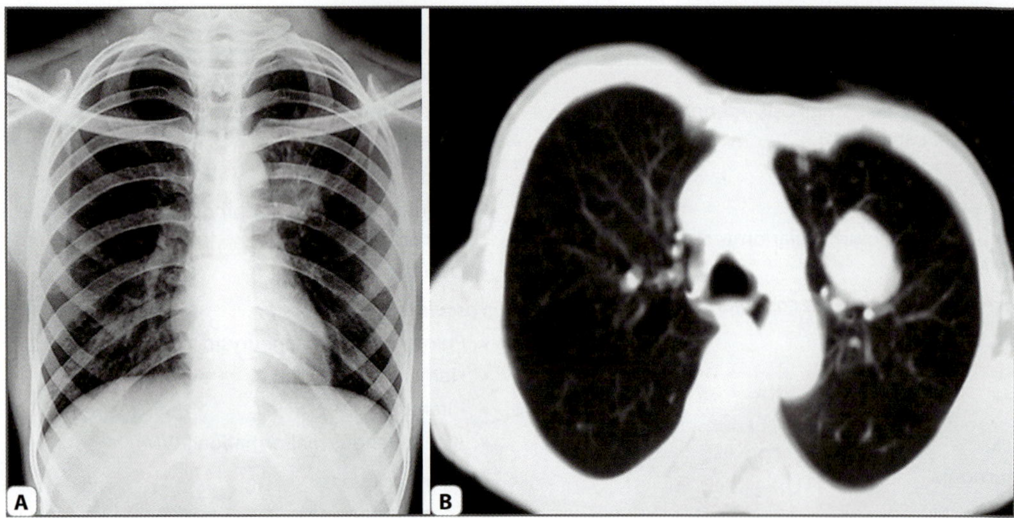

FIGS. 25A AND B: Chest radiograph shows a large nodule with irregular margins in the left upper lobe. Larger the lesion the more likely it is to be malignant—bronchogenic carcinoma.

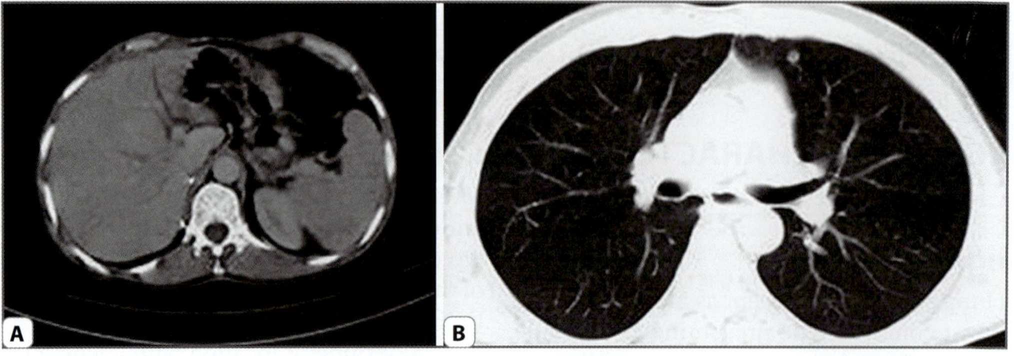

FIGS. 26A AND B: Follow-up CT scan (A) in a post-operative case of right renal cell carcinoma showing a small, smoothly marginated round solitary lesion in the left lung. The lesion is seen at the tip of a small artery (feeding vessel sign) (B)—solitary metastasis in renal cell carcinoma.

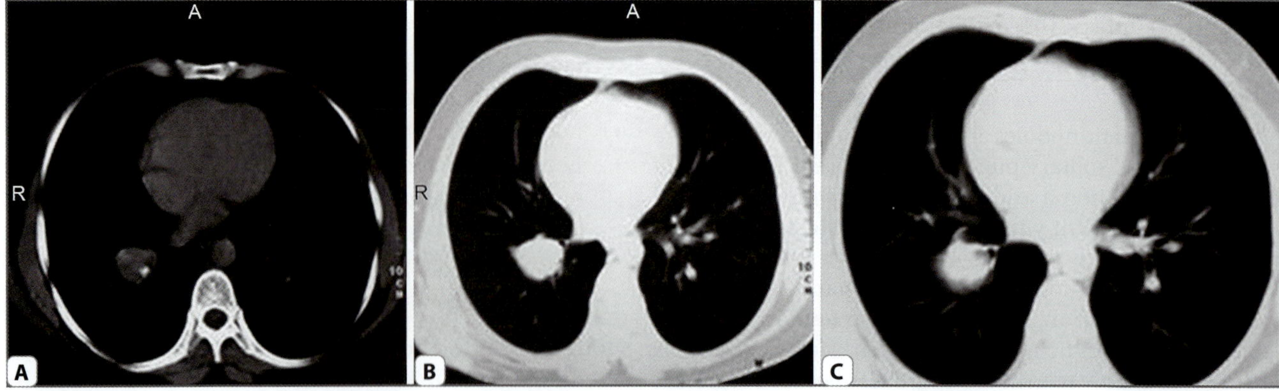

FIGS. 27A TO C: CT sections showing a well-defined rounded lesion in the right lung lying centrally in a perihilar location/vicinity of bronchial bifurcation with eccentric calcification noted within (A). Lung window shows the lesion to have a smooth edge with minimal lobulations (B). The right lower lobe bronchus shows the characteristic widening as it approaches the tumor (C)—bronchial carcinoid.

Benign Neoplasms

Pulmonary Hamartoma

It is a benign pulmonary mass composed of cartilage, myxomatous connective tissue, fat, marrow, bone, smooth muscle in different amounts. 90% of the hamartomas have a peripheral location. These are seen as well-defined, round or lobulated nodules with a characteristic "popcorn calcification" owing to the cartilaginous and osseous component.[120] CT detects fat as areas with negative attenuation values. The presence of fat and calcification within a well-defined nodule is virtually diagnostic of a pulmonary hamartoma **(Figs. 28A to C)**.[121]

Other Benign Tumors

These may arise from epithelial or mesenchymal tissue. Carney's triad is a condition comprising of multiple pulmonary chondromas, extra-adrenal paragangliomas and gastric epitheloid leiomyosarcoma. This condition is seen in women <35 years of age, the presence of multiple cartilage tumors in the lung should warrant a search for the other tumors which are more lethal than chondromas.[122]

Infective Causes

Granuloma

The commonest cause of granuloma is tubercular though other causes include histoplasmosis, cryptococcosis, coccidioidomycosis. These are seen as a solitary nodule 1–3 cm in diameter with a well-defined smooth regular margin and often showing calcification **(Figs. 29 A to C)**. The patterns of calcification seen in a granuloma include amorphous, punctate, fleck-like or laminar, often subpleural in location, granulomas rarely show cavitation. Cavitation when seen should suggest reactivation.

Hydatid Cyst

Caused by *Echinococcus granulosus*, the hydatid cyst is seen as a sharply demarcated, well-defined round or oval lesion with a homogenous soft tissue density on radiographs **(Figs. 30A and B)**. The cysts occur more commonly in mid and lower lobes. An air-fluid level, water lily sign and rising sun sign are seen in cases of rupture of the hydatid cyst.

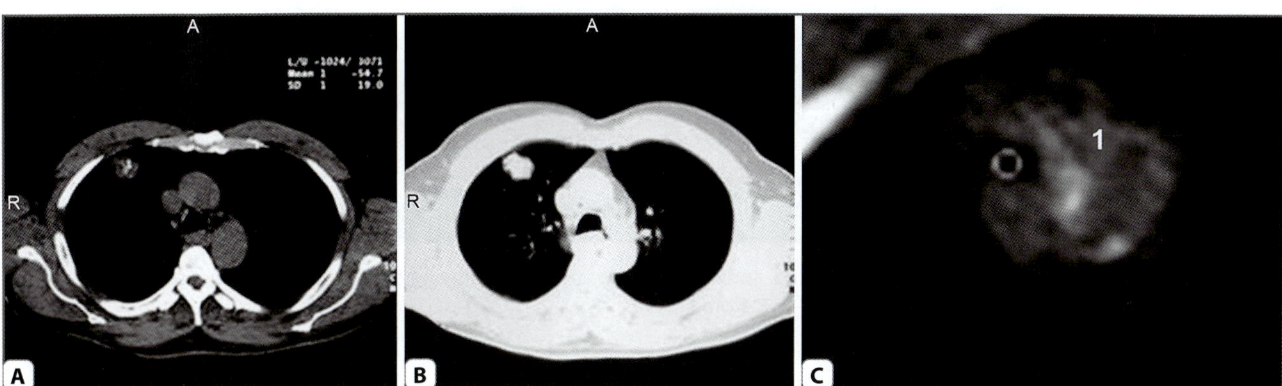

FIGS. 28A TO C: CT chest mediastinal (A) and lung parenchymal (B) window settings revealing a well-defined nodular lesion in the right upper lobe. The lesion shows fat attenuation (negative attenuation) values within. Magnified view of the lesion (C) showing the fat clearly and small specks of calcification in the lesion—pulmonary hamartoma.

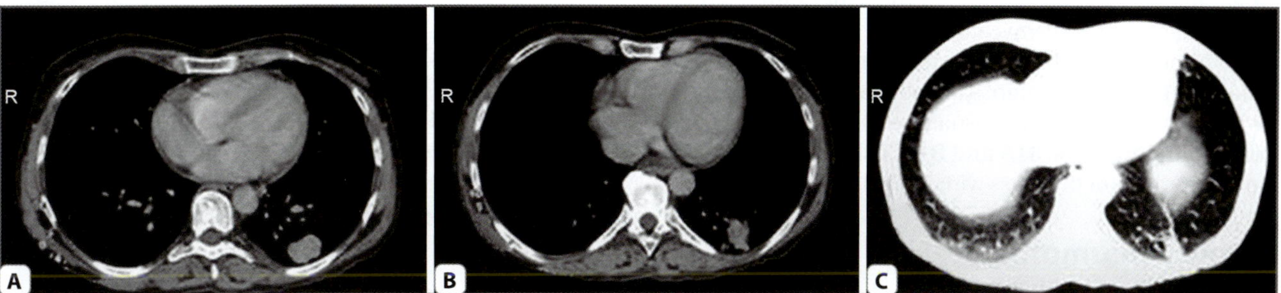

FIGS. 29A TO C: CT scans showing a single well-defined lesion 2 cm in size in a subpleural location with no evidence of cavitation (A). The lesion shows evidence of multiple fibrotic strands around it (B and C)—tuberculoma.

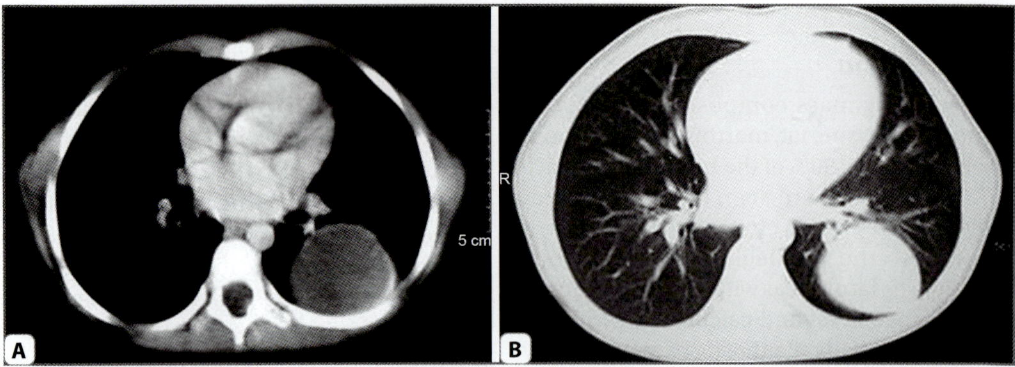

FIGS. 30A AND B: CT scan chest mediastinal (A) and lung windows (B) showing an oval, sharply marginated homogenous fluid density cystic lesion in the left lower lobe—hydatid cyst.

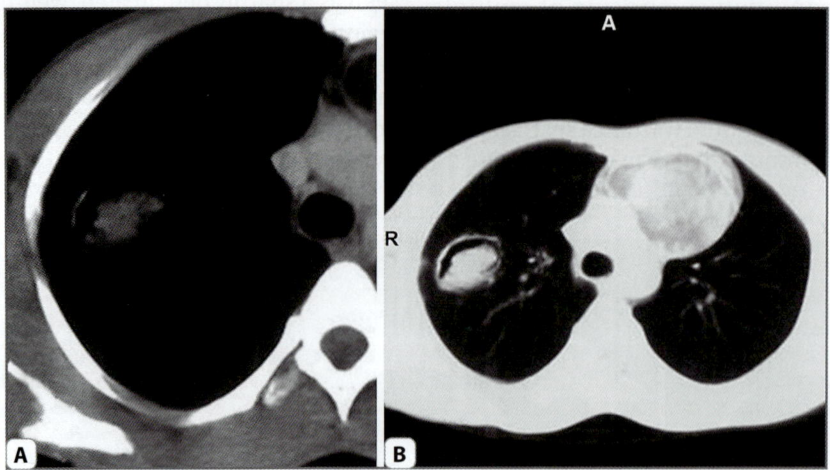

FIGS. 31A AND B: CT sections of the chest mediastinal and lung windows (A and B) showing the "air meniscus sign" seen as air crescent between the mass and the cavity in the right lung—mycetoma.

Mycetoma/Fungal Ball

A mycetoma results from saprophytic invasion of a pre-existing cavity. The causes of the cavity in the majority of the cases are tubercular, but sarcoidosis, bronchiectasis, bulla, histoplasmosis, etc. may also result in a cavity in which the fungal mass develops. Matting of the aspergillus hyphae results in a fungal ball/mycetoma seen as an intracavitary mass in the upper lobe or superior segment of lower lobe usually. "Air-crescent sign" (air between the wall of the cavity and the fungal ball) is usually seen and is a diagnostic imaging finding **(Figs. 31A and B)**. CT shows a sponge like the appearance of the mass with irregular air spaces.

Round Pneumonia

Round pneumonias are more commonly seen in children in cases of *Streptococcus* infection. Other causative organisms include: *K. pneumoniae, S. aureus, M. tuberculosis* and fungi. On imaging round pneumonia appears as a focal round wedge-shaped opacity in a peripheral location typically in the posterior lower lobe **(Figs. 32A and B)**. These have a predominant posterior distribution owing to the supine sleeping position of children while the gravity dependent passage of bacteria loaded fluid into the most dependent bronchus accounts for the lower lobe distribution. The underdeveloped pores of Kohn and the absence of canals of Lambert in children account for the sharp margins of the round pneumonia in contrast to the ill-defined margins of pneumonia seen in adults.[123] The centrifugal pattern of spread of the inflammation results in the lesion margin being sharply demarcated from the unaffected lung parenchyma **(Figs. 33A to C)**.

Lung Abscess

The etiology can be pyogenic, anaerobic bacteria or mycobacterial. Radiographs show an abscess as an ill-defined opacity with surrounding consolidation. An air-fluid level is seen in cases of communication with the bronchus. Contrast enhancement CT shows the abscess as a hypodense lesion with thick enhancing walls, shaggy margins and an air fluid level **(Figs. 34A to C)**.

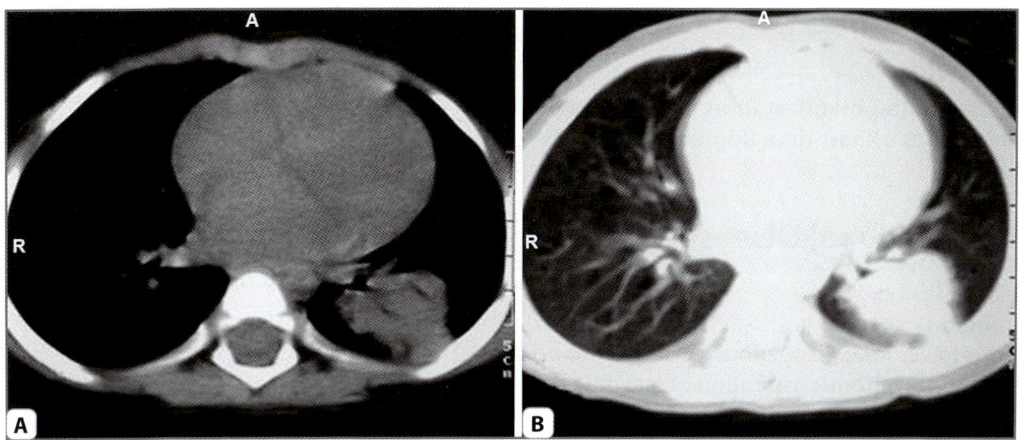

FIGS. 32A AND B: CT scan in a 2-year-old child showing a peripherally located wedge shaped opacity with air bronchogram within in the left lower lobe located posteriorly. The opacity is based against a focally thickened pleura—round pneumonia.

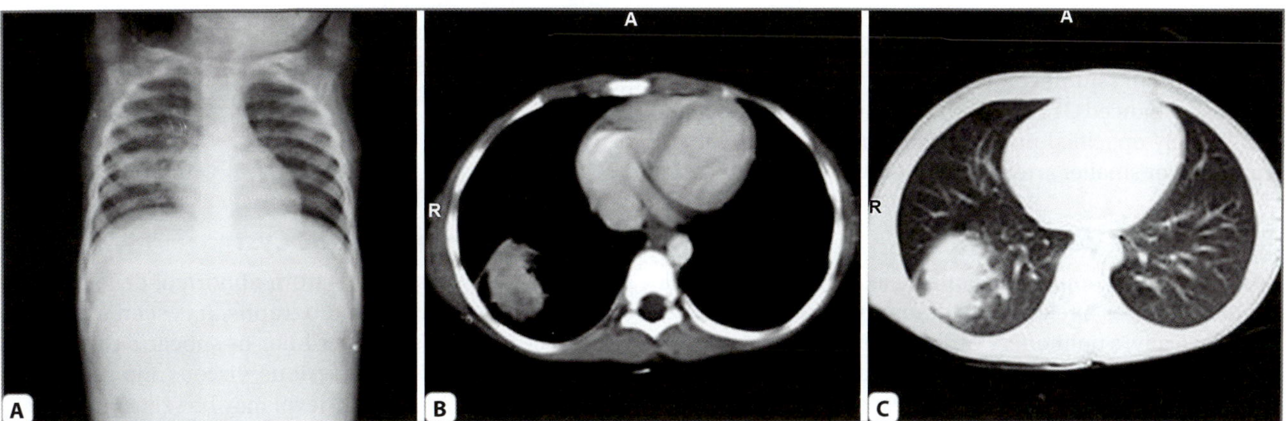

FIGS. 33A TO C: Chest radiograph (A) in a child showing a focal round nodule in the right lung. CT sections (B and C) showing an area of spherical consolidation in the right lower lobe with associated pleural thickening—round pneumonia.

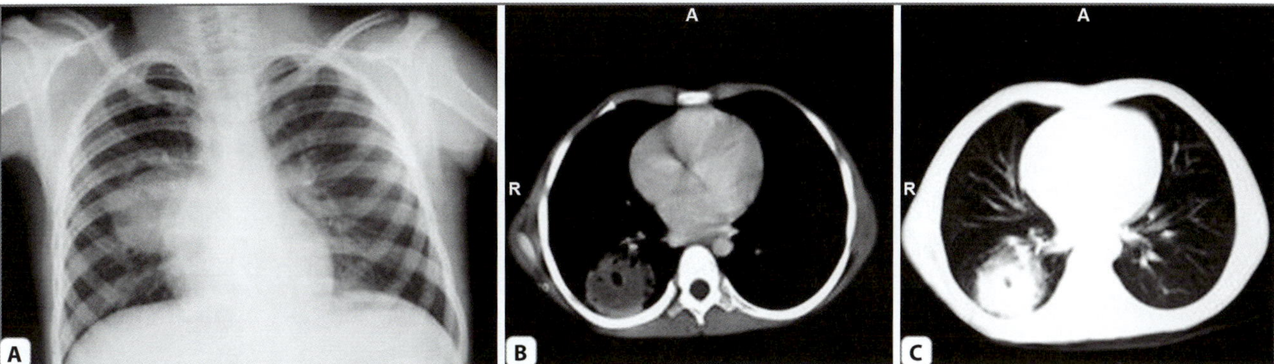

FIGS. 34A TO C: Chest radiograph (A) showing a focal round lesion in the right lung. A small air loculus is seen within. CT sections (B and C) showing a low attenuation lesion (i.e., fluid attenuation) lesion with enhancing wall. Multiple air loculi are seen in the center and in the periphery of the lesion (B). The margins are mildly irregular with surrounding consolidation (C)—lung abscess.

Inflammatory Nodules

Rheumatoid Nodules

These are an uncommon manifestation of rheumatoid arthritis, may be seen as solitary or multiple nodules in the lung parenchyma.[124]

Airway or Inhalational Disease

Lipoid Pneumonia

Lipoid pneumonia is seen as an ill-defined nodule or mass in posterior lower lobe. Exogenous variety of lipoid pneumonia results from chronic aspiration of fat while the endogenous form occurs due to accumulation of lipid rich cellular debris distal to bronchial obstruction.

Vascular Lesions

Pulmonary Artery Aneurysm

Pulmonary artery aneurysm can present as a lung nodule.[125] Rasmussen aneurysm is seen in tuberculosis and is a mycotic aneurysm developing in the infectious cavity. Contrast enhanced CT is diagnostic as the aneurysm is seen as a densely opacified nodular lesion in relation to lobar, segmental or smaller arteries **(Figs. 35A to C)**.

Pulmonary Vein Varix

A varix can result from a congenital defect of the wall, mitral valvular diseases or elevated pulmonary venous pressure. Radiologically, a pulmonary varix is seen as a round or oval density adjacent to the left atrium. Usually asymptomatic, a pulmonary varix can enlarge in response to high atrial pressure with resultant rupture and hemorrhage.

Arteriovenous Malformation

Arteriovenous malformation (AVM) is characterized by an enlarged artery feeding the nodule and a draining vein. Radiographs reveal the AVM as a well-circumscribed nodule with a lobular outline, usually seen in the lower lobe, in a subpleural location. Contrast enhanced CT reveals rapid enhancement and washout in the pulmonary AVM corresponding to the opacification and washout of the main pulmonary artery and right ventricle.[126]

Pulmonary Infarction

A pulmonary infarct is seen as a wedge-shaped opacity in contact with the pleural surface known as Hampton's hump **(Figs. 36A and B)**. A halo sign due to adjacent hemorrhage or low attenuating areas due to necrosis may be seen. On contrast administration, feeding vessels may be seen and the periphery of the infarct may enhance owing to collateral flow. Cavitation of a pulmonary infarct occurs with infection of the bland infarct or with septic emboli. Pulmonary infarcts decrease in their size slowly over months what has been described as the "melting sign".[127]

Congenital Lesions

Pulmonary Bronchogenic Cyst

A bronchogenic cyst results from abnormal development of the lung bud. On the radiographs, it is seen as a well-circumscribed mass in a perihilar or subcarinal location. The fluid in the cyst can be serious, viscous and gelatinous or hemorrhagic. An air fluid level may be seen if the cyst is infected.

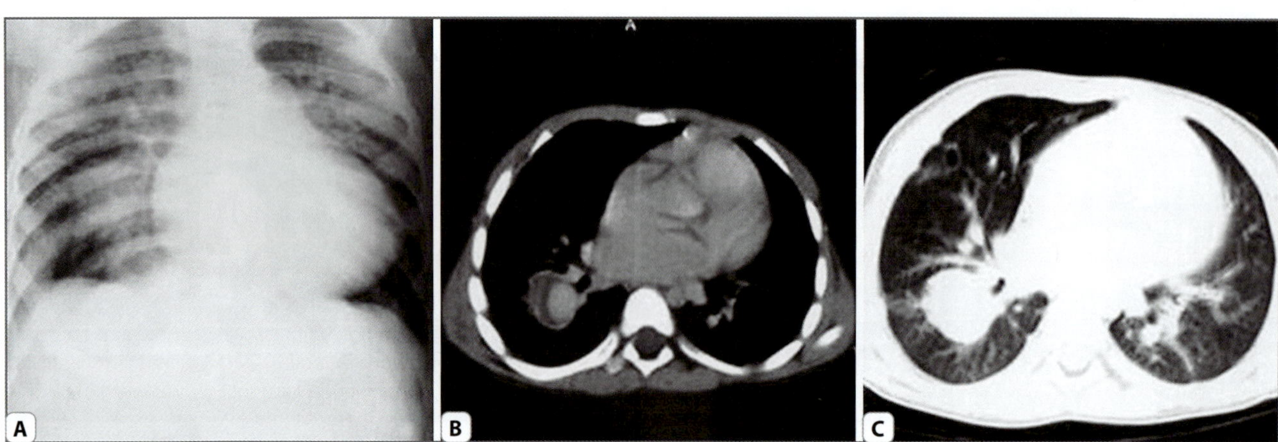

FIGS. 35A TO C: Chest radiograph (A) showing a sharply marginated solitary lesion located centrally in a perihilar location in the right lung (A). CT sections (B and C) showing an enhancing nodule in relation to a right interlobar pulmonary artery. A crescentic hypodensity is seen in the periphery of the lesion symptom of thrombus—pulmonary artery aneurysm.

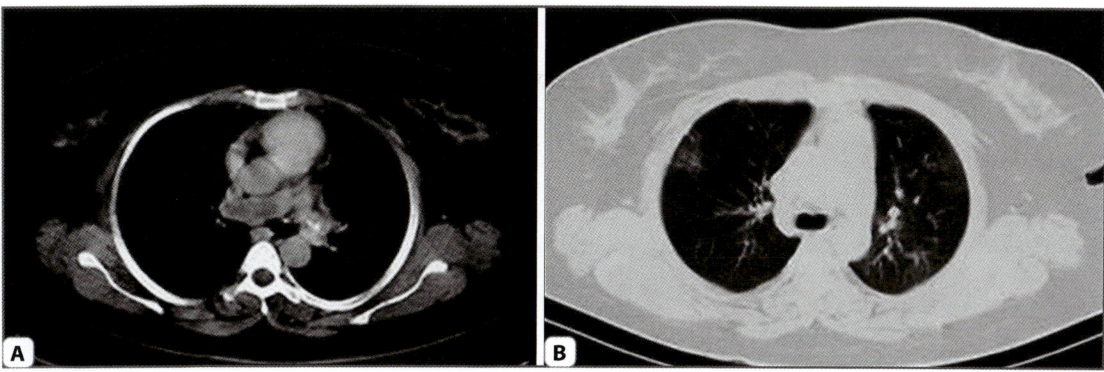

FIGS. 36A AND B: Contrast enhanced CT (A) in a case of DVT showing a filling defect in the right pulmonary artery suggestive of thrombus. Lung parenchyma (B) shows a wedge shaped pleural based opacity with surrounding halo symptoms of Hampton's hump in the right lung—pulmonary infarction.

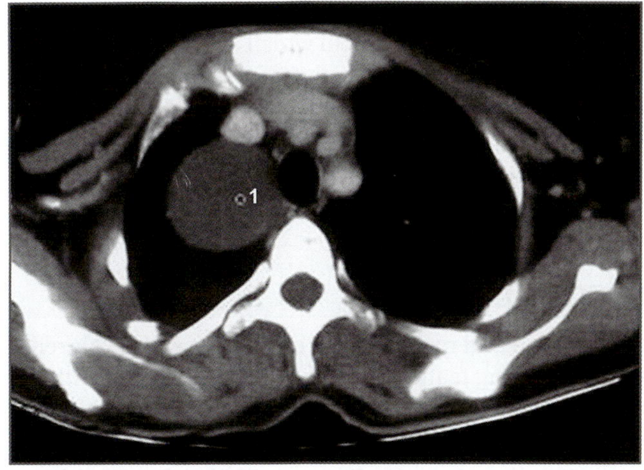

FIG. 37: CT scan showing a well circumscribed cystic density lesion adjacent to the trachea on the right side. The cyst wall is thin and smooth—bronchogenic cyst.

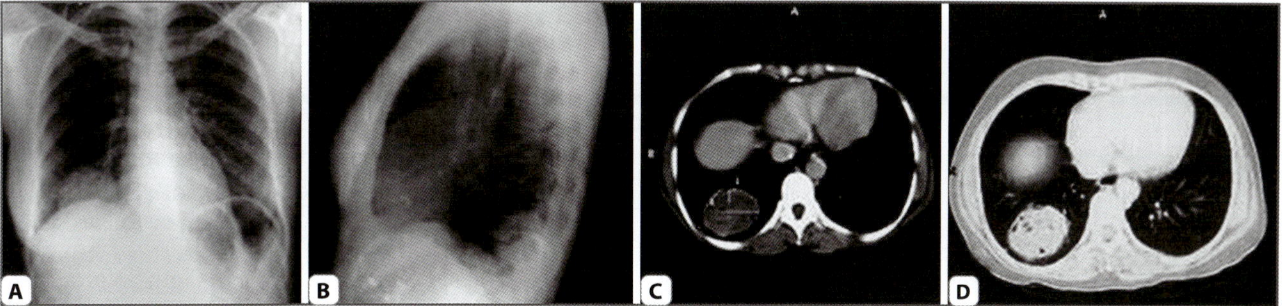

FIGS. 38A TO D: Chest radiograph frontal (A) and lateral projection (B) in a 35-year female with recurrent chest infections showing a well-defined sharply marginated lesion in the posterior basal segment of the right lower lobe. CT sections (C and D) showing a hypodense well-circumscribed lesion with multiple air foci suggesting communication with adjacent bronchi due to infection—pulmonary intralobar sequestration.

On CT, a variable density of the cyst ranging from water to soft tissue may be seen. The wall of the cyst is usually thin and smooth **(Fig. 37)**.

Sequestration

A disorganized area of pulmonary parenchyma without normal pulmonary arterial or bronchial communication is called "sequestrated lung". It is of two types intralobar and extralobar. Intralobar, the more common form, occurs usually in the posterior basal segment of the left lower lobe adjacent to the diaphragm **(Figs. 38A to D)**.[128] The intralobar form has a normal pulmonary venous drainage and infections are common in this form. The extralobar variety is more commonly associated with other congenital anomalies, has its own pleural covering and is separate with a systemic venous drainage.

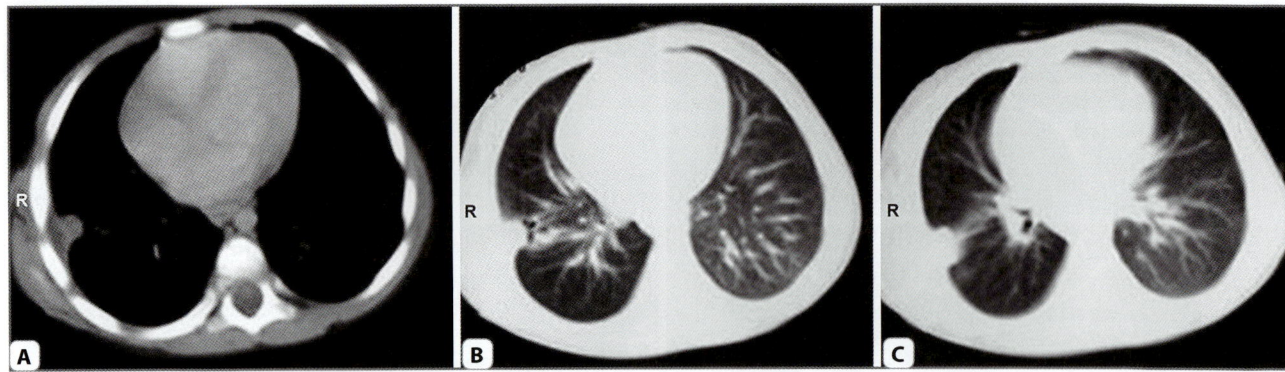

FIGS. 39A TO C: CT sections showing a peripherally located wedge shaped opacity against thickened pleura (A). There is distortion and displacement of vessels adjacent to the opacity. The vessels are more numerous than normal in this portion (B) and have a characteristic curvilinear configuration (C)—round atelectasis.

Miscellaneous

Round Atelectasis

Round atelectasis is a type of chronic atelectasis resembling a mass lesion. It is most often associated with asbestos related pleural disease, but it may occur in association with other conditions like tuberculosis, other infections, Dressler syndrome and mesothelioma. According to one of the suggested mechanisms, the common event is pleural thickening and pleural exudates with the resultant effusion causing passive atelectasis of the adjacent lung. Fibrinous adhesions develop between the pleural surface of the atelectatic lung and the adjacent parietal pleura. Another explanation is that as the pleural fibrosis matures, it retracts causing infolding and atelectasis of the lung parenchyma.[129] On imaging, round atelectasis is seen as a peripheral opacity which is oval or wedge shaped. It is based against a thickened pleura with the edge pointing toward the hilum being ill-defined and irregular. Distortion, displacement of the blood vessels and bronchi which appear pulled toward the lesion forms a characteristic imaging appearance called the "comet tail" or "crow feet" appearance **(Figs. 39A to C)**. Air bronchograms and calcification may be seen.[130] Round atelectasis may show contrast enhancement. Though mostly static, it may shrink and rarely resolve spontaneously.

CONCLUSION

The workup and management of patients with SPNs relies on the imaging features and the clinical findings with the aim to differentiate benign lesions from small malignant tumors. One should strive not only to identify small malignant tumors where resection results in high survival rates, but also to spare patients with benign disease from unnecessary surgery.

REFERENCES

1. Bankier AA, MacMahon H, Colby T, et al. Fleischner Society: Glossary of terms for Thoracic Imaging. Radiology 2024;310(2):e232558.
2. Holin SM, Dwork RE, Glaser S, et al. Solitary pulmonary nodules found in a community wide chest roentgenographic survey. Am Rev Tuberc. 1959;79:427-39.
3. Bray F, Laversanne M, Sung H, et al. Global cancer statistics 2022: GLOBOCAN estimates of incidence and mortality worldwide for 36 cancers in 185 countries. CA Cancer J Clin. 2024;74(3):229-63.
4. Choi Y, Gil BM, Chung MH, et al. Comparing attenuations of malignant and benign solitary pulmonary nodule using semi-automated region of interest selection on contrast-enhanced CT. J Thorac Dis. 2019;11(6):2392-401.
5. Austin JH, Garg K, Aberle D, et al. Radiologic implications of the 2011 classification of adenocarcinoma of the lung. Radiololgy. 2013;266:62-71.
6. Beigelman-Aubry C, Hill C, Grenier PA. Management of an incidentally discovered pulmonary nodule. Eur Radiol. 2007;17:449-66.
7. Heitzman ER, Markarian B, Raasch BN, et al. Pathways of tumor spread through the lung: Radiologic correlations with anatomy and pathology. Radiology. 1982;144:3-14.
8. Zwirewich CV, Vedal S, Miller RR, et al. Solitary pulmonary nodule: High resolution CT and radiologic pathologic correlation. Radiology. 1991;179:469-76.
9. Khan A, Herman PG, Vorwerk P, et al. Solitary pulmonary nodule: comparison of classification with standard, thin section and reference phantom CT. Radiology. 1991;179:477-81.
10. Huston J III, Muhm JR. Solitary pulmonary opacities: plain tomography. Radiology. 1987;163:481-5.
11. Hill CA. "Tail" signs associated with pulmonary lesions: critical rappraisal. AJR. 1982;139:311-6.

12. Chen SW, Price J. Focal organizing pneumonia mimicking small peripheral adenocarcinoma on CT scans. Australas Radiol. 1998;42:360-3.
13. Li F, Sone S, Abe H, et al. Malignant versus benign nodules at CT screening for lung cancer: Comparison of thin section CT findings. Radiology 2004;233:793-8.
14. Libby DM, Smith JP, Altorki NK, et al. Managing the small pulmonary nodule discovered by CT. Chest. 2004;125: 1522-9.
15. Park CM, Goo JM, Lee HJ, et al. Nodular ground glass opacity at thin section CT: histologic correlation and evaluation of change at follow up. Radiographics 2007;27:391-408.
16. Berger WG, Erly WK, Krupiniski EA, et al. The solitary pulmonary nodule on chest radiography: can we really tell if the nodule is calcified? AJR. 2001;176:201-4.
17. Grewal RG, Austin JH. CT demonstration of calcification in carcinoma of the lung. J Comput Assist Tomogr. 1994;18: 867-71.
18. Mahoney MC, Shipley RT, Corcoran HL, et al. CT demonstration of calcification in carcinoma of the lung. AJR. 1990;154:255-8.
19. Swensen SJ, Morin RL, et al. CT reconstruction algorithm selection in the evaluation of solitary pulmonary nodules. J Comput Assist Tomogr. 1995;19:932-5.
20. Ko JP, Naidich DP. Lung nodule detection and characterization with multislice CT. Radiol Clin North Am. 2003;41:575-97.
21. Woodring JH, Fried AM. Significance of wall thickness in solitary cavities of the lung: A follow up study. AJR. 1983;140:473-4.
22. Honda T, Kondo T, Murakami S, et al. Radiologic implications of the 2011 classification of adenocarcinoma of the lung. Radiology. 2013;266(1):62-71.
23. Travis WD, Brambilla E, Noguchi M, et al. Diagnosis of lung adenocarcinoma in resected specimens, implication of the 2011 International Association for the study of Lung Cancer/ American Thoracic Society/European Respiratory Society classification. Arch Pathol Lab Med. 2013;137(5):685-705.
24. Park CM, Goo JM, Lee HJ, et al. CT findings of atypical adenomatous hyperplasia in the lung. Korean J Radiol. 2006;7(2):80-6.
25. Goo JM, Park CM, Lee HJ. Ground glass nodules on CT as imaging biomarkers in the management of lung adenocarcinoma. Am J Roentgenol. 2011;196:533-43.
26. Tsutani Y, Miyata Y, Nakayama H, et al. Prognostic significance of using solid versus whole tumour size on high resolution computed tomography for predicting pathologic malignant grade of tumours in clinical stage IA of lung adenocarcinoma: a multicentric study. J Thorac Cardiovasc Surg. 2012;143(3): 607-12.
27. Truong MJ, Ko JP, Rosi SE, et al. Update in the evaluation of the solitary pulmonary nodule. Radiographics. 2014;34: 1658-79.
28. Garland LH. Bronchial carcinomas: lobar distribution of lesions in 250 cases. Calif Med. 1961;94:7-8.
29. Swensen SJ, Viggiano RW, Midthun DE, et al. Lung nodule enhancement at CT: multicentre study. Radiology. 2000;214:73-80.
30. Winer Muram HT, Jennings SG, Tarver RD, et al. Volumetric growth rate of stage I lung cancer prior to treatment: serial CT scanning. Radiology. 2002;223:798-805.
31. Quinn D, Gianlupi A, Broste S. The changing radiographic presentation of bronchogenic carcinoma with reference to cell types. Chest. 1996;110:1474-9.
32. Swensen SJ, Silverstein MD, Ilstrup DM. The probability of malignancy in solitary pulmonary nodules: Application to small radiographically in determinate nodules. Arch Int Med. 1997;157:849-55.
33. Kundel HL. Predictive value and threshold detectability of lung tumors. Radiology. 1981;139(1):25-9.
34. Bueno J, Landeras L, Chung JH. Updated Fleischner Society guidelines for managing incidental pulmonary nodules: common questions and challenging scenarios. Radiographics. 2018;38(5):1337-50.
35. Zerhouni EA, Stitik FP, Siegelman SS, et al. CT of the pulmonary nodule: a cooperative study. Radiology. 1986;160(2):319-27.
36. Webb WR. Radiologic evaluation of the solitary pulmonary nodule. AJR. 1990;154:701-8.
37. Bankier AA, MacMahon H, Goo JM, et al. Recommendations for measuring pulmonary nodules at CT: a statement from the Fleischner Society. Radiology. 2017;285(2):584-600.
38. Rampinelli C, Cicchetti G, Cortese G, et al. Management of incidental pulmonary nodule in CT: a survey by the Italian College of Chest Radiology. La Radiologia Medica. 2019;124:602-12.
39. Gaeta M, Blandino A, Scribano E, et al. Computed tomography halo sign in pulmonary nodules: frequency and diagnostic value. J Thorac Imaging. 1999;14:109-13.
40. Primack SL, Hartman TE, Lee KS, et al. Pulmonary nodules and the CT halo sign. Radiology 1994;190:513-5.
41. Lee Ks, Kim Y. Han J, et al. Bronchioloalveolar carcinoma: clinical, histopathologic and radiologic findings. Radiographics 1997;17:1345-57.
42. Kuriyama K,Tateishi R, Doi O, et al. Prevalence of air bronchograms in small peripheral carcinomas of the lung on thin section CT: Comparison with benign tumors. AJR. 1991;156: 921-4.
43. Kuii M, Templeton PA, White CS, et al. Evaluation of the air bronchogram sign on CT in solitary pulmonary lesions. J Comput Assist Tomogr. 1996;20(6):983-6.
44. Milne EN, Zerhouni EA. Blood supply of pulmonary metastases. J Thorac Imaging. 1987;2:15-23.
45. Mori K, Saitou Y, Tominaga K, et al. Small nodular lesions in the lung periphery: New approach to diagnosis with CT. Radiology. 1990;177:843-9.
46. Singh SP. The positive bronchus sign. Radiology. 1998;209: 251-2.
47. Snoeckx A, Reyntiens P, Desbuquoit D, et al. Evaluation of the solitary pulmonary nodule: size matters, but do not ignore the power of morphology. Insights imaging. 2018;9:73-86.
48. Soubani AO. The evaluation and management of solitary pulmonary nodule. Postgrad Med J. 2008;84:459-66.
49. Wang YX, Gong JS, Suzuki K, et al. Evidence based imaging strategies for solitary pulmonary nodule. J Thorac Dis. 2014;6(7):872 87.
50. Alpert JB, Ko JP. Management of incidental lung nodules: current strategy and rationale. Radiol Clin N Am. 2018;56(3):339-51.
51. Godoy MC, Naidisch DP. Subsolid pulmonary nodules and the spectrum of peripheral adenocarcinomas of the lung:

recommended interim guidelines for assessment and management. Radiology. 2009;253:606-22.

52. Yankelevitz DF, Heneschke CI. Does 2 year stability imply that pulmonary nodules are benign? AJR. 1997;168:325-8.
53. Ko JP, Bagga B, Gozansky E, et al. Solitary pulmonary nodule evaluation: pearls and pitfalls. Semin Ultrasound CT MRI. 2022;43(3)230-45.
54. Revel MP, Lefort C, Bissery A, et al. Pulmonary Nodules: Preliminary Experience with Three dimensional evaluation. Radiology. 2004;231:459-66.
55. Kim H, Park CM, Woo S, et al. Pure and part solid pulmonary ground glass nodules : measurement variability of volume and mass in nodules with a solid portion less than or equal to 5 mm. Radiology. 2013;269:585-93.
56. Petrou M, Quint LE, Nan B, et al. Pulmonary nodule volumetric measurement variability as a function of CT slice thickness and nodule morphology. AJR. 2007;188:306-12.
57. Zhang L, Yankelevitz PF, Carter D, et al. Internal growth of non-solid lung nodules: radiologic-pathologic correlation. Radiology. 2012;263(1):279-86
58. de Hoop B, Gietema H, Vande Vorst S, et al. Pulmonary ground glass nodules: increase in mass as an early indicator of growth. Radiology. 2010;255:199-206.
59. Qureshi NR, Shah A, Eaton RJ, et al. Dynamic contrast enhanced CT in nodule characterization: how we review and report. Cancer Imaging. 2016;16:1-5.
60. Weir-McCall JR, Joyce S, Clegg A, et al. Dynamic contrast–enhanced computed tomography for the diagnosis of solitary pulmonary nodules: a systematic review and meta-analysis. Eur Radiol. 2020;30:3310-23.
61. Zhang M, Kono M. Solitary pulmonary nodules: Evaluation of blood flow patterns with dynamic CT. Radiol. 1997;205: 471-8.
62. Yamashita K, Matsunobe S, Tsuda T, et al. Solitary pulmonary nodule: Preliminary study of evaluation with incremental dynamic CT. Radiol. 1995;194:399-405.
63. Swensen SJ, Brown LR, Colby TV, et al. Lung nodule enhancement at CT: Prospective findings. Radiol. 1996;201: 447-55.
64. Murayama S, Murakami J, Hashimoto S, et al. Noncalcified pulmonary tuberculomas: CT enhancement patterns with histological correlation. J Thorac Imaging. 1995;10:91-5.
65. Jeong YJ, Lee KS, Jeong SY, et al. Solitary Pulmonary Nodule: Characterization with Combined wash in and washout features at Dynamic Multi detector Row CT. Radiol. 2005;237:675-83.
66. Yi CA, Lee KS, Kim EA, et al. Solitary pulmonary nodules: dynamic enhanced multi detector row CT study and comparison with vascular endothelial growth factor and microvessel density. Radiol. 2004;233:191-9.
67. Gadgeel SM, Ramalingam S, Cummmings G, et al. Lung cancer in patients <50 years of age: the experience of an academic multidisciplinary program. Chest. 1999;115: 1232-6.
68. Guyatt GH, Newhouse MD. Are active and passive smoking harmful? Determination of causation. Chest. 1985;88: 445-51.
69. Bach PB, Kaltan M, Thornquist MD, et al. Variations in lung cancer risk among smokers. J Natl Canc Inst. 2003;95:470-8.
70. Lee PN. Relation between exposure to asbestos and smoking jointly and the risk of lung cancer. Occup Environ Med. 2001;58:145-53.
71. Erasmus JJ, Mc Adams HP, Connolly JE. Solitary pulmonary nodules: Part-II. Evaluation of the indeterminate nodule. Radiographics. 2000;20:59-66.
72. Gurney JW, Lyddon DM, Mckay JA. Determining the likelihood of malignancy in solitary pulmonary nodules with Bayesian analysis Part II. Application. Radiology. 1993;186: 415-32.
73. Black WC, Armstrong P. Communicating the significance of radiologic test results: the likelihood ratio. AJR. 1986;147:1313-8.
74. Soardi GA, Perandini S, Molton M, et al. Assessing probability of malignancy in solid solitary pulmonary nodules with a new Bayesian calculator:improving diagnostic accuracy by means of expanded and updated features. Eur Radiol. 2015;25(1):155-62.
75. Sim YT, Poon FW. Imaging of solitary pulmonary nodule- a clinical review. Quant Imaging Med Surg. 2013;3:316-26.
76. Nomori H, Wattanbe K, Ohtsuka T, et al. Evaluation of F-18 fluorodeoxyglucose (FDG) PET scanning for pulmonary nodules less than 3 cm in diameter with special reference to CT images. Lung Cancer. 2004;45:19-27.
77. Lowe VJ, Fletcher JW, Gobar C, et al. Prospective investigation of PET in lung nodules (PIOPILN), J Clin Oncol. 1998;16: 1075-84.
78. Huber KF, Buonocore E, Gould HR, et al. Differentiating benign from malignant lung lesions using quantitative parameters of FDG PET images. Clin Nucl Med. 1996;21: 941-49.
79. Shimizu K, Ikeda N, Tuboi M, et al. Percutaneous Ct guided fine needle aspiration for lung cancer smaller than 2 cm and revealed by ground glass opacity at CT. Lung Cancer. 2006;51(2):173-9.
80. Moore EH. Needle aspiration lung biopsy: A comprehensive approach to complication reduction. J Thorac Imaging. 1997;12:259-71.
81. Martin MD, Henry TS, Berry MF, et al. ACR Appropriateness Criteria® Incidentally Detected Indeterminate Pulmonary Nodule. J Am Coll Radiol. 2023;20(11):S455-70.
82. Ohno Y, Hatabu H, Takenaka D, et al. Solitary pulmonary nodules: potential role of dynamic MR imaging in management: initial experiences. Radiol. 2002;224:503-11.
83. Kono M, Adachi S, Kusumoto M, et al. Clinical utility of Gd–DTPA - enhanced magnetic resonance imaging in lung cancer. J Thorac Imaging. 1993;8:18-26.
84. Guckel C, Schnabel K, Deimling M, et al. Solitary pulmonary nodules: MR evaluation of enhancement patterns with contrast enhanced dynamic snapshot gradient echo imaging. Radiol. 1996;200:681-6.
85. Ohno Y, Kauczor HU, Hatabu H, et al. MRI for solitary pulmonary nodule and mass assessment: current state of the art. J Magn Reson Imaging. 2018;47(6):1437-58.
86. Mohakud S, Das R, Bag ND, et al. A prospective observational study of diagnostic reliability of semiquantitative and quantitative high b-value diffusion-weighted MRI in distinguishing between benign and malignant lung lesions at 3 Tesla. Indian J Radiol Imaging. 2024;34(01):6-15.

87. Satoh S, Kitazume Y, Ohdama S. Can malignant and benign pulmonary nodules be differentiated with diffusion weighted MRI? AJR. 2008;191:464-70.
88. Broncano J, Steinbrecher K, Marquis KM, et al. Diffusion-weighted imaging of the chest: a primer for radiologists. RadioGraphics. 2023;43(7):e220138.
89. Bhalla AS, Garg A. Diffusion-Weighted MRI: Potential Tool for Pulmonary Nodule Characterization. Indian J Radiol Imaging. 2024;34(01):1-2.
90. Usuda K, Ishikawa M, Iwai S, et al. Pulmonary nodule and mass: superiority of MRI of diffusion-weighted imaging and T2-weighted imaging to FDG-PET/CT. Cancers. 2021;13(20):5166.
91. Lei Q, Wan Q, Liu L, et al. Values of Apparent Diffusion Coefficient and Lesion-to-Spinal Cord Signal Intensity in Diagnosing Solitary Pulmonary Lesions: Turbo Spin-Echo versus Echo-Planar Imaging Diffusion-Weighted Imaging. Biomed Res Int. 2021;2021(1):3345953.
92. Chae EJ, Song JW, Seo JB, et al. Clinical utility of Dual. Energy CT in the evaluation of solitary pulmonary nodules: Initial Experience. Radiology. 2008;249(2):671-81.
93. Perrella A, Bagnacci G, Di Meglio N, et al. Thoracic diseases: technique and applications of dual-energy CT. Diagnostics. 2023;13(14):2440.
94. Zhu X, Zhu L, Song D, et al. Comparison of single-and dual-energy CT combined with artificial intelligence for the diagnosis of pulmonary nodules. Clin Radiol. 2023;78(2):e99-105.
95. Kundu K, Kumar A, Malik R, et al. The Role of CT Perfusion in Differentiating Benign Versus Malignant Focal Pulmonary Lesions. Cureus. 2024;16(7):e63618.
96. Zhu B, Zheng S, Jiang T, et al. Evaluation of dual-energy and perfusion CT parameters for diagnosing solitary pulmonary nodules. Thorac Cancer. 2021;12(20):2691-7.
97. Liang G, Yu W, Liu SQ, et al. The value of radiomics based on dual-energy CT for differentiating benign from malignant solitary pulmonary nodules. BMC Med Imaging. 2022;22(1):95.
98. Koo CW, Kline TL, Yoon JH, et al. Magnetic resonance radiomic feature performance in pulmonary nodule classification and impact of segmentation variability on radiomics. Br J Radiol. 2022;95(1140):20220230.
99. Ather S, Kadir T, Gleeson F. Artificial intelligence and radiomics in pulmonary nodule management: current status and future applications. Clinical radiology. 2020;75(1):13-9.
100. Liu JA, Yang IY, Tsai EB. Artificial intelligence (AI) for lung nodules, from the AJR special series on AI applications. Am J Roentgenol. 2022;219(5):703-12.
101. de Margerie-Mellon C, Chassagnon G. Artificial intelligence: A critical review of applications for lung nodule and lung cancer. Diagn Interv Imaging. 2023;104(1):11-7.
102. Girvin F, Ko JP. Pulmonary Nodules: Detection, Assessment and CAD. AJR. 2008;191:1057-69.
103. Kim RY, Oke JL, Pickup LC, et al. Artificial intelligence tool for assessment of indeterminate pulmonary nodules detected with CT. Radiology. 2022;304(3):683-91.
104. Nam JG, Hwang EJ, Kim J, et al. AI improves nodule detection on chest radiographs in a health screening population: a randomized controlled trial. Radiology. 2023;307(2):e221894.
105. Wormanns D, Kohl G, Klotz E, et al. Volumetric measurements of pulmonary nodules at multi-row detector CT: in vivo reproducibility. Eur Radiol. 2004;14:86-92.
106. MacMohan MB, Austin JHM, Gamsu G, et al. Guidelines for management of small pulmonary nodules detected on CT scans: A statement from the Fleischner Society. Radiology. 2005;237:395-400.
107. Patel VK, Naik SK, Naidich DP, et al. A practical approach to the diagnosis and management of solitary pulmonary nodules: part 2-pretest probability and algorithm. Chest. 2013;143(3):840-6.
108. Naidich DP, Bankier AA, McMohan H, et al. Recommendations for the management of subsolid pulmonary nodules detected at CT: a statement from the Fleischner Society. Radiol. 2013;266:304-17.
109. Vasquez M, Carter D, Brambilla E, et al. Solitary and multiple resected adenocarcinomas after CT screening for lung cancer: histopathologic features and their prognostic implications. Lung Cancer. 2009;64(2):148-54.
110. MacMahon H, Naidich DP, Goo JM, et al. Guidelines for management of incidental pulmonary nodules detected on CT images: from the Fleischner Society 2017. Radiology. 2017;284(1):228-43.
111. Kazerooni EA, Armstrong M, Amorosa JK, et al. ACR CT accreditation program and lung cancer screening program designation. J Am Coll Radiol. 2016;13(2 Suppl):R 30-34.
112. Christensen J, Prosper AE, Wu CC, et al. ACR lung-RADS v2022: assessment categories and management recommendations. J Am Coll Radiol. 2024;21(3):473-88.
113. Martin MD, Kanne JP, Broderick LS, et al. RadioGraphics Update: Lung-RADS 2022. RadioGraphics. 2023;43(11):e230037.
114. Nam JG, Goo JM. Evaluation and management of indeterminate pulmonary nodules on chest computed tomography in asymptomatic subjects: the principles of nodule guidelines. Semin Respir Crit Care Med. 2022;43(06):851-61.
115. Armstrong P. Basic patterns in lung disease. In: Hansell DM, Armstrong P, Lynch DA, McAdams HP, (Eds). Imaging of Disease of the Chest. Philadelphia: Mosby. 2005;69-141.
116. Hirakata K, Nakata H, Haratake J. Appearance of pulmonary metastases on high resolution CT scans. Comparison with histopathologic findings from autopsy specimens. AJR. 1993;161:37-43.
117. Choplin RH, Kawanmoto EH, Dyer RB, et al. Atypical carcinoid of the lung: Radiographic features. AJR. 1986;146:665-8.
118. Muller NL, Miller RR. Neuroendocrine carcinomas of the lung. Seminar Roentgenol 1990;25:96-104.
119. Au V, Leung AN. Radiologic manifestations of lymphoma in the thorax. AJR. 1997;168:93-8.
120. Gjevre JA, Myers JL, Prakash UB. Pulmonary hamartomas: Mayo Clin Proc. 1996;71:14-20.
121. Siegelman SS, Khouri NF, Scott WW, et al. Pulmonary hamartoma: CT findings. Radiol. 1986;160:313-7.
122. Carney JA. The triad of gastric epithelioid leiomyosarcoma pulmonary chondroma and functioning extra adrenal paraganglioma: A five-year review. Medicine (Baltimore). 1983;62:159-69.
123. Celebi S, Hacimustafaoglu M. Round pneumonia in children. Ind J Paed. 2008;75:523-5.

124. Cortet B, Flipo RM, Remy Jordin M, et al. Use of high-resolution computed tomography of the lungs in patients with rheumatoid arthritis. Ann Rheum Dis. 1995;54:815-9.
125. Ferratti GR, Thony F, Link KM, et al. False aneurysm of the pulmonary artery induced by a Swan Ganz catheter: Clinical presentation and radiologic management. AJR. 1996;167: 941-5.
126. Spear BS, Sully L, Lewis CT. Pulmonary arteriovenous fistula presenting as spontaneous hemothorax. Thorax. 1975;30: 355-6.
127. Burkill GJ, Bell JR, Padley SP. Survey on the use of pulmonary scintigraphy, spiral CT and conventional pulmonary angiography for suspected pulmonary embolism in the British Isles. Clin Radiol. 1999;54:807-10.
128. Frazier AA, Rosado de Christenson ML, Stoker JT, et al. Intralobar sequestration: Radiologic pathologic correlation. Radiographics. 1997;17:725-45.
129. Carvalho PM, Carr DH. Computed tomography of folded lung. Clin Radiol. 1990;41:86-91.
130. O' Donovan PB, Schenk M, Lim K, et al. Evaluation of the reliability of computed tomographic criteria used in the diagnosis of round atelectasis. J Thoracic Imaging. 1997;12:54-8.

Priyanka Naranje, Mukesh Kumar Yadav, Chandan Jyoti Das

CHAPTER

13 Imaging of Pulmonary Neoplasms

INTRODUCTION

Lung cancer is amongst the most common and most lethal cancers around the world. It represents about 13% of the new cancer cases and up to 21% of the cancer deaths.[1,2] In India, lung cancer accounts for 6.9% of all newly diagnosed cancer cases and 9.3% of all cancer-related deaths across both genders. It is the most prevalent cancer and the leading cause of cancer-related mortality among men, with the highest incidence rates reported in Mizoram for both males and females (age-adjusted rates of 28.3 and 28.7 per 100,000 population, respectively).[3]

Overall, 5-year survival with this cancer is less than 15%. Most lung cancers are directly attributed to smoking. Reported highest incidence in smokers is 362 cases per 100,000 per year while the same in non-smokers is up to 21 cases only.[4, 5] Passive smoking increases the risk of lung cancer by up to 30%. Exposure to nickel, cobalt, asbestos, radiation, and pesticides also increase the risk of lung cancer. Lung is also the most common site of metastatic involvement from other extrathoracic malignancies; 20–54% of extrathoracic malignancies have pulmonary metastatic disease.[4] Synchronous and metachronous second lung malignancy occurs in about 2% of patients with lung cancer.[6]

A wide variety of imaging techniques are currently available for detection, diagnosis, and management of pulmonary neoplasms. Chest radiography is the primary imaging modality for detection of lung nodules and masses. Computed tomography (CT) and positron emission tomography (PET) are most commonly used imaging modalities for further characterization, to define extent and for pre-treatment staging of the lung malignancies. Imaging is also required to assess the response to nonsurgical treatment and for follow up in treated patients. MRI has an evolving role in evaluation of lung malignancies and is occasionally used as a problem-solving modality and in assessment of treatment response. Ultrasonography (USG) has limited utility in lung cancer assessment, however, it may be used for guided biopsy in cases of large peripheral tumors abutting the pleura/chest wall. Artificial intelligence algorithms and radiomics are emerging technologies with potential applications in lung cancer imaging.

THE WHO CLASSIFICATION

Pulmonary neoplasms are classified pathologically according to 5th edition of the World Health Organization (WHO) classification 2021 which provides a standardized terminology for lung cancer **(Box 1)**.[7] The 2015, followed by 2021 WHO classification book brought significant updates, driven by advancements in genetics and molecular-targeted therapies. The incorporation of immunohistochemistry and molecular testing throughout the classification has enabled more advanced methods for pathological diagnosis. These developments have led to a more accurate pathological and genetic classification of lung tumors, facilitating improved therapeutic approaches. For example, epidermal growth factor (EGFR) mutations, anaplastic lymphoma kinase (ALK) rearrangements and ROS1 are found in adenocarcinoma, and these are effective targets for specific drugs such as EGFR tyrosine kinase inhibitors (Erlotinib, Gefitinib) or ALK inhibitors (crizotinib) in patients with advanced lung adenocarcinoma. Similarly, a pneumocyte marker such as thyroid transcription factor (TTF)-1 is desired to address primary versus metastatic adenocarcinoma.

CLINICAL FEATURES

Depending on the location, extent, size and histopathology of the tumor, various clinical manifestations are seen. Systemic symptoms of weight loss, anorexia and fever are common. Cough and hemoptysis are the most common clinical features of lung cancers. Hemoptysis may be streaky or massive at the presentation. Central tumors may present with wheeze and recurrent pneumonia

BOX 1: The 2021 WHO classification of lung tumors.

Epithelial tumors

- Papillomas:
  - Squamous cell papilloma, NOS
  - Squamous cell papilloma, inverted
- Adenomas:
  - Sclerosing pneumocytoma
  - Bronchiolar adenoma/ciliated muconodular papillary tumor
- Precursor glandular lesions:
  - Atypical adenomatous hyperplasia
  - Adenocarcinoma in situ—mucinous/non-mucinous
- Adenocarcinomas
- Minimally invasive adenocarcinoma *(*mucinous / non-mucinous*)*
- Invasive nonmucinous adenocarcinoma:
  - Lepidic adenocarcinoma
  - Acinar adenocarcinoma
  - Papillary adenocarcinoma
  - Micropapillary adenocarcinoma
  - Solid adenocarcinoma
- Invasive mucinous adenocarcinoma
- Squamous precursor lesions:
  - Squamous cell carcinoma in situ, mild/moderate/severe squamous dysplasia
- Squamous cell carcinomas:
  - Squamous cell carcinoma, NOS/ keratinizing/ nonkeratinizing
  - Lymphoepithelial carcinoma
- Large cell carcinomas
- Sarcomatoid carcinomas:
  - Pleomorphic carcinoma
  - Carcinosarcoma
- Other epithelial tumors:
  - NUT carcinoma
  - Thoracic SMARCA4-deficient undifferentiated tumor[a]
- Salivary gland-type tumors:
  - Pleomorphic adenoma
  - Adenoid cystic carcinoma
  - Epithelial-myoepithelial carcinoma
  - Mucoepidermoid carcinoma
- Myoepithelioma/ carcinoma.

Lung neuroendocrine neoplasms

- Precursor lesion:
  - Diffuse idiopathic neuroendocrine cell hyperplasia
- Neuroendocrine tumors:
  - Carcinoid tumor:
    - Typical carcinoid/neuroendocrine tumor, grade 1
    - Atypical carcinoid/neuroendocrine tumor, grade 2
    - Neuroendocrine carcinomas:
  - Small cell carcinoma

Continued

Continued

Tumors of ectopic tissues

- Melanoma
- Meningioma

Mesenchymal tumors specific to the lung

- Pulmonary hamartoma
- Chondroma
- Diffuse lymphangiomatosis
- Pleuropulmonary blastoma
- Intimal sarcoma
- Congenital peribronchial myofibroblastic tumor
- Pulmonary myxoid sarcoma with EWSR1-CREB1 fusion
- PEComatous tumors:
  - Lymphangioleiomyomatosis
  - PEComa, benign/malignant

Hematolymphoid tumors

- MALT lymphoma
- Diffuse large B-cell lymphoma, NOS
- Lymphomatoid granulomatosis, NOS/ grade 1–3
- Intravascular large B-cell lymphoma
- Langerhans cell histiocytosis
- Erdheim–Chester disease

Source: This table is modified from WHO Classification of Tumours, Thoracic Tumours, 5th edition. pages 2–3, IARC, 2021.

due to bronchial obstruction. Advanced lung tumors with locoregional invasion of the pleura, chest wall or mediastinum may manifest with chest pain, brachial plexus neuropathy, Horner syndrome, phrenic or recurrent laryngeal nerve palsy, dysphagia or SVC obstruction. Besides, there are several paraneoplastic syndromes that may be associated with lung cancer such as Eaton-Lambart syndrome, subacute cerebellar degeneration, encephalomyelopathy, Cushing syndrome, hypertrophic pulmonary osteoarthropathy. Some small peripheral lung cancers may be asymptomatic and only be detected incidentally or on screening. Signs and symptoms due to metastasis could be bone pain, neurologic symptoms or pathological fracture.

IMAGING MODALITIES

Conventional chest radiography and cross-sectional imaging techniques such as computed tomography (CT), magnetic resonance imaging (MRI) and PET-CT play a role in the detection, diagnosis, and management of pulmonary parenchymal neoplasms. USG including CEUS has specific utility in guided sampling of the peripheral based lung tumors.[8]

Chest radiography (PA view) is the primary modality for detection of the lung cancer **(Fig. 1A)**.[9] Any solitary pulmonary nodule (rounded opacity <3 cm) or mass (opacity > 3 cm with any shape/margins) in an adult may be a lung cancer unless it is proved otherwise.

CT is more accurate for detection of abnormality and it is a modality of choice for characterization of pulmonary neoplasms.[9,10] CT forms an integral imaging technique for staging the lung cancers.[11] Advanced CT techniques such as dynamic perfusion CT,[12] dual energy CT[13] and dual-energy spectral CT imaging[14] as well as software based texture analysis[15] are new methods under evaluation for the characterization of lung tumors and help in distinguishing benign from malignant lesions. A routine CT protocol for the evaluation of suspected lung cancer should consist of a contrast-enhanced CT (CECT) of chest and upper abdomen including liver and adrenals.

PET provides functional information and hence it is generally more precise for overall evaluation of the disease extent. PET is not useful in T staging as its resolution is inferior and CECT is sufficient for this purpose. FDG uptake is also variable in tumors like invasive mucinous adenocarcinoma, carcinoid and small cell lung cancer and this may result in high false negative results on PET.[16-18] Conversely, false positive results may be seen in benign conditions like tuberculosis and sarcoidosis.[19]

PET is recommended as a single test for comprehensive preoperative evaluation of local and distant disease spread, with overall staging accuracy of > 90%.[20, 21] It is especially useful for mediastinal lymph node staging, differentiating benign from malignant pleural effusions[22] and detection of bone metastases.[23] In some patients, inflammatory lymph nodes may show PET uptake and cause false positive PET results. Similarly, because of the resolution issue, lymph nodes < 5 mm cannot be reliably evaluated on PETCT.[24]

PET is also useful in monitoring of patients undergoing nonsurgical management. Modern conformal radiotherapy techniques require accurate delineation of the tumor volume for the treatment plans. PET-CT is now preferred for radiotherapy planning as it can differentiate the viable tumor from adjacent necrotic tissues or consolidations and hence, more accurate than CT based planning.[25] This characteristic of PETCT is also useful for planning image guided biopsies from viable area of the tumor.

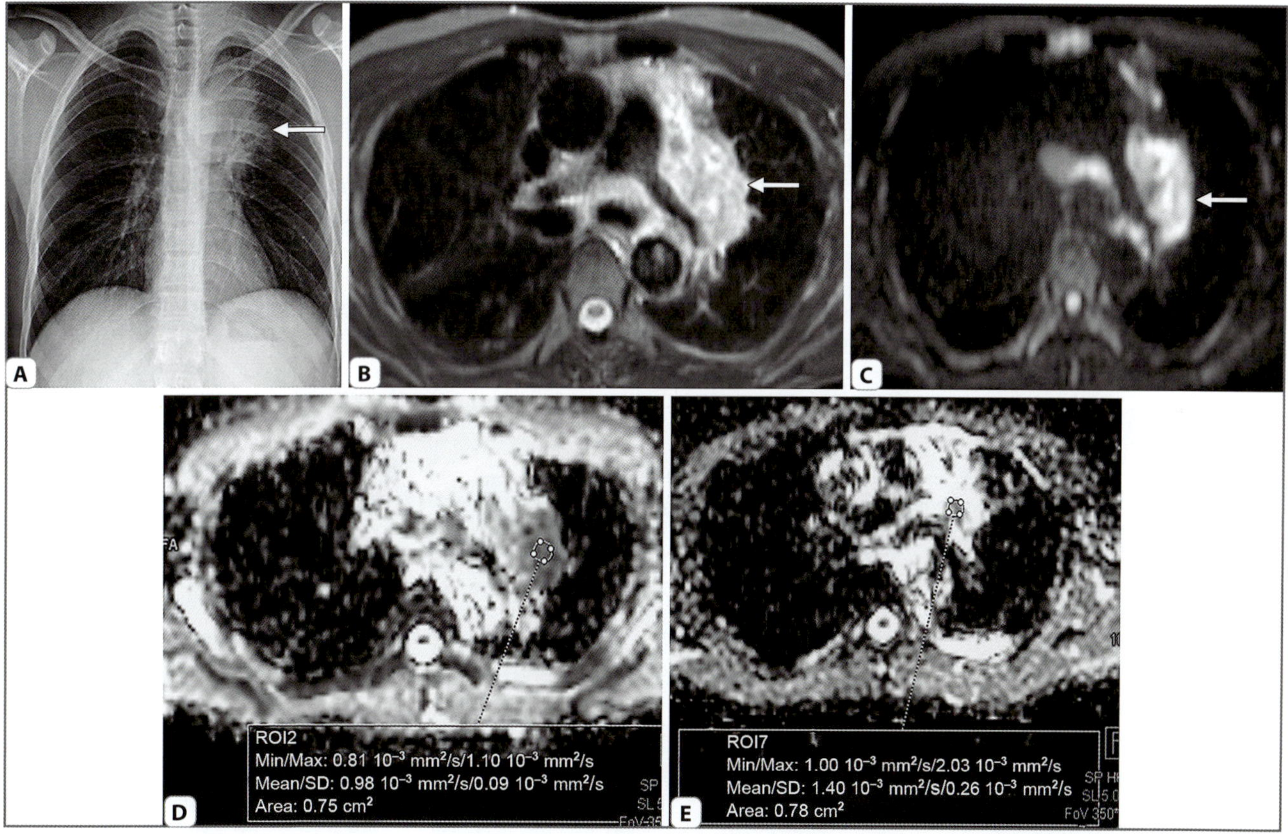

FIGS. 1A TO E: Diffusion weighted MRI in carcinoma lung: (A) Frontal chest radiograph showing mass in the left upper lobe extending in region of aortopulmonary window in a case of adenocarcinoma; (B) STIR axial image shows hyperintense mass in left upper lobe with mediastinal invasion; (C) Pre-chemotherapy DWI at b-1000 value, shows hyperintense signal in the region of mass with hypointense signal on corresponding ADC map; (D) ADC map shows a value of 0.98×10^{-3} mm²/s suggestive of restricted diffusion; (E) Post-chemotherapy there is reduction in the size of the tumor with increase in the ADC value suggestive of good response to chemotherapy.

For the assessment of response to chemotherapy, SUV monitoring is also more accurate and correlates better with patient survival than the RESIST size criteria used for conventional imaging techniques.[26,27] PET-CT is also useful to detect recurrences in treated patients, as it is more accurate in differentiating post-treatment changes from recurrences. However, radiation changes can sometimes show FDG uptake. To avoid false positive results, PET should be deferred until six months after the radiotherapy.

Magnetic Resonance Imaging

Owing to the recent advances made in overcoming the challenges in MR acquisition of lung, current status of MRI is increasing in detection, characterization of pulmonary nodules, tumor, node, metastasis (TNM) staging and tumor response assessments.[28] DWI as well as dynamic contrast enhanced MRI have shown to be useful in distinguishing benign and malignant lung nodules. Using a cutoff ADC value of 1.1×10^{-3} mm^2/s, a sensitivity of 70% and specificity of 97% using a b value of 1000 s/mm^2 was seen in one study.[29] DWI can be used for early assessment of tumor response post chemotherapy **(Figs. 1B to E)**. Similarly, there are various dynamic MRI techniques for distinguishing malignant nodules from benign nodules, with reported sensitivities ranging from 94% to 100%, specificities from 70% to 96%, and accuracies >88%.[30,31] MRI useful for brachial plexus involvement in superior sulcus tumors and assessment of chest wall, diaphragmatic pleura, great vessel and cardiac involvement.[32]

Imaging Features

Imaging features of the lung cancer are discussed under following headings: Peripheral tumors and central tumors.

Peripheral Tumors

Peripheral tumors are those arising beyond the segmental bronchi. Most commonly presents as nodule or mass with following characteristics.

Shape: Majority are spherical or oval in shape **(Fig. 2A)**. Superior sulcus tumors may resemble apical pleural thickening **(Fig. 2B)**.

Margins: It may be well-defined or ill-defined. Uneven rate of growth in different parts of the tumor may produce lobulations **(Fig. 3A)**. One or more strands may be seen extending from the main mass into surrounding lung giving rise to spiculated appearance which is termed as "corona radiata" **(Fig. 3A)**. Spiculations represent either tumor extension or desmoplastic reaction to the tumor. Spiculated margin is a useful sign to differentiate lung cancer from benign pulmonary nodules, although it may be rarely seen in granuloma and organizing pneumonia as well. A sharply defined spherical smooth edged nodule due to a carcinoma is rare. Sometimes, one or more linear strands may extend from a peripheral mass to the pleura known as "pleural tail" **(Fig. 3B)**. It can be seen in both benign and malignant lesions and hence it is not helpful in differentiating between the two.

Cavitation: Best seen on CT. Most commonly seen in squamous cell carcinoma histology, however, may be seen in any type of lung cancer. The wall of the cavity is usually >8 mm thick, may be smooth or more commonly is irregular and nodular **(Figs. 4A to C)**. Fluid levels may be seen within the cavity. It develops due to central necrosis, liquifection and emptying of the contents in the airways. Rarely, the cavity is seen as an air crescent, similar to the fungal ball. This appearance is caused by the air around an intracavitary tumor.

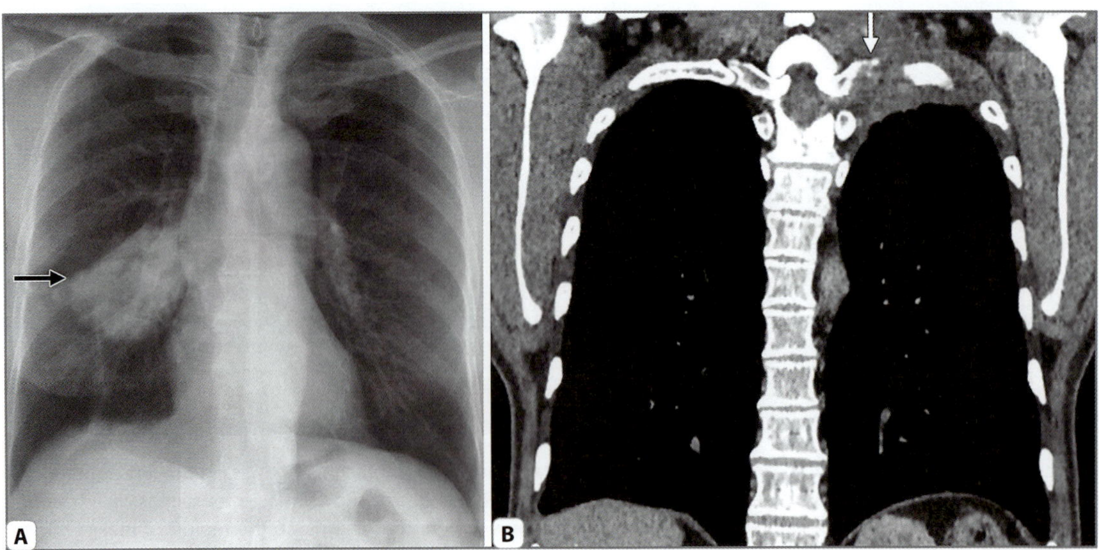

FIGS. 2A AND B: (A) Frontal chest radiograph showing an oval-shaped mass (arrow) in right parahilar location in a case of squamous cell carcinoma; (B) Coronal CT image showing plaque like thickening in the left apical region with adjacent rib erosion (white arrow) suggestive of superior sulcus tumor.

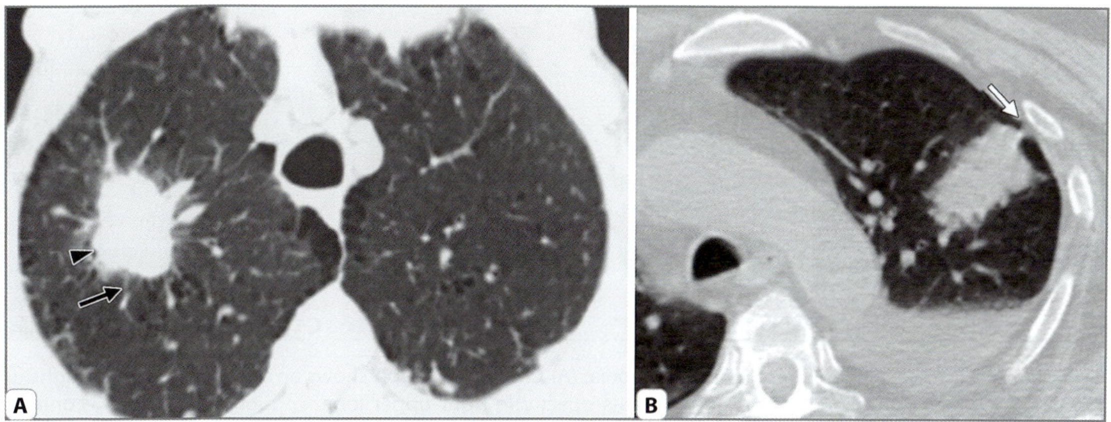

FIGS. 3A AND B: Corona radiata: (A) Axial CT image in a case of adenocarcinoma showing mass with multiple spiculations (arrow) as well as lobulations (arrowhead); (B) A small pleural tail is seen extending from the mass to pleura (arrow).

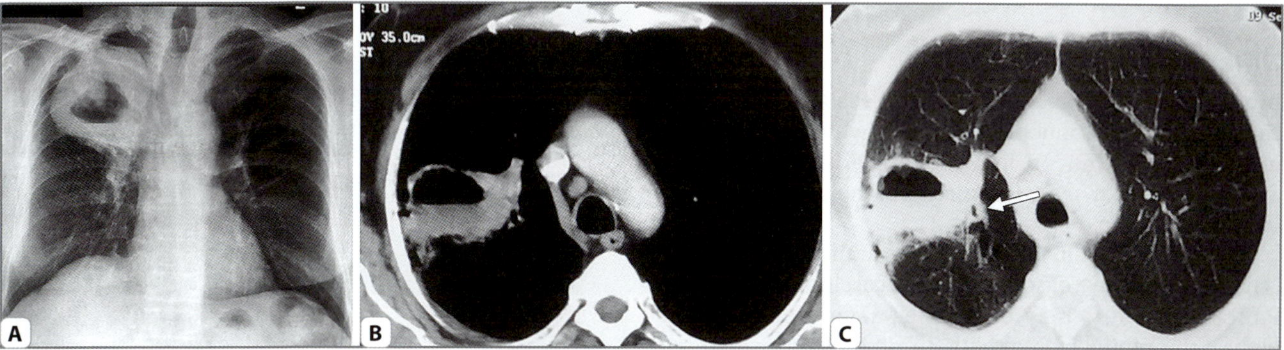

FIGS. 4A TO C: Squamous cell carcinoma: (A) Chest radiograph shows large cavitary lesion in right upper lobe with thick nodular walls and an air-fluid level; (B and C) CT scan of same patient shows right upper lobe cavity with irregular and nodular enhancing wall thickening with air fluid level. There is abrupt cut-off of bronchus at the tumor margin (arrow).

Calcification: Calcifications are rarely seen in lung cancers on chest radiographs; however, CT may demonstrate it in 6–10% patients.[33] These represent either preexisting granulomatous calcifications engulfed by the tumor or dystrophic calcifications developed in the areas of tumor necrosis. The dystrophic tumor calcification is usually amorphous **(Fig. 5)** or cloudy in appearance and located centrally while engulfed calcifications tend to be located at the periphery of the tumor. Tumor calcification may be seen in any type of bronchogenic carcinoma and there is no predilection for any specific histological subtype.[34]

Consolidation pattern: Atypical presentation can be tumors with entirely ill-defined margins resembling consolidation/pneumonia on chest radiographs **(Figs. 6A and B)**, e.g., lepidic predominant adenocarcinoma [formally called bronchiolo-alveolar carcinoma (BAC)], invasive mucinous adenocarcinoma (formally called mucinous BAC). Persistent or recurrent consolidation at same site, air bronchograms, bubble-like lucencies or pseudocavitation, expansion of the consolidated lobe, Golden S sign, dilated fluid filled bronchi are the features on CT scan or chest X-ray suspicious of malignancy.

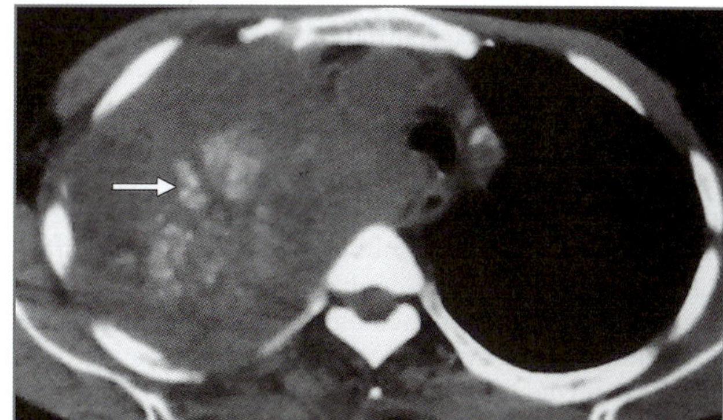

FIG. 5: Calcifications in lung cancer: NCCT shows large lung mass with fine, amorphous tumoral calcifications in a case of squamous cell carcinoma.

Ground glass attenuation nodule: A feature of adenocarcinoma in situ, atypical adenomatous hyperplasia or minimally invasive adenocarcinoma which may present as pure ground glass nodule **(Fig. 6C)** or part solid nodule and these tend to be slow growing tumors with better

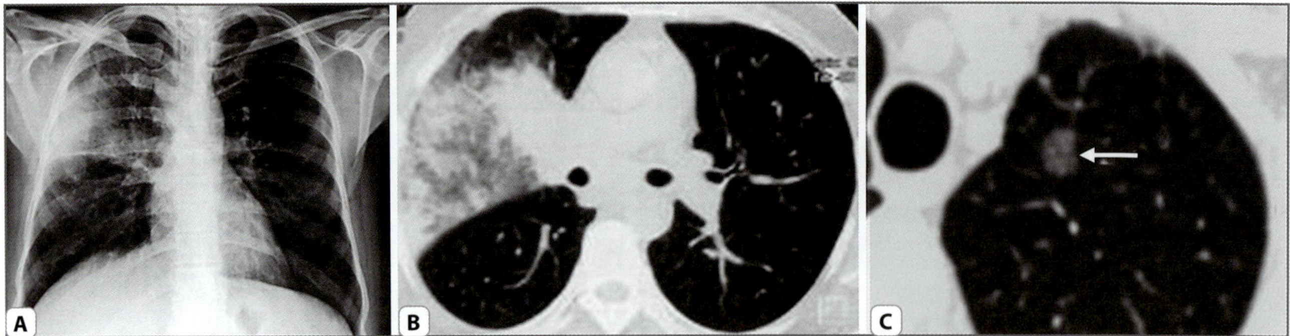

FIGS. 6A TO C: Lung cancer seen as non-resolving pneumonia: (A) Chest radiograph shows an airspace opacity in right upper lobe; (B) Corresponding CT shows consolidation and ground glass opacity in right upper lobe. Endobronchial biopsy confirmed lepidic predominant adenocarcinoma; (C) Adenocarcinoma in situ presenting as focal ground glass nodule in a different patient (arrow).

prognosis.[35] GGO surrounding a solid tumor may represent hemorrhage or inflammation or edema.

Other Findings

Bronchial carcinoma in segmental or distal bronchi may cause retention of mucoid secretions which is known as bronchocele or mucocele. On chest radiographs, these appear as tubular/oval densities with their stem pointing toward the hilum.

An abrupt cut-off of the bronchus at the tumor margin is highly suggestive of squamous cell carcinoma **(Fig. 4C)**. Pancoast tumors may present as asymmetric apical pleural thickening with or without rib erosions which are better delineated on CT. Old tubercular fibrosis does not predispose to lung cancer. In so-called scar carcinomas, the fibrous reaction follows, rather than precedes the carcinoma.

Growth rate: The round or oval shape of the opacity and slow growth on serial radiographs should raise the suspicion for malignancy. Growth rate of non-small cell lung cancer (NSCLC) is highly variable and related to histological subtype and smoking history, but not the presence of symptoms at diagnosis.[36,37] Lung cancers usually have doubling time between 1 and 18 months and a 26% increase in the diameter is equal to the doubling of tumor volume. Most lung cancers double in volume in 4–8 months; however, invasive mucinous adenocarcinomas tend to grow more slowly, and may even metastasize. Significant growth may be detected in as early as 2 months in smokers.

Central Tumors

Chest Radiograph Findings

Hilar enlargement: The cardinal imaging finding of a central tumor on chest radiograph is presence of hilar enlargement with or without distal collapse/consolidation of the lung. The hilar enlargement may be due to central tumor itself, enlarged lymph nodes, consolidation or combination of these **(Fig. 7)**.

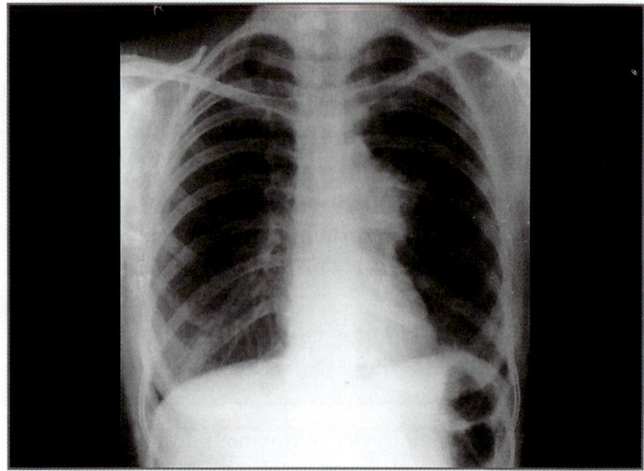

FIG. 7: Central lung cancer: Frontal chest radiograph shows increased density and enlargement of left hilum. Associated elevation of left hemidiaphragm is suggestive of mediastinal invasion and phrenic nerve palsy.

Dense hilum sign: Sometimes, a small mass overlying the hilum may produce only an asymmetrically increased density of the hilum and this should raise a suspicion of tumor and a CECT is indicated.

Distal collapse: It is seen as homogenous pulmonary opacity with volume loss, confined to one lobe. Air bronchogram, however, is usually absent **(Figs. 8A to D)**. Displacement of the fissure toward the collapsed lung. "Golden S sign" in right upper lobe collapse occurs due to central mass limiting the expected movement of the fissure and hence the medial aspect of fissure shows bulging contour. If there is retention of mucous in the collapsed lung bronchi, it may not lead to volume loss and rather an enlarged lobe "drowned lung" may be visualized.

Consolidation: Inhomogenous opacity persistent or recurrent in same lobe should raise a suspicion of central obstructing mass.

Contrast-enhanced CT Findings

Central lung cancers are seen as mildly enhancing soft tissue masses whereas distal collapse shows significant enhancement. Distended fluid filled bronchi may be seen as fluid bronchogram within the enhancing collapsed lung distal to the mass. Such an appearance should prompt a bronchoscopy, even when tumor is not visualized on CT. Delineation of the tumor separately from distal collapse consolidation cannot always be made on CT **(Figs. 8B and C)**. This may pose a difficulty in the confident initial diagnosis of lung cancer on CT. PETCT can demonstrate the central mass with FDG uptake separate from collapse. Accurate tumor delineation is an important requirement for radiotherapy planning. Dynamic perfusion CT can help distinguishing between tumor mass and collapsed lung as well as demonstrate viable tumor tissue separate from necrotic non-viable area, thereby guiding proper CT guided needle placement for biopsy **(Figs. 9A to D)**.

RADIOLOGICAL CHARACTERISTICS BY CELL TYPE

Amongst the common subtypes of the lung cancers, adenocarcinoma accounts for 38.5% of the cases, squamous cell carcinoma 20–25%, small cell carcinoma 11–15% and large cell carcinoma 2.9–8% of cases.[38,39]

Adenocarcinoma

Adenocarcinomas are typically peripherally located tumor. These can either present as a localized ground glass opacity or as solid nodule or mass. They are usually less than 4 cm in diameter and cavitation is rare (seen in only 4–6% lesions).[40] Adenocarcinomas are frequently associated with enlarged hilar and mediastinal lymph nodes, though not as massive as seen in small cell carcinomas. Pleural effusion is a feature of adenocarcinoma.

Invasive mucinous adenocarcinoma: Formally known as mucinous bronchioloalveolar carcinoma (BAC). It may

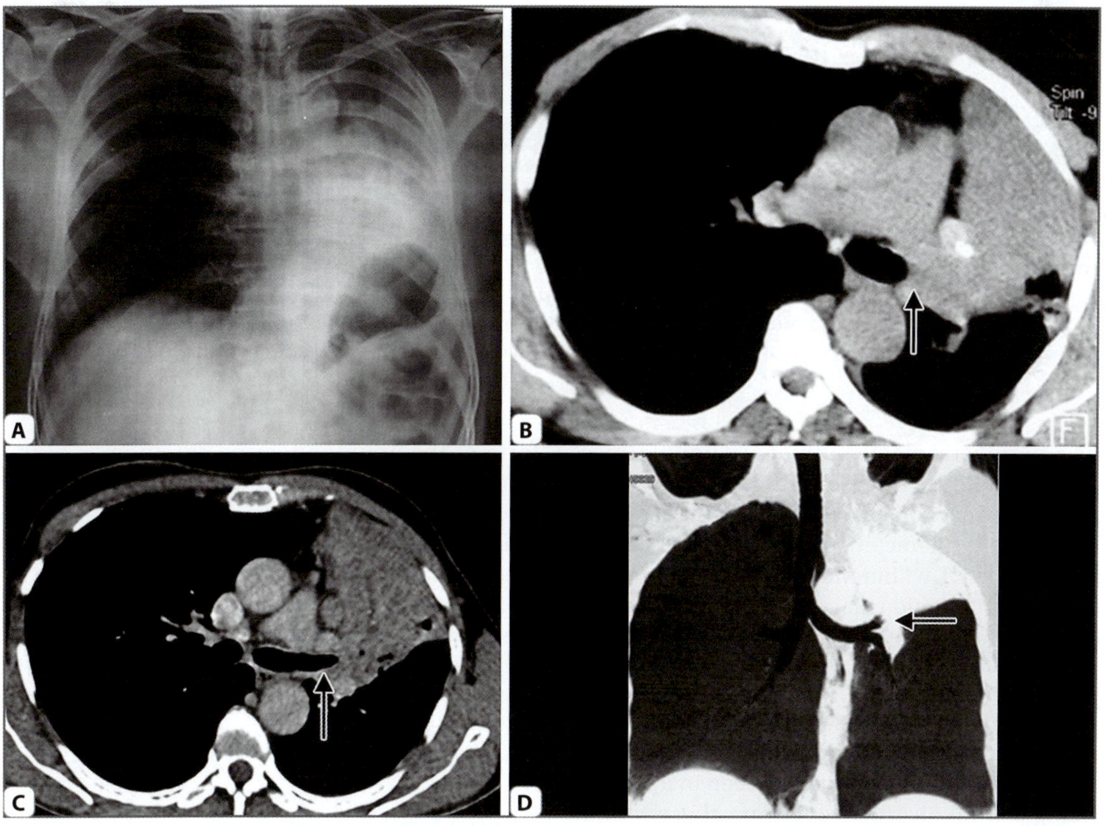

FIGS. 8A TO D: Central lung cancer with lobar collapse: (A) Chest radiograph shows signs of collapse of the left upper lobe with ipsilateral mediastinal shift; (B) Corresponding CT shows ill-defined mass occluding the left upper lobe bronchus (arrow) with distal collapsed lung. Endobronchial biopsy revealed squamous cell carcinoma; (C) CT scan of another patient showing cut off of left upper lobe bronchus (arrow), left upper lobe collapse with no identifiable tumor. Bronchoscopy and biopsy confirmed squamous cell carcinoma; (D) Minimum intensity projection image in same patient, shows cut off of the bronchus (arrow).

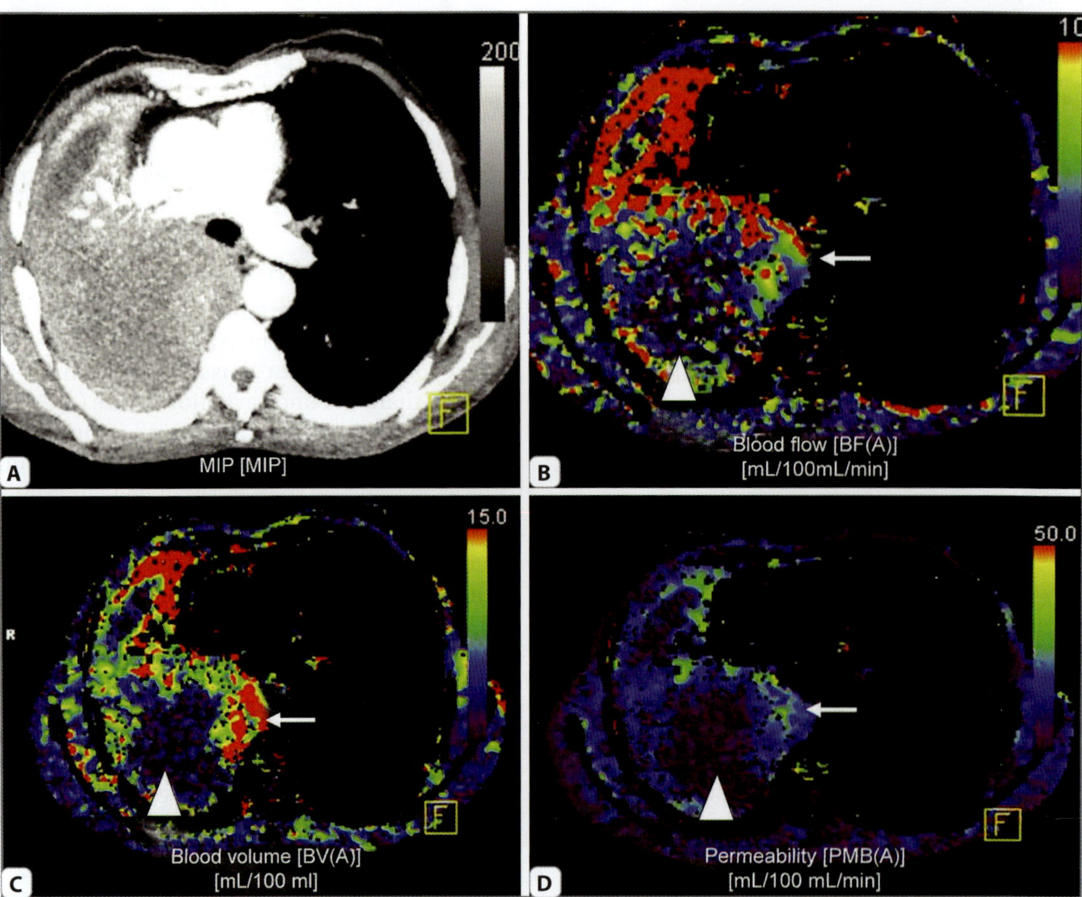

FIGS. 9A TO D: Dynamic perfusion CT lung: (A) MIP CT image shows heterogenous mass in right lung and viable tumor tissue could not be confidently identified. CT perfusion blood flow color coded image (B) and blood volume image (C) shows increased blood flow and blood volume (areas depicted in red/yellow color) in the medial aspect of the mass suggestive of viable tumor tissue (white arrows). Minimal blood flow and volume in the central and lateral aspect of the mass suggesting necrosis (arrowhead); (D) Permeability images show mildly increased permeability in medial aspect of the mass. CT-guided biopsy revealed adenocarcinoma.

present as a peripheral single pulmonary nodule/mass or multicentric or diffuse disease **(Figs. 10A and B)** or a localized parenchymal consolidation form in decreasing order of incidence.[41] Characteristic bubble-like lucencies can be identified on CT within the mass.[40] Sometimes, air bronchograms and cavitation may also be seen.[42] Hilar and mediastinal lymphadenopathy is uncommon.

Squamous Cell Carcinoma

These are more often centrally located within the lung and may attain greater size. Cavitation is seen in up to 82% cases.[40] Being central obstructive lesions, these tumors frequently produce segmental or lobar lung collapse **(Figs. 8B and C)**.[43]

Small Cell Lung Cancer

This tumor is characterized by a high growth fraction and rapid doubling time. It represents the most malignant form of the neuroendocrine carcinomas of the lung. It is associated with poor prognosis as 60–70% of patients present with metastatic disease at the time of diagnosis.[44] These tumors most often present with massive enlarged mediastinal or hilar lymphadenopathy **(Figs. 11A and B)**. A large noncontiguous centrally located mass can be seen within the lung parenchyma and it rarely cavitates. Mediastinal invasion is common and seen in upto 68 % of cases[44, 45] on CT. Sometimes only conglomerate mediastinal nodal mass may be present without detection of primary lung tumor.

Large Cell Carcinoma

It is a poorly differentiated non-small cell carcinoma and is diagnosed in the absence of histopathologic features for adenocarcinoma or squamous cell carcinoma and presence of a large cell morphology. These are high grade tumors with rapid growth rate and tend to metastasize early to the mediastinum and brain.

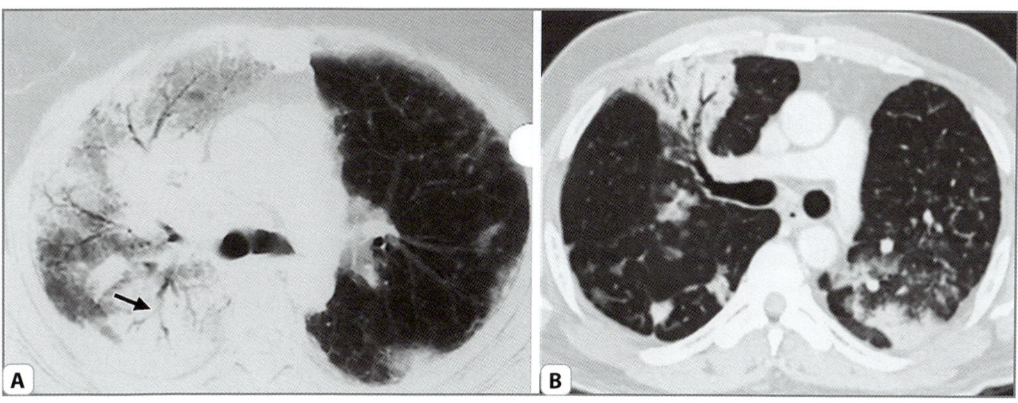

FIGS. 10A AND B: Invasive mucinous adenocarcinoma (formally known as invasive bronchoalveolar carcinoma): (A) CT shows pneumonic form of cancer with extensive airspace opacities with characteristic stretching and narrowing of the bronchi (arrow) due to mass effect of the tumor; (B) Another patient showing multicentric pattern of disease.

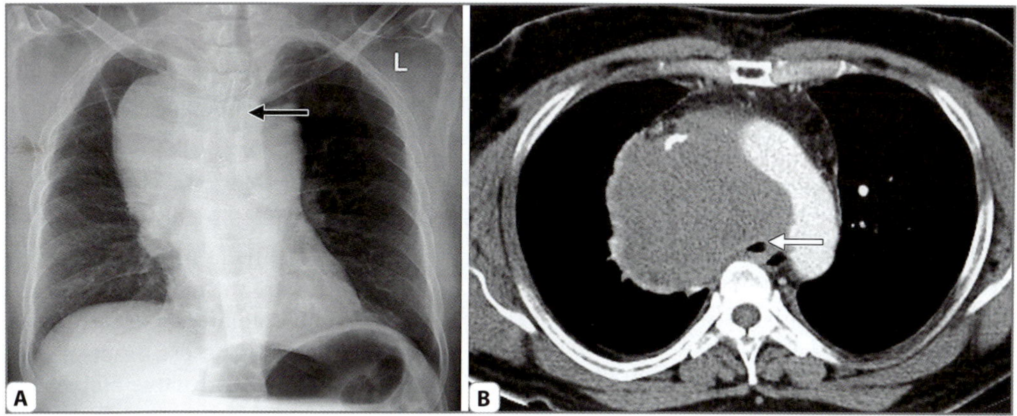

FIGS. 11A AND B: Small cell carcinoma presenting as mediastinal mass: (A) Chest radiograph showing large mediastinal mass. A tracheal stent is seen as the mass was causing severe narrowing of the tracheal lumen; (B) Pre-procedural CT shows large mediastinal lymphadenopathy with compression of SVC and trachea (arrow). No separate mass could be identified within the lungs.

SAMPLING FOR SUSPECTED LUNG CANCER

In a suspected lung cancer, if a patient is producing sputum, the cytology assessment can often establish the diagnosis of malignancy. However, since the inception of the 2021 WHO classification and new targeted treatment options, immunohistochemistry of small biopsies or even cytology is indicated for further typing of the tumor. Bronchoscopy is used for evaluation and biopsy of most lung cancers. It is most useful for central tumors and diagnostic yield ranges from 81–90% for visible tumors.[46] Peripheral lesions can also be sampled using indirect bronchoscopic methods such as lavage, brushes, biopsy forceps or radial EBUS guided biopsy.[47]

CT guided transthoracic FNAC or core biopsy **(Fig. 12A)** is accurate for the tumors not amenable to bronchoscopic visualization. However, non-diagnostic or nonspecific benign results are not reliable and repeat biopsy must be performed in these situations. Major complications include pneumothorax, hemotharax, hemoptysis, infection and air embolism. Peripheral lung tumors can be accessed under ultrasound guidance **(Fig. 12B)** and in case of necrotic tumors, a contrast enhanced ultrasound may be used to differentiate between active areas and nonviable areas before sampling thereby increasing the accuracy of core needle biopsy.[8] CT or ultrasound guided biopsies are useful to obtain samples from metastatic sites of the lung cancer. In some patients with resectable disease on imaging, preoperative lymph node staging may be performed with mediastinoscopy and lymph node sampling and sometimes, with endoscopic or endobronchial ultrasound guided FNAC of mediastinal lymph nodes. Pleural effusions require thoracocentesis to determine if these are malignant. Video assisted thoracoscopic surgery (VATS) is frequently used for diagnosis, staging and occasionally, resection of the lung cancer.[48,49]

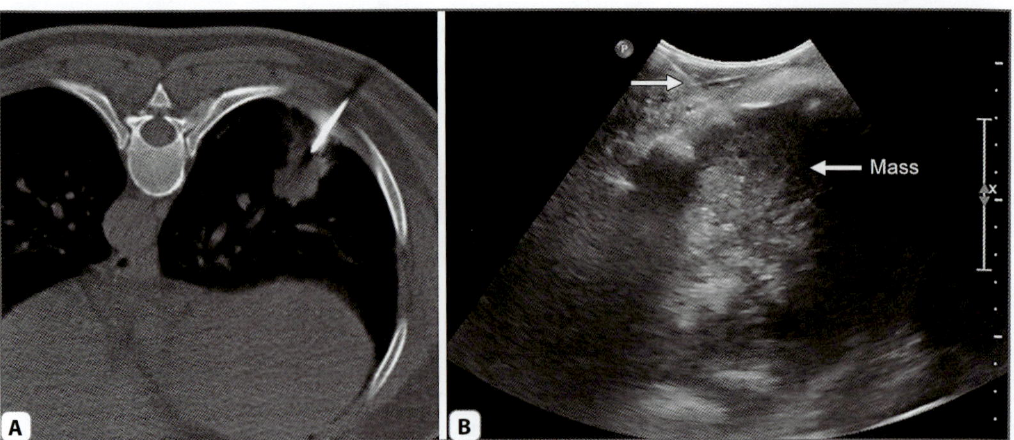

FIGS. 12A AND B: CT and USG guided biopsy of lung mass: (A) Prone CT image showing a coaxial needle in situ within a peripheral lung mass through which multiple biopsy cores were taken which revealed adenocarcinoma; (B) USG image of a large peripheral lung mass showing needle advanced through intercostal space (arrow) within the mass. Biopsy revealed squamous cell carcinoma.

STAGING OF LUNG CANCER

The TNM system remains the best prognosticator of lung cancer outcome and guides the treatment strategies. The 8th edition of Union for International Cancer Control and the American Joint Committee on Cancer (UICC/ AJCC) TNM staging system of lung cancer[50,51] was published in January 2017 based on the recommendations of International Association for Study of Lung cancer (IASCL) **(Tables 1 and 2)**. This system is used to stage NSCLC, SCLC and bronchial carcinoids. The Proposed 9th edition of TNM Classification **(Table 3)** for lung cancer has also been slated to take effect in 2025 as it has been adopted by AJCC and UICC.[52]

Imaging Modalities for the Staging of Lung Cancers

Chest radiographs and thin section CECT of the thorax and upper abdomen, including liver, and supraclavicular areas, are the basic imaging required for staging lung cancer. Multiplanar reconstructions are essential for the assessment of relationship of the tumor with the fissure, adjacent cardiovascular structures and exact localization prior to surgery. CT is the primary modality to assess the resectability of the tumor and for assessing the treatment options. However, the accuracy of the CT staging is poor when compared with surgico-pathological staging.[53] For tumor size measurement, the largest long-axis diameter must be measured using multiplanar reformation. Performance of CT alone for T staging is significantly lower than PET-CT, and precise T stages are provided in 68% and 86% respectively.[54] PET-CT is recommended gold standard for N staging of the lung cancer as CT, though highly sensitive for detection of lymph nodes, has low specificity for lymph node characterization into benign or malignant.[54,55] Also, CT data should be analyzed in conjunction with other modalities such as bone scan or PETCT for accurate M staging.

Salient Points

T Staging

- It includes measuring tumor size (largest long-axis diameter), invasion into adjacent structures and identification of satellite/separate nodule.
- It may be difficult to assess exact size of the tumor in presence of a postobstructive atelectasis/pneumonia and such lesion are considered T2.
- T1 and T2 tumors are most amenable for curative surgical resection. Parietal extension (T3) (rib bone lysis, extrapleural extension) is not a contraindication for surgery and some candidates may benefit from surgical intervention. Though conventionally T4 tumors are unresectable, some cases of T4 tumors may also be eligible for surgery (after a multidisciplinary discussion).[54]

Tracheobronchial Invasion

On CT, the bronchial invasion (T2) or tracheal invasion (T4) is seen as fixed smooth/nodular thickening of their wall. A bronchoscopic correlation is indicated whenever CT detects this finding.

Mediastinal Invasion

- Parietal pericardium/phrenic nerve involvement—T3
- Invasion of heart/great vessels/diaphragm/ mediastinum/trachea/carina/esophagus/recurrent laryngeal nerve/vertebral body are categorized under T4.
- On CT/MRI, criteria for vascular invasion include complete circumferential encasement of a vessel **(Figs. 13A and B)** or presence of an intravascular enhancing focus of tumor. Loss of fat planes with the

TABLE 1: TNM descriptors.

T	Primary tumor
Tx	Cannot be assessed; malignancy in sputum/bronchial washings and not in imaging/bronchoscopy
T0	No tumor evidence
Tis	Carcinoma in situ
T1	≤ 3 cm surrounded by lung/visceral pleura, not involving main bronchus
T1a(mi)	Minimally invasive adenocarcinoma
T1a	≤ 1 cm
T1b	Between 1 to 2 cm
T1c	> 2 to ≤ 3 cm
T2	>3 and < 5 cm or Involves main bronchus without carina involvement or Visceral pleural invasion or Atelectasis/postobstructive pneumonitis extending to hilum
T2a	>3 to ≤ 4 cm
T2b	>4 to ≤ 5 cm
T3	> 5 to ≤ 7 cm, or Separate tumor in same lobe as primary mass, or Direct invasion of chest wall/ parietal pleura/ superior sulcus)/pericardium/phrenic nerve
T4	> 7 cm, or Separate tumor in different lobe of ipsilateral lung, or Invasion of mediastinum/trachea/carina/esophagus/heart/great vessels/diaphragm/ recurrent laryngeal nerve/spine
N	**Regional lymph node**
N0	No nodal involvement
N1	Ipsilateral hilar nodes and intrapulmonary nodes
N2	Ipsilateral mediastinal and/or subcarinal nodes
N3	Contralateral mediastinal or hilar; ipsilateral/contralateral scalene/ supraclavicular nodes
M	Distant metastasis
M0	No distant metastasis
M1	Distant metastasis is present
M1a	Nodule/Mass in contralateral lung; pleural/pericardial deposits/malignant effusion
M1b	Single extrathoracic metastasis
M1c	Multiple extrathoracic metastases, in one/more organs

adjacent tissue may not represent actual invasion and such tumors may also be amenable for resection.

- If contact of the mass with the mediastinal vessel is > 3 cm or > 90° or there is parietal stiffness of the vessels, then it can be suggested as nonresectable; however, these findings needs surgical confirmation and hence

TABLE 2: Stage groups.

		N0	N1	N2	N3
T1 M0	T1a T1b T1c	IA1 IA2 IA3	IIB IIB IIB	IIIA IIIA IIIA	IIIB IIIB IIIB
T2/M0	T2a T2b	IB IIA	IIB IIB	IIIA IIIA	IIIB IIIB
T3M0		IIB	IIIA	IIIB	IIIC
T4M0		IIIA	IIIA	IIIB	IIIC
TXM1	M1a M1b M1c	IVA IVA IVB	IVA IVA IVB	IVA IVA IVB	IVA IVA IVB

TABLE 3: What's new in 9th TNM edition.

	Changes in 9th TNM when compared to 8th edition
T component	No changes
N component	• Subdivision of N2: • N2a – metastasis to a single station • N2b – multiple N2 stations
M component	• Subdivision of M1c: • M1c1 – Multiple metastases in a single organ system • M1c2 – Metastasis to multiple organ systems
Staging groups	T1N1 – Staging IIA T1 N2a – Stage IIB T1N2b – Stage IIIA T2/T3 N2a – Stage IIIA T2/T3 N2b or T4N2a/b – Stage IIIB Any T, Any N, M1c1/c2 – Stage IV B

a patient should not be deferred surgery on the basis of these imaging findings.

- Involvement of pulmonary veins or left atrium would be seen as hypodense filling defects within the intensely enhancing vessel/atrial chamber and it is categorized into T4 stage.

Pleural Invasion

- Crossing of the fissure by the mass classifies it into T2 **(Fig. 14A)**
- Involvement of parietal pleura makes it T3 lesion
- Distant or non-contiguous nodular pleural thickening—metastatic
- On CT, presence of definite pleural invasion is attributed when there is extension of tumor into the soft tissues beyond the pleura or associated rib bone lysis. Loss of extrapleural fat plane is also a sign of pleural invasion **(Fig. 14B)**. Mere presence of pleural effusion or contact with the pleura are not the signs for pleural invasion and diagnostic pleural fluid aspiration for malignant cytology or VATS guided pleural biopsy should be done to confirm the pleural involvement if it affects the therapy planning.

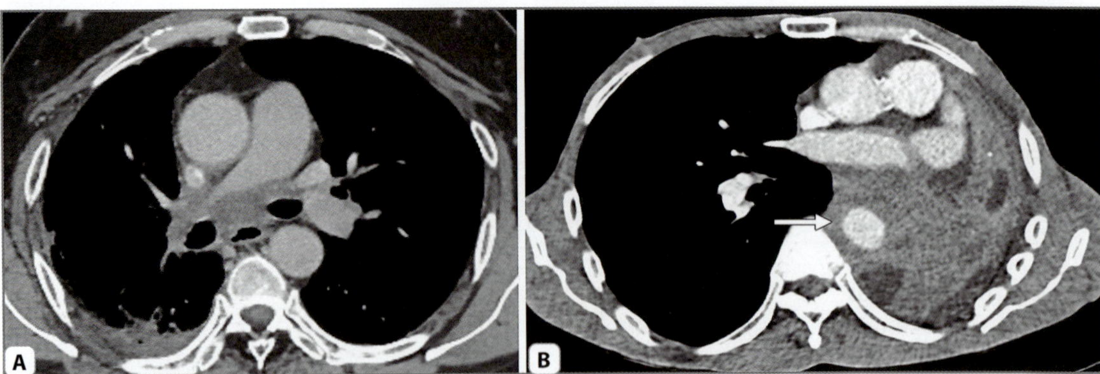

FIGS. 13A AND B: T4 tumors: (A) Central mass causing narrowing and circumferential involvement of right pulmonary artery suggestive of invasion; (B) Large left lung mass with circumferential invasion of aorta (arrow).

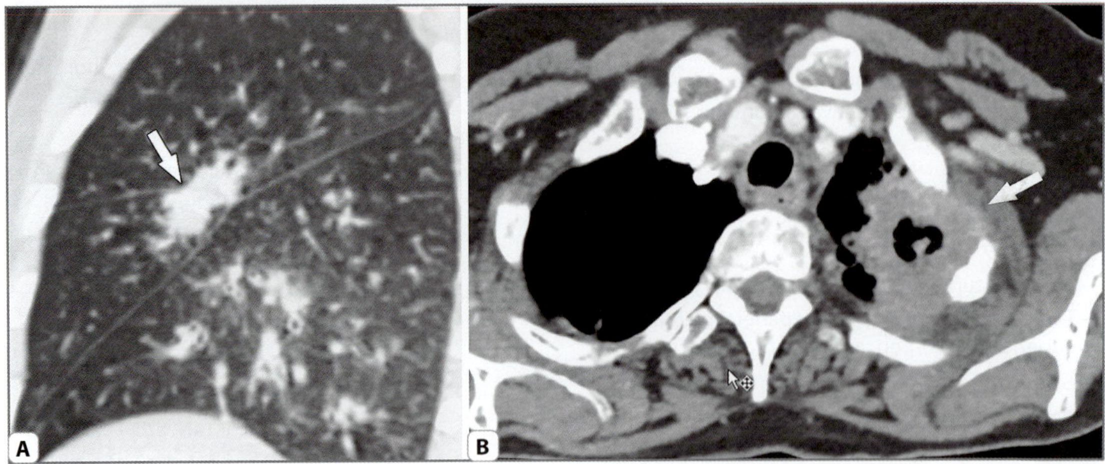

FIGS. 14A AND B: Invasion of fissure: (A) Sagittal CT image shows crossing of the horizontal fissure by a spiculated mass sign of invasion and T2 tumor; (B) Tumor is abutting the pleura with loss of extrapleural fat plane; a sign of chest wall invasion.

Chest Wall Invasion

Presence of extrapleural tumor tissue or extension into the ribs confirms the chest wall invasion and these are categorized as T3 lesions **(Figs. 15A and B)**.

MRI and PET-CT may be required for better delineation of chest wall invasion **(Fig. 15C)** as well as in cases of diaphragmatic involvement.

If a Pancoast's tumor demonstrates involvement thoracic nerve roots, then it is a T3 stage. If it involves subcalvian vessels, vertebra, shows intraspinal extension **(Fig. 15D)** or involvement of lower cervical nerve roots (C8 and above) or cords of the brachial plexus, then T stage for such tumors would be classified as T4.

Satellite Nodules

Tumor with separate nodules in the same lobe is classified as T3.

Tumor with an ipsilateral nodule in another lobe—T4 Tumor with a nodule contralateral to the primary tumor—M1.

CT is highly sensitive to detect the nodules however lacks specificity. However, the presence of separate nodule in same lobe as that of tumor is an indicator of poor prognosis and usually represents tumor nodule.

Lymphangitic Carcinomatosis

This finding has not been addressed in TNM staging criteria; however, it is important to identify this because presence of diffuse or more than one lobe involvement by lymphangitis carcinomatosis (LC) is a contraindication to surgery. Still, if the same lobe as that of tumor is affected then it is not a contraindication.

On CT, it appears as nodular peribronchovascular and septal thickening which represents the perilymphatic extension of tumor nodules **(Fig. 16)**.

N Staging

On CECT, a hilar lymph node of >7 mm and mediastinal lymph node of >10 mm are considered involved. However, some studies have shown 40% normal sized lymph nodes

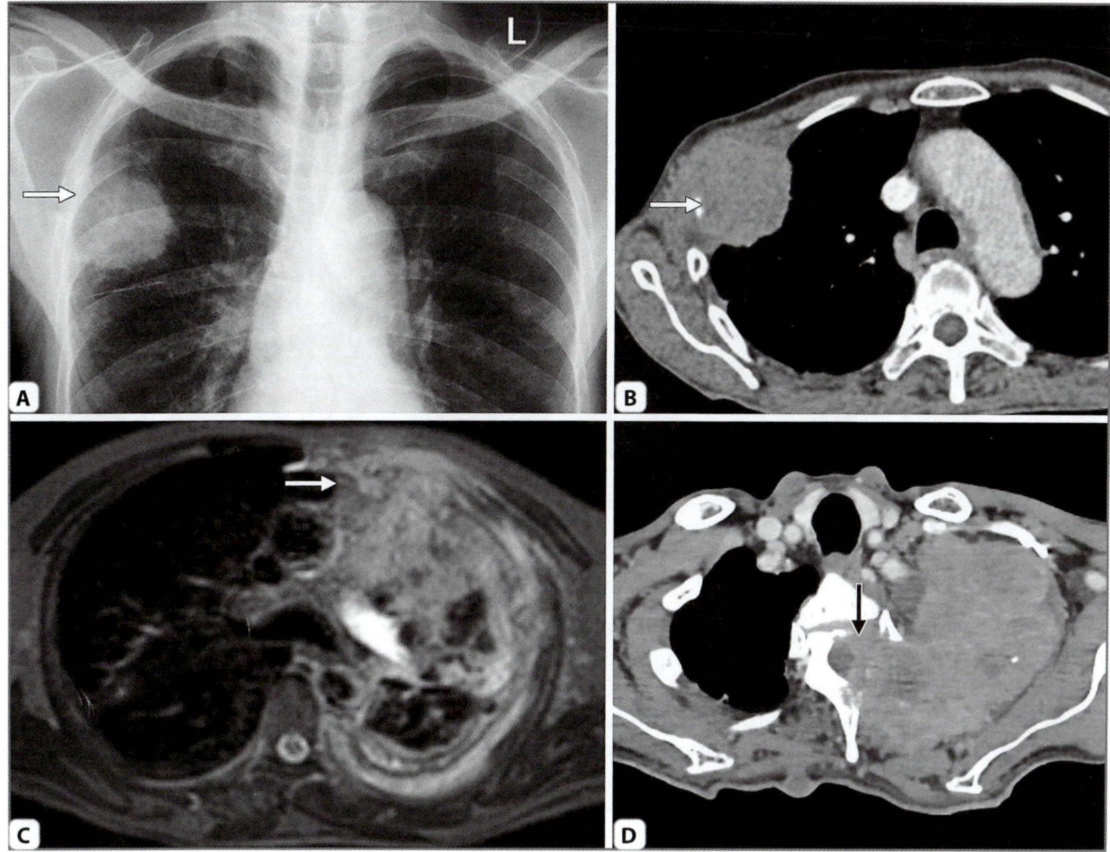

FIGS. 15A TO D: Chest wall invasion. (A) Frontal chest radiograph showing peripheral mass with nonvisualization of anterior end of second and third ribs; (B) CT shows a large right lung mass with contiguous invasion of the chest wall with rib destruction and extrathoracic soft tissue component (arrow); (C) Axial STIR MRI shows extension of the left upper lobe mass into the anterior chest wall muscles infiltrating the deep fibers of pectoralis muscle; (D) Intraspinal extension of left Pancoast's tumor makes it T4 lesion.

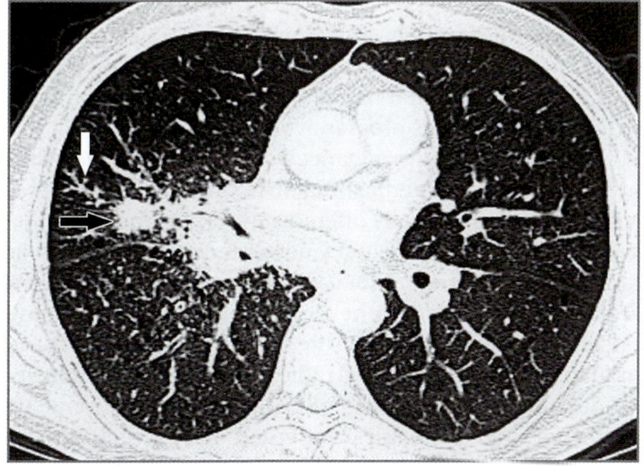

FIG. 16: Lymphangitis carcinomatosis. HRCT image showing a spiculated mass (black arrow) in right parahilar region adjacent peribronchovascular thickening and nodules (white arrow), also extending in right lower lobe.

up to 7 mm to be metastatic (such findings more commonly found in adenocarcinomas).

It should be reported according to 1-14 mediastinal lymph nodal stations described by IASLC.[51]

PET-CT is the gold standard for N staging with a high negative predictive value (>90%).

M Staging

- *M1a:* Intrathoracic metastasis—pleural or pericardial nodules, contralateral lung nodule, malignant pleural/ pericardial effusion **(Fig. 17)**.
- *M1b:* Single metastatic lesion in an extrathoracic organ/ non-regional lymph node.
- *M1c:* Multiple metastasis.

Most common organs involved by metastasis include brain, bones, liver and adrenals **(Fig. 18)**. Liver is most commonly involved in small cell lung cancers and sometimes in cases of diffuse metastasis CT may not demonstrate any nodular lesions. Adrenal incidentalomas

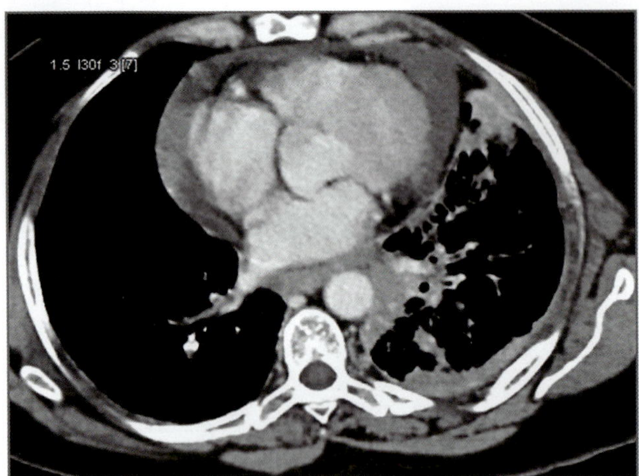

FIG. 17: Malignant pericardial and pleural effusion. CT axial image showing irregular left pleural thickening and mild pericardial effusion in a case of lung adenocarcinoma.

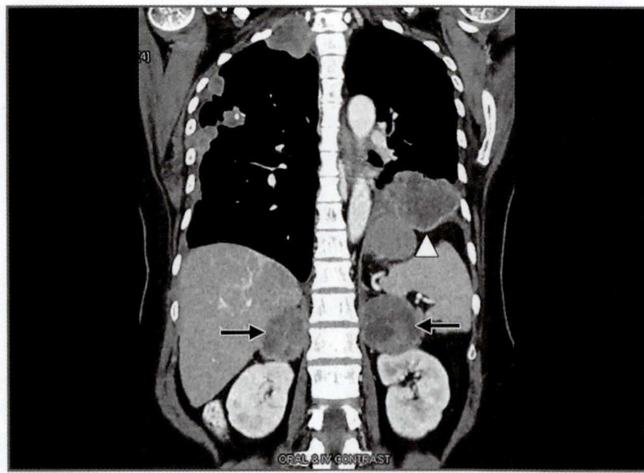

FIG. 18: Adrenal metastasis in disseminated adenocarcinoma lung (right apical tumor). Coronal CT image showing heterogenous enhancing masses in bilateral suprarenal locations suggestive of adrenal metastasis (arrows). Note is also made of left invasive diaphragmatic metastatic deposit (arrowhead).

and metastasis may not be differentiated based on single phase CT alone and may require further imaging in the form of MRI/PETCT and at times even sampling. On CECT, peripheral irregular enhancement of the nodule with central necrotic area is highly suggestive of adrenal metastasis over an adenoma. CT and PET-CT are adequate in demonstration of the metastatic lesions, and histological confirmation should be done in most of the cases.

The CT report must always contain the TNM staging. If there is doubt about the correct T, N or M category then one should assign a lower category as well as stage.

TREATMENT OF LUNG CANCER

If detected in early stage, surgery remains mainstay of treatment for lung carcinoma in the form of either lobectomy, bilobectomy or pneumonectomy.Well defined lesions, away from fissures and no contiguous organ infiltration are the ideal lesions for surgery. However, tumors near carina, chest wall infiltration, or early mediastinal invasion can also be operated if there is no lymphadenopathy or metastatic lesions. Sleeve resection of tracheobronchial tree, chest wall reconstruction etc. are the adjunctive procedures in addition to primary surgery for such difficult lesions. A vast number of these patients will also receive chemo or radiotherapy or both. Involvement of trachea, pulmonary artery, aorta become contraindication for surgery. Hence, the involvement of these structures should be clearly documented in radiological reports.

Chemotherapy for carcinoma lung is different for different histological type of malignancy (squamous, adeno or small cell, etc.). The choice of chemotherapeutic agents also vary depending upon the presence or absence of many specific receptors, e.g., epidermal growth factor receptor (EGFR). Main therapeutic agents are cisplatin, etoposide, or gemcitabine, etc.[56] For some large (not disseminated) tumors chemotherapy may shrink the tumor to make it surgically resectable in follow-up period.

Conventionally for the cytotoxic drugs given for treatment of lung malignancies, Response Evaluation Criteria in Solid Tumors (RECIST) criteria are used for evaluating treatment response. It is suggested to read the recent RECIST criteria described by Eisenhauer EA et al.[57,58] and use this for assessing tumor response. However, for some newer (non-cytotoxic) chemotherapeutic agents the conventional RECIST criteria are not suitable as these drugs don't cause reduction in size. For these drugs newer evaluation criteria are being followed in randomized controlled trials (RCTs) which incorporate other imaging features like decrease in enhancement, increasing necrotic component etc. For such lesions even the presence of a few new lesions and initial increase in size of lesions are not strictly considered as progressive disease.

Patients with more advanced stage malignancies with invasion of major mediastinal structure or contralateral lymph nodes are usually offered supportive and palliative radiotherapy. There are many newer techniques to deliver radiotherapy in a more focused way to only the diseased area and avoiding adjacent normal lung thereby reducing radiation induced damage to the surrounding organs. These modalities are image guided radiotherapy (IGRT), intensity modulated radiation therapy (IMRT), conformational 3D radiotherapy and respiratory gated 4D CT techniques, etc.[59] Heart, esophagus and spinal cord are few of the more radiosensitive organs which need to be preserved more diligently and hence it is important on the part of the reporting radiologist to clearly define involvement of these structures by the neoplastic lesions so that during RT planning the treating radiotherapist is better equipped to avoid injury to these structures.

Radiofrequency ablation (RFA) is another option for those patients who have limited diseases but surgically unfit due to medical comorbidities.[60-64] Excellent results can be achieved for tumors < 3–4 cm sizes. The complications of RFA can be pneumothorax, hemoptysis, pleural effusion, lung abscess etc. Another potential use of RFA is for treatment of isolated metastatic lesion in adrenal gland.[65]

Few newer minimally invasive treatments are also being evaluated for lung cancers. Microwave, cryotherapy and irreversible electrophoresis are few of these. Main advantages cited for microwave are relatively uniform ablation zone, larger ablated area, lack of heat sink effects and lesser ablation time. These characteristics appear to make microwave more suitable for achieving complete ablations in patients with larger lesions or lesions closer to larger blood vessels.[66,67]

Similarly for cryotherapy main perceived advantages are suitability for lesions near large vessels or near hila and lesser pain during the procedure. Another advantage of cryotherapy over RFA is that real time evaluation of ablation site is feasible during the procedure enabling better treatment optimization.[68,69]

In addition, combined synergistic effects of cryotherapy and immunotherapy are also being evaluated and encouraging results are seen in early studies.[70]

SCREENING FOR LUNG CANCER

Screening for lung cancers was started based on the premise that if detected in early stage (stage 1A) there are high survival rates for 5 years in these patients. In many previous randomized clinical trials (RCTs) which used chest X-ray and/or sputum cytology for screening in chronic smokers, there was detection of many early stage cancers, however there was no proven benefit regarding mortality rates.[71]

More recently many RCTs are going on in US and Europe (e.g., Mayo CT screening project, PLCO (Prostate, Lung, Colorectal and Ovary) and Early Lung Cancer Action Project (ELCAP) using low dose CT protocol (25–30 mAs). As CT is more efficient in detecting smaller nodules as compared to chest X-rays, the likelihood of detection of lung malignancies at earlier stages is more with CT as a screening tool.[72] Few of these studies have evaluated the parameters and concluded that screening with CT for lung malignancies in high risk patient profile (age 55–80 and chronic smokers) provides significant decrease in mortality rates.[73] Many of the societies have recommended that screening should be done in all elderly smokers (55/60 to 80 years) who smoke >30 pack cigarette per year. They have recommended strict criteria regarding definition of nodules, reporting format as well as guidelines for pathological evaluation and the treatment algorithms for such detected lesions in screening programs and are to be reported using Lung -RADS.[74] The nodules detected during screening are typically smaller in size and represent less advance malignancies. Majority of these lesions will ultimately prove to be benign. High false positivity for these nodules to be cancers is a particular disadvantage. This problem is even more severe in areas with high prevalence of granulomatous diseases, e.g., in India. Careful evaluation of all the characteristics of these screening detected nodules is necessary to reduce the number of unnecessary biopsy or thoracotomy. A nodule which is smaller than 8 mm is usually followed and subjected to biopsy when it shows suspicious growth pattern for malignancy. For larger lesions PET and CT guided biopsies are performed.

Till now there is no state sponsored lung screening program in India. This is partly attributed to high prevalence of granulomatous disease tuberculosis in our country in which imaging findings may mimic early cancers resulting in significant anxiety and resultant more invasive tests to prove the exact nature of these nodules; and partly due to lack of availability of sufficient imaging, pathology as well as surgical services which have got overburdened from various other diseases utilizing the already existing meager health care resources.[75,76]

FOLLOW-UP IMAGING

Follow-up imaging for lung malignancies is done to detect treatment response. If a patient has been treated with surgery and complete resection was feasible, then follow up imaging is done to detect recurrence and metastatic lesions. If a patient has been treated with chemotherapeutic agents, then follow-up imaging is done to detect early responses.

This helps in deciding whether to continue with the same treatment regime or should change it early to try other regimens. With few newer non-cytotoxic chemotherapeutic agents, the clinical question of interest is to find whether there is progression or not. If there is no progression, then the same agent will continue for further treatment otherwise a decision will be taken to change the agent quite early in the course of treatment. Similarly, imaging is also done to detect complications due to treatments. If the patient is asymptomatic then chest X-ray and clinical examination are sufficient. There is no standard protocol to follow these patients on CT, some centers do not prefer any follow up if patient is asymptomatic while other centers prefer every 6 monthly follow up.[77,78] Other expected changes are pleural thickening , crowding of ribs, ipsilateral mediastinal shift, etc.

Radiologists should be familiar with expected changes in imaging after some treatment. In the initial phase after lobectomy, there is presence of postoperative cavity with air fluid level **(Figs. 19A to C)**. The pneumothorax may be large in the initial phase of postoperative time. In due course of time the cavity disappears with absorption of fluid and compensatory hyperinflation of the residual lobes.

Post-radiotherapy changes are seen as acute or chronic changes. In acute radiation pneumonitis there is the appearance of ground glass opacities within three months of completion in the radiation portal area. In chronic

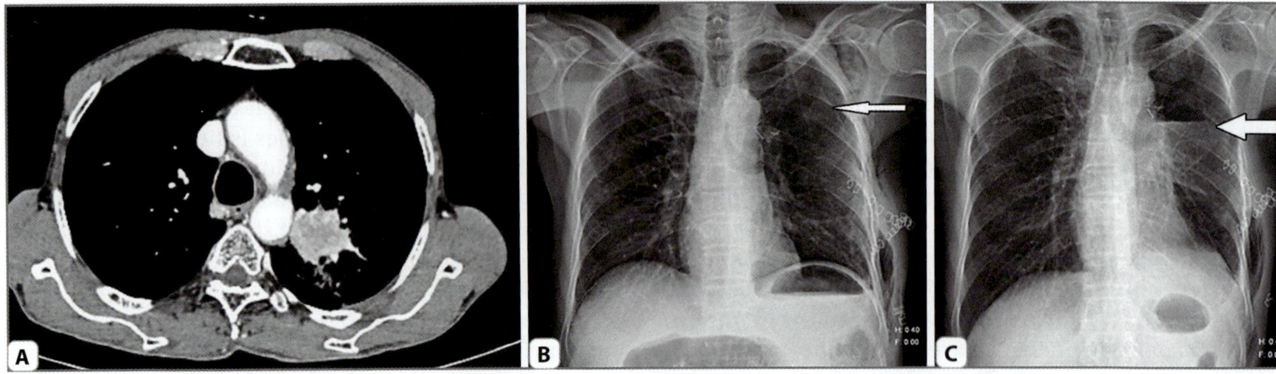

FIGS. 19A TO C: Normal post-lobectomy appearance: (A) CT shows a stage IIA lobulated mass for which a left upper lobectomy was done; (B) Chest radiograph shows mild pneumothorax on postoperative day 4; (C) Postoperative day 14 radiograph shows air fluid level in the pleural cavity in left upper zone which is normal finding after lobectomy

phase other changes are seen like consolidation, fibrosis, bronchiectasis or volume loss.[79,80] The area of involvement shrinks with passage of time. The changes of radiation pneumonitis need to be differentiated from infective etiology. Infections usually conform to lobar or segmental anatomy; on the contrary the radiation changes conform to the radiation field and may even cross fissures. However, for proper evaluation of these postradiation changes the radiologist should have complete information regarding the radiation field, type of radiation technique used, e.g., IGRT, IMRT or conformal RT.[81,82] Small pericardial or pleural effusions are quite common after radiation therapy and they usually develop up to initial 9 months and resolve themselves by 12–16 months.

Other changes seen in the post-treatment period are drug toxicity and infections, both of which may give a similar radiological appearance. One of the commonly given drugs, Geftinib, causes interstitial pulmonary fibrosis. [83,84] Almost all chemotherapeutic agents given in patients with NSCLC can cause lung fibrosis. The main imaging findings are ground glass opacity, fibrosis and interstitial opacities.

RECURRENT LUNG CANCER

In lung cancer patients who have been treated, recurrences are more common at distant site as compared to the loco regional site.[78] The imaging findings in recurrence are usually similar to original tumors. The main imaging features of recurrent lesions are either developing mass or lymphadenopathy. Other features suspicious of recurrence are increasing hydropneumothorax in postpneumonectomy patients, or appearance of a new air fluid level. Because of significant distortion of normal bronchial anatomy following lobectomy and post radiotherapy fibrotic changes, interpretation of CT examination in these patients become particularly challenging. Still there are few features which make one suspicious of recurrence are, emergence of new pulmonary nodule, or new bronchial stenosis, new or increasing soft tissue at hilum or enlarging mediastinal or hilar lymph nodes.[83] Similarly, new appearance of pleural effusion after 6 months of radiotherapy also is a suspicious finding which needs aspiration to exclude recurrent lesion. In the areas of postradiation pneumonitis, new opacification of previously dilated and patent bronchi is also an important clue for recurrence of the disease.[85] When recurrence is suspected, PET is the most sensitive modality to diagnose the recurrence.[86]

RARE LUNG MALIGNANCIES

Other uncommon lung malignancies are sarcomas and pulmonary blastomas. Few of these sarcomas are quite benign in the course of disease, e.g., endobronchial fibrosarcoma and leiomyosarcoma. Other sarcomas which are quite aggressive in clinical behavior are rhabdomyosarcoma, osteosarcoma, chondrosarcoma, angiosarcoma and malignant fibrous histiocytoma, myxoid sarcoma, etc. **(Figs. 20A and B)**. Sometimes there are sarcomatous components in non-small cell lung carcinoma (NSCLC) which are classified as carcinosarcoma, which have imaging appearance similar to non-small cell lung cancer. Out of these the angiosarcomas have a characteristic enhancement on CT as well as MRI. Kaposi sarcomas are common in AIDS patients which show multiple nodular flame shaped opacities or linear peribronchial opacities. Other findings associated with Kaposi sarcoma are ground glass opacities secondary to hemorrhage, lymphadenopathy or pleural effusion.[87] Pulmonary blastomas are usually found in children with solid masses having extensive cystic changes. Another separate entity pleuropulmonary blastoma show solid cystic masses which may mimic congenital lung lesion like cystic adenomatoid malformation or sequestration.[88] Pulmonary blastoma arises from germ cell and classified under carcinosarcoma. These are usually found in children and young adults. On imaging, these are seen as single or multiple peripheral solid lung masses with cystic changes, cavitation and occasionally, calcifications.[89] Pleuropulmonary blastoma

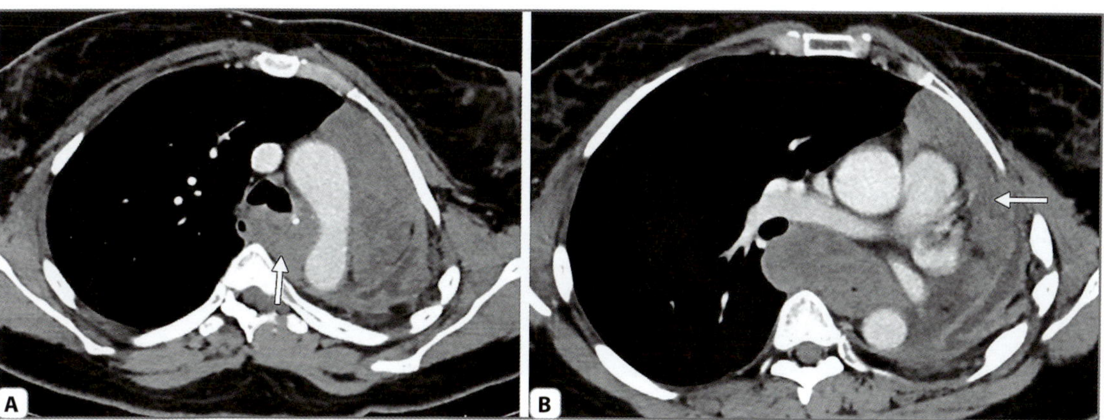

FIGS. 20A AND B: Myxoid sarcoma. Axial CT images of a 34-year-old female showing heterogenous infiltrating mass (arrow) involving the left main bronchus with contiguous mediastinal extension and complete collapse of left lung (arrow). Endobronchial biopsy was suggestive of myxoid sarcoma.

is a separate entity seen in early childhood. These arise from primitive blastomatous tissues and develop in pre-existing congenital lung lesions like cystic adenomatoid malformation, sequestration or bronchogenic cysts. On imaging, these are seen as cystic-solid masses.[90]

PULMONARY LYMPHOMA PRIMARY

Pulmonary Lymphoma

Most primary pulmonary lymphomas commonly arise from mucosa-associated lymphoid tissue commonly called MALT lymphoma, comprising up to 90% of cases although it is a fairly rare disease. The rest of the pulmonary lymphomas include diffuse large B-cell non-Hodgkin's lymphoma (NHL) followed by Hodgkin lymphoma (HL) usually from direct extension of mediastinal disease to involve parenchyma.[91]

There is lymphangitic spread at the periphery of these lesions leading to invasion of the adjacent pleura, vessels, and airways.[92] Main imaging findings on CT include nodules, masses, and/or nodular/mass like areas of ground-glass attenuation or consolidation (CT angiogram sign) with air bronchograms around bronchovascular distribution, hilar and mediastinal lymphadenopathy. Pleural effusion is uncommonly seen. They appear FDG avid in PET/CT scan in 50% cases. Patients tend to present around the 6th decade former or active smokers and has been associated with multiple autoimmune diseases such as Sjögren syndrome, rheumatoid arthritis, common variable immunodeficiency, concurrent lymphoid interstitial pneumonitis (LIP), chronic inflammation from smoking, and infections such as HIV and hepatitis C.[92,93]

The imaging picture on CT can be mimicked by sarcoidosis as it tends to show peribronchovascular distribution. Similarly, polyangiitis (formerly Wegener granulomatosis), perilymphatic spread of metastatic disease and infection showing peribronchial consolidation can mimic MALT lymphoma. Clinical presentation and laboratory parameters can be helpful in narrowing the differential diagnosis.

Diagnosis is made usually by transbronchial, CT-guided percutaneous transthoracic biopsy or at times with a surgical biopsy. Immunohistochemical studies are required for definitive diagnosis to confirm a monoclonal B-cell population, which is positive for pan-B-cell antigens like CD19, CD20 and PAX-5.[94]

Treatment is usually with chemotherapy or immunotherapy (rituximab) with options of surgery and radiation therapy for localized disease. MALT lymphoma tends to recur in the lung in up to 50% cases within the first years after diagnosis. Although regional involvement of hilar lymph nodes does not affect prognosis, but presence pleural effusion or amyloid within the tumor signifies poorer prognosis.[94,95]

Secondary Pulmonary Lymphoma (SPL)

All the different forms of lymphoma may secondarily involve the lungs, but the mature B-cell neoplasms are the most frequent. Although a greater proportion of patients with HL rather than NHL have lung involvement, more NHL SPL is seen in clinical practice because NHL is more prevalent. Lymphomatous involvement of the lung itself is often asymptomatic and non-specific. However, B-symptoms of HL are more often related to the presence of mediastinal lymphadenopathy.

Imaging findings are varied and nonspecific and include nodules <1 cm in diameter, solitary or multiple, mass/mass-like consolidation, bronchovascular thickening mimicking lymphangitis carcinomatosa, air bronchograms (NHL > HL) **(Figs. 21A and B)**. Mediastinal lymphadenopathy with nodules/masses with or without air bronchograms are the commonest HRCT features.[96] In HL, there is contiguous spread of the disease from the adenopathy to

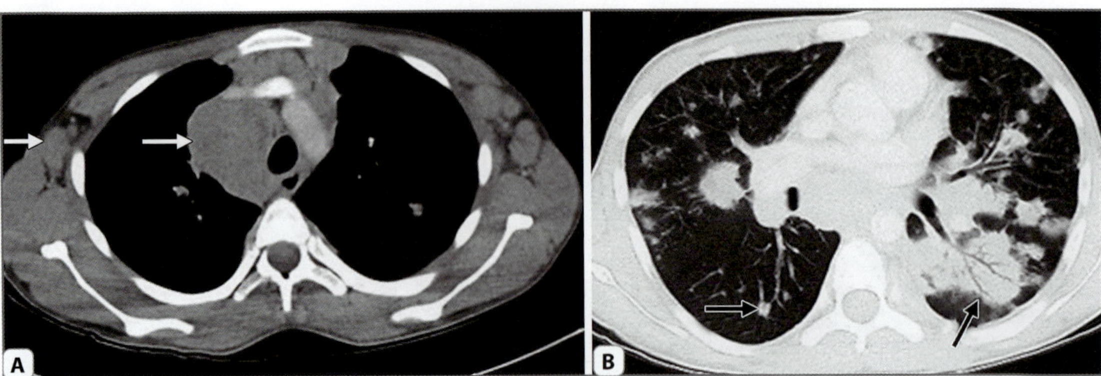

FIGS. 21A AND B: Secondary pulmonary involvement by lymphoma (nodular form): (A) Axial CT image mediastinal window shows homogenous enlarged lymph nodes in mediastinum and bilateral axillae in a case of non-Hodgkins's lymphoma; (B) Multiple irregular lung nodules with air bronchograms (arrows) are seen in both lungs suggestive of lymphomatous involvement.

involve parenchyma whereas isolated lung disease without mediastinal involvement can occur in NHL.

Acquired Immunodeficiency Syndrome-related Lymphoma (ARL)

Lymphoma is the second most common tumor occurring in patients with AIDS, after Kaposi's sarcoma. Most patients are symptomatic, presenting with cough and shortness of breath. This subset of patients usually develops aggressive B-cell lymphomas.[97,98]

Imaging findings include well-defined pulmonary nodules (0.5–5 cm) with or without cavitation or a large solitary pulmonary nodule/mass (2–5 cm). Pleural effusions is commonest thoracic manifestation followed by pericardial effusions, consolidation and/or ground-glass opacity. Combinations of nodules, effusions, and adenopathy in a HIV positive patient is highly suggestive of ARL.[97,99]

Post-transplantation Lymphoproliferative Disorder (PTLD)

The PTLD is a lymphoid/plasmacytic proliferation that occurs following solid organ or hematopoietic stem cell transplantation, manifesting as a spectrum of disorders ranging from polyclonal benign proliferations to monoclonal and monomorphic aggressive lymphomas.

The etiology of PTLD is thought to be closely associated with EBV infection. PTLD is seen in less than 2% of all transplant cases and there is a clear association with the specific organ transplanted, with the highest incidence in lung transplantation (6–9%), followed by heart, liver and renal transplant. The majority of cases of PTLD occur within 2 years of transplantation, but it may be seen as early as 60 days post-transplant.[100]

The clinical presentation is variable and includes fever, lymphadenopathy, and abdominal pain with diarrhea, a mononucleosis-like syndrome and weight loss.

B-cell NHL is the most common type of lymphoma associated with PTLD. The commonest imaging findings of PTLD are well defined usually multiple nodules (size range 0.3–5 cm), "halo sign" around nodules, patchy/focal consolidation or ground-glass opacity, more peribronchial/subpleural than diffuse distribution of nodules and lymphadenopathy.[101-103]

PULMONARY NEUROENDOCRINE NEOPLASMS

Pulmonary neuroendocrine neoplasms constitute approximately 20–25% of all invasive primary lung cancers. The WHO in 2015 has grouped pulmonary neuroendocrine neoplasms into three histologic grades: Typical carcinoid as low-grade malignant neoplasm, atypical carcinoid as intermediate grade, and large cell neuroendocrine carcinoma (LCNEC) and small cell lung carcinoma (SCLC) as high-grade malignancies.[104,105]

Carcinoid Tumors

The respiratory tract is the second most common location after gastrointestinal tract, accounting for 20–30% of carcinoids.[106] They are indolent neoplasms with the potential to metastasize. Typical carcinoid is the least aggressive carcinoid type whereas atypical carcinoid is a more aggressive with 57% of affected patients present with lymph node metastases.[107]

Typical carcinoid is defined as a well-differentiated neoplasm with neuroendocrine histologic features, measuring 5 mm or more, exhibiting < 2 mitoses per 10 high-power fields (HPF) or 2 mm^2, and no necrosis. The carcinoid is classified as atypical carcinoid when there are 2 to 10 mitoses per 10 HPF or necrosis, which is often punctate.[104] Most carcinoids are vascular lesions, and 30% of cases exhibit calcification.[108]

Most affected patients are adults, although carcinoids are the most common malignant primary lung neoplasm untill young adulthood.

Most patients with centrally located neoplasms, present with symptoms such as recurrent infections, cough, hemoptysis, and wheezing whereas peripheral tumors are asymptomatic and hence detected late.[105] Patients may present with Cushing syndrome and Carcinoid syndrome particularly patients with liver metastases. Carcinoid syndrome is characterized by skin flushing, bronchoconstriction, intractable diarrhea, and right-sided heart disease.[109]

Imaging Findings

Carcinoids show a centrally located (hilar or perihilar), well-defined solitary 2–5 cm nodule more common in occur in the right lung (60%).[110] Atypical carcinoid tends to be larger and more peripheral than typical carcinoid.[111] Consider atypical carcinoid rather than typical carcinoid in older patients with well-defined peripheral nodule or central mass associated with lymph node or distant metastases. Multidetector CT demonstrates soft-tissue nodule located adjacent to airway and may be completely endoluminal **(Figs. 22A and B)**, partially endoluminal, or may abut the airway. Positive "bronchus sign" demonstrating bronchus leading directly to the tumor may suggest the diagnosis. CT may demonstrate variable degrees of tumor enhancement differentiating it from adjacent atelectasis **(Figs. 22A and B)** or consolidation.[74] Calcification may be seen. CT is also useful for detection of lymphadenopathy and metastases in the liver, bone, or adrenal glands.[112]

MR imaging usually shows lesions with high T2 and STIR (short inversion time inversion-recovery) signal intensity and intense enhancement during the systemic circulatory phase. Indium 111 octreotide or lanreotide (short- and long-acting somatostatin analogs) scintigraphy can be useful for localization of occult tumors. 68 Gallium DOTANOC scan is currently used to image the primary as well as lymph node metastasis (more sensitive investigation).[113]

The diagnosis of carcinoid tumor requires microscopic evaluation of tissue, which can be obtained with bronchoscopy or CT guided biopsy or thoracotomy.[114]

Large Cell Neuroendocrine Carcinoma

The LCNEC is defined as a high-grade NSCLC with neuroendocrine histologic features, more than 10 mitoses per 10 HPF (median, 70 mitoses per 10 HPF), and necrosis. Most patients with LCNEC are heavy smoker male, with a mean age of 65 years (range, 44–82 years). Presenting symptoms are like other lung masses whereas paraneoplastic syndromes are rare. The diagnosis of LCNEC is by surgical lung biopsy.

Imaging Findings

At imaging, LCNEC typically manifests as a large (13–92 mm), peripheral mass indistinguishable from other lung cancers and typically exhibits well-defined lobular margins.[115] Approximately one-fifth of LCNECs are centrally located and may be associated with pressure symptoms.[116] Necrosis, heterogeneous or peripheral enhancement, calcification, hilar and mediastinal lymphadenopathy.

Small Cell Lung Carcinoma

It is the most common neuroendocrine lung neoplasm, representing 15–20% of invasive lung malignancies.[117]

Small cell lung carcinoma is characterized by its small cell size, scant cytoplasm, finely granular nuclear chromatin, absent or faint nucleoli, extremely high mitotic rates (>10 mitoses per 10 HPF; median, 80 mitoses per 10 HPF), and extensive necrosis. The diagnosis is often established by image-guided or bronchoscopy biopsy. A panel of immunohistochemical stains including CD56, TTF-1, and Ki-67 is typically used to differentiate SCLC from other lung masses. The Ki-67 proliferation index is most helpful in separating SCLC from carcinoids.[105] SCLC occurs almost exclusively in smokers, and affected patients present with cough, hemoptysis, chest pain, and dyspnea. Constitutional symptoms, symptoms related to SVC invasion or extrapulmonary metastases. Patients with SCLC may also present with endocrine and nonendocrine paraneoplastic syndromes like SIADH and Cushing syndrome, Eaton-Lambert syndrome, and encephalomyelitis.

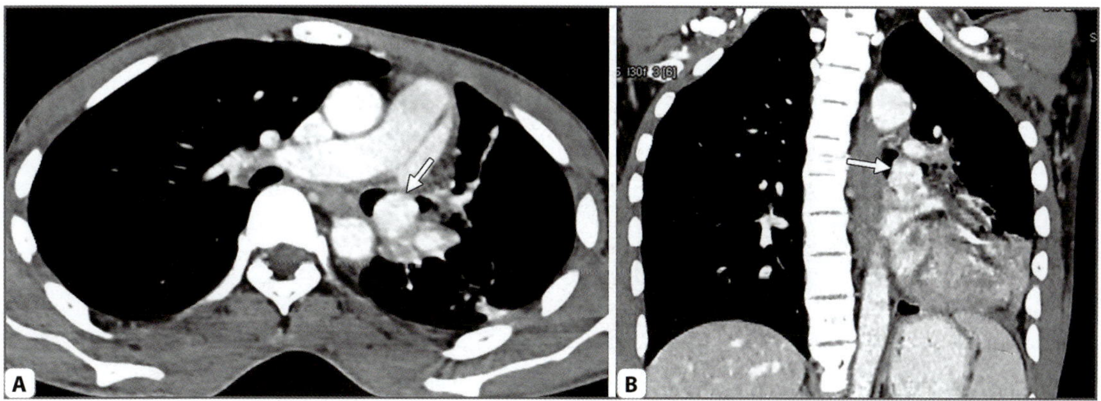

FIGS. 22A AND B: Typical carcinoid: (A and B) Intensely enhancing endoluminal nodule is seen in left main and lower lobe bronchus (arrow) with partial collapse of left lower lobe.

Imaging Findings

On CT, SCLC typically manifests as a large central or mediastinal mass which are combination of the primary and associated lymphadenopathy. Bronchus cut-off sign, calcifications and pleural effusion may be present. The primary tumor may not be visible at times due to mediastinal lymphadenopathy. Encasement or invasion of mediastinal structures, pleural effusion, pericardial thickening, pleural nodules, and metastases to the liver, adrenal glands, and bones may be seen.[44,118]

Diffuse Idiopathic Pulmonary Neuroendocrine Cell Hyperplasia

It is a preinvasive lesion of neuroendocrine group of tumors. On CT, it may present as mosaic attenuation secondary to expiratory air-trapping due to proliferation of neuroendocrine cells within bronchial/bronchiolar epithelium. Sometimes, it may manifest as multiple lung nodules or tumorlets (<5 mm).[119]

Pulmonary Metastases

The lung metastasis is extremely common due to its high blood or lymphatics supply and through hematogenous and lymphatic routes. Lymphangitis carcinomatosis is a special form of lung metastasis where lymphatics in interlobular septa are clogged with tumor cells and appear nodular thickening of sepate on HRCT images. The most common cancers that metastasize to the lungs include breast, colon, kidney, uterus, and head and neck are the most common primary sites with pulmonary metastasis.[120] Cancers like choriocarcinoma, osteosarcoma, testicular tumor, melanoma, Ewing tumor, and thyroid carcinoma also frequently metastasize to the lung.[121] The early diagnosis of pulmonary metastases is crucial for treatment planning as well as for prognostication. MDCT is the most common imaging modality used for detection of possible pulmonary metastases. Typically, metastases appear well circumscribed soft tissue attenuation, rounded lesions, more often in the periphery of the lung of variable size, a feature which is of some use in distinguishing them from a granuloma. A prominent pulmonary vessel (feeding vessel sign) can be seen heading into a metastasis **(Fig. 23A)**. The usual radiologic findings of pulmonary metastasis include multiple peripherally located round variable-sized nodules (hematogenous metastasis) and diffuse thickening of the interstitium (lymphangitic carcinomatosis). Among cases of multiple nodules detected with CT, 73% were reported to be pulmonary metastases. The unusual radiologic features include cavitation **(Fig. 23B)** (squamous cell carcinoma, most often from the head and neck or from the lung), hemorrhage around the metastatic nodules (choriocarcinoma, angiosarcoma) **(Fig. 23C)**, pneumothorax (osteosarcoma), calcification (osteosarcoma **(Figs. 24A to C)**, chondrosarcoma, papillary thyroid carcinoma), air-space pattern, tumor embolism, endobronchial metastasis, solitary mass, dilated vessels within a mass, and sterilized metastasis. Innumerable small metastases (miliary pattern) may be seen in malignant melanoma, osteosarcoma, renal cell carcinoma, thyroid carcinoma and trophoblastic disease. Conversely, pulmonary metastasis may be single in colorectal carcinoma, malignant melanoma, skeletal sarcoma and testicular carcinoma. Adenocarcinoma metastases, rather than displace or destroy adjacent lung parenchyma, may grow in a lepidic fashion (spread along alveolar walls) resulting in pneumonia-like consolidation/air bronchograms.

Pulmonary Hamartoma

Hamartoma is the most common, slowly growing benign mesenchymal pulmonary neoplasm and represents about 6% of SPN detected on a chest X-ray.[122] It consists of connective tissue elements such as fat, calcification, muscle, lymphatics. On CT, hamartomas typically manifest as well-circumscribed peripheral solitary pulmonary nodules or masses with smooth or lobular borders **(Fig. 25)**. 10% are central and endobronchial. Calcification is more common

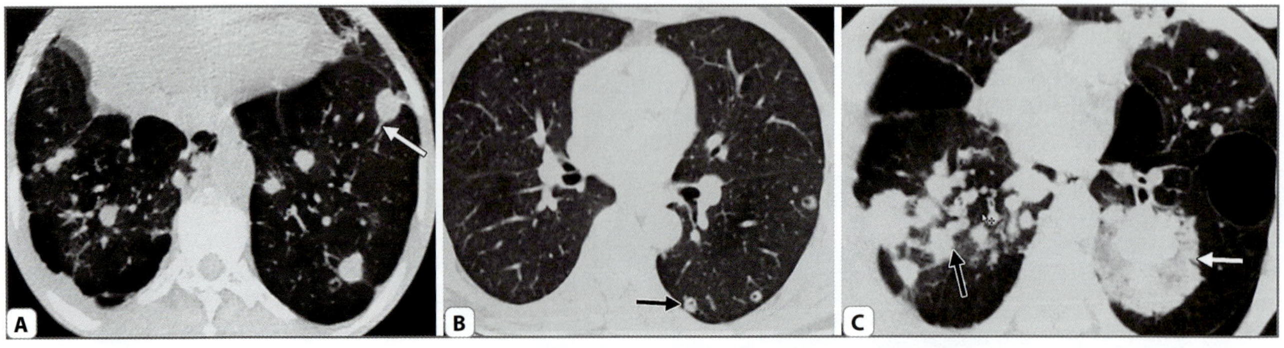

FIGS. 23A TO C: Pulmonary metastases: (A) CT lung window shows multiple well-defined nodules (arrow) predominantly in peripheral lung with feeding vessel sign; (B) Cavitary metastases: CT of the patient with supraglottic squamous cell cancer shows multiple lung metastases in left lung showing cavitation (arrow); (C) Hemorrhagic metastases: CT of the patient with renal cell carcinoma shows multiple lung masses with ground glass opacities around them (arrows), secondary to hemorrhages.

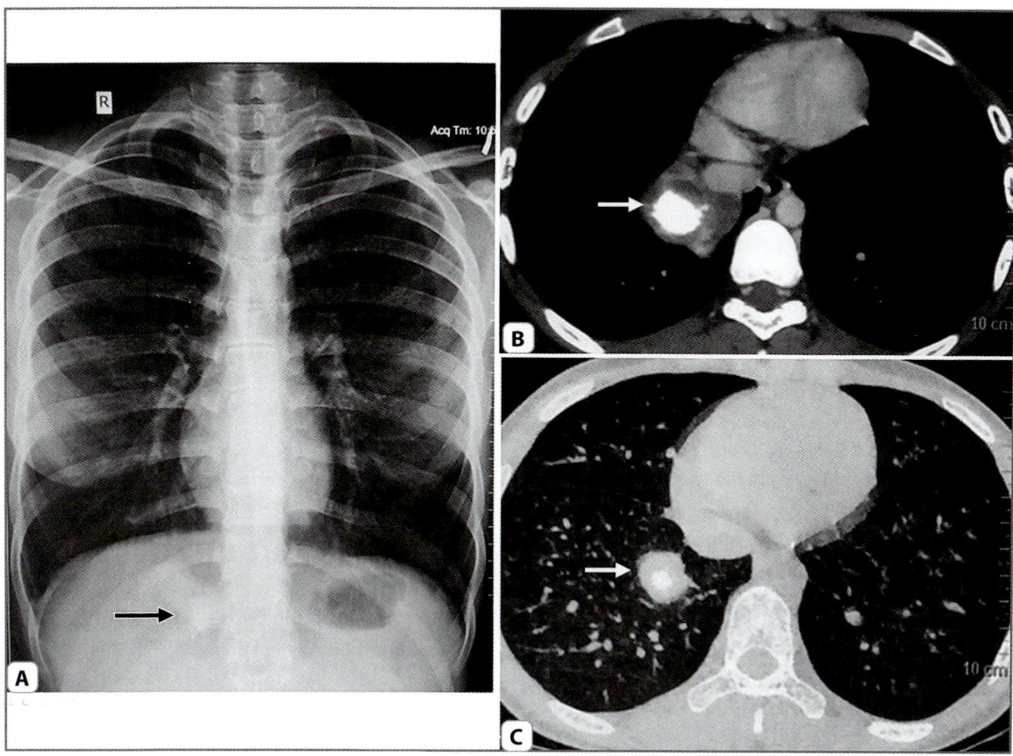

FIGS. 24A TO C: Calcified/ossified lung metastasis; (A) Chest radiograph showing a dense nodular radio-opacity below the right hemidiaphragm (arrow); (B and C) CT shows a soft tissue nodule in right lower lobe (arrow) with central chunky calcification suggestive of metastasis in a case of osteosarcoma of femur.

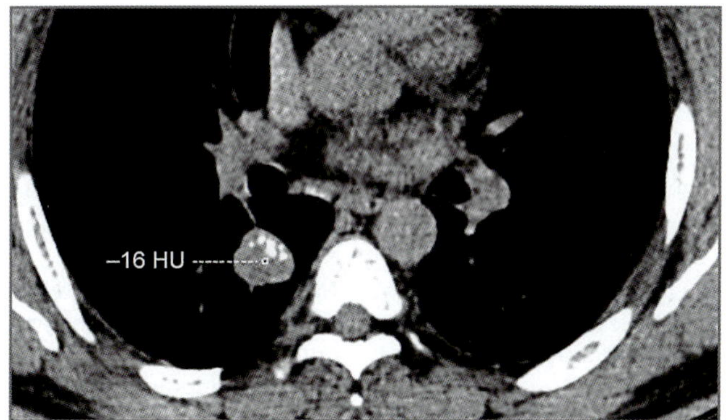

FIG. 25: Pulmonary hamartoma. A non-contrast CT axial image shows a well-defined nodule in peripheral aspect of right lower lobe with internal calcification and fat attenuation suggestive of pulmonary hamartoma.

in larger lesions and is much better visualized on CT than on radiography. Although a characteristic popcorn pattern of calcification has been described, it is only present in 10–15% of cases. Internal fat, identified by Hounsfield units of -20 to -120 on CT, is present in 60% of cases. Identification of both internal fat and calcium is virtually diagnostic of a hamartoma.[123] Following the administration of intravenous contrast, most lesions demonstrate heterogeneous enhancement.

CONCLUSION

In conclusion, imaging is an integral part of management protocol for pulmonary neoplasms. A thorough knowledge of available imaging modalities and judicious utilization of these is necessary for optimal patient care. Chest radiography and CT are most commonly used modalities. MRI can be used as a problem-solving tool. Survival in carcinoma lung depends on stage; early detection and diagnosis can help in achieving surgical cure. Here, the cross-sectional imaging plays a key role in the assessment of malignancy. CT, being less expensive and more widely available than MRI, is more likely to remain as a principal modality for evaluation of this disease. PET-CT helps for further characterization and assessment of extent of disease. It is important that radiologists are familiar with the 8th and upcoming 9th TNM staging system for accurate assessment of prognosis and treatment planning. FNAC, biopsy and image guided ablations (e.g., RFA/microwave) for lung tumors are major interventions performed, which need meticulous planning using various imaging modalities.

REFERENCES

1. Siegel RL, Miller KD, Wagle NS, Jemal A. Cancer statistics, 2023. CA Cancer J Clin. 2023;73(1):17-48.
2. Bade BC, Dela Cruz CS. Lung Cancer 2020: Epidemiology, Etiology, and Prevention. Clin Chest Med. 2020;41(1):1-24.
3. Malik PS, Raina V. Lung cancer: prevalent trends & emerging concepts. Indian J Med Res. 2015;141(1):5-7.
4. Jamil A, Kasi A. Lung Metastasis. StatPearls. Treasure Island (FL): StatPearls Publishing Copyright © 2025, StatPearls Publishing LLC.; 2025.
5. Ettinger DS, Akerley W, Bepler G, Blum MG, Chang A, Cheney RT, et al. Non-small cell lung cancer. J Natl Compr Canc Netw. 2010;8(7):740-801.
6. Xue X, Liu Y, Pan L, Wang Y, Wang K, Zhang M, et al. Diagnosis of multiple primary lung cancer: a systematic review. J Int Med Res. 2013;41(6):1779-87.
7. Nicholson AG, Tsao MS, Beasley MB, Borczuk AC, Brambilla E, Cooper WA, et al. The 2021 WHO Classification of Lung Tumors: Impact of Advances Since 2015. J Thorac Oncol. 2022;17(3):362-87.
8. Dong Y, Mao F, Wang WP, Ji ZB, Fan PL. Value of Contrast-Enhanced Ultrasound in Guidance of Percutaneous Biopsy in Peripheral Pulmonary Lesions. Biomed Res Int. 2015;2015:531507.
9. Batra P, Brown K, Aberle DR, Young DA, Steckel R. Imaging techniques in the evaluation of pulmonary parenchymal neoplasms. Chest. 1992;101(1):239-43.
10. De Wever W, Verschakelen J, Coolen J. Role of imaging in diagnosis, staging and follow-up of lung cancer. Curr Opin Pulm Med. 2014;20(4):385-92.
11. Madani MH, Riess JW, Brown LM, Cooke DT, Guo HH. Imaging of lung cancer. Curr Probl Cancer. 2023;47(2):100966.
12. Tacelli N, Santangelo T, Scherpereel A, Duhamel A, Deken V, Klotz E, et al. Perfusion CT allows prediction of therapy response in non-small cell lung cancer treated with conventional and anti-angiogenic chemotherapy. Eur Radiol. 2013;23(8):2127-36.
13. Zhang LJ, Yang GF, Wu SY, Xu J, Lu GM, Schoepf UJ. Dual-energy CT imaging of thoracic malignancies. Cancer Imaging. 2013;13:81-91.
14. Hou WS, Wu HW, Yin Y, Cheng JJ, Zhang Q, Xu JR. Differentiation of lung cancers from inflammatory masses with dual-energy spectral CT imaging. Acad Radiol. 2015;22(3):337-44.
15. Dennie C, Thornhill R, Sethi-Virmani V, Souza CA, Bayanati H, Gupta A, et al. Role of quantitative computed tomography texture analysis in the differentiation of primary lung cancer and granulomatous nodules. Quant Imaging Med Surg. 2016;6(1):6-15.
16. Heyneman LE, Patz EF. PET imaging in patients with bronchioloalveolar cell carcinoma. Lung Cancer. 2002;38(3):261-6.
17. Erasmus JJ, Macapinlac HA. Low-sensitivity FDG-PET studies: less common lung neoplasms. Semin Nucl Med. 2012;42(4):255-60.
18. Jiang Y, Hou G, Cheng W. The utility of 18F-FDG and 68Ga-DOTA-Peptide PET/CT in the evaluation of primary pulmonary carcinoid: A systematic review and meta-analysis. Medicine (Baltimore). 2019;98(10):e14769.
19. Chang JM, Lee HJ, Goo JM, Lee HY, Lee JJ, Chung JK, et al. False positive and false negative FDG-PET scans in various thoracic diseases. Korean J Radiol. 2006;7(1):57-69.
20. Fischer B, Lassen U, Mortensen J, Larsen S, Loft A, Bertelsen A, et al. Preoperative staging of lung cancer with combined PET-CT. N Engl J Med. 2009;361(1):32-9.
21. De Leyn P, Dooms C, Kuzdzal J, Lardinois D, Passlick B, Rami-Porta R, et al. Revised ESTS guidelines for preoperative mediastinal lymph node staging for non-small-cell lung cancer. Eur J Cardiothorac Surg. 2014;45(5):787-98.
22. Gupta NC, Rogers JS, Graeber GM, Gregory JL, Waheed U, Mullet D, et al. Clinical role of F-18 fluorodeoxyglucose positron emission tomography imaging in patients with lung cancer and suspected malignant pleural effusion. Chest. 2002;122(6):1918-24.
23. Song JW, Oh YM, Shim TS, Kim WS, Ryu JS, Choi CM. Efficacy comparison between (18)F-FDG PET/CT and bone scintigraphy in detecting bony metastases of non-small-cell lung cancer. Lung Cancer. 2009;65(3):333-8.
24. Lardinois D, Weder W, Hany TF, Kamel EM, Korom S, Seifert B, et al. Staging of non-small-cell lung cancer with integrated positron-emission tomography and computed tomography. N Engl J Med. 2003;348(25):2500-7.
25. Greco C, Rosenzweig K, Cascini GL, Tamburrini O. Current status of PET/CT for tumour volume definition in radiotherapy treatment planning for non-small cell lung cancer (NSCLC). Lung Cancer. 2007;57(2):125-34.
26. Hicks RJ. Role of 18F-FDG PET in assessment of response in non-small cell lung cancer. J Nucl Med. 2009;50(Suppl 1):31S-42S.
27. Usmanij EA, de Geus-Oei LF, Bussink J, Oyen WJ. Update on F-18-fluoro-deoxy-glucose-PET/computed tomography in nonsmall cell lung cancer. Curr Opin Pulm Med. 2015;21(4):314-21.
28. Koyama H, Ohno Y, Seki S, Nishio M, Yoshikawa T, Matsumoto S, et al. Magnetic resonance imaging for lung cancer. J Thorac Imaging. 2013;28(3):138-50.
29. Mori T, Nomori H, Ikeda K, Kawanaka K, Shiraishi S, Katahira K, et al. Diffusion-weighted magnetic resonance imaging for diagnosing malignant pulmonary nodules/masses: comparison with positron emission tomography. J Thorac Oncol. 2008;3(4):358-64.
30. Schaefer JF, Schneider V, Vollmar J, Wehrmann M, Aebert H, Friedel G, et al. Solitary pulmonary nodules: association between signal characteristics in dynamic contrast enhanced MRI and tumor angiogenesis. Lung Cancer. 2006;53(1):39-49.
31. Kono R, Fujimoto K, Terasaki H, Müller NL, Kato S, Sadohara J, et al. Dynamic MRI of solitary pulmonary nodules: comparison of enhancement patterns of malignant and benign small peripheral lung lesions. AJR Am J Roentgenol. 2007;188(1):26-36.
32. Hochhegger B, Marchiori E, Sedlaczek O, Irion K, Heussel CP, Ley S, et al. MRI in lung cancer: a pictorial essay. Br J Radiol. 2011;84(1003):661-8.
33. Grewal RG, Austin JH. CT demonstration of calcification in carcinoma of the lung. J Comput Assist Tomogr. 1994;18(6):867-71.

34. Khan AN, Al-Jahdali HH, Allen CM, Irion KL, Al Ghanem S, Koteyar SS. The calcified lung nodule: What does it mean? Ann Thorac Med. 2010;5(2):67-79.
35. Aoki T, Tomoda Y, Watanabe H, Nakata H, Kasai T, Hashimoto H, et al. Peripheral lung adenocarcinoma: correlation of thin-section CT findings with histologic prognostic factors and survival. Radiology. 2001;220(3):803-9.
36. Mackintosh JA, Marshall HM, Yang IA, Bowman RV, Fong KM. A retrospective study of volume doubling time in surgically resected non-small cell lung cancer. Respirology. 2014;19(5):755-62.
37. Nakahashi K, Shiono S, Nakatsuka M, Endo M. Prognostic impact of the tumor volume doubling time in clinical T1 non-small cell lung cancer with solid radiological findings. J Surg Oncol. 2022;126(7):1330-40.
38. Dela Cruz CS, Tanoue LT, Matthay RA. Lung cancer: epidemiology, etiology, and prevention. Clin Chest Med. 2011;32(4):605-44.
39. Zhang Y, Vaccarella S, Morgan E, Li M, Etxeberria J, Chokunonga E, et al. Global variations in lung cancer incidence by histological subtype in 2020: a population-based study. Lancet Oncol. 2023;24(11):1206-18.
40. Hollings N, Shaw P. Diagnostic imaging of lung cancer. Eur Respir J. 2002;19(4):722-42.
41. Wang T, Yang Y, Liu X, Deng J, Wu J, Hou L, et al. Primary Invasive Mucinous Adenocarcinoma of the Lung: Prognostic Value of CT Imaging Features Combined with Clinical Factors. Korean J Radiol. 2021;22(4):652-62.
42. Qi L, Jia J, Zhang G, Liu J, Li F, Chen J, et al. Radiological Features of Primary Pulmonary Invasive Mucinous Adenocarcinoma Based on 312 Consecutive Patients. Clin Respir J. 2024;18(8):e13820.
43. Takahashi M, Nitta N, Takazakura R, Nishimoto Y, Furukawa A, Murata K. Many faces of squamous cell carcinoma of the lung: its wide spectrum of radiological findings. Curr Probl Diagn Radiol. 2003;32(2):45-65.
44. Carter BW, Glisson BS, Truong MT, Erasmus JJ. Small cell lung carcinoma: staging, imaging, and treatment considerations. Radiographics. 2014;34(6):1707-21.
45. Ganti AKP, Loo BW, Bassetti M, Blakely C, Chiang A, D'Amico TA, et al. Small Cell Lung Cancer, Version 2.2022, NCCN Clinical Practice Guidelines in Oncology. J Natl Compr Canc Netw. 2021;19(12):1441-64.
46. Acharya K V, B U, Shenoy A, Holla R. Utility of Various Bronchoscopic Modalities in Lung Cancer Diagnosis. Asian Pac J Cancer Prev. 2017;18(7):1931-6.
47. Zhan P, Zhu QQ, Miu YY, Liu YF, Wang XX, Zhou ZJ, et al. Comparison between endobronchial ultrasound-guided transbronchial biopsy and CT-guided transthoracic lung biopsy for the diagnosis of peripheral lung cancer: a systematic review and meta-analysis. Transl Lung Cancer Res. 2017;6(1):23-34.
48. Ikeda N, Saji H, Hagiwara M, Ohira T, Usuda J, Kajiwara N. Recent advances in video-assisted thoracoscopic surgery for lung cancer. Asian J Endosc Surg. 2013;6(1):9-13.
49. Berfield KS, Farjah F, Mulligan MS. Video-Assisted Thoracoscopic Lobectomy for Lung Cancer. Ann Thorac Surg. 2019;107(2):603-9.
50. Kay FU, Kandathil A, Batra K, Saboo SS, Abbara S, Rajiah P. Revisions to the Tumor, Node, Metastasis staging of lung cancer (8th edition): Rationale, radiologic findings and clinical implications. World J Radiol. 2017;9(6):269-79.
51. Detterbeck FC, Boffa DJ, Kim AW, Tanoue LT. The Eighth Edition Lung Cancer Stage Classification. Chest. 2017;151(1):193-203.
52. Detterbeck FC, Woodard GA, Bader AS, Dacic S, Grant MJ, Park HS, et al. The Proposed Ninth Edition TNM Classification of Lung Cancer. Chest. 2024;166(4):882-95.
53. Lewis JW, Jr., Pearlberg JL, Beute GH, Alpern M, Kvale PA, Gross BH, et al. Can computed tomography of the chest stage lung cancer? Yes and no. Ann Thorac Surg. 1990;49(4):591-5; discussion 5-6.
54. Beigelman-Aubry C, Dunet V, Brun AL. CT imaging in pre-therapeutic assessment of lung cancer. Diagn Interv Imaging. 2016;97(10):973-89.
55. Owens C, Hindocha S, Lee R, Millard T, Sharma B. The lung cancers: staging and response, CT, (18)F-FDG PET/CT, MRI, DWI: review and new perspectives. Br J Radiol. 2023;96(1148):20220339.
56. Hirsch FR, Scagliotti GV, Mulshine JL, Kwon R, Curran WJ, Jr., Wu YL, et al. Lung cancer: current therapies and new targeted treatments. Lancet. 2017;389(10066):299-311.
57. Eisenhauer EA, Therasse P, Bogaerts J, Schwartz LH, Sargent D, Ford R, et al. New response evaluation criteria in solid tumours: revised RECIST guideline (version 1.1). Eur J Cancer. 2009;45(2):228-47.
58. Sun JM, Ahn MJ, Park MJ, Yi JH, Kim TS, Chung MJ, et al. Accuracy of RECIST 1.1 for non-small cell lung cancer treated with EGFR tyrosine kinase inhibitors. Lung Cancer. 2010;69(1):105-9.
59. Ezhil M, Vedam S, Balter P, Choi B, Mirkovic D, Starkschall G, et al. Determination of patient-specific internal gross tumor volumes for lung cancer using four-dimensional computed tomography. Radiat Oncol. 2009;4:4.
60. Simon CJ, Dupuy DE, DiPetrillo TA, Safran HP, Grieco CA, Ng T, et al. Pulmonary radiofrequency ablation: long-term safety and efficacy in 153 patients. Radiology. 2007;243(1):268-75.
61. Sano Y, Kanazawa S, Gobara H, Mukai T, Hiraki T, Hase S, et al. Feasibility of percutaneous radiofrequency ablation for intrathoracic malignancies: a large single-center experience. Cancer. 2007;109(7):1397-405.
62. Lencioni R, Crocetti L, Cioni R, Suh R, Glenn D, Regge D, et al. Response to radiofrequency ablation of pulmonary tumours: a prospective, intention-to-treat, multicentre clinical trial (the RAPTURE study). Lancet Oncol. 2008;9(7):621-8.
63. Lanuti M, Sharma A, Digumarthy SR, Wright CD, Donahue DM, Wain JC, et al. Radiofrequency ablation for treatment of medically inoperable stage I non-small cell lung cancer. J Thorac Cardiovasc Surg. 2009;137(1):160-6.
64. Zhao Q, Wang J, Fu YL, Hu B. Radiofrequency ablation for stage <IIB non-small cell lung cancer: Opportunities, challenges, and the road ahead. Thorac Cancer. 2023;14(32):3181-90.
65. Mayo-Smith WW, Dupuy DE. Adrenal neoplasms: CT-guided radiofrequency ablation—preliminary results. Radiology. 2004;231(1):225-30.
66. Yao W, Lu M, Fan W, Huang J, Gu Y, Gao F, et al. Comparison between microwave ablation and lobectomy for stage I non-small cell lung cancer: a propensity score analysis. Int J Hyperthermia. 2018;34(8):1329-36.

67. Han X, Yang X, Huang G, Li C, Zhang L, Qiao Y, et al. Safety and clinical outcomes of computed tomography-guided percutaneous microwave ablation in patients aged 80 years and older with early-stage non-small cell lung cancer: A multicenter retrospective study. Thorac Cancer. 2019;10(12):2236-42.
68. Ye X, Fan W, Wang H, Wang J, Wang Z, Gu S, et al. Expert consensus workshop report: Guidelines for thermal ablation of primary and metastatic lung tumors (2018 edition). J Cancer Res Ther. 2018;14(4):730-44.
69. McDevitt JL, Mouli SK, Nemcek AA, Lewandowski RJ, Salem R, Sato KT. Percutaneous Cryoablation for the Treatment of Primary and Metastatic Lung Tumors: Identification of Risk Factors for Recurrence and Major Complications. J Vasc Interv Radiol. 2016;27(9):1371-9.
70. Feng J, Guiyu D, Xiongwen W. The clinical efficacy of argon-helium knife cryoablation combined with nivolumab in the treatment of advanced non-small cell lung cancer. Cryobiology. 2021;102:92-6.
71. Marcus PM, Bergstralh EJ, Fagerstrom RM, Williams DE, Fontana R, Taylor WF, et al. Lung cancer mortality in the Mayo Lung Project: impact of extended follow-up. J Natl Cancer Inst. 2000;92(16):1308-16.
72. Wood DE, Kazerooni EA, Baum SL, Eapen GA, Ettinger DS, Hou L, et al. Lung Cancer Screening, Version 3.2018, NCCN Clinical Practice Guidelines in Oncology. J Natl Compr Canc Netw. 2018;16(4):412-41.
73. Lancaster HL, Heuvelmans MA, Oudkerk M. Low-dose computed tomography lung cancer screening: Clinical evidence and implementation research. J Intern Med. 2022;292(1):68-80.
74. Christensen J, Prosper AE, Wu CC, Chung J, Lee E, Elicker B, et al. ACR Lung-RADS v2022: Assessment Categories and Management Recommendations. J Am Coll Radiol. 2024;21(3):473-88.
75. Vora A, Balamugesh T, Behera D, Kumar P, Tiwaskar M, Mehta P, et al. Screening for Lung Cancer in India: Expert Opinion Statement. J Assoc Physicians India. 2024;72(5):e1-e16.
76. Lam DC, Liam CK, Andarini S, Park S, Tan DSW, Singh N, et al. Lung Cancer Screening in Asia: An Expert Consensus Report. J Thorac Oncol. 2023;18(10):1303-22.
77. Younes RN, Gross JL, Deheinzelin D. Follow-up in lung cancer: how often and for what purpose? Chest. 1999;115(6):1494-9.
78. Bogot NR, Quint LE. Imaging of recurrent lung cancer. Cancer Imaging. 2004;4(2):61-7.
79. Hanania AN, Mainwaring W, Ghebre YT, Hanania NA, Ludwig M. Radiation-Induced Lung Injury: Assessment and Management. Chest. 2019;156(1):150-62.
80. Arroyo-Hernández M, Maldonado F, Lozano-Ruiz F, Muñoz-Montaño W, Nuñez-Baez M, Arrieta O. Radiation-induced lung injury: current evidence. BMC Pulm Med. 2021;21(1):9.
81. Koenig TR, Munden RF, Erasmus JJ, Sabloff BS, Gladish GW, Komaki R, et al. Radiation injury of the lung after three-dimensional conformal radiation therapy. AJR Am J Roentgenol. 2002;178(6):1383-8.
82. Aoki T, Nagata Y, Negoro Y, Takayama K, Mizowaki T, Kokubo M, et al. Evaluation of lung injury after three-dimensional conformal stereotactic radiation therapy for solitary lung tumors: CT appearance. Radiology. 2004;230(1):101-8.
83. Munden RF, Swisher SS, Stevens CW, Stewart DJ. Imaging of the patient with non-small cell lung cancer. Radiology. 2005;237(3):803-18.
84. Hotta K, Kiura K, Tabata M, Harita S, Gemba K, Yonei T, et al. Interstitial lung disease in Japanese patients with non-small cell lung cancer receiving gefitinib: an analysis of risk factors and treatment outcomes in Okayama Lung Cancer Study Group. Cancer J. 2005;11(5):417-24.
85. Libshitz HI, Sheppard DG. Filling in of radiation therapy-induced bronchiectatic change: a reliable sign of locally recurrent lung cancer. Radiology. 1999;210(1):25-7.
86. Kandathil A, Sibley RC, III, Subramaniam RM. Lung Cancer Recurrence: (18)F-FDG PET/CT in Clinical Practice. AJR Am J Roentgenol. 2019;213(5):1136-44.
87. Bhatia K, Ellis S. Unusual lung tumours: an illustrated review of CT features suggestive of this diagnosis. Cancer Imaging. 2006;6:72-82.
88. Manivel JC, Priest JR, Watterson J, Steiner M, Woods WG, Wick MR, et al. Pleuropulmonary blastoma. The so-called pulmonary blastoma of childhood. Cancer. 1988;62(8):1516-26.
89. Kunisaki SM, Lal DR, Saito JM, Fallat ME, St Peter SD, Fox ZD, et al. Pleuropulmonary Blastoma in Pediatric Lung Lesions. Pediatrics. 2021;147(4).
90. Leung SS, Donuru A, Kandula V, Parekh MR, Saul D. Multimodality Imaging of Pleuropulmonary Blastoma: Pearls, Pitfalls, and Differential Diagnosis. Semin Ultrasound CT MR. 2022;43(1):61-72.
91. Kligerman SJ, Franks TJ, Galvin JR. Primary Extranodal Lymphoma of the Thorax. Radiol Clin North Am. 2016;54(4):673-87.
92. Kurtin PJ, Myers JL, Adlakha H, Strickler JG, Lohse C, Pankratz VS, et al. Pathologic and clinical features of primary pulmonary extranodal marginal zone B-cell lymphoma of MALT type. Am J Surg Pathol. 2001;25(8):997-1008.
93. Huang H, Lu ZW, Jiang CG, Li J, Xu K, Xu ZJ. Clinical and prognostic characteristics of pulmonary mucosa-associated lymphoid tissue lymphoma: a retrospective analysis of 23 cases in a Chinese population. Chin Med J (Engl). 2011;124(7):1026-30.
94. Ahmed S, Kussick SJ, Siddiqui AK, Bhuiya TA, Khan A, Sarewitz S, et al. Bronchial-associated lymphoid tissue lymphoma: a clinical study of a rare disease. Eur J Cancer. 2004;40(9):1320-6.
95. Lee KS, Kim Y, Primack SL. Imaging of pulmonary lymphomas. AJR Am J Roentgenol. 1997;168(2):339-45.
96. Mentzer SJ, Reilly JJ, Skarin AT, Sugarbaker DJ. Patterns of lung involvement by malignant lymphoma. Surgery. 1993;113(5):507-14.
97. Blunt DM, Padley SP. Radiographic manifestations of AIDS related lymphoma in the thorax. Clin Radiol. 1995;50(9):607-12.
98. Hamilton-Dutoit SJ, Pallesen G, Franzmann MB, Karkov J, Black F, Skinhøj P, et al. AIDS-related lymphoma. Histopathology, immunophenotype, and association with Epstein-Barr virus as demonstrated by in situ nucleic acid hybridization. Am J Pathol. 1991;138(1):149-63.
99. Bazot M, Cadranel J, Benayoun S, Tassart M, Bigot JM, Carette MF. Primary pulmonary AIDS-related lymphoma: radiographic and CT findings. Chest. 1999;116(5):1282-6.

100. Bates WD, Gray DW, Dada MA, Chetty R, Gatter KC, Davies DR, et al. Lymphoproliferative disorders in Oxford renal transplant recipients. J Clin Pathol. 2003;56(6):439-46.
101. Carignan S, Staples CA, Müller NL. Intrathoracic lymphoproliferative disorders in the immunocompromised patient: CT findings. Radiology. 1995;197(1):53-8.
102. Tang VK, Vijhani P, Cherian SV, Ambelil M, Estrada YMRM. Primary pulmonary lymphoproliferative neoplasms. Lung India. 2018;35(3):220-30.
103. Yoon GY, Kim MY, Huh JR, Jo KW, Shim TS. Posttransplant Lymphoproliferative Disorder of the Thorax: CT and FDG-PET Features in a Single Tertiary Referral Center. Medicine (Baltimore). 2015;94(31):e1274.
104. Rekhtman N. Neuroendocrine tumors of the lung: an update. Arch Pathol Lab Med. 2010;134(11):1628-38.
105. Travis WD. Advances in neuroendocrine lung tumors. Ann Oncol. 2010;21(Suppl 7):vii65-71.
106. Pinchot SN, Holen K, Sippel RS, Chen H. Carcinoid tumors. Oncologist. 2008;13(12):1255-69.
107. Gustafsson BI, Kidd M, Chan A, Malfertheiner MV, Modlin IM. Bronchopulmonary neuroendocrine tumors. Cancer. 2008;113(1):5-21.
108. Jeung MY, Gasser B, Gangi A, Charneau D, Ducroq X, Kessler R, et al. Bronchial carcinoid tumors of the thorax: spectrum of radiologic findings. Radiographics. 2002;22(2):351-65.
109. Fox DJ, Khattar RS. Carcinoid heart disease: presentation, diagnosis, and management. Heart. 2004;90(10):1224-8.
110. Chong S, Lee KS, Chung MJ, Han J, Kwon OJ, Kim TS. Neuroendocrine tumors of the lung: clinical, pathologic, and imaging findings. Radiographics. 2006;26(1):41-57; discussion-8.
111. Soga J, Yakuwa Y. Bronchopulmonary carcinoids: An analysis of 1,875 reported cases with special reference to a comparison between typical carcinoids and atypical varieties. Ann Thorac Cardiovasc Surg. 1999;5(4):211-9.
112. Rosado de Christenson ML, Abbott GF, Kirejczyk WM, Galvin JR, Travis WD. Thoracic carcinoids: radiologic-pathologic correlation. Radiographics. 1999;19(3):707-36.
113. Caplin ME, Baudin E, Ferolla P, Filosso P, Garcia-Yuste M, Lim E, et al. Pulmonary neuroendocrine (carcinoid) tumors: European Neuroendocrine Tumor Society expert consensus and recommendations for best practice for typical and atypical pulmonary carcinoids. Ann Oncol. 2015;26(8):1604-20.
114. Detterbeck FC. Management of carcinoid tumors. Ann Thorac Surg. 2010;89(3):998-1005.
115. Jung KJ, Lee KS, Han J, Kwon OJ, Kim J, Shim YM, et al. Large cell neuroendocrine carcinoma of the lung: clinical, CT, and pathologic findings in 11 patients. J Thorac Imaging. 2001;16(3):156-62.
116. Oshiro Y, Kusumoto M, Matsuno Y, Asamura H, Tsuchiya R, Terasaki H, et al. CT findings of surgically resected large cell neuroendocrine carcinoma of the lung in 38 patients. AJR Am J Roentgenol. 2004;182(1):87-91.
117. Rudin CM, Brambilla E, Faivre-Finn C, Sage J. Small-cell lung cancer. Nat Rev Dis Primers. 2021;7(1):3.
118. Kalemkerian GP. Staging and imaging of small cell lung cancer. Cancer Imaging. 2012;11(1):253-8.
119. Benson RE, Rosado-de-Christenson ML, Martínez-Jiménez S, Kunin JR, Pettavel PP. Spectrum of pulmonary neuroendocrine proliferations and neoplasms. Radiographics. 2013;33(6):1631-49.
120. Shroff GS, Benveniste MF, Carter BW, de Groot PM, Wu CC, Viswanathan C, et al. Imaging of Metastases in the Chest: Mechanisms of Spread and Potential Pitfalls. Semin Ultrasound CT MR. 2017;38(6):594-603.
121. Seo JB, Im JG, Goo JM, Chung MJ, Kim MY. Atypical pulmonary metastases: spectrum of radiologic findings. Radiographics. 2001;21(2):403-17.
122. Gleeson T, Thiessen R, Hannigan A, Murphy D, English JC, Mayo JR. Pulmonary hamartomas: CT pixel analysis for fat attenuation using radiologic-pathologic correlation. J Med Imaging Radiat Oncol. 2013;57(5):534-43.
123. Siegelman SS, Khouri NF, Scott WW, Jr., Leo FP, Hamper UM, Fishman EK, et al. Pulmonary hamartoma: CT findings. Radiology. 1986;160(2):313-7.

Ashu Seith Bhalla, Smita Manchanda

CHAPTER

14

Imaging of the Large Airways

INTRODUCTION

Airway is divided into the upper airway (above the thoracic inlet) and the lower airway (below the thoracic inlet). The lower airway is further divided into the large and small airways. This chapter focuses on the large airways.

Large airways is a term used for airways which are more than 2 mm in diameter. This includes:

- *Central airway*: Trachea and main bronchi
- *Peripheral airway*: Lobar, segmental, and proximal subsegmental bronchi

Small airways refer to the distal airways, which are small in size (< 2 mm in diameter) and lack cartilage and submucosal glands.

ROLE OF IMAGING

Imaging plays a key role in diagnosis and planning management. The main role of imaging **(Box 1)** is to detect and localize the lesion (with respect to carina), delineate the exact length of the lesion (for stent placement as a therapeutic option), measure the degree of airway narrowing, and lastly to give a specific diagnosis, if possible.

BOX 1: Role of imaging in evaluation of the tracheobronchial tree.

- Detection
- Localization – proximal and distal extent
- *Etiology*: Extrinsic or intrinsic (mural or intraluminal)
- Length for abnormal segment
- Diffuse/focal
- *Obstruction*: Fixed or dynamic
- Degree of narrowing
- Specific diagnosis if possible

The current role of the various imaging modalities is detailed below.

IMAGING MODALITIES

Chest Radiograph

Plain frontal and lateral chest radiographs are useful in acute obstructions such as foreign body and aspiration. These may occasionally demonstrate large masses involving the central airways. Areas of severe narrowing may also be appreciated. The effects of airway disease on the lung, i.e., consolidation, atelectasis or hyperinflation is well seen on plain films. Signs of bronchiectasis are also well described on plain radiographs **(Fig. 1)**. However, largely radiographs are unable to provide enough information for diagnosis or preoperative planning of patients **(Box 2)**.

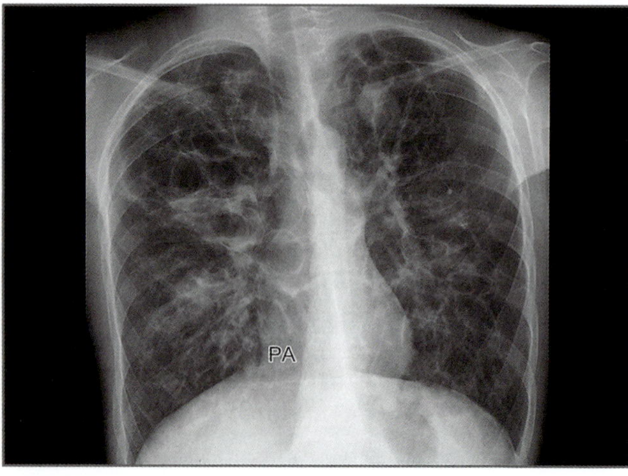

FIG. 1: Plain radiograph showing cystic lucencies and tram track linear opacities in bilateral lung fields in a case of cystic fibrosis.

Digital Tomosynthesis and Dual-energy Chest X-ray

Digital tomosynthesis (DTS) is a new technique using digital radiography and flat-panel detectors, which is based on the principle of geometric tomography.[1] DTS images represent sections through the anatomy that are generated and reconstructed from a set of projection radiographs. Because it removes overlapping clutter, there is improved visualization of thoracic abnormalities compared to radiography and better coronal plane resolution **(Fig. 2)**. The radiation dose to patients is less than that of chest CT.[2] The demonstration of the central airways is considered to be superior or equivalent compared with radiography.[1] In terms of airway evaluation this technique is useful in suspected cases of foreign body.

Dual-energy subtraction chest radiography is an imaging technique which is based on the principle that calcium selectively attenuates lower energy photons in an X-ray beam. This produces two separate images; of the soft tissues of the thorax and of the bones and has predominantly used for nodule imaging. However, it has also been described for the assessment of airway narrowing due to masses or lymphadenopathy and post intubation or subglottic stenosis.[3]

BOX 2: Systematic evaluation on chest radiograph.

- Tracheal caliber
- Mediastinal widening
- Asymmetric lung aeration
- Lung collapse/consolidation
- Length of tracheal narrowing
- Radio-opaque foreign body
- Cardiac size
- Position of the aortic arch

Computed Tomography

Computed temography (CT) is the investigation of choice for initial evaluation of suspected tracheobronchial tree pathology and for follow-up of these cases.[4] In the current generation of scanners, there is volumetric CT acquisition in a single breath hold and precise delineation of the entire tracheobronchial tree, including the distal airways can be done.[5]

Acquisition

Scans are routinely performed in deep inspiration in supine position. In a single breath hold of 3–4 seconds, the entire chest can be scanned without respiratory motion artifacts. Cardiac gating is not recommended and is not usually done.[4,6]

Expiratory scanning is essential for assessing dynamic component and air trapping. Although visualization of airways per se does not require contrast administration, IV contrast may prove helpful in some conditions, e.g., differentiating a central mass from atelectatic lung.

CT acquisition technique has been summarized in **Box 3**. Until recently axial imaging by CT scan was the accepted standard modality for diagnostic work up for suspected airway pathology. However, CT has significantly enhanced the imaging of airways. The numerous reconstruction techniques have virtually revolutionized the way that CT images are viewed and interpreted.[5,7]

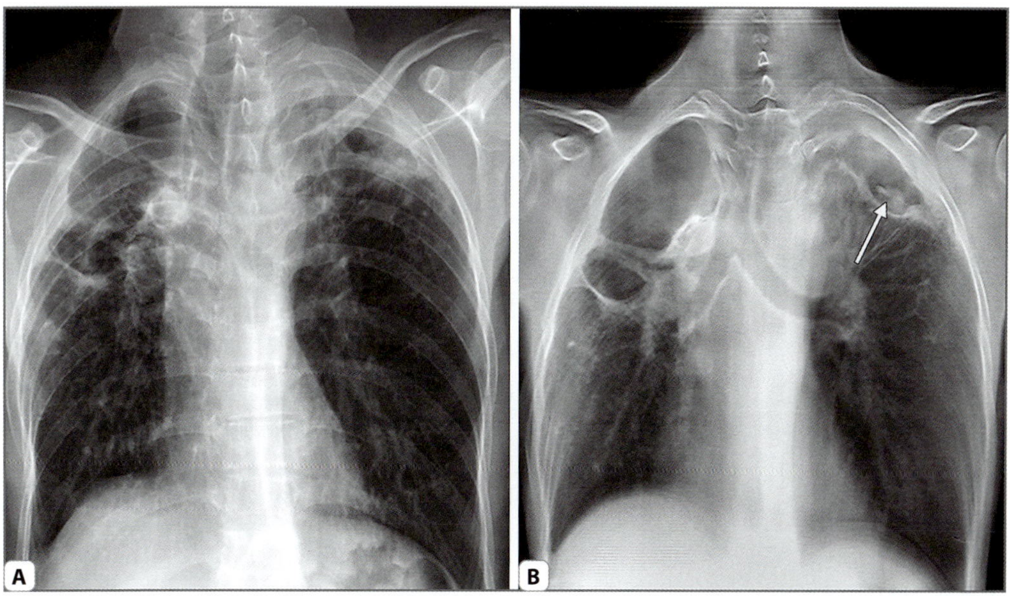

FIGS. 2A AND B: Digital tomosynthesis. Plain radiograph (A) reveals fibrocavitary lesions in bilateral upper lobes with suspicious fungal ball in left upper lobe cavity. DTS image (B) better depicts the central airways and fungal ball (arrow) as it removes overlapping clutter.

BOX 3: CT acquisition technique.[7,8]

- Tube potential and tube current appropriate to patient size
- Use of tube current modulation
- *Scan area*: From the lung apices to the costophrenic sulci
- *Position*:
  - At isocenter to minimize radiation dose and optimize image quality
  - Supine
  - Prone (in specific cases)
- *Phase*:
  - Deep inspiration
  - Paired inspiratory and expiratory: For dynamic assessment of central airways, air trapping
  - Expiratory (end expiration):
    - Obtained throughout the lung fields or at selected 3–5 levels
    - Low dose (30–40 mAs)
- Thin overlapping 0.5–1 mm sections acquired
- *Field of view*:
  - Scan FOV: appropriate to patient size at time of image
  - Reconstructed FOV: limited to the lungs with optimal spatial resolution for each patient (Lung window)
- Data sets:
  - 5 mm width every 5 mm reconstruction interval at lung and mediastinal window settings
  - 1 mm width at 10 mm interval high resolution scans
  - Thin reconstruction at 1–1.5 mm slice thickness
- Retention of the radiation dose report in the radiological record

Source: Adapted from Bankier AA, et al. (2008)[6] & Beigelman AC, et al. (2009)[7]

Of great concern is the potential of added risk resulting from increased radiation exposure especially when paired inspiratory-expiratory CT is performed. Cine imaging also has the potential for high radiation exposure.

The problem of additional radiation exposure can be reduced by routinely using reduced milliamperage whenever, feasible. This is especially true in young patients and those likely to require multiple follow-ups.

Diagnostic images of acceptable quality can be obtained with 80–100 mAs, and use as low as 40 mAs has been reported in thin patients. For the expiratory scans, a low-dose (30–40 mAs) technique should be used. Radiation exposure can be reduced further by using dose modulation techniques.

Acquisition for Dynamic Evaluation of the Airway

There are various techniques described for the evaluation of suspected tracheobronchomalacia/excessive dynamic airway collapse (EDAC); using either expiratory scans or coughing maneuvers.[9] These include:

- Paired end-inspiratory and end-expiratory MDCT: scans at end inspiration and incremental scans at end expiration.
- Paired end-inspiratory and dynamic expiratory MDCT: scans at end inspiration and during expiration.
- Cine MDCT combined with a coughing maneuver: scans beginning at end inspiration which is followed by coughing movements.

Image Reconstruction

The various techniques available in MDCT scanners include multiplanar reconstructions (MPRs), maximum intensity projections (MIPs), minimum intensity projections

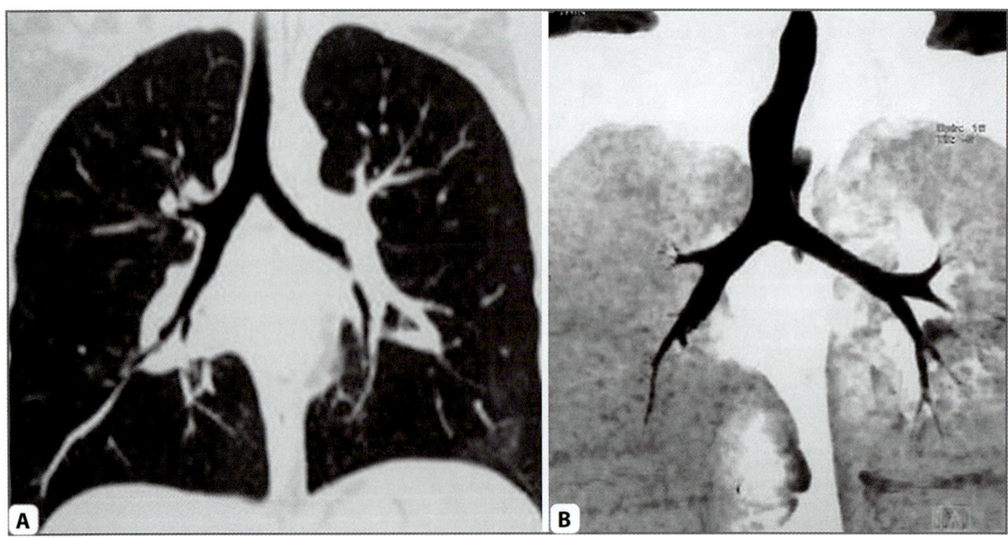

FIGS. 3A AND B: Coronal MPR (A) and coronal minIP (B) showing trachea, main bronchi and lobar bronchi.

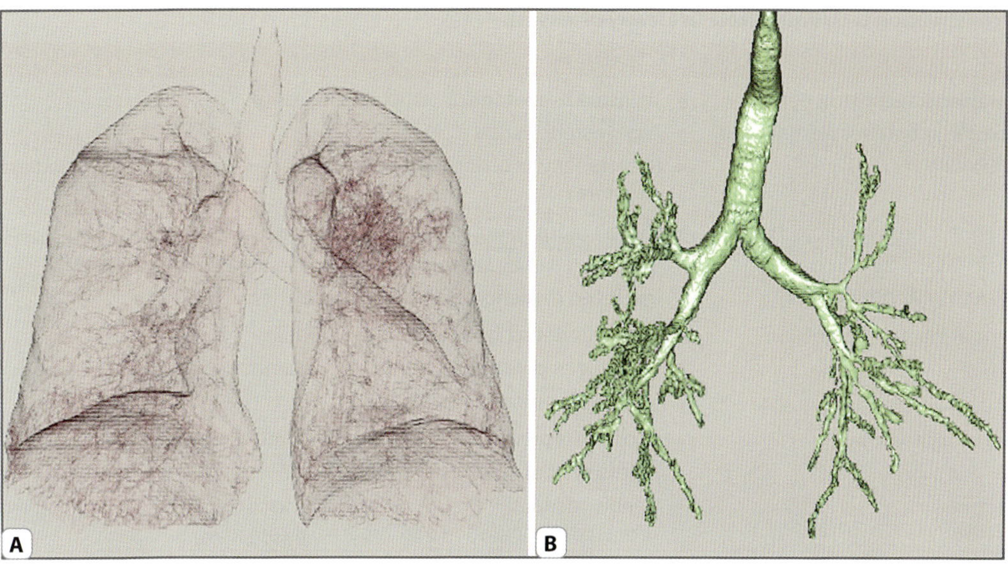

FIGS. 4A AND B: VRT Images. Volume rendered images of the lungs and airways (A) . The entire tracheobronchial tree is displayed in a volume rendered image in B.

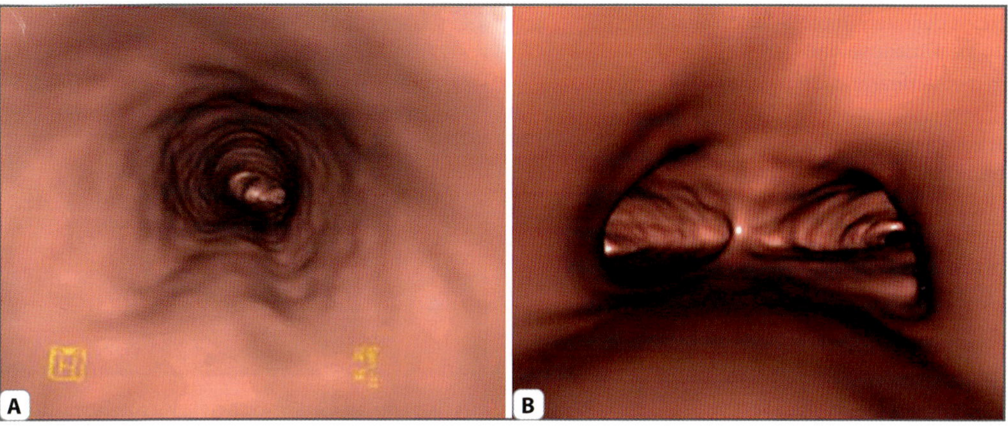

FIGS. 5A AND B: Virtual bronchoscopy images showing endoluminal view of normal trachea (A) and carina (B).

(minIPs) **(Fig. 3)**, volume rendered techniques **(Fig. 4)**, and internal rendering or virtual bronchoscopy (VB)[7,10-12] **(Fig. 5)** and the role of numerous reconstruction techniques is described in **Table 1**.

Quantitative CT Assessment of Airways

The lumen and area of airways can be measured quantitatively on CT images. With the use of MDCT scanners oblique reconstructions can be made in the axis and perpendicular to the axis of the airway.[13] In the current scanners, qualitative and semiquantitative assessment of emphysema and the emphysema subtypes, quantitative evaluation of emphysema using bronchial wall thickness, density histograms, and pulmonary vasculature can be done on the inspiratory scans. The expiratory scans allow image matching and the analysis of functional small airway disease using parametric response mapping.[14]

It is believed that in COPD, the innate variability of the tracheobronchial tree might be associated with the susceptibility to pathological involvement of conducting airways and hence the resultant airflow obstruction.[14]

Smooth muscle hypertrophy, mucous gland expansion, and airway wall fibrosis lead to slow airway wall thickening and luminal narrowing of lumen also known as the process of airway remodeling. The quantitative metrics used to measure airway size include direct measurement of the airway wall thickness and the airway wall area percent [WA% = (total area of airway - area of airway lumen)/total area of airway × 100].[15,16] The Pi10 and Pi15 (square roots of wall areas of theoretical airways with internal perimeters of 10 and 15 mm, respectively) provide the summary measures of airway size. With worsening disease and increase in airflow obstruction, there is a significant increase in WA%.

TABLE 1: CT reconstruction techniques (role in airway diseases).

Name	Technique	Role
MPR	• Multiplanar reconstruction • Evaluate in both mediastinal and lung window	• To visualize anatomical structures in reality • Airway stenosis • Resectability of bronchogenic carcinoma as well as hilar and mediastinal structures
minIP	• Minimum intensity projection • Thick slabs of 25–35 cm used to demonstrate entire TB tree	• Overall morphology of the tracheobronchial tree • Detecting airway stenosis (overestimates degree of narrowing) • Improved depiction of ground-glass pattern
MIP	Maximum intensity projection	• Improves detection of pulmonary nodules • Bronchiolar diseases, especially for patients with so-called tree-in-bud opacities • Size and location of vessels
VB	Virtual bronchoscopy	• Accurate reproduction of major endoluminal abnormalities • Assessment of airway stenoses • Unable to identify the causes of bronchial obstruction or detect mild stenosis, submucosal infiltration and superficial spreading tumors

BOX 4: Role of CT in evaluation of airway pathology.

- Workhorse of airway imaging
- Reconstructions definitely improve lesion evaluation compared to axial images alone
- MPR in both mediastinal and lung windows—length of stenosis
- VB does not have a distinct diagnostic utility, useful where fibreoptic bronchoscopy is not available or not feasible
- minIP, volume rendered images useful in overall depiction of airway anatomy
- Excellent for congenital anomalies
- Limitations of CT
  - Lesions < 2–3 mm not detected
  - Difficult to differentiate between mucosal and submucosal lesions

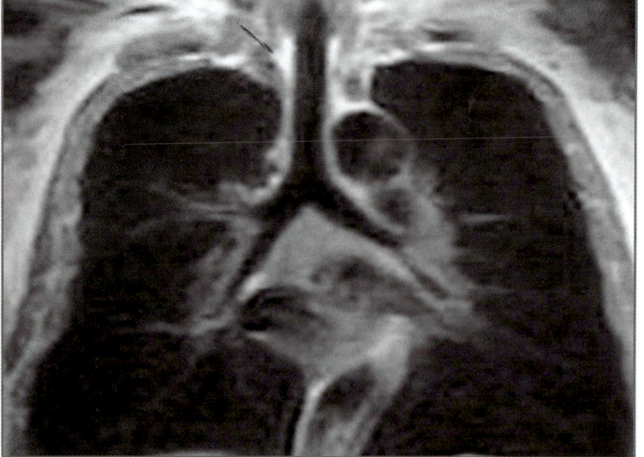

FIG. 6: MRI showing normal airway on T1-weighted sequence coronal image.

Box 4 summarizes the current role of CT in evaluation of airway pathology.

Endoscopic Ultrasound

Over the past decade, there has been a growing interest in the use of endoscopic ultrasound (EBUS) to diagnose to the central and peripheral lesions of tracheobronchial tree. EBUS has the unique capability to differentiate various layers of the bronchial wall.[17] Also pathologic changes both in and adjacent to airways can be assessed. Vessels can be readily identified and differentiated from lymph nodes. It has hence found a significant role in guided transbronchial needle aspiration (TBNA) of mediastinal nodes currently, the major limitation of EBUS guided TBNA is its high cost, and the need for special configuration of endoscopic probes to provide consistent positioning adjacent to bronchial walls.[4]

Magnetic Resonance Imaging

Magnetic resonance imaging (MRI) provides adequate visualization of the tracheobronchial tree upto lobar bronchi.[18] This is best seen on the coronal T1 TSE (turbo spin echo sequence) **(Fig. 6)**. Mediastinal and hilar masses are also well evaluated on MRI with the superior depiction of vascular or cardiac invasion. MRI has also been used to demonstrate air trapping. There is an increasing use in those requiring repeated imaging such as cystic fibrosis and ABPA. The presence of mucus with high T1 SI and low T2 SI has been found to be highly specific for the diagnosis of ABPA in cystic fibrosis **(Box 5)**.[19]

There are numerous studies using MRI for air trapping in COPD patients. Dynamic, time resolved MRI can be used to visualize the expiratory airway collapse (up-to the lobar level) and the expiratory scans can be used to evaluate small airway obstruction.

MRI using hyperpolarized noble gases (^{129}Xe, ^{3}He) is used to directly show the large airways along with the peripheral lung ventilation. Indirect airway dysfunction can be demonstrated as perfusion deficits due to the hypoxic vasoconstriction of dependent lung volumes on dynamic contrast-enhanced MRI.[20]

Ultrashort echo-time (UTE) MRI uses a radial k-space acquisition technique which is more resistant to motion artifacts and provides higher quality sharper images with fewer artefacts. UTE MRI has also been described to evaluate the airway dynamics quantitatively.

NORMAL AIRWAY ANATOMY

The trachea is a cartilaginous and fibromuscular tube extending from the inferior aspect of cricoid cartilage to the carina, measuring 10–12 cm in length. It is divided into intra and extrathoracic parts. It contains 16–22 cartilaginous rings, which are incomplete posteriorly. The posterior portion of the tracheal wall, lying between the open ends of the tracheal cartilages, is a thin fibromuscular membrane termed posterior tracheal membrane.[21]

BOX 5: Suggested MRI protocol for central airway evaluation.

- T1-weighted gradient sequence
  - With fat supression (pre and post contrast): Axial
  - Without fat supression: Axial, coronal
- T2-weighted fast spin echo sequence
  - With fat supression: Axial
  - Without fat supression: Axial
- T2-weighted sequence HASTE: Coronal
- Diffusion weighted sequence: Axial (b values of 0, 400, 800) (in cases of masses)

There is marked variability in the cross-sectional appearance of the trachea, which may appear rounded or oval (most common) or horseshoe shaped trachea with flat posterior tracheal membrane (in about 25% of normal individuals).[21] Tracheal diameter can vary widely in anatomically normal persons. In men, tracheal diameter ranges from 13 to 25 mm (mean 19.5 mm) and in females it is slightly less, ranging from 10 to 21 mm in the coronal plane (average 17.5 mm). In children's variations in tracheal diameter at different levels can be as much as 20%. During forced expiration, there is invagination of the posterior tracheal membrane, and the lumen becomes horseshoe shaped.

There is dichotomous branching with approximately 23 generations of branches from trachea to alveoli.

ANATOMIC VARIANTS

In adults, the most commonly encountered anomalies are either anomalous or supernumerary bronchi.[4] Other anomalies include agenesis, congenital bronchial atresia, bronchogenic cysts or even congenital lobar obstruction. A clinically useful modified classification has been proposed by Wu et al.[22] for these anomalies.

1. *Anomalies arising from normal higher order bronchial divisions*: These include accessory superior segmental bronchi and axillary bronchi supplying lateral aspect of right upper lobe.
2. *Anomalies arising from sites typically lacking branches:* This group refers to tracheal bronchi, accessory cardiac bronchi and bridging bronchi.

   The commonest amongst these is the "tracheal or pig bronchus", seen in upto 1–2% of normal individuals.[23] Tracheal bronchus arises on the right side exclusively, and on endoscopy may be confused with tracheal diverticula or tracheoceles. CT readily identifies these **(Fig. 7)**.

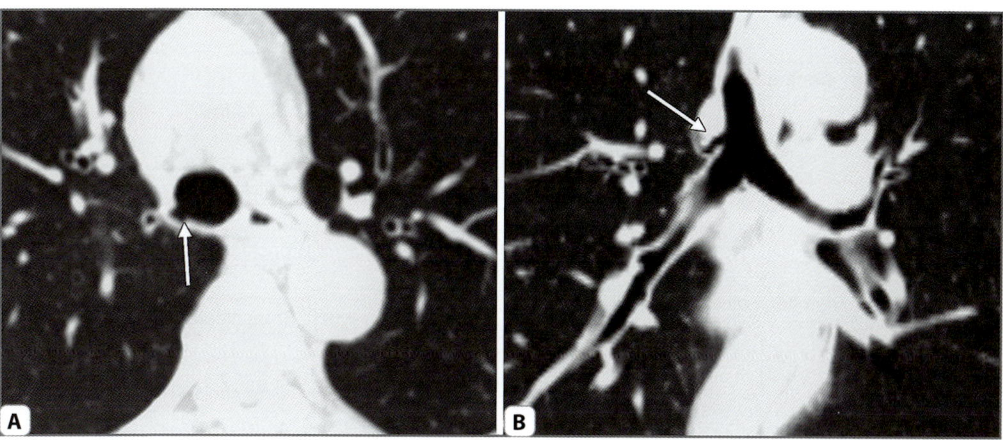

FIGS. 7A AND B: Tracheal bronchus. Axial (A) and coronal MPR (B) in lung window show the right upper lobe bronchus (arrow) arising directly from the trachea.

The "cardiac bronchus" usually arises from the bronchus intermedius, the origin being opposite and distal to origin of upper lobe bronchus **(Fig. 8)**. It is variable in size and in many cases is a blind ending stump, which does not aerate any lung parenchyma.

3. *Anomalies associated with abnormalities of situs.* In this category, reversal of the right and left sided airways is the most commonly encountered form. Less frequent anomalies include bronchial isomerism, in which pattern of airway branching and pulmonary location is identical in both the lungs.

TRACHEOBRONCHIAL TREE PATHOLOGIES

Pathologies affecting the tracheobronchial tree can be broadly considered in three categories—those affecting the central airways, the peripheral airways and others involving the small airways. The levels of lower airway pathologies are described in **Flowchart 1**. Central airways and peripheral airway pathologies are described in the subsequent sections.

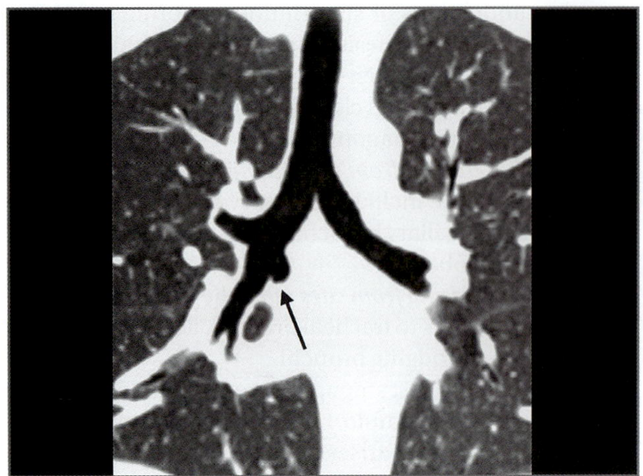

FIG. 8: Cardiac bronchus. Blind ending bronchial stump (arrow) arising medially from the bronchus intermedius.

Central Airways

Central airway obstruction can occur because of extrinsic or intrinsic causes (which are further divided into mural and intraluminal causes). These are detailed in **Table 2**.

Extrinsic

A diverse variety of mediastinal masses or mass like lesions can cause extrinsic compression of the airways. These have been described in detail elsewhere.

Intrinsic Mural

Congenital

Tracheobronchomalacia

Tracheobronchomalacia (TBM) is characterized by weakness of the tracheobronchial walls and/or supporting cartilage. This results in a dynamic obstruction of the airway because of excessive collapse during expiration.[9,24] CT diagnosis **(Fig. 10)** can only be made in paired scans (end inspiration and expiratory scan/during coughing) as described above in CT acquisition. It may be congenital or acquired due to prior intubation, trauma, prolonged extrinsic compression **(Fig. 11)**, infection or chronic inflammation.[25] It is discussed in detail under the section of Expiratory central airway collapse (ECAC) below.

Tracheal stenosis

Congenital subglottic or tracheal stenosis occurs because of incomplete recanalization of the laryngotracheal tube. The various types of congenital tracheal stenosis include hypoplasia, funnel-shaped and segmental stenosis.[26]

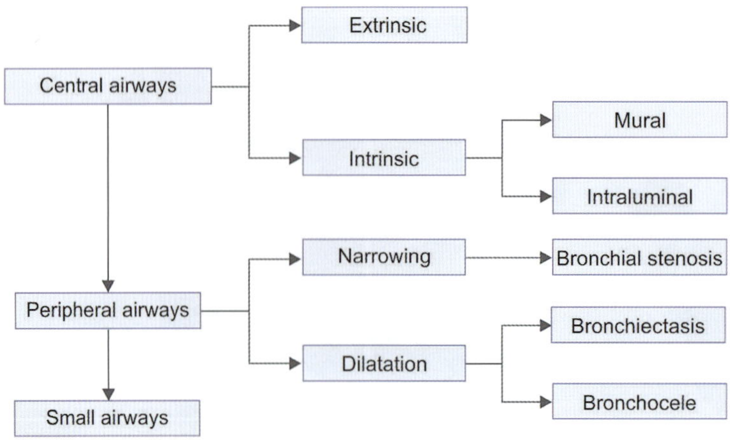

FLOWCHART 1: Levels of lower airway pathologies.

TABLE 2: Etiology of central airway obstruction.

Etiology	Extrinsic	Intrinsic	
		Mural	Intraluminal
Congenital	• Vascular compression • Bronchopulmonary foregut malformations • Thoracic deformity • Vascular malformations	• Tracheobronchomalacia • Tracheal stenosis	
Inflammatory/ Infective	• Lymph nodes **(Fig. 9)** • Mediastinal abscess/cellulitis • Fibrosing mediastinitis	• Tuberculosis/fibrotic stricture • Vasculitis • Relapsing polychondritis • Post-intubation stricture • Sarcoidosis • IgG4-related disease	• Granulation tissue • Broncholithiasis
Masses	• Lymphoma • Germ cell tumor • Vascular malformations		• Malignant tumors • Benign tumors
Miscellaneous		• Expiratory central airway collapse (ECAC)/ tracheomalacia • Tracheopathia osteochondroplastica • Amyloidosis	• Mucus plugs • Foreign body • Clots

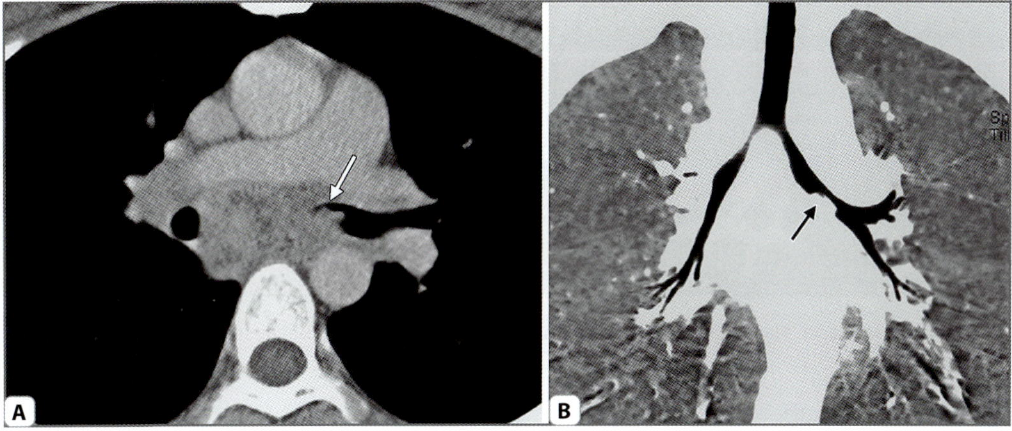

FIGS. 9A AND B: Extrinsic involvement by TB lymph nodes. Axial CT (A) and min-IP (B) show necrotic subcarinal nodes extending into the left main bronchus (arrow).

Inflammatory/Infective

Infections/fibrotic stricture

Inflammatory tracheal stenosis due to tuberculosis: Tubercular stenosis **(Fig. 12)** is an endo-bronchial complication of pulmonary tuberculosis that can develop acutely at the time of infection or can become manifest years later. Endobronchial tuberculosis has been reported in 10–37% of patients with pulmonary parenchymal tuberculosis.[27] Tuberculosis typically involves the distal trachea and proximal main stem bronchi **(Fig. 13)**; isolated tracheal disease is rare.[28] Granulation tissue formation and subsequent fibrosis involving the airway causes luminal narrowing. Unlike active tuberculosis, which involves both mainstem bronchi equally, fibrotic TB usually involves the left main bronchus, perhaps because of its greater length. Evidence of associated mediastinal inflammation, in the form of enlarged mediastinal nodes or increased attenuation of mediastinal fat, may also be identified. CT findings are seldom specific. Findings that help differentiate tuberculosis from bronchogenic carcinoma include longer circumferential involvement and the absence of an intraluminal mass.[29] Focal infection may be responsible for tumor-like lesions when it produces granulation or endoluminal masses.

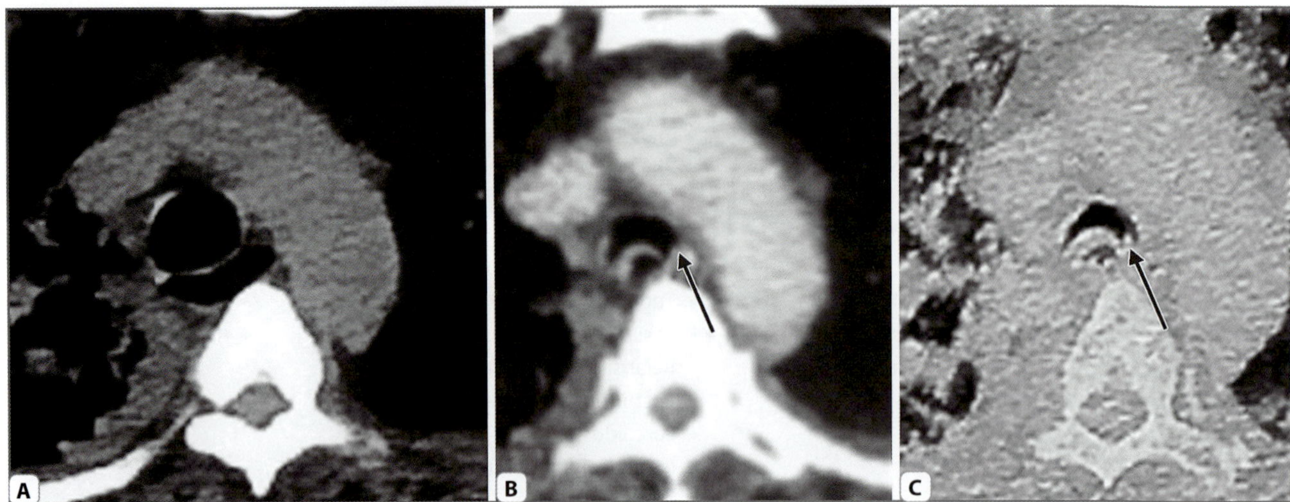

FIGS. 10A TO C: Tracheomalacia. Axial end inspiration CT (A) shows normal appearance of trachea with collapse of the lumen during expiration with abnormal flattened anterior tracheal cartilage and exaggerated bowing of the posterior membrane (component of EDAC) (arrow in B and C).

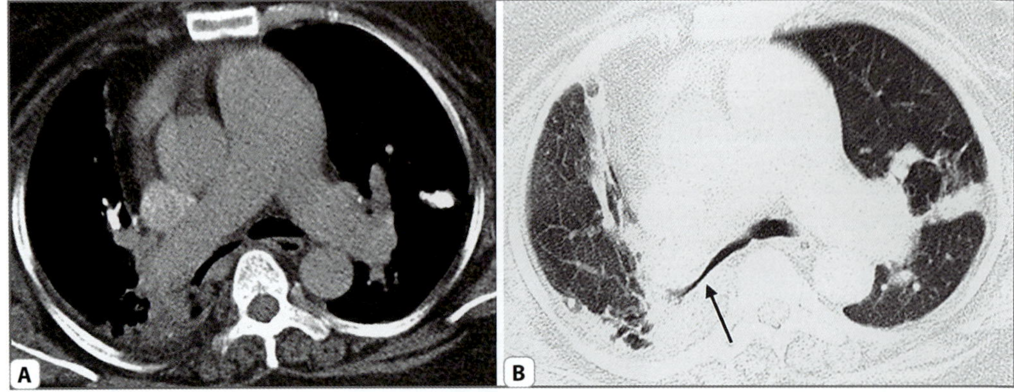

FIGS. 11A AND B: Bronchomalacia. Narrowing of the bronchus intermedius (arrow) because of chronic compression by enlarged pulmonary artery.

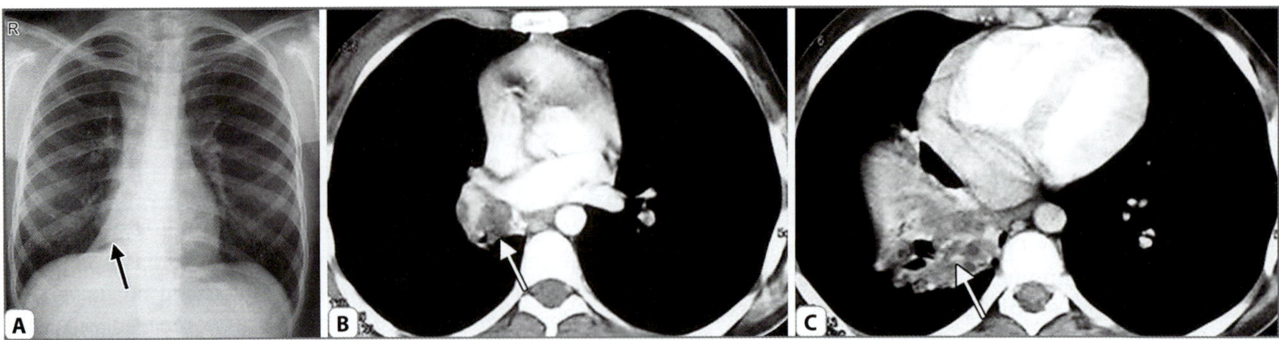

FIGS. 12A TO E: *Continued*

Continued

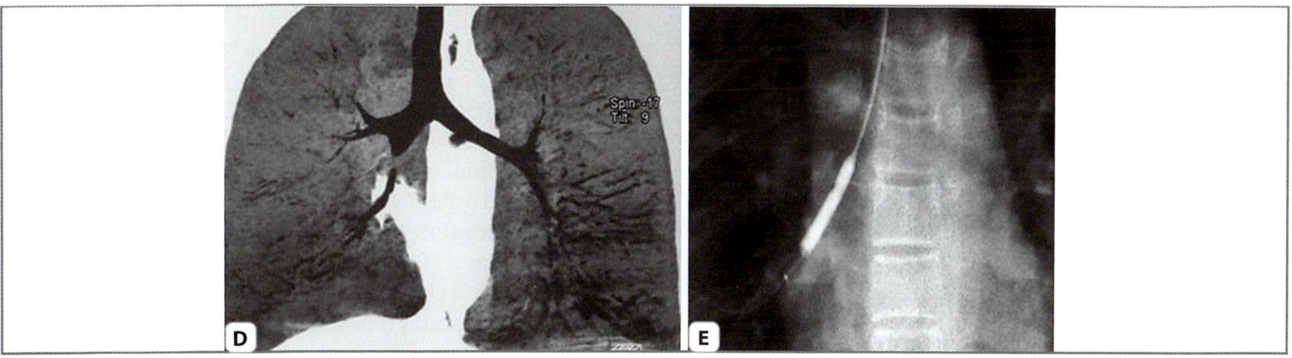

FIGS. 12A TO E: Tubercular stricture. Chest radiograph (A) of a 19-year-old girl showing collapse of right lower lobe (black arrow). Axial CT (B, C) and coronal min-IP (D) demonstrates necrotic right hilar nodes (white arrows) narrowing the bronchus intermedius and lower lobe bronchus (black arrow). (E) balloon dilatation of the stricture was performed.

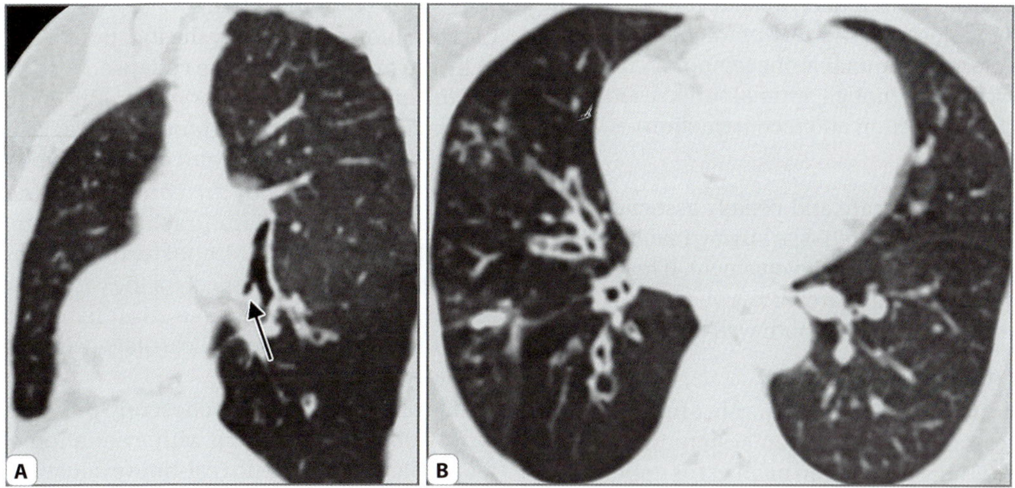

FIGS. 13A AND B: Post tubercular bronchostenosis. Sagittal MPR (A) and axial CT (B) show narrowing of right middle lobe bronchus (arrow) with bronchiectatic changes in middle and lower lobes.

Fungal infections (aspergillosis): Airway disease caused by aspergillus takes many forms, including saprophytic colonization, tracheobronchitis, ulcerative tracheobronchitis with or without pseudomembrane formation, and necrotizing (invasive) aspergillosis,[30] the latter being further divided into acute and chronic airway invasive forms. Multifocal or diffuse tracheobronchial wall thickening, causing luminal narrowing is seen on CT.

Rhinoscleroma: Rhinoscleroma is an insidious infectious granulomatous disease caused by Klebsiella rhinoscleromatis.[31] The involvement is characteristically of the upper respiratory tract; trachea and proximal bronchi may occasionally be involved. CT findings include diffuse nodular tracheobronchial wall thickening, causing luminal narrowing with mediastinal or hilar lymphadenopathy.[32]

Vasculitis

Granulomatous polyangiitis: Airway involvement in granulomatous polyangiitis (GPA) includes bronchial stenosis, inflammation and pseudotumors.[33] Often, no correlation is seen between c-ANCA levels and the presence of tracheobronchial inflammation.

Relapsing polychondritis

Relapsing polychondritis is a multisystem disease of unknown etiology characterized by recurrent inflammation of cartilage of nose, external ear, peripheral joints, larynx, trachea and bronchi.[34] It is commonly seen in the 3rd and 6th decades with initial involvement of larynx and subglottic trachea. Distal trachea and bronchi may be involved as the disease progresses. An acute inflammatory infiltrate in the cartilage and perichondrial tissue is seen on pathology.

CT findings include increased airway wall attenuation in association with smooth tracheal or bronchial wall thickening. The increased attenuation may appear as frank calcification in later stages. There is characteristic sparing of the posterior membranous portion of the trachea.[35]

Post-intubation stenosis

Among acquired strictures, the most common cause is injury resulting from intubation. Although investigators have estimated that complications occur in upto 10–15% of patients after intubation and upto 40% patients with tracheostomies, the incidence of serious complications after intubation has decreased dramatically since the introduction of high-volume/low-pressure tubes.[36] The two principal sites for post-intubation stenoses are at the stoma or at the level of the endotracheal tube or tracheostomy tube balloon. Strictures result from pressure necrosis, which causes ischemia and subsequent scarring **(Fig. 14)**. Other complications of intubation include tracheal rupture and tracheo-brachiocephalic artery or tracheoesophageal fistulas. Stent placement remains one temporary option for treating such strictures, though optimal surgical technique is laryngotracheal resection and reconstruction.

Sarcoidosis

Tracheal involvement is rare and usually associated with laryngeal disease.[27] In sarcoidosis, airway involvement is usually in the form of bronchial involvement. It may be seen in upto 65% of patients with sarcoidosis on high resolution CT in the form of nodular or smooth wall thickening.[37]

IgG4-related disease

IgG4-related disease is a systemic fibroinflammatory disease and can involve any organ system in the body. Airway disease is unusual and can manifest as upper airway mass or diffuse tracheal thickening and tracheobronchial narrowing/stenosis. Bronchiectasis can occur due to fibrotic changes in the lung and resultant traction bronchiectasis.[38]

Miscellaneous

Expiratory central airway collapse

Expiratory central airway collapse (ECAC) is the exaggerated tracheobronchial narrowing during expiration. It includes both TBM and excessive dynamic airway collapse (EDAC).[39] The etiopathogenesis of the two entities is different with TBM occurring due to cartilaginous weakening, whereas EDAC is characterized by membranous malacia.[40] The tracheal cartilage is normal and there is excessive invagination of the lax posterior membrane into airway lumen during expiration in EDAC.

EDAC is usually associated with atrophy of smooth muscle fibers of the trachealis muscle in the membranous portion of the trachea.

Tracheobronchomalacia

Classification of TBM is by the location of the abnormality or by the morphology of the collapse.[39]

- *The location of the abnormality*: This includes tracheomalacia (only trachea), bronchomalacia (only bronchi), or TBM (both trachea and bronchi involved).
- *The morphology of the collapse*: This includes the crescent type (anterior tracheal cartilage, is abnormal with decreased anteroposterior dimension), saber-sheath type (lateral aspects of the cartilage are weakened with narrow transverse dimension) and (diffuse abnormality of tracheal cartilage with circumferential narrowing).

Flexible dynamic bronchoscopy provides an extent of airway abnormality along with evaluation of degree and morphology of TBM with real-time evaluation and is hence, the investigation of choice for TBM.

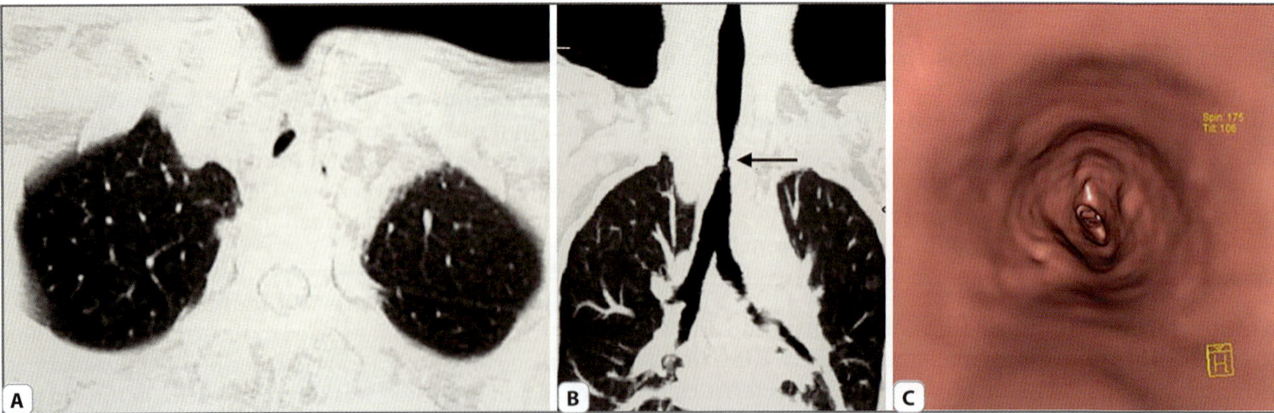

FIGS. 14A TO C: Post-intubation stenosis. Axial CT (A) coronal MPR (B) and VB (C) showing a tracheal stricture. Patient had a past history of prolonged intubation.

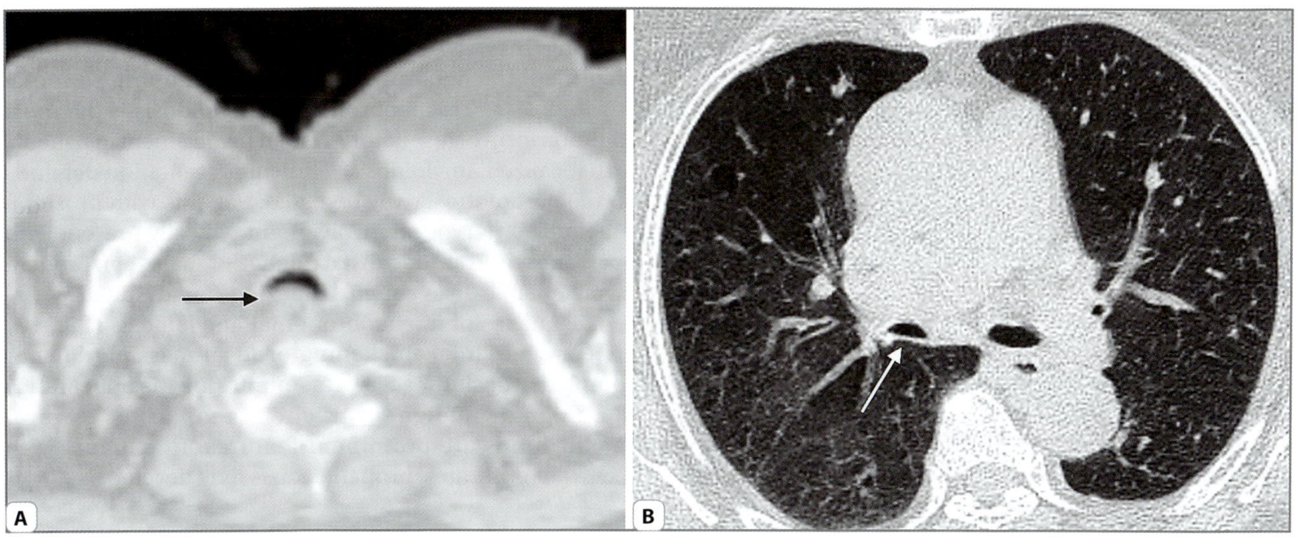

FIGS. 15A AND B: Excessive dynamic airway collapse (EDAC). Axial CT image in forceful exhalation showing excessive bowing of the posterior membrane with preserved integrity of the anterior cartilage of the trachea and right main bronchus.

Excessive dynamic airway collapse

EDAC is also known as membranous or posterior malacia. The tracheal cartilage has a normal configuration with excessive inner bulging of the posterior membrane **(Fig. 15)**. EDAC represents obstructed peripheral airways and is considered a marker of the severity of COPD or asthma rather than a distinct pathology.[39]

Etiology: There is an increase in transmural pressure gradient because of the low pressure in small airways in COPD patients and high pleural pressure in expiration. This increased gradient results in collapse of the large airways during expiration (central airways are downstream from the small airways during expiration). Since the posterior membrane is the weakest point this collapse causes the characteristic appearance of EDAC.

Role of imaging in EDAC

CT protocol: The central airways are imaged during two different phases of respiration which include the end inspiratory phase (suspended end inspiration) and the dynamic expiratory phase (imaging during forceful expiration and not end expiration as is routine for small airway disease). This has been detailed above under CT Acquisition.

Imaging interpretation: Dynamic CT helps in better assessment of the airways in ECAC and can also help surgeons and interventional pulmonologists to plan therapeutic interventions including 3D printed tracheal splints. The following parameters[39] can be evaluated:

- *Assessment of tracheal collapsibility*: The inner wall of the airway is traced using an electronic tracing tool/advanced workstation and cross-sectional area of the airway lumen is measured on end inspiratory and dynamic expiratory CT images. The percentage of the collapsibility of trachea is then measured using the equation:

$$LC = 100\,(1 - [LAe/LAi])$$

(where, LC is percentage of luminal collapse, LAe represents luminal area during dynamic expiration, and LAi represents luminal area at end inspiration).

These measurements are done at 1 cm above the aortic arch and 1 cm above the carina. In addition, the site of maximal narrowing should also be included. Grading of the severity of expiratory collapse is as follows: mild (70–80%), moderate (81–90%) and severe (>90%).[39]

- *Assessment of tracheal morphologic characteristics in TBM*: The tracheal index is the ratio of coronal to sagittal diameter of the trachea (normal ratio is approximately 1).[39] Routinely alteration of this tracheal index is evident on subjective evaluation, although the tracheal index can also be calculated. Due to weakness of the anterior cartilage, there is an increase in the tracheal index and a lunate shape of the trachea. Lateral cartilage malacia has a decrease in the tracheal index with a narrow transverse diameter and a resultant saber-sheath trachea.
- *Air trapping and ECAC*: In patients with ECAC, expiratory air trapping is commonly observed and is usually multifactorial. It is believed that small-airway diseases may predispose to EDAC because of the associated respiratory dynamics. However, ECAC could also lead to air trapping because of the impaired airway clearance which is a result of the associated chronic inflammation of small airways.

Tracheopathia osteoplastica

Tracheopathia osteoplastica is characterized by multiple small osteocartilaginous growths in the submucosa of the inner anterior and lateral walls of the trachea. It is usually seen in asymptomatic elderly males. On CT scan, multiple, small (1–5 mm sized) irregular nodules, which are occasionally calcified, can be seen protruding into the tracheal lumen**(Fig. 16)**.

Amyloidosis

Amyloidosis entails a number of entities characterized by deposition of an autologous fibrillar protein and associated protein derivatives in extracellular tissue. Amyloidosis can be either primary (frequently associated with multiple myeloma or Waldenstrom macroglobulinemia) or secondary (in the setting of chronic inflammatory diseases including TB, cystic fibrosis, bronchiectasis, etc.). Within the lung, three types of localized amyloidosis have been identified: tracheobronchial, nodular and diffuse septal amyloidosis.[41] Tracheobronchial amyloidosis is the most common form of respiratory system involvement in patients with localized amyloidosis. Clinical presentation depends on the part of the airway involved. Patients with proximal subglottic or laryngeal involvement typically present with hoarseness and stridor, distal trachea or mainstem bronchi involvement causes cough, wheezing, and dyspnea.

CT images of tracheobronchial amyloidosis **(Fig. 17)** appear as nodular thickening or focal mass partially or completely occluding airways, mimicking the appearance of benign or malignant tracheal neoplasms.[42] Mural calcifications are prominent features. In patients with recurrent infiltrates, bronchiectasis may develop.

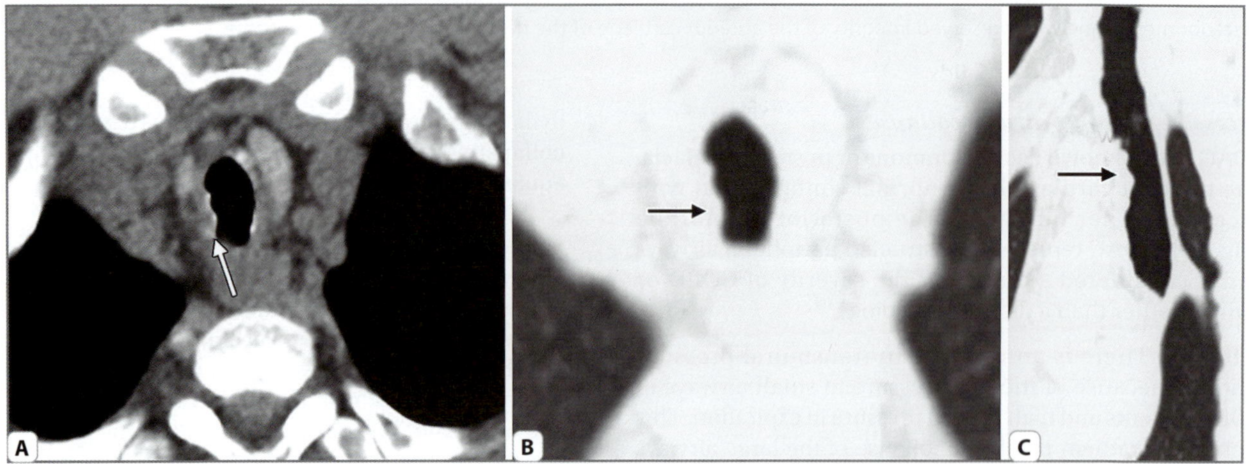

FIGS. 16A TO C: Tracheopathia osteoplastica. Axial CT (A and B) and sagittal MPR (C) showing multiple, small soft tissue nodules along the inner tracheal aspect with sparing of the posterior tracheal wall.

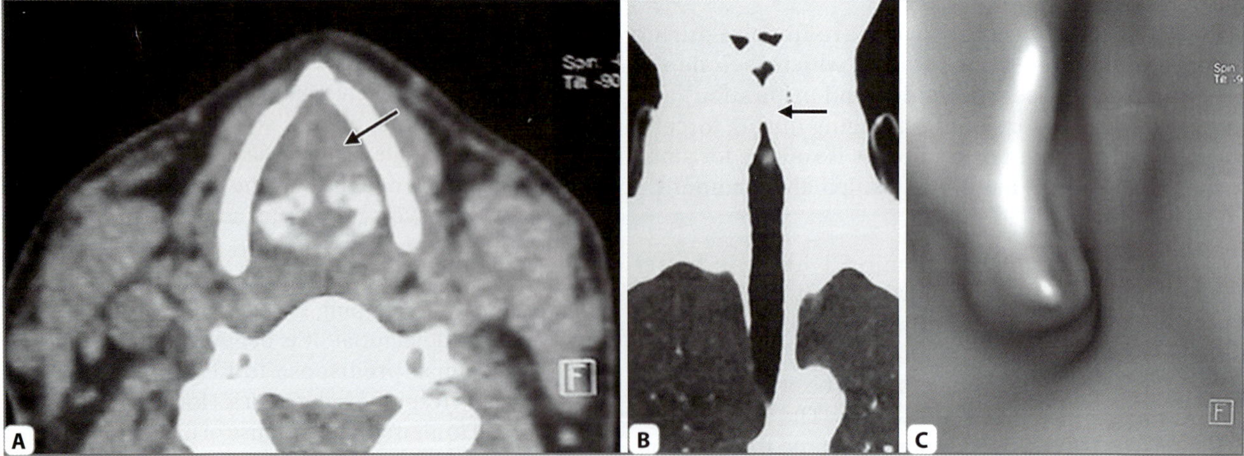

FIGS. 17A AND B: Amyloidosis. MDCT reveals diffuse wall thickening of the laryngeal wall and vocal cords with obliteration of the lumen (arrow).

Intraluminal

Inflammatory/Infective

Granulation tissue

Chronic inflammation of infective/non-infective nature can result in non-specific granulation tissue forming bronchial obstructive lesions.

Broncholithiasis

In this condition, calcified lymph nodes erode into the tracheobronchial tree and it is a complication of granulomatous lymphadenitis. Patients may expectorate or aspirate the calcified material. On CT **(Fig. 18)**, a calcified focus is seen within the bronchial lumen without any mass. Peribronchial lymph node calcification may be seen and postobstructive abnormalities are often associated.[4,43]

Masses/Neoplasms of Tracheobronchial Tree

Primary tracheal neoplasia accounts for only 1–2% of all respiratory tract tumors.[44] In adults, most (60–90%) of these tumors are malignant,[45] whereas benign tumors represent the majority of lesions in children.

Primary tumors include epithelial and mesenchymal neoplasms of which the most common are squamous cell carcinoma (SCC) and adenoid cystic carcinoma (ACC) with occasional cases of carcinoid and mucoepidermoid carcinoma. The most common benign lesions are hamartomas and bronchial papillomas. Secondary neoplasms are either metastases, or direct infiltration by adjacent mediastinal tumors (carcinomas lung, thyroid or esophagus).[44]

Clinical presentation is usually non-specific with a significant overlap between the imaging appearances of benign and malignant lesions. The main role of imaging **(Fig. 19)** is in delineation of tumor extent within the lumen, airway wall, and surrounding structures before treatment planning.

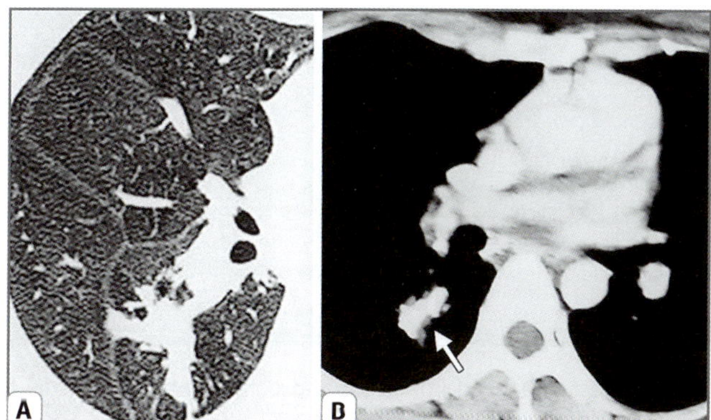

FIGS. 18A AND B: Broncholith. A branching tubular opacity is seen in the right lower lobe (A) of a 32-year-old woman with past history of tuberculosis. (B) On mediastinal window, the lesion is seen to be calcified (arrow).

Malignant tumors

Primary tracheal cancer is rare and seen commonly in middle aged/elderly males smokers. The prognosis of patients is poor, with the 5-year survival rate being 5–35%.[46]

Squamous cell carcinoma: Squamous cell carcinoma is usually seen in smokers with up to one third of the cases associated with other malignant lesions of the respiratory tract.[47] In approximately 10% of patients, these tumors are multifocal and extend into the mainstem bronchi or adjacent esophagus, resulting in esophago-bronchial fistula.[47] CT demonstrates a polypoid intraluminal mass of soft tissue density with irregular, smooth, or lobulated contours **(Fig. 20)**.[44] The relationships of the tumor with the tracheal wall vary from localized eccentric pedunculated lesions to circumferential invasion.

Adenoid cystic carcinoma: Adenoid cystic carcinomas are low-grade malignancies that typically arise from the tracheobronchial mucous glands, most frequently on the posterolateral tracheal wall. These show a marked propensity for local, submucosal and perineural invasion. Unlike squamous cell carcinoma, no known association exists between smoking and development of ACC. CT appearances **(Fig. 21)** include soft tissue attenuating intraluminal mass which may infiltrate the mediastinal fat or localized stenosis because of circumferential wall thickening.[48]

Mucoepidermoid carcinoma: Mucoepidermoid carcinoma arises from the minor salivary glands lining the tracheobronchial tree.[49] Patients are less than 40 years old and usually present with obstructive airway symptoms. On CT, it is seen as a smooth, oval or lobulated, mildly enhancing endobronchial mass, often smoothly oval or lobulated.[50] Punctate calcifications are occasionally seen.

Malignancies of trachea or esophagus can also lead to the formation of acquired tracheo-esophageal fistulas **(Fig. 22)**.

Carcinoid tumors: Carcinoid tumors are neuroendocrine tumors, which arise from bronchial, or bronchiolar epithelium. They present a histologic spectrum of low-grade to high-grade neoplasms, with the highest grades merging with small cell carcinoma.[4] Most endobronchial carcinoids are central in location arising in the main, lobar, or segmental bronchi. On CT **(Figs. 23 and 24)**, they appear as a hilar mass or an endobronchial lesion. Classical findings have been described of a well-defined round or lobulated tumor causing narrowing of the adjacent airway, associated with eccentric calcifications.[51] These often show intense enhancement.

Endobronchial metastases: Metastases to the bronchus can also present like an endobronchial mass. The metastases are usually from carcinoma breast, colon and kidney.

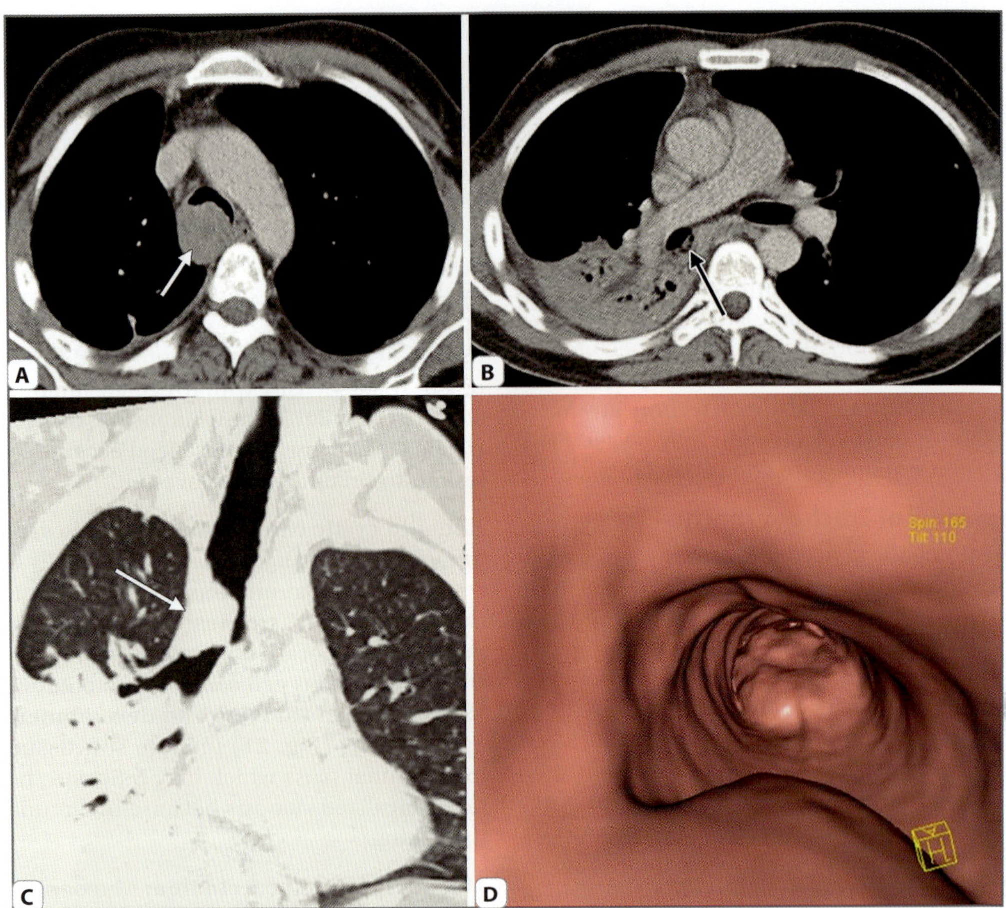

FIGS. 19A TO D: Tracheal mass. Axial CT (A, B) coronal MPR (C) and VB (D) showing a mass involving the trachea (white arrow). In addition, a low density lesion with air bubbles is seen in the right lower lobe with distal collapse suggestive of a mucous plug (black arrow in B).

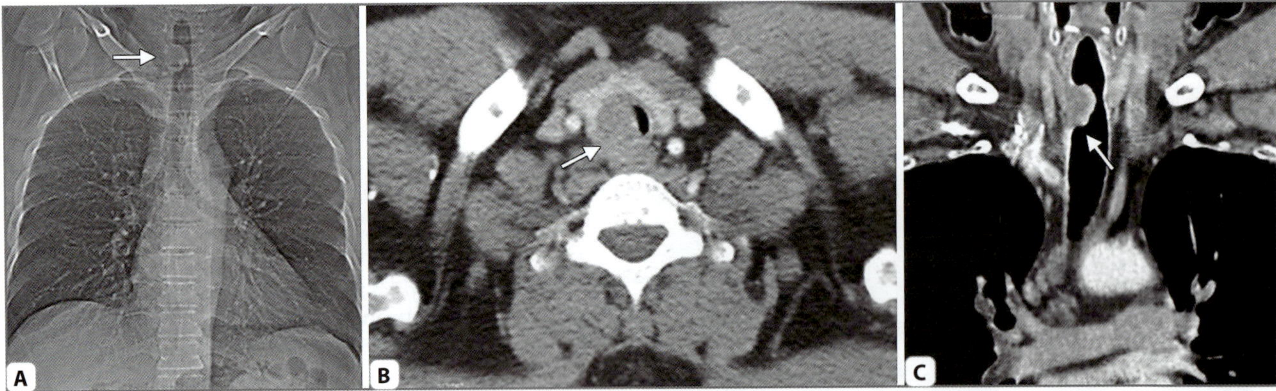

FIGS. 20A TO C: Tracheal squamous cell carcinoma. CT scout (A), axial contrast-enhanced image (B) and coronal MPR (C), reveal a polypoidal, lobulated tracheal mass (arrow) focally involving about 180 degrees of the tracheal wall.

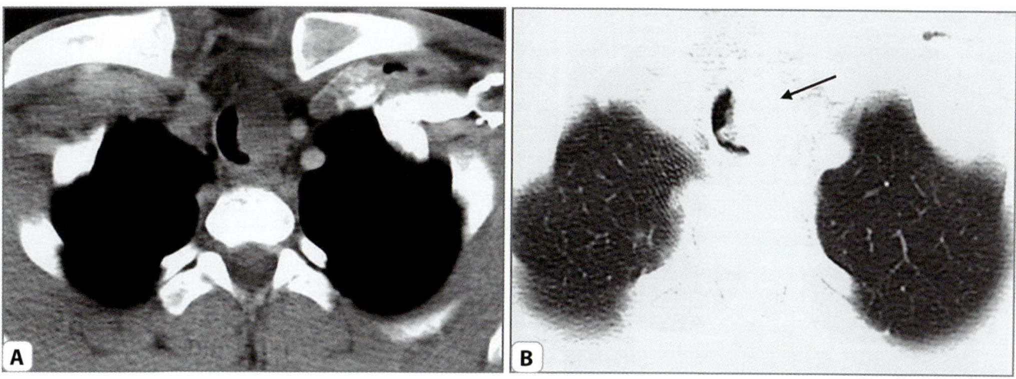

FIGS. 21A AND B: Tracheal adenoid cystic carcinoma. Axial contrast enhanced CT in mediastinal window (A) and lung window (B) showing an irregular, soft tissue mass (arrow) with focal tracheal wall involvement. CT appearances of different tracheal tumors show significant overlap.

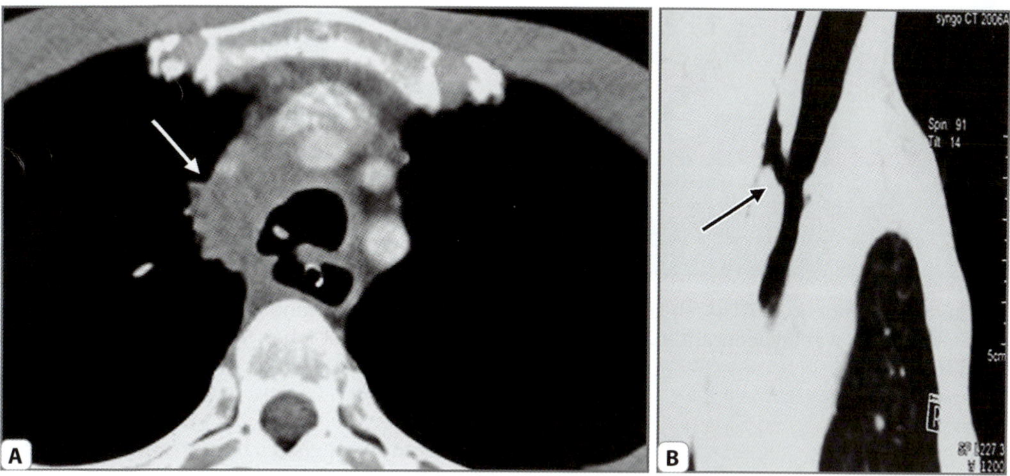

FIGS. 22A AND B: Tracheo-esophaegeal fistula. Axial CECT (A) showing necrotic mediastinal nodes (white arrow) with a communication between trachea and esophagus. Sagittal MPR demonstrates the fistula (black arrow) well (B).

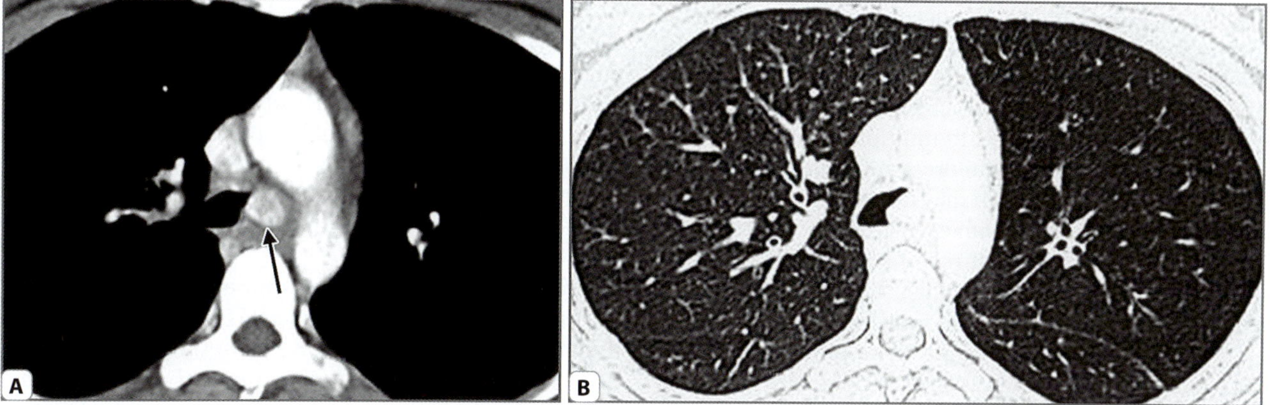

FIGS. 23A AND B: Carcinoid tumor. CT showing an intensely enhancing mass (arrow) involving the left main bronchus with hyperlucent left lung.

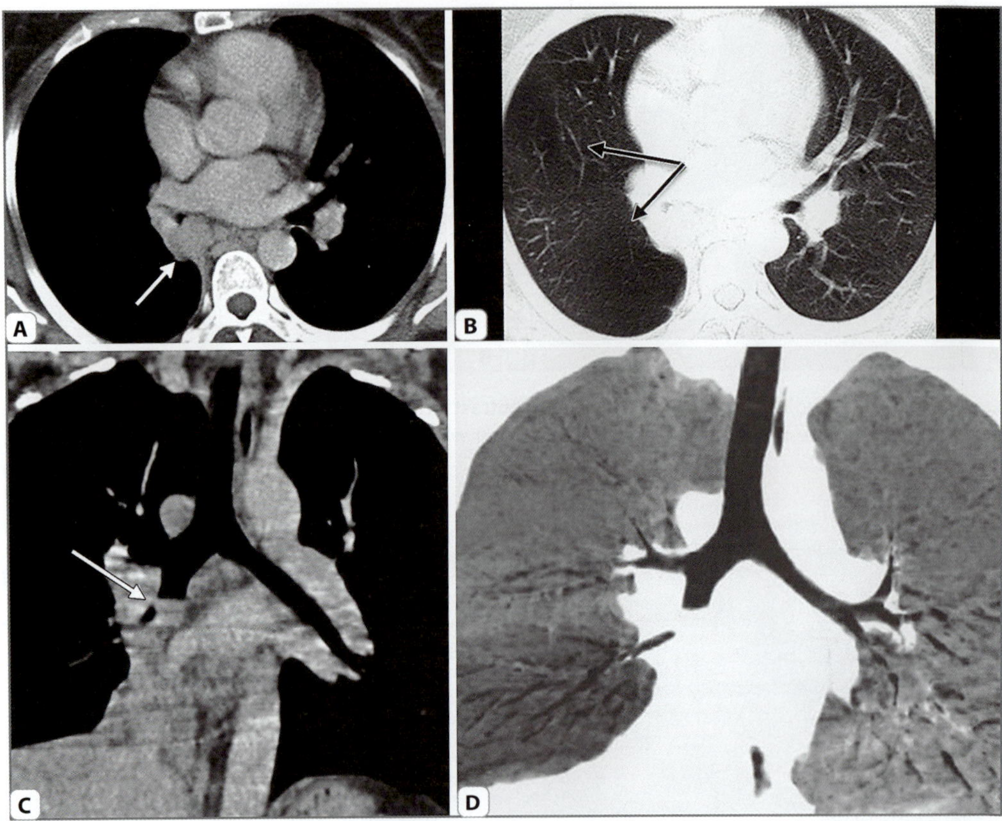

FIGS. 24A TO D: Carcinoid tumor. Axial CT (A, B) coronal MPR (C) and min IP (D) showing a lobulated mass (white arrow) involving the right bronchus intermedius with hyperlucent (black arrow) right middle and lower lobes. MinIP shows the cranio-caudal extent of airway involvement the best.

Benign tumors

Benign tumors of the central airways are rare.[44] They can be of epithelial, mesenchymal, neural or composite origin. These tumors appear in clinical practice as the differential diagnosis of malignant lesions that are much more common.

Most common amongst these is the "squamous cell papilloma". These most often occur in middle-aged male smokers, and typically involve the larynx or bronchi, tracheal involvement being uncommon. Involvement, when present, is limited to tracheal wall.[44] Papillomatosis is a condition associated with multiple papillomas. This condition typically affects children and young adults and is often limited to the larynx. It may involve the intrathoracic airways and also present with cavitating lung nodules and is referred to as "recurrent respiratory papillomatosis" (RRP) **(Fig. 25)**. These lesions have a high propensity for recurrence and even malignant transformation.[52]

CT appearance may suggest the pathology of the neoplasm. Fat attenuation is seen in lipoma or hamartochondroma, while calcification may occur in hamartoma, chondroma or carcinoid. Presence of both fat and calcification suggests a hamartoma. High contrast-enhancement is seen in carcinoid, hemangioma, glomus tumor or fibroma.

Miscellaneous

Mucus plugs, foreign body and clots

Mucus is the most common soft tissue mass within the airways. On CT scan **(Figs. 19 and 26)**, it is of low attenuation, non-enhancing, may contain small air bubbles and is not associated with cartilaginous ring disruption. Typically seen in the dependent portions of the airway, it can move after coughing.

Other miscellaneous causes of focal airway narrowing include foreign bodies **(Figs. 27 and 28)** and blood clot **(Fig. 29)**.

Prolonged increased intraluminal pressure can lead to the formation of acquired tracheal **(Fig. 30)** and bronchial diverticula **(Fig. 31)**. Usually, these are seen in COPD patients with chronic cough. Tracheal diverticulum is typically seen as an air-filled outpouching from the right posterolateral tracheal wall.

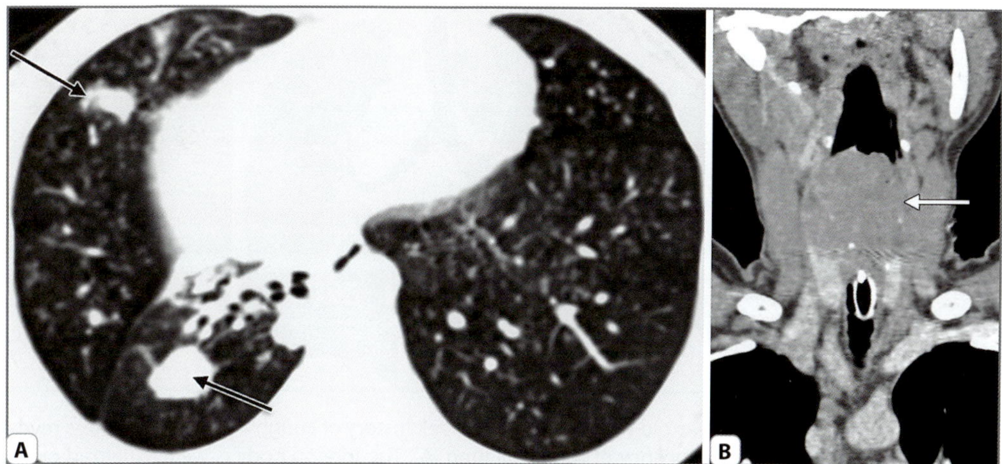

FIGS. 25A AND B: Recurrent respiratory papillomatosis. Multiple lung nodules (black arrow) and transglottic carcinoma (white arrow) in a young male with recurrent respiratory papillomatosis. The right lower lobe bronchiectasis is because of recurrent infections due to aspiration.

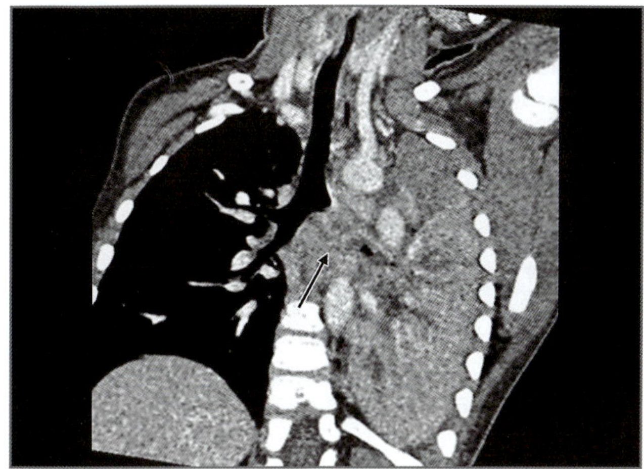

FIG. 26: Mucus plug. A fluid attenuating lesion is present in the left main bronchus (arrow) of an elderly male, with distal collapse of the left lung. These plugs can be successfully cleared bronchoscopically.

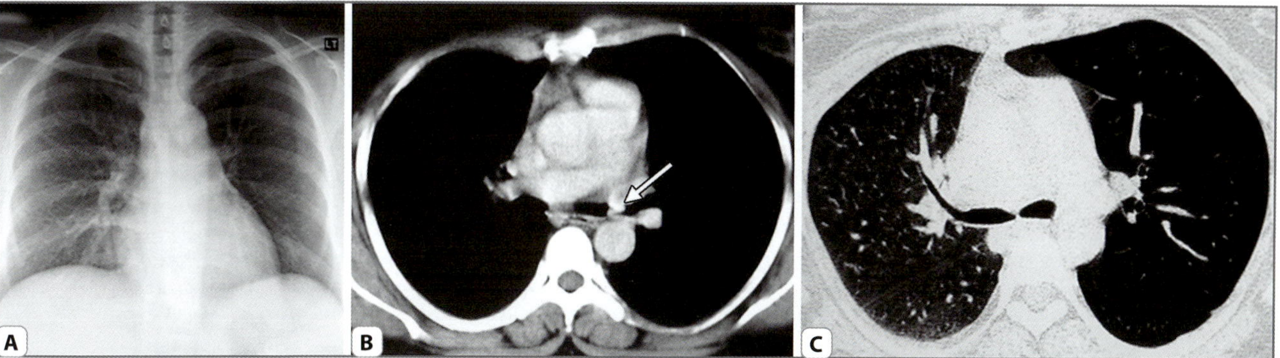

FIGS. 27A TO C: Foreign body. (A) Chest radiograph of a middle-aged man with history of dyspnea and wheezing reveals a hyperlucent left lung field. CT scan (B, C) reveal a dense foreign body (white arrow in B) in the left main bronchus causing distal air trapping.

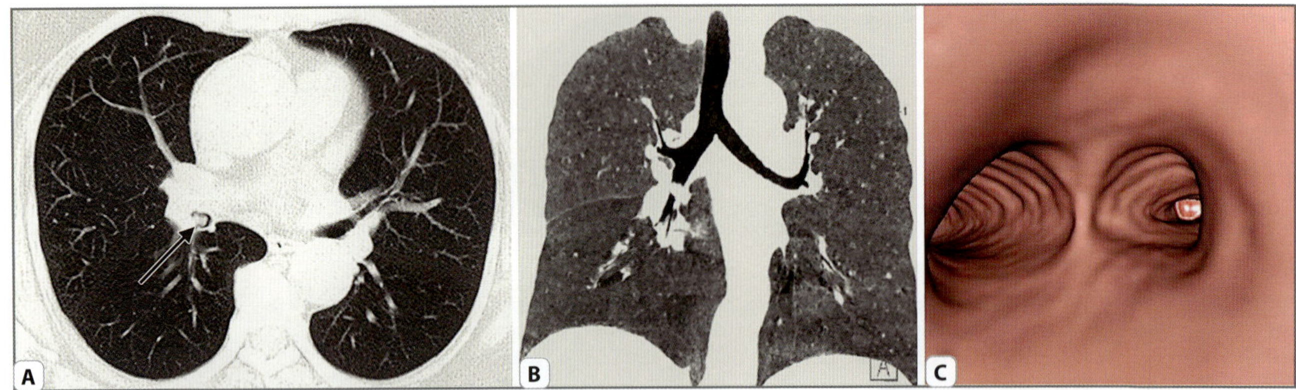

FIGS. 28A TO C: Foreign body. MDCT of a 65-year-old woman with one week history of cough and breathlessness reveals a low-density lesion in the bronchus intermedius with subtle lucency of the distal lung (A). The foreign body is well-visualized on the minIP (B) and VB (C). The left-right orientation is reverse of an axial image on VB to simulate FB. Two days later the patient coughed out a chickpea.

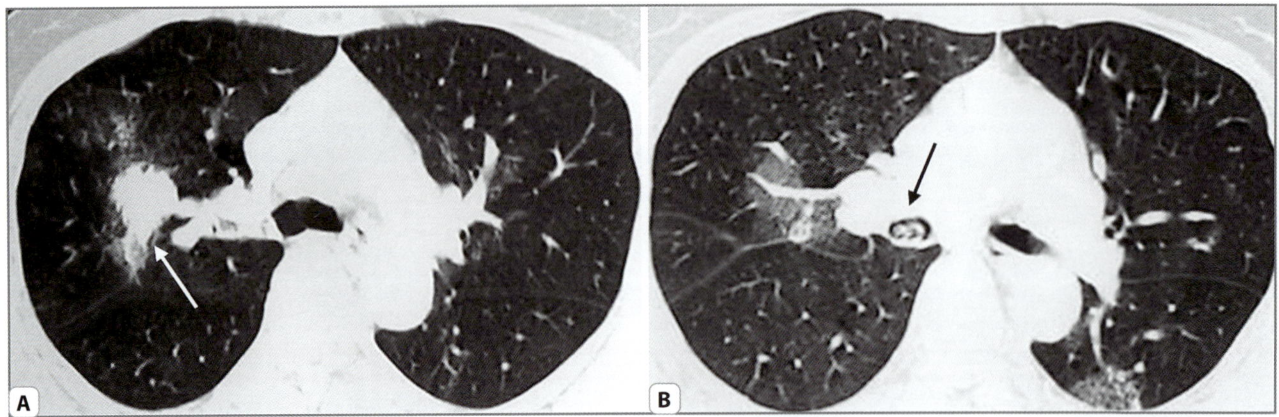

FIGS. 29A AND B: Blood clot. An elderly male presenting with hemoptysis. CT reveals a malignant mass in right upper lobe with surrounding hemorrhage (white arrow), and a blood clot (black arrow) in the right upper lobe bronchus. A blood clot resembles a mucous plug on imaging.

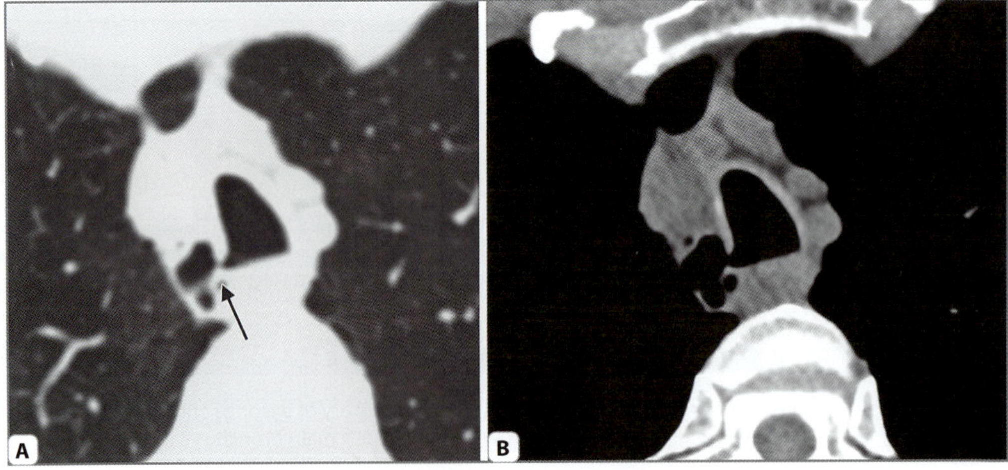

FIGS. 30A AND B: Tracheal diverticulum. Air-filled outpouching from the right posterolateral tracheal wall with small focal communication (arrow).

Peripheral Airways

Bronchiectasis

Definition and Pathophysiology

Bronchiectasis is the localized, irreversible dilatation of the cartilage-containing airways or bronchi. It usually results from bronchial wall injury, bronchial lumen obstruction, and traction from adjacent fibrosis.[53] Obstruction and fibrosis are readily apparent on imaging. Bronchial wall injury and subsequent bronchiectasis can occur because of infection and, impaired host defense leading to recurrent infections, exaggerated immune response, congenital structural defects of the bronchial wall, and extrinsic insults damaging the airway wall.[54] Underlying mechanism of mucus plugging and superimposed bacterial colonization is common to these conditions.

Dilatation is classified by its gross appearance as tubular (cylindric), varicose, or cystic (saccular). These types are discussed in **Table 3** and shown in **Figure 32**.

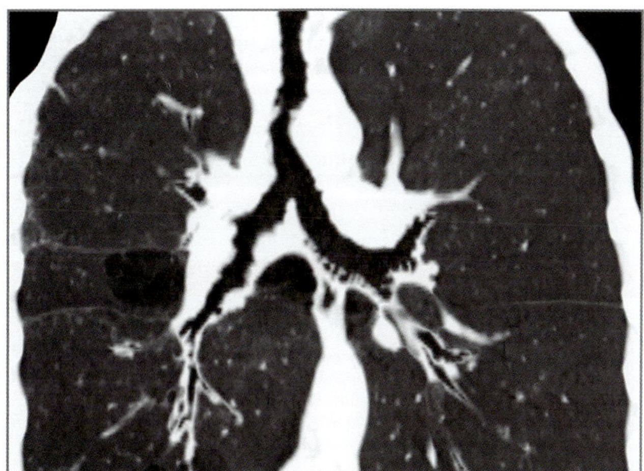

FIG. 31: Bronchial diverticulae. Multiple small diverticulae along the bilateral main and segmental bronchi with bronchial wall thickening and emphysematous changes in bilateral lung fields in a case of COPD.

Clinical Features

Symptoms can be very nonspecific varying from mild cough or minimal dyspnea to chronic cough, abundant sputum production, progressive dyspnea, and repeated pulmonary infections. Chronic hypoxemia and hypercarbia can lead to digital clubbing, anemia, and weight loss. Other associated symptoms or manifestations include sinusitis, hemoptysis and pulmonary hypertension.[54]

Diagnosis is usually confirmed by spirometry and high-resolution computed tomography (HRCT). The diagnostic workup may include a sweat electrolyte test, serum immunoglobulin levels, or serum aspergillus antibody and precipitin, or even genetic testing according to the age of presentation and symptoms.

Imaging Findings (Figs. 1 and 33)

The imaging findings on conventional radiography are due to the bronchial wall thickening and are detailed in **Table 4**.

HRCT is reliable to diagnose bronchiectasis. The key imaging features are due to bronchial dilatation and bronchial wall thickening and are detailed in **Table 5**. Bronchial wall thickening is seen in all cases of bronchiectasis, except those caused by congenital cartilage deficiency (William-Campbell syndrome, Mounier-Kuhn syndrome) or in allergic bronchopulmonary aspergillosis (ABPA).[54]

TABLE 3: Types of bronchiectasis.

Type of bronchiectasis	Luminal dilatation	Wall thickening
Cylindrical	Uniform	Smooth
Varicose	Alternating areas of dilatation and constriction (beaded appearance)	Irregular
Cystic	Uniform dilated bronchus	Thick-walled bronchus terminates in a thick-walled cyst

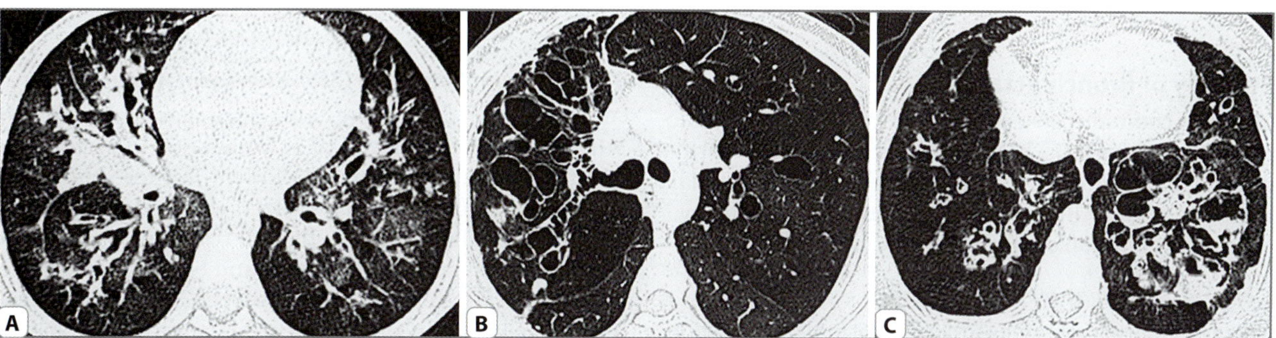

FIGS. 32A TO C: Types of bronchiectasis. (A) Bilateral cylindrical bronchiectasis, (B) Varicose bronchiectasis in right upper lobe (C) Cystic bronchiectasis and air-fluid levels in left lower lobe.

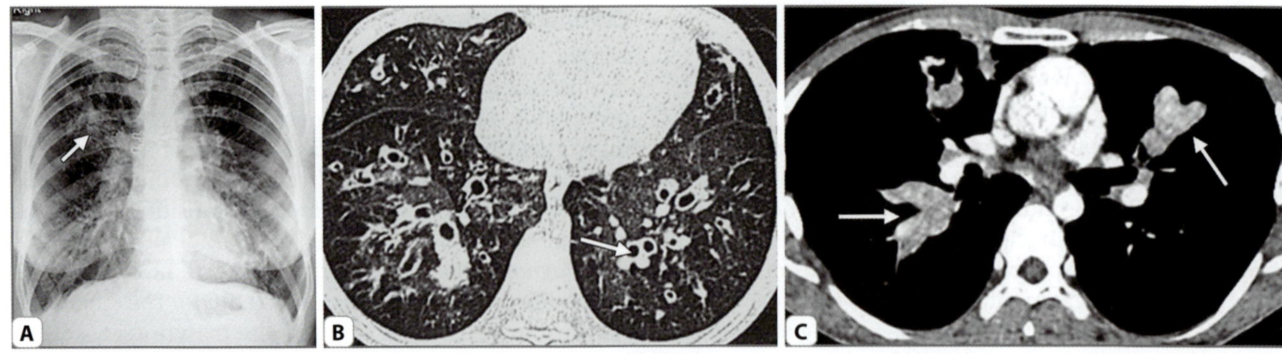

FIGS. 33A TO C: Chest radiograph (A) features of bronchiectasis. Ill defined perihilar linear opacities and "tram-track" lesions (arrow). CT signs of bronchiectasis: Signet ring sign (arrow in B), Tram track sign (arrowhead in B), branching dense tubular structures (arrow in C).

TABLE 4: Key radiographic features of bronchiectasis.

Imaging finding	Etiology
Ill-defined perihilar linear densities with indistinctness of the margins of the central pulmonary arteries	Bronchial wall thickening
Ill-defined ring shadows (Bronchus seen end on)	Bronchial wall thickening
Tramlines or parallel lines along expected course of bronchi	Bronchial wall thickening in severe bronchiectasis
Elongated opacities + calcified	Mucus plugging
Air-fluid levels in thick-walled cysts with surrounding consolidation	Superadded infection
Hyperinflation	Increased lung volume

TABLE 5: Key HRCT findings of bronchiectasis.

Imaging finding	Etiology
Internal luminal diameter of one or more bronchi > diameter of adjacent artery	Bronchial dilatation
Lack of normal tapering of a bronchus	Bronchial dilatation
Visible bronchus abutting mediastinal pleura	Bronchial dilatation
Visible bronchus within 1 cm of pleura	Bronchial dilatation
Signet ring sign	*Jewel*: artery abutting the *Ring*—thick-walled dilated bronchus on axial view
Tram-track sign	Parallel, thickened walls of a dilated bronchus on a longitudinal section
Branching dense tubular structures	Mucus plugging of dilated bronchi and bronchioles
Centrilobular nodules, in a "tree-in-bud" pattern	Mucus-filled bronchiolectasis
Mosaic attenuation and air trapping	Coexisting constrictive bronchiolitis

Etiology of Bronchiectasis

The most common cause is postinfectious, followed by idiopathic bronchiectasis; bronchiectasis related to abnormal mucociliary clearance (cystic fibrosis and primary ciliary dyskinesia) and ABPA and systemic immunodeficiency.[55] Few of the common etiologies are discussed below.

Congenital airway wall abnormality

There is abnormal physiologic clearing of mucoid excretions in congenital defects of cartilage, collagen, or other components of the bronchial wall. This predisposes to repeated infections and progressive bronchial dilatation.

Tracheobronchomegaly (Mounier-kuhn disease)

An uncommon disease presenting in males, in the 4th and 5th decades, it is believed to be congenital in origin. The common associations include Ehlers-Danlos syndrome, Marfan syndrome, and generalized elastosis (cutis laxa). Tracheobronchomegaly is characterized by pathological thinning of the muscle, cartilage, and elastic tissue of the airway walls. There is increased distensibility of the tracheal and bronchial walls, with uniform dilatation of the tracheal and bronchial lumina predisposing to recurrent infections in the dependent lungs. On CT scan, a tracheal diameter of > 3 cm in both coronal and sagittal planes, along with central bronchiectasis but without airway wall thickening, is observed **(Figs. 34)**.[54]

Williams-campbell syndrome

Williams-Campbell syndrome is a rare disease characterized by defects in the cartilage of the fourth-, fifth-, and sixth-generation bronchi. It may be congenital or acquired, likely as a sequela of prior adenovirus (measles and pertussis) infections. On CT imaging, there is cystic bronchiectasis distal to the third-generation bronchi, with ballooning on inspiratory CT and collapse on the expiratory phase.[56]

Congenital bronchial atresia

There is congenital focal obliteration of the lumen of a segmental bronchus. This results in focal bronchiectasis and air trapping more distally. Usually identified as an incidental finding on a chest radiograph as an ovoid, tubular, or branching density. CT shows the characteristic bronchial, branching nature, and distal air trapping **(Fig. 35)**. It should be differentiated from an acquired mucocele which is caused by focal scarring of a segmental bronchus (infective) or from an endobronchial lesion.[57] In case of an acquired mucocele an endobronchial neoplasm should be excluded.

Acquired wall abnormalities

Inflammation of the bronchial wall because of chronic infections, inhalational injury, and cellular infiltration in the setting of graft-versus-host disease can cause damage to the bronchial wall.

Mucociliary clearance abnormalities

In cystic fibrosis, the consistency of mucus is abnormal whereas primary ciliary dyskinesia and immotile ciliary syndrome are characterized by abnormalities of the structure and function of the cilia of the airway epithelium.

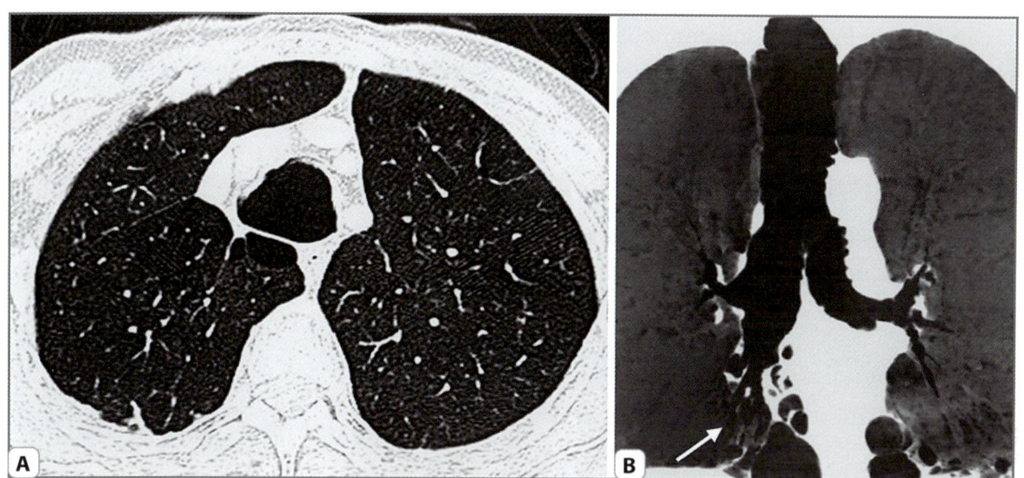

FIGS. 34A AND B: Mounier-Kuhn disease. CT reveals dilatation of the trachea and major bronchi. Bronchiectasis is seen in right lower lobe (arrow).

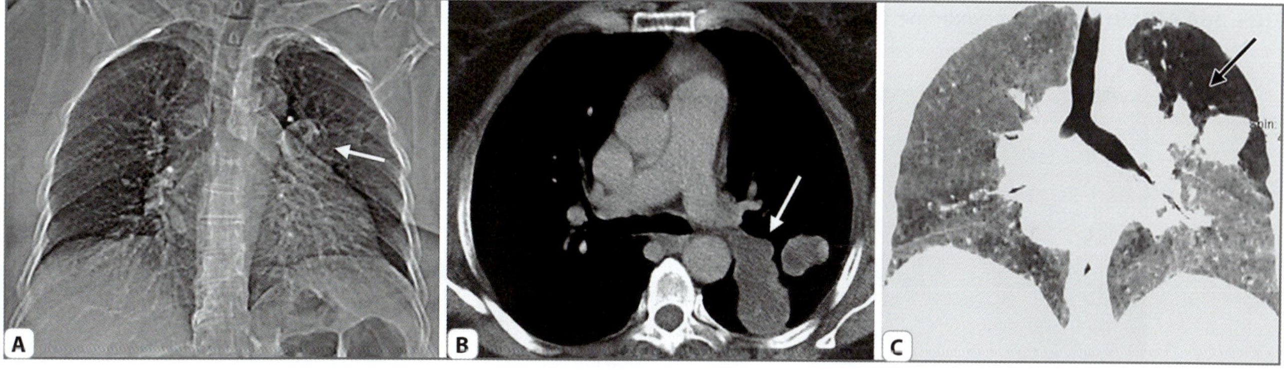

FIGS. 35A TO C: Congenital bronchial atresia. CT scout film (A) shows a well-defined left parahilar opacity (arrow). Mediastinal window (B) reveals a fluid- filled branching, tubular lesion (arrow) in the posterior segment of left upper lobe. MinIP (C) demonstrates the distal hyperinflation (arrow).

This leads to ineffective mucus clearance and secondary colonization of the airway lumina by bacteria and repeated episodes of infections. There is upper lobe involvement in cystic fibrosis whereas in primary and acquired ciliary dyskinesia the bronchiectasis is worse in the lower lungs.[58] Numerous scoring systems are available with the Bhalla score being commonly used.[59] It assesses the radiological severity of bronchiectasis and the course of pulmonary exacerbation in patients of cystic fibrosis.

Primary ciliary dyskinesia (PCD) or immotile ciliary syndrome is caused by a defect in structure and function of the airway cilia and causes progressive bronchiectasis. Kartagener syndrome **(Fig. 36)** or triad (situs inversus, bronchiectasis, and sinusitis) is seen in half of the PCD patients.[60,61] Bronchiectasis in PCD is primarily in the lingular, middle and lower lobes of the lung.

Hyperimmune response

Hyperimmune response to internal or external antigens with inflammation of the airway wall and subsequent bronchiectasis can be seen in ABPA, inflammatory bowel disease, rheumatoid arthritis, Sjögren's disease and granulomatous polyangiitis.

Allergic bronchopulmonary aspergillosis is a hypersensitivity reaction to aspergillus fumigatus antigens seen commonly in patients with atopic rhinitis, asthma, or CF. Patients present with fever, wheeze and expectoration of brown mucus plugs. Elevated serum IgE level, eosinophilia on peripheral blood smears, or positive skin reaction to aspergillus antigen are seen on clinical evaluation. Mycelia can sometimes be identified in the expectorated mucus plugs. Imaging characteristically shows migratory consolidation early in the disease, usually involving the upper lobes. On HRCT **(Fig. 37)**, there is central and upper lobe bronchiectasis, varicose or cystic subtypes. Inspissated mucus in the dilated central bronchi gives the classic finger in-glove appearance on the chest radiographs in more chronic cases.[54,58] There is atelectasis or hyperinflation of the lung distal to the impacted bronchi. In up to 20% of the patients, high-attenuation mucus may be seen.[61]

Complications of Bronchiectasis

The complications of bronchiectasis include respiratory failure, recurrent pneumonias, lung abscess, empyema, septicemia, cardiac failure and secondary amyloidosis.

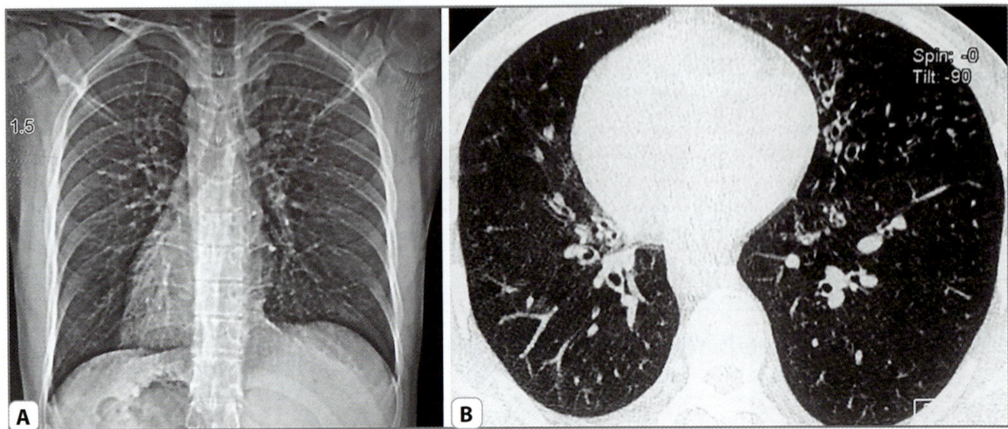

FIGS. 36A AND B: Kartagener syndrome. CT scout film (A) shows situs inversus. HRCT chest (B) reveals bilateral central bronchiectasis.

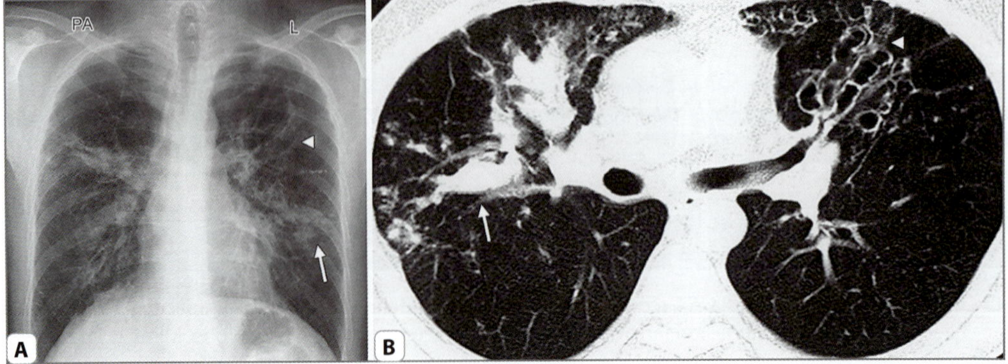

FIGS. 37A AND B: Allergic bronchopulmonary aspergillosis (ABPA). Chest radiograph (A) and CT scan (B) showing classical central, tubular bronchiectasis (arrowhead) with mucous plugging giving "finger-in-glove" appearance (arrow).

CONCLUSION

Tracheobronchial lesions include a wide range of abnormalities and MDCT is the modality of choice. Axial images should always be used with MPR and 3D reconstruction images for evaluating tracheobronchial disorders. MPR images are a useful adjunct and minIP gives good overview of airway. Virtual bronchoscopy can guide the bronchoscopist and may avoid bronchoscopy especially in children.

REFERENCES

1. Chou SSH, Kicska GA, Pipavath SN, Reddy GP. Digital Tomosynthesis of the chest: Current and Emerging Applications. RadioGraphics. 2014;34:359-72.
2. Dobbins JT 3rd, McAdams HP, Godfrey DJ, Li CM. Digital tomosynthesis of the chest. J Thorac Imaging. 2008;23(2): 86-92.
3. Gupta A, Kikano EG, Bera K, et al. Dual energy imaging in cardiothoracic pathologies: A primer for radiologists and clinicians. Eur J Radiol Open. 202120;8:100324.
4. Nadich P et al. Airways. In Naidich DP, Webb WR, Muller NC, Vlahos L, Krinsky GA eds. Computed Tomography and Magnetic Resonance of the thorax 4th edn 2007. Lippincott Williams, and Wilkins, Philadephia, USA 2007;453-556.
5. Sundarakumar DK, Bhalla AS, Sharma R, et al. Multidetector CT evaluation of central airways stenoses: Comparison of virtual bronchoscopy, minimal-intensity projection, and multiplanar reformatted images. Indian J Radiol Imaging. 2011;21(3):191-4.
6. Bankier AA, O'Donnell C, Boiselle PM. Respiratory instructions for CT examinations of the lungs: A hands on guideline. Radiographics 2008;28:919-31.
7. Beigelman AC, Brillet PY, Grenier PA. MDCT of the Airways: Technique and Normal Results Radiol. Clin N Am. 2009;47(2):185-201.
8. American College of Radiology. ACR–SABI-SPR-STR practice parameter for the performance of thoracic computed tomography (CT). https://www.acr.org/-/media/acr/files/practice-parameters/ct-thoracic.pdf. Accessed on January 2, 2025.
9. Lee EY, Litmanovich D, Boiselle PM. Multidetector CT. Evaluation of Tracheobronchomalacia Radiol. Clin N Am. 2009;47(2):261-69.
10. Boiselle PM, Reynolds KF, Ernst A. Multiplanar and three-dimensional imaging of the central airways with multidetector CT. AJR Am J Roentgenol. 2002;179:301-08.
11. Hooper KD, Iyriboz AT, Wise SW, et al. Mucosal details at CT virtual reality: Surface versus volume rendering. Radiology 2000;214:517-22.
12. Boiselle PM, Lynch DA. Anatomical airway imaging methods. In: Boiselle PM, Lynch DA, (Eds). CT of the airways. Totowa (NJ): Humana Press 2008:75-94.
13. Fetita CI, Preteux F, Beigelman-Aubry C, et al. Pulmonary airways: 3D reconstruction from multislice CT and clinical investigation. IEEE Trans Med Imaging. 2004;23:1353-64.
14. Bhatt SP, Washko GR, Hoffman EA, et al. Imaging Advances in Chronic Obstructive Pulmonary Disease. Insights from the Genetic Epidemiology of Chronic Obstructive Pulmonary Disease (COPDGene) Study. Am J Respir Crit Care Med. 2019;199(3):286-301.
15. Grydeland TB, Dirksen A, Coxson HO, et al. Quantitative computed tomography measures of emphysema and airway wall thickness are related to respiratory symptoms. Am J Respir Crit Care Med. 2010;181:353-9.
16. Kim V, Davey A, Comellas AP, et al. COPDGene® Investigators. Clinical and computed tomographic predictors of chronic bronchitis in COPD: a cross-sectional analysis of the COPD Gene Study. Respir Res. 2014;15:52.
17. Tanaka F, Muro K, S Yamasaki, et al. Evaluation of tracheobronchial wall invasion using transbronchial ultra sonography (EBUS). Eur J Cardio Throac Surg. 2000;17:570-74.
18. Hochhegger B, de Souza VVS, Marchiori E, et al. Chest magnetic resonance imaging: a protocol suggestion. Radiol Bras. 2015;48(6):373-80.
19. Dornes G, Berger P, Refait J, et al. Allergic Bronchopulmonary aspergillosis in cystic Fibrosis: MR Imaging of Airway Mucus Contrasts as a Tool for Diagnosis. Radiology. 2017;285(1): 261-9.
20. Biederer J. MR imaging of the airways. Br J Radiol. 2023;96(1146):20220630.
21. Gamsu G, Webb WR. Computed tomography of the trachea: Normal and abnormal. AJR Am J Roentgenol. 1982;139: 321-26.
22. Wu Ju, White CS, Meyer CA, et al. Variant bronchial anatomy-CT appearance and classification. AJR Am J Roentgenol. 1999;172:741-44.
23. Landing BH, Dixon LG. Congenital malformation and genetic disorders of the respiratory tract. Am Rev Respir Dis. 1979;120:151-85.
24. Fraser RS, Colman N, Müller NL, et al. Upper airway obstruction. In: Fraser RS, Colman N, Müller NL, Pare PD, editors. Synopsis of diseases of the chest. 3rd edition. Philadelphia: BW Saunders. 2005:631-34.
25. Carden KA, Boiselle PM, Waltz DA, et al. Tracheomalacia and tracheobronchomalacia in children and adults: An in-depth review. Chest. 2005;127:984-1005.
26. Sundarakumar DK, Bhalla AS, Sharma R, et al. Multidetector computed tomography imaging of congenital anomalies of major airways: A pictorial essay. World J Radiol. 2011;3(12):289-97
27. Swensen SJ, Aughenbaugh GL, Douglas WW, Myers JL. High-resolution CT of the lungs: Findings in various pulmonary diseases. AJR Am J Roentgenol. 1992;159:971-72.
28. Arora A, Bhalla AS, Jana M, et al. Overview of airway involvement in tuberculosis. J Med Imaging Radiat Oncol. 2013;57:576-81
29. Moon WK, Im JG, Yeon KM, et al. Tuberculosis of the central airways: CT findings of active and fibrotic disease, AJR Am J Roentgenol. 1997;169:649-53.

30. Franquet T, Serrano F, Giménez A, et al. Necrotizing aspergillosis of large airways. CT findings in eight patients. J Comput Assist Tomogr. 2002;26:342-45.
31. Yigla M, Ben-Izhak O, Oren I, et al. Laryngotracheobronchial involvement in a patient with nonendemic rhinoscleroma. Chest. 2000;117(6):1795-98.
32. Grenier PA, Beigelman AC, Brillet PY. Nonneoplastic Tracheal and Bronchial Stenoses. Radiol Clin N Am. 2009; 47(2):243-60.
33. Cordier JF, Valeyre D, Guillevin L, et al. Pulmonary Wegener's granulomatosis. A clinical and imaging study of 77 cases. Chest. 1990;97:906-12.
34. Trentham DE, Le CH. Relapsing polychondritis. Ann Intern Med. 1998;129(2):114-22.
35. Behar JV, Choi YW, Hartman TA, et al. Relapsing polychondritis affecting the lower respiratory tract. AJR Am J Roentgenol. 2002;178(1):173-77.
36. Stark P. Imaging of tracheobronchial injuries. J Thoracic Imaging. 1995;10:206-19.
37. Lenique F, Brauner MW, Grenier P, et al. CT assessment of bronchi in sarcoidosis: Endoscopic and pathologic correlations. Radiology. 1995;194(2):419-23.
38. Wheeler S, Andeen N, Reddy R. Isolated IgG4 related disease of the trachea. Respir Med Case Rep. 2024 28;49:102031.
39. Aslam A, De Luis Cardenas J, Morrison RJ, et al. Tracheobronchomalacia and Excessive Dynamic Airway Collapse: Current Concepts and Future Directions. Radiographics. 2022;42(4):1012-27.
40. Bankier AA, MacMahon H, Colby T, et al. Fleischner Society: Glossary of Terms for Thoracic Imaging. Radiology. 2024;310(2):e232558.
41. O'Regan A, Fenlon HM, Beamis Jr JF, et al. Tracheobronchial amyloidosis. The Boston University experience from 1984 to 1999. Medicine. 2000;79:69-79.
42. Kim HY, Im JG, Song KS, et al. Localized amyloidosis of the respiratory system: CT features. J Comput Assist Tomogr. 1999;23:627-31.
43. Conces DJ, Tarver RD, Vix VA. Broncholithiasis: CT features in 15 patients. AJR Am J Roentgenol. 1991;157:249-53.
44. McCarthy MJ, Rosado-de-Christenson ML. Tumors of the trachea. J Thorac Imaging. 1995;10(3):180-98.
45. Macchiarini P. Primary tracheal tumors. Lancet Oncol 2006;7:83-91.
46. Honings J, van Dijck JA, Verhagen AF, et al. Incidence and treatment of tracheal cancer: A nationwide study in the Netherlands. Ann Surg Oncol. 2007;14(2):968-76.
47. Grillo HC, Mathisen DJ, Wain JC. Management of tumors of the trachea. Oncology. 1992;6:61-67.
48. Kwak SH, Lee KS, Chung MJ, et al. Adenoid cystic carcinoma of the airways: Helical CT and histopathologic correlation. AJR Am J Roentgenol. 2004;183(2):77-81.
49. Yousem SA, Hochholzer L. Mucoepidermoid tumors of the lung. Cancer 1987;60(6):1346-52.
50. Kim TS, Lee KS, Han J, et al. Mucoepidermoid carcinoma of the tracheobronchial tree: Radiographic and CT findings in 12 patients. Radiology. 1999;212(3):643-48.
51. Naidich DP. CT/MR correlation in the evaluation of tracheobronchial neoplasia. Radiol Clin North Am. 1990;28:555-71.
52. Marchiori E, de Araujo Neto C, Meirelles GSP, et al. Laryngotracheobronchial papillomatosis: findings on computed tomography scans of the chest. J Bras Pneumol. 2008;34(12):1084-9
53. Shoemark A, Ozerovitch L, Wilson R. Etiology in adult patients with bronchiectasis. Respir Med. 2007;191:1163-70.
54. Nejad CJ, Bhalla S. Bronchiectasis. Radiol Clin N Am. 2009;47(2):88-306.
55. Muller NL, Fraser RS, Lee KS, et al. Diseases of the lung-radiologic and pathologic correlations, 1st edition. [chapter 15]. Philadelphia: Lippincott Williams and Wilkins. 2003:280-1.
56. Hartman TE, Primack SL, Lee KS, et al. CT of bronchial and bronchiolar diseases. Radiographics. 1994;14:991-1003.
57. Kinsella D, Sissons G, Williams MP. The radiological imaging of bronchial atresia. Br J Radiol. 1992;65:681.
58. Martinez S, Heyneman LE, McAdams HP, et al. Mucoid impactions: Finger-in-glove sign and other CT and radiographic features. Radiographics. 2008;28:1369-82.
59. Bhalla M, Turcios N, Aponte V, et al. Cystic fibrosis: scoring system with thin-section CT. Radiology. 1991;179(3):783-8.
60. Brown DE, Pittman JE, Leigh MW, et al. Early lung disease in young children with primary ciliary dyskinesia. Pediatr Pulmonol. 2008;43:514-16.
61. Agarwal R, Khan A, Garg M, Aggarwal AN, Gupta D. Pictorial essay: Allergic bronchopulmonary aspergillosis. Indian J Radiol Imaging. 2011;21:242-52.

Radhika Batra, Swati Gupta, Alpana Manchanda

CHAPTER

15

Small Airway Imaging

INTRODUCTION

Small airways refer to the small membranous and respiratory bronchioles (internal diameter <2 mm) which lack cartilage and submucosal glands in their walls.[1] According to the Fleischner Society: glossary of terms for thoracic imaging, small airway disease is an umbrella term which summarizes diseases of the peripheral airways. The definitions of the term vary. Some radiologists consider small airways as those with an internal diameter of less than or equal to 2 mm and a wall thickness of less than 0.5 mm. Others regard the level of the bronchiole as the demarcation between central and peripheral airways. Although the two definitions are not consistent, the first one appears more practical and is more commonly used in literature.[2]

High-resolution computed tomography (HRCT) of the chest plays an essential role in the diagnosis of small airway disease and provides a detailed evaluation of the lung parenchyma and the interstitium. On CT examination, these diseases can manifest as peribronchiolar and/or bronchiolar abnormalities, including tree-in-bud opacities, centrilobular micronodules, air trapping, bronchiolectasis, oligemia, or a combination of these findings.[3]

ANATOMY

A basic knowledge of the anatomy of the secondary pulmonary lobule (SPL) is essential for recognizing small airway disease. A SPL is the smallest structural unit of the lung parenchyma, encased in a connective tissue sheath. It has an irregular polyhedral or pyramidal shape, with length ranging from 5 to 25 mm. There are 3–25 acini within a SPL. The central portion of the SPL contains bronchioles and their accompanying pulmonary arterioles and lymphatic vessels which are also known as the "core structures" or "centrilobular structures". The connective tissue surrounding the lobule contains veins and additional lymphatic vessels. The lobule also features an internal support system, the intralobular interstitium. CT imaging can effectively reveal the three main components of a normal secondary pulmonary lobule—the central structures, the region containing the acini, and the connective tissue sheath that forms the interlobular septa.[2]

There is dichotomous branching in the airways with about 23 divisions from the trachea to the alveoli.[4] Bronchi are conducting airways with cartilage in their walls, while bronchioles are airways which do not have cartilage. Small bronchi give rise to membranous bronchioles. Membranous bronchioles conduct air whereas respiratory bronchioles supply alveoli and provide gas exchange. The terminal bronchiole is the last purely conducting membranous bronchiole and does not participate in gas exchange. It is roughly 0.7 mm in diameter, and gives rise to respiratory bronchioles. A respiratory bronchiole is the largest bronchiole which participates in gas exchange. It gives rise to alveolar ducts and alveoli. The interalveolar pores of Kohn and the canals of Lambert are important collateral channels, the former provide direct communication between alveoli and the latter between membranous bronchioles and adjacent alveoli.[5,6]

In normal lung these airways offer minimal resistance, however, their combined cross-sectional area is so extensive that even slight abnormalities in the small airways can significantly impact lung function. Normal bronchioles are not visible on HRCT chest and visible bronchiolar abnormalities suggest underlying small airways inflammation and/or fibrosis.

IMAGING OF SMALL AIRWAY DISEASE

HRCT chest is an essential tool for diagnosing small airway disease. Thin-section images with high spatial

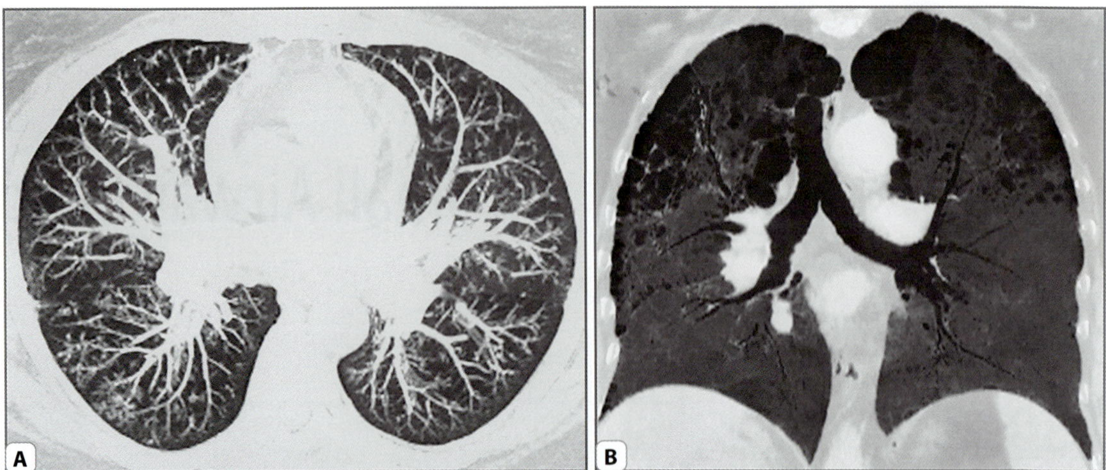

FIGS. 1A AND B: Axial MIP image (A) demonstrates multiple centrilobular nodules in right lower lobe. Coronal MinIP (B) image demonstrates paraseptal and centriacinar emphysema in bilateral lungs, more marked in upper lobes.

(MIP: maximum intensity projection; MinIP: minimum intensity projection)

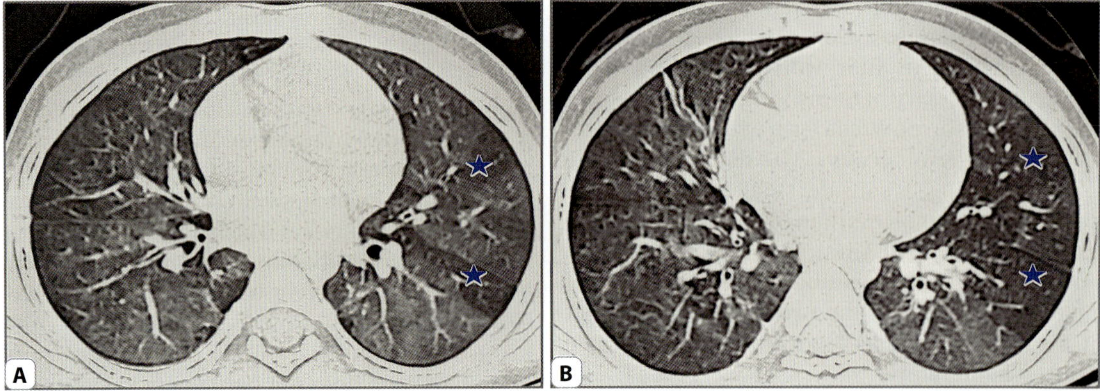

FIGS. 2A AND B: In a patient with bronchial asthma, axial CT chest images in lung window in inspiration (A) and expiration (B) show geographic areas of hypoattenuation suggestive of air trapping bilaterally (★ in A and B), which are accentuated on expiratory scan (B).

resolution (typically 1–1.5 mm thick to minimize partial volume averaging) enable precise identification of abnormalities. Multiplanar volume reconstructions can be made. Maximum intensity projection (MIP) and minimum intensity projection (MinIP) images highlight voxels with the highest and lowest attenuation values, respectively. MIPs enhance the detection of pulmonary nodules, including small centrilobular nodules, tree-in-bud opacities, and poorly defined centrilobular nodules, while MinIPs are particularly useful for identifying traction bronchiectasis and mosaic attenuation **(Figs. 1A and B)**.[5-7] For patients suspected of having small airway disease, the imaging evaluation should also include expiratory phase scans to assess for air trapping **(Figs. 2A and B)**.

DIRECT AND INDIRECT SIGNS OF SMALL AIRWAY DISEASE

The small airways are generally not visible on HRCT, they become visible at the centre of the SPL as increased soft tissue density in or around the bronchiole and bronchiolar wall thickening. This can be seen as centrilobular or tree-in-bud nodules. Bronchiolectasis which is dilatation of bronchioles can also be seen and is associated with a chronic fibrotic process in the subpleural lung.

Centrilobular nodules may be solid or ground glass attenuation and are distributed in the centre of the SPL, several millimeters from the pleural surfaces, fissures and interlobular septa. The most common cause is infections

BOX 1: Causes of tree-in-bud pattern.

- *Infection*:
  - Bacterial:
    - *Mycobacterium tuberculosis*
    - *M. avium* intracellulare complex
    - *Staphylococcus aureus*
    - *Haemophilus influenzae*
  - Fungal:
    - *Aspergillus*
  - Viral:
    - Cytomegalovirus
    - Respiratory syncytial virus
- *Congenital disorders*:
  - Cystic fibrosis
  - Kartagener syndrome
- *Aspiration*
- *Inhalation*:
  - Toxic fumes and gases
- *Allergic bronchopulmonary aspergillosis*
- *Connective tissue disorders*:
  - Rheumatoid arthritis
  - Sjögren syndrome
- *Neoplasms*:
  - Gastric cancer
  - Breast cancer
  - Ewing sarcoma
  - Renal cancer

(bacterial, viral, mycobacterial). Other causes include smoking related respiratory bronchiolitis, hypersensitivity pneumonitis and follicular bronchiolitis. The tree-in-bud pattern consists of multiple small clusters of soft tissue attenuation connected to multiple branching linear structures of similar caliber which originate from a single stalk. **Box 1** enlists the various causes of tree-in-bud pattern.

Indirect signs of small airway disease include mosaic attenuation and air trapping. Mosaic attenuation refers to areas of differing attenuation on CT lung. Air trapping is seen on end-expiratory CT scans as sharply defined areas with less than expected increase in attenuation and a lack of volume reduction as in a normal lung.[8,9]

BRONCHIOLITIS

Bronchiolitis refers to a small airway disease which can be classified according to etiology and histologic features. The two forms of bronchiolitis include cellular bronchiolitis and constrictive bronchiolitis.[10] In cellular bronchiolitis inflammatory cells are the predominant histopathological finding. Cellular infiltration in peribronchial alveoli manifests as poorly defined centrilobular nodules which may be solid or ground glass attenuation on HRCT. Constrictive bronchiolitis is a fibrotic process with luminal narrowing by collagenous fibrosis and scarring which may be subtle or result in complete luminal obliteration.[5]

Cellular Bronchiolitis

Infectious Bronchiolitis

Infectious bronchiolitis (IB) results from the inflammation of bronchioles due to infections which may be caused by viruses, bacteria or fungi. Inflammatory infiltrates in the airway wall and adjacent alveoli are seen on histology. Certain histologic findings may suggest a specific diagnosis such as the presence of hyphae indicates infection due to *Aspergillus* while acid fast bacilli may be seen in *Mycobacterium tuberculosis* infection.

Chest radiographs may be normal or show bilateral nodular or reticulonodular opacities. Thickening of walls of the airway and peribronchial consolidations are common in children. On CT scan IB is characterized by centrilobular nodules, branching tree-in-bud opacities and bronchial wall thickening.[11,12] The nodules may be patchy and asymmetric and either unilateral or bilateral. Although presence of tree-in-bud nodules is highly suggestive of IB it is not specific and may be seen in various other non-infectious conditions including aspiration, cystic fibrosis.[11-13]

Chronic IB is more frequently seen in adults. The presence of bronchiectasis primarily affecting right middle lobe and lingula suggests a chronic nontuberculous *Mycobacterium* infection while presence of other findings such as cavitary lesions suggests *Mycobacterium tuberculosis* **(Figs. 3A and B)**.[14,15]

Follicular Bronchiolitis

Follicular bronchiolitis (FB) is a cellular bronchiolitis which is characterized by peribronchial and peribronchiolar lymphoid follicles with germinal centers along bronchial walls on histology. The conditions associated with FB include immunologic disorders such as Sjögren syndrome, autoimmune hemolytic anemia, chronic active hepatitis, primary biliary cirrhosis, myasthenia gravis, immunodeficiency such as HIV/AIDS, allergy, asthma and allogenic bone marrow transplantation.

FB usually occurs in middle aged adults but may be seen in children who are immunocompromised. The presenting symptoms include progressive worsening dyspnea and cough. Pulmonary function tests reveal a mixed pattern of obstructive and restrictive functional abnormality. The treatment consists of corticosteroids.

On chest radiographs, FB presents with hyperinflation, small nodules and bilateral reticular or reticulonodular opacities, however, the findings may be subtle. HRCT chest demonstrates diffuse poorly defined centrilobular nodules. Other findings include peribronchial and subpleural nodules, patchy ground glass opacities, bronchial wall thickening and patchy areas of low attenuation.[16]

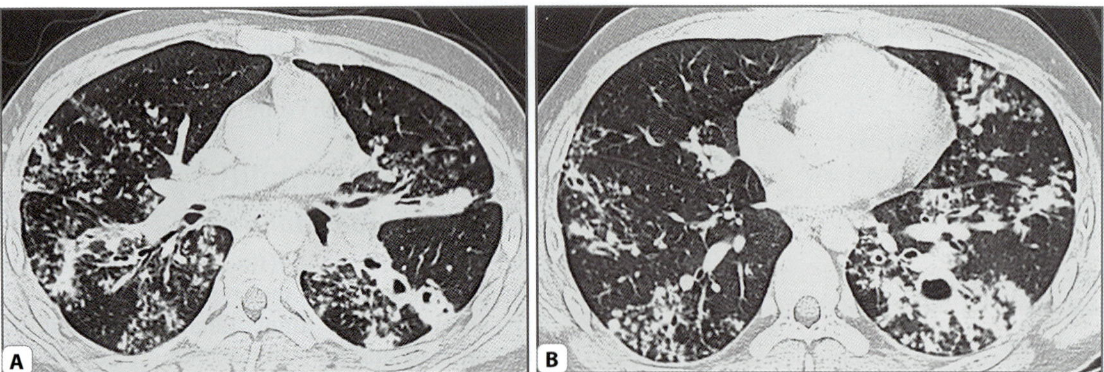

FIGS. 3A AND B: Axial CT chest images in lung window show cavitary lesions in left lower lobe with centrilobular nodules and tree-in-bud opacities in bilateral lungs suggestive of *Mycobacterium tuberculosis* infection.

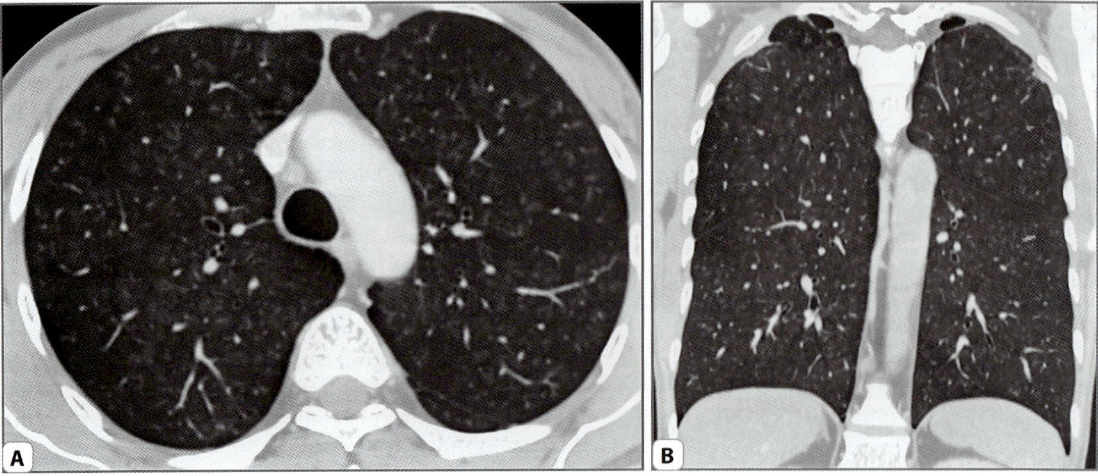

FIGS. 4A AND B: Axial (A) and coronal (B) CT chest images in lung window in an adult male patient with history of active cigarette smoking demonstrate innumerable centrilobular ground-glass nodules in bilateral lungs suggestive of respiratory bronchiolitis.

Respiratory Bronchiolitis

Respiratory bronchiolitis (RB) and RB-associated ILD (RB-ILD) are associated with smoking. They are characterized by submucosal inflammation and fibrosis of the respiratory bronchioles alongwith the presence of fine pigment laden pulmonary macrophages in the airway lumen.

Patients with RB are usually asymptomatic while those with RB-ILD present with cough and progressive shortness of breath. Pulmonary function tests reveal a restrictive or mixed (obstructive and restrictive) pattern of disease. On CT, ill-defined centrilobular nodules and patchy ground glass opacities with upper lobe predominance are seen in RB **(Figs. 4 and 5)**. RB-ILD is characterized by centrilobular nodules in upper lobes with findings being more marked as compared to RB. Additional findings may include reticular opacities representing mild pulmonary fibrosis in lower lobes, bronchial wall thickening and emphysema. Histological abnormalities are reversible with cessation of smoking which is recommended for these patients.[17,18]

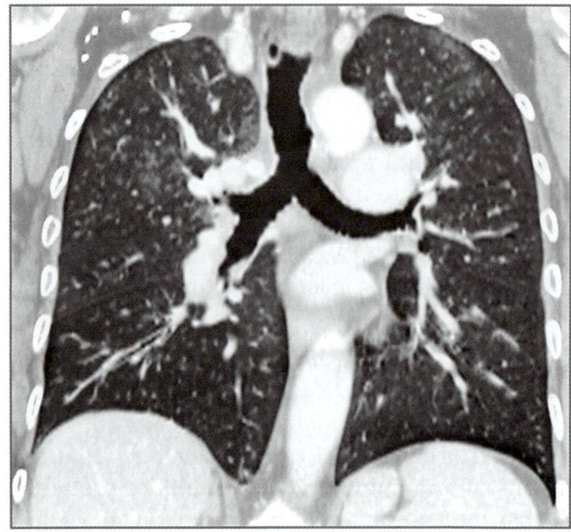

FIG. 5: Coronal CT chest image in lung window in another adult male patient with history of active cigarette smoking demonstrates centrilobular ground-glass nodules bilaterally with upper lobe predominance-respiratory bronchiolitis.

Diffuse Panbronchiolitis

Diffuse panbronchiolitis (DPB) is a progressive form of cellular bronchiolitis which is characterized by inflammation of the respiratory bronchioles. On histology, DPB is characterized by transmural infiltration of the bronchiolar interstitium and peribronchial tissue by foamy macrophages, lymphocytes and plasma cells; the terminal bronchioles may be ectatic.

It is almost exclusively seen in Asians, especially in adults of Japanese, Korean or Chinese origin. Middle aged men are commonly affected and no association with smoking is known. Presenting symptoms include productive cough, dyspnea, sinusitis and purulent sputum. Colonization of the respiratory tract by *Pseudomonas aeruginosa* is frequently seen in affected patients. Pulmonary function tests reveal marked obstruction and mild restrictive disease. Treatment includes long term low dose erythromycin or other macrolides. The long-term prognosis is poor with progression of bronchiectasis.

Chest radiographs reveal diffuse nodules, reticulonodular opacities with lower lobe predominance and mild-to-moderate hyperinflation. In early stages, HRCT chest shows tree-in-bud pattern while in later stages bullae, air trapping and mosaic attenuation can be seen.[19] The imaging features may overlap with those of other inflammatory airway diseases including follicular bronchiolitis and constrictive bronchiolitis.

Hypersensitivity Pneumonitis

Hypersensitivity pneumonitis (HP) results from an immune mediated reaction to inhaled organic and inorganic antigens. The organism or protein complex lodges in the terminal and respiratory bronchioles and induces non-necrotizing granulomas with adjacent peribronchiolar metaplasia of variable severity. In the subacute phase patients present with cough and dyspnea which has an insidious onset.

On HRCT chest, centrilobular nodules are seen, which are ground glass nodules located in the center of the secondary pulmonary nodule. These are more profuse in the nonfibrotic form of HP **(Figs. 6A and B)**. Upper and mid zone predominance of the nodules may be seen. The "three-density sign" is considered to be most specific for HP and is characterized by the presence of all three attenuations including ground glass opacification, decreased attenuation and areas of normal attenuation **(Figs. 7A to C)**.[20-22] The "three-density sign" was formerly known as the "head cheese sign". Pulmonary edema and diffuse air space opacification are seen in acute HP.

Imaging features in fibrotic HP include reticular or ground glass opacities associated with tractional bronchiectasis or bronchiolectasis, lobar volume loss and honey combing **(Figs. 8A and B)**. Presence or absence of fibrosis has implications for treatment and prognosis; therefore, the American Thoracic Society's recent guidelines recommend that HP should be subclassified based simply on the presence or absence of histological or radiological evidence of fibrosis.[20]

Aspiration Bronchiolitis

Aspiration bronchiolitis (AB) is characterized by chronic inflammation of bronchioles which results from recurrent aspiration of foreign particles. Patients with oropharyngeal dysphagia, neurologic disorders and gastroparesis are prone to be affected. Presenting complaints include chronic cough, wheezing and fever, however, many patients may be asymptomatic. Histologically, it is characterized by chronic mural inflammation and scarring of bronchioles with foreign body giant cells.

Chest radiographs show nodular opacities which may be unilateral or bilateral and hyperinflation.[23,24] HRCT chest demonstrates disseminated centrilobular branching nodules with tree-in-bud pattern along with adjacent areas of lobular consolidation. The lower lobes and posterior segments of upper lobes are usually affected **(Figs. 9A to C)**. Central bronchi may show the presence of aspirated material. Bronchial wall thickening and bronchiectasis may be seen with recurrent aspiration.

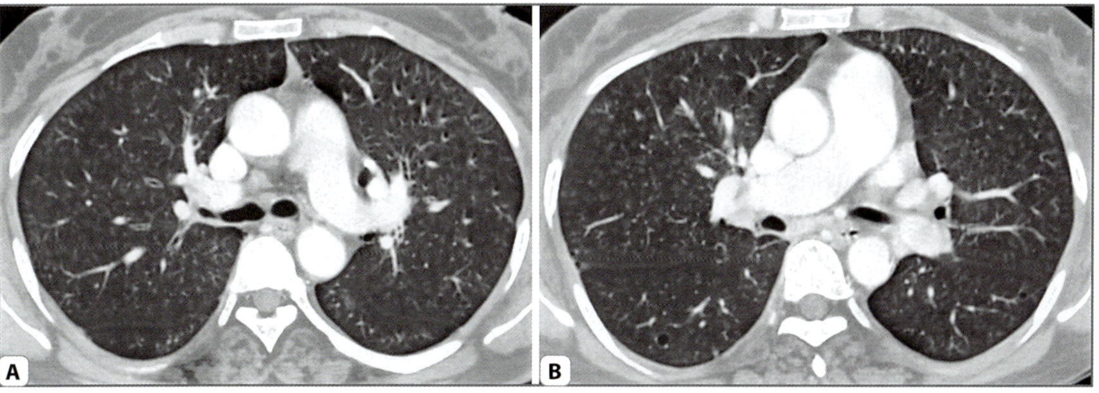

FIGS. 6A AND B: Axial chest CT images (lung window) of an adult woman with pet birds demonstrate numerous centrilobular ground-glass nodules diffusely involving both lungs: subacute hypersensitivity pneumonitis.

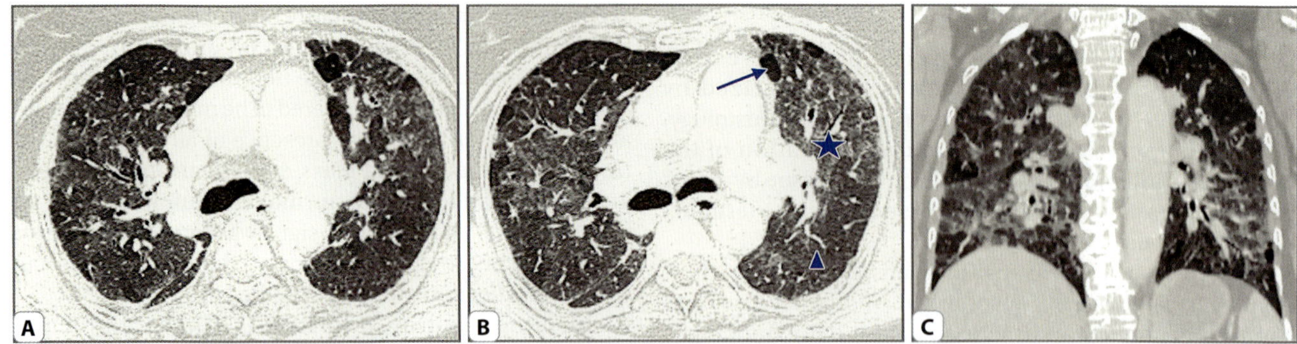

FIGS. 7A TO C: Axial (A and B) and coronal (C) chest CT images in lung window demonstrate the "three-density-sign" of hypersensitivity pneumonitis with sharply demarcated areas of three different attenuations—normal lung, areas of ground glass opacities and areas of hyperlucent lung corresponding with air trapping (▲, ✶ and ⟶ in B).

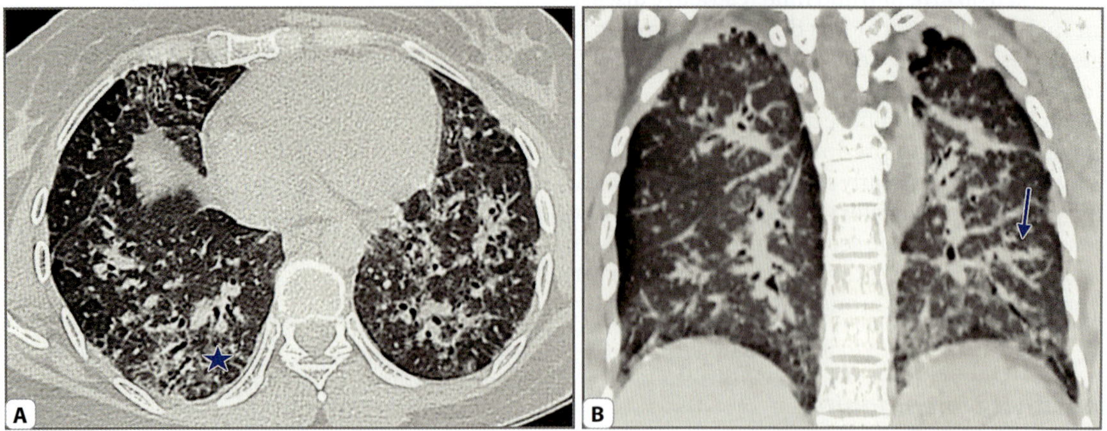

FIGS. 8A AND B: In a case of fibrotic hypersensitivity pneumonitis axial (A) and coronal (B) CT chest images in lung window show reticular (✶ in A) and fibrotic opacities (⟶ in B) in bilateral lungs with tractional bronchiectasis and few areas of air trapping.

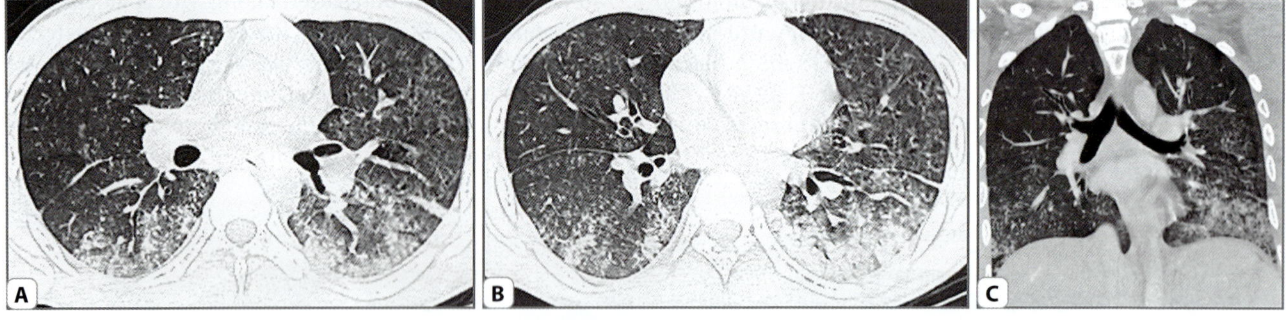

FIGS. 9A TO C: Axial (A and B) and coronal (C) CT chest images in lung window show multiple centrilobular nodular opacities and areas of consolidation in dependent areas of bilateral lungs in a patient with aspiration bronchiolitis.

Table 1 lists the differential diagnosis for cellular bronchiolitis.

Constrictive Bronchiolitis

Constrictive bronchiolitis (CB) is an irreversible disorder which is characterized by submucosal fibrosis resulting in narrowing or occlusion of bronchioles. Histologically there is concentric luminal inflammation and fibrosis of bronchioles, accumulation of fibroblasts and fibroproliferation results from injury to respiratory epithelium. CB can be caused by childhood infection, inhalational lung disease, lung transplant rejection, graft-versus-host disease in stem cell transplant recipients and connective tissue disorders.

The presenting symptoms in patients with CB include dyspnea and chronic cough. The symptoms follow a lower respiratory tract infection in postinfectious cases.

TABLE 1: Differential diagnosis for cellular bronchiolitis.

Cause	Imaging features	Clinical features
Infectious bronchiolitis	• Tree-in-bud opacities • Focal or multifocal involvement • *Cavitation*: Tuberculosis	• Infectious symptoms • History of immunocompromise • History of bronchiectasis
Follicular bronchiolitis	• Focal/multifocal or diffuse nodules • May be seen with other ILD (CTD related)	• Mostly develops with underlying systemic disorder • CTD • HIV • Common variable immunodeficiency
Respiratory bronchiolitis	• Bilateral and diffuse involvement with upper-lobe predominance • Other diseases related to smoking (emphysema, DIP, LCH)	History of smoking
Diffuse panbronchiolitis	• Nodules and bronchial wall thickening • Progression to bronchiectasis, air trapping and cysts/bullae	• Asian descent • Chronic sinusitis • *Pseudomonas aeruginosa* or *Haemophilus influenzae* may be present in sputum
Hypersensitivity pneumonitis	• Mostly diffuse, symmetric nodules • Air trapping and ground glass opacities may be present	• Mostly nonsmokers • History of exposure
Aspiration bronchiolitis	• Tree-in-bud opacities • Dependent portions of lungs • Focal or multifocal involvement	• Predisposing factors to aspiration • Oropharyngeal dysfunction • Head and neck malignancies

TABLE 2: Differential diagnosis for constrictive bronchiolitis.

Cause	Imaging features	Clinical features
Infection	Hyperlucency of lobe or lung with air trapping, reduced vascularity and bronchiectasis	Childhood airway infection, usually viral
Connective tissue disease	Air trapping	• Known CTD, usually rheumatoid arthritis; also seen with scleroderma, lupus erythematosus, Sjögren syndrome • Progressive dyspnea, cough
Inhalational	• Air trapping • Bronchiectasis may be seen	Smoke inhalation from burning of synthetic building materials
Lung transplantation	Air trapping	Risk factors include acute cellular rejection, primary graft dysfunction, gastroesophageal reflux disease and respiratory infections
Stem cell transplantation	Air trapping	Affected patients develop graft-versus-host disease
DIPNECH	• Air trapping • Nodular bronchial wall thickening • Small parenchymal nodules	Middle aged or elderly females

The condition follows a progressive chronic course over weeks or months. Pulmonary function tests show airflow obstruction with a mixed restrictive and obstructive pattern. CB can progress to cor pulmonale and right heart failure.

Chest radiographs are usually normal and may show only mild hyperinflation, sometimes, nodular and reticular pulmonary opacities can be seen. CT demonstrates a pattern of mosaic attenuation where geographic areas of mixed lung attenuation are seen. The lucent areas result from air trapping and are accentuated on expiratory scan images. There is a decrease in the size of vascular structures in the areas of low attenuation due to hypoxic vasoconstriction. Bronchial wall thickening or bronchiectasis may be seen. Tree-in-bud opacities or centrilobular nodules are usually absent.[3] **Table 2** lists the differential diagnosis for constrictive bronchiolitis.

Postinfectious Constrictive Bronchiolitis

Constrictive bronchiolitis may result as sequelae of recurrent childhood viral pneumonias. Swyer–James–Macleod syndrome is a condition with unilateral small lung with diffuse or lobar pulmonary hyperlucency due to constrictive bronchiolitis and hypoplasia of pulmonary arteries which results from repeated insult to lung parenchyma from childhood pneumonias.[25] CB may also be a sequela to endobronchial tuberculosis, *Mycoplasma pneumoniae* or *Pneumocystis jiroveci* infection in patients with AIDS.

Chest radiographs may be normal or may show hyperinflation or scarring from prior infection. CT demonstrates focal areas of scarring and bronchiectasis from prior infection with hyperinflation on inspiratory CT **(Figs. 10A to C)**.

Connective Tissue Disorders

Constrictive bronchiolitis may be seen in association with connective tissue disorders such as rheumatoid arthritis, polymyositis, dermatomyositis, SLE, scleroderma and Sjögren syndrome. Chest radiograph may be normal or show hyperinflation. CT shows mosaic pulmonary attenuation. Other manifestations of connective tissue disorders such as interstitial lung disease, rheumatoid nodules, esophageal abnormalities and pleural effusion may also be seen **(Figs. 11A to C)**.

Inhalational Injury

Exposure to toxic fumes from burning of synthetic building materials which produce gases such as nitrogen dioxide, sulfur dioxide, acrolein, formaldehyde and acetaldehyde can result in constrictive bronchiolitis.

Post-transplant

Bronchiolitis obliterans syndrome occurs as a complication of lung transplantation. It is a chronic allograft rejection and is associated with decreased pulmonary function. The most sensitive and specific feature is air trapping on expiratory HRCT chest in patients post-transplant although the degree of air trapping does not correlate with severity of rejection. Bronchiolitis obliterans syndrome occurs in approximately 50% of patients with lung transplant and in 5% of hematopoietic stem cell transplant recipients.

Constrictive bronchiolitis is also a manifestation of graft-versus-host disease associated with hematopoietic stem cell transplantation. As in other causes of chronic bronchiolitis, air trapping is the predominant finding on imaging.[3]

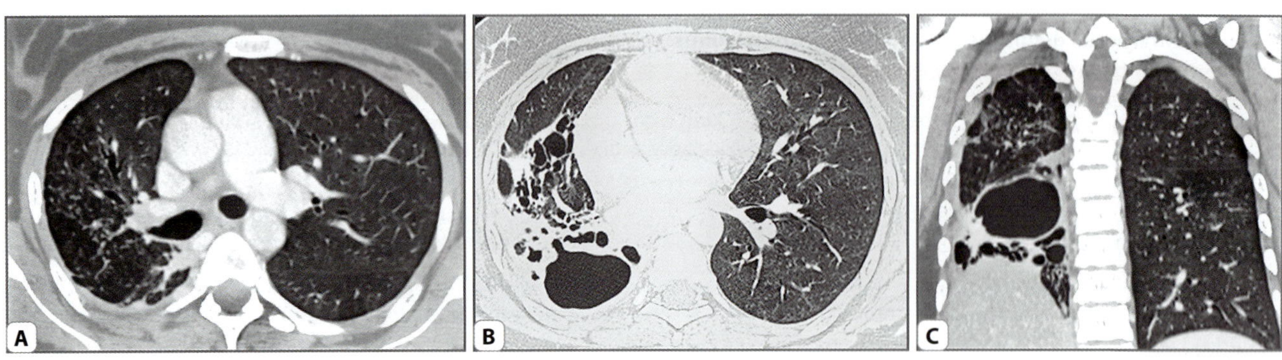

FIGS. 10A TO C: Axial (A and B) and coronal (C) CT chest images in lung window show cystic bronchiectasis in right lung. The right lung also shows decreased attenuation and evidence of volume loss. Few centrilobular nodules seen in right upper lobe.

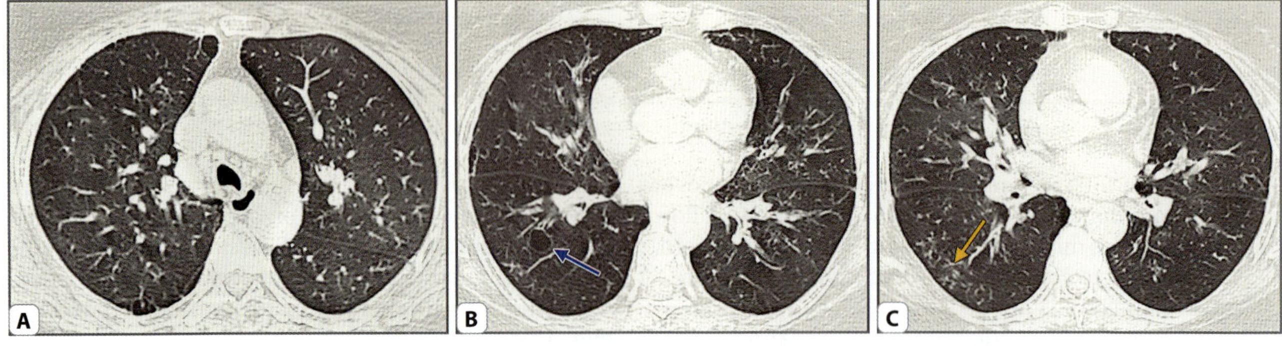

FIGS. 11A TO C: In a lady with rheumatoid arthritis, axial CT chest images in lung window show mosaic attenuation bilaterally; areas of hypoattenuation suggestive of air trapping are noted. Few centrilobular nodules (⟶ in C) and a lung cyst (⟶ in B) are seen in right lower lobe.

Diffuse Idiopathic Pulmonary Neuroendocrine Cell Hyperplasia

Diffuse idiopathic pulmonary neuroendocrine cell hyperplasia (DIPNECH) is usually seen in middle aged and older women and is not associated with smoking. Patients may be asymptomatic or present with nonproductive cough, dyspnea and wheezing. Pulmonary function tests reveal an obstructive or mixed obstructive and restrictive ventilation defect. The disease is slowly progressive and usually not fatal.

Plain radiographs are often normal or may demonstrate hyperinflation or small pulmonary nodules. On CT, multiple small solid or ground glass pulmonary nodules are seen. The nodules may enlarge slowly or remain stable. Mosaic attenuation can also be seen with areas of air trapping on expiratory images.[3]

CHRONIC OBSTRUCTIVE PULMONARY DISEASE

Chronic obstructive pulmonary disease (COPD) is characterized by chronic airflow obstruction due to chronic bronchitis, emphysema or both. It is a progressive disease which presents with dyspnea and chronic cough. Advances in imaging allow quantitative and qualitative analysis of the lung parenchyma and related airways, vascular and extrapulmonary manifestations of COPD. Imaging helps in prognostication of disease and also to guide pharmacological and nonpharmacological interventions.

Chest radiographs in emphysema reveal hyperlucent lungs with flattening of diaphragm, vascular pruning, widening of intercostal spaces and narrowed, vertical cardiac silhouette. Bullae may be seen which appear as well demarcated hyperlucent areas which are devoid of vascular markings **(Fig. 12)**. Hyperinflation can result in increased retrosternal space and anteroposterior diameter of chest (barrel chest) on lateral chest radiographs. Increased bronchovascular markings, also referred to as "dirty lungs" may be seen due to chronic bronchitis which is often concomitant with emphysema **(Fig. 13)**.[26] Advances in chest radiography include dark field radiographic imaging and dynamic radiography for pulmonary functional imaging. Dark field radiography relies on scattering of X-rays at tissue interfaces, highlighting the alveolar microstructure in lungs. In emphysematous lungs, the damaged alveoli lead to increased scattering resulting in dark areas on the dark field image, indicating the extent of emphysema. Dynamic chest radiography enables the acquisition of sequential chest radiographs at lower radiation exposure while subjects are either standing or sitting. This method allows for the evaluation of diaphragm and thoracic cage movements, as well as lung ventilation and perfusion. Lung ventilation is assessed by observing changes in local pixel values during breathing.[27]

CT scan imaging is an accurate imaging method for the characterization of COPD. It helps in diagnosing emphysema and also in detecting the type, extent and distribution of emphysema. Volumetric full chest scan is performed in full inspiration with slice thickness of 1–1.25 mm and reconstructed with a high spatial frequency or sharpening algorithm. Coronal and sagittal reconstructions can be obtained. Maximum intensity projection images can help in detection of nodules while minimum intensity projection images can help to show the presence and extent of emphysema. Airway disease

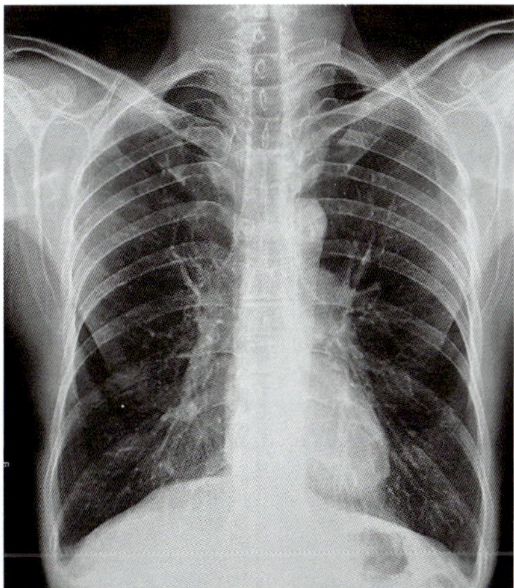

FIG. 12: Chest radiograph posteroanterior (PA) view shows emphysematous lungs bilaterally which appear hyperinflated and hyperlucent. Note is made of flattening of diaphragm and tubular heart shadow.

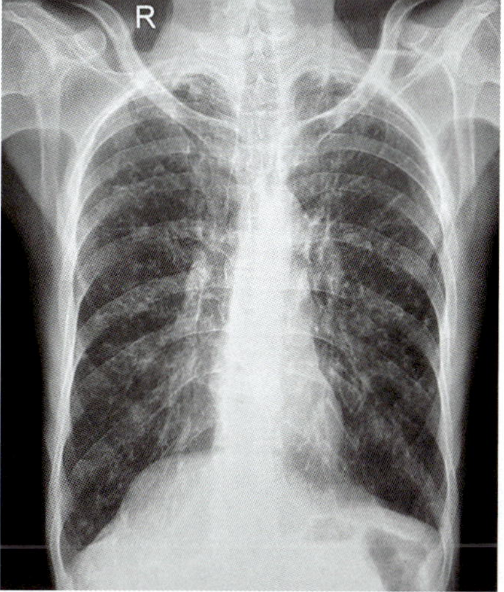

FIG. 13: Chest radiograph posteroanterior (PA) view shows hyperinflated lungs bilaterally with prominent bronchovascular markings referred to as "dirty lungs" in a patient with chronic bronchitis. Note is made of flattening of diaphragm and tubular heart shadow.

may manifest as bronchial wall thickening, bronchiectasis, centrilobular nodules, air trapping or a combination of these findings **(Figs. 14A and B)**. End-expiratory imaging can be used to assess air trapping.

Emphysema can be classified into three major subtypes, which include centrilobular, paraseptal and panacinar emphysema. These subtypes may coexist **(Figs. 15A to C)**. Centrilobular or centriacinar emphysema is the most common type and is associated with cigarette smoking. Pathologically, the central portion of the acinus is destroyed. On CT, they may appear to arise from the centre of the secondary pulmonary lobule. Centrilobular emphysema usually affects the upper lobes and superior segments of lower lobes and the central lungs more affected than the peripheral lungs. Mild-to-moderate centrilobular emphysema is characterized by multiple round or oval low attenuation areas which are several millimetres in size and predominantly scattered in upper and inner lung zones. As opposed to lung cysts, these areas of low attenuation do not have definable walls and are bordered by normal lung parenchyma. They may coalesce to form larger lucencies with well-defined and thin walls formed by adjacent compressed lung parenchyma. The presence of preserved lung parenchyma around large airways and vessels helps in identifying that emphysema has originated in the centrilobular portion.

Paraseptal or distal acinar emphysema affects the subpleural upper lungs including perifissural and peribronchovascular lung parenchyma. This type may not be associated with smoking. Pathologically, there is destruction of distal portion of the acinus—alveolar ducts and sacs. On CT, paraseptal emphysema is seen as subpleural and peribrochovascular areas of low attenuation varying from few millimeters to one centimeter in diameter, separated by thin intact interlobular septa. In contrast, honeycombing is multi-layered, more frequent at the lung bases, has thicker walls and is associated with fibrosis and architectural distortion. Pneumothorax from blebs and bullae may be seen in young patients.

Panacinar or panlobular emphysema affects the lower lung zones and is usually associated with alpha-1 antitrypsin deficiency. Other causes may include Swyer–James syndrome and injection of talc containing substances (mostly seen with drug abuse). Pathologically, there is uniform enlargement of the entire acini. On CT, they appear as extensive areas of uniform low attenuation and result in greater degree of hyperinflation than centrilobular emphysema.

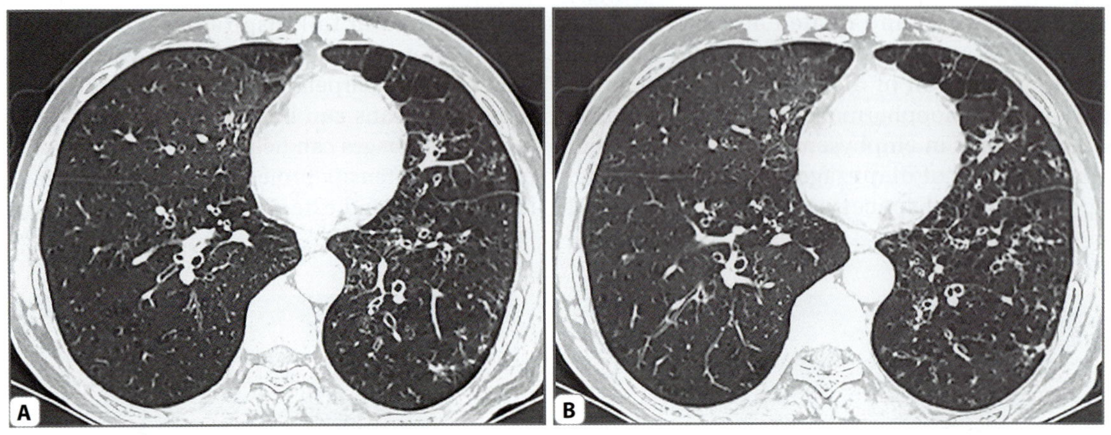

FIGS. 14A AND B: Axial chest CT (lung window) in an elderly man shows centriacinar emphysematous changes in bilateral lungs with centrilobular nodules in lingula and left lower lobe.

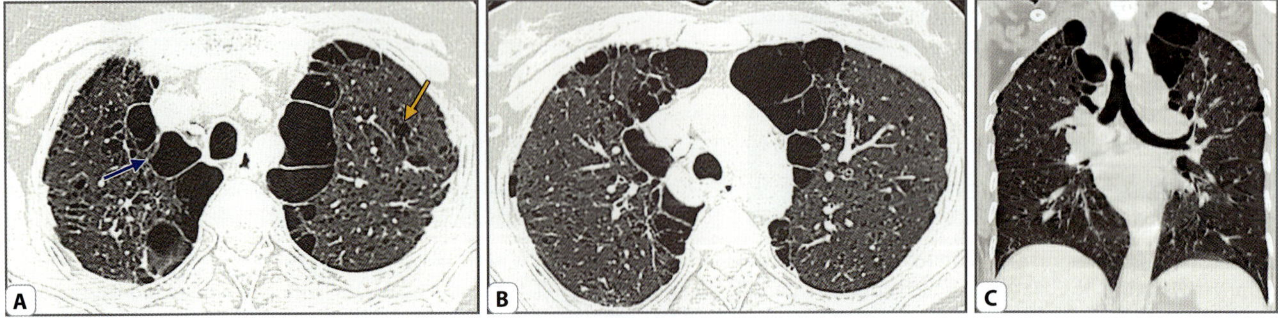

FIGS. 15A TO C: Axial (A and B) and coronal (C) chest CT images in lung window show paraseptal (⟶ in A) and centriacinar emphysematous (⟶ in A) changes in bilateral lungs.

On CT, emphysema can be seen as focal, regional or diffuse areas of low attenuation. On inspiratory CT scan a reduced tissue density due to emphysema is represented by lower pixel values, i.e., a low attenuation area (LAA) or low attenuation volume (LAV). Low attenuation area percent (LAA%) or low attenuation volume percent (LAV%) are defined as percentage of all LAAs to the total lung area or the percentage of all LAVs to the total lung volume and are associated with symptoms, decline in FEV_1, exacerbations and mortality. A LAA% (or LAV%) of 5% is considered the threshold for detecting clinically relevant emphysema **(Fig. 16)**.[28]

Quantitative Assessment of Emphysema

The primary methods for quantifying emphysema on CT scans are the threshold technique and histogram analysis. Both approaches rely on the fact that emphysematous lung tissue exhibits lower attenuation compared to normal lung parenchyma. Since their introduction, several variations of these techniques have emerged, driven largely by advancements in CT technology and image processing software including 3D assessment of lung density, enabled by the rapid image acquisition capabilities of multidetector CT, which allows for the evaluation of the entire lung volume.

Threshold technique: In this method, emphysema is identified when the attenuation values of pixels in a region of interest fall below a predetermined Hounsfield unit (HU) threshold. A threshold of –950 HU has been shown to correlate well with pulmonary function tests and pathological findings when performing thin-section CT with 10 mm intervals. Other threshold values between –900 and –980 HU have also been used, with the optimal value depending on various factors such as scanning parameters.

Histogram analysis: This technique detects emphysema by examining the attenuation values of pixels in relation to a predefined percentile. The characteristic enlargement of distal airspaces and the destruction of alveolar walls in emphysema lead to a reduced ratio of the surface area of distal airspace walls to lung volume (AWUV). Unlike the threshold technique, which uses an absolute HU value as a marker for emphysema, histogram analysis can underestimate emphysema severity if other conditions (such as pulmonary masses or consolidations) cause a shift in the overall histogram distribution toward higher Hounsfield values.[26]

Recent advancements in lung MRI technology enable the assessment of lung function without the risks associated with radiation exposure. *Oxygen-enhanced pulmonary MRI* provides insights into regional oxygen transfer across the alveolar membrane by using inhaled oxygen as a contrast agent. This technique has been shown to correlate with pulmonary function in patients with COPD. However, because oxygen inhalation produces only minimal changes in signal intensity, multiple acquisitions or longer acquisition times are often necessary, especially for whole-lung imaging.

In *hyperpolarized noble gas MRI*, emphysema can be quantified by measuring the apparent diffusion coefficient (ADC) using inhaled hyperpolarized ^{3}He or ^{129}Xe gas. These gases diffuse within the lung microstructure during breath-hold at inspiration. Additionally, ventilation defects can be visualized and quantified as the ventilation defect percentage (VDP), which has been found to predict future exacerbations in COPD patients.[29,30]

Coregistered chest CT and functional MRI, using parametric response mapping, have further demonstrated that areas with normal CT but low MRI ventilation (indicative of small airway disease) and those with normal CT but high ADC (suggesting mild emphysema) are negatively correlated with FEV_1 and DLCO in both

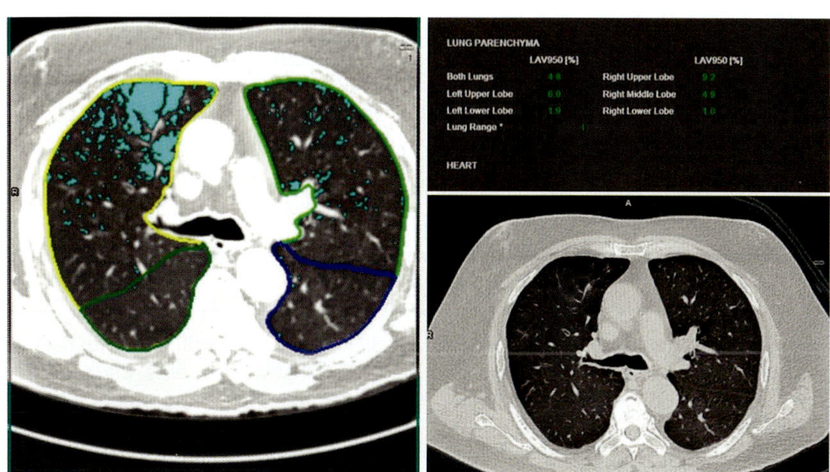

FIG. 16: Axial CT images in lung window show low attenuation volume percent (LAV%) of 4.8%, which is just below the threshold for clinically significant emphysema.

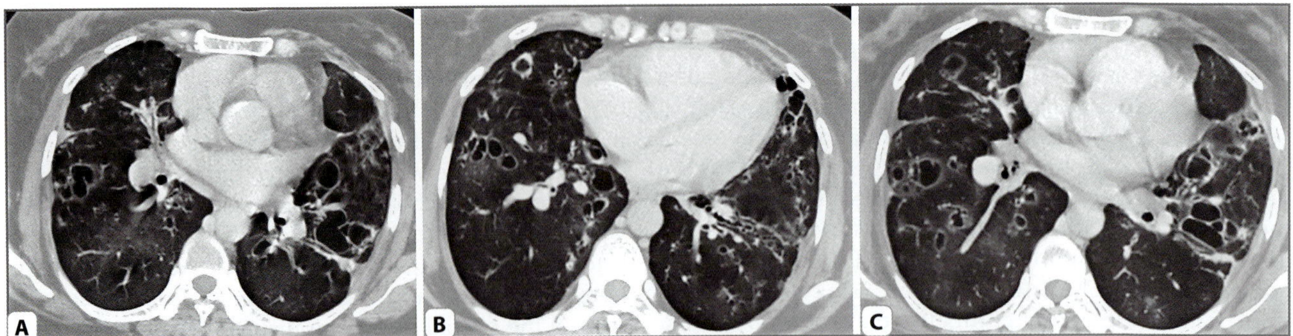

FIGS. 17A TO C: In a lady with bronchial asthma, axial CT chest images in lung window show cystic bronchiectasis and bronchiolectasis bilaterally with peribronchial thickening (A and B). Geographic areas of hypoattenuation suggestive of air trapping also noted bilaterally which are accentuated on expiratory scan (C). Few centrilobular nodules seen in right middle and left lower lobes.

smokers with and without COPD. The *combination of CT and hyperpolarized ^{3}He MRI* also allows the detection of localized ventilation defects, which can occur alongside mucus plugging that obstructs the airway lumen.

Hyperpolarized ^{129}Xe MRI enables detailed evaluation of ventilation defects and the efficiency of gas transfer from the alveoli to the blood. This process involves the inhaled hyperpolarized ^{129}Xe gas first dissolving in the lung parenchyma, plasma, and subsequently in red blood cells, revealing impaired diffusion capacity in COPD patients.

Inert fluorine-19 gases, which are naturally abundant, allow for ventilation imaging via MRI without the need for gas hyperpolarization.[31] For perfusion imaging, both contrast-enhanced MR angiography and non-contrast-enhanced perfusion MRI are utilized. Time-resolved contrast-enhanced MR angiography provides a comprehensive assessment of pulmonary vascular structure and parenchymal perfusion within a single examination.

ASTHMA

Asthma is characterized by airway inflammation and obstruction which is reversible. Pathologically, there is bronchial and bronchiolar wall thickening due to inflammation, smooth muscle hyperplasia, edema, mucus production, and eosinophilic infiltration. Bronchiectasis may be seen in cases with long-standing disease. Patients present with cough, shortness of breath, wheezing and feeling of chest tightness. Pulmonary function tests show airway obstruction during an episode of asthma, but return to normal between attacks.

The chest radiographs in patients with asthma show subtle findings which include increased lung volume, hyperlucency, mild bronchial wall thickening and mild prominence of hilar vasculature due to transient pulmonary hypertension. Complications though uncommon include pneumonia, atelectasis, pneumomediastinum and pneumothorax. Radiographic abnormalities are more commonly seen in children with asthma.

CT is not indicated in routine assessment of patients with asthma, but is useful in the evaluation of complications such as allergic bronchopulmonary aspergillosis (ABPA) or in diagnosing emphysema in smokers with asthma. HRCT may show mild bronchial wall thickening or dilatation of small bronchi. Mucoid impaction and tree-in-bud opacities can be seen. Mosaic attenuation may be seen with patchy air trapping on expiratory scans **(Figs. 17A to C)**.

SUMMARY

Small airway disease encompasses a spectrum of inflammatory and fibrotic pulmonary diseases which affect the small conducting airways. There may be direct signs such as centrilobular nodules and branching tree-in-bud nodules and indirect signs such as mosaic attenuation of small airway disease on HRCT chest. The imaging findings should be interpreted keeping the clinical picture in context so as to reach an accurate diagnosis.

REFERENCES

1. Tomashefski JF, Farver CF. Anatomy and histology of the lung. In: Tomashefski JF(Ed). Dail and Hammar's pulmonary pathology, 3rd edition. New York: Springer; 2008. pp. 20-48.
2. Bankier AA, MacMahon H, Colby T, Gevenois PA, Goo JM, Leung ANC, et al. Fleischner Society: Glossary of Terms for Thoracic Imaging. Radiology. 2024;310(2):e232558.
3. Rodriguez K, Hariri LP, VanderLaan P, Abbott GF. Imaging of Small Airways Disease. Clin Chest Med. 2024;45(2):475-88.
4. Biegelman-Aubry C, Hill C, Guibal A, Savatovsky J, Grenier PA. Multi-detector row CT and postprocessing techniques in the assessment of diffuse lung disease. Radiographics. 2005;25:1639-52.

5. Cagle PT, Roggli VL. Pathology of small airways. In: Tomashefski JF(Ed). Dail and Hammar's pulmonary pathology, 3rd edition. New York: Springer; 2008. pp. 886-910.
6. Abbott GF, Rosado-de-Christenson ML, Rossi SE, Suster S. Imaging of small airways disease. J Thorac Imag. 2009;24(4):285-98.
7. Pipavath SJ, Lynch DA, Cool C, Brown KK, Newell JD. Radiologic and pathologic features of bronchiolitis. Am J Roentgenol. 2005;185:354-63.
8. Lynch DA. Imaging of small airways disease and chronic obstructive pulmonary disease. Clin Chest Med. 2008;29:165-79.
9. Hansell DM. Small airways disease: detection and insights with computed tomography. Eur Respir J. 2001;17:1294-313.
10. Visscher DW, Myers JL. Bronchiolitis: the pathologist's perspective. Proc Am Thorac Soc. 2006;3:41-7.
11. Berniker AV, Henry TS. Imaging of small airways diseases. Radiol Clin North Am. 2016;54(6):1165-81.
12. Hochhegger B, Langer FW, Irion K, Souza A, Moreira J, Baldisserotto M, et al. Pulmonary acinus: understanding the computed tomography findings from an acinar perspective. Lung. 2019;197(3):259-65.
13. Poletti V, Costtable U. Bronchiolar disorders: classification and diagnostic approach. Semin Respir Crit Care Med. 2003;24:457-64.
14. Aquino SL, Gamsu G, Webb WR, Kee ST. Tree-in-bud pattern: frequency and significance on thin section CT. J Comput Assist Tomogr. 1996;20:594-9.
15. Kwon YS, Koh WJ. Diagnosis and treatment of non-tuberculous mycobacterial lung disease. J Korean Med Sci. 2016;31(5):649-59.
16. Tashtoush B, Okafor NC, Ramirez JF, Smolley L. Follicular bronchiolitis: a literature review. J Clin Diagn Res. 2015;9(9):OE01-5.
17. Sieminska A, Kuziemski K. Respiratory bronchiolitis-interstitial lung disease. Orphanet J Rare Dis. 2014;9:106.
18. Kumar A, Cherian SV, Vassallo R, Yi ES, Ryu JH. Current concepts in pathogenesis, diagnosis, and management of smoking-related interstitial lung diseases. Chest. 2018;154(2):394-408.
19. Poletti V, Casoni G, Chilosi M, Zompatori M. Diffuse panbronchiolitis. Eur Respir J. 2006;28(4):862-71.
20. Matar LD, McAdams HP, Sporn TA. Hypersensitivity pneumonitis. Am J Roentgenol. 2000;174:1061-6.
21. Silva CIS, Churg A, Muller NL. Hypersensitivity pneumonitis: spectrum of high-resolution CT and pathologic findings. Am J Roentgenol. 2007;188:334-44.
22. Raghu G, Remy-Jardin M, Ryerson CJ, Myers JL, Kreuter M, Vasakova M, et al. Diagnosis of hypersensitivity pneumonitis in adults. An official ATS/JRS/ALAT clinical practice guideline. Am J Respir Crit Care Med. 2020;202(3):e36-69. Erratum in: Am J Respir Crit Care Med. 2021;203(1):150-1. Erratum in: Am J Respir Crit Care Med. 2022;206(4):518.
23. Teel GS, Engeler CE, Tashijian JH, duCret RP. Imaging of small airways disease. Radiographics. 1996;16:27-41.
24. Barnes TW, Vassallo R, Tazelaar HD, Hartman TE, Ryu JH. Diffuse bronchiolar disease due to chronic occult aspiration. Mayo Clin Proc. 2006;81:172-6.
25. Lucaya J, Gartner S, Garcia-Pena P. Spectrum of manifestations of Swyer-James-MacLeod syndrome. J Comput Assist Tomogr. 1998;22(4):592-7.
26. Sayegh K, Pressacco J, Kovacina B, Digumarthy S, Semionov A. Imaging of Emphysema: A Comprehensive Review. COPD - Pathology, Diagnosis, Treatment, and Future Directions. IntechOpen; 2023. Available from: http://dx.doi.org/10.5772/intechopen.1002748
27. Ohkura N, Tanaka R, Watanabe S, Hara J, Abo M, Nakade Y, et al. Chest Dynamic-Ventilatory Digital Radiography in Chronic Obstructive or Restrictive Lung Disease. Int J Chron Obstruct Pulmon Dis. 2021;16:1393-9.
28. Tanabe N, Nakagawa H, Sakao S, Ohno Y, Shimizu K, Nakamura H, et al. Lung imaging in COPD and asthma. Respir Investig. 2024;62(6):995-1005.
29. Woods JC, Conradi MS. ^{3}He diffusion MRI in human lungs. J Magn Reson. 2018;292:90-8.
30. Kirby M, Pike D, Coxson HO, McCormack DG, Parraga G. Hyperpolarized (3)He ventilation defects used to predict pulmonary exacerbations in mild to moderate chronic obstructive pulmonary disease. Radiology. 2014;273(3):887-96.
31. Gutberlet M, Kaireit TF, Voskrebenzev A, Lasch F, Freise J, Welte T, et al. Free-breathing Dynamic 19F Gas MR Imaging for Mapping of Regional Lung Ventilation in Patients with COPD. Radiology. 2018;286(3):1040-51.

Nidhi Prabhakar, Akshay Kumar Saxena,
Kushaljit Singh Sodhi, Veenu Singla

CHAPTER

16

Radiographs and Computed Tomography in Intensive Care Unit Patients

INTRODUCTION

Imaging of chest in patients in the intensive care unit (ICU) is a challenging job. Rapid and accurate interpretation of radiological investigations in these patients can make a significant contribution to the management of these critically sick patients. Since most of these patients are on life support devices, portable chest radiography is the most performed radiological investigation. This is supplemented by portable ultrasonography and computed tomography (CT) in selected patients.

CHEST RADIOGRAPH

A chest radiograph is the most requested radiology examination in the ICU. It is an essential supplement to physical examination, which is difficult to perform properly in an ICU setting, as most of these patients are uncooperative, unconscious, and intubated.[1] Chest radiography is an economically viable investigation that can be performed rapidly with ease at the bedside of a critically ill patient. It can help in the diagnosis of several cardiopulmonary diseases. It is also used to evaluate monitoring and support devices.[2] Usually, upright posteroanterior and lateral views are performed for chest radiography. However, in the ICU, an anteroposterior (AP) supine radiograph is mostly performed using a portable X-ray unit (portable radiography).

Earlier, it was very common to get chest radiographs of ICU patients daily, especially those on mechanical ventilation. It was thought to be useful for identifying misplaced life support devices or new lung pathologies that might not be detected clinically. However, some studies have demonstrated that daily radiographs are not required. Studies have indicated the same duration of hospital stay in both patient subsets with daily radiography versus those in which it was done only for clinical indications.[3] The American College of Radiology (ACR) in 2013 published the "appropriateness" criteria and recommended that routine daily chest radiographs are not indicated.[4,5] ACR in 2020 published three circumstances under which the chest radiograph is indicated: (1) When the patient is admitted or transferred to ICU, (2) when a patient is clinically worsening, or (3) following an invasive support device placement.[6]

Interpretation of chest radiographs for patients admitted in the ICU is a difficult task as the radiograph is not usually of optimum quality. The portable radiograph is taken with the patient usually in supine position, and there is inconsistency in the technique from day to day. Patients are often critically ill and are monitored and supported by various medical devices, which make it still more difficult to obtain a good quality chest radiograph. In case of any doubts, repeat chest radiograph can be done by putting the patient in different oblique positions.[7] Digital radiography in place of conventional portable chest radiography has gained acceptance in most centers because of consistent film quality and wide latitude of exposure possible with this technique, which decreases the need for repeat examinations.

A systematic approach is required to correctly interpret chest radiographs in the ICU. The following points should be noted while evaluating the chest radiograph: (1) The technical quality, (2) the location of all support and monitoring devices and any related complications, (3) the cardiovascular status of the patient, (4) abnormal lung opacities, (5) signs of barotrauma, (6) pleural effusion or pneumothorax, and (7) comparison with previous studies if available.[8]

With the development of digital radiology techniques, clinicians can review imaging studies without visiting the radiology department. This may lead to inadvertent errors in interpretation. Hence, collaboration between intensivists and radiologists is important for optimal ICU care of critically ill patients. Intensivists find it difficult to leave the

ICU to review cases with radiologists. Virtual rounds over the internet can be effective in these kinds of situations.[8]

COMPUTED TOMOGRAPHY

While CT scan is known to provide superior diagnostic information for chest diseases, its use for patients admitted to ICU has remained limited. This is because the patients admitted to the ICU are dependent on life support devices, and their transportation to CT scan room is hazardous. However, recent studies unequivocally reveal the potential of CT scans to provide superior diagnostic information and have an impact on patient management. CT scans have been shown to change the therapeutic decision of patients in more than half of the cases. CT scan is also important for the evaluation of cerebral complications in ICU patients.[9,10]

Computed tomography plays an invaluable role in the management of ICU patients; however, the benefits need to be more than the risks of patient exposure to ionizing radiation and contrast material. In addition, there is an additional risk of transporting sick patients out of the ICU. Nowadays some institutes have portable CT scanners, but they are not so common. In a study of 134 patients in the ICU, the most common indications for CT were found to be pulmonary embolism, abnormal findings on chest radiographs, and hypoxia. The common findings that were seen on CT included lung consolidations, other lung parenchymal abnormalities, and pleural effusion.[11] CT scan allows clear evaluation of the parenchyma of the lung. Any nonspecific opacities seen on a chest radiograph can be diagnosed on CT. It is also important to note that the visualized lower neck and upper abdomen can give clues and should be evaluated while reporting the chest CT. CT scans expose the patient to approximately 6 mSv of radiation compared to 0.1 mSV from a chest radiograph. However, radiation concerns should not dissuade the use of CT in a critically sick patient.[8]

IMAGING OF CARDIOPULMONARY COMPLICATIONS IN INTENSIVE CARE UNIT PATIENTS

Common cardiopulmonary complications, which can be visualized on imaging in patients of ICU, are atelectasis, aspiration, pneumonia, hydrostatic pulmonary edema, acute respiratory distress syndrome (ARDS), and barotrauma. By careful attention to the imaging pattern, the timing of the changes, and the clinical setting, these entities may be correctly diagnosed. Role of CT scan in imaging patients of pulmonary thromboembolism is discussed in detail elsewhere in this book.

Atelectasis

The most common cause of pulmonary opacities in the ICU is atelectasis, which is frequently seen in postoperative and intubated patients. It often appears quickly and changes quickly. If unresolved in several days, secondary infection should be suspected. The most common locations of atelectasis are the left lower lobe, right lower lobe, and right upper lobe. It is usually subsegmental. Atelectasis is classified as obstructive, cicatricial, compressive, or adhesive. Obstructive atelectasis, which occurs due to impaired mucociliary clearance, retained secretions, and altered consciousness, is the most commonly seen type of atelectasis in an ICU setting. If only the distal airways are blocked, peripheral areas of atelectasis are seen with crowding of bronchi and air bronchograms. However, if larger airways are obstructed, air bronchograms may not be visualized. A common cause of large airway obstruction leading to acute lung collapse is mucus impaction **(Figs. 1A and B)**. If acute lobar collapse is seen without an air bronchogram within the atelectatic area, mucoid impaction is usually the cause. This predicts a favorable response after bronchoscopy. Compressive atelectasis is caused due to mass effect on lungs, with pleural fluid being the most

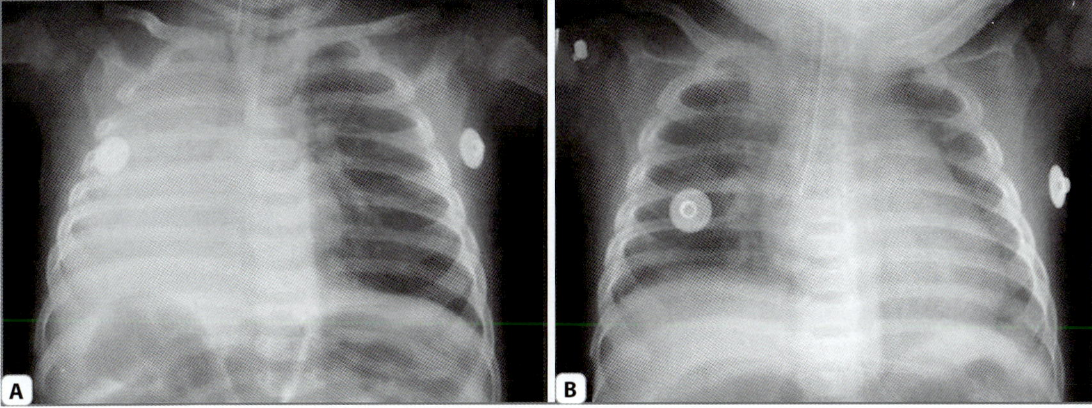

FIGS. 1A AND B: Atelectasis: (A) Chest radiograph of a child on mechanical ventilation reveals complete collapse of right lung. (B) Suction via the endotracheal tube followed by chest radiograph after few hours reveals re-expansion of the right lung.

common cause. Cicatricial atelectasis occurs secondary to lung fibrosis. Adhesive atelectasis is seen in premature neonates due to inadequate production of surfactant. On CT, atelectasis is seen as areas of collapse with evidence of volume loss such as crowding of airways and vessels. Lung atelectasis shows higher attenuation on postcontrast CT compared to areas of consolidation due to pneumonia. This can help in differentiating the two entities.[2]

Aspiration Pneumonitis

A depressed state of consciousness and a nasogastric tube, which disrupts the esophagogastric sphincter, are the most frequent predisposing factors to aspiration pneumonia in an ICU patient. Aspiration can occur despite the inflated cuff of the endotracheal tube and has varying clinical presentation. Mild cases may not be clinically apparent, while severe cases may cause respiratory distress. Aspirated contents may obstruct airway, chemical pneumonitis, or infective pneumonia.[12]

Chest radiography often shows patchy ground glass or nodular opacities with areas of consolidation. These findings are seen in the dependent parts of the lungs (posterior segments of the upper lobes, and the superior, posterior basal segments of lower lobes).[2] These changes often occur within a few hours after aspiration and progress in the next 24–48 hours after which they regress. Persistence of opacities beyond this time is suggestive of aspiration pneumonia **(Fig. 2)**. On CT, patchy ground-glass opacities (GGOs), nodules, and areas of consolidation in the dependent parts of the lung are seen in cases of aspiration pneumonitis. Centrilobular nodules seen in the dependent regions on CT scans are highly suggestive of aspiration.[12]

Pneumonia

Pulmonary infections are commonly seen in the patients who are admitted in the ICU. Colonization of the upper airway is almost universal with prolonged hospitalization. The respirators and endotracheal tubes may act as a source and distributor of infected material. Aspiration is another risk factor for patients developing pneumonia.[12] This diagnosis is made when there is a combination of fever, leukocytosis, and sputum production, which is rich in white cell count and bacteria. Mixed anaerobic bacteria are the most common cause of pneumonia in the ICU patients. However, in ventilated patients, aerobic gram-negative bacteria are also an important cause. Pneumonia is seen as an area of focal or multifocal consolidation on chest radiography and CT **(Figs. 3A and B)**. The infiltrates usually progress over several days, but their radiographic appearance is seldom as rapid as in atelectasis, aspiration, or pulmonary edema.[2] Air bronchogram is usually seen. Lung infection secondary to septicemia may appear as nodules (which are peripheral and may be cavitary) or wedge-shaped peripheral lesions on imaging.

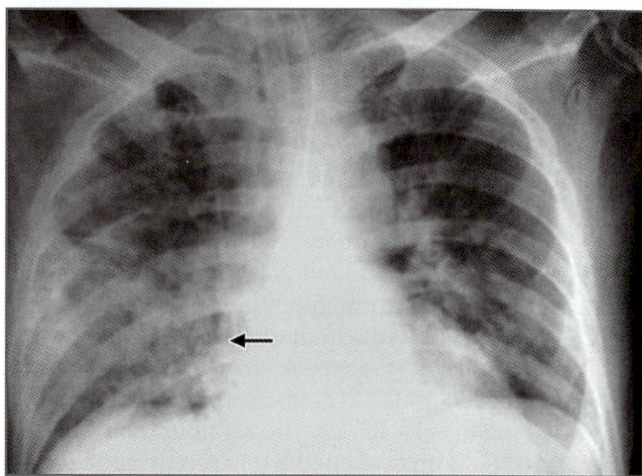

FIG. 2: Aspiration pneumonia: Chest radiograph showing patchy alveolar opacities predominantly involving the right lower zone (arrow).

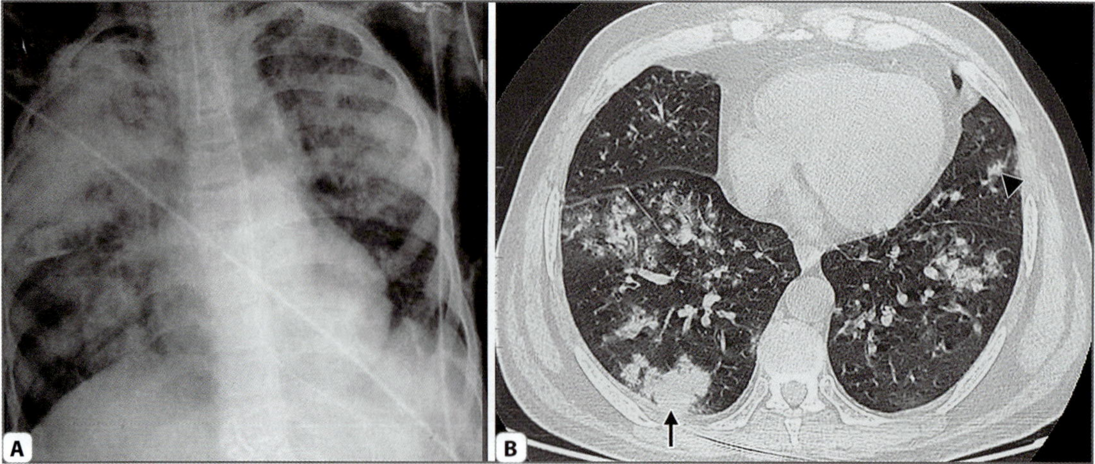

FIGS. 3A AND B: Pneumonia: (A) Chest radiograph in a 12-year-old male child shows patches of consolidation in both lungs suggestive of pneumonia. The patient was a diagnosed case of Bruton's disease. (B) Computed tomography chest in a 50-year-old male patient shows multiple nodules (arrowhead) and areas of consolidation (arrow) in bilateral lungs suggestive of pneumonia.

Hydrostatic Pulmonary Edema

Hydrostatic pulmonary edema in an ICU patient may be due to various etiologies, which include renal failure, cardiac failure, and overhydration.[12] The progression is often rapid, and the response to therapy is equally rapid. The earliest change is congestion of vessels due to an increase in capillary hydrostatic pressure. As the pressure rises, lymphatics get congested, and fluid accumulates in the interstitium around vessels and airways. This mechanism initially protects the lung against alveolar edema, which is caused due to leakage of fluid in the alveoli. These sequences of changes can be appreciated in chest radiography. The first phase is "redistribution," which is characterized by distension of upper lobar pulmonary veins. Subsequently, the prominence of hila and loss of their definition is seen, followed by the appearance of septal lines (Kerley A and B) in the lower lobes. Peribronchovascular thickening with hazy margins and thickening of interlobar fissures is seen in the later stage. Redistribution is only seen when there is chronic pulmonary venous hypertension. Cardiomegaly and pleural effusion are other findings seen on imaging.[13] Early alveolar edema is seen as diffuse, poorly defined GGOs predominantly in perihilar and lower regions. This can progress to air space consolidation. The diagnosis and management of hydrostatic pulmonary edema are commonly based on radiographic findings in appropriate clinical settings. However, recognizing the appearance of hydrostatic pulmonary edema on CT is also important, as edema may be seen on chest CT done for other indications.[14] The high-resolution computed tomography (HRCT) findings include GGOs, smooth interlobular septal thickening, consolidation, increased vascular diameter, peribronchovascular thickening, and pleural fluid **(Figs. 4A and B)**. The distribution of these findings is usually central and gravitational. Mitral regurgitation patients may have pulmonary edema, which is not central, but asymmetric and localized to the right upper lobe.[2]

Noncardiogenic Pulmonary Edema

Noncardiogenic pulmonary edema is also called increased permeability edema. It is difficult to differentiate radiologically from hydrostatic pulmonary edema, and the two conditions may sometimes coexist. The etiology of noncardiogenic pulmonary edema is diverse and includes thoracic (e.g., pneumonia, pulmonary contusion, and aspiration) as well as extrathoracic pathologies (e.g., sepsis, shock, systemic inflammatory response syndrome, extrathoracic trauma, and drug toxicity). Pathologically, there is diffuse alveolar damage secondary to the injury to alveolar capillaries and epithelium. The severe form of diffuse alveolar damage is ARDS. The "Berlin definition" as created by ARDS definition task force, defined ARDS as "respiratory failure (1) Occurring within 1 week of a known clinical insult or new or worsening symptoms, (2) with opacities involving two or more quadrants on imaging (frontal radiograph or CT), (3) not attributable to cardiac failure or volume overload, and (4) having arterial partial pressure of oxygen to fraction of inspired oxygen (PaO_2/FiO_2) ratio of <300 mm Hg." These levels were further classified as mild ARDS (PaO_2/FiO_2 ratio of 200–300 mm Hg), moderate ARDS (PaO_2/FiO_2 ratio of 100–200 mm Hg) or severe ARDS (PaO_2/FiO_2 ratio of <100 mm Hg). The term "acute lung injury" is now no longer used and has been replaced by "mild ARDS."[15,16]

The course of ARDS is a continuum of findings, which is frequently classified into proliferative, exudative, and fibrotic phases. The radiographic findings frequently lag behind the onset of respiratory failure, and chest radiographs may not be helpful in the first few hours of

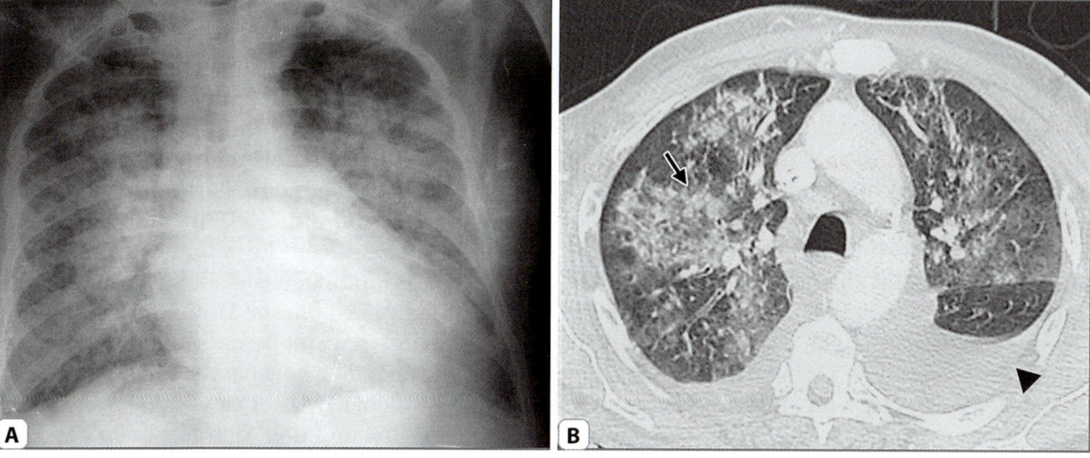

FIGS. 4A AND B: Hydrostatic pulmonary edema: (A) Chest radiograph of a postrenal transplant patient shows cardiomegaly and bilateral pulmonary consolidation with predominantly perihilar distribution. (B) Computed tomography chest in another chronic renal failure patient shows areas of ground-glass opacities and consolidation, predominantly in perihilar location (arrow) involving bilateral lungs suggestive of pulmonary edema. In addition, bilateral pleural effusion is seen (arrowhead).

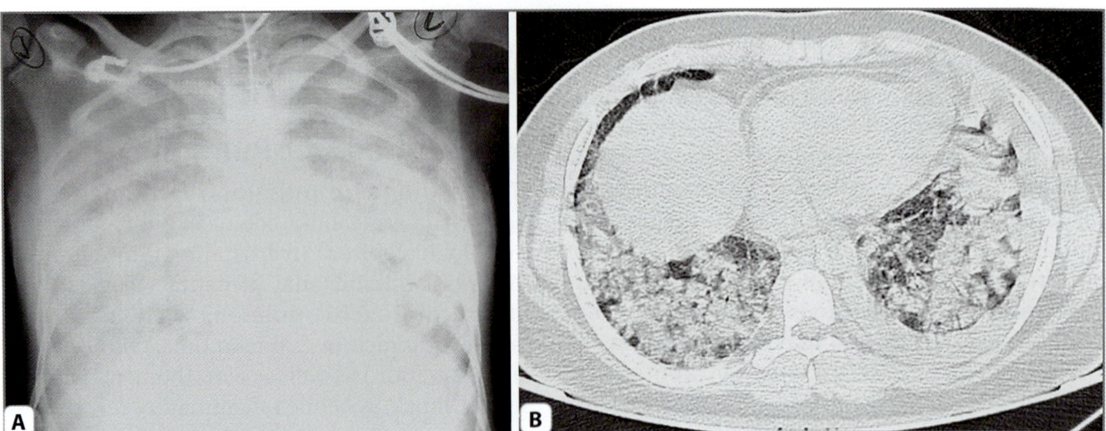

FIGS. 5A AND B: Acute respiratory distress syndrome: (A) Chest radiograph of a 7-year-old child shows bilateral diffuse air space consolidation. (B) CT chest of a 25-year-old male, admitted in ICU and in sepsis, shows multiple areas of consolidation in bilateral lungs, predominant in the lower lobes due to ARDS. In addition, mild left empyema was noted.

(ARDS: acute respiratory distress syndrome; CT: computed tomography; ICU: intensive care unit)

illness. Pulmonary opacities coalesce to cause diffuse pulmonary opacification on radiographs or CT **(Figs. 5A and B)**. These opacities can last for a variable duration (days to months), which depends on the cause, severity, treatment, and presence of associated complications such as aspiration and/or pneumonia. Chest radiograph findings may resemble hydrostatic pulmonary edema; however, patchy and peripheral distribution are seen in noncardiogenic edema vis-à-vis cardiogenic pulmonary edema. Radiographic changes are also slow in ARDS. The heart size is frequently normal in ARDS compared to hydrostatic pulmonary edema. When ARDS is caused by extrathoracic causes, the more symmetric pattern of GGOs is predominant, and when ARDS is secondary to thoracic diseases, asymmetric GGOs and consolidation patches are predominant. The prevalence of fibrotic changes early in the disease predicts a bad prognosis. The most common finding in survivors of ARDS is anterior fibrotic opacities.[17]

Pulmonary Embolism

In critically ill patients, there are numerous risk factors such as cardiac disease, obstructive airway disease, indwelling catheters, and prolonged bed rest, which predispose the patient to pulmonary embolism. The diagnosis of pulmonary embolism can be very difficult when multiple factors can lead to respiratory distress. The most common chest radiographic findings are normal radiograph, pleural effusion, elevated hemidiaphragm, cardiac enlargement, pulmonary artery enlargement, peripheral consolidation, and peripheral atelectasis **(Figs. 6A and B)**.[18] These radiographic signs are nonspecific. In a patient with sudden onset respiratory distress, a normal radiograph is usually suggestive of pulmonary embolism. Ventilation-perfusion scanning is of limited value in a critically ill patient as other accompanying conditions, such as pneumonia, obstructive airway disease, and pulmonary edema, make definitive interpretation difficult in most patients. CT pulmonary angiography is the modality of choice for the radiological evaluation of patients with pulmonary embolism. This topic is discussed in detail elsewhere in this book.

Barotrauma

Barotrauma is a well-recognized complication of mechanical ventilation in the lungs. The most recognized manifestation of barotrauma is the occurrence of extra-alveolar air collection due to the air leak phenomenon. The overall incidence of barotrauma is approximately 3% in mechanically ventilated patients. Incidence varies depending on the presence of underlying lung diseases.[19]

Pulmonary Interstitial Emphysema

Pulmonary interstitial emphysema (PIE) occurs due to increased alveolar pressure causing rupture of the alveolar wall followed by dissection of air along the pulmonary interstitium up to the hilum (Macklin effect).[20] The air can subsequently reach the mediastinum and pleural cavity to cause pneumomediastinum and pneumothorax. Radiographic findings of PIE include multiple lung cysts of variable size, lucent lines that are directed toward the hilum, air around large vessels, subpleural air, intraseptal air, and subpleural cysts. However, these findings may be subtle and may not be detected on radiography in the absence of opacified lung parenchyma. On CT, perivascular and peribronchial cysts or air within interlobular septa are seen. The "line and dot" sign has been described on CT, which is due to air in the interstitium. The bronchovascular bundles are seen as "lines or dots" within the air lucencies **(Figs. 7A and B)**.[21]

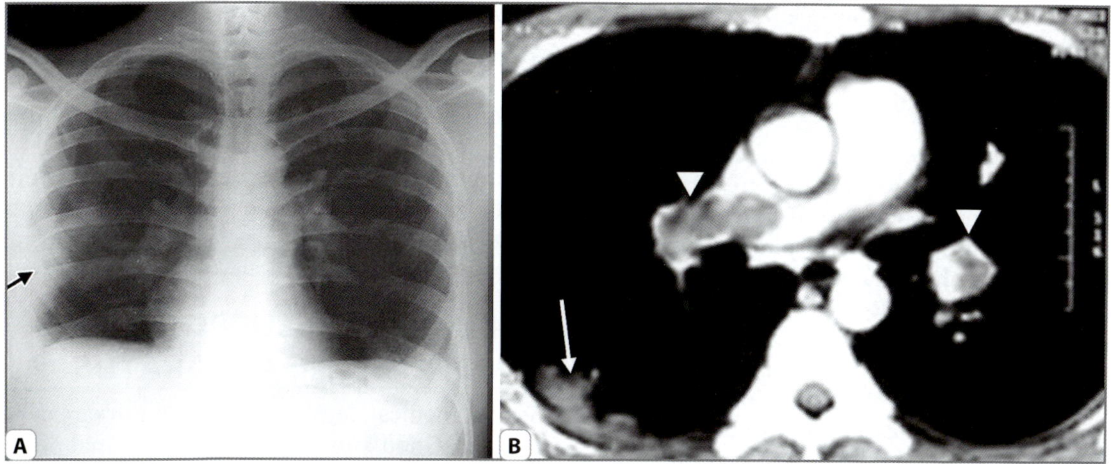

FIGS. 6A AND B: Pulmonary thromboembolism: (A) Chest radiograph of a 32-year-old male patient presenting with sudden onset shortness of breath. The right mid and lower zones show an ill-defined peripheral opacity (black arrow). (B) Computed tomography pulmonary angiography in the same patient shows thrombi in right and left main pulmonary arteries (white arrowheads). Infarction is seen in right lower lobe (white arrow).

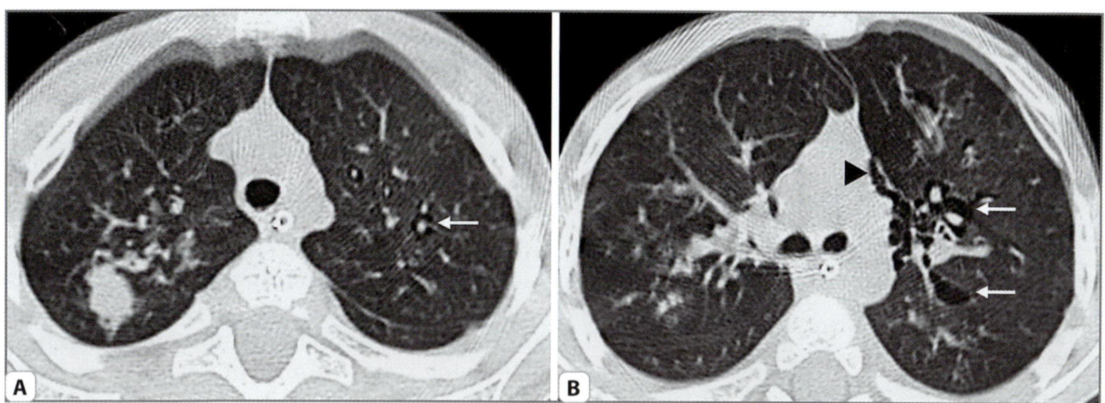

FIGS. 7A AND B: Pulmonary interstitial emphysema: (A and B) CT chest of a 7-month-old child showing air-filled cystic structures in pulmonary interstitium (arrows). The pulmonary vessels appear as line and dot-like structures within the interstitial air. These findings are suggestive of pulmonary interstitial emphysema. Pneumomediastinum (arrowhead) is also seen. In addition, few nodules and consolidation areas are seen in the right lung.

Pneumomediastinum

Pneumomediastinum signifies the presence of extraluminal air in the mediastinum. When occurring due to barotrauma, it may be accompanied by PIE. The radiographic findings in pneumomediastinum depend on the visualization of air outlining the normal anatomic structures in the mediastinum. These signs are the thymic sail sign, "ring around the artery" sign, double bronchial wall sign, continuous diaphragm sign, tubular artery sign, and extrapleural sign. It is sometimes difficult to distinguish pneumomediastinum from pneumopericardium and medial pneumothorax. False-positive diagnosis of pneumomediastinum may be made due to the Mach band effect, which manifests as apparent radiolucency adjacent to convex border structures. In addition, normal anatomic structures (e.g., anterior junction line, major fissure) may occasionally mimic pneumomediastinum.[22,23]

Pneumothorax

The most common life-threatening emergency in patients on mechanical ventilation is pneumothorax because of barotrauma. It may or may not always be preceded by pneumomediastinum. Although of great clinical significance, the diagnosis of pneumothorax is often missed on the radiographs. This is because apicolateral accumulation of air is rather uncommon in the supine films.[24] Air preferentially accumulates in the anteromedial and subpulmonic recesses in the supine position.[24] The anteromedial air collection may cause a sharp outline of contiguous mediastinal structures. Subpulmonic pneumothorax presents as a relatively lucent area in the left or right upper abdominal quadrant. Sometimes, the only radiographic sign of subpulmonic pneumothorax is the deep lateral costophrenic angle (deep sulcus sign).[25] The air can also collect in apicolateral, posteromedial, interlobar fissures, and inferior pulmonary ligament.[24] The position of air collection is also modified by underlying lung diseases.

Tension Pneumothorax

Tension pneumothorax develops when a one-way valve is formed between the lung and pleural cavity. This leads to an increase in intrathoracic pressure due to accumulation of air in the pleural cavity during each respiratory cycle. Rapid progressive collapse of the ipsilateral lung and contralateral shift of mediastinum occur. Venous return is obstructed, causing cardiac arrest.[26] Characteristic radiological features include flattening or inversion of the hemidiaphragm and contralateral mediastinal shift **(Fig. 8)**.[12] Loculated tension pneumothorax is a complication of respiratory therapy in ARDS patients in which there is an accumulation of air, usually in an inferior subpulmonic or paracardiac location. This may occur even if there is an ipsilateral chest tube. The only radiographic evidence of loculated tension pneumothorax may be a subtle degree of mediastinal shift, slight flattening of the cardiac border, and change of contour or depression of the diaphragm, which may be apparent only after comparison with previous radiographs. This loculated tension pneumothorax may lead to severe pulmonary and cardiovascular compromise even from a small volume of pneumothorax, and rapid drainage is required. On a few occasions, the diagnosis of tension pneumothorax in an ARDS patient may only be apparent on a CT scan.[27]

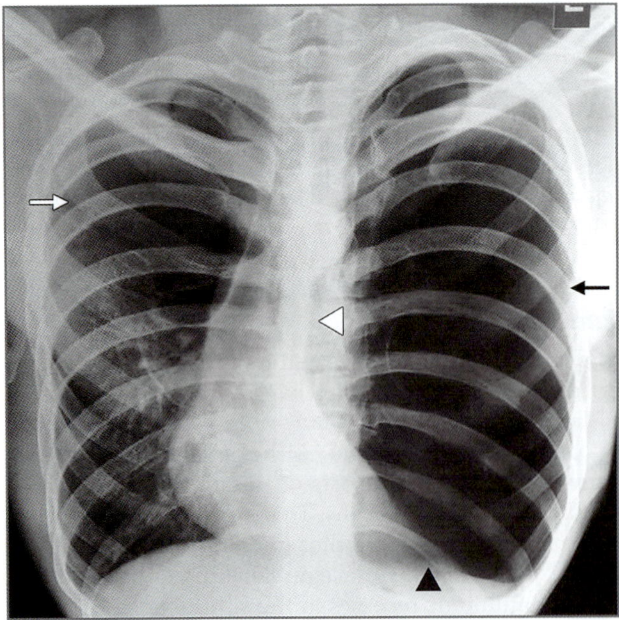

FIG. 8: Tension pneumothorax: Chest radiograph shows tension pneumothorax on the left side (black arrow) with complete collapse of left lung, flattening of the left diaphragm (black arrowhead), and contralateral mediastinal shift (white arrowhead). Large emphysematous bullae are seen on the right side in the upper zone (white arrow).

Subcutaneous Emphysema

Air can travel from the mediastinum along the fascial planes into the subcutaneous tissues of the neck, chest wall, and abdominal wall. The underlying pneumothorax may be difficult to detect in the supine radiograph, and sometimes the air in the chest wall in patients receiving mechanical ventilation is the first radiographic sign of barotrauma in them.

IMAGING OF SUPPORT AND MONITORING APPARATUS

Several medical devices are used in the care of patients in the ICU. Good knowledge of their normal positions and complications is of vital importance to the radiologist and critical care physician.

Endotracheal and Tracheostomy Tube

Endotracheal intubation is done to provide short-term ventilatory support. Following endotracheal intubation, a radiograph should be obtained to ensure proper endotracheal tube placement. The ideal location for the tube tip is the mid trachea, approximately 4 ± 1 cm above the carina, in a neutral head position **(Figs. 9A and B)**. Flexion or extension of the neck can alter the position by as much as 2 cm caudally or cranially, respectively. Tubes placed too high may lead to inadvertent extubation or damage to the larynx. Tubes placed too deeply may irritate the carina or enter the main bronchus (usually right side).[12] Apart from localizing the endotracheal tube tip, the chest radiograph may also show contralateral atelectasis, ipsilateral hyperinflation, and features of barotrauma. Following repositioning of the tube, re-expansion of the contralateral lung may take several hours to days. Endotracheal balloon cuff should not be inflated beyond the diameter of the trachea else it can lead to rupture or tracheal stenosis (as chronic complication) **(Fig. 9C)**. Esophageal intubation is usually clinically apparent and leads to the introduction of large amounts of air in the gastrointestinal tract.[2]

A tracheostomy is done to provide long-term ventilation support. The tip of the tracheostomy tube should be placed at the T3 level, approximately. The diameter of the tracheostomy tube should be approximately two-thirds of the tracheal diameter, and the cuff should not dilate the tracheal wall. Pneumomediastinum may be noted sometimes even after uncomplicated tracheostomy tube placement.[2]

Chest Tube

Chest tubes may be malpositioned in approximately 10% of cases. Chest tube side holes are seen as interruptions of the tube's radiopaque line on chest radiography. All these side holes must be located within the pleural space. If the tube is inserted into the lung parenchyma, a lung contusion may occur. This is seen as a new opacity adjacent to the chest tube on either radiography or CT. Sometimes, malpositioned chest tubes can injure the heart, major blood vessels, diaphragm, or upper abdominal organs.[2] Hence, a critical assessment of chest tube placement should be done to differentiate correct placement from aberrant position.

Venous Catheter

The tip of the central venous line should be within the superior vena cava (SVC), beyond the venous valves, to decrease the risk of thrombosis **(Figs. 10A and B)**. The presence of a catheter tip in the lower SVC or at the cavoatrial junction is associated with reduced thrombosis around the catheter.[28] However, the tip should not be within the atria to avoid arrhythmias and cardiac perforation. Aberrant positioning of the venous catheters intra-arterially (usually subclavian artery or common carotid artery) is usually apparent because it leads to bright red oxygenated blood flowing from the catheter. However, in patients with sepsis and hypotension, this may not be so apparent. On an AP radiograph, if the venous catheter is noted above the level of clavicles, subclavian artery placement should be suspected.

Pneumothorax following subclavian vein catheterization is not uncommon because of the proximity of the apical pleura to the subclavian vein. Another complication is extravascular fluid collection. Widening of the mediastinum following catheterization usually indicates mediastinal fluid or blood accumulation due to venous laceration or extravenous insertion of the catheter. Rapidly developing pleural effusion may also occur due to faulty position.

Swan–Ganz Catheter

The flow-directed balloon-tipped Swan-Ganz catheter measures the pulmonary capillary wedge pressure, pulmonary artery pressure, and cardiac output. The Swan-Ganz catheter tip should be either within the right main pulmonary artery, left main pulmonary artery, or proximal interlobar pulmonary arteries. On the radiograph, the catheter should be seen in the main pulmonary artery and not extending beyond the major hilar vessels as the distal location of the catheter may result in arterial occlusion and rupture. The chest radiograph should be scrutinized for any knots, which may complicate catheter removal.[12] Other complications like those seen in venous catheter placement

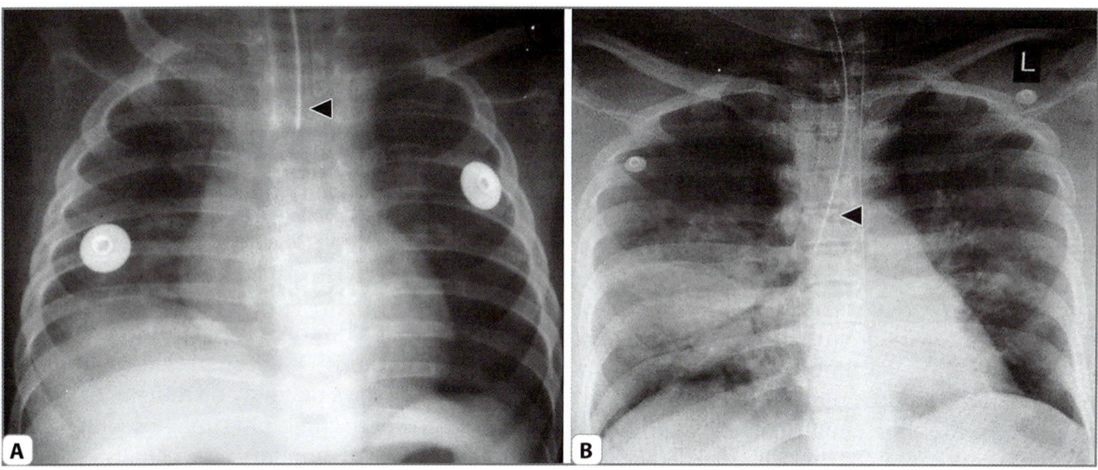

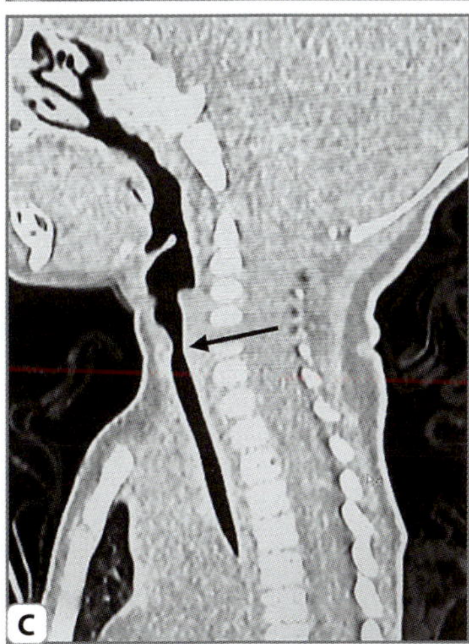

FIGS. 9A TO C: Endotracheal tube position: Chest radiographs showing (A) correct and (B) abnormal (right bronchial) positions of the endotracheal tube (arrowheads). (C) Subglottic stenosis (arrow) seen as a complication of endotracheal intubation in another patient.

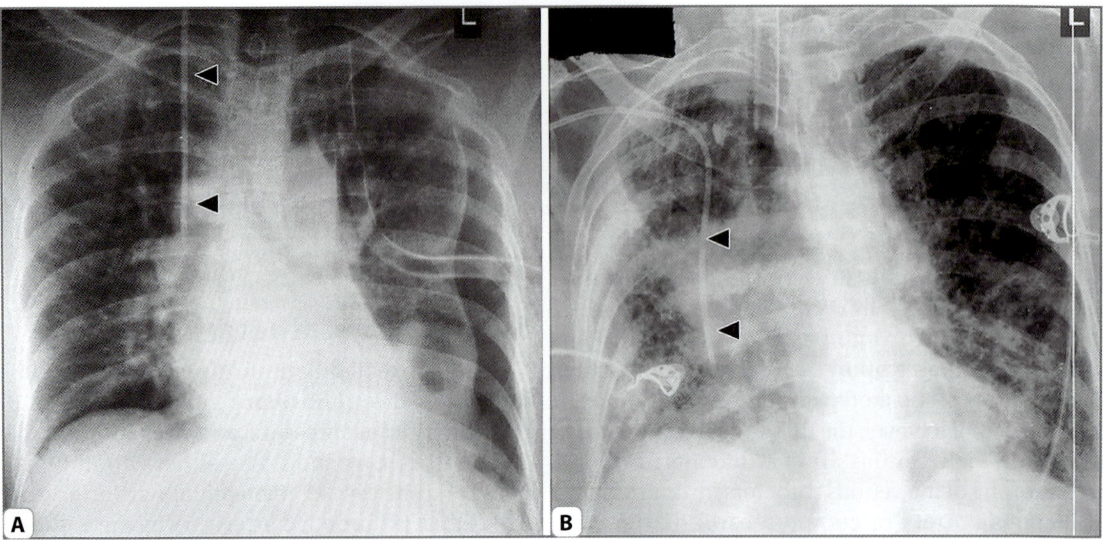

FIGS. 10A AND B: Central venous catheter position: Chest radiographs showing (A) correct and (B) deep positions of the venous catheters (arrowheads).

such as dysrhythmias, cardiac perforation, pneumothorax, or hemothorax may be also seen.

Artificial Intelligence in the Intensive Care Unit

Artificial intelligence (AI) is important in every aspect of our modern life. Its role in the ICU has also grown steadily.[29] With the availability of health data and accelerating computational abilities to analyze them, there is an increasing opportunity to define health and disease status. This ability has its use in real-time diagnosis and patient management. However, the ICU environment involves challenges, and to achieve these goals, the obstacles are many, as direct time-critical clinical applications are required. These machine learning-based AI techniques to define states and predict events are common in all aspects of modern life; however, their usage in acute critical care medicine needs additional care. Several studies have shown the utility of AI in the interpretation of chest radiographs in the ICU.[30-32] In a study that involved the training of deep neural network on 297,541 publicly available patient images, which was then used to evaluate radiographs and CT scans of 166 patients. There was a minor level of performance difference between board-certified radiologists and the algorithm. The authors concluded that there was high potential to reduce the missed findings in AI-based assisted reading settings.[30] Another study also involved AI in which 11-year data of bedside chest radiographs of a university was used, and the reports by 98 radiologists were used to quantify the severity of disease patterns. Reports were used to train a neural network to identify the radiographic findings of cardiomegaly, pulmonary congestion, pleural effusion, parenchymal opacities, and atelectasis. A total of 193,566 radiographs were divided into training, validation, and test sets. The neural network showed higher agreement with the majority vote of an expert panel of six radiologists than each individual radiologist.[31]

CONCLUSION

Radiology is an important part of the care of critically ill patients in the ICU. These patients can be affected by several pathologies that may be difficult to differentiate by imaging; however, combining imaging with history, clinical examination, and laboratory tests usually guides the correct diagnosis and helps in planning further management for the patient. Chest radiographs should be interpreted systematically, particularly the location of invasive devices, and any associated complications should be mentioned. Chest radiograph is not a sensitive imaging modality, and the findings obtained are nonspecific. CT is a more sensitive and specific imaging modality that can help diagnose nonspecific findings on chest radiographs. Collaboration between radiologists and intensivists is required for optimal management of ICU patients.

REFERENCES

1. Rubinowitz AN, Siegel MD, Tocino I. Thoracic imaging in the ICU. Crit Care Clin. 2007;23(3):539-73.
2. Bentz MR, Primack SL. Intensive care unit imaging. Clin Chest Med. 2015;36(2):219-34.
3. Krivopal M, Shlobin OA, Schwartzstein RM. Utility of daily routine portable chest radiographs in mechanically ventilated patients in the medical ICU. Chest. 2003;123(5): 1607-14.
4. Amorosa JK, Bramwit MP, Mohammed TLH, Reddy GP, Brown K, Dyer DS, et al. ACR appropriateness criteria routine chest radiographs in intensive care unit patients. J Am Coll Radiol. 2013;10(3):170-4.
5. Halpern SD, Becker D, Curtis JR, Fowler R, Hyzy R, Kaplan LJ, et al. An official American Thoracic Society/American Association of Critical-Care Nurses/American College of Chest Physicians/Society of Critical Care Medicine policy statement: the Choosing Wisely® top 5 list in critical care medicine. Am J Respir Crit Care Med. 2014;190(7):818-26.
6. Expert Panel on Thoracic Imaging, Laroia AT, Donnelly EF, Henry TS, Berry MF, Boiselle PM, et al. ACR Appropriateness Criteria® intensive care unit patients. J Am Coll Radiol. 2021;18(5S):S62-72.
7. Villasana-Gomez G, Toussie D, Kaufman B, Stojanovska J, Moore WH, Azour L, et al. Chest intensive care unit imaging: pearls and pitfalls. Clin Chest Med. 2024;45(2):213-35.
8. Toy D, Siegel MD, Rubinowitz AN. Imaging in the intensive care unit. Semin Respir Crit Care Med. 2022;43(6):899-923.
9. Aliaga M, Forel JM, De Bourmont S, Jung B, Thomas G, Mahul M, et al. Diagnostic yield and safety of CT scans in ICU. Intensive Care Med. 2015;41(3):436-43.
10. Dorenbeck U, Bein T, Strotzer M, Geissler A, Feuerbach S, Traeger K. Thoracic computed tomography in intensive care patients – evaluation of clinical usefulness. Anasthesiol Intensivmed Notfallmed Schmerzther. 2002;37(5):273-9.
11. Moloney F, Fama D, Twomey M, O'Leary R, Houlihane C, Murphy KP, et al. Cumulative radiation exposure from diagnostic imaging in intensive care unit patients. World J Radiol. 2016;8(4):419-27.
12. Hill JR, Horner PE, Primack SL. ICU imaging. Clin Chest Med. 2008;29(1):59-76.
13. Cardinale L, Priola AM, Moretti F, Volpicelli G. Effectiveness of chest radiography, lung ultrasound and thoracic computed tomography in the diagnosis of congestive heart failure. World J Radiol. 2014;6(6):230-7.
14. Storto ML, Kee ST, Golden JA, Webb WR. Hydrostatic pulmonary edema: high-resolution CT findings. Am J Roentgenol. 1995;165(4):817-20.
15. ARDS Definition Task Force, Ranieri VM, Rubenfeld GD, Thompson BT, Ferguson ND, Caldwell E, et al. Acute respiratory distress syndrome: the Berlin definition. JAMA. 2012; 307(23):2526-33.
16. Sweeney RM, McAuley DF. Acute respiratory distress syndrome. Lancet. 2016;388(10058):2416-30.
17. Desai SR, Wells AU, Rubens MB, Evans TW, Hansell DM. Acute respiratory distress syndrome: CT abnormalities at long-term follow-up. Radiology. 1999;210(1):29-35.
18. Elliott CG, Goldhaber SZ, Visani L, DeRosa M. Chest radiographs in acute pulmonary embolism. Results from the International Cooperative Pulmonary Embolism Registry. Chest. 2000;118(1):33-8.
19. Anzueto A, Frutos-Vivar F, Esteban A, Alía I, Brochard L, Stewart T, et al. Incidence, risk factors and outcome of barotrauma in mechanically ventilated patients. Intensive Care Med. 2004;30(4):612-9.
20. Wintermark M, Schnyder P. The Macklin effect: a frequent etiology for pneumomediastinum in severe blunt chest trauma. Chest. 2001;120(2):543-7.
21. Donnelly LF, Lucaya J, Ozelame V, Frush DP, Strouse PJ, Sumner TE, et al. CT findings and temporal course of persistent pulmonary interstitial emphysema in neonates: a multiinstitutional study. AJR Am J Roentgenol. 2003;180(4): 1129-33.
22. Zylak CM, Standen JR, Barnes GR, Zylak CJ. Pneumomediastinum revisited. Radiographics. 2000;20(4):1043-57.
23. Bejvan SM, Godwin JD. Pneumomediastinum: old signs and new signs. AJR Am J Roentgenol. 1996;166(5):1041-8.
24. Tocino IM, Miller MH, Fairfax WR. Distribution of pneumothorax in the supine and semirecumbent critically ill adult. AJR Am J Roentgenol. 1985;144(5):901-5.
25. Gordon R. The deep sulcus sign. Radiology. 1980;136(1):25-7.
26. Watts BL, Howell MA. Tension pneumothorax: a difficult diagnosis. Emerg Med J. 2001;18(4):319-20.
27. Gobien RP, Reines HD, Schabel SI. Localized tension pneumothorax: unrecognized form of barotrauma in adult respiratory distress syndrome. Radiology. 1982;142(1):15-9.
28. Cadman A, Lawrance JA, Fitzsimmons L, Spencer-Shaw A, Swindellet R. To clot or not to clot? That is the question in central venous catheters. Clin Radiol. 2004;59(4):349-55.
29. Beam K, Sharma P, Levy P, Beam AL. Artificial intelligence in the neonatal intensive care unit: the time is now. J Perinatol. 2024;44(1):131-5.
30. Rueckel J, Kunz WG, Hoppe BF, Patzig M, Notohamiprodjo M, Meinel FG, et al. Artificial intelligence algorithm detecting lung infection in supine chest radiographs of critically ill patients with a diagnostic accuracy similar to board-certified radiologists. Crit Care Med. 2020;48(7):e574-83.
31. Khader F, Han T, Müller-Franzes G, Huck L, Schad P, Keil S, et al. Artificial intelligence for clinical interpretation of bedside chest radiographs. Radiology. 2023;307(1):e220510.
32. Tanaka K, Nakada TA, Takahashi N, Dozono T, Yoshimura Y, Yokota H, et al. Superiority of supervised machine learning on reading chest X-rays in intensive care units. Front Med (Lausanne). 2021;8:676277.

Atin Kumar, Shivanand Gamanagatti, Amarinder Singh Malhi

CHAPTER

17

Imaging in Thoracic Trauma

INTRODUCTION

Thoracic injury is the third most common injury in the trauma patient after head and extremity injury. The mortality from thoracic injury with related complications ranges from 15–77% especially in the setting of multisystem trauma.[1] Thoracic injuries can potentially affect airway and breathing which are the two most important components responsible for early mortality in patients with torso trauma. The mode of injury can be blunt trauma or penetrating trauma. The chest wall remains intact in blunt trauma whereas its integrity is breached in penetrating trauma resulting in communication between the external environment and internal contents of the thorax, even if only transiently. Blunt trauma due to motor vehicle collision is the most common cause.

ROLE OF IMAGING

Imaging plays an important role in the diagnosis of injuries due to thoracic trauma. After ensuring the hemodynamic stability of the patient, chest radiograph is obtained as the initial imaging evaluation during the primary survey.

Chest Radiograph

It is usually obtained in the supine anteroposterior projection. It is a useful adjunct to rule out immediate life-threatening conditions such as large pneumothorax, massive hemothorax, and hemomediastinum (mediastinal widening). Besides, it is also useful to detect lung injuries, osseous trauma and the position of various internal catheters, lines and tubes. However, it has multiple limitations including suboptimal patient positioning, magnification and distortion of mediastinum, overlap of soft tissue and lung parenchyma, inability to detect air-fluid level in the supine position besides being less sensitive in characterizing mediastinal and lung parenchymal injuries.

Ultrasound

Ultrasound of the chest is done as an extension of the focussed assessment with sonography in trauma (eFAST). This is also done alongwith the chest radiograph during the primary survey of the patient as part of initial evaluation and resuscitation. It is used to detect hemothorax, pneumothorax and hemopericardium. Pneumothorax is diagnosed on ultrasound by detecting loss of "lung sliding sign". When the chest is evaluated by ultrasound in a healthy patient, the parietal and visceral pleura are seen opposed to each other and appear as a bright echogenic line. This is the first air interface and acts as a barrier for the ultrasound beam. Beyond this line, the ultrasound beam is not able to penetrate and gets reflected back. Hence, only reverberation artefacts and comet tail artefacts are seen deeper to this interface. With respiratory movements, the visceral pleura slides in a craniocaudal direction in relation to the parietal pleura. The ultrasound detects it as an inner bright echogenic line moving up and down. The reverberation artefacts and the comet tail artefacts also move with this line. This has been described as "lung sliding sign". When there is pneumothorax, the parietal and visceral pleura get separated by air. Now the ultrasound beam encounters air just after the parietal pleura and the first air interface is, therefore, the parietal pleura rather than visceral pleura. The beam is not able to penetrate beyond this and therefore the visceral pleura or the lung parenchyma which are deeper are not visualized. In this scenario, the echogenic bright line does not move with respiration as the air column in the pleural space is static. This leads to loss of "lung sliding sign". This is a marker of pneumothorax. It should be looked for in the most nondependent area like beneath the second intercostal space in parasternal location. The reverberation and the comet tail artefacts are also not well seen in pneumothorax.

Computed Tomography

It is the modality of choice for detection of pulmonary, pleural, mediastinal and osseous abnormalities in the setting of thoracic trauma. However, it is done after the patient has been stabilized hemodynamically. The current indications in patients of thoracic trauma include significant findings on a chest radiograph or eFAST, penetrating chest injury, suspicion of mediastinal vascular injury (aortic injury), significant osseous injuries on radiograph especially upper rib fractures or flail segments.[2] It is also done in patients with dangerous mechanism of injury even when the chest radiograph and eFAST are normal. The CT is done as a part of torso imaging protocol combined with abdomen. At our center, we routinely do the CT chest in the arterial phase to look for vascular injuries. A negative contrast CT examination virtually rules out any significant thoracic injury.

The following section describes the radiographic and CT findings of major lung parenchymal, pleural, mediastinal, diaphragmatic, and chest wall injuries.

PULMONARY PARENCHYMAL INJURIES

Pulmonary Contusion

Pulmonary contusions are the most common cause of pulmonary opacifications in blunt chest trauma with a prevalence of 17–70%.[2,3] The causative force is direct injury to the lung parenchyma at the site of impact or in the opposite portion of the lung (contrecoup injury). It represents a combination of parenchymal edema and hemorrhage secondary to alveolar membrane disruption. Patients may be asymptomatic (50%) or may have hemoptysis, fever, tachypnea, hypoxia and hypercarbia. The initial chest radiograph may be normal, but the findings usually are evident within 6 hours. The contusion appears as unilateral or bilateral, ill-defined, focal or multifocal, patchy airspace opacity which is not confined by fissural boundaries (nonsegmental distribution). They are usually seen in the lung periphery adjacent to the site of lung trauma and frequently have associated bony injuries of ribs or spine except in pediatric patients where they often occur without overlying bony injuries. Lung bases are a preferred site due to increased basilar mobility. Air bronchograms are usually absent due to blood filling the airways. The maximal radiographic opacity is seen within 24–72 hours after which it gradually clears completely over the next 3–10 days.

Computed tomography is more sensitive than chest radiograph for detection of pulmonary contusions.[4] In CT also it appears as ill-defined areas of ground glass opacity which readily cross pleural fissures **(Figs. 1A and B)**. The peripheral 1–2 mm of lung may show sparing especially in pediatric population. Recently, CT has been used to quantify the volume of contusion to predict the clinical course and outcome. Miller et al.[5] found contusion volume to be a direct predictor of subsequent development of acute respiratory distress syndrome (ARDS).

Pulmonary Laceration

Pulmonary laceration represents a tear of lung parenchyma secondary to penetrating injury, lung perforation from rib fractures or shearing forces caused by inertial deceleration. Clinically, it may manifest as hemoptysis. The lacerations are more common in children and young adults because of the greater flexibility of the chest wall causing higher likelihood of lung getting injured with blunt trauma.[6] They

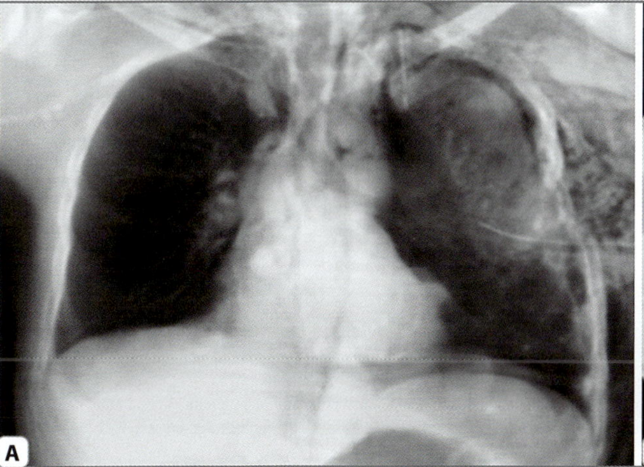

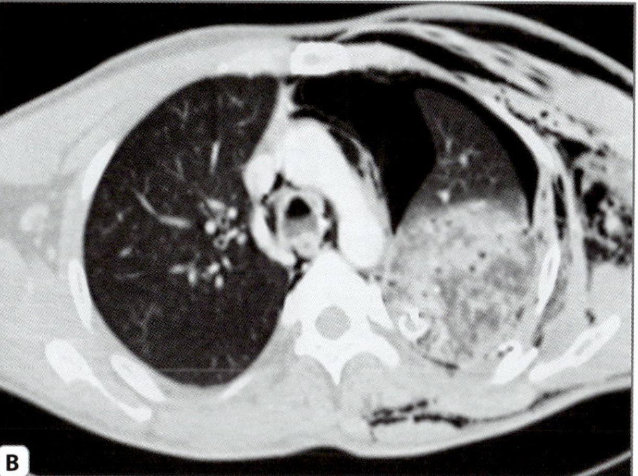

FIGS. 1A AND B: Pulmonary contusion. Thick coronal multiplanar reconstruction (A) and axial (B) CT images show homogenous ground glass density in the left upper lobe of lung consistent with pulmonary contusion. Note presence of left pneumothorax and pneumomediastinum.

are not frequently identified on the initial chest radiograph because they get obscured by surrounding contusions. A chest CT is significantly more sensitive to detect and evaluate the extent of the pulmonary laceration than a conventional chest radiograph. Lacerations are usually ovoid. Radiologically, lacerations appear as ovoid lucent areas because of the elastic recoil of the lung with a thin rim of hyperdensity, representing a pseudomembrane. The laceration cavity may be filled with air (traumatic pneumatocele), blood (traumatic hematocele) or both with air and blood (traumatic hematopneumatocele). On CT, when air filled, they appear as localized air collections within areas of contusion **(Fig. 2)**. After clearing of the adjacent lung contusion, they are seen as thin-walled cysts filled with air or blood. The lacerations resolve slowly over a period of 3 weeks to a year. They may persist as a pulmonary nodule containing blood clots.

Lacerations have been described to be of four types based on the mechanism of injury. Type 1 is due to compression rupture and is the most common type. They are usually seen in the central parts of the lung **(Figs. 2A and B)**. Type 2 is due to compression shear and are most often seen in the paraspinal location **(Figs. 2C and D)**. Type 3 are due to penetration of lungs by a fractured rib at the periphery of the lung. Type 4 are the most uncommon type seen due to adhesion tears at a site of pre-existing adhesions at the periphery of the lung. It is not usually evident on imaging but seen only on surgery or autopsy.

Larger lacerations which are completely filled are often described as hematomas.[2] The hematoma obscures underlying anatomy in contrast to a contusion in which the underlying alveolar and interstitial tissues remain intact.

Potential complications include infection leading to pulmonary abscess, increased size of laceration or development of bronchopleural fistula when the laceration communicates with a bronchus and pleural surface.[3,7] The abscess appears as thick-walled cavity with irregular inner margins and an air-fluid level. Bronchopleural fistula leads to persistent air leak which does not respond to chest tube placement. Abscess and bronchopleural fistula often require surgical or percutaneous drainage if the medical therapy fails.

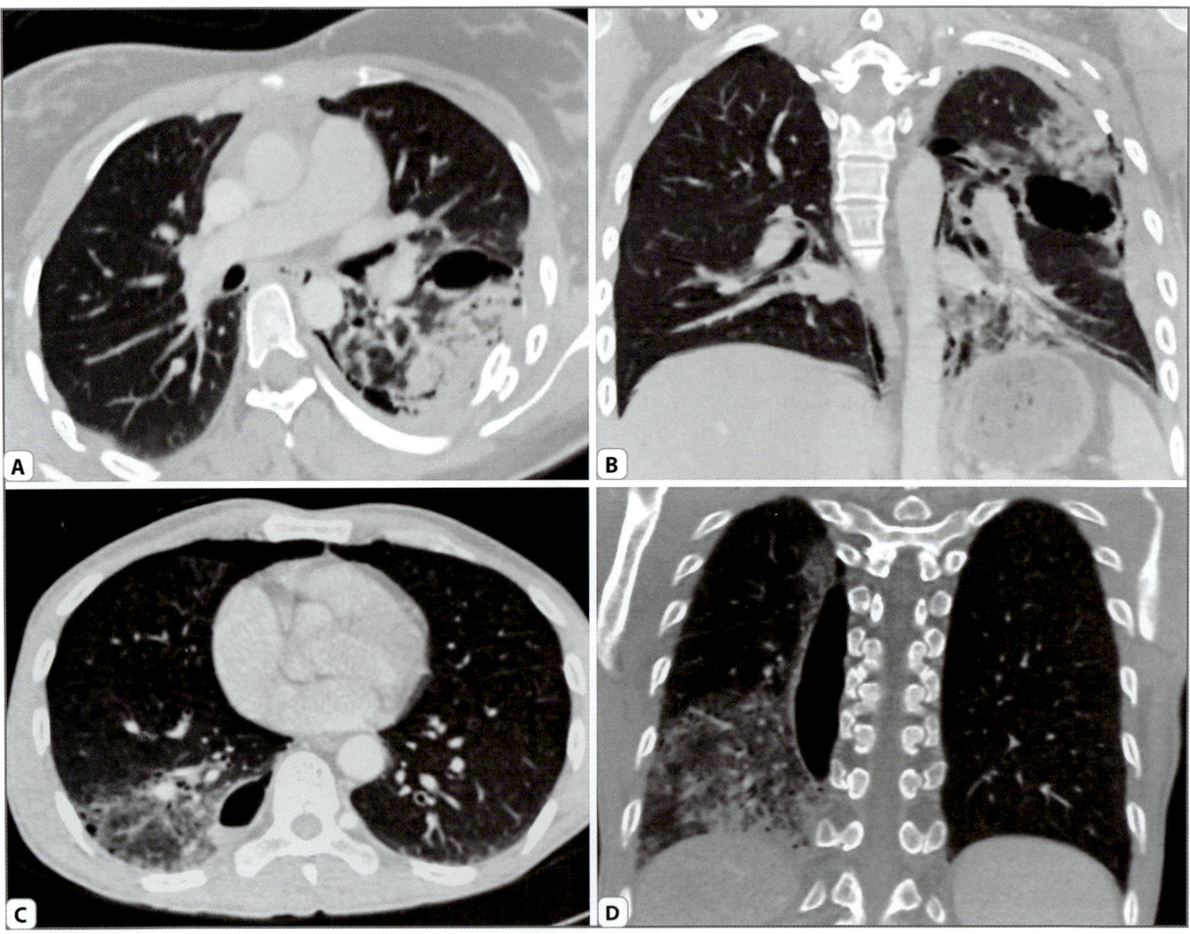

FIGS. 2A TO D: Pulmonary laceration. Axial (A) and coronal multiplanar reconstruction (B) CT images show an air-filled ovoid lesion in central part of left lung parenchyma (type 2 laceration). Note the adjacent ground glass density representing contusion. Axial (C) and coronal multiplanar reconstruction (D) CT images in a different patient show a type 2 laceration containing air and blood in the right paraspinal location with adjacent contusion and a small pneumothorax.

Aspiration Pneumonitis

Aspiration pneumonitis is a frequent finding seen in post-traumatic patients, especially those with head or maxillofacial injuries. It is important to differentiate aspiration pneumonitis from contusion because the management for the two entities is different. Aspiration produces "tree-in-bud" poorly defined centrilobular opacities usually in the dependent portions of the lung in contrast to contusions which appear as ill-defined areas of ground glass opacity not respecting fissural boundaries with likely associated lacerations appearing as cysts **(Fig. 3)**. The CT "tree-in-bud" appearance of aspiration reflects aspirated material filling the distal small airways, whereas the confluent ground glass opacity of contusion represents injury to the localized parenchymal area. The most frequently involved lung segments in aspiration include the superior and posterior basilar segments of the lower lobes and the posterior segments of the upper lobes. The classical "tree-in-bud" opacities are not easily visualized after few hours as they become confluent resulting in consolidative appearance except along the periphery where some isolated filled terminal bronchioles often persist.

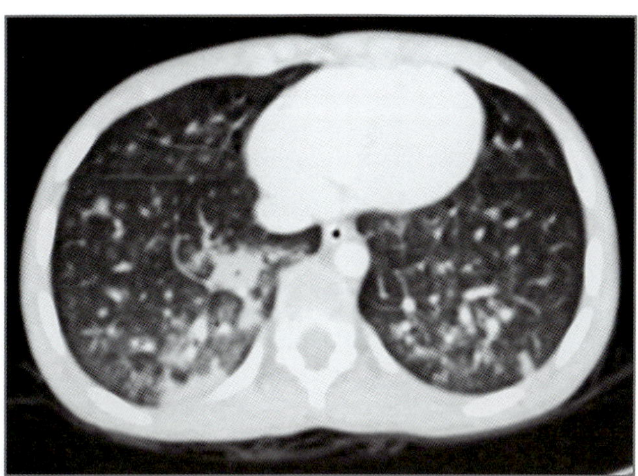

FIG. 3: Aspiration pneumonitis. Axial CT image shows poorly defined centrilobular nodules with some having "tree-in-bud" configuration in the apical segment of the right lower lobe.

Atelectasis

Lung collapse in the trauma patient can be separated broadly into the categories of obstructive, compressive, passive, and adhesive atelectasis. Obstructive atelectasis occurs due to obstruction of the airway by mucus plug, foreign body, blood or airway rupture. Compressive atelectasis occurs from mass effects of large contusions or traumatic lung cysts. Passive atelectasis occurs secondary to pneumothorax or hemothorax which disrupts the inherent elastic recoil properties of the lung **(Figs. 4A and B)**. It is the most common form seen in the setting of trauma. Adhesive atelectasis is caused by decreased surfactant production secondary to pulmonary contusion. Air bronchograms are often seen in all forms of atelectasis except from a central bronchial obstructive cause.

Radiologically, atelectasis appears as a dense homogenous opacity with signs of volume loss such as fissure deviation, bronchovascular crowding, ipsilateral hilar or mediastinal shift and elevated diaphragm. On contrast enhancement, the collapsed part shows greater enhancement due to crowded pulmonary vasculature compared to consolidation. These above findings help to differentiate atelectasis from contusion or consolidation.

Traumatic Lung Herniation

This uncommon entity occurs when a pleura covered part of lung herniates through a defect in the chest wall.[3,6] It is usually associated with a rib fracture. It is important to recognize this condition because if left untreated the herniation may increase secondary to positive pressure ventilation.

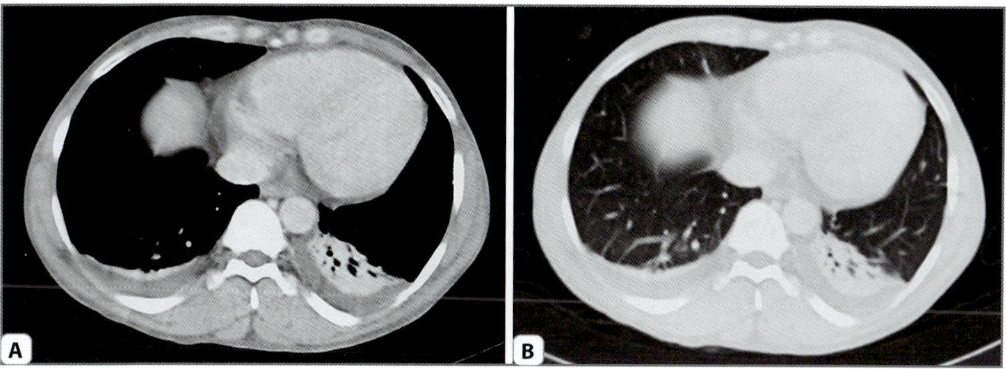

FIGS. 4A AND B: Atelectasis. Axial chest CT images in mediastinal (A) and lung (B) window show passive atelectasis of left lower lobe segment with air bronchogram within secondary to pleural fluid. Also seen in right pleural fluid.

PLEURAL INJURIES

Pneumothorax

Pneumothorax is seen in 30–40% of all blunt chest trauma patients.[2] It is usually caused by alveolar rupture due to sudden increase in intrathoracic pressure associated with pleural tear. It may also be secondary to rib fracture with rib piercing the pleura and the lung. The diagnosis is first made on a chest radiograph. However, 30–50% pneumothoraces are missed on the radiographs which are usually taken in supine position in the setting of trauma.[6] These can be seen on CT and are called as "occult pneumothoraces". In the supine position air collects anteriorly and medially in the anterior costophrenic sulcus. The signs of pneumothorax on a supine chest radiograph are described in **Box 1**.

On an upright chest radiograph pneumothorax is seen as thin, sharply defined line that represents the visceral pleura. Lung markings are not seen beyond this line. False positive cases may be due to skin folds, large bullae, overlying tubes and catheters, bedding, scapular margin mimicking the pneumothorax. The correct diagnosis can be made by an upright expiratory chest radiograph or CT.

As described earlier in this chapter, eFAST has been increasingly used to detect pneumothorax and has shown very high sensitivity in experienced hands. Loss of "lung sliding sign" confirms pneumothorax. The clinical significance of a small pneumothorax which remains undetected on the chest radiograph or the eFAST is very low and does not warrant further radiographs in additional views except if the patient is on ventilation where even a small pneumothorax can quickly become life-threatening due to positive pressure ventilation. CT is highly sensitive for detecting the pneumothoraces **(Fig. 6)**. Even evaluation of an abdominal CT often detects pneumothorax because of the tendency of the air to collect in the anterior costophrenic sulcus in the supine patient.

Chest tube placement is usually required in patients who are symptomatic, have >20% pneumothorax, in patients who are on ventilator or are likely to be put on ventilator or who have to undergo a lengthy operative procedure. If the pneumothorax is persistent and does not completely respond to treatment including a chest tube placement,

BOX 1: Signs of pneumothorax on supine chest radiograph.

- Abnormally increased lucency in the lower chest or upper abdomen **(Fig. 5)**
- The "deep sulcus" sign—abnormally wide and deep costophrenic sulcus
- The "double diaphragm" sign—when air outlines the dome and anterior insertion of diaphragm
- Sharply outlined diaphragmatic or cardiac border
- Depression of hemidiaphragm

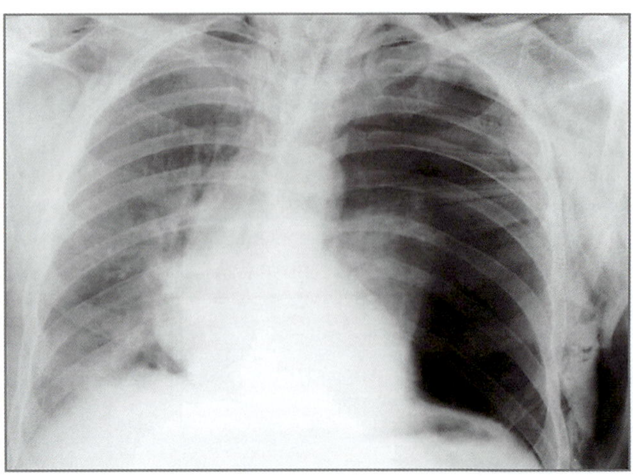

FIG. 5: Pneumothorax. Chest radiograph shows left sided pneumothorax with clear visualization of lung border and deep sulcus sign. Also note subcutaneous emphysema along the pectoralis muscle.

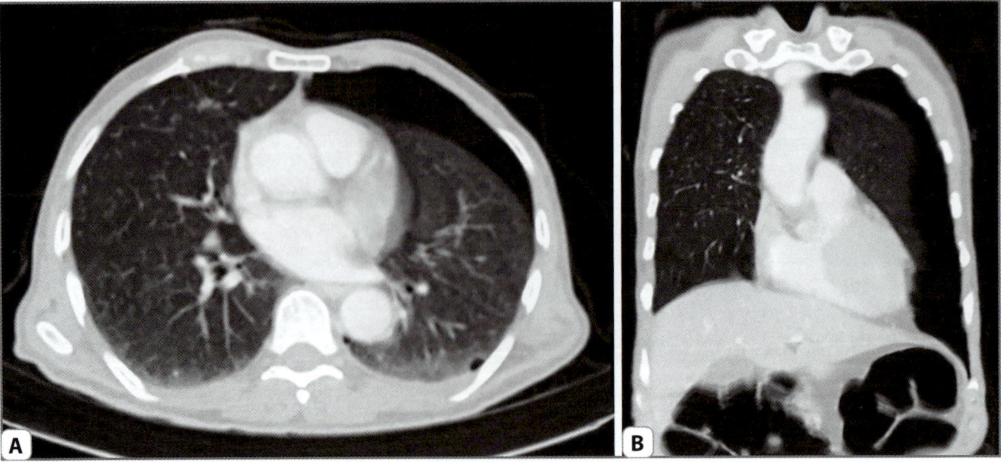

FIGS. 6A AND B: Pneumothorax. Axial (A) and coronal reformatted coronal (B) chest CT image shows mild left sided pneumothorax.

then malpositioned chest tube, tracheobronchial injury or a bronchopleural fistula needs to be ruled out on imaging.

Tension pneumothorax develops when the intrapleural pressure exceeds that of the atmosphere. This serious condition occurs when the pulmonary or bronchial injury acts as a one-way valve with air entering into pleural space without exit. This leads to pulmonary and cardiac compromise. It is a clinical diagnosis. However, there are signs to suggest tension pneumothorax on a radiograph **(Figs. 7A and B)**. These have been enumerated in **Box 2**. If suspected, it warrants an immediate rapid decompression with a large bore needle followed by a chest tube placement.

Hemothorax

Hemothorax is seen in approximately 50% of patients of blunt thoracic trauma, especially those caused by penetrating trauma.[2,3] Source of bleeding is injury to pleura, lung parenchyma, mediastinum, diaphragm or with injuries to liver and spleen with associated diaphragmatic injury. Decubitus chest radiograph can detect as less as 5 mL of fluid in pleural space whereas blunting of costophrenic angle is seen on upright radiograph when approximately 200 mL of fluid accumulates in the pleural space. Progressive increase leads to the "meniscus" sign, i.e., concave upward sloping of the fluid in the costophrenic angle **(Fig. 8)**. An air-fluid level indicates hemopneumothorax. However, in the setting of trauma since most often it is the supine radiograph which is acquired, the hemothorax is seen as increased opacity of the ipsilateral hemithorax with mediastinal shift to contralateral side **(Figs. 9A and B)**. eFAST is used to detect hemothorax with high sensitivity.

Computed tomography is highly sensitive for small amounts of pleural fluid and is also helpful in its characterization. A Hounsfield unit (HU) value of 35–70 represents hemothorax whereas HU less than 15 typically is seen in sympathetic pleural effusion which is seen in patients with hepatic, splenic or pancreatic injuries.

Other uncommon causes of pleural fluid in the setting of trauma include chylothorax which may occur secondary to injury to the thoracic duct, bilious effusion which is caused by biliopleural fistula secondary to hepatic and diaphragmatic injury and urinothorax which occurs secondary to renopleural fistula.

BOX 2: Signs of tension pneumothorax on chest radiograph.

- Widening of lateral diameter of thorax
- Contralateral mediastinal shift
- Flattening or inversion of ipsilateral diaphragm
- Collapsed lung in the hilar region
- Deep sulcus sign
- Widening of intercostal spaces

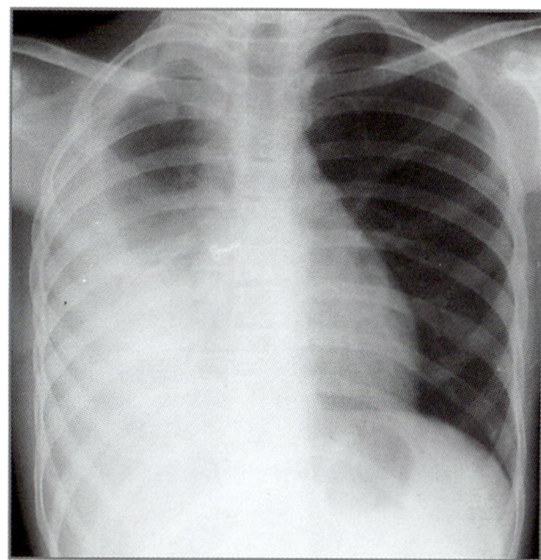

FIG. 8: Hemothorax. Chest radiograph in erect position shows right sided pleural fluid with meniscus sign.

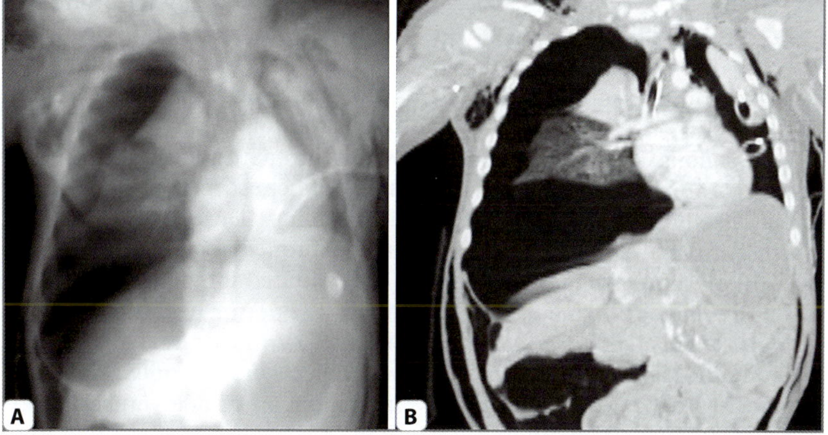

FIGS. 7A AND B: Tension pneumothorax. Coronal thick (A) and thin (B) multiplanar reconstruction CT images show right sided tension pneumothorax with inversion of right diaphragm, collapsed left lung and mediastinal shift toward right.

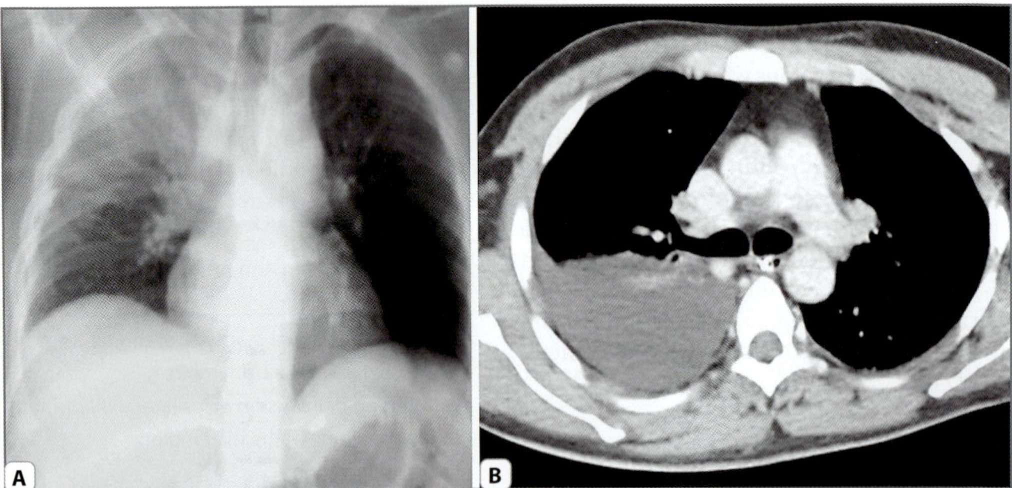

FIGS. 9A AND B: Hemothorax. Computed tomography (CT) thick coronal multiplanar reconstruction image (A) shows appearance of pleural fluid in supine patient appearing as diffuse haze of right hemithorax. CT axial image (B) shows moderate amount of right pleural fluid in dependent position. The fluid appears of high density signifying hemothorax.

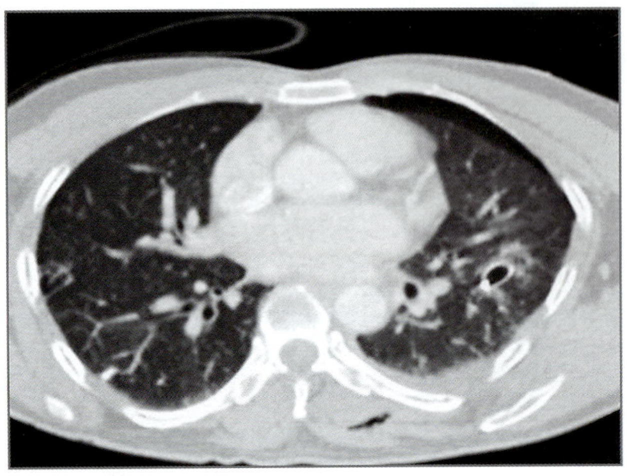

FIG. 10: Malpositioned chest tube. Axial CT image shows the tip of chest tube lying within lung parenchyma. Note small pneumothorax on left side.

However, any fluid detected in the pleural cavity at presentation in a post-traumatic patient is considered as hemothorax unless proven otherwise and managed accordingly.

Source of bleeding can be venous which is usually self-limiting or arterial which usually progresses on follow-up imaging. Arterial bleed may also be seen on CT as active contrast extravasation usually from an intercostal artery. It is also important to note the placement of the chest tube on CT. A malpositioned tube impinging into mediastinum, displaced into fissure or outside the pleura or in the lung parenchyma should be communicated to the clinician **(Fig. 10)**. A chest tube in the fissure may adequately drain a pneumothorax but is less effective for a hemothorax.

INJURIES OF THE MEDIASTINUM

Tracheobronchial Injury

Tracheobronchial injuries are uncommon injuries occurring in 1–3% of blunt chest trauma and 2–9% of patients with penetrating chest trauma.[8] Penetrating injury accounts for 70% of tracheobronchial injuries and rest is from blunt trauma, iatrogenic from intubation or tracheostomy, foreign body aspiration, inhalation. Penetrating injuries most commonly involve the cervical part of trachea whereas blunt injury most commonly involves the intrathoracic part.[9] Right main stem bronchus is injured more commonly than the left side due to less protection from surrounding structures. The bronchial injuries usually occur within 2.5 cm of the carina whereas the tracheal injuries usually occur >2 cm above the carina.[10]

Clinically, the diagnosis of tracheobronchial injury is often delayed in many patients because the airway column is maintained by the peribronchial tissue. Tracheal and proximal bronchial injuries result in pneumomediastinum whereas distal bronchial injuries result in pneumothorax. On chest radiograph, presence of significant pneumomediastinum, persistent pneumothorax and atelectasis with increasing subcutaneous emphysema despite adequate chest tube placement should raise a doubt of airway injury. The classical radiological signs described for tracheobronchial injury are enumerated in **Box 3**.

Computed tomography with multiplanar reconstructions is superior to radiograph for detection of airway injury. The most direct sign on CT is demonstration of wall defects or deformity **(Figs. 11A and B)**. The tracheal lacerations are usually vertical and longitudinal and located at the junction of cartilaginous and membranous portion

BOX 3: Radiological signs of tracheobronchial injury.

- "Double wall" sign—due to intramural air within the proximal airway[2]
- "Fallen lung" sign—inferior falling of collapsed lung in the dependent portion due to complete disruption of the central airway
- "Bayonet" sign—tapered air filled bronchus[6]

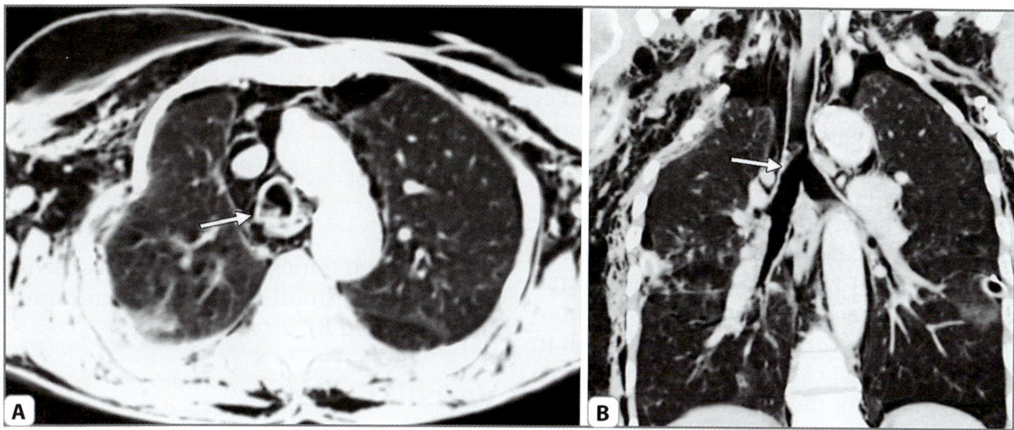

FIGS. 11A AND B: Tracheal injury. Axial (A) and coronal multiplanar reconstruction; (B) CT images show irregularity of right posterolateral wall of lower trachea (arrows) with formation of a luminal flap representing tracheal injury. Note the extensive pneumomediastinum and subcutaneous emphysema.

of the trachea whereas bronchial lacerations occur parallel to the cartilaginous rings. The indirect signs on imaging include an abnormal configuration of endotracheal balloon cuff, pneumomediastinum or pneumothorax and distal atelectasis. Multiplanar images with three-dimensional volumetric images as well as virtual bronchoscopy aid in the diagnosis of tracheobronchial injuries.

Esophageal Injury

Iatrogenic trauma due to endoscopic procedures is the most common cause for esophageal injury followed by penetrating trauma, toxic ingestions, emetic injury (Boerhaave's syndrome) and rarely blunt trauma. Early diagnosis and treatment are important as esophageal injury is associated with high morbidity and mortality. Radiological signs of esophageal perforation include cervical and mediastinal emphysema, pleural effusion, abnormal mediastinal contour due to leakage of fluid, hematoma or mediastinitis, leakage of oral contrast material into mediastinum or pleural space, and esophageal wall thickening. Mid to distal esophageal rupture causes right pleural effusion whereas lower esophageal or rupture of injury at gastroesophageal (GE) junction causes left pleural effusion. Contrast esophagography (radiographic or CT) followed by flexible esophagoscopy may be required to confirm and evaluate the site of injury **(Fig. 12)**.

Rarely, a traumatic tracheoesophageal, fistula may be formed. It is usually secondary to long-term use of an endotracheal or nasogastric tube.

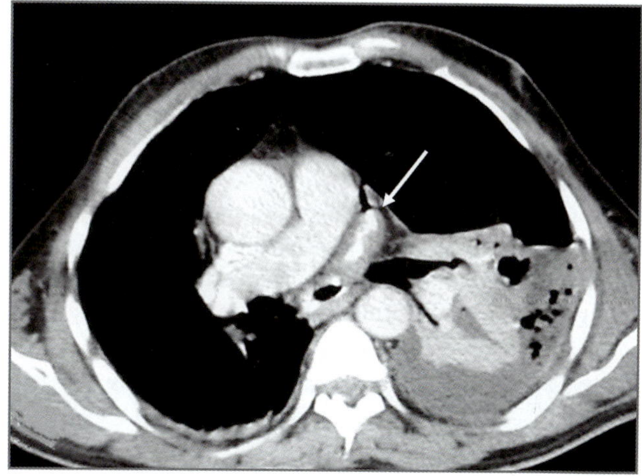

FIG. 12: Esophageal injury. Axial chest CT image shows a leak of oral contrast (arrow) into mediastinum from a tear in the esophagus. Also seen is left pleural fluid with atelectasis of left lower lobe.

Pneumomediastinum

Pneumomediastinum can be due to intrathoracic and extrathoracic sources. Intrathoracic sources include injury to lung, tracheobronchial tree or esophagus whereas extrathoracic sources include head and neck and anterior retroperitoneum. The mediastinum and retroperitoneum communicate through the aortic and esophageal hiatus and at sternocostal attachments of diaphragm. Pneumomediastinum is not itself a dangerous condition but a sign of potentially more serious other injuries.

The most common cause of pneumomediastinum is air from rupture of alveoli due to increased alveolar pressure secondary to trauma. The leaked air dissects along the bronchovascular sheath and spreads into mediastinum. This phenomenon is known as "Macklin effect".[11] The pneumomediastinum may increase in size with positive pressure ventilation. The CT appearance of Macklin effect is that of streaks of air along the bronchovascular bundles (similar to that seen in pulmonary interstitial emphysema) along with pneumomediastinum.

Pneumomediastinum is visualized on anteroposterior chest radiograph as a lucency bordered by a thin white pleural line coursing along the pericardium and lateral mediastinum **(Fig. 13)**. It needs to be differentiated from pneumopericardium and pneumothorax. Pneumopericardium appears as more ovoid in shape than linear and does not extend above the level of aortic arch respecting the boundaries of the pericardium. Also, the pericardium can be visualized in pneumopericardium. Medial pneumothorax may mimic pneumomediastinum but are usually associated with rib fractures and other evidence of pneumothorax. Also, visualization of apparent septae favors a pneumomediastinum. Repeating the imaging in decubitus position confirms the diagnosis as the mediastinal air does not change in location whereas pneumothorax and pneumopericardium would show change in location of air. The pneumomediastinum may dissect into neck and soft tissues on increasing in size. The radiographic signs of pneumomediastinum are described in **Box 4**.

False-positive pneumomediastinum may be caused by "Mach effect", where a thin linear lucency outlines the dense opaque cardiac silhouette. This is due to visual perception of edge enhancement and occurs at the level of the retina.

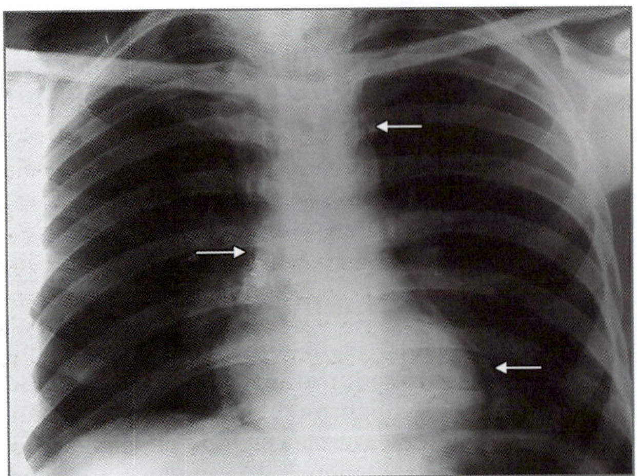

FIG. 13: Pneumomediastinum. Chest radiograph shows air outlining the mediastinum (arrows) on both sides. The air is seen above the level of the aortic arch also (upper left arrow).

BOX 4: Radiological signs of pneumomediastinum on chest radiograph.

- "Double bronchial wall" sign—visualization of both sides of bronchial wall due to air accumulating adjacent to bronchial wall
- "Continuous diaphragm" sign—visualization of entire diaphragm from medial to lateral due to air trapped posterior to the pericardium at base
- "Tubular artery" sign—air outlining the medial side of aorta with lung air outlining the lateral side
- "Ring around the artery" sign—air outlining the pulmonary artery
- Elevation of the thymus especially in children

Computed tomography is the most sensitive modality for detecting small amount of pneumomediastinum **(Figs. 14A and B)**.

Vascular Injury

Traumatic aortic injury is an important cause of morbidity and mortality in patients with blunt thoracic trauma. Early recognition and treatment are of utmost importance as early medical and definitive surgical treatment can improve survivability in these patients. The sites of aortic injury in descending order of frequency are—proximal descending aorta at isthmus (90–95%), ascending aorta including aortic root, aortic arch and distal descending aorta.[12] It causes mediastinal hemorrhage especially in the periaortic region due to bleeding from small veins in the area or from vasa vasorum of the aorta.

Plain chest radiograph is the first investigation after initial resuscitative efforts. The findings on chest radiograph for possible traumatic aortic injury are shown in **Box 5**.

Mediastinal widening has a high sensitivity (90–100%) for mediastinal hematoma and associated aortic injury but the specificity is low (60%). False-positive diagnosis may be due to variety of causes including supine position, expiratory film, atelectasis, pleural effusions or lung injuries obscuring mediastinal margins, mediastinal tumors and mediastinal hemorrhage due to nonaortic causes like spinal fracture or spinal ligamentous injury. A negative plain chest radiograph has a high negative predictive value of 90%. It should, however, be noted that rarely the radiograph may also be normal in aortic injury especially in intimal injuries.

Multislice CT with CT angiography is now the investigation for choice for detecting aortic injuries. It has replaced catheter angiography for screening for aortic injury. Catheter angiography is reserved for doubtful cases and for interventional treatment. The American College of Radiology (ACR) appropriateness criteria recommend using CT angiography for evaluation of all suspected cases of traumatic aortic injury.[13] CT has been reported to have sensitivity of 100% and specificity of 96% for diagnosing aortic injury.[7] Multiplanar reconstructions (MPR) with

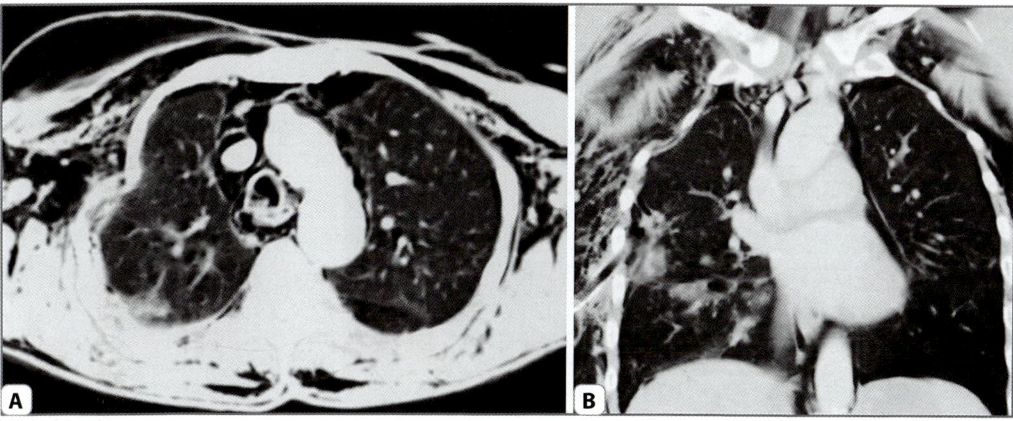

FIGS. 14A AND B: Pneumomediastinum. Axial (A) and coronal multiplanar reconstruction (B) CT images in a patient with tracheal injury (same patient as in **Fig. 11**) show extensive air in the mediastinum. The coronal image (B) shows the air to be present above the level of aortic arch and also tracking along the descending aorta inferiorly.

BOX 5: Chest radiograph signs for possible aortic injury.

- Mediastinal widening
- Depression of the left mainstem bronchus
- Blurring of aortic contour
- Thickening of right or left paratracheal stripe
- Shift of trachea and nasogastric tube to the right
- Left hemothorax (effusion)
- Left apical pleural cap

volume rendering, and virtual angioscopy have been shown to aid in the detection of small rents. The signs of aortic injury on CT are enumerated in **Box 6**.

There are various classifications for grading the severity of aortic injuries based on the direct signs.[14] The most commonly followed is Society for Vascular Surgery (SVS) classification. Grade 1 is intimal flap, grade 2 is intramural hematoma, grade 3 is pseudoaneurysm and grade 4 is aortic rupture. The Harborview classification divides the injuries into three categories: minimal, moderate, and severe. "Minimal" aortic injury encompasses the type 1 and 2 of SVS classification and includes intimal tear and thrombus of <10 mm **(Figs. 15A and B)**. "Moderate" aortic injury includes intimal tears >10 mm or external contour abnormality (pseudoaneurysm). Active contrast extravasation signifying aortic rupture is categorized as "severe" aortic injury. This categorization is useful for management decisions. The "minimal" injuries do not require any active intervention and may or may not require follow-up imaging. The "moderate" injuries require a semi-elective repair after controlling other major injuries. The most preferred method is by thoracic endovascular aortic repair (TEVAR) by putting an aortic stent graft. The "severe" injuries require an immediate aortic repair **(Figs. 16A to C)**.

Non-aortic vascular injury may also occur in thoracic trauma. These include injury to aortic arch branches, internal mammary artery, pulmonary artery and venous injuries. The spectrum of injuries includes intimal tears, dissection, pseudoaneurysm, partial or total occlusion and arteriovenous fistula.

BOX 6: Signs of traumatic aortic injury on CT.

- *Direct signs*:
  - Active contrast extravasation
  - Pseudoaneurysm formation
  - Abrupt change in aortic diameter caliper
  - Aortic dissection
  - Intimal flaps or filling defects **(Figs. 15A and B)**
  - Aortic wall irregularity
- *Indirect signs*:
  - Indistinctness of mediastinal fat planes
  - Mediastinal hematoma
  - Periaortic hematoma

Cardiac and Pericardial Injury

The diagnosis of blunt cardiac injury relies on a high degree of clinical suspicion. Elevated cardiac enzymes with alterations in ECG findings in the setting of blunt thoracic trauma should raise a doubt of cardiac injury. Transthoracic echocardiography is the most appropriate modality for evaluation of cardiac injury. If it is equivocal, then transesophageal echocardiography or cardiac MRI can be used as problem-solving tool. If contrast CT of the thorax has been done for evaluation of thoracic trauma, cardiac and pericardial injury manifestations include pericardial effusion/hemopericardium, pneumopericardium, contrast extravasation into pericardium or a decreased area of myocardial enhancement **(Figs. 17A and B)**.

Pericardial injury is most commonly on the left side of pericardium parallel to phrenic nerve followed by diaphragmatic surface of pericardium. A large pericardial tear can cause cardiac herniation and death.

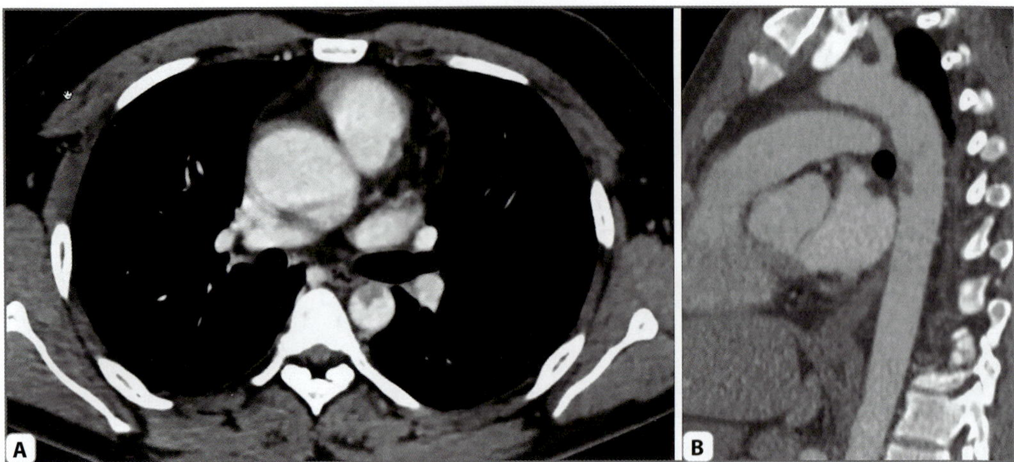

FIGS. 15A AND B: Minimal aortic injury. Axial (A) and coronal MPR (B) CT images show a small <10 mm mural thrombus attached to anterior wall of aortic isthmus.

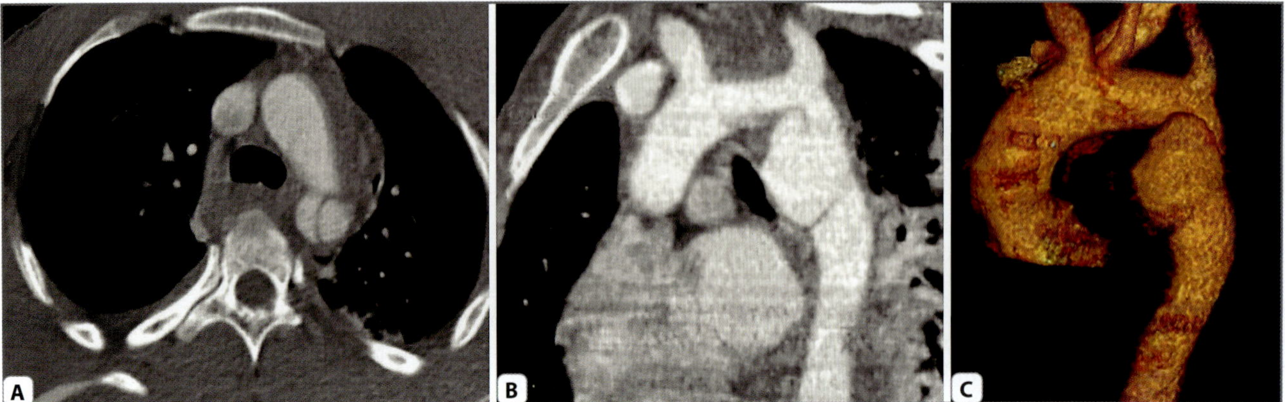

FIGS. 16A TO C: Moderate aortic injury. Axial (A), sagittal MPR (B) and volume rendered 3D (C) CT images show a dissecting pseudoaneurysm at aortic isthmus with surrounding hematoma.

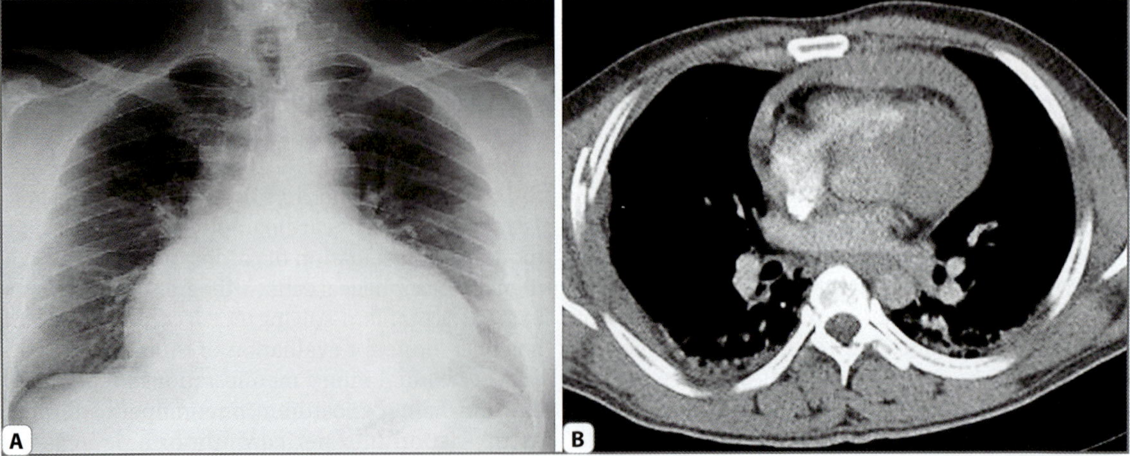

FIGS. 17A AND B: Hemopericardium. Chest radiograph (A) shows an enlarged flask shaped cardiac silhouette representing pericardial fluid. Axial CT image (B) in a different patient shows the hemopericardium. The patient was found to have ventricular wall injury peroperative.

INJURY OF DIAPHRAGM

Diaphragmatic rupture and subsequent herniation of abdominal contents into thorax is nine times more common on left side than right due to the protective effect of the liver. On the right side most injuries to the diaphragm go unrecognized during the acute phase. In the interval phase, the abdominal viscus may not have herniated, or the patient may have acclimatized to the presence of abdominal contents in the thorax. In the later phase, obstruction or strangulation presents with severe abdominal or chest pain. The injury may also be evident at a later stage in those patients who were earlier on positive pressure ventilation and have now been extubated. Chest radiograph may reveal nonspecific findings that include an indistinct or elevated hemidiaphragm, pleural effusion, atelectasis with shift of the mediastinum to the contralateral side, hemothorax, pneumothorax or lower rib fractures. Specific findings are visualization of bowel loops or solid masses above the diaphragm and loss of the normal diaphragmatic contour. Detection of a nasogastric tube above the left hemidiaphragm is also a strong indicator. Contrast studies (barium meal or enema) can be used to clearly delineate the herniation.

The advent of MDCT with multiplanar reconstructions significantly improved the sensitivity of CT in detecting diaphragmatic injuries and has made it as the modality of choice. The various CT signs of diaphragmatic injury are given in **Box 7**.[15,16]

The "collar" sign refers to the narrowed waist of a herniated intra-abdominal organ due to compression at the neck (diaphragm tear). In a healthy individual, the intra-abdominal organs such as spleen and stomach are seen to be separated by the costal margin by a layer of the diaphragm on cross-sectional imaging. However, if these organs have herniated through the diaphragm into the chest, then they appear to lie directly in contact with the posterior thoracic wall without the diaphragm intervening between them **(Figs. 18A and B)**. This has been described as the "dependent viscera" sign. The "dependent viscera" sign and the "collar" signs are reported to be 100% specific.[17] MRI also has been reported to be highly sensitive in detecting diaphragmatic rupture.[18]

INJURY OF CHEST WALL

Rib fractures occur in approximately 50% of all blunt chest trauma and are the most common skeletal manifestation of injury. Isolated rib fractures are usually not clinically significant. However, multiple and bilateral rib fractures signify severe trauma and act as external manifestation of coexisting thoracic or abdominal injuries. Fractures of the first three ribs occur after severe trauma and are associated with injuries of brachial plexus or subclavian vessels. Fractures of the lower three ribs are associated with intra-abdominal visceral organ injuries to kidney, spleen and liver. Further, due to the pain and immobility associated with rib fractures, the underlying lung is more prone to atelectasis and pneumonia. Rarely traumatic lung herniation, as described previously, can also occur. Chest radiography is much less sensitive than CT in detecting rib fractures. CT with three-dimensional volume rendering best depicts the rib fractures.[19]

BOX 7: Signs of diaphragmatic injury on CT.

- Focal diaphragmatic discontinuity or elevation
- Focal diaphragmatic thickening (retraction)
- Herniated abdominal contents into thorax
- "Collar" sign
- "Dependent viscera" sign

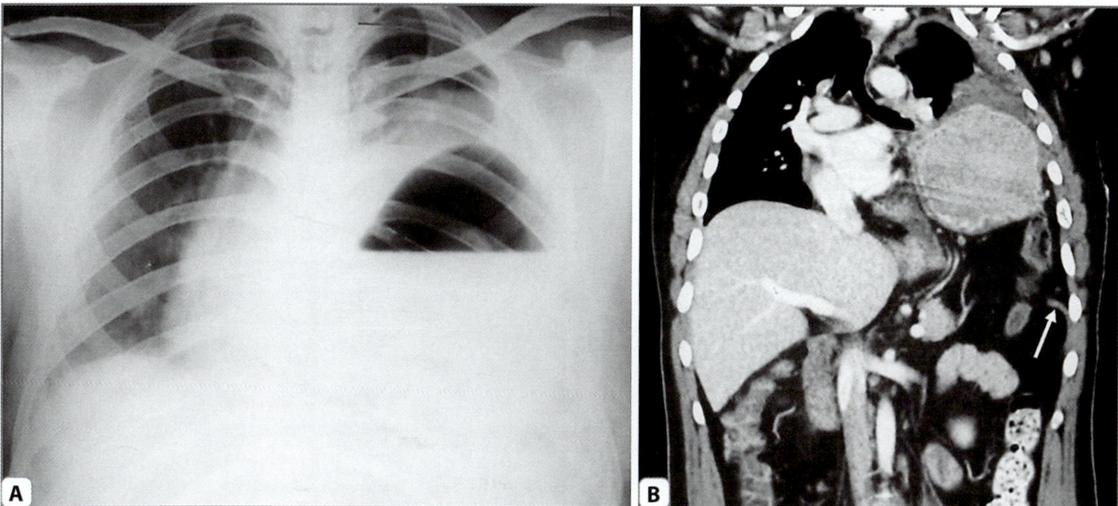

FIGS. 18A AND B: Diaphragmatic injury. Erect chest radiograph (A) shows indistinct left hemidiaphragm outline with large air-fluid level (of stomach) in left thoracic cavity with mediastinal shift toward right. Coronal MPR CT image (B) shows the left diaphragmatic hernia with thickened and retracted torn diaphragm (arrow).

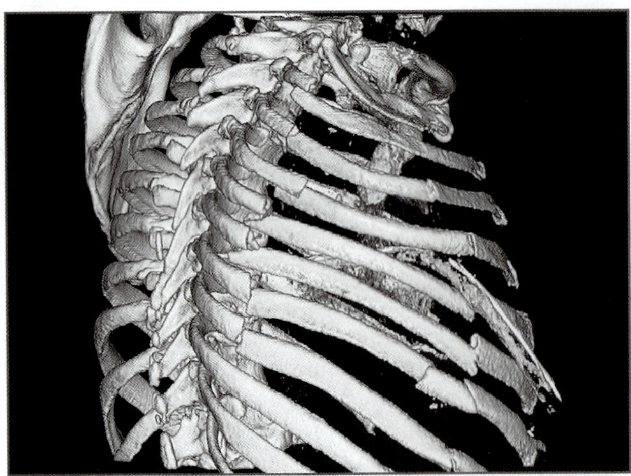

FIG. 19: Flail chest. Three-dimensional volume rendered CT image shows fractures of multiple ribs on right side with many ribs fractured at two places at lateral and posterior ends.

Flail chest occurs when there are atleast two sites of fractures on each of three or more consecutive ribs creating a flail segment which moves paradoxically with respiratory motion **(Fig. 19)**. It signifies significant chest trauma and is associated with atelectasis and pneumonia and often requires ventilator support or surgical intervention.

Sternal fractures are uncommon. The fracture typically involves the manubrium or body. CT is the most sensitive for detection followed by lateral chest radiograph **(Figs. 20A and B)**. A retrosternal hematoma may be seen. A significantly displaced sternal fracture may be associated with underlying cardiac injury.

Fractures of the clavicle are classified according to their location. Group 1 fractures are most common (80%) and involve the mid-part of clavicle; group 2 fractures (15%) involve the lateral third of clavicle; and group 3 fractures (5%) involve the medial third of the clavicle **(Figs. 21A and B)**. Most fractures are managed conservatively

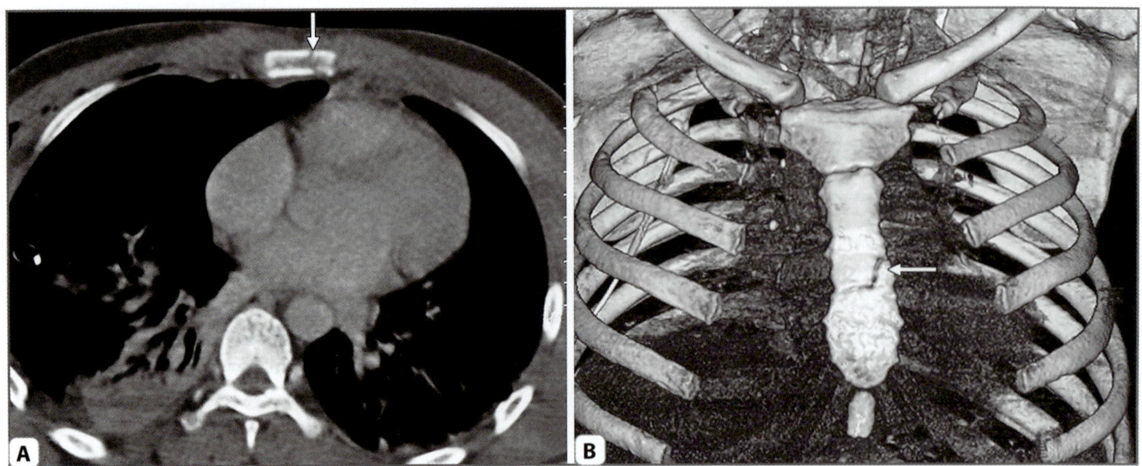

FIGS. 20A AND B: Sternal fracture. Axial (A) and volume rendered three-dimensional (B) CT images show fracture of mid body of sternum.

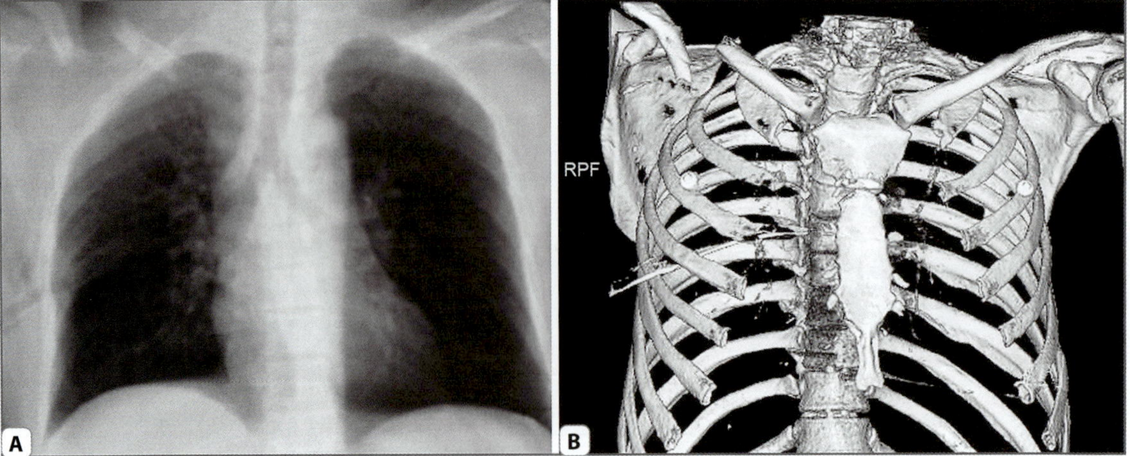

FIGS. 21A AND B: Clavicle fracture. Thick MPR (A) and volume rendered three-dimensional (B) CT images show fracture of mid-part of right clavicle.

although the surgical rate for distal third fractures is more as they have a high rate of nonunion.

Sternoclavicular dislocations can be anterior or posterior. Anterior dislocation of clavicle is more common. It is usually not associated with significant injuries and is managed conservatively. Posterior dislocation of clavicle at sternoclavicular joint is more serious as the clavicle can cause injury of trachea, esophagus and mediastinal blood vessels.

Scapular fractures are seen with severe trauma and are usually associated with vascular and neurological injuries. Most fractures occur at the body or neck of scapula. They are usually managed conservatively except for displaced glenoid intra-articular fractures and juxta-articular fractures which require surgical management. Rarely there may be scapulothoracic dissociation in which scapula is displaced laterally. Multiplanar CT reconstructions are best to visualize the fracture fragments.

Spinal fractures may also be associated with thoracic trauma. The spinal fractures are easily seen on the multiplanar reconstructions of the CT done for chest. The fractures may be associated with significant neurological deficits in up to 60% of patients. MRI is indicated in patients with spinal trauma and associated neurological deficit for characterization of the spinal cord damage.

CONCLUSION

Diagnostic imaging quickly gives important information on the extent and type of thoracic injuries from blunt and penetrating trauma. The chest radiograph is the "first look" imaging modality and has a role in detecting some immediate life-threatening conditions like tension pneumothorax and massive hemothorax. Ultrasound is also used as a first line investigation for detecting hemothorax, pneumothorax and hemopericardium. Multislice CT has become the definitive modality which detects and characterizes the full extent of spectrum of thoracic trauma. MRI does not have any significant role in the setting of acute trauma except for evaluation of spinal cord in spinal injuries.

REFERENCES

1. Lomoschitz FM, Eisenhuber E, Linnau KF, et al. Imaging of chest trauma: radiological patterns of injury and diagnostic algorithms. European Journal of Radiology. 2003;48:61-70.
2. Lewis BT, Herr KD, Hamlin SA, Henry T, Little BP, Naeger DM, et al. Imaging Manifestations of Chest Trauma. Radiographics. 2021;41(5):1321-34.
3. Miller LA. Chest wall, lung, and pleural space trauma. Radiol Clin North Am. 2006;44:213-24.
4. Costantino M, Gosselin MV, Primack SL. The ABC's of thoracic trauma imaging. Semin Roentgenol. 2006;41(3):209-25.
5. Miller PR, Croce MA, Bec TK, et al. ARDS after pulmonary contusion: accurate measurement of contusion volume identifies high-risk patients. J Trauma. 2001;51:223-30.
6. Kaewlai R, Avery LL, Asrani AV, et al. Multidetector CT of blunt thoracic trauma. Radiographics. 2008;28(6):1555-70.
7. Rivas LA, Fishman JE, Múnera F, et al. Multislice CT in thoracic trauma. Radiol Clin North Am. 2003;41(3):599-616.
8. Bagga B, Kumar A, Chahal A, Gamanagatti S, Kumar S. Traumatic Airway Injuries: Role of Imaging. Curr Probl Diagn Radiol. 2020;49(1):48-53.
9. Durso AM, Caban K, Munera F. Penetrating Thoracic Injury. Radiol Clin N Am. 2015;53:675-93.
10. Sangster GP, González-Beicos A, Carbo AI, et al. Blunt traumatic injuries of the lung parenchyma, pleura, thoracic wall, and intrathoracic airways: multidetector computer tomography imaging findings. Emerg Radiol. 2007;14:297-310.
11. Wintermark M, Wicky S, Schnyder P, et al. Blunt traumatic pneumomediastinum: using CT to reveal the Macklin effect. AJR Am J Roentgenol. 1999;172:129-30.
12. Fishman JE. Imaging of blunt aortic and great vessel trauma. J Thorac Imaging. 2000;15:97-103.
13. Demehri S, Rybicki FJ, Desjardins B, et al. ACR Appropriateness Criteria: Blunt chest trauma—suspected aortic injury. Emerg Radiol. 2012;19:287-92.
14. Gupta S, Kumar A, Kaur T, Gamanagatti S, Kumar A, Gupta A, et al. Current updates in acute traumatic aortic injury: radiologic diagnosis and management. Clin Exp Emerg Med. 2022;9(2):73-83.
15. Panda A, Kumar A, Gamanagatti S, et al. Traumatic diaphragmatic injury: a review of CT signs and the difference between blunt and penetrating injury. Diagn Interv Radiol. 2014;20(2):121-8.
16. Polireddy K, Hoff C, Kinger NP, Tran A, Maddu K. Blunt thoracic trauma: role of chest radiography and comparison with CT - findings and literature review. Emerg Radiol. 2022;29(4):743-55.
17. Stanescu AL, Gross JA, Bittle M, et al. Imaging of blunt abdominal trauma. Semin Roentgen. 2006;41(3):196-204.
18. Barbiera F, Nicastro N, Finazzo M, et al. The role of MRI in traumatic rupture of the diaphragm. Our experience in three cases and review of the literature. Radiol Med. 2003;105(3):188-94.
19. Marro A, Chan V, Haas B, Ditkofsky N. Blunt chest trauma: classification and management. Emerg Radiol. 2019;26(5):557-66.

Anjali Prakash, Rashmi Dixit, Sapna Singh

CHAPTER

18

Imaging of Pleura

INTRODUCTION

The pleura is a serous membrane of mesodermal origin that envelops the lungs, mediastinum, diaphragm and rib cage. It is composed of two layers—parietal and visceral. The lung is covered with visceral pleura, the parietal pleural covers the mediastinum, diaphragm and inner surface of thoracic cage. The layers are in continuity, both at the hilum and below, where they form the pulmonary ligament. The parietal pleura is divided into costal pleura, diaphragmatic pleura, mediastinal and cervical pleura, based on its relationship to various regions of the thoracic cavity. The visceral and parietal pleural are separated by a potential space that normally contains only a few mL of fluid. As the thickness of the pleural space and its visceral and parietal pleura measures about 0.2–0.44 mm, it is only seen when parallel to the X-ray beam or outlined by air, extrapleural fat or fascia. The pleura is appreciated as:

- The major, minor or accessory fissures, all of which (with the exception of azygos fissure) consists of two invaginated sheets of visceral pleura.
- The junctional lines, which consists of four sheets of pleura (two parietal and two visceral), which are often more than a hairline thickness as both (particularly posterior) may contain fibrofatty tissue.

The vascular supply of the parietal pleural is from the systemic circulation, whereas the visceral pleural is supplied by branches of the pulmonary arteries and to a lesser extent by bronchial arteries. Lymphatic drainage of the visceral pleural is by a lymphatic plexus that covers the surface of the lung, just beneath the visceral pleural. This elaborate plexus connects to the bronchial lymphatics that drain centrally along the bronchovascular bundles to the pulmonary hilum. The parietal pleural is the primary drainage route for the pleural space and is lymphatically connected to the intercostal, internal mammary and mediastinal lymph node chains.

IMAGING MODALITIES

Chest radiograph is the initial screening radiological investigation when pleural disease or pulmonary disease is suspected. Chest frontal, lateral, decubitus views are helpful in detecting small amount of pleural effusion. Expiratory films may be required to visualize a small pneumothorax. The drawback is its limited ability to differentiate benign from malignant pleural disease. It is important to differentiate pleural from extrapleural disease and pulmonary disease.

Extrapleural masses usually displace the overlying parietal and visceral pleura resulting in an obtuse angle between the lesion and chest wall. Associated abnormalities include soft tissue mass or rib destruction. They are sharply marginated at the point they contact lung and displace pulmonary vessels away from them.

Pleural masses, arising from visceral or parietal pleura, usually remain confined to pleural space. The presence of an obtuse angle is common, unless the lesion is large. Large pleural lesions may have an acute angle, where they meet the chest wall, although some pleural thickening is seen adjacent to them. Pleural lesions are also sharply marginated and displace pulmonary vessels away from them.

A peripherally placed pulmonary lesion will have acute angle with the pleural surface, unless there is pleural invasion, which could result is an obtuse angle. Pulmonary lesions are often ill defined along their inner aspect and may engulf, rather than displace vessels **(Table 1)**.

TABLE 1: Radiological differentiation of pleural, extrapleural and pulmonary lesion.

Features	Pulmonary	Pleural	Extrapleural
Incomplete border sign (radiograph)	Absent	Present	Present
Angle with chest wall	Acute	Obtuse	Obtuse
Epicenter	In lung	Along chest wall	Along chest wall
Pulmonary vasculature	Engulfs	Displace	Displace
Extrapleural fat displacement	–	Outwards	Inwards
Rib erosion	Unusual	Unusual	Usual

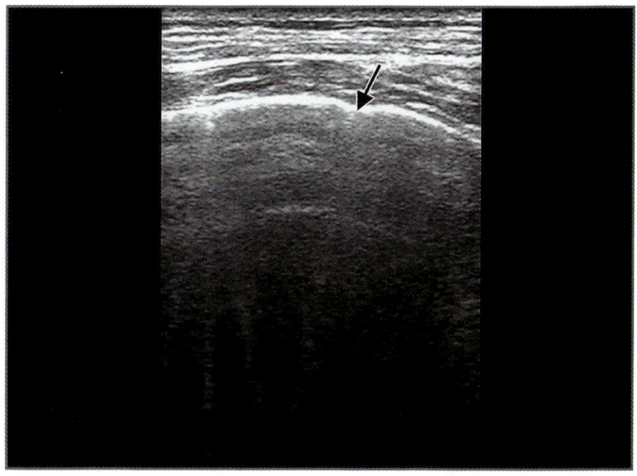

FIG. 1: Chest ultrasound direct intercostal approach: Echogenic line depicting the lung pleura interface.

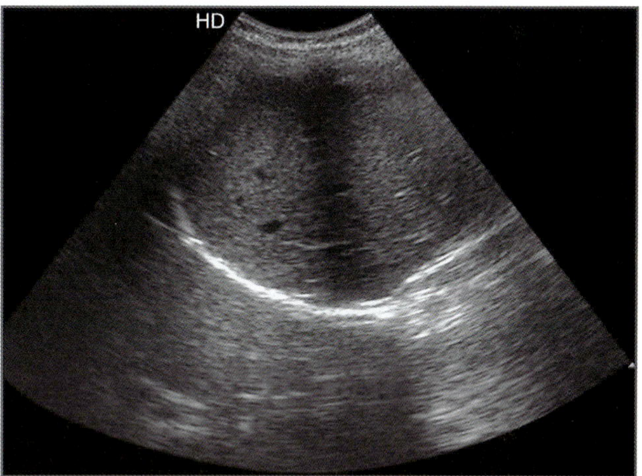

FIG. 2: Ultrasound of chest-abdominal approach-mirror image of liver seen above the diaphragm implying the presence of air-filled lung.

Ultrasonography is an efficient, "point of care" imaging modality for evaluation of the chest wall and pleura because of the superficial location. It has low cost, bedside availability and involves no radiation. The indications and uses of chest ultrasound examination for pleural disease are:

- To clarify the nature of unknown pleural densities
- To detect pleural effusion and to guide thoracocentesis and drainage, especially in minimal or loculated effusion
- To differentiate subpulmonic effusion from subphrenic fluid accumulation
- To detect pneumothorax in emergency setting
- To localize pleural tumors/thickening and guide biopsy of the pleura

Pleura is a superficial structure and hence seen with a high frequency linear transducer applied directly over the chest—the direct intercostal approach. A sector probe (3.5 MHz) may be used for the lower aspect of pleura via the abdominal approach, with the liver and spleen providing an acoustic window. Normal pleura is identified just below the ribs and is seen on ultrasound as an echogenic line just beneath the chest wall **(Fig. 1)**. The air-filled lung covered by visceral pleura reflects the ultrasound beam producing the echogenic line that moves with respiration. This normal movement of lung surface is called "gliding sign". This echogenic line represents the visceral pleura, with the parietal pleura appearing as a weakly echogenic, less distinct line, often obscured by artifacts. Using the abdominal approach, the diaphragm is seen as a bright curving echogenic line. An air-filled lung above it will cause specular reflection and mirror image reflection of liver or spleen on the left side **(Fig. 2)**. The presence of this mirror image implies the presence of an air-filled lung and the absence of pleural fluid above the diaphragm.

CT is the modality of choice in evaluating diseases of the pleura, especially pleural tumors. It is particularly helpful in determining chest wall, mediastinum and diaphragmatic involvement. CT allows differentiation of benign from malignant pleural disease except in very early disease. It can display anterior and paravertebral pleural plaques, areas not well seen on chest radiographs.

For complete evaluation of the pleural surfaces the patient is scanned contiguously from the thoracic inlet to the L3 level. Pleural enhancement is best demonstrated with a delayed scan time of 45–60 seconds.

On HRCT, the pleura may be identified when it forms the fissures. Depending on its obliquity to the imaging plane, a fissure appears as a thin, high density line or band. On conventional CT, the fissure is appreciated as an avascular band. Peripherally on CT and HRCT, there is a thin line–the intercostal stripe separating the lung margin and the fat lying inside the internal intercostal muscle **(Fig. 3)**. This line (the lung chest wall interface) connects the inner aspect of the ribs and is 1–2 mm thick. It comprises the two layers of pleura.

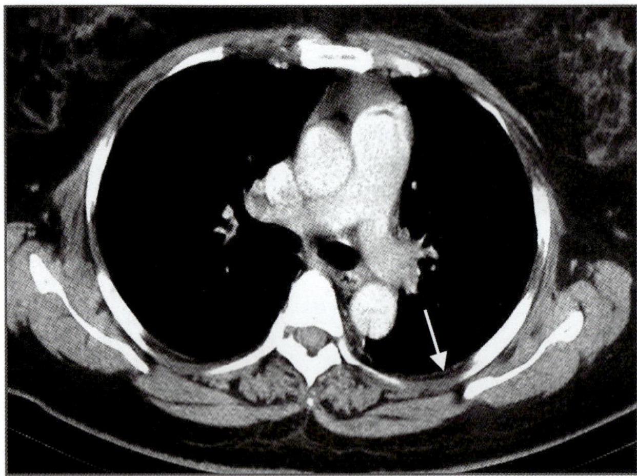

FIG. 3: CT—A thin white stripe (marked with arrow) between adjacent ribs represents the intercostal stripe, primarily representing the innermost intercostal muscle. This is anatomically absent in the paravertebral region.

1. *Subparietal pleural fat*: Separates parietal pleura from endothoracic fascia. This is very thin in most locations, but can be markedly thickened over the lateral or posterolateral ribs, resulting in extrapleural fat pads.
2. *Endothoracic fascia*: This fibroelastic fascia covers the surface of the intercostal muscles and intervening ribs, blends with the perichondrium and periosteum of the costal cartilages. Posteriorly, it is continuous with the prevertebral fascia that covers the vertebral bodies and intervertebral discs.

MRI suffers from the drawback of a poor signal to noise ratio in lung, cardiac and respiratory motion artefacts and susceptibility artifacts at air tissue boundaries. However, it is sometimes used as a problem solving tool.

Diffusion imaging (DWI) helps to noninvasively characterize various types of effusion. Diffusion weighted imaging can differentiate benign from pleural malignant disease with a cut-off ADC threshold being 1.52×10^{-3} mm^2/s. This has a sensitivity of 71.4% and specificity of 100%. In cases where ADC is indeterminate, dynamic contrast enhanced MRI improves the diagnostic confidence.[1]

MRI also plays an important role in the evaluation of extent of pleural neoplasm especially in areas like lung apices and diaphragm.

FDG-PET is complementary to CT in the evaluation of pleural tumors. It has an important role in staging pleural mesothelioma.

PLEURAL PATHOLOGY

Pleura may be affected by the following pathologies which may be linked to each other:
- Effusion
- Pneumothorax
- Pleural thickening
- Tumor
- Tumor like conditions

PLEURAL EFFUSION

Fluid moves across the capillary membranes of the visceral pleura into the pleural space and is then reabsorbed by the lymphatic system. Changes in capillary permeability, hydrostatic and oncotic pressure or lymphatic function affects the balance between the formation and resorption of pleural fluid leading to accumulation of fluid in the pleural space.

The pleural fluid may be transudate, exudate, blood or chyle. All types of pleural effusion are radiographically identical, though clinical and biochemical features may help limit the differential diagnosis. Most pleural effusion are classified as exudates or transudates based on their chemical composition which is usually defined by thoracocentesis. The criteria most commonly used to separate transudative from exudative effusion are known as Light's criteria.[2] Pleural fluid is considered an exudate if one or more of the following criteria are met.
1. A ratio of pleural fluid protein to serum protein higher than 0.5.
2. A ratio of pleural fluid lactate dehydrogenase (LDH) to serum LDH level that exceeds 0.6.
3. A pleural fluid LDH level more than two-thirds the upper limit of normal serum LDH.

Exudative effusion reflects the presence of a pleural abnormality associated with increased permeability of pleural capillaries. These effusions have high protein content. Common causes of exudative effusion include pneumonia with parapneumonic effusion, empyema, TB, pleuritis, neoplasm, pulmonary embolism, drug reaction, etc.

Transudative effusion is unassociated with pleural disease. It usually results from systemic abnormalities causing an imbalance in the hydrostatic and osmotic forces governing pleural fluid formation. These are low in protein and are usually bilateral. Common causes include CHF, pericardial disease, liver cirrhosis, renal disease, and hypoalbuminemia.

Bilateral effusions are usually transudates as they are secondary to generalized causes such as hypoproteinemia. Some bilateral effusions may be exudates, e.g., those associated with metastatic disease, lymphoma, rheumatoid disease, systemic lupus erythematosus (SLE). Right-sided effusions are typically associated with ascitis, heart failure and liver abscess. Effusions associated with pancreatitis, pericarditis, esophageal rupture and aortic dissection tend to be left sided. The various causes of pleural effusion are enumerated in **Box 1**.

Massive effusions are most commonly due to malignant disease, especially metastatic (lung or breast), but may also

BOX 1: Causes of pleural effusion.

Transudative effusion:
- Congestive heart failure
- Cirrhosis
- Nephrotic syndrome
- Hypoalbuminemia
- Hypothyroidism
- Peritoneal dialysis
- Ovarian hyperstimulation syndrome

Exudative effusion:
- Malignant neoplasms
- Pulmonary thromboembolism
- Empyema
- Collagen vascular diseases
- Benign asbestos pleural effusion-BAPE
- Chylothorax
- Hemothorax

occur in heart failure, cirrhosis, tuberculosis, empyema and trauma.

Specific Causes of Pleural Effusion

Congestive Heart Failure

Congestive heart failure (CHF) is the most common cause of transudative effusion, though exudative effusions may also occur. Pleural fluid accumulates in CHF because pulmonary interstitial fluid (due to edema) crosses into the pleural space. Bilateral effusions are seen is 70% of cases, if unilateral, it is usually right sided. A large unilateral pleural effusion should suggest an alternative diagnosis.

Renal Disease

Pleural effusion is seen with renal disease due to various causes.

- Renal failure with overhydration may result in transudative effusion, usually bilateral.
- Nephrotic syndrome may cause transudative effusions due to increased hydrostatic pressure and hypoalbuminemia resulting in decreased oncotic pressure.
- Uremia may result in fibrinous pleuritis and a bloody exudative effusion that is often unilateral and large. Pleural thickening may also be seen.
- Hydronephrosis due to retroperitoneal lesion may result in ipsilateral pleural effusion—which is rich in creatinine.
- Effusion may result from peritoneal dialysis, fluid enters the pleural space via diaphragmatic defects.

Radiation (Therapeutic)

Approximately 5% of patients having chest radiation develop a small exudative pleural effusion. This is usually in association with radiation pneumonitis the effusion being on the same side as that of radiation, develops within 6 months of radiation. It resolves slowly with time.

Dressler's Syndrome

It occurs in a few patients postmyocardial infarction or cardiac surgery. It occurs 2–3 weeks after the event and is associated with chest pain, fever, dyspnea. Radiographs show pleural effusion (85%) lung consolidation and pericardial effusion. It is thought to be an immunologically mediated response. They are usually bilateral, when unilateral, it is usually left sided.

Pulmonary Embolism

Pleural effusion occurs in 30% of patients with pulmonary embolism. Usually associated with infarction, exudates (75%) are more common than transudates.

Pericardial Disease

Pleural effusion is common in patients with inflammatory pericardial disease. They are left sided in 70%. In patients with constrictive pericarditis, effusions or CHF may result from elevated left or right sided venous pressure.

Meigs's Syndrome

Pleural effusion with ascitis and ovarian fibroma is the classical triad of Meigs's syndrome. Other ovarian tumors may show similar presentation. It may be exudative or transudative. Resection of the tumor results in resolution of pleural effusion and ascitis.

Pancreatitis

Pleural effusion is associated with acute and chronic pancreatitis. The effusion shows high amylase levels. In acute pancreatitis, exudative effusion is seen, mostly on left side. In chronic pancreatitis, effusions are large and indolent. The pleural effusion is probably secondary to fistula formation following ductal rupture.

Chylothorax may result from rupture of thoracic duct or of a prominent lymphatic channel. Lymph may also accumulate as a result of oozing from pleural lymphatics or due to passage of chylous ascites via diaphragm. Chylous effusion is associated with neoplastic etiology in majority[3] of cases, seen in patients with lymphoma, metastatic neoplasm. Chylothorax also develops following thoracic surgery chest trauma, inflammatory mediastinal lymph node disease, and in some developmental anomalies such as lymphangioma, lymphangioleiomyomatosis. Traumatic chylothorax resolves over time as the thoracic duct heals. Reduction in lymph flow may be helpful. Ligation of duct is curative.

Chylous effusion contains intestinal lymph (i.e., chyle), which is high in protein and fatty acids and is low in cholesterol. It looks milky on naked eye examination.

Chylothorax does not have a low CT number despite the presence of fat as it is rich in proteins. A chylous effusion can show high signal intensity on T1WI. Pseudochylous or chyliform effusion contains cholesterol, but not chyle. It may be seen in patients with chronic inflammatory disease like to TB, rheumatoid arthritis. Chylous effusions may remain chronic for years.

Hemothorax

It refers to pleural fluid having a hematocrit of over 50% of blood hematocrit. On CT, hemothorax results in fluid with high attenuation (mostly >50 HU) containing a dense clot or a fluid-fluid level, with the densest fluid posteriorly. Most of cases are traumatic in origin, others may be spontaneous, including rupture of aneurysm/dissection, pulmonary or pleural neoplasm, coagulopathy. Treatment includes drainage. Organization of hemothorax results in fibrosis and calcification. A resolving exudative effusion or hemothorax may deposit a clot of fibrin within the pleural space termed as fibrin body or pleural mouse. These appear 1–2 cm in diameter, mimicking a solitary nodule, localized to pleural space and are sometimes seen to move with change in patient position. They resolve or may remain stable for years.

IMAGING IN PLEURAL EFFUSION

Plain Radiographs

The radiological signs of a pleural effusion depend on the posture of the patient and distribution of fluid which may be free or loculated. The pleural space extends inferiorly below the visible lung, in relation to the diaphragm and ribs. A small amount of pleural fluid is not visible on erect radiograph as it collects under the lung. These small **subpulmonic** effusions are detected by ultrasound or CT.

In an upright subject at least 175 mL of fluid must be present to result in blunting of the lateral costophrenic angle on the frontal radiograph and rarely as much as 500 mL may be present without blunting **(Fig. 4)**. On a lateral decubitus film, as little as 10 mL fluid may be seen. The classical signs of pleural effusion include—homogenous opacification of lower chest with obliteration of costophrenic angle and the hemidiaphragm. The upper margin of the opacity is concave to the lung and is higher laterally than medially. The highest point of the "meniscus" reflects the true level of fluid **(Fig. 5)**. This is because the X-ray beam traverses a greater thickness of fluid at the periphery due to circumferential configuration of the pleural space around the air-containing lung. Above and medial to the meniscus, there is a hazy increase in opacityowing to fluid behind and in front of the lungs.

Massive effusion can cause dense opacification of the hemithorax with contralateral mediastinal shift **(Fig. 6) (Box 2)**. Shifted structures include the trachea, the heart, the azygoesophageal recess, producing a paravertebral retrocardiac density convex to the lung. The absence of mediastinal shift with a large effusion should raise the possibility of obstructive collapse of the ipsilateral lung or extensive pleural malignancy such as seen with mesothelioma or metastatic carcinoma.

Fluid entering into fissures may produce other opacities like middle lobe step or broad band with a curvilinear inner margin extending from midlung to chest wall, often becoming denser as it passes laterally.

On the frontal radiograph, fluid extending into the posterolateral major fissure typically results in an arcuate opacity, sharply defined medially and inferiorly. Fluid extending into the lateral aspect of the minor fissure and

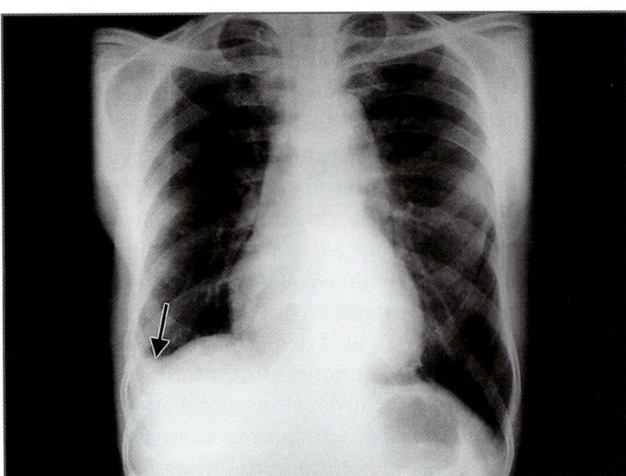

FIG. 4: X-ray of chest PA view—blunting of right costophrenic angle-pleural effusion.

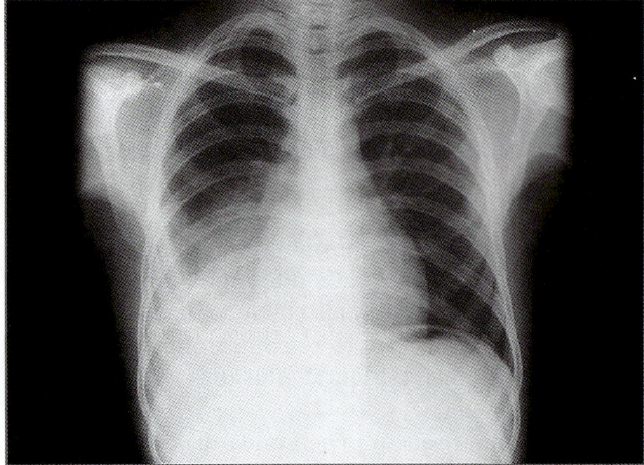

FIG. 5: X-ray of chest PA view—homogeneous opacification of right lower zone with obliteration of the right costophrenic angle and the hemidiaphragm. The upper margin of the opacity is concave and extends higher laterally "meniscus sign"—Pleural effusion.

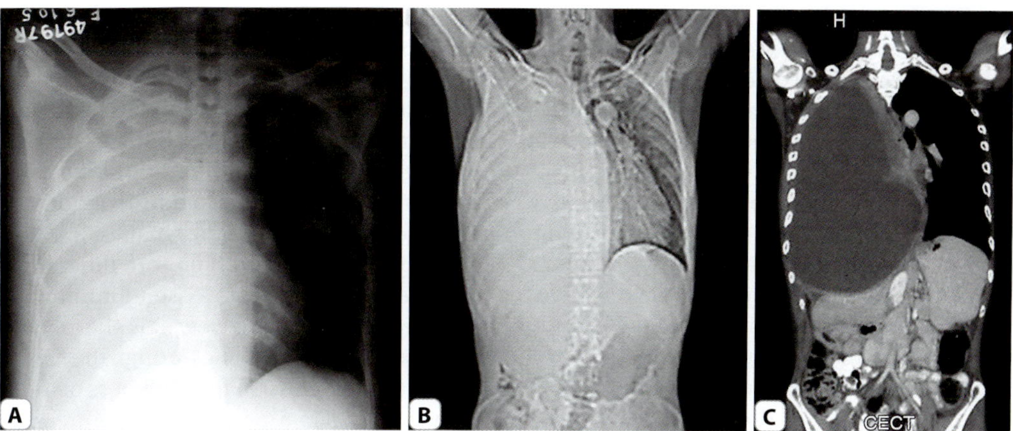

FIGS. 6A TO C: X-ray of chest (A) Opaque hemithorax without shift of the mediastinum—scanogram (B) and coronal MPR (C) opaque hemithorax with shift of mediastinum and inversion of right hemidiaphragm in another patient.

BOX 2: Causes of opaque hemithorax.

- Pleural effusion
- Consolidation
- Collapse
- Massive tumor
- Fibrothorax
- Pneumonectomy
- Lung agenesis

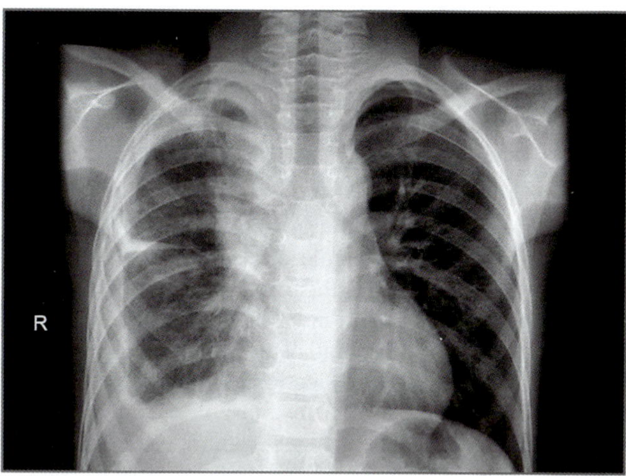

FIG. 7: Right pleural effusion is seen with associated mediastinal lymphadenopathy. Fluid is entering the minor fissure resembling a "rose thorn".

slightly separating the lobes, result in an opacity resembling a rose thorn (the thorn sign—**Fig. 7**).

As the lung is fixed medially, medial pleural fluid collections are usually smaller and more difficult to recognize. Medial fluid collection may be seen when effusions are large. More often, these accumulate in the posterior gutters, with thickening of the paravertebral stripe. The fluid collection may be triangular simulating lower lobe collapse.

Pleural fluid may accumulate in the subpulmonic space, allowing the lung base to float superiorly on a frontal radiograph. Subpulmonic effusion presents as a "high hemi diaphragm" with an unusual contour that peaks more laterally **(Fig. 8)**. On the left side, 2 cm of separation of the lung base from the top of the stomach bubble is taken as evidence of subpulmonic effusion, although distance may be variable. Most subpulmonic effusion are mobile with postural change. These are often transudates. On the lateral view, a subpulmonic effusion elevates the posterior lung, flattening its under surface, insinuates into the major fissure resulting in focal triangular thickening of the fissures, flattens the inferior contour of the lung anterior to the fissure which then angles sharply downward. Fluid may accumulate between the lung and visceral pleura, a common finding in patients of heart failure. This is called "lamellar effusion" and is not a true pleural effusion

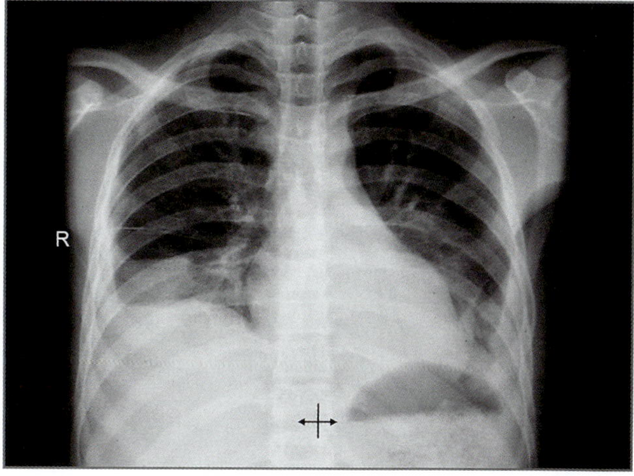

FIG. 8: Bilateral pleural effusion. Raised right hemidiaphragm with a lateralized apex suggestive of subpulmonic effusion.

because it lies outside the pleural sac. It is a manifestation of waterlogged lung interstitium and is often accompanied by septal lines. Lamellar effusion is seen as vertical band of soft tissue density between the lung and chest wall above the costophrenic angle, this remains fixed with postural change **(Fig. 9)**.

Supine and semi-erect radiographs are less sensitive in showing pleural effusion. Signs of effusion on a supine radiograph are a hazy veil like opacity affecting the whole or lower part of hemithorax with preserved vascular opacities in the overlying lung **(Fig. 10)**. Additional signs include haziness of the diaphragmatic margins blunting of the costophrenic angle, a pleura apical cap which disappears in an upright film, thickening of the minor fissure and widening of the paraspinal interface. The lack of an air bronchogram and preserved vascular markings differentiate it from parenchymal disease such as pneumonia.

Loculated Pleural Fluid (Encysted/Encapsulated)

Fluid can loculate between visceral pleural layers in fissures or between visceral and parietal layers, usually against the chest wall. Loculated effusion usually occurs in association with exudative effusion, high in protein, such as those that occur in empyema, hemothorax or chylothorax.

The appearance of loculated pleural fluid on chest radiograph varies with its location and the radiographic projection used. It is sharply marginated when the surface is parallel to the X-ray beam and ill-defined when viewed en-face **(Figs. 11A and B)**. A collection loculated in the lateral pleural space will appear sharply marginated on the frontal radiograph and ill-defined on lateral film. For the effusion loculated anteriorly or posteriorly, the converse is true.

Fissural interlober loculation, seen particularly in heart failure produces the "pseudotumor" or the "phantom" tumor which can recur in the same place on repeated occasions. Pleural pseudotumors are transudates. Besides congestive cardiac failure these are seen with renal failure and in cirrhotic patients. In the presence of pleural effusion, the elastic recoil of the lung causes each lobe to retract toward the hilum. This widens the fissure and can draw fluid into the fissure even in nondependent locations. The middle lobe, because it is the smallest lobe, has the greatest tendency to retract, and therefore the minor fissure is the most likely fissure to have a pseudotumor.[4]

Viewed in the lateral view, it is sharply marginated and biconvex, with a tail passing through the fissure. The en-face appearance depends on the thickness of the effusion. If it is relatively thin, it may produce a vague area of radio-opacity. If it has a certain thickness, it may appear clear edged and mass-like. Sometimes encysted fluid in the right lower oblique fissure may be confused with middle lobe collapse. Features that favor a collapsed, consolidated middle lobe collapse include nonhomogeneity, a straight or concave border in the lateral view, and a wedgelike outline with the base reaching the sternum. The presence of a dependent pleural effusion aids in recognizing a pleural pseudotumor. Fluid collections are rounded or lenticular and may show a tapering triangular opacity or "beak" at the point they merge with the fissure. Fluid collections in the minor fissure appear sharply marginated and lenticular on both frontal and lateral views. Collection in the major fissure may be ill-defined on the frontal view.

Ultrasound of Pleural Effusion

Ultrasonography is extremely sensitive to the presence of fluid, detecting even small amounts accurately. It is helpful in detecting subpulmonic and subphrenic effusion by noting the position and movement of diaphragm. USG is also useful in opaque hemithorax, to differentiate solid

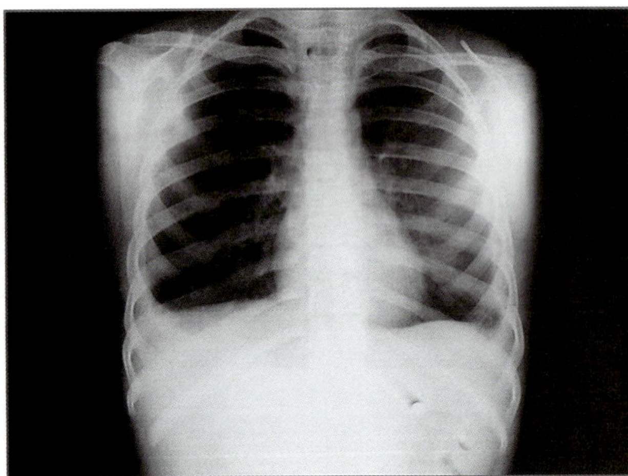

FIG. 9: Bilateral lamellar effusion with blunting of the costophrenic angles.

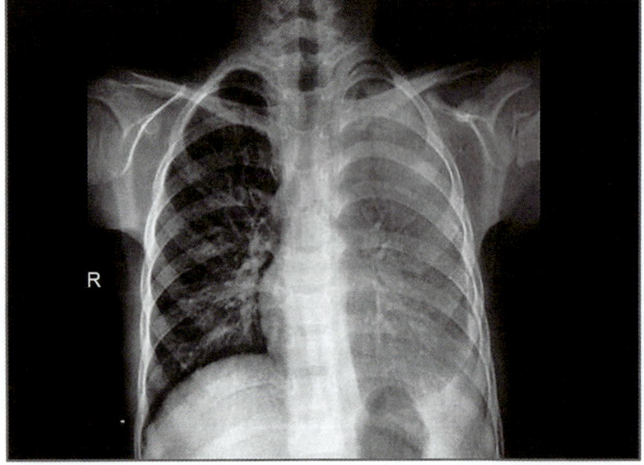

FIG. 10: X-ray of chest: AP view (supine) shows a veil like opacification of the left hemithorax with preserved vascular markings due to pleural effusion.

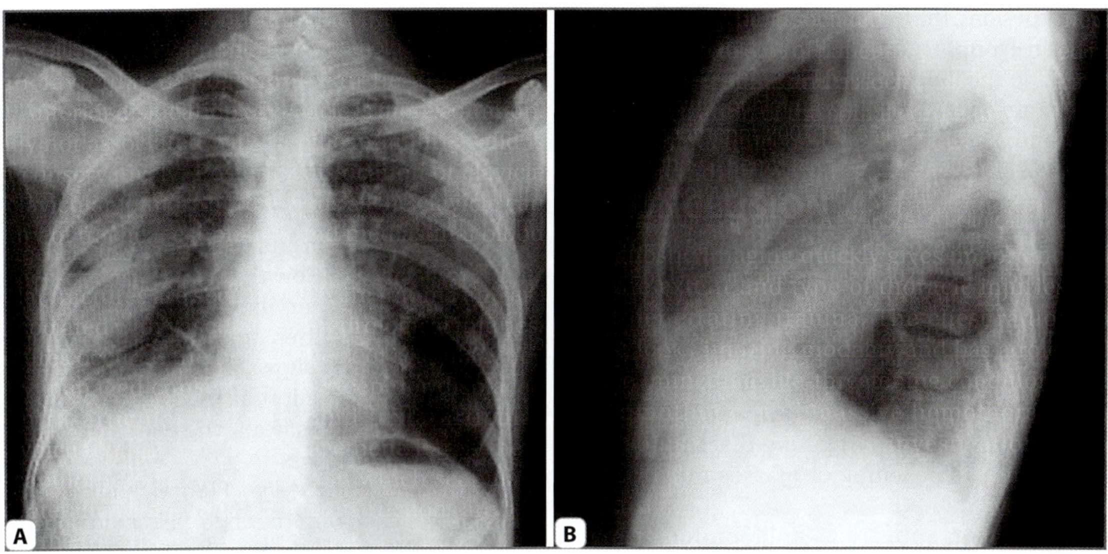

FIGS. 11A AND B: X-ray of chest PA (A) and lateral (B)—opacities bilaterally with sharper medial margin and fading toward periphery-loculated fluid.

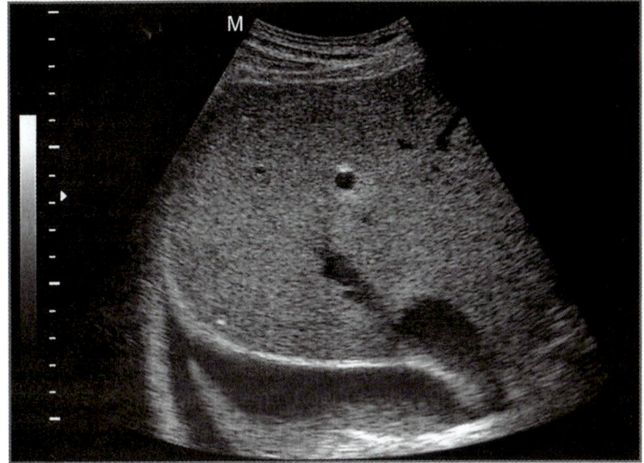

FIG. 12: Anechoic fluid in the right pleural space—seen on transabdominal ultrasound. Note absence of mirror image of liver.

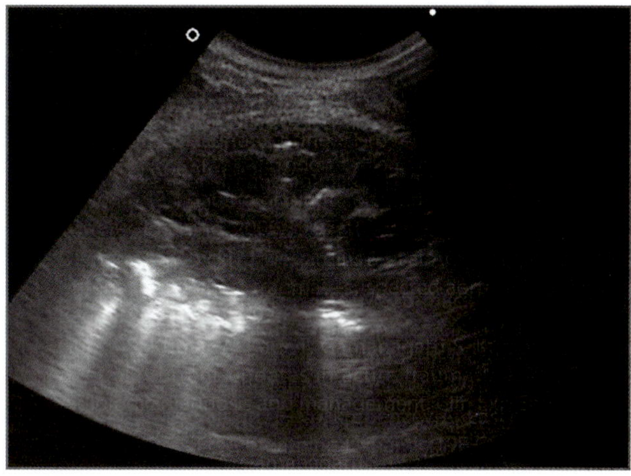

FIG. 13: Ultrasound of chest shows multiseptated collection in the right pleural cavity.

from fluid lesion and is mandatory before performing thoracocentesis of an opaque hemithorax.

The US image of pleural effusion is characterized by echo free space between the visceral and parietal pleura **(Fig. 12)**. Visceral pleura is identified by movement of echogenic line with breathing, parietal pleura is identified by its position approximately 1 cm deep to ribs. The rough estimate of the amount of fluid can be made by measuring the maximum perpendicular distance between the lung surface and chest wall. The patient is supine and measurement is done in full inspiration. A 20-mm width has a mean volume of 380 ± 130 mL, 40 mm width would correspond to 1,000 ± 330 mL.[5]

The sonographic characteristics of effusion may be helpful in differentiating transudates from exudates.[6] Pleural fluid, especially when it is a transudate is echo-free, though occasionally an exudate may also be anechoic. Exudative and hemorrhage effusions may be echogenic, complex and septated **(Fig. 13)**. The septae may be profuse giving rise to honeycomb appearance. These may not be well-appreciated on CT and may pose difficulty in tube drainage. Other sonographic features may be helpful in assessing the nature of pleural effusion such as associated consolidation favors empyema, while pleural nodules favor malignancy.

Ultrasound can be used to distinguish between pleural fluid, solid pleural or extrapleural lesions and peripheral lung lesions. Features that help distinguish a fluid from a solid echogenic lesion include changes in shape with breathing, the presence of septa and fibrous strands and the movement of the components, induced by breathing. In peripheral lung lesions, the presence of fluid bronchograms and vessels on Doppler identify consolidation. Color Doppler signal in the fluid collection in the pleural space during respiratory or cardiac cycle is a pointer toward the presence of fluid. Patients with pleural thickening do not show this sign **(Fig. 14)**.[7]

Computed Tomography of Pleural Effusion

The CT is sensitive in detecting pleural fluid and can distinguish between free and loculated fluid, identifying the extent and location of the loculation. It also allows differentiation of pleural from parenchymal pathology and the evaluation of underlying lung disease. Pleural morphology such as thickening or masses may also be studied by CT.

A pleural effusion appears as a dependent, sickle shaped opacity with a lower CT number than any adjacent pleura thickening or mass **(Fig. 15)**. Most pleural effusions are near water attenuation on CT, ranging up to 20–30 HU regardless of cause. CT attenuation numbers alone do not allow a reliable distinction between an exudate and a transudate.[8] Distinguishing between the two is important for clinical management. The differentiation has to be made on the basis of thoracocentesis. The appearance of parietal pleura on CECT is of value in predicting the nature of pleural fluid collection. Visibility of enhancement of the parietal pleura indicates that it is thickened (enhancing pleura is thickened pleura) the presence of thickened parietal pleura is indicative that the fluid is an exudate. This is seen in up to 60% of exudative effusions and its accuracy in predicting the presence of exudates is nearly 100%. If pleural thickening is not present, an associated effusion may be a transudate or exudate.

CT findings of fluid loculation include a localized collection, an elliptical or lenticular shape/rather than crescentic, a nondependent location (i.e., anterior, lateral, or posterolateral) **(Figs. 16 and 17)**. If air is present within a loculated effusion, multiple septations may be seen, resulting in multiple localized air collections or air fluid levels.

PLEURAL EFFUSION OR ASCITES

Subpulmonic effusion and pleural fluid in the costophrenic angle can be seen below the lung bases on CT and mimic ascites. The parallel curvilinear configuration of the pleura and peritoneal cavities at the level of perihepatic and perisplenic recesses allows fluid in either cavity to appear as a crescentic collection displacing liver or spleen away from the adjacent chest wall. The two can be distinguished by certain signs.[9,10]

1. *The "displaced crus" sign:* Pleural fluid collections in the posterior costophrenic angle lie medial and posterior to the diaphragm and causes lateral displacement of the

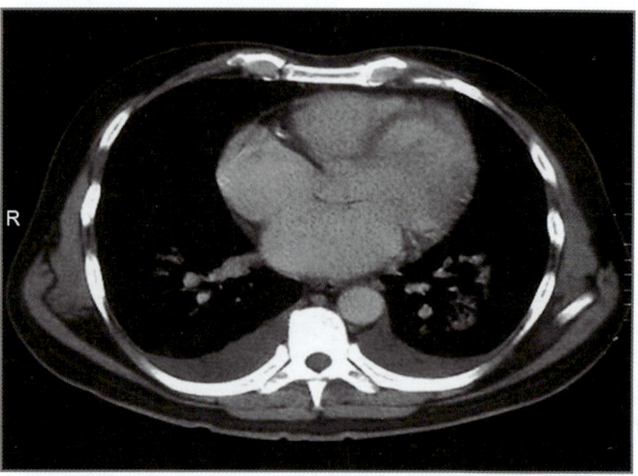

FIG. 15: CT-sickle shaped opacity seen in dependent location—bilateral pleural effusion.

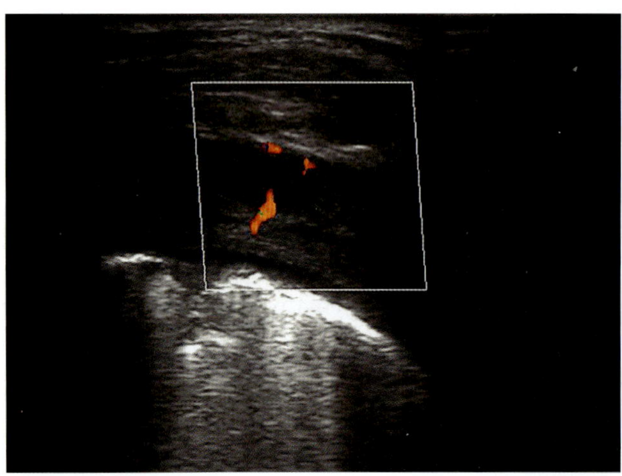

FIG. 14: Color Doppler depicting the "color fluid sign".

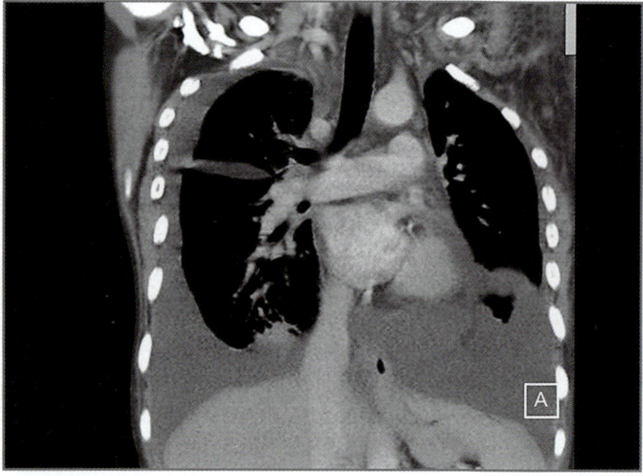

FIG. 16: Coronal MPR—bilateral pleural effusion, also tracking in the horizontal fissure.

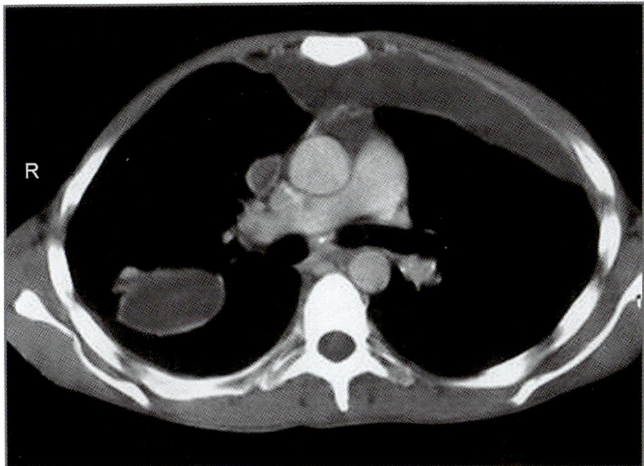

FIG. 17: CECT of chest—loculated fluid along the chest wall anteriorly and horizontal fissure.

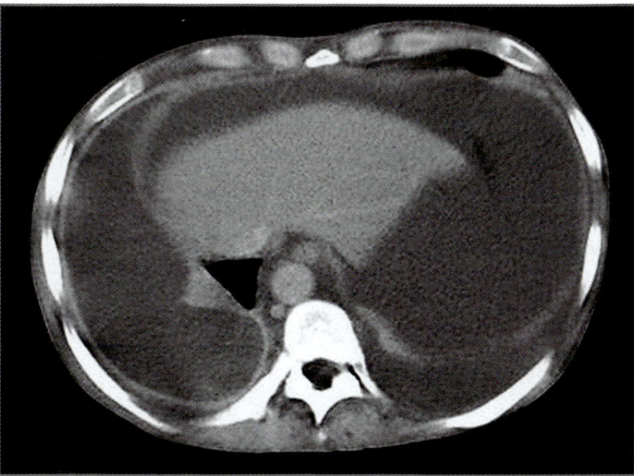

FIG. 18: Pleural effusion and ascitis in the same patient. Pleural fluid is seen medial and posterior, and lateral to the crus of the diaphragm. Crus is displaced away from the vertebral body, better appreciated on the left side ascitis does the reverse. The displaced crus and diaphragm sign.

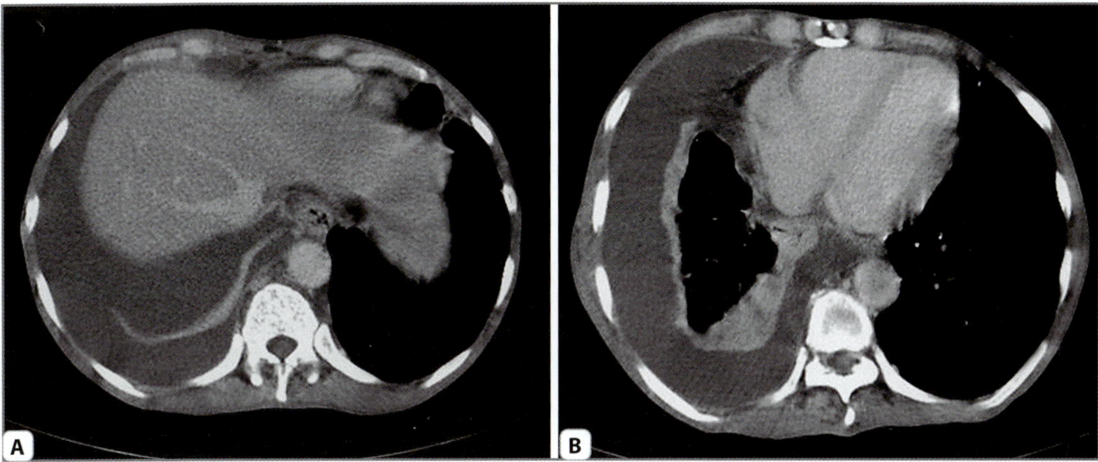

FIGS. 19A AND B: CT shows posterior edge of the right lower lobe as an arcuate density surrounded by fluid anteriorly and posteriorly resembling the diaphragm: (A) On sequential cephalad scan; (B) This is contiguous with the remainder of the lower lobe.

crus—away from adjacent vertebral body, ascitis does the reverse **(Fig. 18)**.

2. *The "diaphragm sign":* The most reliable sign to localize fluid is to identify its relationship to the diaphragm, if visible. The diaphragm is seen as uniform curvilinear structure of muscle density, fluid posterior or lateral to the diaphragm is pleural. A large pleural effusion will allow the lower lobe to float anteriorly and lose volume. On CT the posterior edge of the lower lobe, when surrounded by fluid, both anteriorly and posteriorly can appear to represent the diaphragm—pseudodiaphragm **(Figs. 19A and B)**. On sequential scans at more cephalad levels, the density of atelectatic lower lobe becomes thicker, merges with the rest of lower lobe and often contains air-bronchograms.
3. *The "bare area sign"*: Ascitic fluid is excluded from the bare area between coronary ligaments on the posterior aspect of the liver as the peritoneal space does not extend into this region. Pleural fluid can be seen in the entire posterior costophrenic sulcus **(Figs. 20A and B)**.
4. *The "interface sign"*: Pleural fluid can be distinguished from ascitis by the clarity of the interface of the fluid with diaphragm. With pleural fluid, the interface is hazy, whereas with ascitis it is sharp.

MRI of Pleural Effusion

Pleural fluid has a low signal on T1 and a high signal on T2-weighted images. Exudates give a higher signal than transudates on T2WI. A chylous effusion shows signal intensity similar to subcutaneous fat on T1W images. In the

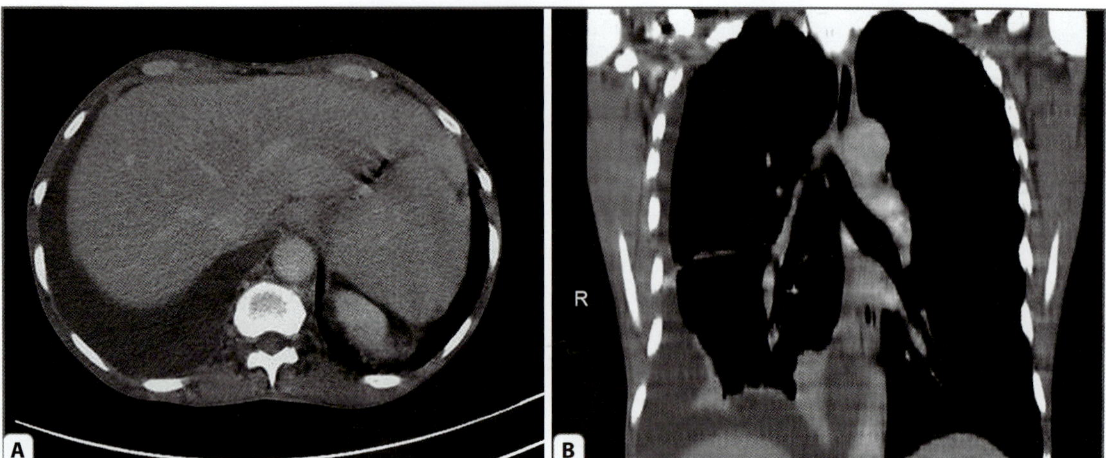

FIGS. 20A AND B: CT–axial (A), MPR (B), shows the pleural fluid occupying the entire posterior costophrenic sulcus, ascitis is excluded from this space due to lack of peritoneal reflection—bare area sign. Note that the interface with liver is hazy—interface sign.

subacute and chronic stage hematomas show a bright signal on T1WI, surrounded by a dark rim caused by hemosiderin.

MRI may be used to differentiate transudates from exudates. A gradual enhancement on delayed images of malignant pleural effusions after intravenous administration of GD-DTPA, in patients with lung cancer has been reported. Signal enhancement of the pleura indicates the presence of exudates while absence of the same suggests transudate. Noninvasive characterization of pleural effusion by means of DWI with single shot EPI technique may obviate the need for thoracocentesis with its associated patient morbidity. Most transudative effusions are isointense, while exudative effusions are hyperintense on DWI with b factor of 500 and 1,000 s/min **(Figs. 21A to E)**. The ADC of exudative effusion is significantly lower than those of transudative effusions. The higher the protein content of pleural fluid, the less is the diffusion. The cellular content of exudates may also contribute to ADC values. At a cut off value of 3.6×10^{-3} mm^2/s, ADC has a sensitivity of 71% and a specificity of 63% for differentiating transudative from exudative effisions.[11,12]

Parapneumonic Effusion with Empyema

Pleural fluid accumulates in approximately 40% of patients with pneumonia. This is diagnosed by thoracocentesis and culture of the aspirated fluid. The term "parapneumonic" effusion is used and it is classified into three stages of empyema. Progression from one stage to another does not necessarily take place.[13-18]

Simple Parapneumonic Effusion (Exudative Stage)

Simple parapneumonic effusion results from increased permeability of the visceral pleura occurring in association with pulmonary inflammation in patients with pneumonia. Effusions in this stage are usually sterile exudates and have a normal glucose level (> 40–60 mg/dL) and pH (>7.2). They are usually dependent in location, do not show evidence of loculation, show a meniscus on plain radiographs and appear crescent shaped on CT. These usually resolve with antibiotic treatment of pneumonia.

Empyema (Fibrinopurulent Stage)

The term empyema is used when a pleural effusion is infected, although the definition necessitates the presence of pus in the pleural space. Although most occur in association with pneumonia, approximately 10% are unassociated with obvious lung disease.

A large percentage of bacterial empyemas result from anaerobic infections. Common anerobic organisms include bacteroides, *Fusobacterium*. Common aerobic organisms are *Staphylococcus aureus*, *Streptococcus pneumoniae*, *Haemophilus influenzae*. Tuberculosis may also result in empyema.

Empyema is characterized by the presence of infectious organisms in pleural fluid, increased white blood cells and polymorph nuclear cells, fibrin deposition along the pleural surfaces, a tendency for loculation, decreased glucose levels (<40 mg/dL) and (pH <7.2) and increased LDH (>1,000 1U/L).

In a patient who has pneumonia, the presence of localized or loculated pleural effusion strongly suggests the presence of an empyema. On plain radiographs, empyemas often have a lenticular shape and tend to appear larger or better defined in one projection (e.g., frontal) than in other (e.g., lateral). On radiographs, an empyema containing air may be difficult to differentiate from a peripheral lung abscess abutting the chest wall. This distinction can be important to make because empyemas are often treated by tube thoracostomy in addition to systemic antibiotics, whereas most lung abscesses require antibiotics alone.

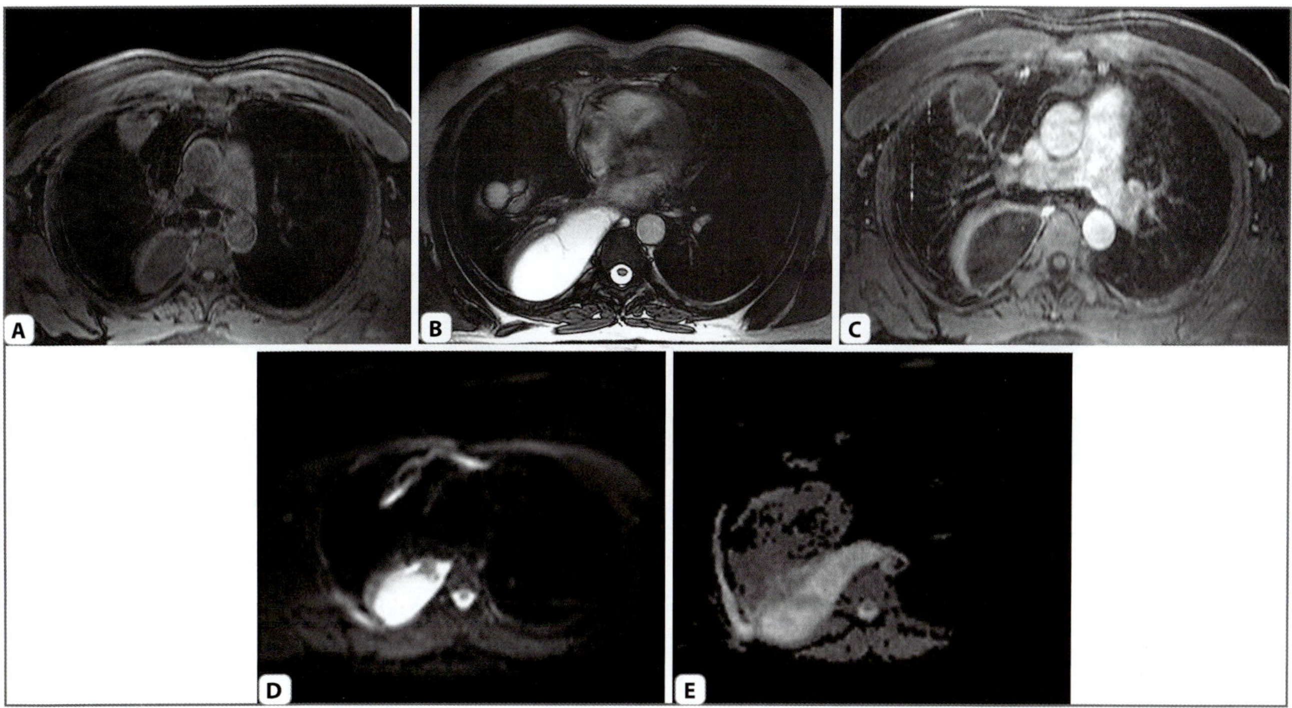

FIGS. 21A TO E: MRI shows loculated fluid collections in the right paraspinal location and along the anterior chest wall, hypointense on T1 (A) and hyperintense on T2W1 (B) On postcontrast scan (C) enhancement of the pleural layers are seen suggestive of an exudate. Diffusion weighted image (D) and ADC map of the same (E).

CT shows characteristic findings of empyema. It is seen in a nondependent location with an elliptical or lenticular shape, with a sharp demarcation from the adjacent lung; the enhancing visceral and parietal pleural surfaces split apart by the fluid collection giving the "split pleura sign" **(Fig. 22)**.

Empyemas show the thickened pleural layers as smooth and of uniform thickness when enhanced by contrast or outlined by air. Empyema compresses and displaces adjacent lung and vessels. In patients with parapneumonic effusion or empyema, extrapleural fat is commonly thickened. The extrapleural fat adjacent to empyema may show increased attenuation with edema of chest wall muscles **(Figs. 23 and 24)**. In contrast to empyema, lung abscesses are round and poorly defined owing to surrounding pneumonia, have shaggy walls or irregular thickness and tend to obliterate bronchi and vessels **(Figs. 25 and 26)**. The differences between a peripherally located lung abscess and empyema are enumerated in **Table 2**. Malignant neoplasms may arise in the walls of chronic long-standing empyemas, mostly in tubercular cavities. Non-Hodgkin's lymphoma, mesothelioma and rarely sarcoma may occur.

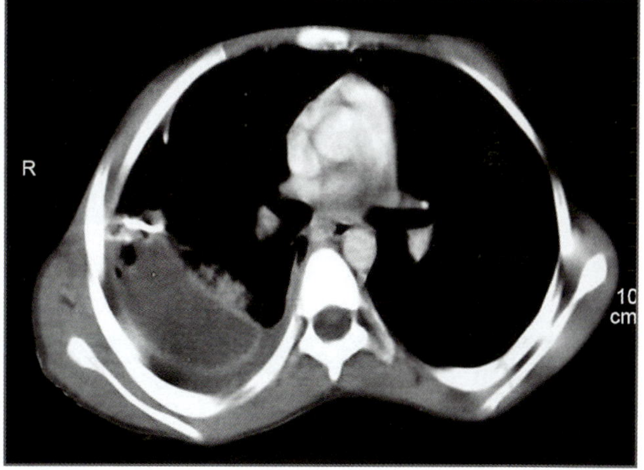

FIG. 22: Empyema CT show loculated collection in the hemithorax with enhancement of the visceral and parietal pleura—split pleura sign.

Organization Stage (Pleural Peel)

In patients with chronic empyema ingrowth of fibroblasts and organization can result in extensive pleural fibrosis and the development of an inelastic fibrotic pleural peel or fibrothorax. This can cause lung restriction and decreased lung volume—the trapped lung **(Fig. 27)**. Plain radiographs and CT show smooth pleural thickening. Extrapleural fat thickening is frequently visible on CT, separating the thickened parietal pleura from the intercostal muscle or rib. On CT a fibrothorax is defined as pleural thickening that extends >8 cm in craniocaudal direction, 5 cm laterally and with a thickness equal or more than 3 cm. Focal or extensive calcification is common with a tubercular etiology. Asbestos

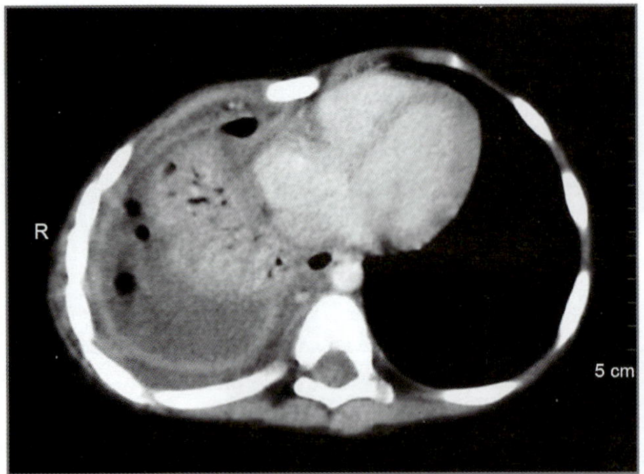

FIG. 23: Thickened enhancing pleura with proliferation of extrapleural fat on the right side. There are air loculi within the pleural cavity (postintervention). Loss of volume with underlying consolidation is also noted.

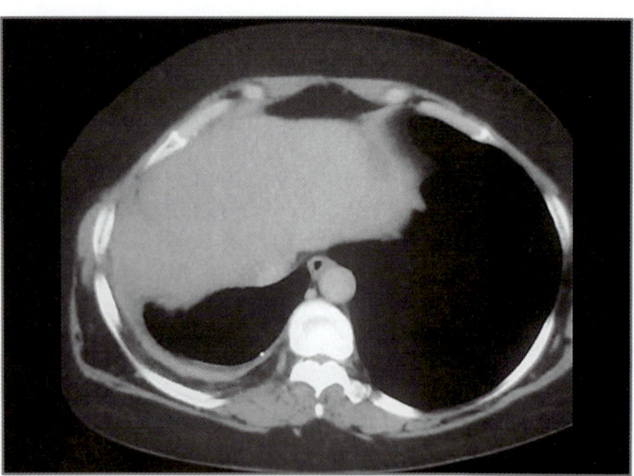

FIG. 24: CT—pleural thickening with proliferation of extrapleural fat.

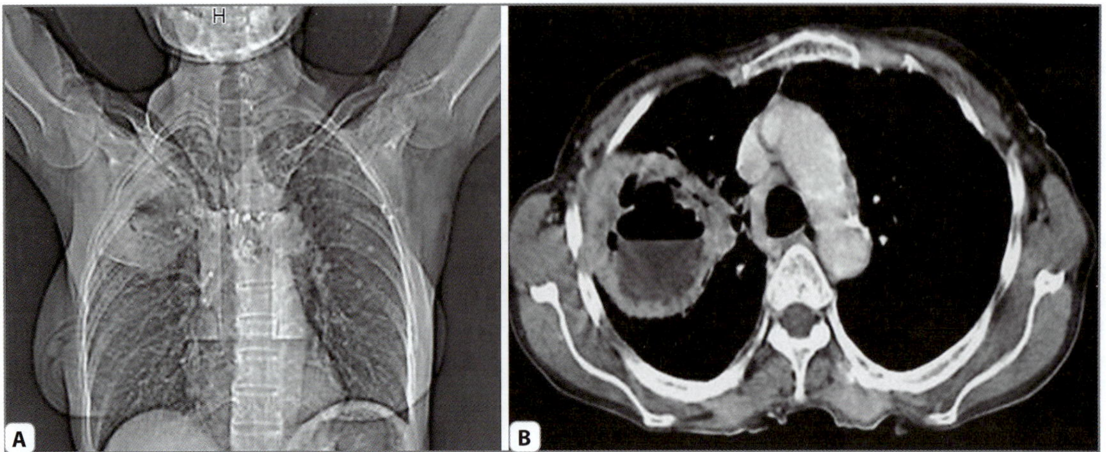

FIGS. 25A AND B: A large opacity with an air fluid level with an acute angle with the chest wall with shaggy inner walls—lung abscess.

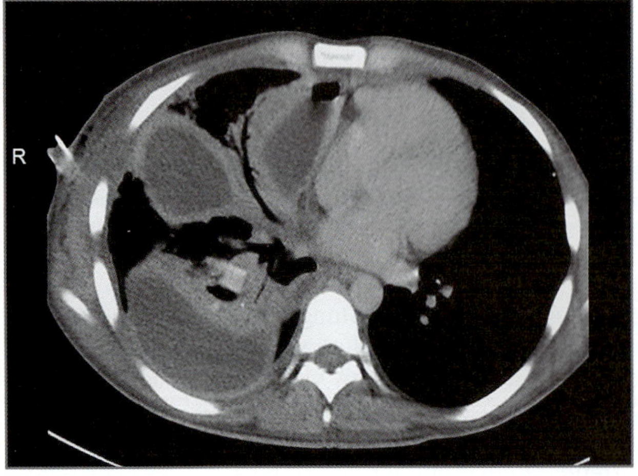

FIG. 26: CT of chest—multiple loculated empyemas.

TABLE 2: Differences between empyema and lung abscess.

Empyema	Lung abscess
Lenticular shape	Round shape
Uniform enhancing wall	Non-uniform thick wall
Compression of adjacent lung	Non-compression of surrounding lung
Obtuse angle with chest wall	Acute angles with chest wall
Separation of pleural layers	–

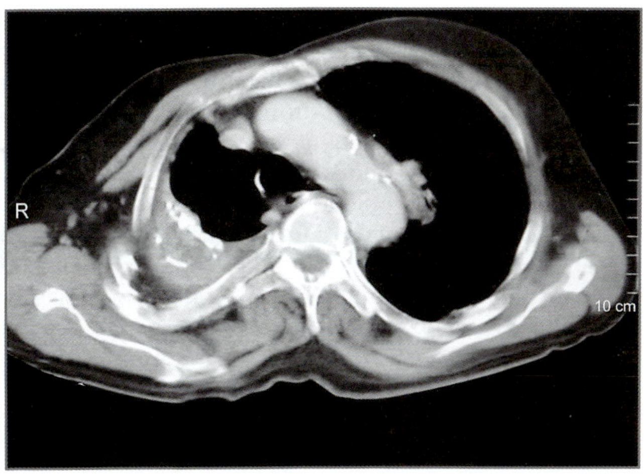

FIG. 27: CECT thorax: Calcified and thickened pleural layers on.

exposure related fibrothorax is usually bilateral and rarely calcified. An important finding in diagnosing pleural peel is reduction in the volume of the affected hemithorax **(Figs. 28A and B)**. A pleural peel may be the result from chronic pleural effusion and inflammation in the absence of infection, e.g., in cases of collagen vascular disease, uremia, etc.

Empyema Necessitans

Empyema can extend from the parietal pleura into the chest wall and surrounding soft tissue and this is called empyema necessitatis or necessitans. The other sites of involvement include esophagus, breast, retroperitoneum, flank and pericardium. Tuberculosis accounts for about 70% of these cases, other organisms like Actinomycosis or Nocardia have also been implicated. CT demonstrates thick-walled fluid collections extending from pleural cavity into the chest wall **(Figs. 29A and B)**.

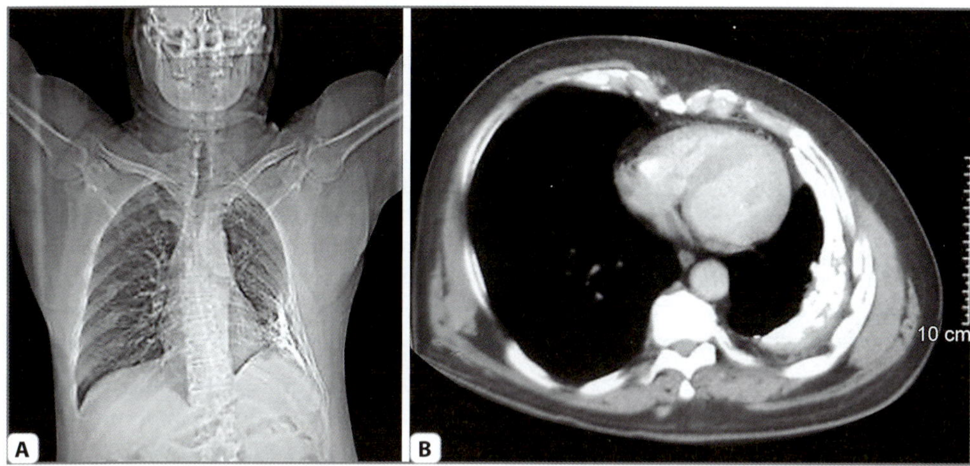

FIGS. 28A AND B: Chest X-ray (A), CT (B)—Loss of volume on the left with extensive pleural thickening with calcification—fibrothorax.

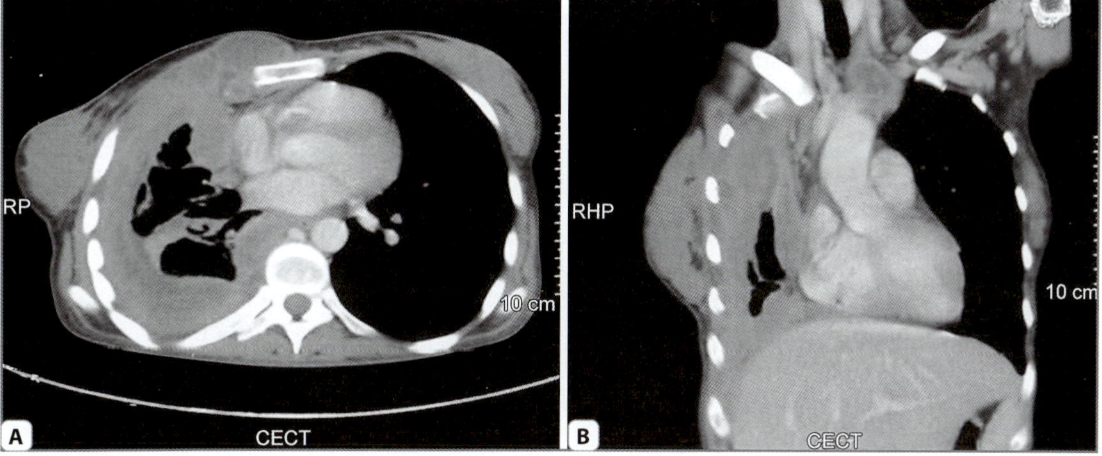

FIGS. 29A AND B: Empyema with direct extension into chest wall—empyema necessitans.

Tube Drainage of Empyema

- Drainage of empyema is required if there is: Thick pus on thoracentesis
- Positive gram stain
- Positive pleural fluid culture
- Pleural fluid glucose <60 mg/dL
- Pleural fluid pH <7.2
- LDH >1,000 IU/L
- No response to antibiotics

Multiple septations within an infected or reactive fluid may be broken down by instillation of fibrinolytic agents such as urokinase. Indications for decortication include persistent sepsis despite appropriate antibiotic therapy and drainage, persistent thick pleural rind that appears to be trapping the underlying lung. CT can be used to determine the adequacy of chest tube drainage, the thickness of the pleural rind, the presence of loculi, and the extent to which the lung is trapped.

After thoracentesis of a large pleural effusion, the re-expanded lung shows edema which persists for a few days. The lung sometimes fails to expand fully, and a pneumothorax may persist. This usually occurs in patients with malignancy and is known as "trapped lung". Metastatic implants on the visceral pleural surface prevent the lung from expanding. A trapped lung can also occur in cases of chronic empyema when a rind of thickened visceral pleura encases and contracts the underlying lung, preventing re-expansion of the lung despite adequate drainage of the empyema fluid. The other cause of persistent pneumothorax or hydropneumothorax is a bronchopleural fistula.

PLEURAL FISTULA

An abnormal communication between the pleural cavity and an adjacent structure is called a pleural fistula. The close proximity of pleura to several intrathoracic structures like bronchi, esophagus, pericardium, the deep pleural recesses and negative pleural pressure make pleura vulnerable for fistulization. The most common causes are iatrogenic, necrotizing infections, malignancy, postradiation therapy. Bronchopleural fistula and esophageopleural are relatively common while nephropleural and subarachnoidpleura, pancreaticopleural fistula are rare. Diagnosis is difficult with visualization of fistula tract being rare. Contrast with IV and compartment specific contrast is the modality of choice for imaging the fistulae.[19]

Bronchopleural fistula (BPF) is a communication between the pleural cavity and the bronchial tree It can involve large airways or peripheral airways where it is also called alveolopleural fistula. A parenchymal pleural fistula (PPF) refers to a fistula between pleura and lung parenchyma. In both these conditions there is a pneumothorax not attributable to trauma. Bronchopleural fistula results from rupture of the visceral pleura with a direct communication with the airway. It may occur following trauma or surgery or in association with necrotizing infections—empyema, TB, septic embolus and infected pulmonary infarct. Gas within a pleural fluid collection, in absence of a recent thoracocentesis is presumptive evidence of empyema and BPF. It differs from pneumothorax in that the communication with the pleural space is via airways rather than the distal air spaces **(Figs. 30A and B)**. MDCT can detect bronchopleural fistula with the same or superior sensitivity as bronchoscopy **(Fig. 31)**.[20]

Postsurgical Bronchopleural Fistula

Following an uncomplicated pneumonectomy, the residual space contains air and fluid and there is ipsilateral mediastinal shift and elevation of the hemidiaphragm. Over 2–4 months, there is gradual resorption of air and increasing fluid accumulation, followed by organization and progressive movement of the mediastinum and

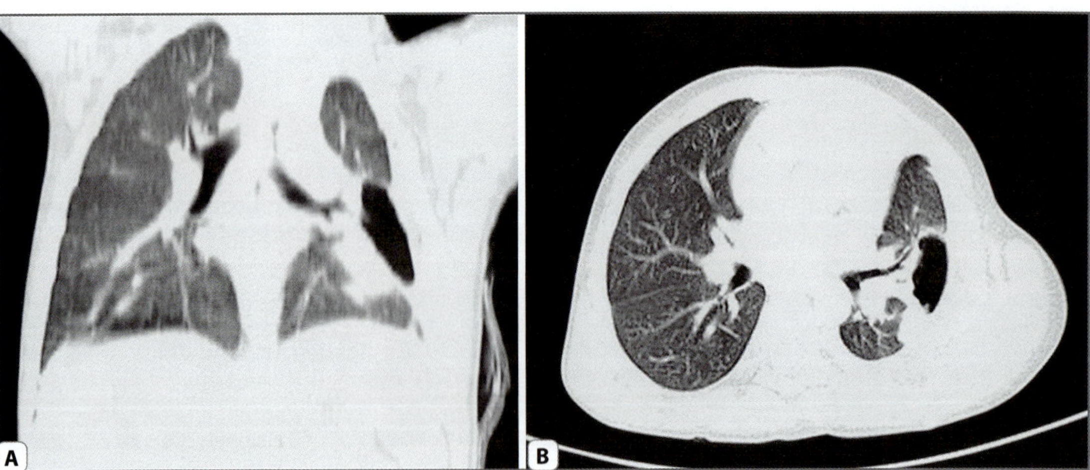

FIGS. 30A AND B: CT chest shows a loculated air containing space in the left pleural cavity that was not draining completely. A segmental bronchus is seen in close proximity to it—bronchopleural fistula.

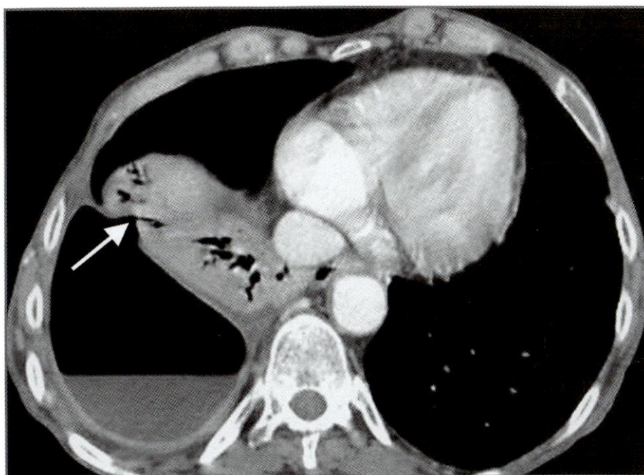

FIG. 31: CT of chest-bronchus in communication with a hydropneumothorax—bronchopleural fistula.

hemidiaphragm, leading to obliteration of the space. BPF arises as an early complication, usually develops 7–10 days later with clinical deterioration, pneumonia, hemopytsis and the sudden expectoration of fluid and a persistent large air leak from the pleural drain. The diagnosis is made radiologically by the following signs:

- Return of the mediastinum to the midline.
- Presence of increasing air and decreasing fluid in the pneumonectomy space.
- Contralateral aspiration pneumonitis. If less than the whole lung has been removed, the main radiological sign is the sudden appearance of air-fluid level within the pleural space.

The delayed appearance of a fistula (>6 months after surgery) means tumor recurrence and is signaled by the appearance of air in the previously air free post-pneumonectomy space.

Infective Bronchopleural Fistula

This occurs in the setting of necrotizing pulmonary infection and is heralded by the appearance of an air-fluid level in the pleural cavity. The mimickers can be air introduced at thoracocentesis, pleuroesophageal fistula, herniated bowel and a subdiaphragmatic abscess.

Subarachnoid pleural fistula: This is seen after surgical or nonsurgical trauma to the thoracic spine at the costovertebral angle A new pleural effusion after a thoracotomy with neurological signs is a pointer and MR myelography is the imaging modality of choice.[19]

Pleuropericardial fistula: It is usually following pericardiocentesis or cardiac procedures such as epicardial ablation. These are of not much clinical significance and heal spontaneously.

Esophagopleural fistula: It follows iatrogenic trauma to esophagus after a surgical procedure. The other causes are malignancy, corrosive ingestion and tubercular mediastinal infection.

BOX 3: Causes of pleural thickening and masses.

Infectious and inflammatory disease and conditions:
- Empyema
- Tuberculosis
- Hemothorax
- Fibrothorax
- Irradiation
- IgG4 related disease

Tumor-like conditions:
- Pleural plaque
- Thoracic splenosis
- Diffuse pleural thickening associated with asbestos exposure
- Diffuse pulmonary lymphangiomatosis (DPL)
- Erdheim chester disease

Benign tumor:
- Benign solitary firous tumor of pleura (SFTP)
- Lipoma

Malignant tumor:
- Metastasis
- Malignant pleural mesothelioma (MPM)
- Lymphoma
- Malignant SFTP

Pancreaticopleural fistula: Necrotizing pancreatitis, pancreatic surgery and trauma can lead to a fistula. Raised level of amylase in the pleural aspirate is diagnostic. Secretin enhanced MRCP may play a role in delineating the tract.

PLEURAL THICKENING

Pleural thickening results from various diseases both neoplastic and inflammatory and is an end stage process. The various causes are enumerated in **Box 3**. Pleural thickening can be unilateral or bilateral, may be focal or diffuse in distribution and may show calcification. Generalized and gross pleural thickening is termed as fibrothorax and may cause significant ventilatory impairment.

On a chest radiograph, pleural thickening appears as a fixed shadow of water density, most commonly located at the dependent parts of the pleural cavity **(Fig. 32)**. En profile, it appears as a band of soft tissue density, with a sharp interface with the lung. En face, it is seen as an ill-defined veil-like shadowing. Blunting of the costophrenic angle and tenting of the diaphragm are noted (On USG, benign pleural thickening is seen as homogeneous echogenic layer inside the chest wall **(Fig. 33)**. Pleural thickening, visible on radiographs and CT primarily affect the parietal pleura **(Box 4)**. On CT it is seen as:

1. A stripe of soft tissue density 1 mm more in thickness, internal to the ribs.
2. A stripe of soft tissue density 1 mm or more in thickness, internal to the innermost intercostal muscle and separated from it by a thin layer of extrapleural fat.

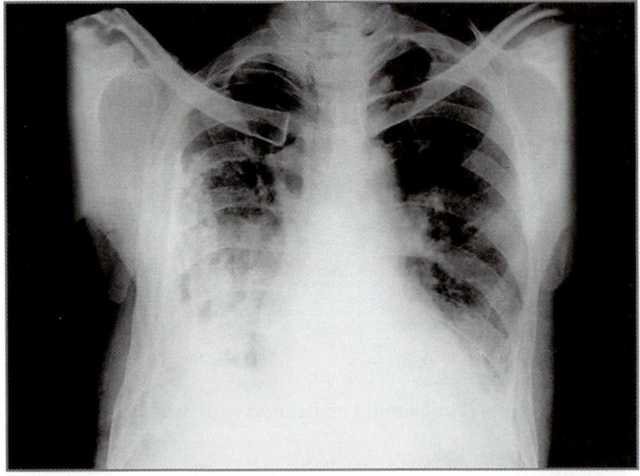

FIG. 32: Chest radiograph—diffuse pleural thickening bilaterally with calcification.

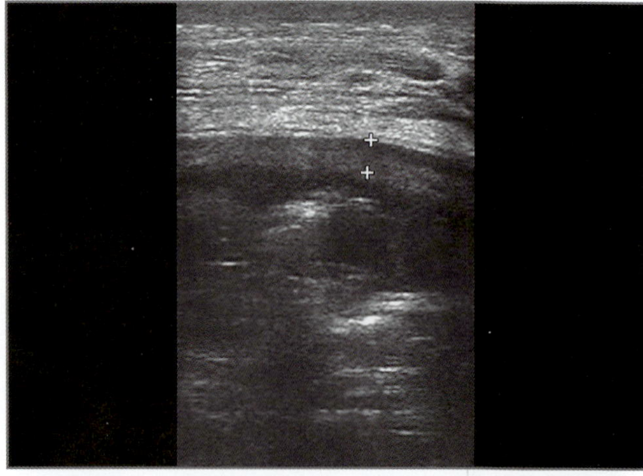

FIG. 33: Ultrasound of chest—pleural thickening with minimal effusion.

BOX 4: Pleural thickening—criteria.

- A stripe of soft tissue density 1 mm more in thickness, internal to the ribs or innermost intercostal muscle
- A distinct stripe in the paravertebral region >1 mm thickness
- Thickening of the normal extrapleural fat layer

3. A distinct stripe in the paravertebral region 1 mm or more in thickness.
4. Thickening of the normal extrapleural fat layer.

Diffuse pleural thickening may be seen unilaterally or bilaterally. The radiographic criteria used for diffuse pleural thickening are coverage of at least 25% of the total chest wall on a chest radiograph (50% if unilateral); and it must extend to a thickness of at least 5 mm in at least one site on the chest radiograph. [21]

CT criteria of diffuse pleural thickening includes, a continuous sheet of pleural thickening >5 cm wide, >8 cm in craniocaudal extent, and >3 mm thick.[21]

Visceral Pleural Thickening

This occurs almost always in association with parietal pleural thickening and effusion, empyema being the most common cause. Visceral pleural thickening alone is uncommon and may be seen in patients with lung disease, such as abscess or fibrosis. Visceral pleural thickening cannot be distinguished from parietal pleural thickening on chest radiographs, although it may appear as:

- Thickening of a fissure
- Separation of lung from adjacent ribs and chest wall, which may occur in association with contiguous lung disease. Both these signs may be seen in pleural effusions.

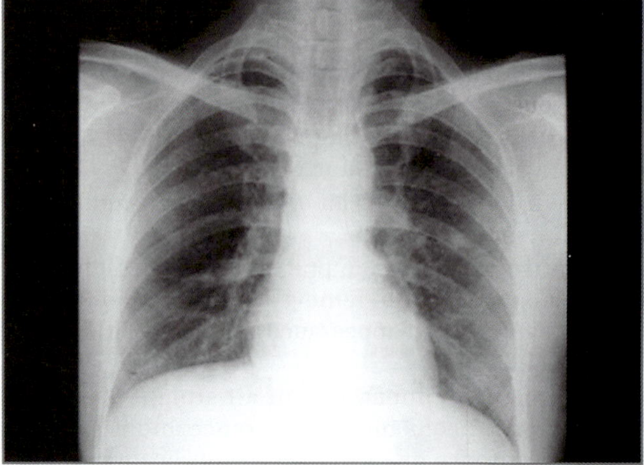

FIG. 34: Right pleural apical cap with soft opacities in left mid zone.

On CT, visceral pleural thickening may appear as either of the following:

- A distinct stripe of soft tissue at the lung surface in patients with pleural effusion and normal lung parenchyma.
- An enhancing stripe at the lung surface in patients with abnormal lung. Thickened visceral pleura enhances more than airless lung.

Pleural Apical Cap and Fibrous Thickening

Fibrous pleural thickening is common at the lung apex.[22] This may be secondary to tuberculosis or represent age related changes of unknown etiology. Apical caps may have a scalloped contour or be associated with tenting toward the lung **(Fig. 34)**. They can be unilateral or bilateral. Apical pleural caps need to be differentiated from companion shadows of upper ribs and from extrapleural fat.

Mimics of Pleural Thickening

Normal structures may mimic the findings of pleural thickening or effusion.

Normal fat pads: Normal extrapleural fat is most abundant over the posterolateral 4th–8th ribs and can be several mm thick that extend into the intercostal space. In contrast to pleural thickening or effusion, normal fat thickening is typically symmetrical, smooth in contour, low in attenuation and unassociated with costophrenic angle blunting. On CT, extrapleural fat appears very low in density.

The subcostalis and transversus thoracis muscles: These are not seen on chest radiograph. On CT, a 1–2 mm thick line is seen internal to one or more ribs, along the posterior chest wall at the level of heart, representing the subcostalis muscle. Anteriorly, at the level of heart, adjacent to lower sternum or xiphoid process, the transversus thoracis muscle is nearly always visible on CT, internal to the anterior ends of ribs or costal cartilages. These muscles are smooth, uniform in thickness and bilateral.

Paravertebral intercostal veins: They may sometimes be seen in the paravertebral regions. Continuity of these opacities with azygous or hemiazygous veins may be visible these do not indent the lung surface, as pleural thickening would.

PLEURA AND ASBESTOSIS[23-26]

Asbestos is a mineral widely used in various industries like construction and ship building. Its use is now regulated as it was labeled as a carcinogen in 1972 by the World Health Organization. Prolonged and improper exposure to Asbestos causes both neoplastic and non-neoplastic thoracic disease. The benign diseases include pulmonary fibrosis called Asbestosis and pleural diseases like pleural plaques, benign asbestos pleural effusion_(BAPE), diffuse pleural thickening and round atelectasis. Neoplastic diseases include lung cancer and malignant mesothelioma BAPE is the earliest sign of asbestos exposure and is usually small and unilateral. Pleural effusions are typically hemorrhagic exudates of mixed cellularity but do not typically contain asbestos fibers. Patients may be asymptomatic or may present with chest pain and dyspnea in the presence of large effusions.

Pleural plaques are the most common manifestation of asbestos inhalation and usually occurs 20–30 years after first exposure, they may occur early within 10 years of exposure. Pleural plaques are seen in 3–14% of dockyard workers and in 58% of insulation workers. The pathogenesis of plaques is uncertain, but is postulated that fibers reach the pleura via lymphatic channels and cause an inflammatory response, which in turn leads to hyaline fibrosis along the parietal pleural surface. They usually arise from the parietal pleura but may arise from the visceral pleura. Plaques are seen over the diaphragmatic dome and the undersurface of the lower posterolateral ribs.

Imaging both by X-ray and CT, shows bilateral, multifocal flat or nodular plaque like pleural thickening with abrupt shouldering. The characteristic sign is holly leaf sign due to irregular margins with calcifications. The diameter of the plaques can vary from several millimeters to 10 cm. Any pleural or pericardial surface can be affected, but asbestos-related pleural plaques are usually in the lower two-thirds of the thorax and are bilateral. Calcification most often affects the parietal and diaphragmatic pleura (virtually pathognomonic) and spares the costophrenic sulci and apices **(Figs. 35A and B)**. The size and number are variable. Calcification may be the only evidence of exposure.

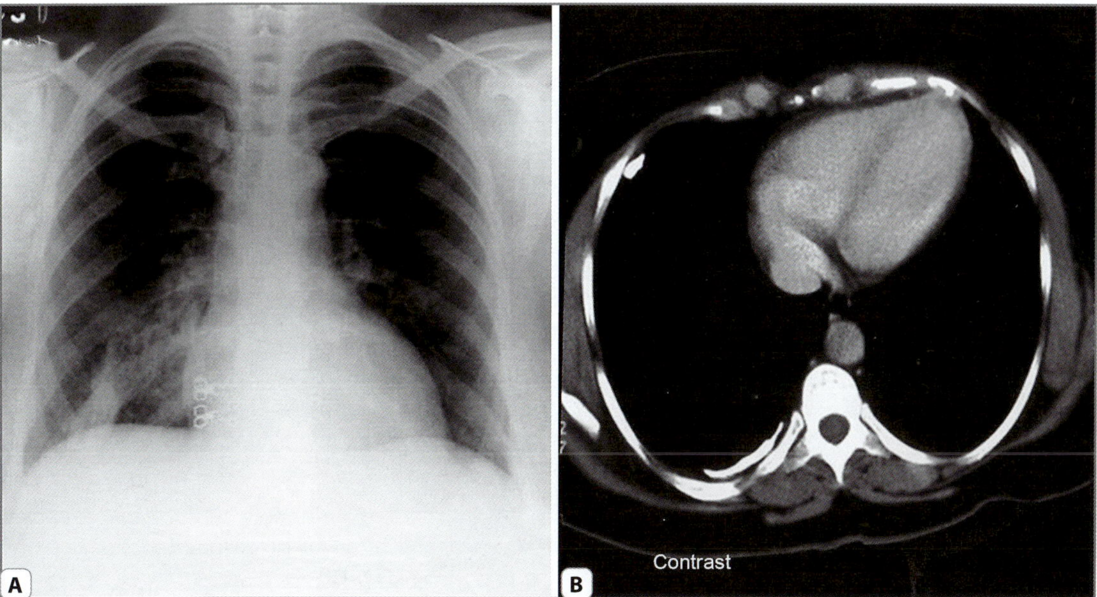

FIGS. 35A AND B: A X-ray of chest (A)—calcified pleural plaque on the right side; (B) CT of chest—calcified pleural plaque seen in the right costal pleura and posteriorly along paraspinal gutter in a patient with history of asbestos exposure.

Patients with pleural plaques are asymptomatic, there is no risk of malignant degeneration, but patients with pleural plaques may have an increased risk of developing mesothelioma and bronchogenic carcinoma compared with a control population matched for exposure but without pleural plaques. The plaques are most useful as a marker of asbestos exposure.

Differential diagnosis includes old tubercular pleuritis or sequlae of hemothorax. In both, the disease is usually unilateral with a sheet-like calcification. Talc pleurodesis demonstrates nodular or linear high attenuation pleural thickening involving both visceral and parietal pleura.

Dense pleural thickening >1 cm in thickness can also follow asbestos exposure. It results from thickening and fibrosis of visceral pleura, which leads to fusion with parietal pleura pleural thickening limited to at least one-fourth of the chest wall with or without involvement of the costophrenic angle may also be seen.

ASBESTOSIS PSEUDOTUMOR (ROUND ATELECTASIS)

The pathogenesis is thought to be due to an inflammatory reaction and fibrosis in the superficial layer of pleura. As the fibrous tissue matures, it contracts, causing pleura to fold into the lung, which in turn causes the atelectasis.

Chest radiograph shows a rounded peripheral "mass" with or without lung distortion. The CT features are of a round or oval mass that abuts the pleura, a "comet tail" of bronchovascular structures going into the mass, and thickening of the adjacent pleura. USG may show an echogenic line that extends into the mass from the pleura, representing the scarred invaginated visceral pleura **(Figs. 36A and B)**.

MRI shows a curved low signal intensity line caused by thickened indentation of visceral pleura. The main differential is malignancy of the lung. Stability or shrinkage of the mass with time suggests benignancy, but biopsy may be required.

PLEURAL CALCIFICATION

This is seen following asbestos exposure, empyema, tuberculosis, and hemothorax. In the later two conditions calcification is irregular and resembles a plaque (**Figs. 37A and B)** or sheet and is contained within thickened pleura. It may occur anywhere but is most common in the lower posterior half of chest and is usually unilateral.

Following tubercular empyema both parietal and visceral pleura may be calcified. These layers are separated by a soft tissue opacity that may contain fluid for many years.

PNEUMOTHORAX

Air within the pleural cavities is referred to as pneumothorax. It is classified as spontaneous or traumatic. The causes of pneumothorax are summarized in **Box 5**.

Spontaneous Pneumothorax

These are classified as primary or secondary.

Primary Spontaneous Pneumothorax

It occurs without an antecedent cause in an otherwise healthy patient. It often occurs at rest, as a result of rupture of an apical subpleural bulla. The peak incidence is in young patients (20–40 years), men (80%), tall and thin patients and smokers (90%). Pain is common and a small pleural effusion is present in 10–20% manifested as an air-fluid level. It may be asymptomatic and detected incidentally. These patients are at increased risk of another pneumothorax.

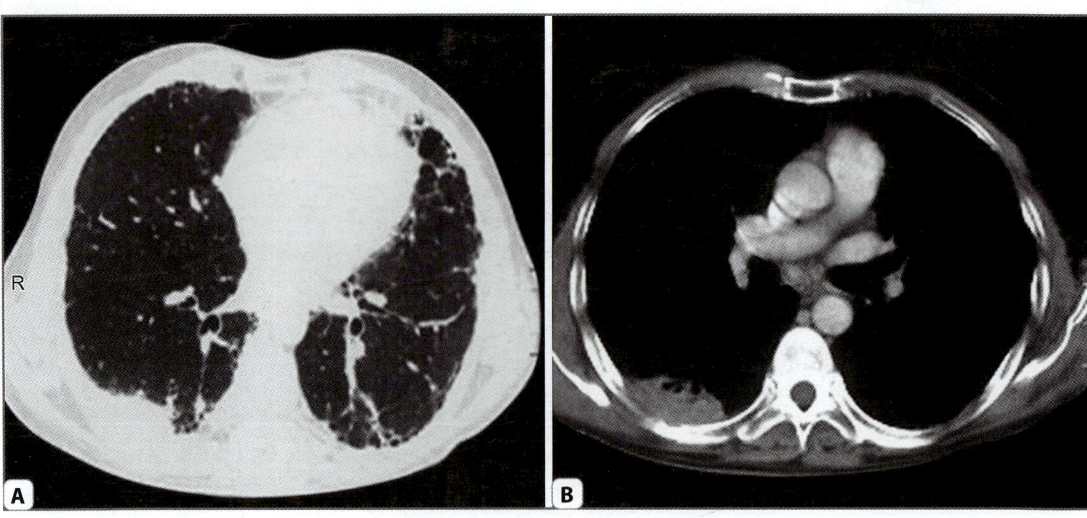

FIGS. 36A AND B: CT of chest shows a peripherally based opacity on the right side with vessels curling up to it—round atelectasis.

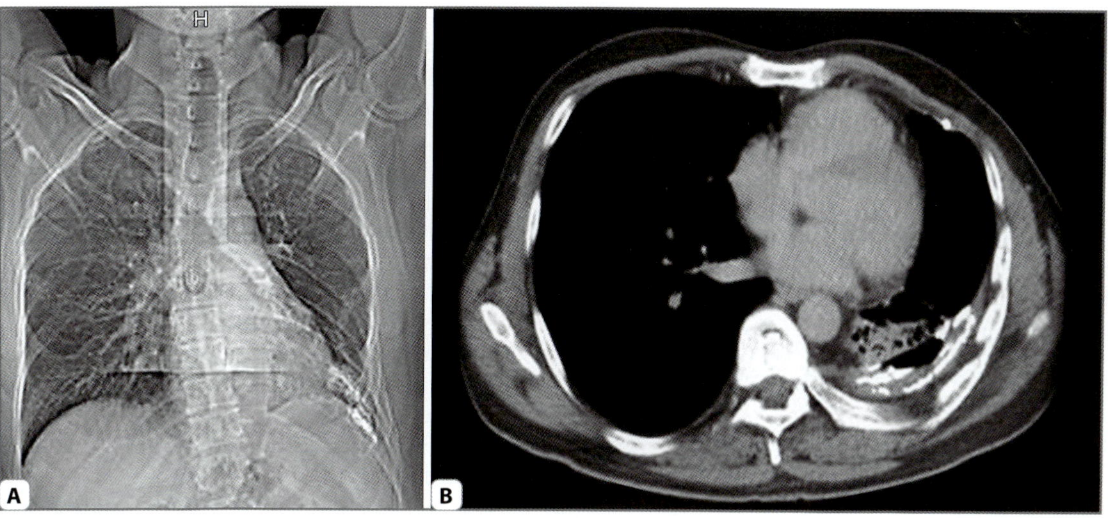

FIGS. 37A AND B: (A) Chest scanogram; (B) CT—pleural calcification with loss of volume—post-tubercular.

BOX 5: Causes of pneumothorax in adult.

Spontaneous
- *Primary spontaneous*:
  - Secondary spontaneous
  - Airflow obstruction—asthma, COPD, cystic fibrosis
  - Pulmonary infection—cavitary pneumonia, tuberculosis, fungal disease, AIDS, pneumatocele
  - Pulmonary infarction
  - Neoplasm—metastatic sarcoma
  - Diffuse lung disease—histiocytosis X lymphangioleiomyomatosis
  - Endometriosis (catamenial pneumothorax)
- *Traumatic*:
  - Noniatrogenic—ruptured esophagus/trachea, closed chest trauma (± rib fracture), penetrating chest trauma
  - Iatrogenic—thoracotomy/ thoracentesis, percutaneous biopsy, tracheostomy, central venous catheterization

Secondary Spontaneous Pneumothorax

It occurs due to an underlying disease like COPD, Langerhans histiocytosis. These are symptomatic and have a high recurrence rate.

Pneumothorax Ex Vacuo

It is a rare cause of secondary spontaneous pneumothorax, occurring in patients with acute lobar collapse due to bronchial obstruction. Sudden collapse results in rapid decrease in intrapleural pressure adjacent to the collapsed lobe. This leads to gas, entering the pleural space. The resulting pneumothorax is seen adjacent to the collapsed lung.

Traumatic Pneumothorax

It can be caused by chest trauma (penetrating/nonpenetrating, accidental or iatrogenic) or in patients on mechanical ventilation. Pneumothoraces with mechanical ventilation (due to high ventilator pressures) occurs due to alveolar rupture leading to interstitial emphysema, pneumomediastinum and rupture of pneumomediastinum into pleural subpleural location. Traumatic pneumothorax requires chest tube drainage.

Catamenial Pneumothorax

Pneumothorax coincident with menstruation is rare. The symptoms start within 48 hours of onset of menses. Air may reach the peritoneum via vagina, uterus or the fallopian tubes. From there it may enter the pleural space via defect or diaphragm, common on the right. Endometrial implants may enter the pleural space by the same route. Endometrial implants involve visceral space and peripheral lung; the breakdown may result in pneumothorax.

IMAGING FINDINGS OF PNEUMOTHORAX

Radiograph

In an *upright patient* air usually collects first above the lung apex. The presence of a visible visceral pleural line is a key to diagnosis. This is visible as a very thin line at the pleural space with an avascular space above or lateral to it and one in the lung below and medial to it **(Figs. 38 and 39)**. Air may enter the fissure, outlining its pleural surface. In absence of underlying lung disease or adhesions; the partially collapsed lung maintains its normal shape. Lung markings are not seen peripheral to the pleural line. The visibility of pneumothorax is accentuated on expiration as there is an increase in volume. Expiratory film or decubitus view with suspected side uppermost may demonstrate a small pneumothorax. Skin folds, hair, clothing, etc., may mimic the walls of bulla and visceral pleural line of pneumothorax. Artefacts and skin folds can be distinguished from

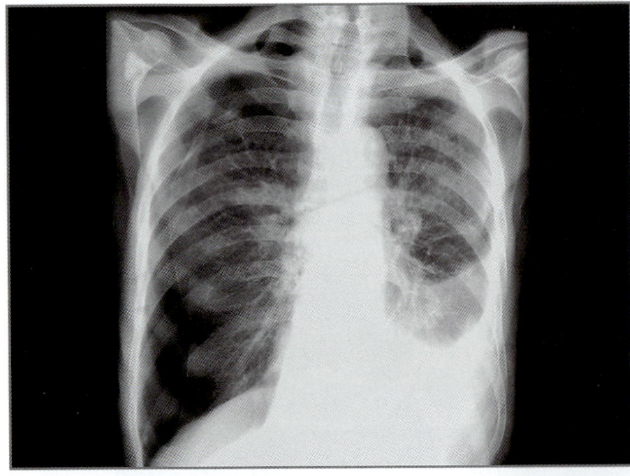

FIG. 38: Right-sided pneumothorax seen on chest skiagram as an avascular space, bounded by the visceral pleural line. Left pleural effusion is also seen.

pneumothorax by extension of these beyond margin of chest cavity laterally located vessels. The margin of the skin fold is usually wider than the thin line of the visceral pleura. A repeat radiograph or an expiratory radiograph may be required in certain situation.

Distinction of a bulla from a pneumothorax is usually based on shape. Pneumothoraces are typically crescent shaped and taper toward the lung base. Bullae are rounded and have inner margin concave to the chest wall and do not conform to the costophrenic angle when they are at the lung base.

In supine patients, free pneumothorax usually collects within the anterior pleural space. A visceral pleural line may be seen medially in some patients mimicking a pneumomediastinum. Pneumothorax in a supine patient may be inferred by the following:

- *Deep sulcus sign*: Costophrenic angle may appear abnormally deep and lucent because of air in the anterolateral pleural space **(Figs. 40 and 41)**.[27]

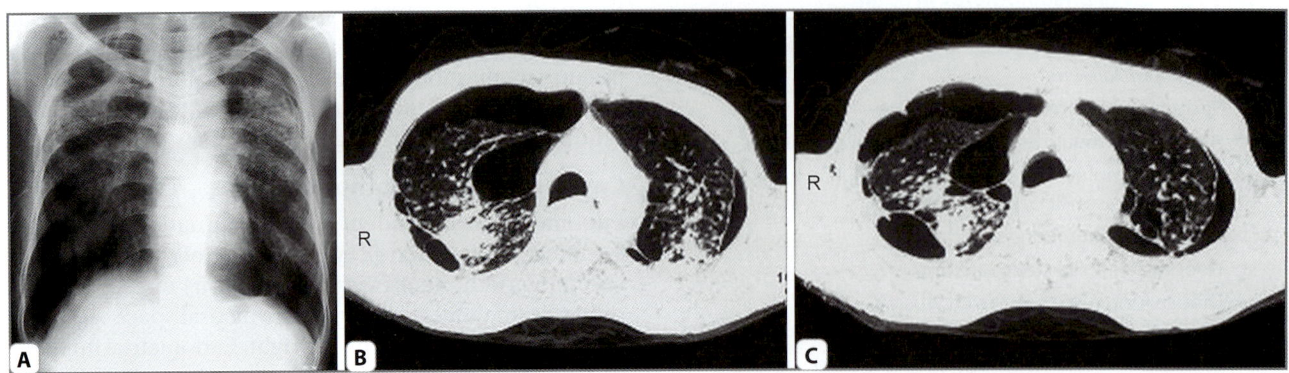

FIGS. 39A TO C: (A) Chest X-ray; (B and C) CT multiple pleural adhesions causing loculation of air—pneumothoraces in a case of silicosis.

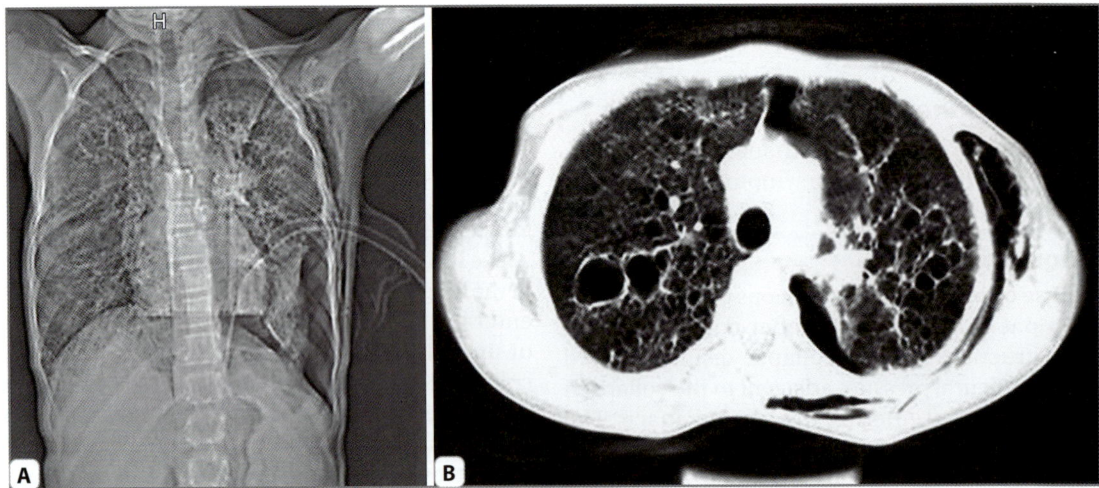

FIGS. 40A AND B: CT-topogram (A) demonstrates the deep costophrenic sulcus on the left and clarity of the left hemidiaphragm due to pneumothorax in a patient of lymhangioleiomyomatosis (B).

FIG. 41: Scanogram—traumatic pneumothorax. Note the clarity of the diaphragm and the deep costophrenic sulcus on the right side.

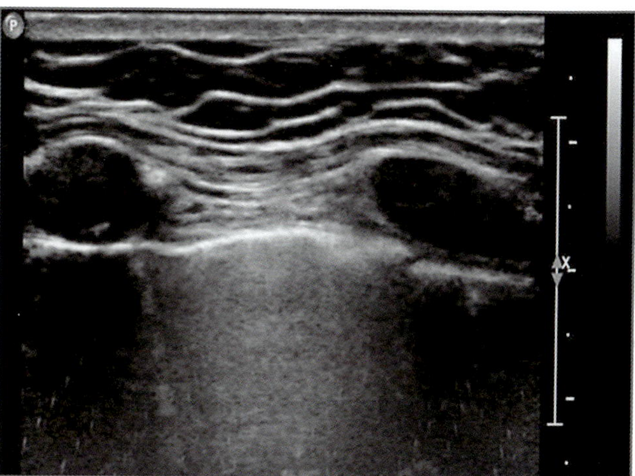

FIG. 42: Ultrasound of chest transverse view intercostal approach—bright pleural line identified between two ribs-bat sign.

- Increased lucency over the chest wall and abdomen
- Visualization of the anterior costophrenic angle as an edge separate from the diaphragm, but parallel to it—the double diaphragm sign
- Increased sharpness of the hemidiaphragm, cardiac border or mediastinum (because it is outlined by air)
- A lumpy appearance at the cardiac apex, due to alteration in the shape of the epicardial fat pat
- Air in the minor fissure

Ultrasonography in Pneumothorax

Ultrasound is now routinely used to detect pneumothorax in emergency settings. Standard lung views are now part *of E-Fast ultrasound (Extended—focused assessment with sonography in trauma).*[28] Ultrasound has higher sensitivity than chest radiograph in the diagnosis of pneumothorax, especially in identifying occult pneumothoraces of traumatic origin.

Technique of Ultrasound to Detect Pneumothorax

A high frequency linear probe is used for analyzing superficial structure such as pleura. Patients are scanned in supine positions, with the probe placed on the anterior chest wall in a sagittal plane at the 2nd intercostal space in the mid clavicular line. Two adjacent ribs are identified by posterior shadowing behind them and bright hyperechoic pleural line in between them. This is termed the "bat sign" **(Fig. 42)**. In the supine position air rises to least dependent part of chest which is anteriorly. In a normal lung the visceral pleura will glide in a to and fro pattern over the parietal pleura with respiration. This is seen on dynamic ultrasound as horizontal sliding movement of pleural line, best seen over apex of lung.[29,30]

M-mode is also used to detect this sliding movement. M-mode cursor is placed over the pleural line. The chest wall above the pleural line forms horizontal—the "waves" and sliding pleural line forms a granular pattern—the "Sand". The resultant image of motionless chest wall and sliding pleura is *seashore sign* **(Fig. 43)**.

Reverberation artifacts are also seen as hyperechoic vertical lines that extend from pleura to edge of screen without fading. These are seen due to acoustic impendence differences.

Sonographic Signs of Pneumothorax

- *The absence of lung sliding in presence of pneumothorax,* visualized pleura will not be identified and movement of pleural line will not be present.[31,32] The M-mode tracing will display one pattern of parallel horizontal lines above and below the pleural line. This is termed the "*barcode sign*" or the *"stratosphere sign"* **(Fig. 44)**. This is an important sign as it has a negative predictive value of almost 100%. The presence of sliding sign rules out pneumothorax. Absence of lung sliding may be seen in other conditions like adult respiratory distress syndrome, pulmonary fibrosis, etc.
- *Comet tail artifacts or B lines*: These reverberation artifacts will be absent in pneumothorax. This is due to the presence of air which does not allow sound to propagate. The negative predictive value of this sign is 98–100%.
- *Lung point sign:*[32,33] This indicates the border of pneumothorax and is useful to assess the size of pneumothorax which has therapeutic implications. At this point sliding and nonsliding lung will be seen together. On M-mode alternate seashore and barcode pattern will be seen. The probe is slowly moved from anterior part to lateral or posterior chest to locate the lung point. The more lateral this point is, the bigger is the pneumothorax.
- *Power slide sign:*[34] Power Doppler is sometimes used to detect sliding movement. This requires the probe

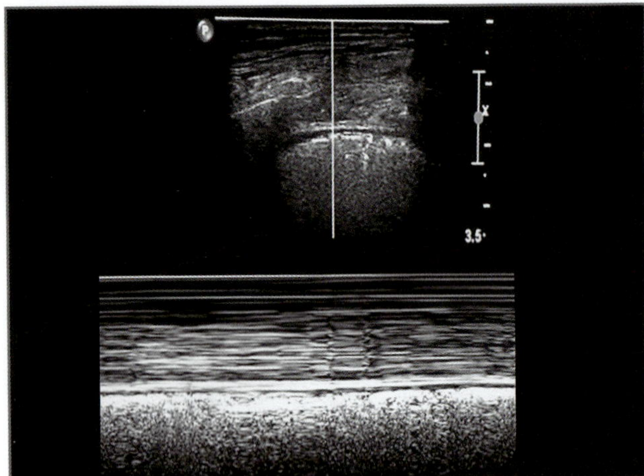

FIG. 43: M-mode—the chest wall above the pleural line forms horizontal—the "waves" and sliding pleural line forms a granular pattern—the "Sand"-seashore sign.

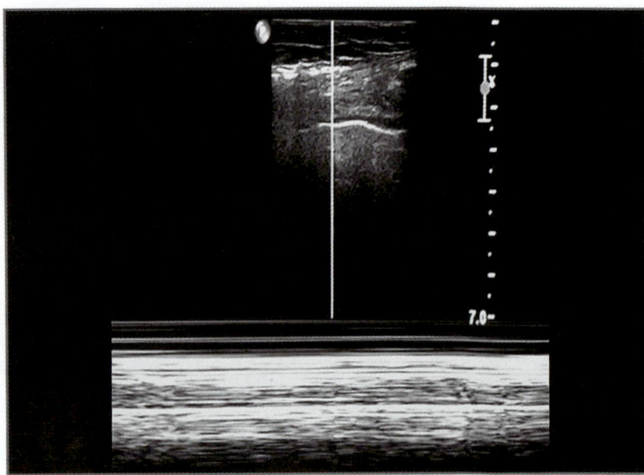

FIG. 44: M-mode tracing displays one pattern of parallel horizontal lines above and below the pleural line—"barcode sign" or the "stratosphere sign".

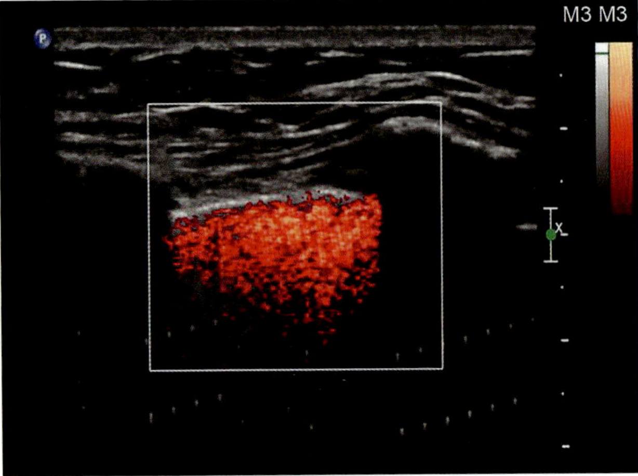

FIG. 45: Power Doppler—depicting normal sliding motion of lung. Absence of this sliding is seen in pneumothorax.

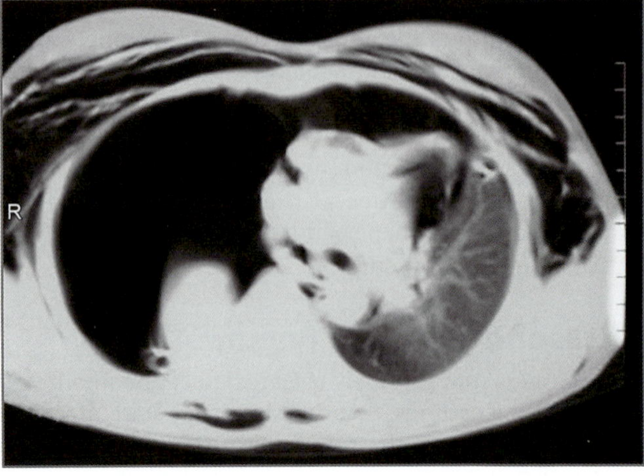

FIG. 46: Large right pneumothorax with passive collapse of the underlying lung, mediastinal shift to the opposite side. Extensive subcutaneous emphysema noted secondary to tube placement.

to be steady and patient motionless to avoid artefacts. Absence of sliding indicates pneumothorax **(Fig. 45)**.

Computed Tomography

CT is extremely sensitive to the presence of air in pleural cavity. Lung Window settings should be used to detect pneumothorax. A pneumothorax is imaged as air in the pleural space outside the lung and visceral pleura **(Fig. 46)**. CT can be used to distinguish bullae from a pneumothorax. Differentiating a medial pneumothorax from a pneumomediastinum may be difficult.

Tension Pneumothorax

This is a life-threatening emergency. It occurs when the pressure in pleural air exceeds atmospheric pressure for a significant part of the respiratory cycle. Tension has an adverse effect on gas exchange and cardiovascular performance causing a rapid deterioration in the patient's condition. It is most often seen in mechanically ventilated patients or in patients of chest trauma.

Tension pneumothorax is difficult to diagnose on chest radiographs **(Box 6)**. Shift of mediastinum away from side of pneumothorax may be seen in any large pneumothorax

BOX 6: Tension pneumothorax.

Life threatening—immediate decompression required

Suggestive radiographic signs:
- Contralateral displacement of mediastinum
- Inferior displacement of the diaphragm
- Hyperlucent hemithorax
- Ipsilateral collapse

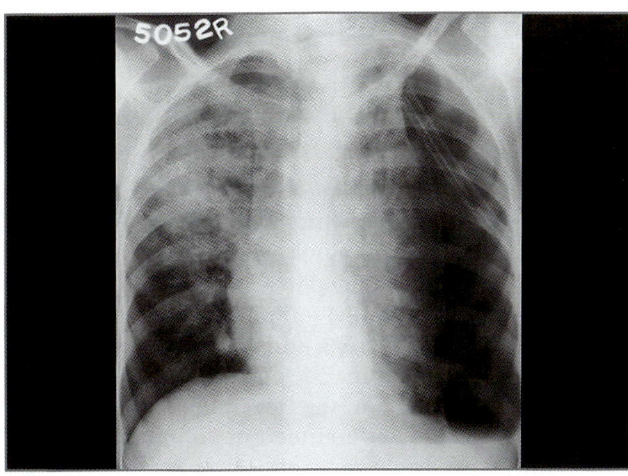

FIG. 47: A chest X-ray—infiltrative opacities right upper and mid zone, with left-sided pneumothorax—shift of the mediastinum to the right and flattening of left hemidiaphragm—tension pneumothorax.

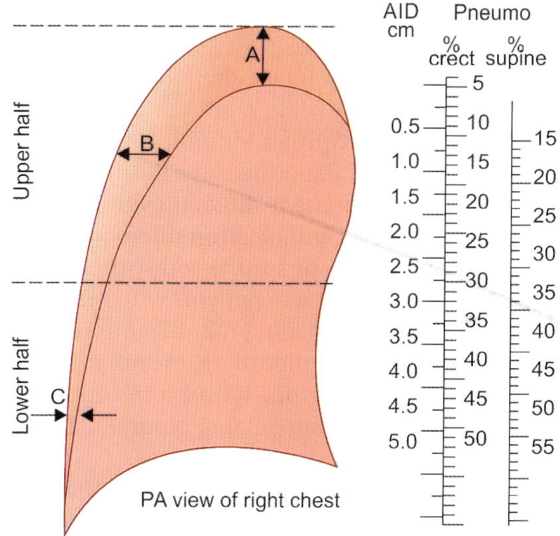

FIG. 48: Illustration depicting the calculation of size of pneumothorax. A = maximum apical interpleural distance, B = interpleural distance at the midpoint of upper half of lung, C = interpleural distance at the midpoint of lower half of lung. Average interpleural distance AID = A+B+C/3 in cm.

(**Fig. 47**). Combination of this with clinical symptom of circulatory compromise is diagnostic. Downward displacement or inversion of hemidiaphragm, is a reliable sign of tension especially in a ventilated patient in whom mediastinal shift is absent. The condition must be urgently treated by immediate decompression of the pleural space.

Size of Pneumothorax

A large pneumothorax may be differentiated from a small pneumothorax by the presence of a visible rim of >2 cm between lung margin and the chest wall at the level of the hilum. Pneumothorax may be calculated as percentage of the pleural space[35] as shown in **Figure 48**. A pneumothorax of >30% is generally considered to require treatment.

PLEURAL NEOPLASM

The pleura may be involved by primary tumor or one of several metastatic neoplasms. Metastatic disease is the most common pleural neoplasm.[34]

Pleural neoplasm may present as pleural effusion or pleural thickening/mass.

MESOTHELIOMA (MALIGNANT PLEURAL MESOTHELIOMA)

Malignant pleural mesothelioma (MPM) is the most common primary neoplasm of the pleura and the second most common malignancy of the pleura after pleural metastasis.[36-40] It is a highly malignant aggressive neoplasm of mesothelial cell origin. It occurs mainly in the pleura or peritoneum, but may arise in the pericardium or tunica vaginalis testis. There is a strong association between development of this neoplasm and asbestos exposure, with approximately 40–80% patients having history of exposure. The incidence of MPM in persons exposed to Asbestos is 10%. The carcinogenicity of asbestos fibers is proportional to the fiber aspect ratio (the ratio of fiber length to width), with the stiff and straight amphibole fibers such as crocidolite, being implicated more in causation of MPM. A latency period of 20–40 years between exposure and development of tumor is seen. Other risk factors for MPM include radiation therapy for malignancies such as lung and breast cancer. Symptoms include non-pleuritic chest pain, dyspnea and weight loss with mean age at presentation of 60 years. Men are affected more than women in a ratio of 4:1 three histological types are seen. Epithelioid MPM is the most common type, representing 55–65% of cases. Epithelioid MPM may be difficult to distinguish from lung and metastatic adenocarcinomas but typically demonstrates a higher degree of nuclear atypia. Sarcomatoid MPM is less common, comprising 10–15% of cases Sarcomatoid MPM includes the desmoplastic variant and may be difficult to distinguish from true sarcomas. Biphasic MPM constitutes 20–35% of cases and includes elements of the epithelioid and sarcomatoid types.[39] Osseous and/or cartilaginous differentiation may be seen rarely. The epithelioid type has a slightly better prognosis and is associated with pleural effusion.

Mesothelioma arises in relation to parietal pleura and is characterized morphologically by gross and nodular pleural thickening, which can involve fissures. Hemorrhagic pleural effusion often occurs. It spreads by local infiltration of the pleura. The tumor can invade both visceral and parietal pleura and frequently extends to adjacent structures, such as chest wall, mediastinum and diaphragm, lymph node spread or metastasis to different organs such as liver, lung and kidneys can occur. The overall survival is related to the extent of the primary tumor.

Diagnosis is made by image guided core biopsies or surgical biopsies as the yield from cytology of pleural fluid aspirate is poor. Spread along biopsy site is well documented the differentiation between mesothelioma and metastatic adenocarcinoma is difficult even with biopsy. Immunohistochemistry and electron microscopy aid the diagnosis. Serum levels of soluble mesothelin-related protein (SMRP) are elevated in patients with MPM.

The most common imaging manifestations of MPM include pleural effusion, pleural thickening, ipsilateral volume loss, local invasion, lymphadenopathy, and metastatic disease. Asbestos-related pleural disease may also be seen

The overall prognosis for patients with MPM is poor, with a median survival of 9–17 months after diagnosis. Patients with epithelioid histology have a greater median survival time than patients with sarcomatoid histology. Disease limited to the parietal pleura, negative surgical margins, and lack of lymph node involvement are associated with better outcomes.

Radiographic Findings of MPM

The most common plain radiographic findings are unilateral pleural effusion (30–95%) and concentric or lobulated pleural thickening **(Figs. 49 to 51)**.

Solid pleural lesions may vary from focal masses to diffuse thickening surrounding and encasing the entire lung surface. Extension into the interlobar fissure is common occurring in 40–86% patients. Distinct pleural masses without effusion are identified in less than 25% of patients. Benign calcified or noncalcified plaques may be present. Because of pleural thickening and mediastinal infiltration, the involved hemithorax may be normal in volume, despite presence of large effusion (the frozen mediastinum sign). The hemithorax may be reduced in volume because of restriction of lung expansion.

Ultrasonography

Ultrasound demonstrates pleural effusion and nodular soft tissue masses. The accuracy of US in detecting invasion of pleura and chest wall is high. Transthoracic ultrasound is used for guiding pleural fluid aspiration and biopsy.

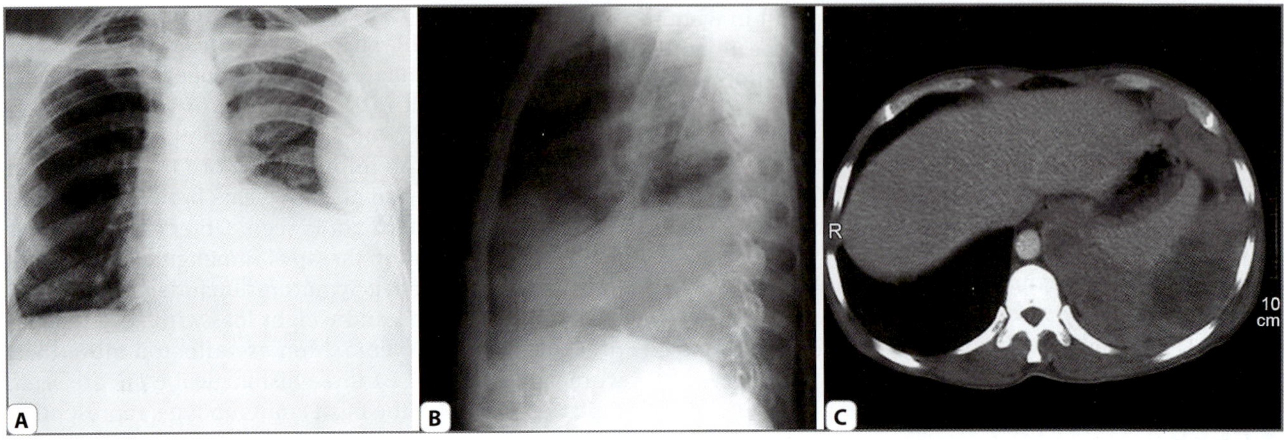

FIGS. 49A TO C: Chest X-ray (A and B), A nodular opacity noted along the left chest wall and lower zone. CT (C) shows, nodular pleural masses all along the pleural surface—malignant pleural mesothelioma.

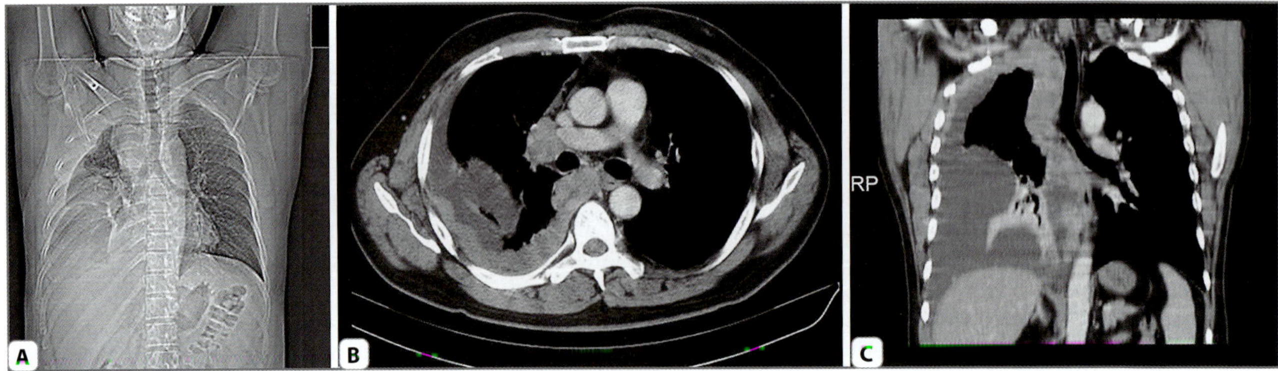

FIGS. 50A TO C: X-ray (A) CT chest (B and C)—circumferential and nodular enhancing pleural tumor with associated effusion.

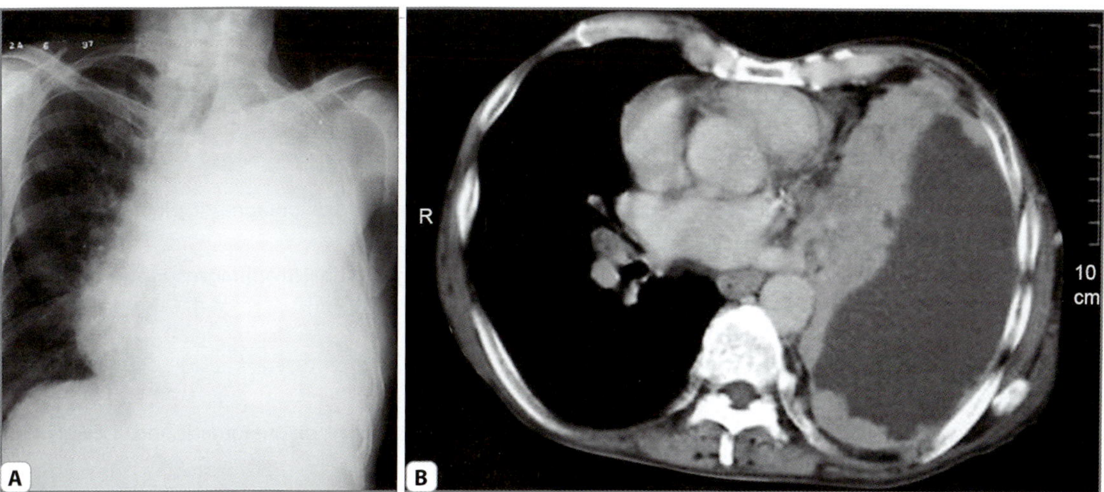

FIGS. 51A AND B: Chest X-ray (A)—opaque left hemithorax with shift of mediastinum to the right. CT scan (B) of the same patient shows nodular, thickened, enhancing pleura with associated effusion, malignant pleural mesothelioma.

Computed Tomography

CT is the primary imaging modality for diagnosis, staging and for assessment of response to therapy in cases of MPM. IV Contrast is recommended, and scanning should commence 60–80 second after contrast to maximize pleural uptake. Images should be reconstructed in 1–2 mm thickness in all three planes. The FOV should include the entire chest and all pleural spaces including the most caudal extent of the posterior costophrenic sulcus. An international consensus group has recommended that CT for a suspected MPM must include chest and abdomen as the pleural space can extend up to L3 level posteriorly.[41]

Major findings include unilateral pleural effusion and nodular pleural thickening. Pleural thickening that is nodular, circumferential, and greater than 1 cm in thickness is highly suggestive of malignant pleural disease, including MPM. Calcified plaques may be seen and are a sign of asbestos exposure; these are not a precursor to mesothelioma. Calcified plaques can be differentiated from osseocartilaginous differentiation of MPM by the morphology as they are linear whereas large or punctuate foci of calcification is seen in the tumor.

In early disease, pleural thickening may appear localized and discontinuous. As the disease progresses, pleural thickening becomes continuous, it increases in thickness and nodularity and the amount of fluid may decrease as pleural layers become fused.

In some cases, pleural effusion may be the only finding. The combination of an unexplained pleural effusion and pleural pain should raise the possibility of mesothelioma. Enhancement of the pleura after contrast administration can help differentiate tumor from adjacent fluid collections. Mesothelioma is visible most frequently along the lateral chest wall. The abnormal hemithorax can appear contracted and fixed with little change in size during inspiration. Thickening of fissures, particularly the lower part of major fissures can reflect tumor infiltration or associated pleural effusion. Involvement of fissures is seen on CT in 85% of cases of mesothelioma.

Malignant pleural mesothelioma may extend into the mediastinal fat and result in the loss of fat and tissue planes between mediastinal structures. Encasement of >50% of the circumference of the trachea or esophagus and obliteration of fat planes are findings suggestive of mediastinal invasion. Involvement of the pericardium, which may be nontransmural or transmural, may result in pericardial effusion, pericardial thickening, pericardial nodules and masses, and/or infiltrating soft tissue mediastinal pleural thickening is seen with extensive disease. MPM may locally invade the chest wall, this appears as loss of normal extrapleural fat planes, invasion of intercostal muscles, rib displacement or bony destruction. The accuracy of CT for identifying transdiaphragmatic extension is limited; the presence of a distinct fat plane between the inferior surface of the diaphragm and the adjacent abdominal organs is a sign which can be used to negate transdiaphragmatic extension.

Mediastinal lymph nodes, specifically paratracheal, hilar, subcarinal, paraesophageal, and paraaortic nodes, that are 10 mm or larger are considered abnormal. Internal mammary, retrocrural, and extrapleural lymph nodes have no specific size criteria, and visualization of these nodes is considered abnormal.

CT may demonstrate intrathoracic and extrathoracic metastatic disease. Pulmonary metastases may manifest as nodules, masses, or lymphangitic carcinomatosis, with thickening and nodularity of the interlobular septa.

There is a TNM international staging system, proposed by the International Mesothelioma Interest Group for diffuse malignant pleural mesothelioma **(Table 3)**.[42-45]

TABLE 3: International Mesothelioma Interest Group TNM staging system.

Category	Definition
T descriptors as per 8th edition of the TNM classification	
Tx	Primary tumor not assessable
T0	No evidence of primary tumor
T1	Tumor involving the ipsilateral parietal pleura (including mediastinal and diaphragmatic pleura) with or without involvement of visceral pleura
T2	Tumor involving each of the ipsilateral pleural surfaces (parietal, mediastinal, diaphragmatic and visceral pleura) with at least one of the following features: • Confluent visceral pleural tumor (including the fissures) • Involvement of diaphragmatic muscle • Invasion of the lung parenchyma
T3	Tumor involving all of the ipsilateral pleural surfaces (parietal, mediastinal, diaphragmatic and visceral pleura) with at least one of the following features: • Invasion of the endothoracic fascia • Extension into the mediastinal fat • Solitary, completely resectable focus invading soft tissues of the chest wall • Nontransmural involvement of the pericardium
T4	Tumor involving all of the ipsilateral pleural surfaces with at least one of the following features: • Diffuse or multifocal invasion of soft tissues of the chest wall • Any rib involvement • Invasion of the peritoneum through the diaphragm • Invasion of any mediastinal organ • Direct extension to the contralateral pleura • Invasion of the spine or brachial plexus • Transmural invasion of the pericardium (with or without pericardial effusion) or myocardium invasion.
N descriptors as per 8th edition of the TNM classification	
Nx	Regional lymph nodes not assessable
N0	No evidence of regional lymph node metastases
N1	Metastases in the ipsilateral bronchopulmonary, hilar, or mediastinal lymph nodes (including the internal mammary, peridiaphragmatic, pericardial fat pad or intercostal lymph nodes)
N2	Metastases in the contralateral bronchopulmonary, hilar, or mediastinal lymph nodes or ipsilateral or contralateral supraclavicular lymph nodes
M descriptors as per 8th edition of the TNM classification	
Mx	Presence of distant metastases not assessable
N0	No evidence of distant metastases
M1	Evidence of distant metastases

	Stage grouping for 8th edition		
Stage	**T**	**N**	**M**
I			
IA	T1	N0	M0
IB	T2, 3	N0	M0
II	T1, 2	N1	M0
III			
IIIA	T3	N1	M0
IIIB	T1-3	N2	M0
	T4	Any N	M0
IV	Any T	Any N	M1

The seventh edition had separate T1a (involvement limited to the ipsilateral parietal pleura) and T1b (if the visceral pleura was also involved) but these were combined following a survival analysis showing no difference between these two groups. The seventh edition also had an extra category for nodal involvement. Intrapleural (previous N1) and extrapleural (previous N2) lymph nodes are now combined into one category (N1) and previous N3 nodes have been moved into the N2 category.

CT criteria of resectability include:
- Preservation of extrapleural fat planes
- Absence of extrapleural soft tissue masses
- Normal CT attenuation values of adjacent structures
- Smooth inferior diaphragmatic surface

CT criteria of unresectability include:
- Multifocal or diffuse invasion of the chest wall
- Invasion of mediastinal structures
- Transmural invasion of pericardium
- Transdiaphragmatic extension
- Involvement of contralateral pleura
- Presence of metastasis

Magnetic Resonance Imaging

MRI due to its excellent soft tissue discrimination plays a complementary role to CT in accurate staging of the tumor. MRI is used to determine the presence and extent of tumor invasion into the diaphragm, chest wall, and mediastinal structures, which aids in determining resectability and surgical decision making. Malignant mesothelioma is intermediate in signal intensity relative to muscle on T1- and T2-weighted imaging, allowing distinction from the chest wall, diaphragm, and pericardium which are usually uniformly low in signal intensity on both T1- and T2-weighted images mesotheliomas enhance on postgadolinium scans. The important technical consideration is to use a large bore magnet and a body coil that includes the posterior costophrenic sulci and the diaphragm in the FOV. A short bore magnet may lead to field inhomogenity when a large FOV is required.

Diffusion MRI can also help to differentiate benign from malignant pleural disease. The presence of hyperintense pleural spots on high b value DW images called as "pleural pointillism" and has a sensitivity of 93% and a specificity of 79%.[46] Pleural pointillism can be used to provide guidance for biopsy or thoracoscopic evaluation. Perfusion MRI is a promising technique for assessment of perfusion, vascularity, and permeability of tumors. Therapeutic effect of chemotherapy can be monitored with perfusion MRI.

Positron Emission Tomography

Functional imaging with FDG-PET has facilitated the noninvasive evaluation of tumor pathophysiology, metabolism and proliferation and is an important adjunct modality in diagnosis and staging of MPM. Most mesotheliomas are FDG avid. Mesothelioma shows moderate to high FDG uptake involving areas of thickened pleura. FDG uptake in MPM is significantly higher than in benign pleural diseases, and greater FDG uptake has been associated with a shorter survival time. Tumors at earlier stage tend to have focal or linear patterns of uptake, whereas the mixed and encasing patterns are indicative of more advanced disease. PET/CT increases the accuracy of overall staging and improves the selection of patients for extrapleural pneumonectomy as it detects more extensive disease and identifies occult distant metastasis.

Whole-body FDG-PET CT imaging encompassing a FOV from the skull base to the proximal thighs, should be done that allows characterization of local intrathoracic disease and the detection of occult metastasis. Both attenuation-corrected (AC) and non-AC fused and unfused image sets should be reviewed particularly for chest wall invasion. In cases where PET CT is being done postintervention (surgery or radiation) adequate time interval should be there to prevent false positives from inflammation due to treatment.

Measurement of tumor burden: Accurate measurement of tumor burden is important for response assessment and for follow-up in cases of MPM. The morphology of multiple sub centimeter pleural nodules and rind like thickening of pleura, the curved surface of the pleura with respiratory artifacts pose a significant technical challenge. mRECIST (version 1.1) for mesothelioma is an adaptation of RECIST to overcome these. It consists of six radial pleural tumor measurements (axial) measurements performed perpendicular to the chest wall through the thickest portion of the tumor deposit for assessment of response tumor deposits chosen for measurement should ideally be located away from the curvature of the diaphragm and apex of the lung, between the levels of the inferior pulmonic vein and aortic arch **(Box 7)**.[41]

The differential diagnosis of malignant mesothelioma includes benign causes of pleural thickening (such as postinfection or diffuse pleural thickening) and pleural metastases, pleural dissemination of thymoma, localized fibrous tumor of the pleura, and epithelioid hemangioendothelioma. The lobulated outline, nodular masses, involvement of mediastinal pleura associated pleural effusion, or evidence of more advanced disease may help differentiate mesothelioma from benign causes of diffuse pleural thickening.

Pleural Metastasis

Metastatic disease accounts for the majority of pleural neoplasms and may present as pleural effusion, nodules or masses. Bronchogenic carcinoma is the most common malignancy to cause malignant pleural effusion, followed by breast cancer and lymphoma. Several extrathoracic primary tumors like ovarian, uterine, gastrointestinal or

BOX 7: Recommendations for MPM measurement on CT and MRI.

Radial pleural measurements (axial measurements performed perpendicular to the chest wall).

Ideal location for pleural measurement:
- Between level of inferior pulmonic vein and aortic arch
- Nondependent (avoid pleural fluid)
- Adjacent to the identifiable anatomical marker for reproducible measurements

pancreatic may metastasize to the pleura. In absence of a recognizable primary, metastatic adenocarcinoma is difficult to diagnose, because of histological similarity to malignant mesothelioma.

Invasive thymoma is an uncommon thoracic primary neoplasm with a propensity for pleural extension. This pleural implantation results in widespread pleural thickening and/or multiple discrete masses. It may be indistinguishable from mesothelioma, especially when the anterior mediastinal component is small.

Malignant effusion is the most frequent manifestation of metastatic pleural disease and is often accompanied by solid tumor deposits of varying size **(Fig. 52)**. They may appear as solitary implant on the costal, diaphragmatic or mediastinal pleura or within the interlobar fissure. Malignant effusions are exudative and show nonspecific appearance on ultrasound. Contrast CT will depict nodules within effusion. Half of the malignant effusions do not show any nodules and absence of these does not exclude malignant etiology of the effusion. The differential diagnosis of pleural metastasis are primary malignancy of the pleura-malignant mesothelioma, tubercular pleuritis, chronic empyema. FDG-PET CT may help in detecting primary neoplasm and malignant pleural involvement, though false positives may occur with empyema and prior talc pleurodesis.

Pleural Lymphoma

Involvement of pleura occurs in both Hodgkin and non-Hodgkin disease. It can be a primary involvement or secondary to lymphoma elsewhere. The lymphomatous deposits arise from lymphatic channels and lymphoid aggregates in the subpleural connective tissue below the visceral pleura. Solid pleural lymphoma occurs as either a solitary nodule or as diffuse tumor infiltration. Associated exudative pleural effusion may be seen due to lymphatic obstruction and resolves with radiation. Marked thickening of extrapleural soft tissue may be seen with associated mediastinal lymph node enlargement.

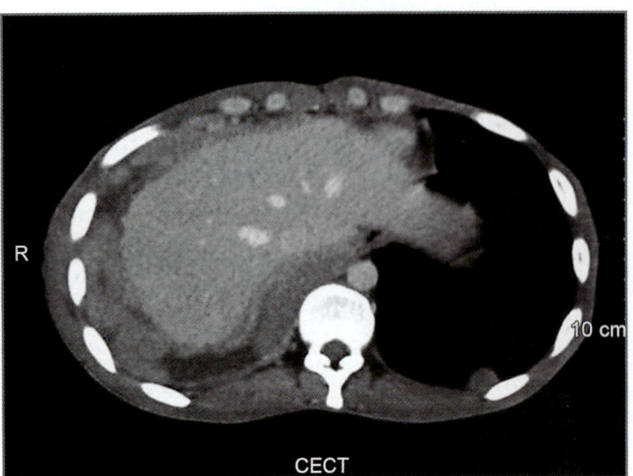

FIG. 52: CT multiple enhancing pleural nodules—metastases.

Primary effusion lymphoma: This is a rare type of non-Hodgkins lymphoma caused by human herpes virus 8 (HHV) in patients with immunodeficiency. Imaging findings are nonspecific with unilateral or bilateral pleural effusion unaccompanied by pulmonary or mediastinal abnormalities. PET CT usually demonstrates high avidity.

Pyothorax associated lymphoma (PAL): This is a rare form of NHL that is seen after a long history of empyema and is associated with Epstein–Barr virus infection. PAL appears as an oval or lenticular shaped soft tissue pleural mass that shows local invasion. The most frequent sites being chest wall and ribs. Symmetrical growth pattern of the mass at the margins of a chronic abscess is a specific imaging feature. Chest wall invasion by lung malignancy or empyema necessitans are close differentials.

Solitary Fibrous Tumor of the Pleura

Solitary fibrous tumor (SFTP) of the pleura was formerly known as benign mesothelioma, but it is not mesothelial in origin, and not always benign (30% are malignant). About 50% of cases are encountered in patients in 6th–7th decade, with no gender predilection. It has no association with asbestos exposure. It is rarely associated with paraneoplastic syndrome such as Doege–Potter syndrome patients are frequently asymptomatic, SFTP is detected incidentally on chest radiographs. It can be associated with hypoglycemia (15%), chest pain or hypertrophic pulmonary osteoarthropathy (one-third of cases). These symptoms resolve with resection.

The SFTP arises from the visceral pleura in about 80%. They appear as solitary, well-circumscribed spherical ovoid, noncalcified lesions, contacting a pleural surface. The size ranges from <2 to 30 cm. They are often pedunculated and as a consequence may show change in position and shape during fluoroscopy.

The SFTP, when small has an obtuse angle at the pleural surface, when large angles can be acute. It can be seen within a fissure, mimicking appearance of loculated fluid. A "beak" or "thorn" sign is often seen on radiographs in patients with a SFTP originating from or projecting into a fissure. Pleural effusion is not usually present. On CT, small tumors it appears as well-defined lobulated pleural mass **(Figs. 53A to C)**. Slight pleural thickening is usually visible adjacent to the mass. This is due to small amount of fluid accumulating at the pleural surface at the point of separation of visceral and parietal pleura by the mass. Larger tumors are more heterogeneous and may be difficult to pinpoint its origin from the pleura. Calcification may be seen in 7–26% of cases. Dynamic contrast enhanced CT shows intense enhancement in areas of high cellularity, while the fibrous component shows slow and delayed enhancement. Malignancy should be considered when the mass exceeds 10 cm in size. On imaging malignant SFTP demonstrate atelectasis, mass effect on the mediastinum and pleural effusion. On MRI, SFTP may show low signal on both T1 and T2 weighted images or may have heterogenous signal

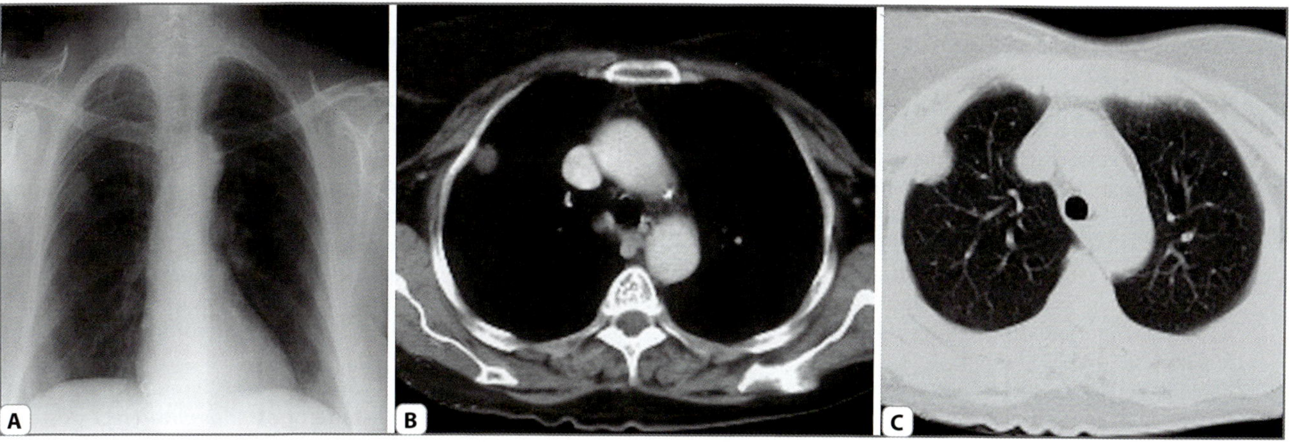

FIGS. 53A TO C: X-ray of chest PA (A) right lateral (B), CT (C)—showing a sharply-defined peripheral upper lube opacity without any other pleural abnormality—benign fibrous tumor.

intensity reflecting the cellularity of these tumors. Surgical excision is the treatment with operative respectability being the most important predictor of clinical outcome. FDG-PET CT can help to differentiate benign from malignant SFTP, with a higher SUV seen in malignant variant.[26,40,47]

Mesenchymal soft tissue tumors, localized malignant pleural mesothelioma and peripheral lung malignancy are the important differential diagnosis. Neurogenic tumors in posterior paraspinal location and anterior mediastinal tumors are the other differential.

Pleural Lipoma

It is rare, though the most common benign tumor of the pleuea. It shows fat attenuation on all modalities.

TUMOR-LIKE CONDITIONS OF THE PLEURA

A tumor-like condition of the pleura is any non-neoplastic lesion of the pleura itself, or within the pleural space, that resembles a tumor.[48] These may be focal or diffuse. Pleural plaque, thoracic splenosis, thoracic endometriosis causing catamenial pneumothorax, and pseudotumor caused by pleural effusion are focal tumor-like conditions of the pleura. Thoracic splenosis is the autotransplantation of splenic tissue into the pleural space after trauma. The diagnosis of thoracic splenosis should be considered in the setting of solitary or multiple left pleural nodules and evidence of remote splenic trauma (i.e., splenectomy or splenules in the left upper quadrant) diffuse tumor-like conditions of the pleura include diffuse pleural thickening and rare conditions such as Erdheim-Chester disease and diffuse pulmonary lymphangiomatosis. Erdheim-Chester disease is classified as non-Langerhans histiocytosis and is characterized by typical skeletal findings of femoral sclerosis, perirenal soft tissue halo. Diffuse pulmonary lymphangiomatosis is a rare condition, demonstrates diffuse pleural thickening, interlobular septal and peribronchovascular interstitial thickening, and mediastinal fat infiltration limited to the thorax.

REFERENCES

1. Coolen J, Keyzer FD, Nafteux P, et al. Malignant pleural disease: Diagnosis by using diffusion weight and dynamic contrast enhanced MR imaging initial experience. Radiology. 2012;263(3):884-92.
2. Parcel JM, Vives. Classic abbreviated and modified Light criteria; Chest. 1999;116:1833-6.
3. Sasson CS, Light RW. Chylothorax & pseudochylothorax. Clin Chest Med. 1985;6:163-71.
4. Walker CM, Takasugi JE, Chung JH, et al. Tumour like conditions of the pleura. Radiographics. 2012;32:971-85.
5. Eibenberger K, dock W, Ammann M, et al. Quantification of pleural effusions: sonography versus radiography. Radiology. 1994;191:681-4.
6. Yang PC, Luh KT, Chang DB, et al. Value of sonography in determing the nature of pleural effusion: analysis of 320 cases. Am J Roentgenol. 1992;159:29-33.
7. Wu RG, Yang PC, Kuo SH. "Fluid colour" sign-a useful indicator for discrimination between pleural thickening and pleural effusion. J Ultrasound Med. 1995;14(10):767-9.
8. Abramowitz Y, Simanovsky N, Goldstein MS, et al. Pleural effusion: Characterisation with CT attenuation values and CT appearance. AJR. 2009;192:618-23.
9. Halvorsen RA, Fedyshin PJ, Korobkin M, et al. Ascitis or pleural effusion? CT differentiation:four useful criteria. Radiographics. 1986;6:135-49.

10. Dwyer RA. The displaced crus: A sign for distinguishing between pleural fluid and ascitis on computed tomography. Comput Assist Tomog. 1978;2:598.
11. Baysal T, Bulut T, Gokirmak M. Diffusion weighted MR imaging of pleural fluid: Differentiation of transudative vs exudative pleural effusions. Eur Radiol. 2004;14:890-6.
12. Ivan N, Arsalan A, Akansel G, et al. Diffusion weighted MRI in the characterization of pleural effusions: Diag Interv Radiol. 2009;15(1):13-8.
13. Chen HJ, Yu YH, Tu CY, et al. Ultrasound in peripheral pulmonary air fluid lesions: Colour Doppler imaging as an aid in differentiating empyema and abscess. Chest. 2009;135(6):1426-32.
14. Kuhlman JE, Singha NK. Complex disease of the pleural space: Radiographic and CT evaluation. Radiographics. 1997;17:63-97.
15. Kuhlman JE. Complex disease of the pleural space: The 10 questions most frequently asked of the radiologist-new approaches to their answers with CT and MR imaging. Radiographics. 1997; 17:1043-50.
16. Stark DD, Federle MP, Goodman PC, et al. Differentiating lung abscess and empyema:radiography and computed tomography. AJRAm J Roentgenol. 1983;141:163-7.
17. Leung AN, Muller NL, Miller RR. CT in differential diagnosis of diffuse pleural disease. AJR Am J Roentgenol. 1990;154:487-92.
18. Neff CC, van Sonnerberg E, Lawson DW, et al. CT followup of empyemas: Pleural peels resolve after percutaneous catheter drainage. Radiology. 1990;176:195-7.
19. Kapoor H, Gulati V Gulati A, Donuru A, et al. Comprehensive Imaging Review of Pleural Fistulas from Diagnosis to Management. RadioGraphics. 2022;42:1940-55.
20. Seo H, Kim TJ, Jin KN, et al. Multi-detector row computed tomographic evaluation of broncho-pleural fistula: correlation with clinical, bronchoscopic and surgical findings. J Comput Assit Tomogr. 2010;34(1):13-8.
21. McLoud TC, Woods BO, Carrington CB, et al. Diffuse pleural thickening in the asbestos-exposed population. AJR Am J Roentgenol. 1985;144:9-18.
22. Renner RR, Pernice NJ. The apical cap. Semin Roentgenol. 1977;12:299-302.
23. Lynch DA, Gamsu G, Aberle DR. Conventional and high-resolution tomography in the diagnosis of asbestos-related diseases. Radiographics. 1989;9:523-51.
24. Cugell DW, Kamp DW. Asbestos and the pleura—a review. Chest. 2004;125(3):1103-17.
25. Roach HD, Davies GJ, Attanoos R. Asbestosis: when the dust settles an imaging review of asbestos related disease. Radiographics. 2002;S167-84.
26. Yamada A,Taiji R, NishimotoY, Takahiro I et al. Pictorial Review of Pleural Disease: Multimodality Imaging and Differential Diagnosis. Radio Graphics. 2024;44(4):e230079.
27. Gordon R. The deep sulcus sign. Radiology. 1980;136:25-7.
28. Kirkpatrick AW, Sirois M1 Laupland KB, et al. Hand held thoracic sonography for detecting post traumatic pneumothoraces: The extended focussed assessment with sonography for trauma (EFAST). J Trauma. 2004;57:288-95.
29. De Luca C, Valentino M, Rimondi M, et al. Use of chest sonography in acute care radiology. J Ultrasound. 2008;11:25-34.
30. Barillari A, Kiuru S. Detection of spontaneous pneumothorax with chest ultrasound in emergency department. Intern Emerg Med. 2010;1:253-5.
31. Lichtenstein DA, Menu Y. A Bedside ultrasound sign ruling out pneumothorax in the critically ill-lung sliding. Chest. 1995;108:1345-8.
32. Lichtenstein D, Meziere G, Biderman P. The lung point: An ultrasound sign specific to pneumothorax. Intensive care Med. 2000;26:1434-40.
33. Lichtenstein DA, Meziere G, Lascols N, et al. Ultrasound diagnosis of occult pneumothorax. Crit care Med. 2005;33:1231-8.
34. Cunnigham J, Kirkpatrick AW, Nicolaous, et al. Enhanced recognition of "lung sliding" with power colour Doppler imaging in the diagnosis of pneumothorax. J Trauma. 2002;52:769-71.
35. Choi BG, Park SH, Yun EH, et al. Pneumothorax size: correlation of supine anteroposterior with erect postero-anterior chest radiograph. Radiology. 1998;209:567-9.
36. Dynes MC, White EM, Fry WA, et al. Imaging manifestations of pleural tumors. Radiographics. 1992;12:1191-201.
37. Wang ZJ, Reddy GB, Gotway MB, et al. Malignant pleural mesothelioma: Evaluation with CT, MR imaging and PET. Radiographics. 2004;(1):105-19.
38. Yanamuro M, Gerbando VH, Gill RR, et al. Morphological and functional imaging of malignant pleural mesothelioma. Eur Radiol. 2007;64(3):355-66.
39. Nickell LT, Licchtenberger JP, Khorashadi L, et al. Multimodality imaging for characterisation, classification and staging of malignant pleural mesothelioma. Radiographics. 2014;341:692-706.
40. Sureka B, Thukral BB, Mittal MK, Mittal A, Sinha M. Radiological review of pleural tumors. Indian J Radiol Imaging 2013;23:313-20.
41. Katz SI, Straus CM, Roshkovan L, et al. Considerations for Imaging of Malignant Pleural Mesothelioma: A Consensus Statement from the International Mesothelioma Interest Group. Journal of Thoracic Oncology. 2022;18(3):278-98.
42. Berzenji L, Van Schil PE, Carp L. The eighth TNM classification for malignant pleural mesothelioma. Translational lung cancer research. 2018;7(5):543-9.
43. American Joint Committee on Cancer. Malignant Pleural Mesothelioma. In: AJCC Cancer Staging Manual. 8th ed. New York, NY: Springer; 2017:457-68.
44. Nowak AK, Chansky K, Rice DC, Pass HI, Kindler HL, Shemanski L, et al. The IASLC Mesothelioma Staging Project: Proposals for Revisions of the T Descriptors in the Forthcoming Eighth Edition of the TNM Classification for Pleural Mesothelioma. J Thorac Oncol. 2016;11(12):2089-99..
45. Rice D, Chansky K, Nowak A, Pass H, Kindler H, Shemanski L, et al. The IASLC Mesothelioma Staging Project: Proposals for Revisions of the N Descriptors in the Forthcoming Eighth Edition of the TNM Classification for Pleural Mesothelioma. J Thorac Oncol. 2016;11(12):2100-11.
46. Coolen J, Keyzer FD, Nafleux P, et al. Malignant pleural mesothelioma: Visceral assessment by using pleural pointillism at diffusion weighted MR imaging. Radiology. 2015;274:576-84.
47. Rosado-de-christenson ML, Abbot GF, Mc Adams HP, et al. Localised Fibrous tumours of the pleura. Radiographics. 2003;23(3):759-83.
48. Walker CM, Takasugi JE, Chung JH, Reddy GP, et al. Tumor like Conditions of the Pleura Radio Graphics 2012;32:971-85.

Ujjwal Gorsi, Arun Sharma, Anupam Lal, Tulika Singh

CHAPTER 19

Imaging of the Diaphragm and Chest Wall

INTRODUCTION

Diaphragm is a thin dome-shaped musculotendinous structure, which serves two important functions: (1) it acts as a physical barrier between the thoracic and abdominal cavities and (2) it is the chief muscle of inspiration. Embryologically, it develops from septum transversum, pleuroperitoneal membranes, dorsal mesentery of the esophagus, and muscular body wall. Diaphragm develops during 4–12 weeks of embryogenesis.[1] The anteriorly placed septum transversum forms the central tendon of the diaphragm. Septum transversum fuses with pleuroperitoneal membranes and esophageal mesentery posteriorly and gets attached to the muscular body wall laterally to form a diaphragm.

The peripheral muscular part of diaphragm arises from the margin of the thoracic outlet and is inserted into a trefoil-shaped central tendon. The muscular fibers arise from three sources and may be grouped into three parts, two slips from the back of the xiphoid (sternal part), muscle fibers arising circumferentially from the inner surfaces of the cartilages and the adjacent parts of lower six ribs of each side interlocking with fibers of the transversus abdominis (costal part), and from the superior three lumbar vertebrae by the right and left crura (lumbar part) that unite anteriorly to the aortic hiatus to form the median arcuate ligament **(Fig. 1)**.[1,2] Lateral to the crura, the diaphragm arises from the arcuate ligaments (medial and lateral), which are the thickened fascia of the quadratus lumborum and psoas. The anterior muscle fibers are shorter than the posterior ones, which give the diaphragm its characteristic dome-shaped configuration.

There are three openings in the normal diaphragm **(Fig. 2)**: (1) aortic hiatus, (2) esophageal hiatus, and (3) the hiatus for inferior vena cava (IVC). Aortic hiatus (osseoaponeurotic opening) is at the level of 12th thoracic vertebra (T12). The aorta, thoracic duct, and azygos and hemiazygos veins course through this hiatus. Decussation of the medial fibers of the right crus at the level of T10 forms an esophageal hiatus, which gives passage to esophagus, vagus,

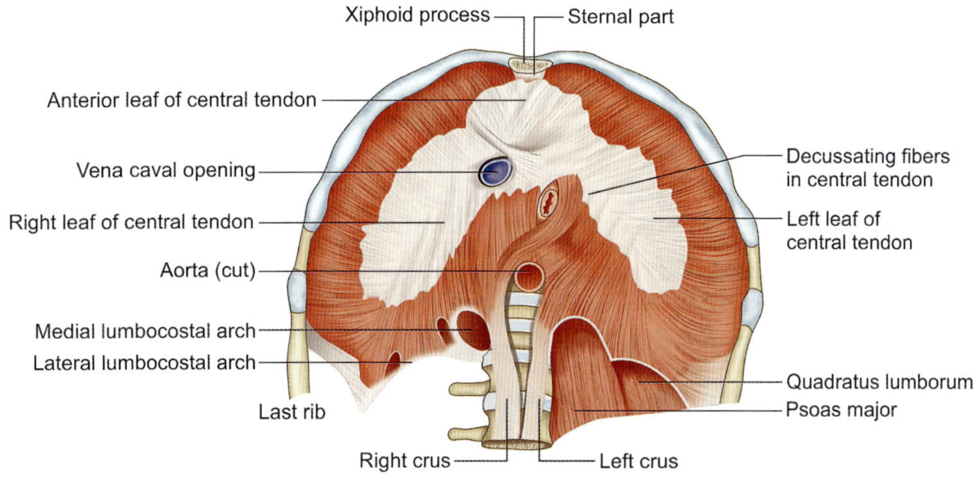

FIG. 1: Schematic diagram of diaphragm as viewed from abdominal aspect.

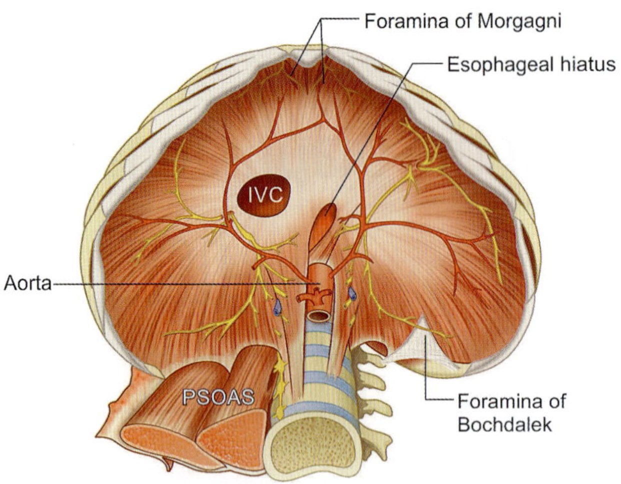

FIG. 2: Schematic diagram of diaphragm showing the hiatuses as viewed from its caudal aspect.

(IVC: inferior vena cava)

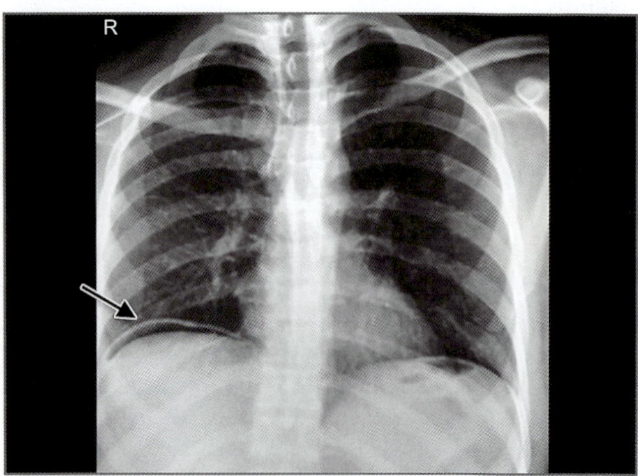

FIG. 3: Chest radiograph showing diaphragm (black arrow) clearly identified because of pneumoperitoneum.

sympathetic nerves, and left gastric vessels. IVC hiatus is in the central tendon at the level of T8–T9 and transmits IVC and branches of the right phrenic nerve. Nerve supply of the diaphragm is from left and right phrenic nerves, which arise from C3 to C5 cervical nerves and have sensory as well as motor function.

FUNCTIONS

The main function of the diaphragm is to act as a muscle for respiration. It contracts along with sternocleidomastoid, scalene, and intercostal muscles, which are the accessory muscles of respiration, during inspiration. This contraction causes expansion of thoracic cavity and reduces the intrathoracic pressure due to which air is drawn into the lungs. During expiration, along with elastic recoil of the lungs, diaphragm relaxes. The diaphragm, by increasing intra-abdominal pressure, helps in urination, defecation, and emesis. In addition, diaphragm helps prevent gastroesophageal reflux as it exerts external pressure at the esophageal opening.[1]

IMAGING MODALITIES

Imaging modalities for diaphragmatic disorders include plain radiography, fluoroscopy, ultrasonography (USG), computed tomography (CT), and magnetic resonance imaging (MRI).

Plain Radiograph

Normal diaphragm is not separately identifiable on a chest X-ray. On a chest X-ray, usually, the top of the abdominal cavity, which normally represents the upper abdominal organs such as the liver, stomach, spleen, or colon with the overlying diaphragm and is opaque on radiograph, is spoken off as diaphragm. It is visualized as a distinct entity only if outlined by air on both sides, i.e., on thoracic and abdominal sides **(Fig. 3)**. On inspiration, the domes of diaphragm are at the level of the 6th rib anteriorly and at or below the 10th rib posteriorly. The right hemidiaphragm is 1.5–2.5 cm higher than the left in most individuals. In about 9%, the two hemidiaphragms are at the same level, and the left hemidiaphragm is up to 1 cm higher than right in a few normal individuals.[3] On the lateral radiograph, both the domes project on each other. The right and left domes can be easily differentiated from each other by the fact that the anterior part of the left hemidiaphragm is mostly obscured by the heart, whereas the right dome can be seen in its entirety. On the left lateral view, the posterior part of the right dome projects under the left dome. The IVC stops at the right hemidiaphragm, while stomach bubble or gas in splenic flexure is in close contact with the left hemidiaphragm. The distance between the dome of diaphragm and the top of the gastric air bubble of the left hemidiaphragm is <1 cm in most individuals (about 88%) and is best demonstrated in the lateral view.[2]

Fluoroscopy

The fluoroscopic sniff test is a real-time fluoroscopic assessment of motor function of diaphragm (excursion). It is commonly used in patients who have breathing difficulties following stroke or in patients who have suffered phrenic nerve palsy to look for the absence of muscular contraction of the diaphragm during inspiration.[1]

Ultrasonography

Ultrasonography is a cheap, portable, easily available, and radiation risk-free imaging modality. Structures above and below the diaphragm can be examined in real time using USG. Structural and functional components of the diaphragm can be assessed with USG even at the bedside. In children and young adults, it is a preferred imaging technique for interrogating the diaphragm. Ultrasound visualizes the lateral and posterior parts of the diaphragm, instead of anteriorly located central tendon, which is examined by fluoroscopy. Transhepatic and trans-splenic sector scanning is the most appropriate technique to visualize the diaphragm **(Fig. 4)**. Pleural disease can also be used as an acoustic window to study the lateral parts of the dome. The diaphragm itself is seen as a thin hypoechoic line. The interface between the diaphragm and liver (or spleen) appears as a thin echogenic line. The interface between the diaphragm and lung appears as a stronger and thicker echogenic band. The diaphragm can be clearly visualized on USG when pleural effusion and ascites are present at the same time. B-mode USG can assess both echogenicity and thickness of the diaphragm, whereas M-mode ultrasound by assessing a specific site over time can evaluate excursion, velocity, and response to phrenic nerve stimulation.[4]

Computed Tomography

The diaphragmatic disorders are usually difficult to assess with CT in axial plane because of the tangential course of the diaphragm to the imaging plane. However, with the arrival of the multidetector CT (MDCT) and the use of multiplanar reconstructions, various diaphragmatic pathologies and injuries can be easily demonstrated **(Fig. 5)**.[5] The costal part of the diaphragm is frequently seen as a stripe of soft tissue between the aerated lung above and fat below. The sternal part is sometimes visualized as linear soft-tissue densities anterior to the heart. The crura appear as smooth linear densities that decussate ventral to the aorta at the cranial level and are located lateral to the aorta at the more caudal level **(Fig. 6)**. Crus of the diaphragm extends up to third lumbar vertebra on the right side and up to second lumbar vertebra on the left side. As the right crus extends far below the left crus, it can be mistaken for a lymph node.

Magnetic Resonance Imaging

Coronal and sagittal MR images provide the best way to evaluate the relationship and involvement of the diaphragm to pathologic processes such as hernia, infection, and tumor.[6] MR can easily identify congenital, acquired, and traumatic diaphragmatic hernias, which commonly present as thoracic masses. In all MRI sequences, diaphragm has signal intensity, which is lower than other skeletal muscles. It is excellent for demonstrating the extent and anatomic relationships of

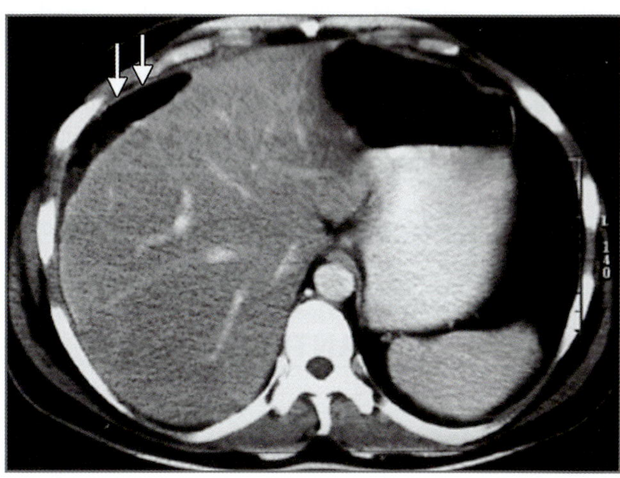

FIG. 5: Axial computed tomography (CT) scan showing diaphragm (white arrows) outlined by air present in the subphrenic abscess.

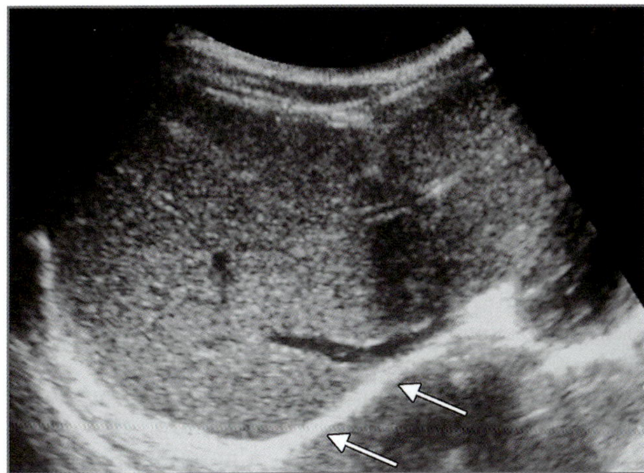

FIG. 4: The transverse ultrasound scan of right hemidiaphragm showing the diaphragm/lung interface as a thick curvilinear echogenic band (white arrows). The triangular hypoechoic band between this and the liver is the peripheral muscular bundles of diaphragm.

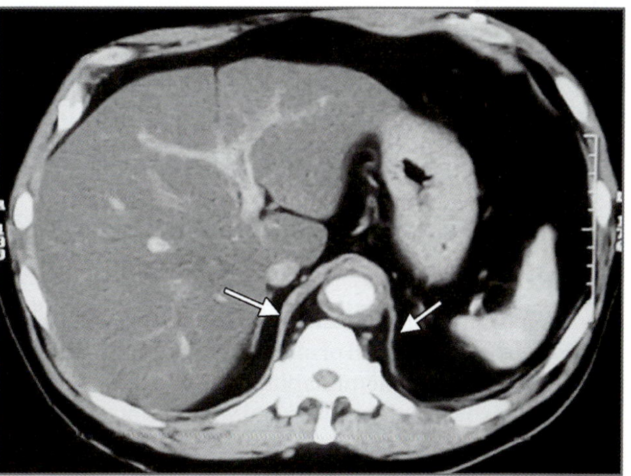

FIG. 6: Axial computed tomography (CT) scan of abdomen showing diaphragmatic crura (white arrows).

juxtadiaphragmatic tumors and can help to identify the location of peridiaphragmatic fluid collections. However, the respiratory motion may impair imaging of the normal diaphragm. In addition to morphologic abnormalities, MRI can be helpful in evaluating functional disorders of the diaphragm. With the advent of faster MRI, such as "gradient recalled echo" (GRE), it is possible to obtain sequential dynamic images of the diaphragm during real-time breathing, which can be viewed as cine loops.[6] This approach allows for the evaluation of diaphragmatic motion without the use of ionizing radiation. MRI allows quantitative evaluation, including the synchronicity, excursion, and velocity of motion of diaphragm.[7]

Radionuclide Scan

The role of radionuclide scans in assessing diaphragmatic pathology is limited. Most of the scans are performed for assessing diaphragmatic integrity in occult cases where the radiologic imaging is equivocal. Intraperitoneal injection of technetium sulfur colloid and subsequent scintigraphy have been shown to be sensitive tests for the diagnosis of diaphragmatic laceration. Radionuclide liver-spleen imaging with ^{99m}Tc sulfur colloid permits assessment of liver and splenic injuries and also their herniation into the thorax in cases of traumatic diaphragmatic hernias.[8]

NORMAL VARIANTS

Scalloping

Scalloping appears as short curves of diaphragm, which are convex upward. It gives a polyarcuate appearance and is seen in approximately 5% of individuals. They are commonly seen on the right side and in patients with pulmonary emphysema or pneumothorax. Muscle slips appear as small curved lines, which are concave upward and are common on the right side. They are commonly seen in tall, thin patients and those with emphysema. Diaphragmatic humps and dromedary diaphragm represent mild forms of eventration with incomplete muscularization of the hemidiaphragm, but there is no muscle defect. They are commonly seen on the right side and anteriorly.

Eventration

Eventration is a congenital anomaly with failure of muscular development of part or all of one or both hemidiaphragms. Total eventration of a hemidiaphragm is more common on the left side, which is often associated with torsion or volvulus of the stomach **(Fig. 7)**. Partial eventration is more common on the right side and frequently involves its anteromedial portion. On chest radiography, partial eventration is seen as a semioval or semicircular homogeneous opacity, which has soft-tissue density arising from the diaphragm.[2,3] On deep inspiration, eventration becomes more apparent as dorsal and lateral parts of the diaphragm move downward, whereas convex segment may remain at the same level or show upward movement. MDCT **(Fig. 8)**, USG, and MRI may be required to differentiate eventration from mediastinal, pericardial, or pleural lesions. Differentiating an eventration involving a large part of a hemidiaphragm from a paralyzed hemidiaphragm and Morgagni hernia with herniation of the liver or fat may not be easy at times. The paralyzed hemidiaphragm often has an adjacent area of atelectatic lung on chest X-ray, whereas large eventration does not. This is due to the fact that an eventration still has some net inspiratory downward movement, while a paralyzed hemidiaphragm has a paradoxical upward motion.

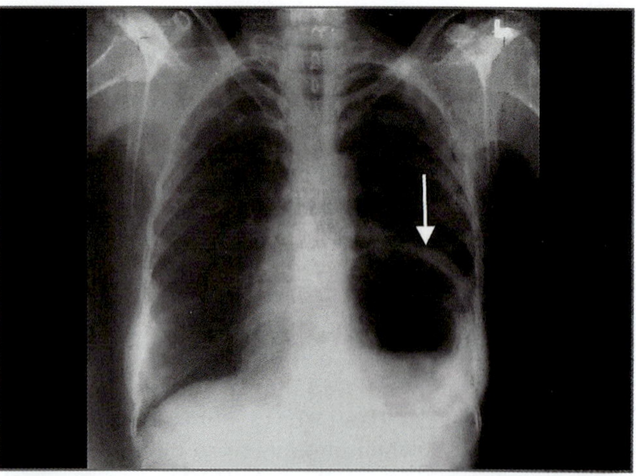

FIG. 7: Chest radiograph showing eventration of the left hemidiaphragm (white arrow) with gastric volvulus.

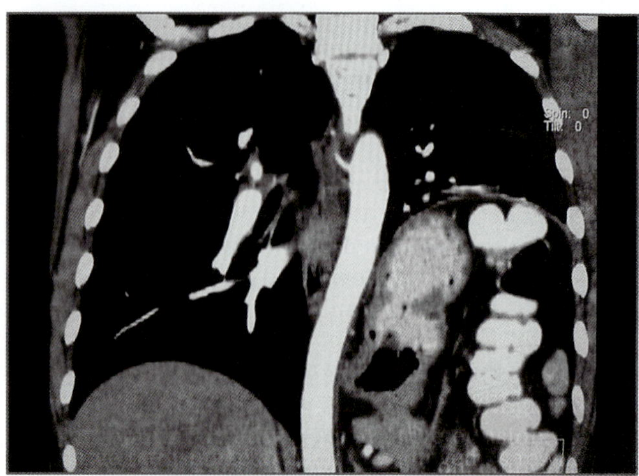

FIG. 8: Coronal reformats of multidetector computed tomography (CT) showing eventration of the left hemidiaphragm with intrathoracic herniation of stomach and colon.

Accessory Diaphragm

It is a partial duplication of a hemidiaphragm, almost always seen on the right side. It courses obliquely backward and upward and gets attached along the 3rd to 7th ribs. Part of the entire lower lobe is contained between the true and accessory hemidiaphragm. On the frontal view of the chest, the entire hemidiaphragm may be elevated, and the heart and mediastinum are shifted to the affected right side. The adjacent right mediastinal margin is indistinct. On the lateral view, the accessory diaphragm appears as an oblique line rising posteriorly.[2]

ELEVATED HEMIDIAPHRAGM

Unilateral Elevation

Causes of a unilateral high hemidiaphragm are eventration, unilateral atelectasis, severe gastric distension, gross hepatomegaly, gross splenomegaly, obstructive emphysema of the contralateral lung, phrenic nerve palsy, subpulmonic effusion, subphrenic abscess, and ipsilateral pulmonary hypoplasia.[2,3]

Bilateral Elevation

Causes of a bilaterally high diaphragm are ascites, pregnancy, hepatosplenomegaly, large intra-abdominal tumors, poor inspiratory effort, and causes of unilateral elevation present bilaterally.[2]

Low-lying Diaphragm

It may be seen in cases of hyperinflated lungs, intrathoracic masses, and large pleural effusions.

Inversion of the Diaphragm

It represents reverse curvature of the diaphragm and can be partial or complete. It can occur with tension pneumothorax, large basal bulla, large pleural effusion, or large tumors. The condition is usually seen on the left side, as the right dome is somewhat protected by the underlying liver. An inverted diaphragm rises actively on inspiration and falls on expiration, resulting in paradoxical movement of the diaphragm and mediastinal shift toward the affected side during inspiration.

Peridiaphragmatic Collections

For localization of peridiaphragmatic collections, identification of the diaphragm is the key factor.[3] Accurate localization of a fluid collection in sub- or supradiaphragmatic location at times may be difficult on cross-sectional imaging. USG, CT, and MRI are helpful in differentiating subdiaphragmatic (ascites) versus supradiaphragmatic (pleural) fluid **(Figs. 9 and 10)**.[9] On axial CT images, a number of CT signs are helpful in differentiating ascites from pleural effusion **(Table 1)**.

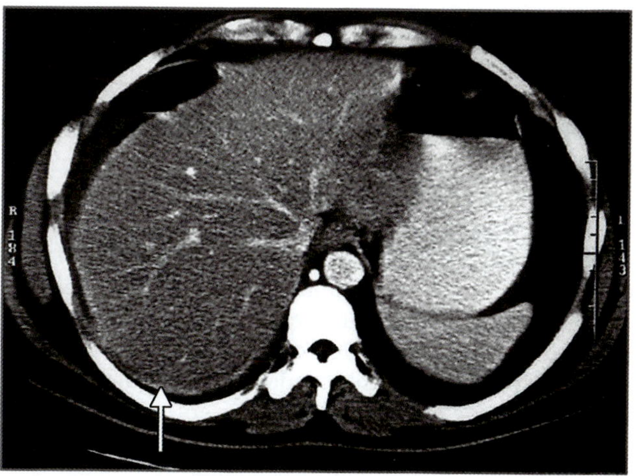

FIG. 9: Axial computed tomography (CT) scan showing fluid collection anterior to the posterior aspect of the diaphragm (white arrow) is subphrenic in location.

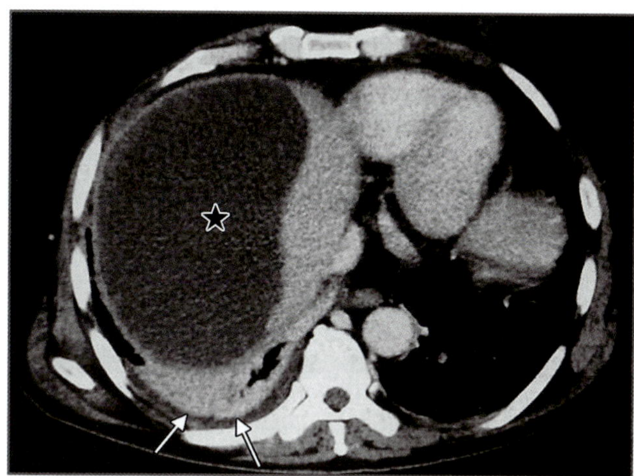

FIG. 10: Axial computed tomography (CT) scan of the abdomen showing right pleural effusion (arrows) and subdiaphragmatic collection (asterisk).

TABLE 1: Differences between ascites and pleural effusion.

Features	Ascites	Pleural effusion
Diaphragmatic circle	Center	Outside
Displaced crus sign	Posteromedial	Anterolateral
Bare area sign	Seen	Not seen
Interface (abdominal viscera)	Sharp	Hazy
Lung	Anterior	Surrounds
Caudally	Increases	Decreases
Cranially	Decreases	Increases

DIAPHRAGMATIC MOVEMENTS

Abnormal movement of the diaphragm during respiration is an important radiologic sign of diaphragmatic or juxtadiaphragmatic disease. Fluoroscopy, ultrasound, and MRI may be employed for assessing diaphragmatic movements.[4,6] The normal amplitude of the motion ranges from 0.8 to 8 cm in normal, healthy, young adults. Most (77%) individuals may show asymmetry of diaphragmatic motion when observed on fluoroscopy, although the difference in excursion is usually <1 cm.[3] Minor asynchronous motion of the hemidiaphragm and even momentary minimal paradoxical movement may be seen. The dome also may move differently from the rest of the diaphragm. In the lateral decubitus position, the dependent hemidiaphragm rises higher than usual, and its respiratory excursion is greatly exaggerated. Abnormal diaphragmatic movement can be classified into three types: (1) paradoxical, (2) complete, or (3) incomplete fixation. Paradoxical movement is the upward movement of the affected hemidiaphragm on inspiration instead of the normal descent, complete fixation is no movement of the affected hemidiaphragm during the respiratory cycle, and incomplete fixation is greatly decreased motion of the affected hemidiaphragm on respiration. These three types of abnormal movement can be seen in various conditions, including paralysis, eventration, subphrenic abscess, traumatic diaphragmatic hernia, unilateral obstructive emphysema, and pneumothorax. Fluoroscopy and real-time USG are reliable in assessing diaphragmatic motion.

DIAPHRAGMATIC WEAKNESS AND PARALYSIS

Weakness or paralysis of diaphragm may be due to central nervous causes or phrenic nerve involvement due to tumor invasion or thoracic surgery.[9] Paralysis of diaphragm is more often unilateral, which is asymptomatic, and is found on imaging incidentally. Bilateral diaphragmatic paralysis is mostly symptomatic and may present with respiratory failure.

On chest radiograph, bilateral diaphragm paralysis is seen as the smooth elevation of both hemidiaphragms and associated reduced volume of the lungs. The costovertebral and costophrenic sulci become narrow and deep. On lateral view, smooth elevation of diaphragmatic position may be better appreciated. At lung bases, linear atelectasis may also be seen. In unilateral diaphragm paralysis, the left hemidiaphragm may lie at or above the right hemidiaphragm. If right hemidiaphragm is paralyzed, it lies more than one interspace higher than the left side. A paralyzed hemidiaphragm is elevated entirely, including the posterior take-off point; this feature helps differentiate it from eventration. On fluoroscopic sniff test, if unilateral diaphragmatic weakness or paralysis is present, during quiet inspiration, deep inspiration, and sniffing, the weak side moves more slowly downward (caudal) or paradoxically upward (with paralysis).[9] The sniff test is not as useful in patients with bilateral paralysis. USG and dynamic MRI are other modalities to assess weakness or paralysis of diaphragm.

DIAPHRAGMATIC HERNIAS

Abdominal viscera can herniate into the thoracic cavity through the diaphragmatic hiatus (sliding and paraesophageal hiatus hernia) or congenital defect (Bochdalek and Morgagni hernia).

Hiatal Hernia

It develops from a weakness or tear (rupture) of the phrenicoesophageal ligament. Sliding hiatus hernias are the most common type (99%) of diaphragmatic hernias. In sliding hernia, the gastroesophageal junction lies above the esophageal hiatus, whereas in paraesophageal hernia, all or portion of the stomach herniates into the chest with gastroesophageal junction lying below the diaphragm. They can be diagnosed by barium examination, but cross-sectional imaging (CT, MRI) may show the size, site, and content of the hernia. A sliding hernia is diagnosed in barium study when the pouch of stomach protrudes >2 cm above the hiatus or three or more gastric folds pass across the hiatus and on CT when the hiatus is wide with diaphragmatic crura separated by >15 mm **(Fig. 11)**. In paraesophageal (rolling) hernia, the stomach herniates through widened esophageal hiatus or occasionally through the separate diaphragmatic gap to lie alongside the lower esophagus.

Between the 8th and 10th weeks of fetal life, the diaphragm forms and the pleuroperitoneal canals close, dividing the coelomic cavity into the abdominal and thoracic cavities. During the same period, the gastrointestinal tract elongates into the umbilical pouch and rotates on its return to the abdominal cavity. The left pleuroperitoneal canal

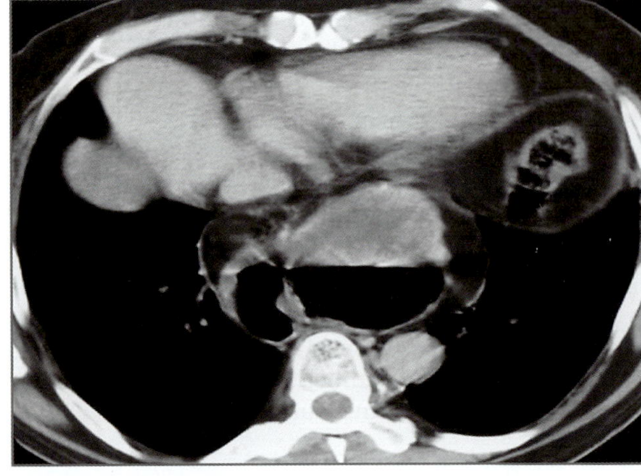

FIG. 11: Axial computed tomography (CT) scan of upper abdomen showing large hiatus hernia.

closes slightly later than the right. The interrelationship of these two important developmental events results in the clinical spectrum of diaphragmatic hernias: Bochdalek hernia (posterolateral defect), Morgagni hernia (retrosternal defect), and intrapericardial hernia (defect of the central tendon).

Bochdalek Hernia

It is the most common congenital hernia and involves the posterior defects in the diaphragm caused by defective fusion or maldevelopment of the pleuroperitoneal membranes. Stomach, bowel, and even spleen or kidney may herniate into the left hemithorax. On the right side, part of the liver may be found above the diaphragm. Bochdalek hernia occurs in one in 2,000–5,000 births with involvement of left hemidiaphragm in 80% of the cases.[10,11] The chest radiograph may show aerated intrathoracic bowel loops and a shift of mediastinum to the opposite side **(Figs. 12 and 13)**. On CT, Bochdalek hernia often presents as fatty or soft-tissue density mass, which abuts the posteromedial aspect of either side of diaphragm. With the advent of CT, however, many small asymptomatic defects are being detected in adults. On the lateral chest radiograph, these hernias are seen as a smooth bulge with an epicenter approximately 4–5 cm anterior to posterior costophrenic angle. Antenatal diagnosis of congenital diaphragmatic hernia on ultrasound is suspected when the fetal heart is displaced either by an intrathoracic solid mass (liver, kidney) or by a fluid-filled structure (stomach, bowel) with decreased abdominal circumference **(Fig. 14)**.[10,11] MRI can also be extremely helpful modality to look for congenital diaphragmatic hernia **(Fig. 15)**. Pulmonary hypoplasia often results from compression of the fetal lung by the herniated viscera.

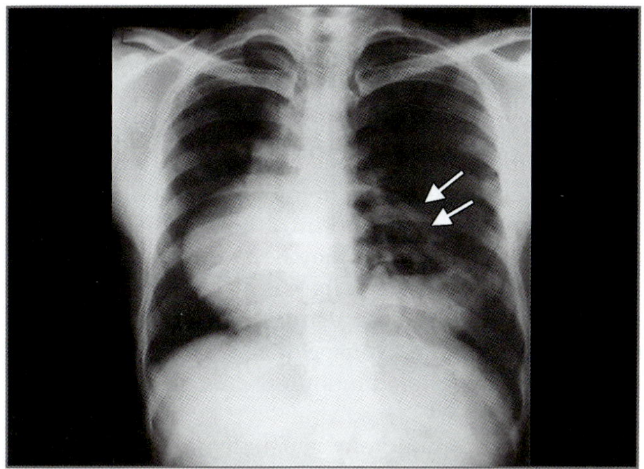

FIG. 12: Bochdalek hernia: Plain radiograph shows herniated bowel loops (white arrows) into the thorax and right mediastinal shift.

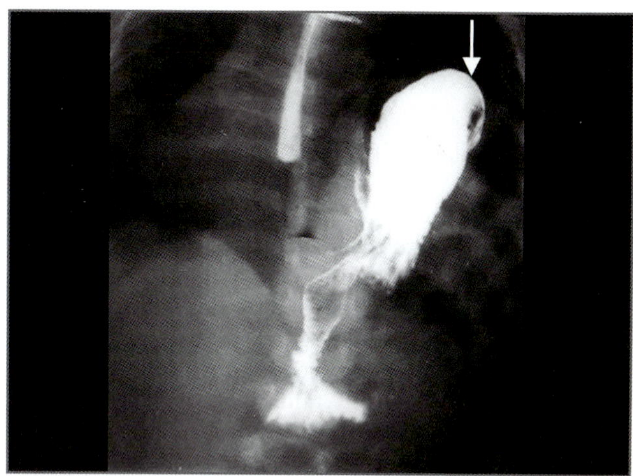

FIG. 13: Bochdalek hernia: Barium study showing herniation of stomach (white arrow) into thorax.

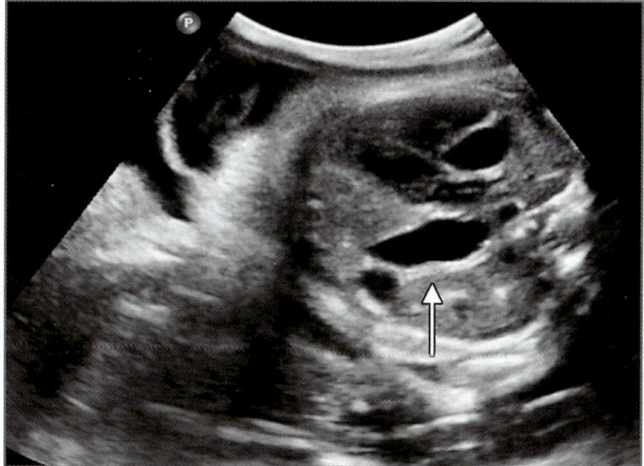

FIG. 14: Congenital diaphragmatic hernia: Antenatal ultrasound showing intrathoracic herniation of stomach (white arrow).

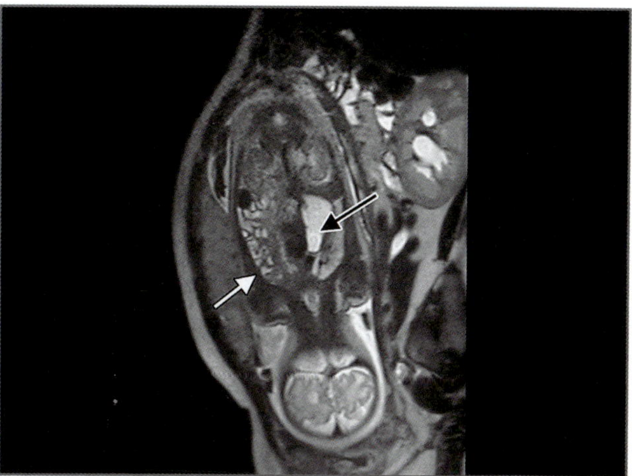

FIG. 15: Bilateral congenital diaphragmatic hernia: Antenatal T2-weighted magnetic resonance (MR) image showing bilateral diaphragmatic hernia with intrathoracic herniation of stomach (black arrow) and bowel loops (white arrow).

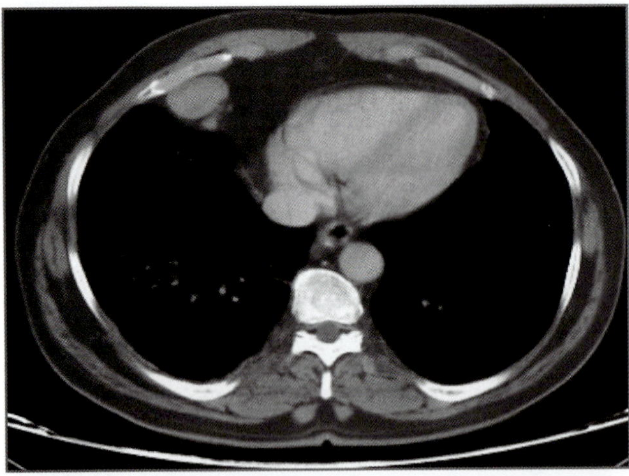

FIG. 16: Morgagni hernia: Axial computed tomography (CT) scan of the abdomen showing fatty lesion with traversing vessels in right paracardiac region.

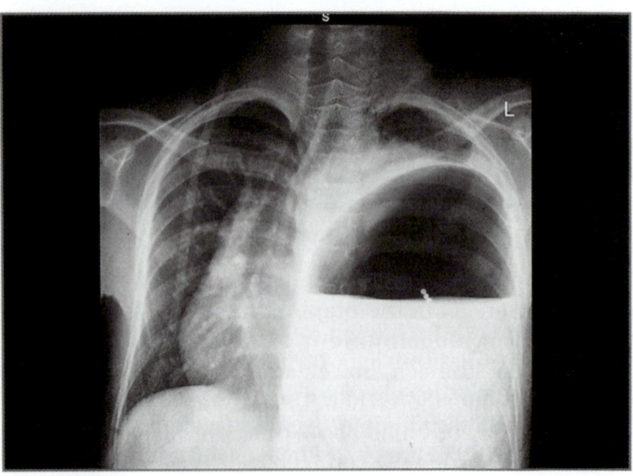

FIG. 17: Chest radiograph with left diaphragm tear showing intrathoracic herniation of the stomach with contralateral mediastinal shift.

Morgagni Hernia

It is commonly seen in adults and is mostly asymptomatic. It is due to the failure of fusion between the fibrotendinous elements of the sternal part and costal part of the developing diaphragm. In Morgagni hernia, peritoneum or abdominal contents pass upward through the foramen of Morgagni in retro- or parasternal location into the thoracic cavity. In Morgagni hernia, a weak area is congenital; however, the herniation of the abdominal contents is often acquired and conditions causing increased intra-abdominal pressure such as severe effort, obesity, and trauma. Morgagni hernia is mostly right-sided because the left-sided defects are covered by heart and pericardium. On the chest radiograph, a Morgagni hernia containing fat or liver presents as a rounded density occupying the right anterior cardiophrenic angle. Herniated organs and diaphragm defects are better evaluated by CT **(Fig. 16)** and MRI.

Intrapericardial Hernia

It results from herniation of abdominal viscera into the pericardial sac through a defect of the central tendon of the diaphragm but is extremely rare.

DIAPHRAGMATIC INJURY

Both blunt and penetrating injuries can injure diaphragm. Diaphragmatic injuries are usually caused by blunt trauma or penetrating injuries. They occur in 0.8–8% after blunt trauma.[12] The confusing clinical and radiographic findings can delay the diagnosis. Tear is left-sided in 70–90% and right-sided in 10–30% of blunt trauma patients. This is attributed to the protection offered by the liver. The stomach is the most commonly herniated organ, but bowel, spleen, liver, and omentum can also herniate into the chest **(Fig. 17)**. The chest X-ray remains valuable in the acute phase for the detection of diaphragmatic injuries, despite its technical limitations, which include supine positioning, use of portable radiography, and limited patient cooperation. Specific diagnostic findings of the injury include the following: asymmetry of a hemidiaphragm or changing hemidiaphragm levels and intrathoracic herniation of the hollow viscus, which may be associated with focal constriction of the viscus at the site of the tear called collar sign. On the left side, nasogastric tube may be seen above the hemidiaphragm.[6] Nonspecific X-ray findings are rib fractures, hemo- or pneumothorax, and atelectasis at the lung bases.

Computed tomography is usually the next imaging modality in trauma patients because of speed and global information provided. MDCT with multiplanar reconstructions is a very valuable diagnostic tool. MDCT features of the diaphragmatic trauma include direct visualization of injury, diaphragm thickening, segmental diaphragm, nonvisualization, viscera herniation **(Figs. 18A and B)**, dependent viscera sign, collar sign, and peridiaphragmatic active contrast extravasation.[12,13] Direct visualization of injury is often possible by depicting the free edge of the disrupted diaphragm. Isolated segmental nonvisualization of the diaphragm is highly sensitive, but this sign must be used with caution when seen in isolation, especially in the elderly, in whom it can be a normal variant. Intrathoracic herniation of viscera has high specificity but has variable sensitivity. If an abdominal structure herniates through a diaphragm rent, the free edges of the diaphragm can constrict the herniated organ and, hence, result in a "collar." The *collar sign* **(Figs. 18A and B)** is an indication of intrathoracic herniation of abdominal contents even when its relative level does not clearly suggest so. When the diaphragm is torn, its constraints are released, and the viscera may lie "dependent" against the posterior chest wall compared to the normal intact diaphragm, which

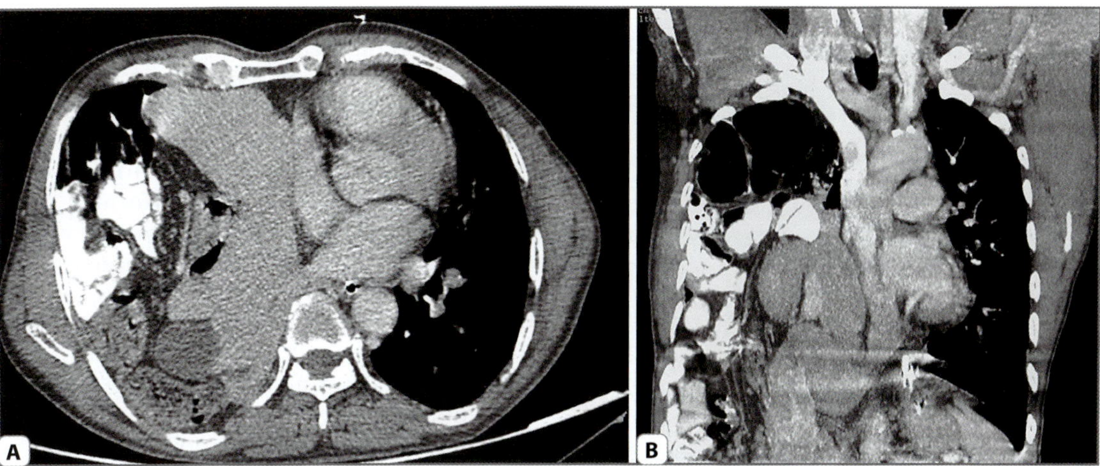

FIGS. 18A AND B: Traumatic right diaphragmatic hernia. (A) Axial and (B) coronal contrast-enhanced computed tomography (CECT) sections show right diaphragmatic hernia with herniation of both hollow and solid viscera.

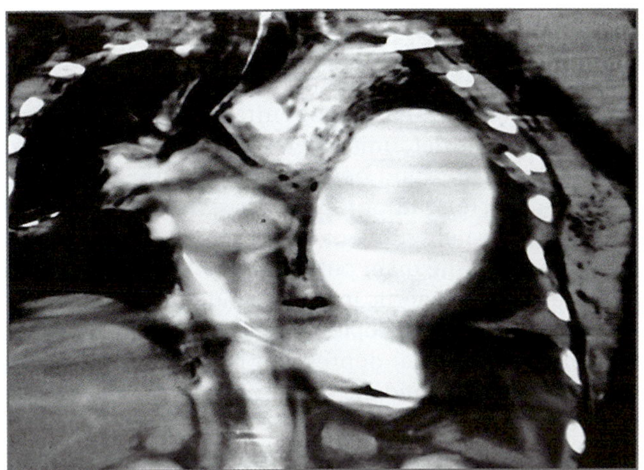

FIG. 19: Collar sign: Multidetector computed tomography (MDCT) with coronal reformation showing intrathoracic herniation of stomach through left diaphragmatic defect with constriction of stomach by the free edges of diaphragm at the site of herniation.

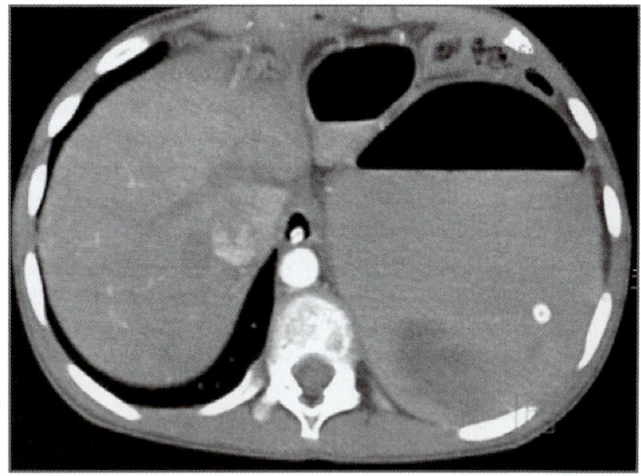

FIG. 20: Dependent viscera sign: Computed tomography (CT) axial sections showing intrathoracic herniation of the stomach through left diaphragmatic rupture and the stomach lying in a dependent position against the posterior ribs.

prevents the upper abdominal viscera from contacting the chest wall **(Fig. 19)**. The diaphragm is considered abnormally thickened by subjective comparison, with the contralateral side or diaphragmatic crus thickness >10 mm. In the presence of injury, intramuscular hematoma, edema, or muscle retraction accounts for the abnormally thick diaphragm.

Magnetic resonance imaging is helpful in equivocal cases of diaphragmatic injury. Direct coronal and sagittal imaging with respiratory and cardiac gating may allow confirmation or exclusion of the diagnosis. Diaphragmatic signal may be interrupted due to the laceration; hence, it confirms a traumatic diaphragmatic injury.[13] Barium studies allow confirmation of herniated intestine or stomach but are limited to evaluation of the hollow viscera. Fluoroscopic demonstration of severely decreased motion is highly suggestive but not diagnostic of injury. USG signs include herniation of viscera, diaphragm disruption, diaphragm nonvisualization, and absent diaphragm excursion during the respiratory cycle **(Fig. 20)**.

TUMORS OF THE DIAPHRAGM

Tumors of the diaphragm are rare. The most common benign solid tumor is a lipoma **(Fig. 21)**. Benign tumors of the diaphragm may be removed surgically if there is a doubt about the diagnosis or if they are symptomatic. Fibroma, angiofibroma, neurofibroma, and neurilemoma are the other benign tumors. The most common primary malignant tumor of diaphragm is rhabdomyosarcoma.[14] Metastatic neoplasms of the diaphragm may be due to direct invasion

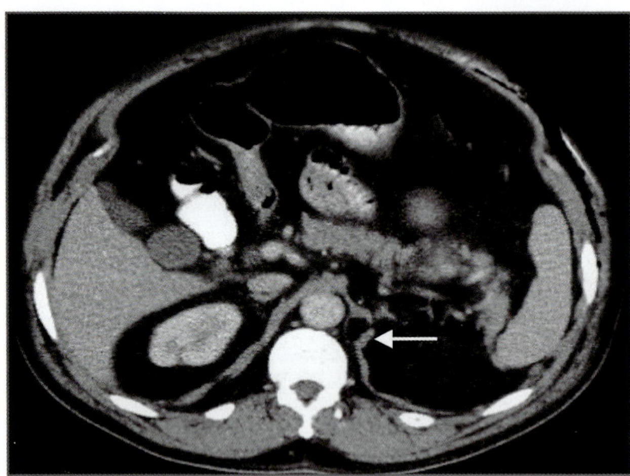

FIG. 21: Lipoma: Computed tomography (CT) axial sections showing well-marginated fat-density lesion in the left crus of the diaphragm (white arrow).

from tumors of adjacent organs. These include tumors of the lung, liver, stomach, colon, pancreas, adrenal, or liver. Cystic lesions of the diaphragm can be acquired or congenital. The most common benign cystic lesions of the diaphragm are bronchogenic or mesothelial cysts.[14] Acquired cysts include simple, fibrous-lined, and post-traumatic cysts. Hydatid disease and tuberculosis rarely cause inflammatory mass of the diaphragm. The majority of patients present with pleuritic chest pain. Radiographically, a mass that abuts the diaphragm is seen. Imaging modalities such as CT and MRI provide a specific diagnosis and look for the extent of the tumor.

CHEST WALL

The chest wall structures are grouped into soft tissue and bony structures on the basis of their radiographic appearances. The soft-tissue structures include muscles of the chest wall, breasts, fat, nerves, blood, and lymphatic vessels. The bony structures include ribs, costal cartilages, sternum, clavicles, and spine. Chest wall may be affected by a variety of disorders affecting these constituents. Chest radiography may be the first imaging study to suggest the presence of a chest wall mass, given its widespread availability and utilization. However, it is difficult to detect, localize, and characterize these disorders by means of conventional radiography alone most of the time, and cross-sectional imaging such as MDCT and MRI helps in the evaluation of these disorders and sometimes allows definitive diagnosis.[15] MDCT and MRI help in knowing the extent and character of the diseases. CT helps in better depiction of small calcifications and bone destruction, whereas MRI helps in marrow involvement and soft-tissue extension. Multiplanar imaging and three-dimensional (3D) reconstructions can be achieved with both modalities. Ultrasound generally provides less detailed information compared to CT and MRI; however, it can be very helpful at times in localizing the lesion. It also helps in differentiating cystic and solid lesions and can characterize cystic lesions. It also provides imaging guidance for aspiration and biopsy when cytological/histopathological diagnosis is required. 2-[fluorine-18] fluoro-2-deoxy-d-glucose (FDG) positron emission tomography (PET)/CT is not performed commonly to evaluate chest wall tumors because many primary and secondary malignancies may demonstrate increased FDG uptake. PET/CT may be used, however, to determine the presence and extent of metastatic disease and assess response to therapy.[16]

Diseases affecting chest wall can be grouped into congenital and developmental anomalies, inflammatory and infectious diseases, and various primary and secondary tumors.[15]

Congenital and Developmental Anomalies

Funnel Chest (Pectus Excavatum or Depressed Sternum)

It is the most common congenital anomaly affecting sternum. In this deformity, sternum is depressed and on each side, ribs extend beyond the sternum anteriorly. Posteroanterior radiograph shows shift of the heart to the left, straightening of the left heart border with a prominence of the main pulmonary artery segment, loss of the descending aortic interface, and an increase in the opacity in the right cardiophrenic angle **(Figs. 22A and B)**.[15] The extent of sternal depression is evaluated easily at lateral radiograph, and the severity can be best quantified with CT. MDCT is usually reserved for the individuals in whom surgery is planned. Severity may be graded using the Haller index. Haller index is a ratio of the maximum internal transverse diameter of the chest divided by the minimum anteroposterior diameter. An index of >3.25 requires correction surgically. Haller index ranges from 1.9 to 2.7 in normal children.[17]

Pigeon Chest (Pectus Carinatum)

It is less common than pectus excavatum. It may be congenital or acquired. In this condition, there is a convex anterior protrusion of the sternum and costochondral joints and results due to disproportionate overgrowth of the costochondral cartilages. It is considered a cosmetic deformity only and may be associated with family history, connective tissue disease, and scoliosis.[18]

Poland Syndrome

In Poland syndrome, there is partial or total absence of pectoralis major muscles with ipsilateral hand and arm anomalies (particularly syndactyly). Radiograph shows an area of hyperlucency on the affected side and an abnormal axillary fold. CT and MRI show the absence of muscles and associated anomalies.[15]

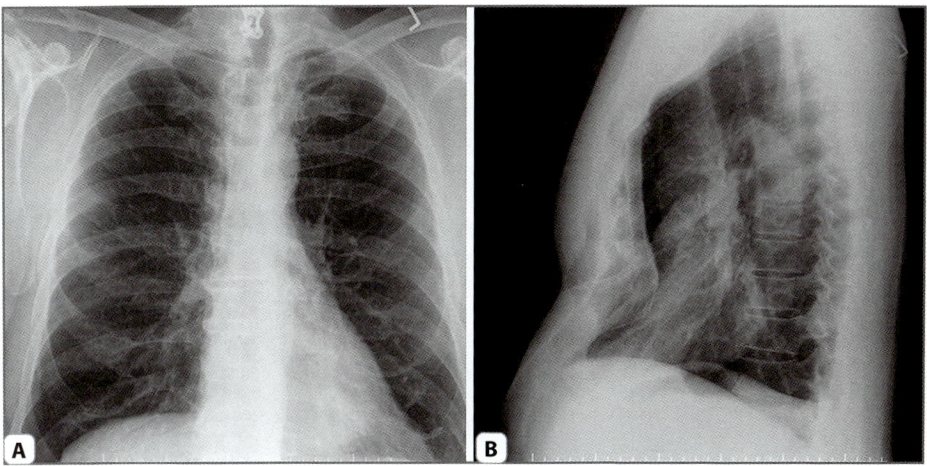

FIGS. 22A AND B: Pectus excavatum. (A) Posteroanterior and (B) lateral chest radiographs showing leftward displacement of the heart and straightening of the left heart border with severe depression of the sternum.

Cervical Rib

Cervical rib commonly originates from the 7th cervical vertebra. It is found in approximately 0.5% of the general population. In 90% of the cases, it is asymptomatic. It is seen as supernumerary rib that articulates with cervical-type transverse process, which is horizontal compared to upward-sloping thoracic transverse process of thoracic vertebra. MDCT helps in showing the relationship between vascular compression and bony deformity.

Clavicles

These may be hypoplastic in a number of syndromes, including cleidocranial dysplasia, Holt–Oram syndrome, pelvic–shoulder dysplasia, some trisomy disorders, and progeria.

Inflammatory and Infectious Diseases

Primary infections of the chest wall are rare and are more common in the setting of trauma, immunosuppression, and diabetes mellitus. They occur more commonly secondary to infectious processes in the lungs or pleural empyema (empyema necessitatis). Other causes are hematogenous spread or iatrogenic (median sternotomy for cardiac surgery).

Cellulitis and Necrotizing Fasciitis

Infections of chest wall soft tissues range from cellulitis to infections of deeper soft tissues, including myositis, osteomyelitis, abscess, and necrotizing fasciitis. Cellulitis often appears more extensive on MRI than on other imaging modalities because of MR imaging's sensitivity to tissue edema. Cellulitis is characterized by a high T2 signal in subcutaneous soft tissues.[19] Necrotizing fasciitis is a serious septic condition more common in immunocompromised, alcoholic, or diabetic patients. It affects subcutaneous fat and the superficial fascia and should not involve the underlying muscles. MRI shows the complete extent of the involvement, and CT may show gas formation. In pyomyositis, predominant involvement is of muscles, and MRI is the best imaging modality to assess intramuscular necrosis.

Pyogenic Osteomyelitis

Osteomyelitis of the chest wall is frequently associated with periosteal elevation, loss of planes of soft tissue, and adjacent soft-tissue masses. Common causative organisms are *Staphylococcus aureus* and *Pseudomonas aeruginosa*. CT and MRI can clearly depict the abnormality **(Figs. 23A and B)**. Median sternotomy is the main surgical approach to a variety of cardiothoracic procedures. Poststernotomy complications can occur in <5% of the cases and include sternal dehiscence, mediastinitis, and osteomyelitis. They manifest usually 1–2 weeks after surgery. CT is a useful modality for detecting and localizing retrosternal abscesses. Acute mediastinitis at CT shows inflammatory tissue replacing mediastinal fat.

Tuberculosis

Chest wall involvement in tuberculosis is commonly due to hematogenous route; however, it may occur as contiguous spread from underlying pleural or pulmonary involvement. It presents as the destruction of bone and/or cartilage with associated soft-tissue mass **(Figs. 24A and B)**, which may show rim enhancement and calcifications.

Fungal Infections

Actinomycosis and aspergillosis may infect the chest wall. Actinomycosis may present as sinuses, massive thickening of the soft tissue, wavy periostitis, and underlying rib destruction. Aspergillosis involving the chest wall is associated with pulmonary involvement and causes permeative osteolytic destruction of underlying ribs.[15]

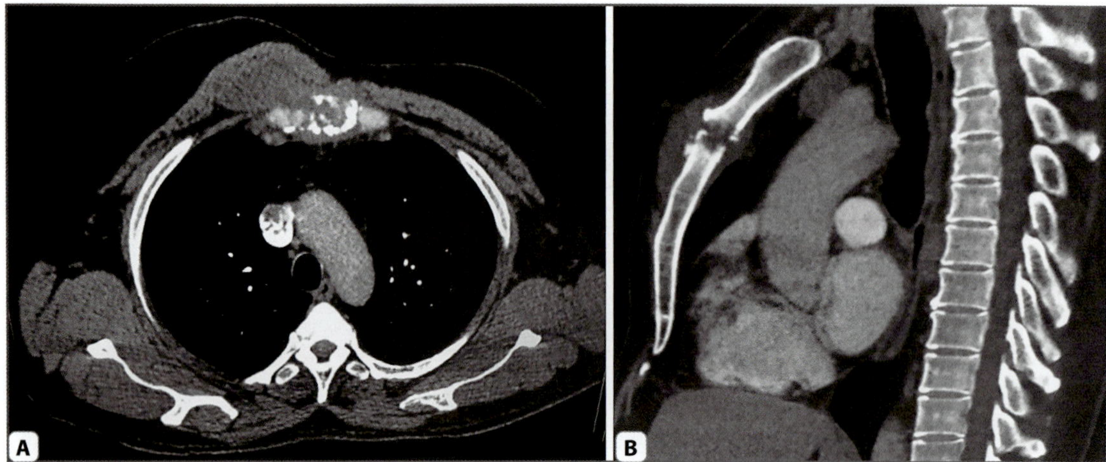

FIGS. 23A AND B: Sternal osteomyelitis. (A) Axial and (B) sagittal multidetector computed tomography (MDCT) showing expansile lytic destruction of sternum with associated soft tissue extending both anterior and posterior to sternum.

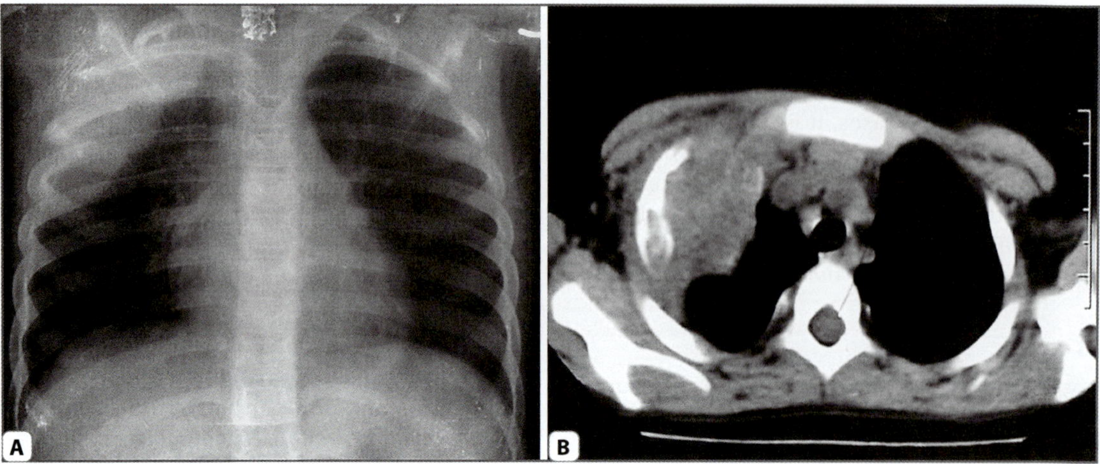

FIGS. 24A AND B: Chest wall tuberculosis. (A) Chest radiograph shows large right upper chest wall soft tissue with destruction of ribs. (B) Computed tomography (CT) shows expansion and destruction of rib with associated soft tissue. Aspiration from the soft tissue confirmed the lesion to be tubercular.

TUMORS OF THE CHEST WALL

Chest wall tumors represent approximately 5% of thoracic tumors.[20] These tumors are typically divided into categories based on the site of origin and tissue composition (osseous or soft tissue) as well as whether they are benign or malignant.[16,21] Greater than 50% of chest wall tumors are malignant, and most of these malignancies represent direct invasion by metastasis from adjacent tumors of the lung, breast, pleura, and mediastinum. The most common primary malignancies of the chest wall are sarcomas, 45% of which arise from soft tissue and 55% of which arise from bone. Once a chest wall mass has been identified, the next step is to determine whether it is malignant or benign. A large soft-tissue mass with invasion into adjacent osseous and/or soft-tissue structures is nearly always malignant. Primary chondrosarcoma or osteosarcoma as well as their metastasis will show characteristic mineralization patterns.[16] Benign osseous neoplasms do not result in extraosseous soft-tissue masses unlike their malignant counterpart and mostly exhibit nonaggressive radiological features.

Benign Osseous Tumors

Benign osseous tumors of the chest wall are less frequently encountered than malignant neoplasms. Most of these lesions are osseous or cartilaginous. *Fibrous dysplasia* presents as fusiform enlargement with cortical thickening and increased trabeculation of involved bones. The ribs are commonly affected, followed by clavicle. This lesion appears lytic or mixed lesion with lytic regions and ground-glass matrix. Osseous erosion is generally not seen.

Osteochondroma

These tumors arise as aberrant growth of normal tissue. These tumors frequently involve costochondral junction of

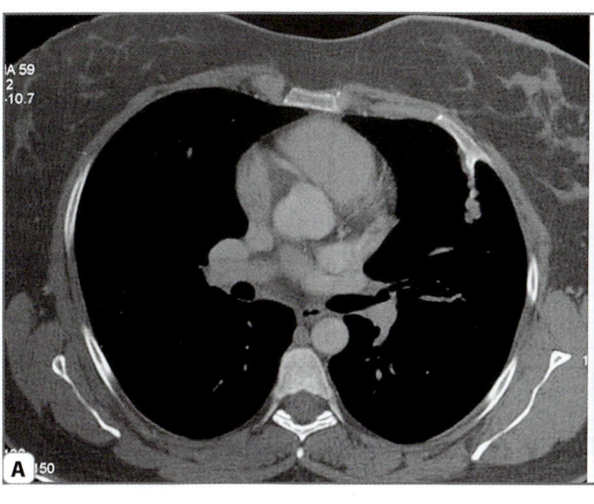

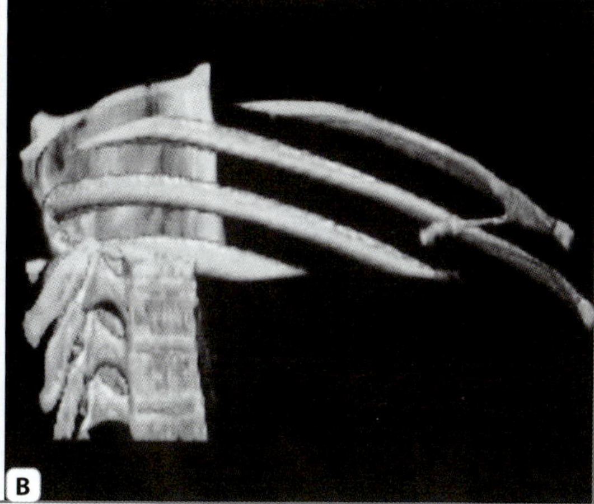

FIGS. 25A AND B: Osteochondroma. (A) Chest CT and (B) 3D bony reformat showing prick-like inward projecting intrathoracic osteochondroma with thickened overlying pleura.

(CT: computed tomography; 3D: three-dimensional)

the ribs. Osteochondromas are pedunculated lesions arising from the surface of the bone **(Figs. 25A and B)**. Evaluation of the associated cartilaginous cap should be carefully evaluated, as caps measuring >3 cm in children and >2 cm in adults raise suspicion for malignant transformation.[22]

Aneurysmal Bone Cyst and Giant Cell Tumor

These may involve a chest wall. In aneurysmal bone cyst (ABC), the most common sites of involvement are posterior elements of the spine, whereas giant cell tumor involves sternum, clavicle, and ribs.

Malignant Osseous Tumors

Malignant osseous tumors of the chest wall account for approximately 55% of all chest wall masses.[20] The most common primary malignancies include sarcomas, such as chondrosarcoma, osteosarcoma, Ewing sarcoma family of tumors (ESFT), as well as multiple myeloma (MM), whereas metastatic disease and direct invasion from intrathoracic malignancies are the most frequent secondary causes.[21]

Chondrosarcomas

Chondrosarcoma is the most common malignant primary tumor of the chest wall. It frequently involves anterior chest wall originating from the costochondral arches or sternum **(Fig. 26)**.[23] Most (90%) of the tumors occur in the ribs, commonly along the upper five, adjacent to costal cartilage. These are primary lesions most of the time; however, approximately 10% arise from benign tumors, which were preexistent. On the chest radiograph, bony destruction, irregular contours, and intratumoral mineralization are present. CT demonstrates well-defined, calcified soft-tissue masses with associated bony changes. MRI also shows characteristic features. On T1-weighted imaging, signal intensity of the lesion matches that of muscle signal intensity and on T2-weighted imaging, it

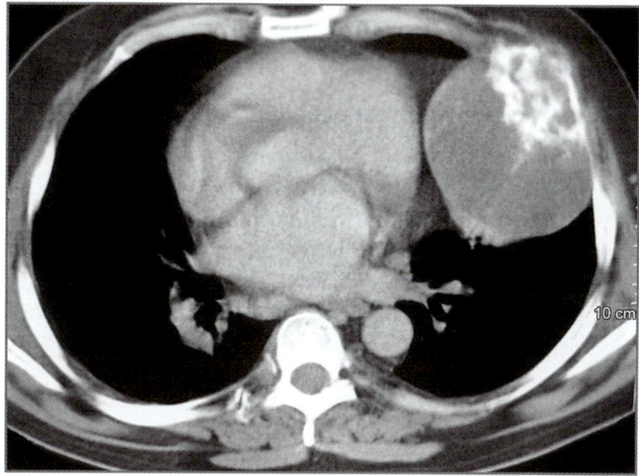

FIG. 26: Chondrosarcoma: Chest computed tomography (CT) showing large expansile mass arising from the rib with matrix calcification and large associated soft tissue.

is equal to or greater than that of fat and shows heterogeneous enhancement postcontrast.

Osteosarcoma

Osteosarcomas account for 10–15% of malignant chest wall tumors.[23] When osteosarcomas arise in a primary fashion from the chest wall, the most frequently affected structures include the ribs, clavicle, and scapula.[23] On T1-weighted images, the nonmineralized regions of osteosarcomas demonstrate variable signal intensity but are often hyperintense to muscle. On T2-weighted images, the nonmineralized regions demonstrate high signal intensity. Tumor mineralization is usually hypointense on both T1- and T2-weighted imaging. Heterogeneous enhancement after the administration of intravenous (IV) contrast is typical.[21]

Ewing Sarcoma

Ewing sarcoma of the chest wall presents either as a solitary mass or as multiple masses with an eccentric growth pattern. Ewing sarcoma can arise from rib, scapula, clavicle, or sternum but may originate from extraskeletal site.[23] These lesions commonly displace adjacent soft-tissue structures instead of encasement or invasion. They may arise in paravertebral region and extend through the vertebral foramina. CT scans show a large ill-defined mass with an inhomogeneous enhancement caused by cystic degeneration. Mass lesions may be accompanied by calcification **(Fig. 27)**. These tumors generally have signal intensity equal to or greater than that of muscle on T1, inhomogeneous high signal intensity on T2-weighted MR images, and show marked enhancement. Small lesions are homogeneous, whereas large lesions have heterogeneous appearance with areas of necrosis and hemorrhage.

Multiple Myeloma

It may involve the vertebral column, ribs, or clavicles and causes multiple osteolytic lesions with discrete margins. At MRI, lesions have low signal intensity on T1-weighted images and T2-weighted images have high signal intensity.

Soft-tissue Tumors

Malignant and benign soft-tissue tumors of the chest wall are a heterogeneous group and can be divided into the following groups based on the tissue of origin: adipocytic, vascular, peripheral nerve sheath, fibroblastic and myofibroblastic, fibrohistiocytic, and cutaneous.[24]

Adipocytic: Lipoma

Lipomas are the most common soft-tissue tumors and present as encapsulated masses composed of adipocytes that are similar to normal fatty tissue found within the chest wall. Lipoma has fat attenuation on MDCT, high signal intensity at T1-weighted imaging, and uniform signal loss at fat-suppressed MRI. Internal septations may be present and appear hypointense on T1-weighted images. After the administration of IV contrast, lipomas do not enhance, although internal septations may enhance when present.[24,25]

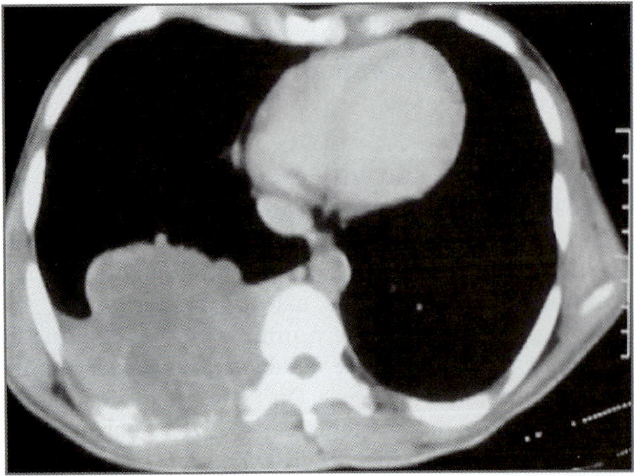

FIG. 27: Ewing sarcoma: Axial computed tomography (CT) sections showing large heterogeneous chest wall lesion with erosion destruction of the posterior rib.

Adipocytic: Liposarcoma

Liposarcomas are the second most common chest wall malignancy of soft-tissue origin. These tumors constitute approximately 15% of all sarcomas, although only 10% involve the chest wall.[23] Well-differentiated liposarcomas are typically composed of 50–75% adipose tissue, which results in high signal intensity on T1-weighted images and low signal intensity on T2-weighted images. Depending on the volume of fat, it may be difficult to distinguish well-differentiated liposarcoma from lipoma. Features that suggest diagnosis of well-differentiated liposarcoma are large tumors (size > 10 cm), thick internal septations, nodular regions of nonadipose tissue, and adipose tissue comprising <75% of the tumor.[26]

Vascular: Hemangioma and Angiosarcoma

Hemangiomas have high signal intensity at T2-weighted imaging, demonstrate variable amounts of internal fat at MDCT and T1-weighted MRI, and frequently contain phleboliths **(Figs. 28A to C)**.[16] In contrast, angiosarcoma is heterogeneous, lacks internal fat, is aggressive, and invades adjacent structures. These tumors may be associated with chronic lymphedema and may exhibit findings related to their origin (such as fibrous thickening, soft-tissue nodules, and fluid collections) adjacent to the chest wall musculature.[23]

Peripheral Nerve Sheath Tumors

Benign nerve sheath neoplasms such as neurofibroma and schwannoma appear as low-attenuating soft-tissue masses, which contain fat or cystic components. The "target" sign, which is characterized by central low signal intensity and peripheral high signal intensity on T2-weighted MR images and central enhancement following the IV administration of gadolinium-based contrast material, and the fascicular sign, characterized by heterogeneous low signal intensity with a ring-like pattern on T2-weighted MR images, are frequently visualized.[16] The "split fat" sign, characterized by fat attenuation around the soft-tissue mass at MDCT, also may be seen. These radiologic signs are typically absent in malignant peripheral nerve sheath tumors, which, when compared with benign nerve sheath neoplasms, demonstrate greater heterogeneity and aggressive behavior and invasion into surrounding structures.[23]

Fibroblastic and Myofibroblastic

Fibromatosis, also known as desmoid tumor, has been reported to primarily arise from the chest wall in 10–28%

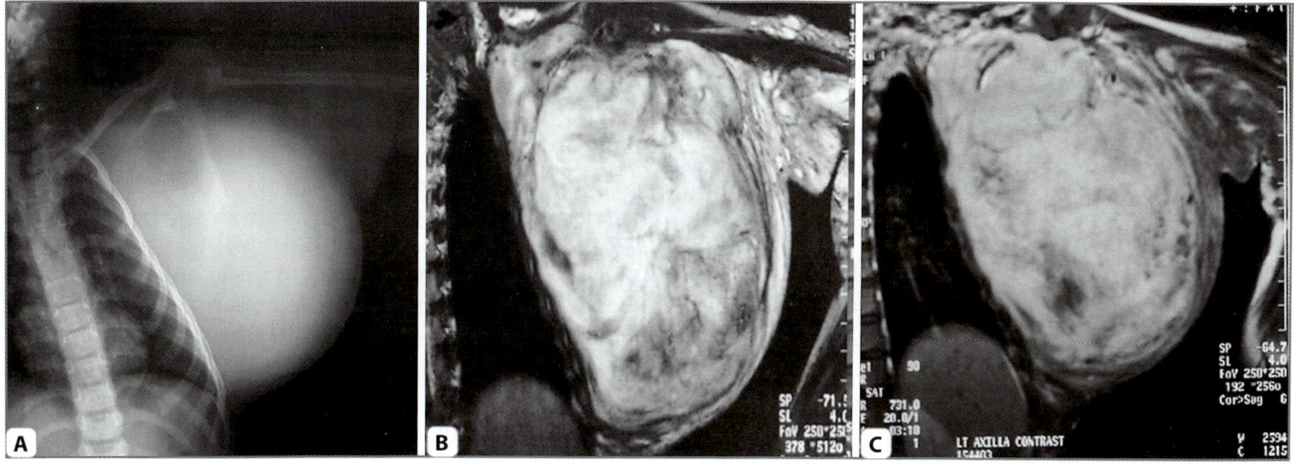

FIGS. 28A TO C: Child with large chest wall hemangioma. (A) Chest radiograph showing large well-circumscribed homogeneous soft-tissue mass along lateral chest wall. (B) Coronal T2 and (C) postcontrast images showing heterogeneously enhancing chest wall lesion.

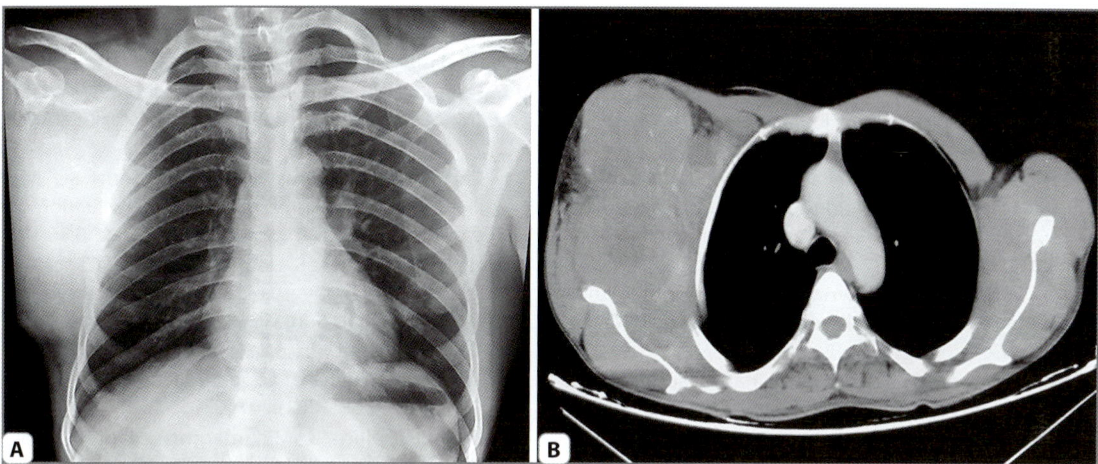

FIGS. 29A AND B: Undifferentiated pleomorphic sarcoma. (A) Chest radiograph showing large well-defined homogeneous mass along the right upper chest wall with no erosion or destruction of underlying bones. (B) Contrast-enhanced computed tomography (CECT) of the chest shows large heterogeneous soft-tissue mass anterior to scapula with no bony involvement.

of cases.[23] Fibromatosis typically manifests as an ill-defined mass that grows in an infiltrative manner. On MRI, lesions have relatively homogeneous low to intermediate signal intensity on T1-weighted images, whereas they appear more heterogeneous on T2-weighted images; low signal intensity bands have been reported in fibromatosis and likely represent dense collagen bundles. Although fibromatosis may demonstrate moderate to marked heterogeneous enhancement, the collagen bundles do not enhance.[21]

Fibrohistiocytic

Undifferentiated pleomorphic sarcoma (UPS), also called malignant fibrous histiocytoma, is classified as a fibrohistiocytic malignancy and represents the most common malignant soft-tissue neoplasm of the chest wall in adults.[26] At MDCT, UPS appears as a soft-tissue mass that involves the deep fascia or skeletal muscle and enhances heterogeneously after IV contrast material administration **(Figs. 29A and B)**. Involvement of adjacent osseous structures is common. Internal mineralization can often be identified in the peripheral aspect of the lesion after treatment. UPS demonstrates low signal intensity and isointense to muscle on T1-weighted MR images. On T2-weighted images, UPS has intermediate-to-high signal intensity and is iso- to hyperintense to fat.

Metastatic Disease

Osseous metastatic disease affecting the chest wall is typically encountered in the setting of extensive metastatic disease elsewhere in the body, but it may be seen early in association with aggressive primary malignancies. These lesions can manifest in many different ways, with some metastases demonstrating imaging characteristics specific to the primary malignancies from which they are derived. Soft-tissue metastatic disease is typically seen only in the setting of extensive metastatic disease elsewhere in the body and is considered an indicator of a poor prognosis.[16]

CHEST WALL INVASION BY THORACIC MALIGNANCY

The chest wall may be directly invaded by aggressive thoracic malignancies—typically lung cancer, breast cancer, pleural tumors, or mediastinal neoplasms. Although MRI and MDCT have been shown to have similar utility in detecting chest wall invasion by lung cancer, MRI is considered to be superior due to better spatial resolution and soft-tissue contrast.[16]

CONCLUSION

Combination of different imaging modalities is needed to evaluate diaphragm and chest wall lesions. Relevant clinical history and comparison with previous imaging studies is very helpful. Chest radiographs and ultrasound are initial modalities, however, MDCT with multiplanar reconstructions and MRI would be needed for characterization and evaluating anatomical extent of various pathologies.

REFERENCES

1. Nason LK, Walker CM, McNeeley MF, Burivong W, Fligner CL, Godwin JD. Imaging of the diaphragm: anatomy and function. Radiographics. 2012;32:E51-70.
2. Felson B. Chest Roentgenology. Philadelphia: WB Saunders; 1973.
3. Adam A, Dixon AK, Gillard JH, Schaefer-Prokop CM. Grainger and Allison's Diagnostic Radiology: A Textbook of Medical Imaging, 6th edition. United Kingdom: Churchill Livingstone/Elsevier; 2014.
4. Sarwal A, Walker FO, Cartwright MS. Neuromuscular ultrasound for evaluation of the diaphragm. Muscle Nerve. 2013;47:319-29.
5. Shackleton KL, Stewart ET, Taylor AJ. Traumatic diaphragmatic injuries: spectrum of radiographic findings. Radiographics. 1998;18:49-59.
6. Gierada DS, Curtin JJ, Erickson SJ, Prost RW, Strandt JA, Goodman LR. Diaphragmatic motion: fast gradient-recalled-echo MR imaging in healthy subjects. Radiology. 1995;194:879-84.
7. Kiryu S, Loring SH, Mori Y, Rofsky NM, Hatabu H, Takahashi M. Quantitative analysis of the velocity and synchronicity of diaphragmatic motion: dynamic MRI in different postures. Magn Reson Imaging. 2006;24(10):1325-32.
8. May AK, Moore MM. Diagnosis of blunt rupture of the right hemidiaphragm by technetium scan. Am Surg. 1999;65:761-5.
9. Kharma N. Dysfunction of the diaphragm: imaging as a diagnostic tool. Curr Opin Pulm Med. 2013;19(4):394-8.
10. Panicek D, Benson C, Gottlieb R, Heitzman E. The diaphragm: anatomic, pathologic, and radiologic considerations. Radiographics. 1988;8(3):385-425.
11. Chavhan G, Babyn P, Cohen R, Langer J. Multimodality imaging of the pediatric diaphragm: anatomy and pathologic conditions. Radiographics. 2010;30(7):1797-818.
12. Iochum S, Ludwig T, Walter F, Sebbag H, Grosdidier G, Blum AG. Imaging of the diaphragmatic injury: a diagnostic challenge? Radiographics. 2002;22:S103-18.
13. Sliker CW. Imaging of diaphragmatic injuries. Radiol Clin North Am. 2006;44:199-211.
14. Kim MP, Hofstetter WL. Tumors of the diaphragm. Thorac Surg Clin. 2009;19:521-9.
15. Jeung MY, Gangi A, Gasser B, Vasilescu C, Massard G, Wihlm JM, et al. Imaging of chest wall disorders. Radiographics. 1999;19:617-37.
16. Carter BW, Benveniste MF, Betancourt SL, de Groot PM, Lichtenberger JP, Amini B. Imaging evaluation of malignant chest wall neoplasms. Radiographics. 2016;36(5):1285-306.
17. Haller JA, Kramer SS, Lietman SA. Use of CT scans in selection of patients for pectus excavatum surgery: a preliminary report. J Pediatr Surg. 1987;22:904-6.
18. Mak SM, Bhaludin BN, Naaseri S, Di Chiara F, Jordan S, Padley S. Imaging of congenital chest wall deformities. Br J Radiol. 2016;89(1061):20150595.
19. Lee TJ, Collins J. MR imaging evaluation of disorders of the chest wall. Magn Reson Imaging Clin North Am. 2008;16(2):355-79.
20. Incarbone M, Pastorino U. Surgical treatment of chest wall tumors. World J Surg. 2001;25(2):218-30.
21. Carter BW, Gladish GW. MR imaging of chest wall tumors. Magn Reson Imaging Clin North Am. 2015;23(2):197-215.
22. Zarqane H, Viala P, Dallaudière B, Vernhet H, Cyteval C, Larbi A. Tumors of the rib. Diagn Interv Imaging. 2013;94(11):1095-108.
23. Tateishi U, Gladish GW, Kusumoto M, Hasegawa T, Yokoyama R, Tsuchiya R, et al. Chest wall tumors: radiologic findings and pathologic correlation part 2. Malignant tumors. Radiographics. 2003;23:1491-508.
24. Nam SJ, Kim S, Lim BJ, Yoon CS, Kim TH, Suh JS, et al. Imaging of primary chest wall tumors with radiologic-pathologic correlation. Radiographics. 2011;31(3):749-70.
25. O'Sullivan P, O'Dwyer H, Flint J, Munk PL, Muller N. Soft tissue tumors and mass-like lesions of the chest wall: a pictorial review of CT and MR findings. Br J Radiol. 2007;80(955):574-80.
26. Kransdorf MJ, Bancroft LW, Peterson JJ, Murphey MD, Foster WC, Temple HT. Imaging of fatty tumors: distinction of lipoma and well-differentiated liposarcoma. Radiology. 2002;224(1):99-104.

Rajendra Kumar Behera, Ashu Seith Bhalla,
Priyanka Naranje, Ankur Goyal

CHAPTER

20

Hemoptysis: Imaging Approach and Interventions

INTRODUCTION

Hemoptysis refers to expectoration of blood from the respiratory tract and is a potentially life-threatening emergency.[1,2] Lungs are supplied by two vascular systems; pulmonary arteries are involved in gas exchange, and bronchial arteries provide oxygenated blood for nourishment.[3] Latter is a high-pressure circulation and is responsible for clinically significant hemoptysis in most of cases.

Bronchial artery embolization (BAE) was first described by Rémy et al. in 1974 as a measure to control hemoptysis.[4] Since then, the technique of BAE has evolved significantly, and its clinical utility has increased manifold. The procedure may be more aptly called *systemic artery embolization* because in addition to the bronchial arteries, the hypertrophied nonbronchial systemic collaterals are also embolized to control hemoptysis. A broader term for *endovascular embolization* would include pulmonary arterial interventions such as *pulmonary artery pseudoaneurysm (PAP) and pulmonary arteriovenous malformation (PAVM) embolization* to control hemoptysis. It is important to note that embolization is a palliative procedure and unless the causative disease is addressed, hemoptysis may recur.

PATHOPHYSIOLOGY AND ETIOLOGY

In majority of cases of noncardiac hemoptysis, the source of bleeding is systemic circulation (bronchial arteries are more commonly responsible than nonbronchial collaterals). This is because the majority of the patients have chronic inflammatory lung disease. This leads to hypoxic vasoconstriction of the pulmonary arterioles in the areas of abnormality, which then incites hypertrophy of systemic arteries. These systemic arteries are recruited in order to participate in gas exchange through anastomoses with the pulmonary vascular system. The hypertrophic bronchial arteries are prone to rupture in the inflamed surroundings and since they are part of high-pressure systemic circulation, this results in clinically significant hemoptysis.

In about 5% of cases, the bleeding is from pulmonary vascular causes (pulmonary arteriovenous malformation, PAP, injury from Swan–Ganz catheter, etc.). Thus, most cases of significant hemoptysis result from systemic arterial source rather than pulmonary circulation.

The common causes of hemoptysis are shown in **Table 1**,[2,5-7] and **Figures 1A to J** show examples of some of

TABLE 1: Noncardiac causes of significant hemoptysis.

Post-tuberculosis (TB) sequelae: Fibrosis and bronchiectasis ~ 30%	*Neoplasms*: Carcinoma, carcinoid, and tracheobronchial lesions
Active TB: ~ 30%	*Vasculitis*: Granulomatosis with polyangiitis, Behçet's disease, and systemic lupus erythematosus (SLE)
Other inflammatory lung diseases: Bronchiectasis/bronchitis/aspergilloma/cystic fibrosis/sarcoidosis/hydatid cyst	*Vascular causes*: Vascular malformations and postbiopsy
Other lung infections: Nontubercular infections and lung abscess	*Miscellaneous*: Pneumoconiosis, chronic obstructive pulmonary disease, and cryptogenic hemoptysis

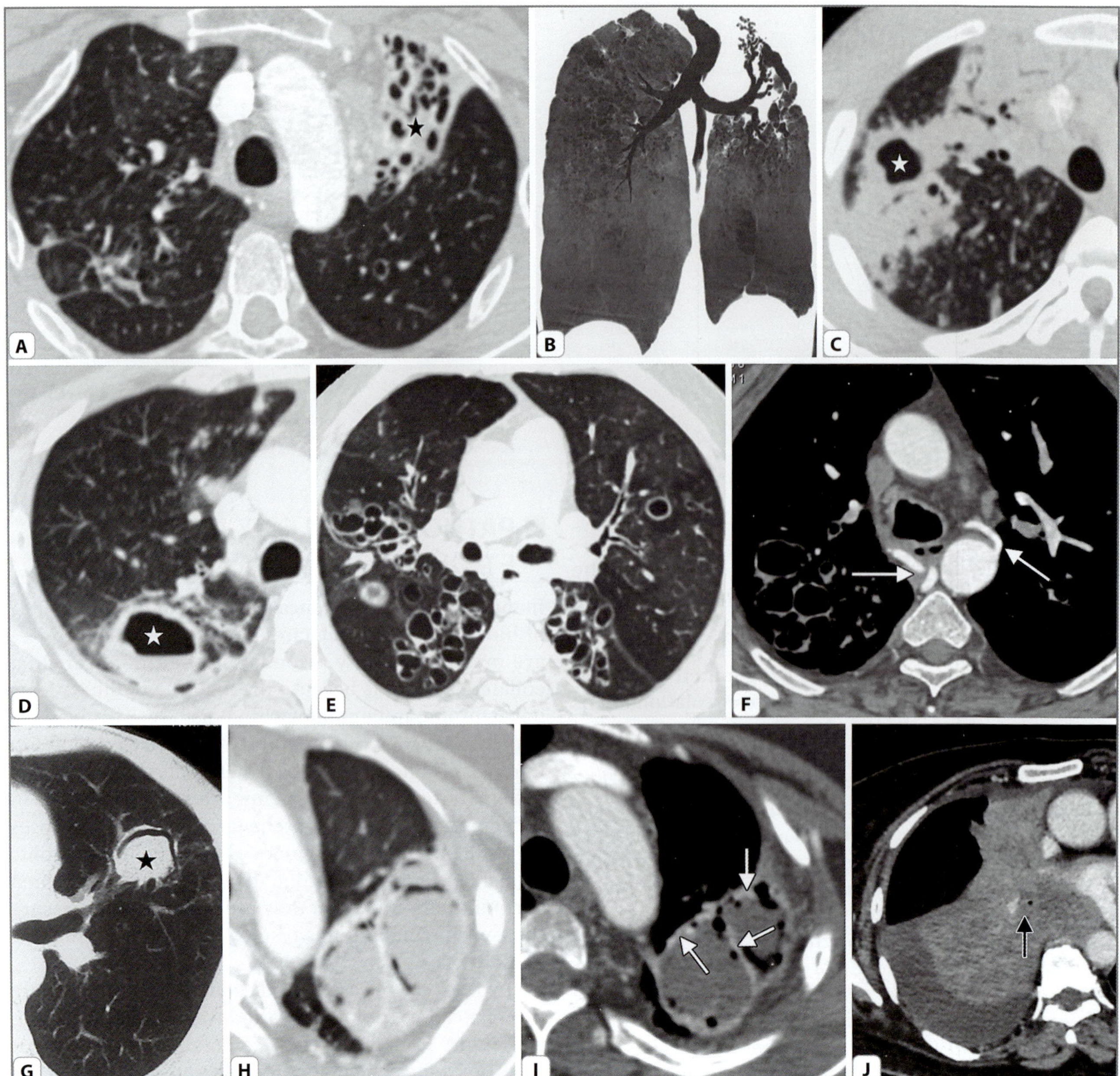

FIGS. 1A TO J: CT images showing common causes of hemoptysis. (A) TB sequelae [fibrobronchiectasis and collapse in the left upper lobe (star) and fibroparenchymal lesions in the right upper lobe]. (B) Coronal MinIP image showing upper lobe predominant post-TB fibrosis with bronchiectasis, volume loss, and cavitation of the left upper lobe. (C) Active TB [thick-walled cavity of the right upper lobe (star) with surrounding dense consolidation and centrilobular nodules]. (D) TB sequelae with superimposed pyogenic bacterial infection [cavity (star) with air-fluid level]. (E and F) Bilateral bronchiectasis with hypertrophied bronchial arteries (white arrows). (G) Thin-walled cavity with aspergilloma (star). (H and I) Chronic cavitary pulmonary aspergillosis with pleural thickening and vascularity in the walls of cavity (white arrows). (J) Carcinoma of lung in the right lower lobe (black arrow) with right pleural effusion.
(CT: computed tomography; MinIP: minimum intensity projection; TB: tuberculosis)

the common causes of hemoptysis. Several of those do not require any interventional radiology management such as vasculitis, diffuse alveolar hemorrhage, and tumors such as carcinoids.

MANAGEMENT APPROACH

Management of hemoptysis depends on the severity of hemoptysis. It can be life-threatening hemoptysis or nonlife-threatening hemoptysis. Life-threatening hemoptysis refers to any hemoptysis > 150 mL in 24 hours or rate of hemoptysis > 100 mL/h and hemoptysis causing airway obstruction, respiratory failure, or hemodynamic instability necessitating blood transfusion.[8] Life-threatening hemoptysis is a respiratory emergency with a high mortality rate of up to 50–100%. Nonlife-threatening hemoptysis can be streaky or nonstreaky hemoptysis.

Life-threatening hemoptysis is managed with urgent measures to secure the airway, hemodynamics, and control the site of bleeding. Nonlife-threatening hemoptysis deals with the evaluation of etiology of hemoptysis and treatment of the underlying cause. For practical purposes, occasional blood-stained sputum (streaky hemoptysis) can usually be managed conservatively, but recurrent episodes of nonstreaky hemoptysis warrant intervention.

Management options of hemoptysis can be surgery, bronchoscopy, or endovascular embolization. BAE is the procedure of choice in life-threatening/massive hemoptysis following stabilization of the patient and nonlife-threatening/massive hemoptysis with hypertrophied bronchial arteries on computed tomography angiography (CTA).[9-11] Early embolization in nonlife-threatening hemoptysis with hypertrophied arteries reduces the hospital stay and chances of recurrence. Pulmonary artery embolization (PAE) is the preferred interventional radiology management option for hemoptysis with a source from the pulmonary circulation.

Surgery is the treatment of choice, if the pulmonary disease is localized and patients have adequate pulmonary reserve without comorbidities. Surgery is also indicated, if the hemoptysis is due to hydatid cyst, mucormycosis, bronchial neoplasms, or mediastinal vascular injuries.[9] Even in surgical candidates, BAE has a role in reducing the intraoperative bleeding, especially if the patient presents in the emergency department with massive hemoptysis.

Death from hemoptysis is rarely due to blood loss. Rather, it is the asphyxia caused by flooding of the airways and alveoli with blood, which is lethal.

PREPROCEDURE DIAGNOSTIC WORKUP

The purpose of a preprocedure workup is to identify the cause and site of hemoptysis. This would not only enable us to exclude the cardiac and neoplastic causes but also to plan the embolization/surgical procedure. **Flowchart 1** depicts the diagnostic approach and management in a case with significant hemoptysis of pulmonary etiology.

Chest Radiograph

It is frequently performed as the first investigation and may be the only investigation feasible in emergency cases. Advantages include wide availability, low cost, and can be done immediately. The American College of Radiology (ACR) recommends a chest radiograph in the evaluation of all patients with hemoptysis because it not only lateralizes the bleeding but may also identify the cause.[12] Radiographs are diagnostic in about 50% of cases.[1]

Computed Tomography

Multidetector computed tomography (CT) is the modality of choice for the evaluation of hemoptysis. Contrast-enhanced CT (CECT) has the capability to detect airway, parenchymal, as well as vascular causes of hemoptysis **(Figs. 1 and 2)**. CT bronchial angiography (CTBA) provides a vascular roadmap by delineating the hypertrophied bronchial and systemic arteries **(Figs. 2A to H)**, while CT pulmonary angiography (CTPA) acquisition can delineate the rarer pulmonary vascular causes of hemoptysis. As per the ACR recommendations, CTBA is the next most appropriate investigation in patients with significant hemoptysis.[12] This technique has the potential to reduce the procedure time as well as improve the outcomes of BAE (by identifying the ectopic and uncommon arterial supply preprocedural). CTA has been found to reduce the rate of vascular catheterization failure in elderly patients.[13] *Split bolus technique* allows

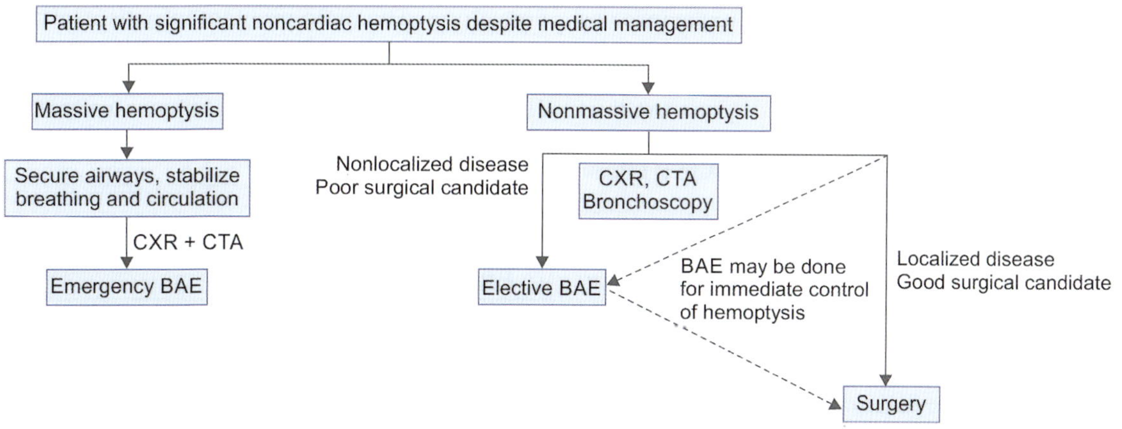

FLOWCHART 1: Approach to a patient with hemoptysis.
(BAE: bronchial artery embolization; CTA: computed tomography angiography; CXR: chest radiograph)

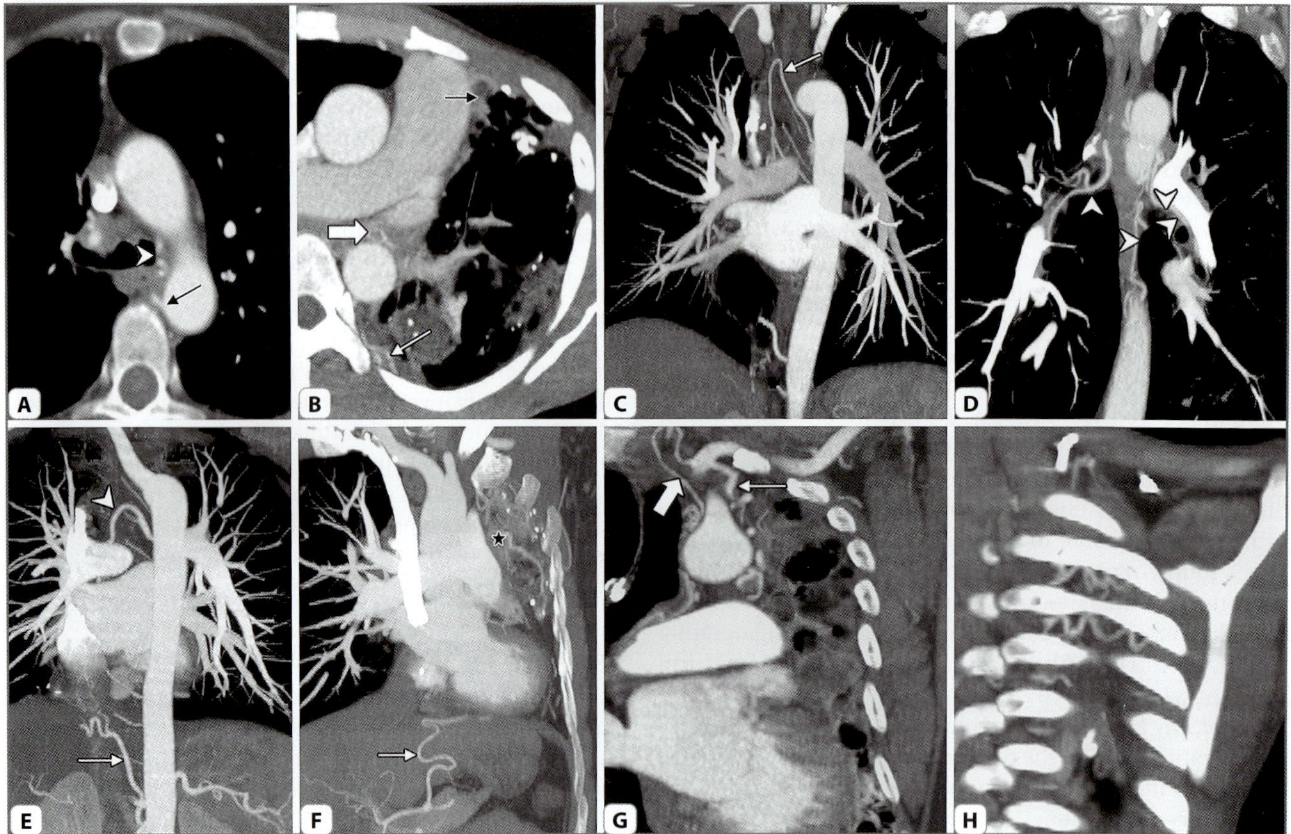

FIGS. 2A TO H: CT angiogram images showing hypertrophied bronchial arteries and NBSC. (A) RT-ICBT arises laterally from the descending aorta (black arrow). Left bronchial artery is seen around the left main bronchus (white arrowhead). (B) Left bronchial artery arises from anterior wall of aorta (solid white arrow). Also noted are NBSC from left internal mammary artery (IMA) (black arrow) and tortuous left posterior intercostal artery (white thin arrow). (C) Combined CT angiogram coronal MIP image showing good opacification of both systemic and pulmonary arterial trees. The entire course of RT-ICBT is well seen (white arrow). (D) Multiple hypertrophied bronchial arteries (white arrowheads). (E) Hypertrophied right bronchial (white arrowhead) and inferior phrenic arteries (thin white arrow). (F) Hypertrophied left inferior phrenic artery (white arrow) and multiple chest wall collaterals (star). (G) Coronal oblique MIP image depicts enlarged left costocervical trunk (solid white arrow) and IMA (thin white arrow). (H) Tortuous hypertrophied left posterior intercostal arteries.

(CT: computed tomography; MIP: maximum intensity projection; NBSC: nonbronchial systemic collateral; RT-ICBT: right intercostobronchial trunk)

evaluation of both systemic and pulmonary vasculature in single contrast injection. Split bolus technique involves the administration of contrast in divided boluses using an automated pressure injector where three-fourths of contrast is administered at 3–5 mL/second, followed by one-fourth of contrast at 3 mL/second followed by saline (volume equals one-fourth of saline) at 3 mL/second **(Figs. 2A to H)**.[14]

Fiberoptic Bronchoscopy

Fiberoptic bronchoscopy (FB) and CTA are complementary in the evaluation of hemoptysis; however, with improvement technique of CTA, it has eliminated the need for pre-embolization FB prior to BAE.[15] CT is more useful to identify the cause, while FB is more accurate in localizing the site of active bleeding. This is especially useful in cases when there is multifocal/bilateral lung disease. FB has the advantage that it can identify the bleeding of endobronchial lesions, enable sampling, as well as interventional pulmonary procedures. The main problem in patients with massive hemoptysis is that blood/clots may fill up the bronchi and preclude further evaluation. Also, the feasibility of FB depends on the local availability as well as the patient condition.

SECTION A: BRONCHIAL ARTERY EMBOLIZATION

Indications of Bronchial Artery Embolization

It may be noted here that bronchial artery abnormalities are much less common in malignancies, acute infection, and vasculitis, whereas in bronchiectasis and postinfective causes, these are usually hypertrophied. Thus, BAE is much more commonly done for nonneoplastic causes.[5,16] Majority of the published data on BAE are from Asia where tuberculosis (TB) (active disease/sequelae) is the most common cause of significant hemoptysis,[4-7,17-19] whereas sarcoidosis and cystic fibrosis are common indications in the West.[20,21] In addition, it is necessary to rule out cardiovascular (mitral stenosis, left heart failure, pulmonary embolism, aneurysm of aorta/pulmonary artery, and iatrogenic injury by Swan-Ganz catheter) and systemic (bleeding diathesis, anticoagulation) causes of hemoptysis.

Relevant Arterial Anatomy

It is important to have a good understanding of the anatomy of the bronchial and commonly hypertrophied nonbronchial arteries, so that the same may be communicated in the radiological report as well as guide management.

Bronchial Arteries

Bronchial arteries are systemic arteries, which course along the branching of the major bronchi. This is a key finding, which helps to distinguish (ectopic) bronchial arteries from nonbronchial systemic collaterals. The bronchial arteries supply the tracheobronchial tree (both intra- and extrapulmonary); regional lymph nodes; visceral pleura; esophagus; and vasa vasorum of aorta, pulmonary artery, and vein.

Origin

Majority of the bronchial arteries are *orthotopic*, i.e., arise from the descending thoracic aorta (DTA) between the superior border of T5 and inferior border of T6 vertebral levels **(Figs. 3A to H)**.[3] Angiographic landmark for the same is 1 cm above and below the crossing of left main bronchus over the DTA or just below the carina.[22] The frequency of orthotopic bronchial arteries varies depending on whether the study is based on CT, digital subtraction angiography (DSA), or postmortem; approximately 65% of patients have orthotopic bronchial arteries.[3] If the origin is anywhere else from DTA or even from a branch of the aorta, but the course is parallel to the bronchial tree, then it is labeled as *ectopic* bronchial artery **(Figs. 4A to I)**. Practically, majority of the bronchial arteries arise from DTA between T4 and T7 vertebral levels. Many variations can, however, occur, and ectopic bronchial arteries may arise from the inferior surface of aortic arch, internal mammary artery (IMA), thyrocervical and costocervical trunk, innominate artery, left subclavian artery (SCA) and inferior thyroid artery, inferior phrenic artery, or abdominal aorta.[23]

Cauldwell and Siekert documented the variations in bronchial artery anatomy by describing nine patterns based on autopsy study of 150 cadavers.[24] Uflacker et al. described 10 patterns of bronchial arterial anatomy based on angiography records of 72 patients.[25] However, what is more relevant is the information regarding number and origin of the hypertrophied bronchial arteries and pattern approach is not that helpful.

Right Side

There are usually two bronchial arteries supplying the right lung. The first arises from DTA as a common intercostobronchial trunk (ICBT), with the third right posterior intercostal artery, and has a posterolaterally lying orifice **(Figs. 2A to H)**. *Right ICBT* (RT-ICBT) is the most consistently seen artery at DSA. The initial course is oblique and upward and can be seen on CT in the retroesophageal region. Then, the trunk divides, with the bronchial component hooking down and paralleling the branching of RT bronchus, while the intercostal component ascends up and then traverses horizontally along the inferior border of the rib **(Figs. 3A to H)**. The second artery is the *common bronchial (CB)* that arises from the anterior surface and supplies both lungs by dividing into right and left bronchial arteries **(Figs. 3A to H)**. Depending upon the parenchymal abnormality, one or both branches may be hypertrophied.

Left Side

On the left side, a separate *left bronchial (LB)* artery is usually present and arises from the anterior left anterolateral surface of the aorta **(Figs. 2 and 3)**. Rarely, the LB artery may arise from the RT-ICBT, but LB arising from left intercostal is not described.

On CT, bronchial arteries can be identified in the retroesophageal, retrotracheal, retrobronchial, or aorto-pulmonary window locations **(Box 1 and Figs. 2A to H)**. Bronchial arteries can communicate with other systemic arteries. Most important of such communication is that of RT-ICBT with anterior medullary artery that contributes to vascular supply of the spinal cord through anterior spinal artery. The *anterior medullary arteries* have a characteristic "hairpin" configuration and follow a vertical course parallel to the spinal cord **(Figs. 4A to I)**.[26] These arteries, when they originate from D9 to D12, may communicate with the great anterior medullary artery (artery of Adamkiewicz). Other less commonly seen communications are with the SCA and right coronary artery.[27,28]

The other type of spinal arteries that may be seen are *radicular arteries*. These are small vessels, which usually arise from the posterior intercostal arteries, do not have the "hairpin" configuration, and supply the dorsal and ventral roots **(Figs. 4A to I)**. Radicular arteries are more commonly seen at DSA and are not considered to be a contradiction to embolization. Medullary arteries, on the other hand, are rarely seen but may give rise to cord ischemia, if inadvertently embolized.[1] Nevertheless, it is advisable to go superselectively beyond the origin of any spinal artery to prevent ominous complications.

Nonbronchial Systemic Collaterals

Nonbronchial systemic collaterals (NBSCs) enter the lung parenchyma through adjacent pleura or the pulmonary

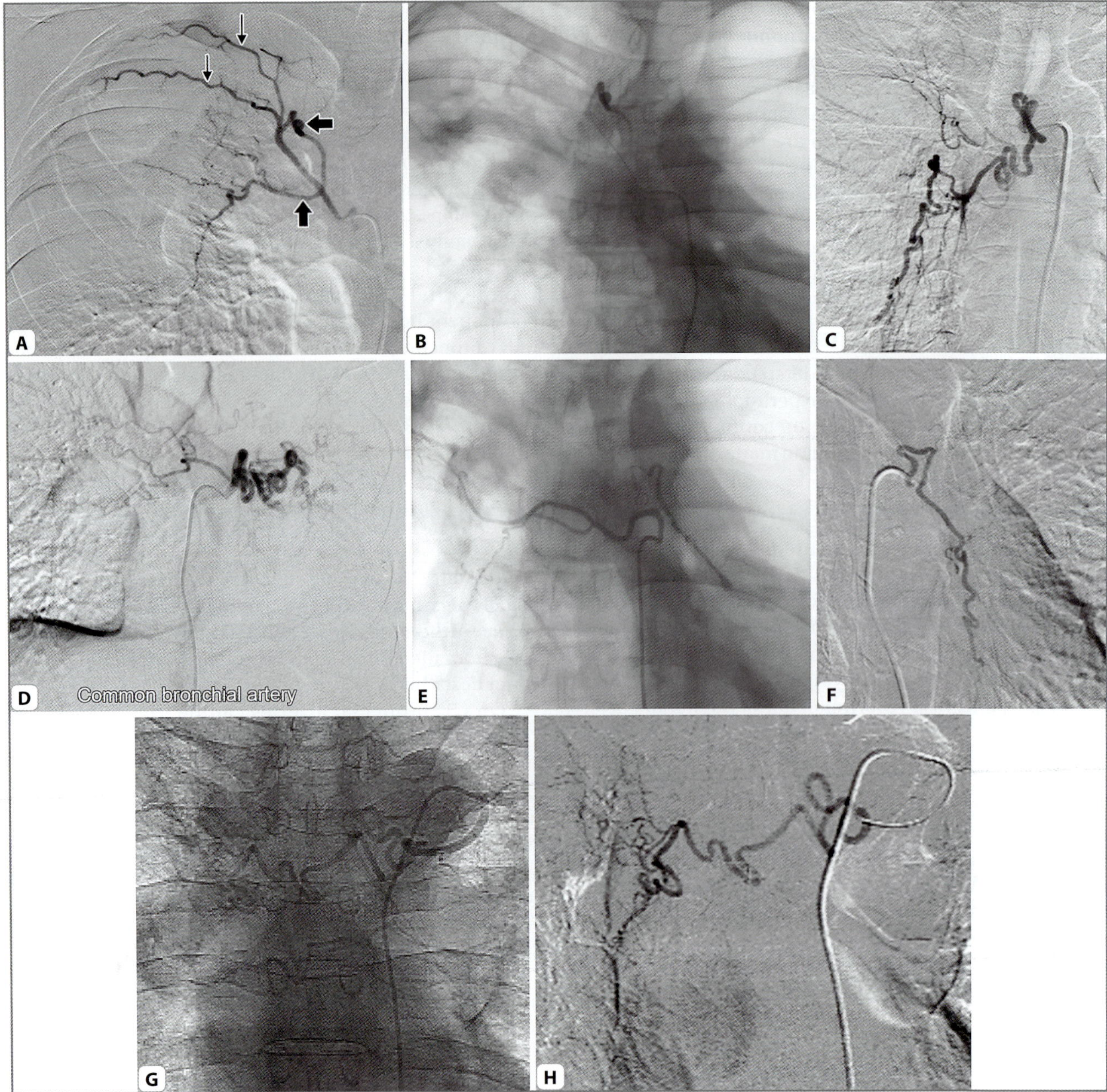

FIGS. 3A TO H: DSA images showing abnormal bronchial arteries. (A) Selective DSA run shows hypertrophied RT-ICBT. The bronchial component is hypertrophied (solid black arrows), while the intercostal component is normal (thin black arrows) at right bronchial (RB). (B) Stasis of contrast after superselective embolization. (C) Hypertrophied RB artery. (D) Common bronchial artery with hypertrophied left component. (E) Common bronchial artery with right component more hypertrophied than left. (F) Hypertrophied left bronchial artery. (G) Ectopic right bronchial artery arising from the arch of aorta. (H) Superselective DSA run through microcatheter shows stable catheter position, just before embolization.

(DSA: digital subtraction angiography; RT-ICBT: right intercostobronchial trunk)

ligament and have a course that does not parallel the bronchial tree. The CT features that suggest the presence of NBSC include pleural thickening and presence of chronic inflammatory disease in the lung apex or base. NBSC may arise from the following:[18,29,30]

- Intercostal arteries in case of peripheral lung/pleural inflammation **(Figs. 2 and 4)**
- Branches of subclavian and axillary arteries (internal mammary, lateral thoracic, costocervical, and cervicothoracic) in case of apical/anterior paramidline lung disease **(Figs. 2 and 4)**
- Phrenic arteries in case of basal lung disease **(Figs. 2 and 4)**
- Rarely left gastric artery

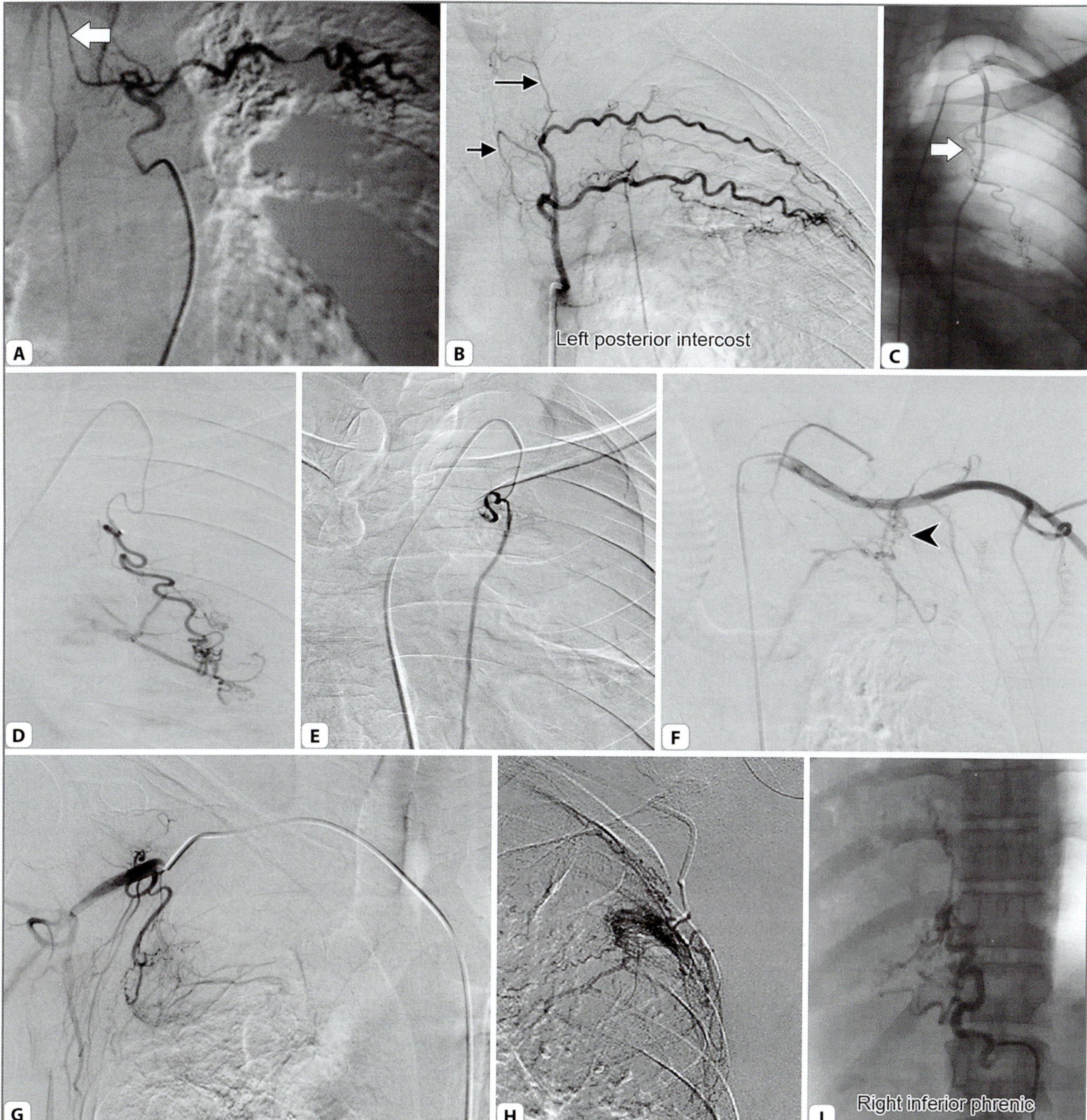

FIGS. 4A TO I: DSA images showing abnormal NBSC and communications with spinal artery. (A) Anterior medullary artery (solid white arrow) arising from left posterior intercostal artery. (B) Radicular arteries (thin black arrows) arise from left posterior intercostal artery. (C) Left subclavian artery (SCA) run shows an abnormal branch arising from LT IMA (solid white arrow). (D) Superselective catheterization of abnormal branch of LT IMA with stable catheter position and check run. (E) Postembolization run of the same. (F) Abnormal costocervical branch of second part of left SCA (black arrowhead). (G) Abnormal pulmonary parenchymal blush from right superior thoracic artery (branch of first part of axillary artery). (H) Superselective catheterization of left superior thoracic artery. (I) Hypertrophied right inferior phrenic artery.

(DSA: digital subtraction angiography; IMA: internal mammary artery; NBSC: nonbronchial systemic collateral)

Normal bronchial arteries have a diameter of <1.5 mm at their origin and 0.5 mm at the level of the entrance into a bronchopulmonary segment. Indicators of abnormal bronchial arteries are[11,17,31] enumerated in **Box 2** and illustrated in **Figures 5A to E**. Systemic collaterals going into abnormal lung parenchyma are considered abnormal irrespective of diameter.

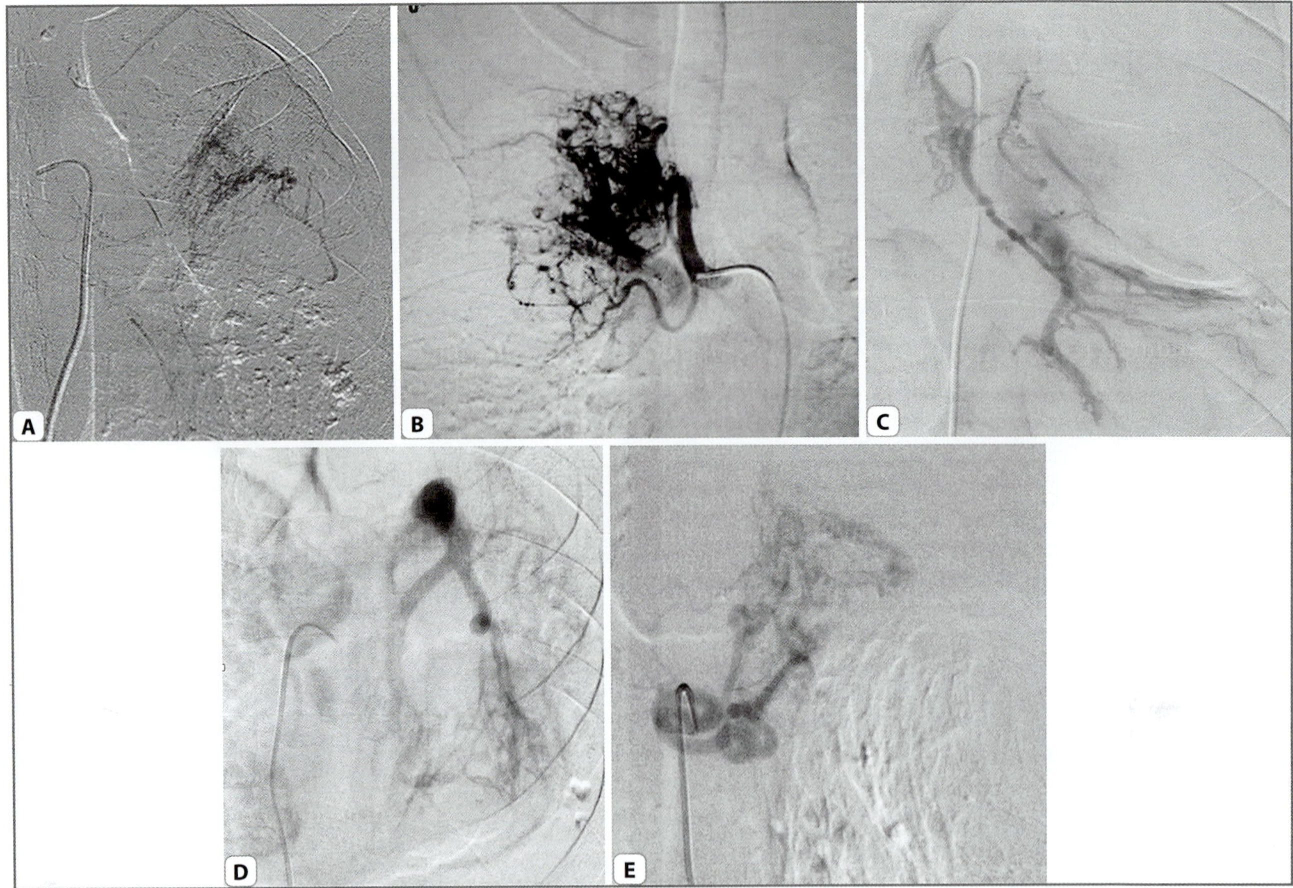

FIGS. 5A TO E: Digital subtraction angiography (DSA) features of abnormal bronchial arteries. (A) Abnormal parenchymal blush. (B) Hypertrophied right bronchial artery with dense vascular blush and shunting. (C) Vascular blush with shunting into pulmonary vein. (D) Delayed phase DSA run depicts shunting into pulmonary artery. (E) Hypertrophied tortuous left bronchial artery with pulmonary arterial shunting.

BOX 1: Tips to identify abnormal bronchial and nonbronchial systemic collaterals (NBSC).

- RT-ICBT arises from the right lateral wall of aorta and courses behind the right main bronchus
- RB or right branch of CB arises anterolaterally from aorta and courses anterior to the RT of main bronchus
- LB arises from the anterior wall of aorta and may course anterior or posterior to the left main bronchus
- Ectopic LB/RB arising from the arch courses anterior to the corresponding bronchus
- Internal mammary arteries are hypertrophied in case disease is localized to anterior segments of upper lobes, RT middle lobe, or lingual
- Right posterior intercostal arteries arise posterolaterally, and left posterior intercostal arteries arise posteriorly from the aorta
- Posterior intercostal arteries are hypertrophied in case of posterior or posterolateral lung involvement
- Inflammatory lung disease close to the lateral chest wall may recruit collaterals from lateral thoracic artery
- Inferior phrenic arteries may hypertrophy in basal lung disease

(CB: common bronchial; LB: left bronchial; NBSC: nonbronchial systemic collateral; RB: right bronchial; RT-ICBT: right intercostobronchial trunk)

Technique of Bronchial Artery Embolization

The first priority in patients with life-threatening hemoptysis is to maintain the airway, optimize oxygenation, and stabilize the hemodynamic status. Blood tests for coagulopathy (prothrombin time, platelet count) and renal dysfunction (blood urea, serum creatinine) need to be done before BAE.

BOX 2: Criteria to identify abnormal bronchial and nonbronchial systemic collaterals (NBSC).

- *Hypertrophy*: Diameter at ostium > 2 mm
- Increased tortuosity
- Bronchial artery traceable up to corresponding hilum on CT
- *DSA features*:
  - Neo- and hypervascularity in the form of abnormal vascular blush and dense soft-tissue staining/parenchymal blush **(Figs. 5A to E)**
  - Shunting into the pulmonary vascular system (arterial or venous) **(Figs. 5A to E)**
  - Extravasation of contrast into the alveoli or bronchial tree
  - Pseudoaneurysm
- Any nonbronchial systemic collateral (NBSC) supplying diseased lung parenchyma is deemed abnormal

(CT: computed tomography; DSA: digital subtraction angiography)

Route

Transfemoral arterial access is routinely used to access the bronchial circulation. Transbrachial/transaxillary access may be helpful in case of increased aortic tortuosity[5,6] and to selectively catheterize branches of subclavian arteries. A long arterial sheath (carotid sheath) may also be used in case of tortuosity of the aortic arch. In case pulmonary angiography needs to be done, then common femoral vein access is used. 6F sheath is commonly used in adults while in young children, 5F access sheath is used.

Thoracic Aortogram

Flush aortogram is not done routinely nowadays due to the availability of CTA. It can be helpful in patients with life-threatening hemoptysis directly taken of embolization. The aim of flush aortogram is to identify all the abnormal bronchial and NBSCs from DTA, so as to facilitate selective catheterization of the same as illustrated in **Figures 6A to E**. The limitation of flush aortogram is that

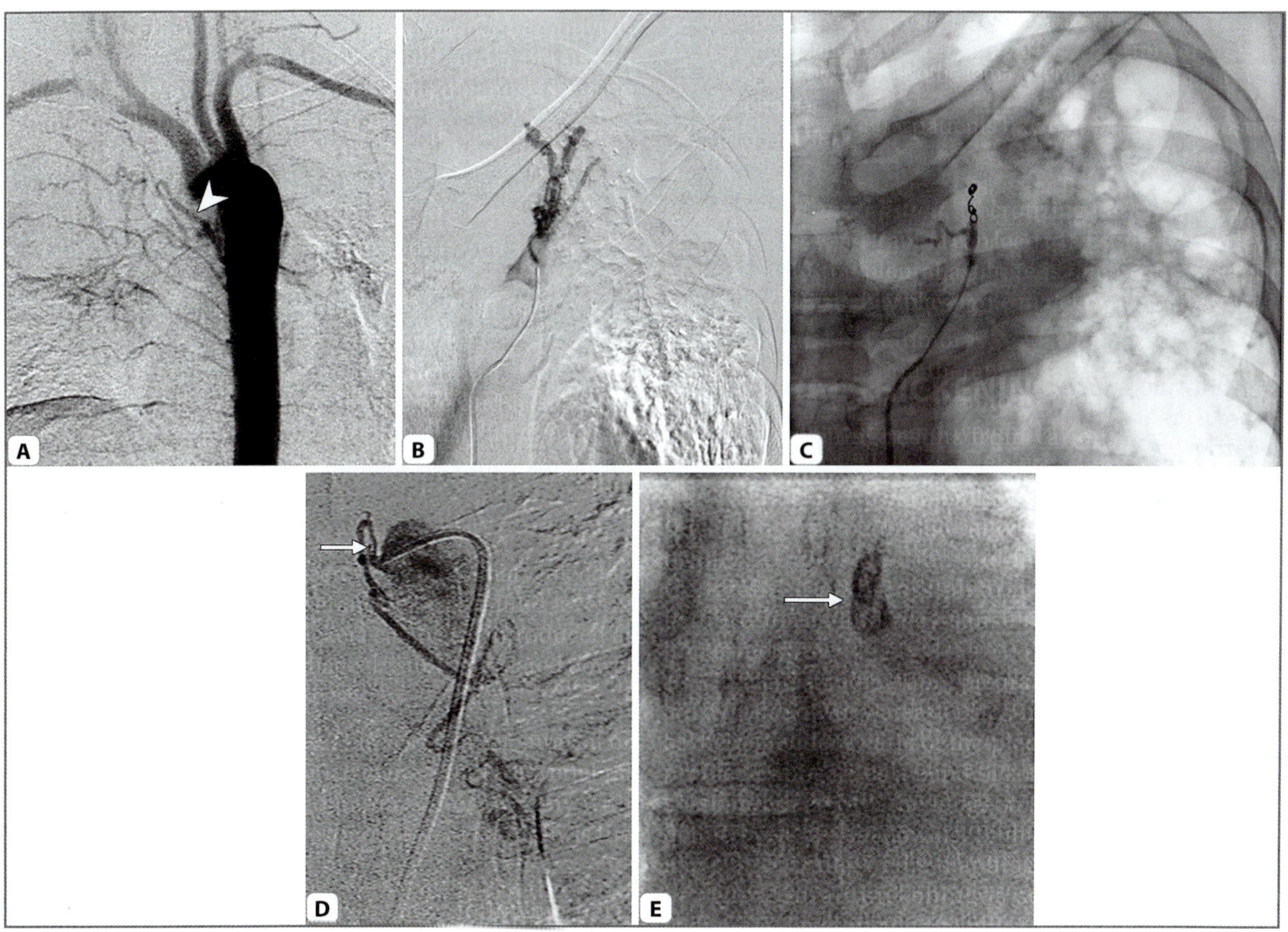

FIGS. 6A TO E: BAE technique and complications. (A) Flush aortogram shows hypertrophied RT-ICBT (white arrowhead). (B) Superselective catheterization of left bronchial artery shows large shunt into the pulmonary vein. (C) Due to large size of the shunt and resultant potential of cerebral embolism, the shunt was blocked using microcoils. (D) DSA run shows shelf-like filling defect at the origin of ectopic left bronchial artery (suggesting dissection), caused by wire manipulation due to acute upward angulation (white thin arrow). (E) Fluoroscopic spot image depicts contrast blob at the origin of this ectopic left bronchial artery (likely representing intramural hematoma in the aortic wall) (white thin arrow).

(BAE: bronchial artery embolization; DSA: digital subtraction angiography; RT-ICBT: right intercostobronchial trunk)

the opacification of subclavian arteries is suboptimal. So, either take separate SCA runs or take the pigtail loop up to proximal arch. Problem with the latter technique is that contrast will unnecessarily go into the head and neck arteries.

Superselective Catheterization

The bronchial arteries are usually hooked using angiographic catheters having more than one curve such as renal double curve (RDC)/cobra catheter **(Table 2)**. Reverse-seeking catheters (such as Simmons) may also be used, especially when there is a sharp upward course from the origin. Once the artery is hooked, then check contrast run is taken. Using this roadmap, the main catheter is secured into the artery, and then microcatheter (2.7 Fr) is advanced through the main catheter (coaxial system). A multipurpose catheter or slip catheter may also be used to go selectively into the artery, by exchanging RDC/cobra over a long (~260 cm) guidewire.

In the case of ICBT, an attempt should be made to superselectively go into the bronchial component, unless the intercostal component is also abnormal **(Figs. 3A to H)**. Care must be taken to look for any contrast opacification of the anterior medullary artery **(Figs. 4A to I)**. Superselective catheterization by microcatheter enables delivery of embolizing agent specifically into the culprit branches with lesser risk of complications and, thus, providing better patient care.[5-7,32] Care should be taken not to create spasm or dissection while negotiating the smaller catheter.

Usually, the bronchial arteries are searched first, followed by any expected NBSC. Intercostal arteries can be searched by directing the RDC catheter posterolaterally for right-sided arteries and posteriorly for left posterior intercostal arteries. SCA branches are evaluated using Picard/vertebral catheter, while phrenic artery may be hooked using RDC or reverse curve (RC) catheter **(Table 2)**. The search for NBSC has been found to reduce the recurrence rates of hemoptysis.[9] A preprocedural CTBA lays down the vascular roadmap for endovascular therapeutic interventions.

Again, an attempt must be made to hook the hypertrophied branch of SCA using the main catheter and then go selectively into it using microcatheter **(Figs. 4A to I)**. If the former is not feasible, then negotiation using microcatheter can be done after keeping the main catheter in SCA itself, provided we use a large bore Tuohy–Borst sidearm adaptor (Y-connector). The latter allows for continuous flushing of the guiding catheter, so as to avoid the formation of thrombus in the dead space. Alternatively, a side hole can be created in a diagnostic catheter (at a distance from the tip), which can serve as an exit for microcatheter. This technique has been described to be helpful in the embolization of proximal subclavian arterial branches, when stable and selective position of the main catheter cannot be achieved.[33] In a similar fashion, catheters with prefabricated side holes can be used in difficult anatomical situations.[34] Before proceeding to the embolization of the target vessel, stability of the catheter tip and absence of backflow into the descending thoracic aorta should be confirmed by means of a test injection using a contrast medium.

TABLE 2: Commonly used catheters for selective cannulation.

Bronchial and intercostal arteries	RDC (double curve), cobra (complex curve), and Simmons (reverse curve)
Subclavian artery and its branches	Picard, vertebral (forward-seeking simple curve angled tip), and headhunter (double curve)
Inferior phrenic artery	RDC, RC, and Simmons

(RC: reverse curve; RDC: renal double curve)

Culprit Arteries

The common culprit bronchial arteries in patients undergoing embolization are RB, RT-ICBT, CB, and LB (in descending order of frequency). Common NBSCs are posterior intercostal artery and IMA. Other branches of SCA (such as superior thoracic, lateral thoracic, costocervical, and cervicothoracic) and inferior phrenic arteries may also be abnormal.

Embolizing Agents

Particulate embolizing materials are commonly used for BAE. Older literature describes the use of a gelatin sponge, but the current agent of choice is polyvinyl alcohol (PVA) particles. Gelatin sponge is readily available and inexpensive. Advantages of PVA over Gelfoam include permanency of embolization (since gelatin sponge gets resorbed) and choice of different sizes **(Table 3)**. Gelfoam has the potential to cause more proximal embolization. Problems with PVA include tendency of the particles to clump in the microcatheter. Microspheres can overcome this problem because of their hydrophilic nature and uniform size.[15] Commonly used size of PVA particles is 300–500 μ, though use of all sizes from 150 to 1,200 μ has been reported in the literature. Particles < 300 μ should ideally not be used because they can pass through the bronchopulmonary anastomoses and result in infarcts.[15] They may lead to occlusion of smaller branches, resulting in bronchial or esophageal necrosis.[26]

Larger particles (500–700 μ) may be indicated in the presence of shunting. Shunting into pulmonary veins is potentially more dangerous than the pulmonary arteries because of the risk of nontarget systemic embolization. PVA/Gelfoam is mixed with contrast and then injected under fluoroscopic guidance. It is important to monitor for slowing of flow and stasis, so as to prevent any backflow/reflux of embolic material. A total of 2 mL/1 mL syringes are routinely used for better precision. Intermittent contrast runs may be taken to look for any vascular anastomoses not previously visible. Always remember to empty the PVA column in the catheter before taking check runs.

TABLE 3: Advantages and drawbacks of various embolizing agents.

Embolizing agents	Advantages	Drawbacks
Polyvinyl alcohol (PVA) particles	• Relatively uniform size • Permanent • Different sizes available	• Tendency to clump • Costly
Microspheres	Better than PVA because do not clump	Costly
Gelfoam	Cheap, readily available	• Heterogeneous particle size • Temporary
Glue	• More permanent than PVA • Useful where significant shunting is there	Needs experienced hands and stable catheter position
Microcoils	• Pseudoaneurysms • Markedly hypertrophied artery with large volume shunt • To protect parent vessel in case superselective catheterization is not feasible	• Preclude future access • Expensive

TABLE 4: Causes of technical and clinical failure of bronchial artery embolization (BAE).

Causes of technical failure	Causes of clinical failure
• Patient not able to breath-hold/constantly coughing/expectorating • Tortuous artery/acute angulation • Proximal/ostial narrowing • Aortic tortuosity may hamper stable • Catheterization of subclavian artery branches • Failure to go beyond the origin of spinal cord branches	• Inability to embolize all culprit arteries • Presence of ectopic bronchial arteries • Pulmonary vascular causes

Polyvinyl alcohol can also be used in conjunction with Gelfoam. Former is used for distal embolization of the abnormal parenchymal bed, and latter is typically used for proximal embolization. Recently, liquid embolic agents [glue, n-butyl-2-cyanoacrylate (NBCA)] have been shown to result in better control of hemoptysis in case of bronchiectasis.[7] This has been attributed to the lower rates of recanalization compared with PVA, but use of glue calls for stable catheter position and need for greater expertise, owing to more chances of complications (distal necrosis and nontarget complications due to reflux are more dangerous). Microcoils have been used uncommonly, and the chief indication is in the case of pseudoaneurysms (provided the microcatheter reaches up to the neck of the aneurysm) and large volume shunts **(Figs. 6A to E)**. Proximal coil embolization precludes repeat access in the case of recurrence of hemoptysis due to distal collateralization.[35,36]

Outcomes

The outcome of any interventional procedure is expressed in terms of technical as well as clinical success. The causes of technical and clinical failure of BAE have been listed in **Table 4**. A preprocedural CT angiogram enhances clinical success by depicting all the abnormal arteries. Few authors suggest a postembolization flush aortogram to avoid missing a pathological vessel. The presence of NBSC is associated with a higher rate of technical failures.[37]

Bronchial artery embolization is very effective in the treatment of acute hemoptysis. *Immediate clinical success* (significant reduction/cessation of hemoptysis within 24 hours of the procedure) is high (70–99%).[2] *Early recurrences* (within 1–3 months) suggest incomplete embolization, i.e., any abnormal vessel has been left untreated. This may be because of a lack of complete search, ectopic origin or NBSC, and too many hypertrophied arteries due to extensive collateralization. In latter scenario, it may be useful to split the embolization into two sessions, starting with the most abnormal arteries first, and bronchial arteries should be done prior to the NBSC.

Late recurrences occur due to recanalization of previously treated arteries or new recruitment of NBSCs.[5,32,37,38] This occurs, if the underlying disease is not simultaneously controlled, thus emphasizing the need to address the underlying disease medically or surgically. Superimposed infection on background TB sequelae, chronic cavitary pulmonary aspergillosis (CCPA), and development of multidrug-resistant TB (MDR-TB) can contribute to recurrence of hemoptysis in previously treated cases.[32,38,39]

Recurrences at long-term follow-up can be as high as 52%, and the probability of recurrence increases with time. The chances of rebleed are more with aspergillomas and cavitary lung disease.[4,25,32,39,40] Recurrences can again be effectively controlled with BAE, and, thus, repeat sessions provide long-term control of hemoptysis.[18,37,38] It has been noted that patients who remain hemoptysis free for 3 years post-BAE have excellent prognosis but those who rebleed and tend to bleed again and again.[18,21] It may be noted here that BAE is a palliative procedure to control hemoptysis and does not treat the underlying cause. Thus, wherever feasible and considered safe, surgery may be considered for definitive treatment.[17,21]

Complications

The most common complication after BAE is transient *chest/back pain*, being reported in up to 34.5% of cases.[2] This is likely related to ischemia of embolized systemic branches and can be severe when intercostal arteries are embolized. Dissection of the bronchial artery or subintimal perforation and wire manipulation may lead to sudden chest pain **(Figs. 6A to E)**. There may be dissection of the aorta as well while negotiating a smaller catheter into its branch **(Figs. 6A to E)**. In such cases, intravenous fluid should be immediately started, and blood pressure should be maintained. Usually, these dissections are nonprogressive, but further catheter/wire manipulation in the vicinity of the injured segment should be avoided. The second most common complication is *dysphagia*, caused by embolization of esophageal branches, with a reported occurrence from 0.7 to 18.2%.[17] Spontaneous resolution of symptoms usually occurs.

The most devastating complication is *spinal cord ischemia* that has been reported to occur in 1.4–6.5% of patients.[11,17] This may lead to transient or permanent paraplegia, and, thus, any doubt of spinal artery anastomosis should become a red flag. The occurrence of this complication can be reduced by using a superselective embolization technique and performing regular check angiograms before and after the administration of embolic agents. *Postembolization syndrome* may occur, and the patient may develop fever, leukocytosis, and chest pain. This is, however, a self-limiting complication seen in up to 30% of cases.[7,9,19,25,37] *Rare complications* include aortic and bronchial necrosis, bronchial stenosis, unilateral diaphragmatic paralysis, pulmonary infarction (especially in patients who have suffered pulmonary artery embolism), left main bronchial-esophageal fistula, and nontarget embolization (colon, coronary, foot, and cerebral circulation).[41-44] In addition, contrast-induced nephropathy, hypersensitivity reactions, and groin hematomas may also occur.

SECTION B: PULMONARY ARTERY EMBOLIZATION

Pulmonary artery embolization is the endovascular management of choice for PAP and PAVMs.

Pulmonary Artery Pseudoaneurysm

Definition

Focal dilatation of segment of pulmonary artery is known as PAP. PAPs are uncommon but important cause of massive hemoptysis. The common causes of PAPs are vasculitis, infection, neoplasm, trauma, and often iatrogenic.[45] Rupture of PAPs leads to the risk of mortality in 50% of patients, and usually death results from aspiration and asphyxia following massive intrapulmonary hemorrhage.[46]

Classification

Pulmonary artery pseudoaneurysms have been classified into four types based on angiographic appearance **(Flowchart 2)**.[47] Type A PAPs are visualized on main pulmonary angiography with patent feeding

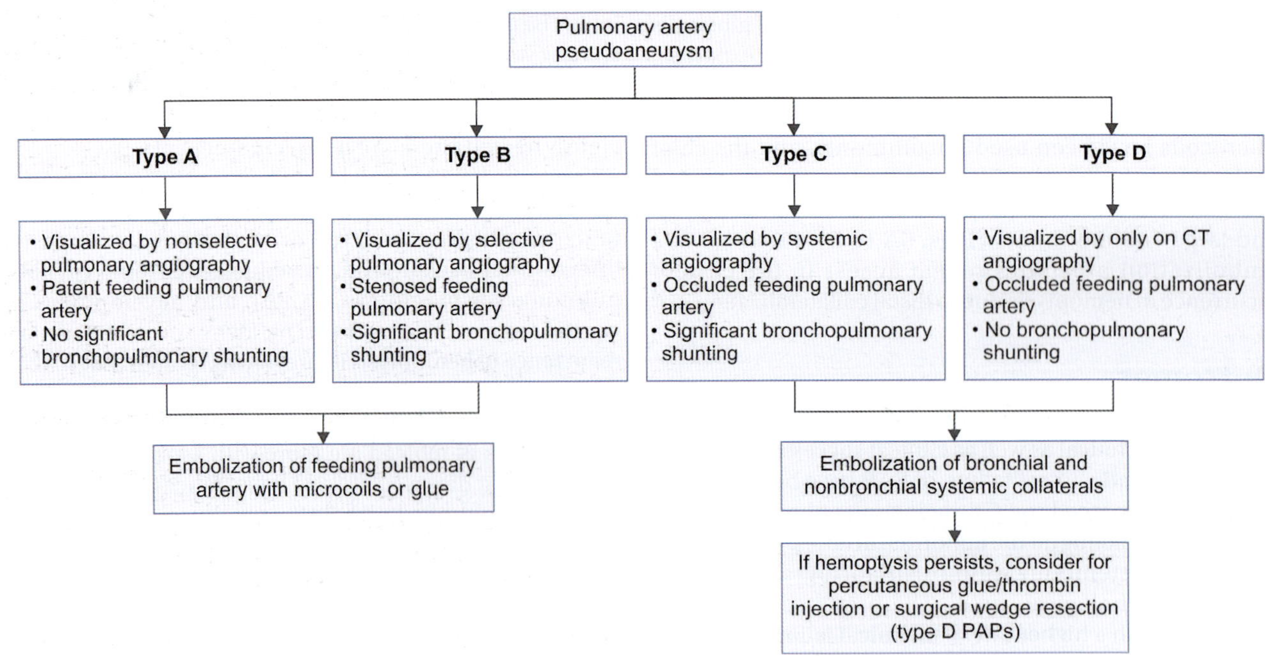

FLOWCHART 2: Types of pulmonary artery pseudoaneurysm and management options.

pulmonary artery branches without significant bronchopulmonary shunt. Type B PAPs have stenosis of feeding pulmonary artery and presence of bronchopulmonary shunt. Type B PAPs are visualized both on pulmonary and systemic angiography. Type C PAPs have occluded feeding pulmonary arteries with bronchopulmonary shut and visualized on systemic angiography and not visualized on pulmonary angiography **(Figs. 7A to F)**. Type D PAPs have occluded feeding pulmonary artery and lack of substantial bronchopulmonary shunt, and these are not visualized on either pulmonary or systemic angiography.

Management

The treatment options for type A and B PAPs are successive embolization of bronchial, other NBSCs, and feeding pulmonary arteries. Type C and D PAPs are treated with embolization of bronchial and other NBSCs to decrease the systemic arterial flow, and persistent PAPs on follow-up CT angiography are usually treated by percutaneous approach or surgical resection.

Pulmonary Arteriovenous Malformation

Definition

Pulmonary arteriovenous malformations are congenital vascular anomalies, which represent the direct communication between the pulmonary artery and a vein through a nidus, without a normal capillary network. PAVMs are often detected incidentally, and it is a rare cause of hemoptysis. Symptoms are mainly due to right-to-left shunting and paradoxical emboli. Hemodynamically significant left-to-right shunting can cause hypoxemia symptoms. Paradoxical emboli can travel anywhere in the body, causing end-organ infarcts (e.g., myocardial infarction, stroke). The different causes of PAVMs are outlined in **Table 5**.[48]

Diagnosis

Computed tomography angiography of the chest is the most commonly used diagnostic modality, typically showing a well-defined soft-tissue nodule with one or more feeding pulmonary arteries and a draining vein. Catheter

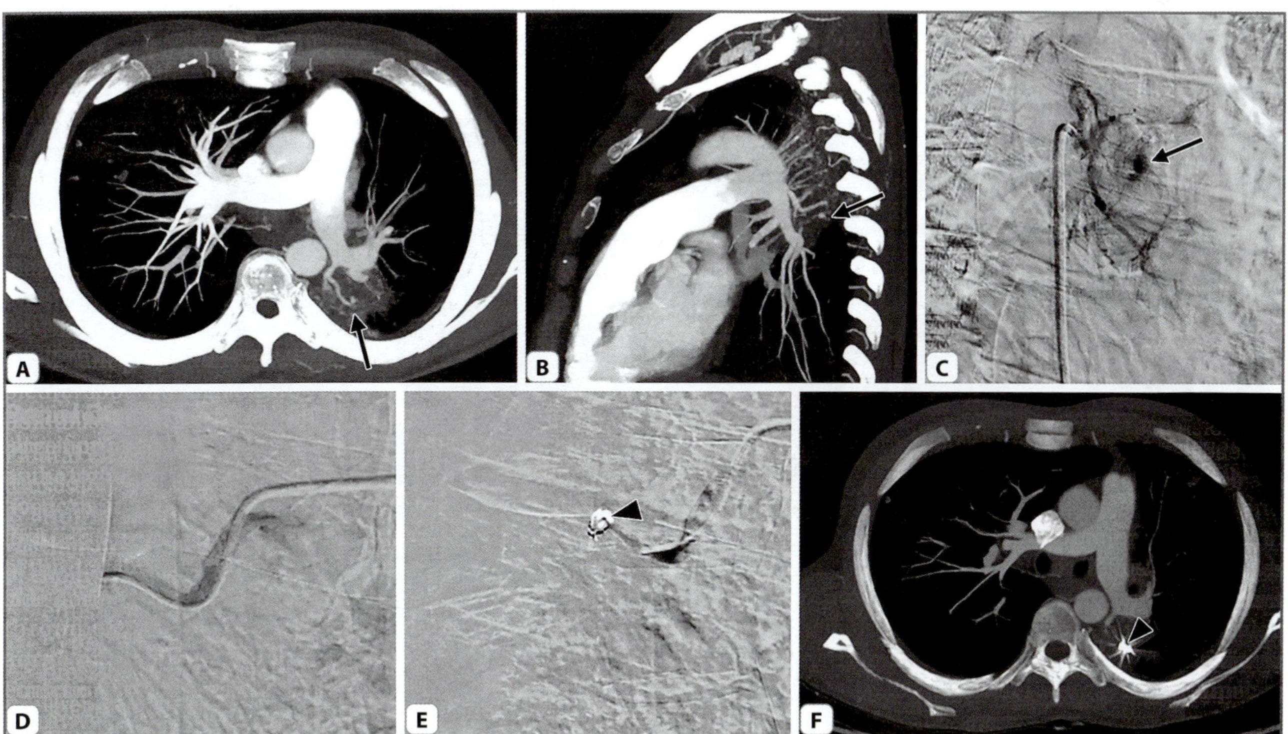

FIGS. 7A TO F: *A case of a 39-year-old male patient with hemoptysis.* (A and B) Axial and sagittal CT images showing pulmonary artery pseudoaneurysm (type C*) (black arrow) arising from the superior segmental branch of left descending pulmonary artery. (C) DSA run shows significant bronchopulmonary shunt from left bronchial artery with opacification of pseudoaneurysm (black arrow), which was embolized with PVA particles. (D) DSA image showing the selective pulmonary angiogram of superior segmental branch of descending pulmonary that does not opacify the pseudoaneurysm. (E) DSA image showing 18-3-3 microcoil in the embolized superior segmental branch of descending pulmonary artery (black arrowhead). (F) Follow-up axial CT image showing coil at the approximate site of pseudoaneurysm and nonopacification of pseudoaneurysm and superior segmental branch of descending pulmonary artery (black arrowhead).

*This is an example of type C pulmonary artery pseudoaneurysm with occluded feeding pulmonary artery having significant bronchopulmonary shunting, as it is visualized on left bronchial angiogram and nonopacified through pulmonary angiography.

(CT: computed tomography; DSA: digital subtraction angiography; PVA: polyvinyl alcohol)

angiography remains the gold standard for diagnosis. Contrast echocardiography is the most sensitive screening test, especially in patients with hereditary hemorrhagic telangiectasia (HHT). During the procedure, agitated saline or air is injected as contrast, and the presence of microbubbles in the left atrium within 3–10 heartbeats indicates the presence of a PAVM.

Classification[49]

- *Simple*: Most common, single segmental feeding artery, which can have single/multiple subsegmental vessels supply the PAVM
- *Complex*: Multiple segmental feeding arteries **(Figs. 8A to G)**
- *Diffuse*: Rare (~5%)

TABLE 5: Causes of pulmonary arteriovenous malformations.[48]

Congenital	80% associated with hereditary hemorrhagic telangiectasia (HHT)*
Acquired	• Postsurgery • Trauma • Hepatopulmonary syndrome (cirrhosis) • Post-Fontan or Glenn surgeries for congenital heart diseases

*Triad of mucocutaneous telangiectasia, recurrent epistaxis, and family history.

Management

Indications of treatment include symptomatic patients, size of feeding artery >2 mm, and increase in size of PAVM.[50] Embolization is the preferred treatment for arteriovenous malformations (AVMs), while surgical intervention is reserved for large lobar AVMs, diffuse AVMs, and complex AVMs unsuitable for embolization. Endovascular embolization is performed using vascular coils or plugs involving the embolization of the main feeding artery. The procedure involves accessing the common femoral vein with a 7F sheath, followed by selective cannulation of the pulmonary artery and superselective catheterization of the feeding arteries. Pushable coils are commonly used, while detachable coils are reserved for small feeding arteries or nidus embolization, where the risk of distal migration is higher. Detachable coils come with various detachment mechanisms, including electrical, mechanical latch, and ball-and-socket systems. Anchoring and scaffolding techniques can be used for stable coil deployment.[50] Balloon inflation can be done to reduce nontarget embolization

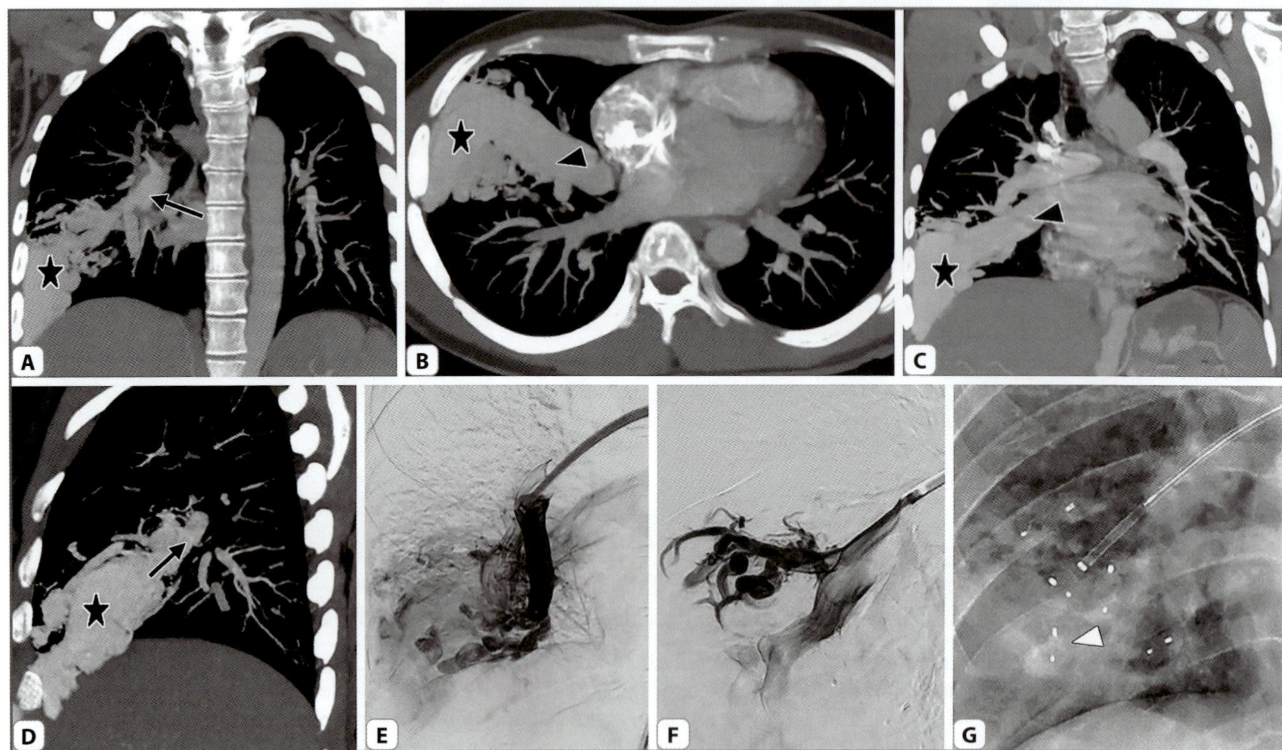

FIGS. 8A TO G: *A case of a 32-year-old male patient with complex pulmonary artery vascular malformation.* (A and B) Axial, (A and C) coronal, and (D) sagittal CT images showing complex pulmonary arteriovenous malformation (black star) in the right lower lobe with supply from multiple segmental branches of right descending pulmonary artery (black arrows) and draining into the right lower pulmonary vein (black arrowheads). (E and F) DSA images of the right descending pulmonary artery angiogram showing multiple feeding segmental branches. (G) The segmental branches superselectively cannulated and five Amplatzer vascular plugs (white arrowhead) of variable size from 8 to 14 mm were deployed in the segmental branches.

(CT: computed tomography; DSA: digital subtraction angiography)

in the high-flow PAVMs. Amplatzer vascular plugs are the preferable embolizing material. Microplugs can be used for smaller feeding arteries ~1.5–3 mm. Common complications include pleuritic chest pain, systemic air embolism, and coil migration.

Follow-up After Treatment

Follow-up is typically performed 3–6 months after embolization to evaluate clinical and radiological response. CECT or contrast-enhanced single-shot whole-thoracic time-resolved magnetic resonance angiography (MRA) can be used for follow-up. Recanalization is defined as a reduction of <70% in the diameter of the nidus or draining vein on CT imaging.[51]

CONCLUSION

Interventional radiology plays a significant role in the management of hemoptysis. BAE is the treatment of choice in acute hemoptysis and can be performed in both emergency as well as elective settings. Knowledge of bronchial and nonbronchial systemic circulation is mandatory to reduce complications and increase technical success. It is imperative to identify hypertrophied bronchial arteries and other systemic collaterals on CTA to enable successful embolization. BAE is a safe and effective procedure and can be done repeatedly for recurrent hemoptysis as well. Pulmonary arterial interventions for the management of PAPs and PAVMs require endovascular embolization.

KEY MESSAGES

- The common diseases leading to significant hemoptysis include TB (sequelae and active disease), bronchiectasis, and aspergillomas.
- Bronchial artery embolization is the procedure of choice for patients presenting in the emergency setting with massive hemoptysis. Also, it is the treatment of choice for immediate control of any amount of hemoptysis in nonsurgical candidates.
- Computed tomography angiogram provides a vascular roadmap, and bronchoscopy helps in localizing the site of active bleeding in diffuse lung disease.
- Superselective catheterization aids in reducing complications.
- Embolizing agent of choice in BAE is PVA particles (300–500) μ. Larger particles may be used in the case of vascular shunts.
- Reactivation TB, MDR-TB, and CCPA patients are more prone to develop recurrence of hemoptysis.
- Pulmonary artery embolization is the procedure of choice in the setting of pulmonary arterial source of hemoptysis likely PAPs and PAVMs.

REFERENCES

1. Yoon W, Kim JK, Kim YH, Chung TW, Kang HK. Bronchial and nonbronchial systemic artery embolization for life-threatening hemoptysis: a comprehensive review. Radiographics. 2002;22(6):1395-409.
2. Panda A, Bhalla AS, Goyal A. Bronchial artery embolization in hemoptysis: a systematic review. Diagn Interv Radiol. 2017;23(4):307-17.
3. Walker CM, Rosado-de-Christenson ML, Martínez-Jiménez S, Kunin JR, Wible BC. Bronchial arteries: anatomy, function, hypertrophy, and anomalies. Radiographics. 2015;35(1):32-49.
4. Rémy J, Voisin C, Dupuis C, Beguery P, Tonnel AB, Denies JL, et al. Treatment of hemoptysis by embolization of the systemic circulation. Ann Radiol (Paris). 1974;17(1):5-16.
5. Bhalla A, Kandasamy D, Veedu P, Mohan A, Gamanagatti S. A retrospective analysis of 334 cases of hemoptysis treated by bronchial artery embolization. Oman Med J. 2015;30(2):119-28.
6. Agmy GM, Wafy SM, Mohamed SAA, Gad YA, Mustafa H, Abd El-Aziz AES. Bronchial and nonbronchial systemic artery embolization in management of hemoptysis: experience with 348 patients. Int Sch Res Not. 2013;2013(1):263259.
7. Woo S, Yoon CJ, Chung JW, Kang SG, Jae HJ, Kim HC, et al. Bronchial artery embolization to control hemoptysis: comparison of N-butyl-2-cyanoacrylate and polyvinyl alcohol particles. Radiology. 2013;269(2):594-602.
8. Singhal R, Babu SKB, Naranje P, Kazimi J, Garg PK, Chandra D, et al. Society of Chest Imaging and Interventions consensus guidelines for the interventional radiology management of hemoptysis. Indian J Radiol Imaging. 2023;33(3):361-72.
9. Anuradha C, Shyamkumar NK, Vinu M, Babu NRSS, Christopher DJ. Outcomes of bronchial artery embolization for life-threatening hemoptysis due to tuberculosis and post-tuberculosis sequelae. Diagn Interv Radiol. 2012;18(1):96-101.
10. Hayakawa K, Tanaka F, Torizuka T, Mitsumori M, Okuno Y, Matsui A, et al. Bronchial artery embolization for hemoptysis: immediate and long-term results. Cardiovasc Intervent Radiol. 1992;15(3):154-8.
11. Wong ML, Szkup P, Hopley MJ. Percutaneous embolotherapy for life-threatening hemoptysis. Chest. 2002;121(1):95-102.
12. Ketai LH, Mohammed TLH, Kirsch J, Kanne JP, Chung JH, Donnelly EF, et al. ACR appropriateness criteria® hemoptysis. J Thorac Imaging. 2014;29(3):W19-22.
13. Khalil A, Fartoukh M, Parrot A, Bazelly B, Marsault C, Carette MF. Impact of MDCT angiography on the management of patients with hemoptysis. AJR Am J Roentgenol. 2010;195(3):772-8.
14. Meena P, Bhalla AS, Goyal A, Sharma R, Kumar A, Srivastva DN, et al. Single-phase split-bolus dual energy computed tomography angiography for evaluation of hemoptysis: a novel application. J Thorac Imaging. 2018;33(6):366-76.

15. Sopko DR, Smith TP. Bronchial artery embolization for hemoptysis. Semin Intervent Radiol. 2011;28(1):48-62.
16. Swanson KL, Johnson CM, Prakash UBS, McKusick MA, Andrews JC, Stanson AW. Bronchial artery embolization: experience with 54 patients. Chest. 2002;121(3):789-95.
17. Ramakantan R, Bandekar VG, Gandhi MS, Aulakh BG, Deshmukh HL. Massive hemoptysis due to pulmonary tuberculosis: control with bronchial artery embolization. Radiology. 1996;200(3):691-4.
18. Tang Y, Goh P, Lin M, Teo N, Shen E, Wong D. Embolization for hemoptysis: a six-year review. Cardiovasc Intervent Radiol. 2002;25(1):17-25.
19. Shao H, Wu J, Wu Q, Sun X, Li L, Xing Z, et al. Bronchial artery embolization for hemoptysis: a retrospective observational study of 344 patients. Chin Med J (Engl). 2015;128(1):58-62.
20. Tom LM, Palevsky HI, Holsclaw DS, Trerotola SO, Dagli M, Mondschein JI, et al. Recurrent bleeding, survival, and longitudinal pulmonary function following bronchial artery embolization for hemoptysis in a U.S. adult population. J Vasc Interv Radiol. 2015;26(12):1806-13.e1.
21. Fruchter O, Schneer S, Rusanov V, Belenky A, Kramer MR. Bronchial artery embolization for massive hemoptysis: long-term follow-up. Asian Cardiovasc Thorac Ann. 2015;23(1):55-60.
22. Tanomkiat W, Tanisaro K. Radiographic relationship of the origin of the bronchial arteries to the left main bronchus. J Thorac Imaging. 2003;18(1):27-33.
23. Sancho C, Escalante E, Domínguez J, Vidal J, Lopez E, Valldeperas J, et al. Embolization of bronchial arteries of anomalous origin. Cardiovasc Intervent Radiol. 1998;21(4):300-4.
24. Cauldwell EW, Siekert RG. The bronchial arteries; an anatomic study of 150 human cadavers. Surg Gynecol Obstet. 1948;86(4):395-412.
25. Uflacker R, Kaemmerer A, Picon PD, Rizzon CF, Neves CM, Oliveira ES, et al. Bronchial artery embolization in the management of hemoptysis: technical aspects and long-term results. Radiology. 1985;157(3):637-44.
26. Marshall TJ, Jackson JE. Vascular intervention in the thorax: bronchial artery embolization for hemoptysis. Eur Radiol. 1997;7(8):1221-7.
27. Furnari ML, Salerno S, Rabiolo A, Caravello V, Pardo F. Bronchial to subclavian shunt in a CF patient. A potential pitfall for embolization. J Cyst Fibros. 2003;2(4):217-9.
28. Van den Berg JC, Overtoom TT, de Valois JC. Case report: bronchial to coronary artery anastomosis—a potential hazard in bronchial artery embolization. Br J Radiol. 1996;69(822):570-2.
29. Keller FS, Rosch J, Loflin TG, Nath PH, McElvein RB. Nonbronchial systemic collateral arteries: significance in percutaneous embolotherapy for hemoptysis. Radiology. 1987;164(3):687-92.
30. Sellars N, Belli AM. Non-bronchial collateral supply from the left gastric artery in massive hemoptysis. Eur Radiol. 2001;11(1):76-9.
31. Zhang H, Jia B, Zeng L, Xiao Z, Shen J, Qian H, et al. Unexpected renal hemorrhage after endovascular repair of complicated type B aortic dissection: two cases report. BMC Surg. 2018;18:100.
32. Shin BS, Jeon GS, Lee SA, Park MH. Bronchial artery embolisation for the management of haemoptysis in patients with pulmonary tuberculosis. Int J Tuberc Lung Dis. 2011;15(8):1093-8.
33. Won JH, Park SI, Park KJ, Oh YJ, Hwang SC. Microcatheter placement through a side hole created in a 5-F catheter into proximal subclavian arterial branches causing hemoptysis. J Vasc Interv Radiol. 2004;15(8):881-4.
34. Miyayama S, Yamashiro M, Okuda M, Yoshie Y, Nakashima Y, Ikeno H, et al. The march of extrahepatic collaterals: analysis of blood supply to hepatocellular carcinoma located in the bare area of the liver after chemoembolization. Cardiovasc Intervent Radiol. 2010;33(3):513-22.
35. Barben J, Robertson D, Olinsky A, Ditchfield M. Bronchial artery embolization for hemoptysis in young patients with cystic fibrosis. Radiology. 2002;224(1):124-30.
36. Saluja S, Henderson KJ, White RI. Embolotherapy in the bronchial and pulmonary circulations. Radiol Clin North Am. 2000;38(2):425-48.
37. Chan VL, So LKY, Lam JYM, Lau KY, Chan CS, Lin AWN, et al. Major haemoptysis in Hong Kong: aetiologies, angiographic findings and outcomes of bronchial artery embolisation. Int J Tuberc Lung Dis. 2009;13(9):1167-73.
38. Lee S, Chan JWM, Chan SCH, Chan YH, Kwan TL, Chan MK, et al. Bronchial artery embolisation can be equally safe and effective in the management of chronic recurrent haemoptysis. Hong Kong Med J. 2008;14(1):14-20.
39. Hwang HG, Lee HS, Choi JS, Seo KH, Kim YH, Na JO. Risk factors influencing rebleeding after bronchial artery embolization on the management of hemoptysis associated with pulmonary tuberculosis. Tuberc Respir Dis (Seoul). 2013;74(3):111-9.
40. Yoo DH, Yoon CJ, Kang SG, Burke CT, Lee JH, Lee CT. Bronchial and nonbronchial systemic artery embolization in patients with major hemoptysis: safety and efficacy of N-butyl cyanoacrylate. AJR Am J Roentgenol. 2011;196(2):W199-204.
41. Ivanick MJ, Thorwarth W, Donohue J, Mandell V, Delany D, Jaques PF. Infarction of the left main-stem bronchus: a complication of bronchial artery embolization. AJR Am J Roentgenol. 1983;141(3):535-7.
42. Girard P, Baldeyrou P, Lemoine G, Grunewald D. Left main-stem bronchial stenosis complicating bronchial artery embolization. Chest. 1990;97(5):1246-8.
43. Chapman SA, Holmes MD, Taylor DJ. Unilateral diaphragmatic paralysis following bronchial artery embolization for hemoptysis. Chest. 2000;118(1):269-70.
44. Munk PL, Morris DC, Nelems B. Left main bronchial-esophageal fistula: a complication of bronchial artery embolization. Cardiovasc Intervent Radiol. 1990;13(2):95-7.
45. Nguyen ET, Silva CIS, Seely JM, Chong S, Lee KS, Müller NL. Pulmonary artery aneurysms and pseudoaneurysms in adults: findings at CT and radiography. Am J Roentgenol. 2007;188(2):W126-34.
46. Poplausky MR, Rozenblit G, Rundback JH, Crea G, Maddineni S, Leonardo R. Swan-Ganz catheter-induced pulmonary artery pseudoaneurysm formation: three case reports and a review of the literature. Chest. 2001;120(6):2105-11.
47. Shin S, Shin TB, Choi H, Choi JS, Kim YH, Kim CW, et al. Peripheral pulmonary arterial pseudoaneurysms: therapeutic

implications of endovascular treatment and angiographic classifications. Radiology. 2010;256(2):656-64.

48. Kuczyńska M, Pyra K, Światłowski Ł, Sobstyl J, Kuklik E, Jargiełło T. Endovascular embolisation strategies for pulmonary arteriovenous malformations. Pol J Radiol. 2018;83:e189-96.

49. White RI, Mitchell SE, Barth KH, Kaufman SL, Kadir S, Chang R, et al. Angioarchitecture of pulmonary arteriovenous malformations: an important consideration before embolotherapy. AJR Am J Roentgenol. 1983;140(4):681-6.

50. Yap CW, Wee BBK, Yee SY, Tiong V, Chua YX, Teo L, et al. The role of interventional radiology in the diagnosis and treatment of pulmonary arteriovenous malformations. J Clin Med. 2022;11(21):6282.

51. Hong J, Lee SY, Cha JG, Lim JK, Park J, Lee J, et al. Pulmonary arteriovenous malformation (PAVM) embolization: prediction of angiographically-confirmed recanalization according to PAVM diameter changes on CT. CVIR Endovasc. 2021;4(1):16.

Harish Bhujade, Naveen Kalra, Mandeep Kang, Anupam Lal, Ujjwal Gorsi

CHAPTER

21

Nonvascular Thoracic Interventions

INTRODUCTION

Image-guided thoracic interventions consist of a wide range of procedures used in the diagnosis and treatment of diseases of the chest. Percutaneous interventional procedures in the chest were actually in use before the advent of imaging. Leyden did the first transthoracic needle lung biopsy in 1882 to confirm pulmonary infections.[1] Lung biopsy continued to be used during the first half of the 20th century for confirming the microbiological diagnosis of infectious lobar consolidation. In 1964, the first fluoroscopically-guided bronchial brush biopsy was described.[2] Around the same time, the technique of transthoracic fine needle sampling in the chest was established by Nordenstrom.[3] Percutaneous mediastinal procedures were adopted on a routine basis after the advent of CT. Percutaneous drainage of fluid collections in the chest was introduced in the late seventies. Better catheter designs and refinement of embolic agents established bronchial artery embolization as an accepted technique in the next decade. Good results with minimally invasive treatment of superior vena cava (SVC) obstruction were achieved with the development of specialized stents. The commonly performed thoracic interventional radiological techniques will be discussed in this chapter. Bronchial artery embolization will be discussed in another chapter.

IMAGE GUIDANCE MODALITIES

Modalities used for image guidance include fluoroscopy, cross-sectional imaging (ultrasound, CT, and MRI) or a combination of both. Uni- or biplanar fluoroscopy was the first imaging technique which was used for the guidance of percutaneous transthoracic needle biopsy (TNB) and percutaneous drainage of fluid collections. The advantages of fluoroscopy include its wide availability, familiarity to most radiologists and real-time control of the procedure. Fluoroscopy may be used in combination with ultrasound for adjusting the tip of catheters introduced into fluid collections. Ultrasound is used for image-guided biopsies of the chest wall, pleural lesions, pulmonary lesions with parietal contact or lesions in the anterior or superior mediastinum. Using this technique, the peripheral pulmonary lesions can be successfully biopsied with very high success rates which are more than 90%.[4] The ultrasound probe should be oriented parallel to the intercostal space as this facilitates the biopsy of the peripheral pulmonary lesions. Other procedures which can be done under ultrasound guidance include percutaneous aspiration and catheter drainage. The advantages of ultrasound guidance are real-time monitoring, lack of ionizing radiation, easy availability, portability and the ability to target non-necrotic part of the lesion. CT guidance provides anatomical display of all the thoracic structures in detail and ensures accurate placement of the needle and drainage catheter. It helps to determine the optimal percutaneous entry point to avoid transgression of the pleural fissure or puncture of bullae, large vessels, bronchi, and the esophagus. Helical CT has not been found superior to sequential scanning.[5] CT fluoroscopy combines the advantages of both cross-sectional imaging and real-time control and is now widely available. High rates of technical success have been reported with sensitivity ranging from 89–95% and specificity of 100%.[6] Studies have shown that using intermittent "quick check" CT fluoroscopy between needle advancements instead of continuous fluoroscopy can reduce the radiation exposure. Recently PET-CT is being used to guide biopsies by providing information about the abnormal metabolic activity of primary neoplasm and metastases. There is scanty literature on usage of MR guidance for thoracic interventions due to limited availability of this modality and the requirement of especially designed needles compatible with MR scanners.

NONVASCULAR INTERVENTIONS

The various percutaneous nonvascular image-guided thoracic interventions are transthoracic needle biopsy, diagnostic thoracocentesis, drainage of fluid collections, pleurodesis, pneumothorax/bulla drainage, lung abscess drainage, pericardial effusion drainage, treatment of secondary pulmonary aspergilloma, endoluminal tracheobronchial stenting and thermal ablation of pulmonary malignancy.

Transthoracic Needle Biopsy of Pulmonary Lesions

Indications

Transthoracic needle biopsy (TNB) is most commonly done for the diagnosis of a solitary pulmonary nodule (SPN). TNB is also used for confirming metastatic lung disease, staging of lung cancer or extrathoracic malignancy, and sampling of suspected focal infections.[7,8]

Patient Evaluation

Before biopsy, every effort should be made to establish the identity of the lesion using noninvasive methods including review of old chest radiographs and thin section CT for nodule characterization. Some clinicians use "pulmonary nodule calculators" based on clinical and radiological risk factors to estimate pretest probability of malignancy. Coagulation parameters should be checked for all patients to exclude bleeding diathesis.

Contraindications

There are no absolute contraindications to TNB. However, percutaneous biopsy should be strictly avoided in suspected vascular lesion (e.g., arteriovenous malformation, pulmonary varix) and hydatid cyst. Bleeding diathesis should be corrected prior to the procedure. Severe pulmonary hypertension is a relative contraindication because of the danger of persistent pulmonary hemorrhage. Emphysematous bullae in the planned biopsy route increases the risk of pneumothorax and should be avoided if possible. Severe pulmonary diseases (FEV less than liter), contralateral pneumonectomy, ventilator dependence and patient's inability to cooperate or hold breath are relative contraindications.

Image Guidance

The choice of image guidance modality is dependent on the availability of various techniques, the skill and preference of the interventional radiologist, and the site, size and other characteristics of the lesion to be targeted. Fluoroscopy is particularly useful for biopsies of nodules in the lower third of the lungs, where large respiratory excursions occur. Orthogonal views of lung nodule and the needle obtained either with a rotating C-arm or a biplane fluoroscopy help confirm proper positioning of the needle tip within the lesion. CT guidance is useful for lesions that are adjacent to hilum or mediastinum (to avoid injury to adjacent vascular structures, bronchi and esophagus), for small lesions and the lesions not clearly seen on fluoroscopy **(Figs. 1A and B)**. The use of US guidance is limited to masses that are apical, juxtadiaphragmatic or adjacent to the chest wall **(Figs. 2 and 3)**. PET-CT guidance may improve the success rate of image-guided biopsies if the functional information obtained from the PET study is used to position the tip of the biopsy needle into the area of highest metabolism **(Figs. 4A to D)**. Endobronchial ultrasound (EBUS) guided biopsy is a safer technique than the percutaneous methods. However, it is expensive, not widely available and is primarily the domain of the interventional pulmonologist.

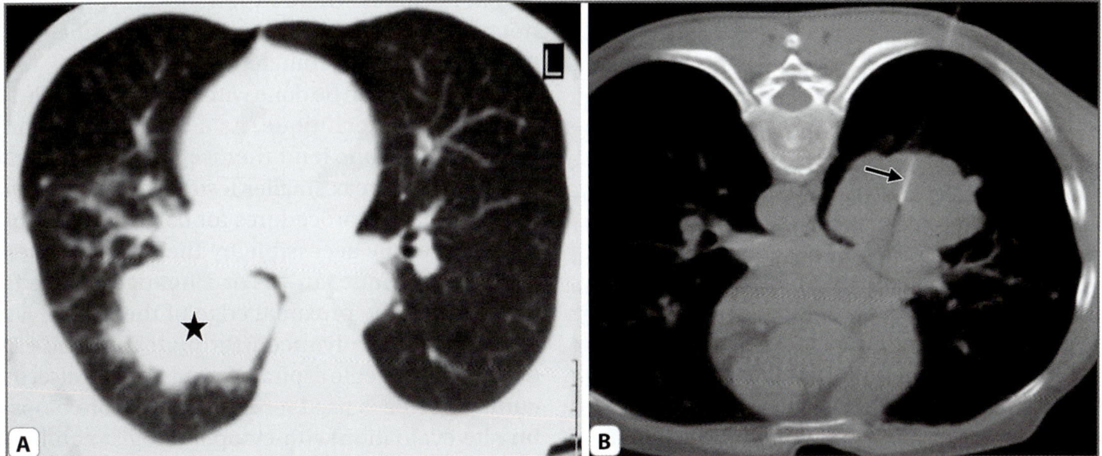

FIGS. 1A AND B: (A) Axial CT section of the chest at lung window settings shows a large mass with spiculated margins in the right hilar region. (B) Axial CT section of the chest in the prone position showing the needle in situ which has been placed in the mass after transgressing the lung parenchyma.

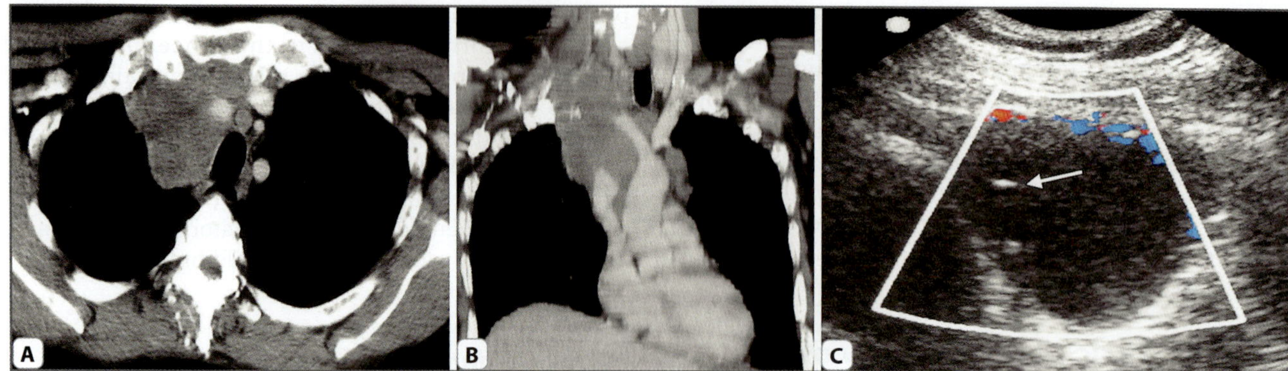

FIGS. 2A TO C: (A) Axial contrast enhanced CT section shows an apical lung mass with loss of fat planes with the trachea and the brachiocephalic artery. (B) Coronal reconstructed image showing the extent of the mass with lymph nodes in the neck region. (C) Color Doppler ultrasound showing the needle in situ (arrow). Doppler ultrasound ensures that there is no vessel in the course of the needle.

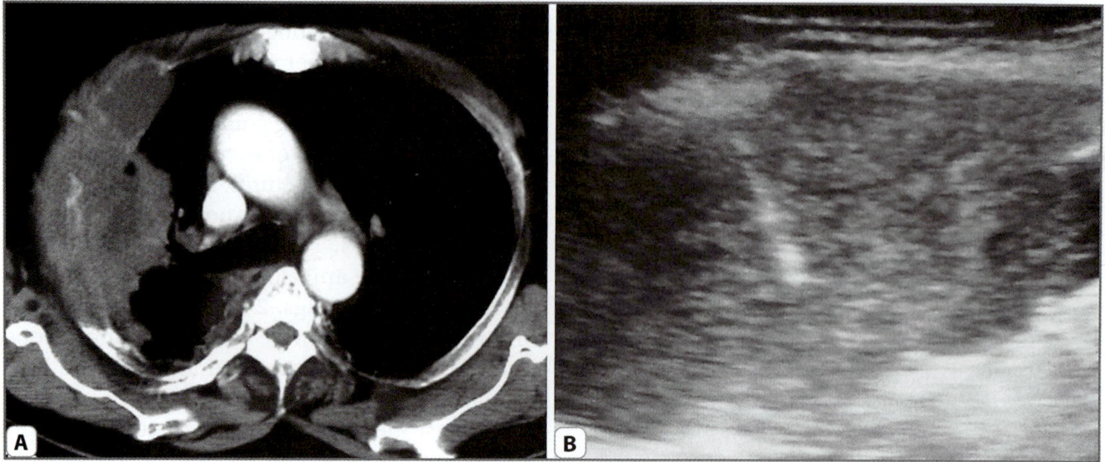

FIGS. 3A AND B: (A) Axial contrast enhanced CT section shows a large peripheral mass with necrotic component in the right upper lobe with chest wall invasion and rib destruction. (B) Ultrasound image shows the entire extent of the needle which has been introduced percutaneously into the mass.

Biopsy Technique

A wide range of needles can be used for percutaneous biopsy procedures. Needles can be classified by their caliber or gauge tip configuration and the mechanism of sample acquisition. Needle sizes can either be smaller gauge (20–25 gauge) or larger gauge (14–19 gauge). Smaller gauge needles result in lesser bleeding and reduce other complications as well. Larger gauge needles on the other hand are easier to direct and provide better samples for cytology and histology. Needles have different angles and bevel of the tip. The Chiba and spinal needles have bevel angle of 25° and 30° respectively. Greene and Franseen needles have 90° tips. Needle tips can also be aspiration (non-cutting) and cutting types. Aspiration needles such as the Chiba, spinal and Greene needles provide cellular material for cytologic evaluation of malignancy. Cutting needles yield pieces of tissue for histological analysis and can be used for the diagnosis of benign lesions, lymphoreticular malignancies, and in hospitals where experienced cytopathologists are not available. Needles can also be classified as manual, spring-loaded or automated.

The biopsy can be done with the single needle technique or the coaxial technique. As a rough guide, large easily accessible lesions lend themselves to the single needle technique whereas smaller lesions or lesions that require lengthy imaging procedures for correct needle placement are more easily accessible by the coaxial system. In the coaxial technique, an 18- or 19-gauge needle is initially advanced to the proximal edge of the lesion. A 22-gauge needle is then advanced through the guide needle to obtain a fine needle aspirate for cytology or else, a 20-gauge cutting needle is used for obtaining a core biopsy. Rapid-on-site evaluation with cytopathologist can increase the diagnostic yield and sample adequacy. Postprocedural chest radiographs, one immediately after the procedure and another 4 hours later, are obtained to rule out

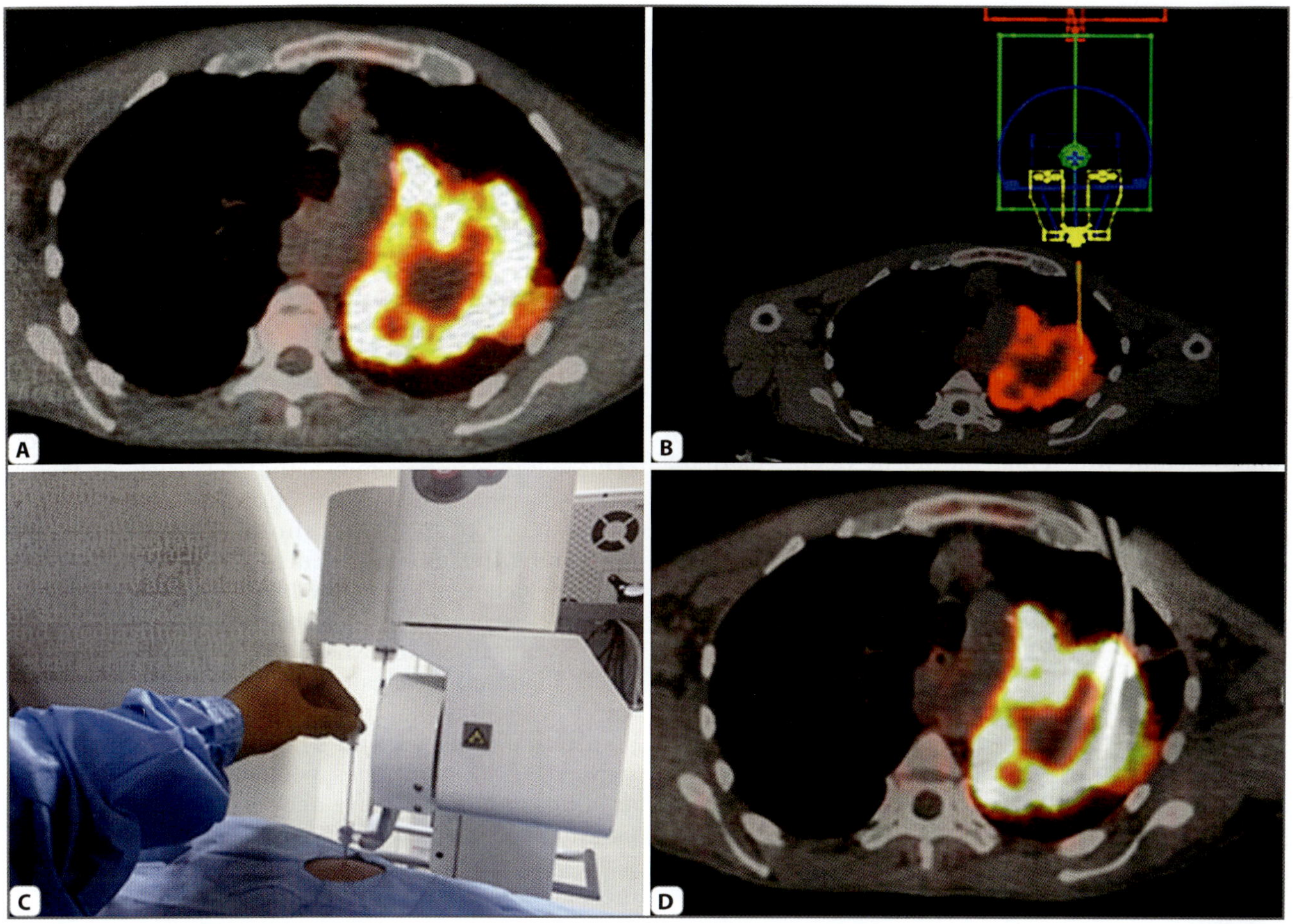

FIGS. 4A TO D: (A) Axial PET-CT functional image showing hypermetabolism in the periphery of the lesion in the left upper lobe of lung consistent with viable cells. (B) Planning of robotic arm assisted trajectory for biopsy needle placement on robotic arm console. (C) Insertion of coaxial biopsy needle along the planned trajectory with the help of robotic arm needle navigation technique. (D) Check scan to confirm the tip of the semi-automated biopsy gun in the hypermetabolic region just before sampling.

(PET-CT: positron emission tomography-computed tomography)

Courtesy: Dr Rajender Kumar Basher and Dr BR Mittal, Department of Nuclear Medicine, PGIMER, Chandigarh, India.

pneumothorax. Use of track embolization via coaxial system has been associated with decreased risk of pneumothorax or bleeding complications.

Complications

The most common complication of percutaneous lung biopsy is bleeding (hemoptysis, chest wall, parenchymal) **(Fig. 5)**. Hemoptysis occurs in about 5% of patients.[8]

Usually, it is minimal manifesting as blood-stained sputum. Rarely, however, it may be massive and may require bronchial artery embolization, balloon occlusion of the affected segmental bronchus or surgical resection.

The most complication requiring intervention is pneumothorax seen in 12–45% of the patients.[9] Having the patient lie with the puncture site dependent approximates the visceral puncture site with the parietal pleural and can decrease the rate of pneumothorax. 2–15% of pneumothoraces require treatment with chest tube

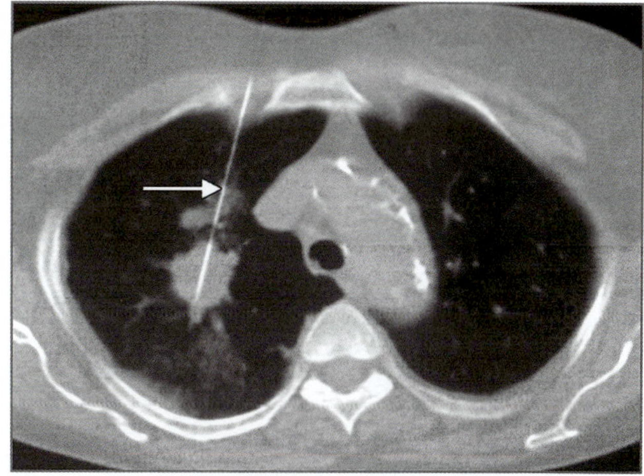

FIG. 5: Axial CT section shows a needle which has been placed in the lung nodule under CT guidance. There is presence of parenchymal hemorrhage along the needle tract (arrow).

placement **(Fig. 6)**. Large or symptomatic pneumothoraces can be treated with image-guided percutaneous placement of a small caliber catheter. The reported fatality rate of percutaneous lung biopsy is about 0.02%. The causes include tension pneumothorax, air embolism and pulmonary hemorrhage. Other uncommon complications include vasovagal reaction, lobar torsion and needle tract metastases. According to guidelines given by the Society of Interventional Radiology, a higher overall complication rate of 10% is acceptable for lung biopsies compared to 2% for all other organ systems.[10]

Results

Transthoracic needle biopsy of lung nodules is a relatively safe procedure with a high diagnostic yield. According to the guidelines for lung biopsy given by the Society of Interventional Radiology, an 85% success rate is acceptable.[10] TNB has an overall sensitivity of 70–100% in most series for the diagnosis of malignancy.[7,8] The yield for benign lesions, however, is 50% or less since benign but nonspecific results are not uncommon; this can be improved by performing both core biopsies and FNA of benign lesions.[11,12]

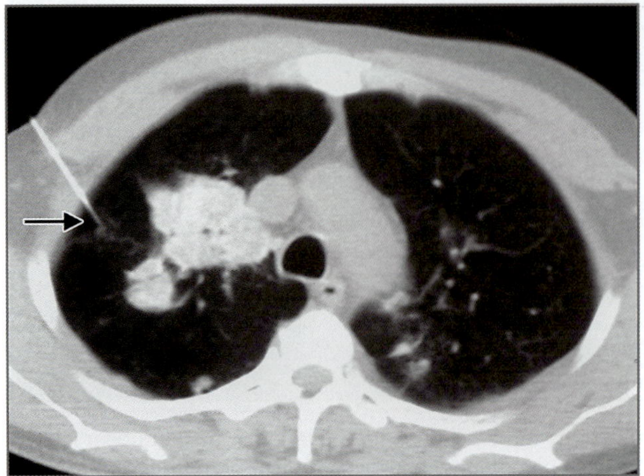

FIG. 6: Axial CT section shows presence of minimal pneumothorax at the site of needle entry. FNAC of the hilar mass was done under CT guidance in this patient (arrow). The pneumothorax was managed conservatively.

(FNAC: fine-needle aspiration cytology)

Transthoracic Needle Biopsy from Other Sites

Mediastinal masses may arise without any associated pulmonary mass and may represent metastatic disease. The best method of biopsy is determined by the location of the mass and its proximity to the vital structures. Biopsy of a mediastinal or hilar mass is usually performed under CT guidance as CT clearly shows the location of the mass and its relation to vital mediastinal structures and allows selection of the optimal biopsy path. Ultrasound guidance can be used for large lesions which are in contact with the chest wall and where a safe acoustic window is available for lesion visualization and needle placement. Anterior mediastinal masses can be accessed by the parasternal **(Figs. 7A and B)**, suprasternal and trans-sternal **(Fig. 8)** approaches, while posterior mediastinal or subcarinal masses are accessed by the posterior paravertebral approach.[13-15] To avoid complications while using the parasternal approach, one should be aware of the anatomical location of internal mammary vessels. A direct mediastinal or extrapleural approach is preferred over a transpulmonary approach, as this reduces the risk of pneumothorax. Saline injection, "salinoma", can be used to widen the paravertebral or substernal extrapleural space for a direct mediastinal approach and is helpful in decreasing the incidence of post-biopsy pneumothorax.[16] A pleural space approach through an existing pleural effusion or an iatrogenically created pneumothorax has

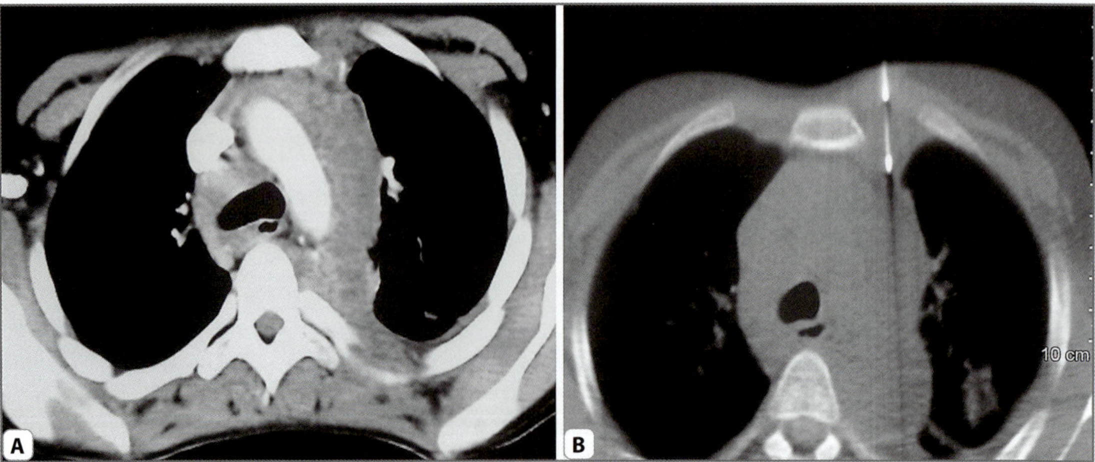

FIGS. 7A AND B: (A) Axial contrast enhanced CT shows conglomerate lymph nodes in the prevascular and precarinal location. (B) CT-guided biopsy was done in this patient by the parasternal approach.

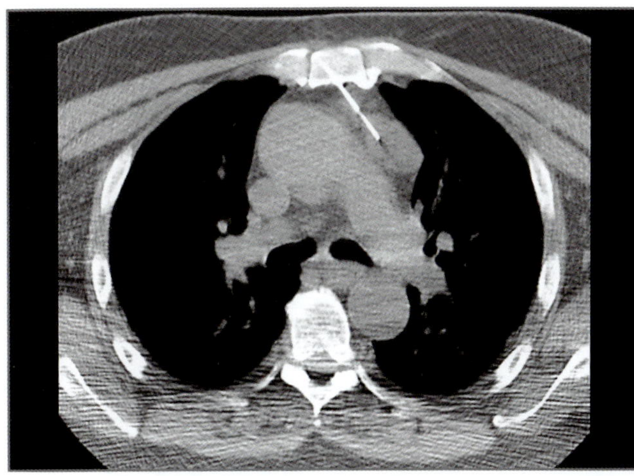

FIG. 8: CT-guided biopsy of the prevascular lymph node being done by the trans-sternal approach.

Courtesy: Dr Sanjay Gupta, MD Anderson Cancer Center, Houston, USA.

also been used for mediastinal biopsies.[17] According to the appropriateness criteria published by the American College of Radiology, nonradiologic mediastinal mass biopsy (bronchoscopically guided transbronchial FNA, transesophageal FNA, mediastinoscopy, thoracoscopy) may be safer and have higher yields compared to radiologic biopsy. However, the choices vary from institution to institution.

Percutaneous Needle Biopsy of the Pleura

Biopsies for diffuse disease are usually done without image guidance. Image-guided pleural biopsy is done for pleural masses or thickening with or without associated pleural fluid, small or loculated pleural effusions where thoracentesis has been nondiagnostic and where there are recurrent pleural effusions of unknown etiology. Most pleural biopsies are done using US guidance, although small pleural lesions require CT guidance for accurate needle placement. Solid masses or pleural thickening can be biopsied with the standard 16–20 gauge biopsy needle. Pleural effusions which are not associated with a discrete mass should be biopsied using a Cope needle system. Ultrasound guidance is able to localize even a small pleural effusion through which a core biopsy can be safely performed thus reducing the risk of pneumothorax. Complications such as pneumothorax, hemothorax, and laceration of diaphragm, liver or spleen have been reported in less than 1% of biopsies.[7]

Localization of a Nodule for Thoracoscopic Resection

Thoracoscopic resection has established itself as an effective method for diagnosing and treating a peripheral lung nodule that is near the visceral pleura. The radiologist can help by marking the lesion with a hook wire. The hook wire is inserted into the lesion through the guide needle of a coaxial system.[7]

Diagnostic Thoracocentesis

The most common indications for diagnostic thoracentesis are the evaluation of suspected infection or malignancy in the pleural space.[18,19] Sonographic guidance is used following a failed unguided thoracocentesis and when effusions are small or loculated. Using an aseptic technique an appropriate size needle (mostly 22 gauge; thicker up to 18 gauge for viscous collection) is inserted at a point where sonography shows the largest fluid dimension, and the fluid is then aspirated. A postprocedure chest radiograph should be done to rule out a pneumothorax. Ultrasound guided diagnostic aspiration is successful in as many as 97% of cases.[20] The yield for cytological examination in documented malignant effusion has been reported to be approximately 50%. Pneumothorax rate is lower (0–3%) than that reported with blind aspiration (3–20%).[21]

Percutaneous Drainage of Pleural Space Fluid Collections

Image-guided percutaneous transthoracic catheter drainage of infected pleural collections is indicated in patients in whom diagnostic thoracocentesis shows frank pus, positive Gram stain on culture or a complicated parapneumonic effusion. Catheter drainage of pleural fluid is also performed for relief of symptoms (dyspnea, cough, pleuritic chest pain).

Empyema is an infected pleural collection caused by pneumonia, bronchiectasis, and/or trauma. Light[22] suggested three stages in the development of empyema. In the acute or exudative stage, although LDH and protein levels are raised, polymorphonuclear leukocytes, pH and glucose are normal. In this stage there is presence of a nonviscous, nonloculated effusion. Most of these collections resolve when appropriate antibiotic therapy is given. The subacute or fibrinopurulent stage is characterized by fall in pH (≤7.00) and glucose (≤40 mg/dL); at this stage, catheter drainage is usually required **(Figs. 9A to C)**. In the third or organizing stage, there is fibrin deposition and a pleural peel form due to adhesion of visceral and parietal pleurae. In this stage, open thoracotomy and decortication are required for effective treatment.[19] Radiologic drainage is most effective in patients who have short duration of symptoms, free flowing or unilocular collections, absence of thick pleural peel and fluid that can be aspirated freely by needle insertion. Shankar et al.[23] found that radiologic drainage was more effective when on ultrasound the empyema was either anechoic or complex with diffusely distributed internal echoes and/or debris and no septations. On the other hand, empyemas which were complex and septated had a lower chance of successful percutaneous

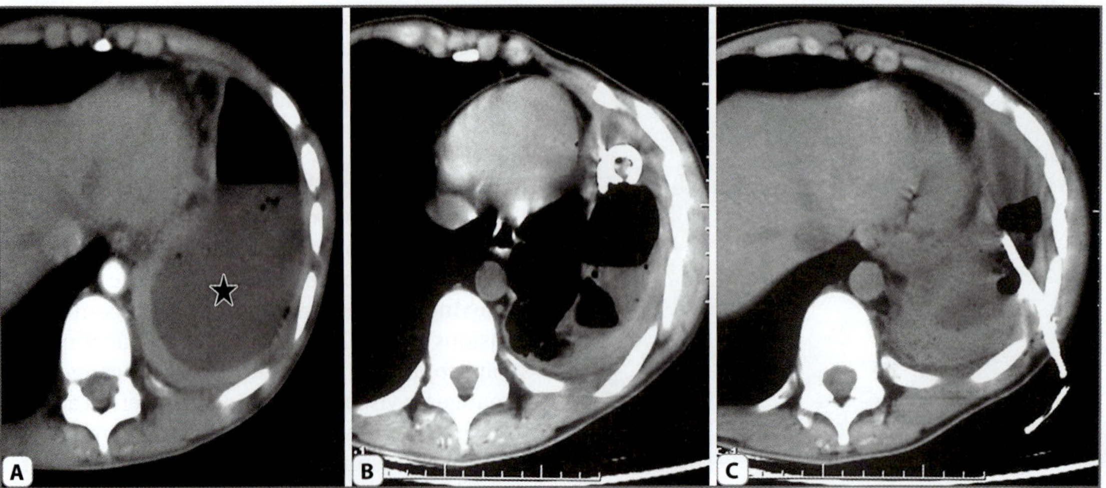

FIGS. 9A TO C: (A) Axial contrast enhanced CT section showing a loculated collection with air-fluid level with enhancing pleura on the left side. (B and C) Axial CT sections done postdrainage show significant resolution of the collection after one week of drainage.

drainage. Postoperative empyemas, particularly those associated with bronchopleural fistula usually require open surgical procedure.

Most commonly, a combination of sonography and fluoroscopy is used for guidance. Fluoroscopy allows continuous monitoring of the course of needle, guidewire and catheter. Sonography is usually used for guidance of initial needle placement, and subsequent guidewire manipulations and catheter placement are performed under fluoroscopic guidance. For large collections, the entire procedure can be safely performed under sonographic control. CT is best used to drain loculated pleural collections, pleural fluid associated with underlying parenchymal fluid consolidation, and small less accessible collections.

Catheters ranging in size from 8–30 French are introduced by the Seldinger or trocar techniques. The catheter is placed in the most dependent part of the collection and is immediately attached to a water-seal pleural drainage system with or without suction. The water-seal system not only allows a unidirectional flow but also permits visual observation of an air-leak. The patient is assessed daily for therapeutic response, amount of drainage, and catheter patency. Periodic imaging is required to assess size of the residual collection and lung re-expansion. Chest radiographs usually suffice for non-loculated collections, but CT scanning may be needed for assessing loculated collections. The drainage catheter is removed when the drainage output is less than 10 mL/day, the patient's fever and leukocyte counts have decreased, and resolution of the pleural collection is documented on imaging.

Poor drainage of pleural fluid and inadequate lung re-expansion may be secondary to improperly positioned or kinked catheter, complex fluid collection, multiple separate locules, a bronchopleural fistula, or airway obstruction. Undrained noncommunicating loculi may require additional catheters. Occasionally, repositioning of catheter or conversion to a large bore catheter may help enhance drainage. A wire advanced through the catheter can be used to disrupt septae in multiseptate collections. Intrapleural administration of fibrinolytic medication (streptokinase, urokinase, or more recently tissue plasminogen activator) may aid in septated or loculated collections. Intrapleural fibrinolytic administration helps dissolve viscous fibrinous material and septations that interfere with drainage. In one protocol, 2–4 mg of tPA in 10–20 mL saline is injected every 8 hours for several days with clamping of the tube after each instillation.[24] The reported clinical success rate is 62–100%.

Retrospective studies of radiologically guided pleural drainage procedures have shown success rates of 72–88%, which compare favorably with success rates of 66–83% reported in surgical literature.[19] Complications including bleeding due to intercostal vessel injury, pneumothorax, bronchopleural fistula, re-expansion pulmonary edema, and bacteremia are uncommon, seen in less than 2% of cases.[18,19]

Pleural Sclerotherapy or Pleurodesis

Recurrent malignant effusions can be managed by instillation of a sclerosing agent into the pleural space. This induces chemical pleurodesis. The procedure is performed by placing a catheter in the pleural space. When the catheter output drops below 100 mL/day and chest imaging shows drainage of fluid and re-expansion of the lung, sclerotherapy is performed. There should be adequate apposition of the visceral and parietal layers of the pleura for sclerosis to be effective. The agents used for this procedure include tetracycline, doxycycline, minocycline, bleomycin, diluted sodium hydroxide and talc.[18,19] A 20–50 mL of 1–2% lidocaine can be instilled into the pleural space before the sclerotic agent for analgesia.

Reported success rates range from 62–90%, and no particular agent has been shown to be superior.[18,19]

Pneumothorax Drainage

The indications for pneumothorax drainage are large volume of the air pocket (>25% of the volume of one hemithorax), an enlarging pneumothorax indicating persistent air leak, tension pneumothorax, a diseased contralateral lung or any sized pneumothorax associated with shortness of breath or severe chest pain.[18,19] Most pneumothoraces drainages can be performed using fluoroscopic guidance. However, CT guidance may be used for small and loculated air collections. The pneumothorax may be approached in two ways, either through the first or second intercostal space in the midclavicular line or through the 4th or 5th intercostal space in the anterior axillary line in females and in males with bulky pectoralis muscles. The anterior approach has the advantage of allowing easier positioning of the catheter tip in the lung apex. The lateral approach allows real-time visualization of the pneumothorax and catheter insertion is then easily performed. Catheters ranging in size from 6 to 16 French are used and are connected to an underwater seal drainage with suction or to a one-way flutter (Heimlich) valve. There is need to confirm the correct catheter placement and reduction in the pneumothorax by doing a chest radiograph immediately after the drainage. The catheter is removed when the lung remains expanded on a follow-up chest radiograph obtained 2 hours after clamping the tube and there is no evidence of air leak. Success rates range from 87 to 93% with majority of pneumothoraces resolving within 24–72 hours.

Lung Abscess Drainage

Lung abscess represents an infected collection of lung parenchyma. Primary abscesses are the result of aspiration and are caused by anaerobic bacteria. Secondary abscesses arise from adjacent infection or by hematogenous spread (e.g., pneumonia, lung cyst, septic emboli). Majority of lung abscesses respond to antibiotics, postural drainage and bronchoscopic lavage. Image-guided percutaneous catheter drainage is used for the treatment of lung abscesses that fail to resolve with medical therapy. A CT scan is done to assess the presence of pleural involvement and to plan a safe transthoracic route for catheter placement. Fluoroscopy, US or CT guidance can be used for performing the procedure. One should avoid traversing normal lungs because of the risk of hemorrhage and bronchopleural fistula formation with empyema. The catheter should transverse the abnormal lung to avoid pneumothorax and collapse of normal lungs. The patient should be positioned to keep the opposite hemothorax nondependent in order to avoid the aspiration of the abscess contents into the normal lung. As lung abscess drainage represents a controlled bronchocutaneous fistula, the size of the drainage catheter should not be more than 12–14 French to avoid large air leaks. The catheter is removed once clinical assessment and chest radiographs indicate resolution of abscess. 73–100% patients show resolution of the abscess after 10–15 days of drainage. However, complete collapse of the cavity may take longer up to 4–5 weeks as abscesses have thick walls.[3]

Mediastinal Abscess Drainage

Mediastinal abscess is a life-threatening infection which occurs subsequent to thoracic surgery or endoscopy. Mediastinal abscesses not considered for surgical drainage can be successfully drained percutaneously or by a transesophageal approach.[25] Drainage is usually done under CT guidance by a parasternal or paraspinous approach to avoid the lung. The few reported series indicate a success rate of 83–100% but 30 days mortality is high.[3]

Pericardial Effusion Drainage

Pericardial effusions require drainage when they impair the diastolic filling of the ventricles. Large pericardial effusions are caused by renal failure, metabolic or immunologic diseases, infection and malignancy. Pericardial catheter drainage is done under ultrasound guidance using a subcostal or subxiphoid approach with or without fluoroscopy. Drainage can also be done under CT guidance by the left anterolateral approach.[26]

Pneumatocele and Bulla Drainage

Percutaneous drainage of an infected or tension pneumatocele or bulla has been performed.[27,28] However, an air–fluid level within a bulla does not indicate infection and a percutaneous diagnostic aspiration should precede catheter insertion in doubtful cases **(Figs. 10A to C)**.

Secondary Pulmonary Aspergilloma

Intracavitatory aspergilloma may present with life-threatening hemoptysis and require surgical resection. However, open thoracotomy may be contraindicated in patients with severe underlying pulmonary pathology. In such patients, transthoracic instillation of amphotericin B has been described. This technique has a reported success rate of 50% for resolution of aspergilloma and 75–100% for acute control of hemoptysis.[29]

Endoluminal Tracheobronchial Stenting

Tracheobronchial airway obstruction can occur due to a malignant or benign cause. Although surgery is the treatment of choice, balloon dilatation or stenting may be done as a palliative treatment in patients who have short life expectancy or extensive airway stenosis. Balloon dilatation results in rapid improvement of the respiratory function.

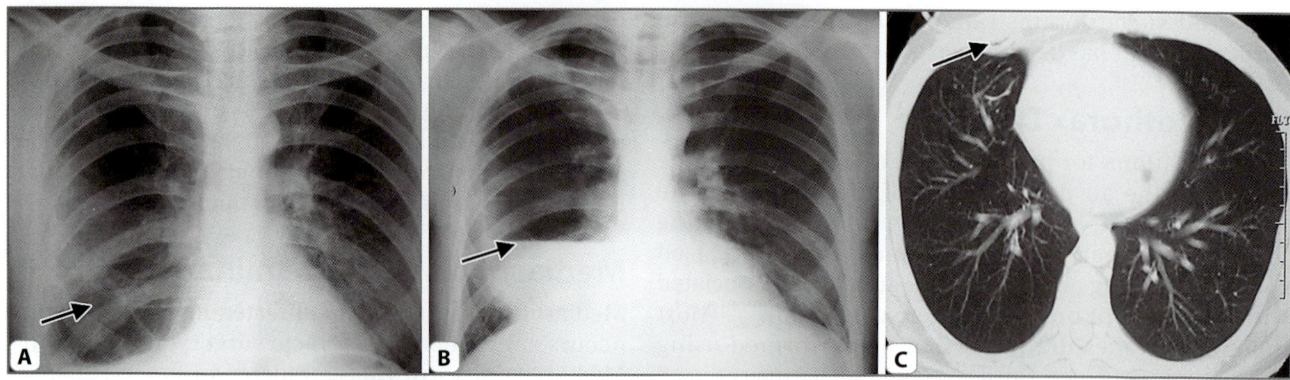

FIGS. 10A TO C: (A) Chest X-ray posteroanterior (PA) view shows multiple emphysematous bullae in the right mid and lower zones (arrow). (B) Chest X-ray PA view shows an air-fluid level in a large bulla in the right mid and lower zones (arrow) on follow-up. (C) Axial CT of the chest at lung window settings postdrainage shows the catheter in situ with resolution of the collection (arrow).

However, relief of symptoms is often short-lasting. Stents can be placed under image guidance or bronchoscopic control or by using a combination of both modalities. Tracheobronchial stenting has been successfully done for symptom palliation in patients with inoperable bronchogenic cancer, esophageal or tracheal tumors and metastatic tumors causing extensive compression or submucosal disease or tracheoesophageal fistula. It has also been done in benign conditions like postintubation or postanastomatic stricture, tracheobronchomalacia, fibrosing mediastinitis, relapsing polychondritis and amyloidosis. Helical CT is used for precise measurement of the diameter of the stenosis and for determining the location of the stenosis. Two types of stents are used: silicone stents (Dumon, Dynamic and others) and metallic stents (balloon expandable stents like Palmaz and Strecker or SEMS, self-expandable stents like Gianturco, Wallstent, Ultraflex). As some of these stents have poor visualization on conventional fluoroscopy, CT fluoroscopy guidance may be used to ensure precise and real-time control on stent deployment. Placement of stents leads to immediate and significant decrease in symptoms and respiratory function improvement in majority (80–95%) of patients. Complications of stent placement are early or late stent migration, infection, tracheobronchial fistula, deformation or breakage of stent and stent obstruction by secretions, granulations or tumor overgrowth.

THERMAL ABLATION OF LUNG LESIONS

The three most commonly used ablative techniques in the lung are radiofrequency ablation (RFA), microwave ablation (MWA) and cryoablation. These ablative techniques are used in the management of inoperable nonsmall cell lung cancer (NSCLC) and in selected patients with pulmonary metastases. Surgical resection is the gold standard for the treatment of stage I NSCLC. Unfortunately, only about one-third of patients are suitable for surgical resection due to various comorbidities or poor cardiopulmonary reserves. Dupuy et al. reported the first clinical experience of percutaneous RFA of lung lesions in the year 2000.[30] RFA is a minimally invasive thermal energy delivery system. It delivers a high frequency alternating current supplied by a radiofrequency generator through a needle electrode placed in the tumor. The application of an alternating current results in ionic agitation and generation of frictional heat which ablates the tumor tissue. As air is a thermal insulator, the aerated lung has high electric impedance. Lung tumors are well suited for RFA as the surrounding normal lung parenchyma acts as an insulator for the heat energy delivered. Hence, less power input is required to achieve adequate ablation. By the same principle, pleural based lesions require more energy to treat and are associated with higher recurrence rates and complications. However, a longer approach traversing atleast 2 cm of aerated lung is recommended even for peripheral tumors to prevent air leak, chest pain, and skin burns. When ablating lung tumors, tract cautery should be avoided to circumvent the risk of bronchopleural fistula formation.

The outcome of ablation is more promising in metastatic disease compared with primary malignancies and in lesions smaller than 3 cm in size. Most centers limit RFA to patients with five or fewer lesions and use 5 cm as the upper limit for size.[31] Contraindications for the procedure include lesions which are close to vessels (within 1 cm), poor lung function, presence of pacemaker and coagulopathy. The lesions are treated in a predetermined order, typically starting with the most dependent lesions as they may be obscured by blood from more anterior lesions as the treatment progresses **(Figs. 11A and B)**. CT done at this time shows the ablated lesion surrounded by ground glass opacity (GGO). The treatment is considered technically complete when the entire tumor is surrounded by GGOs **(Figs. 12A and B)**. Complications of the procedure include pneumothorax,

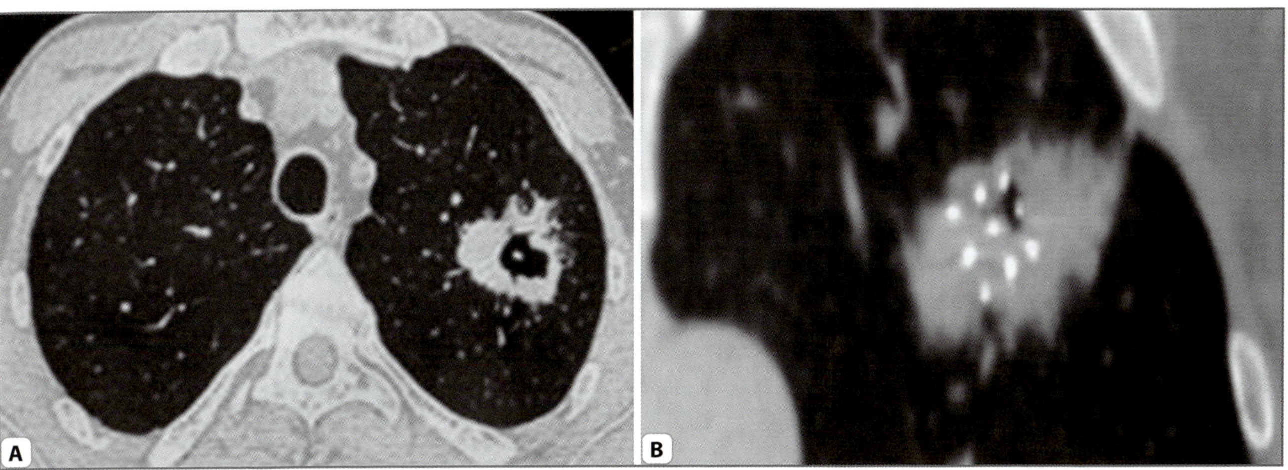

FIGS. 11A AND B: (A) Axial CT in the supine position at lung window settings shows a malignant cavitory nodule in the left upper lobe. (B) Coronal CT section during RF ablation shows the hyperattenuation with increase in the size of the nodule contributed by intraparenchymal hemorrhage.

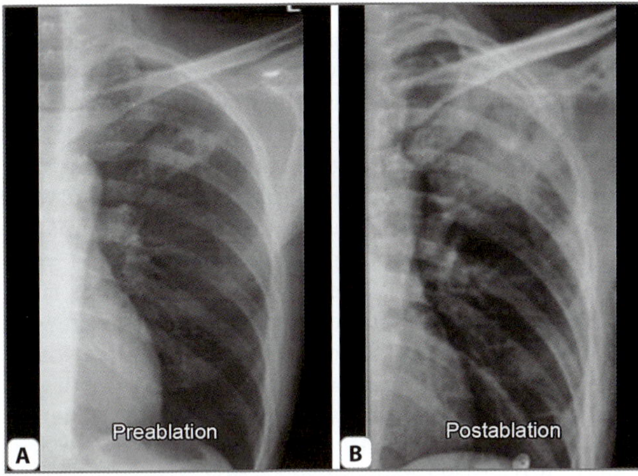

FIGS. 12A AND B: (A) Preablation chest X-ray showing cavitory lesion in left upper lobe. (B) Postablation chest X-ray showing a larger area of opacity due to the surrounding congestion and hemorrhage.

hemothorax, infective complications and tumor ablation syndrome. Symptoms of ablation syndrome include myalgia, fever and productive cough.

Follow-up imaging is done at 1 month and then at 3 months intervals for the first year. The criterion for complete resolution is reduction of the contrast enhancement compared with images taken before the procedure. A CT attenuation higher than 15 HU indicates disease persistence or relapse.[32] The postablation evolution of the lesion on imaging and histology is divided into three phases: early (<1 week), intermediate (1 week to 3 months) and late (>3 months) phases.[33] In the early phase, there are three layers of tissue seen on histology: an inner layer of thermal damage, a middle layer of alveolar congestion and an outer layer of congestion, hemorrhage and both damaged and viable cells. On CT the lesion is surrounded by an inner layer of GGO corresponding to the inner and middle layers on histology, and an outer thin, dense rim corresponding to the outer layer on histology. In the intermediate phase, there is granulation and fibrosis of the necrotic tissue. The size of the ablation zone may still exceed the size of the tumor in this phase. The benign periablational enhancement pattern still persists. In the late phase, the fibrous transformation is completed. The ablated area will be seen as fibrotic, nodular or cavitatory. CT done at this time should be taken as baseline examination in order to evaluate progression or recurrence. Even with PET-CT, an active lesion does not definitely represent tumor in the first three months.[34]

In the RAPTURE study (a prospective, intention-to-treat, multicenter trial), 106 patients (33 patients with primary disease, 73 patients with pulmonary metastases) with 183 lung tumors smaller than 3.5 cm were treated with RFA.[35] The study showed a 1-year overall complete response rate of 88% and a 2-year cancer-specific survival of 92% for primary disease. In another study of pulmonary metastases, RFA was found to be an effective treatment option for nodules less than 2 to 3 cm with a 4-year local efficacy of 89%.[36]

Microwave ablation is now becoming the favored technique for treating lung malignancies. It uses electromagnetic energy which is at a much higher frequency than RFA (300 MHz to 300 GHz). It delivers all the benefits of RFA and has several advantages.[37] The ablative zone is larger and is less susceptible to heat sink effect. The various benefits include consistently higher intratumoral temperatures, an improved convection profile, the capability of using multiple applicators, larger tumor ablation volumes and no need for grounding pads. Tumors smaller than 2 cm in maximal diameter are treated with a single applicator and tumors 2 cm or larger are treated with multiple antennae each powered by individual microwave generators. The

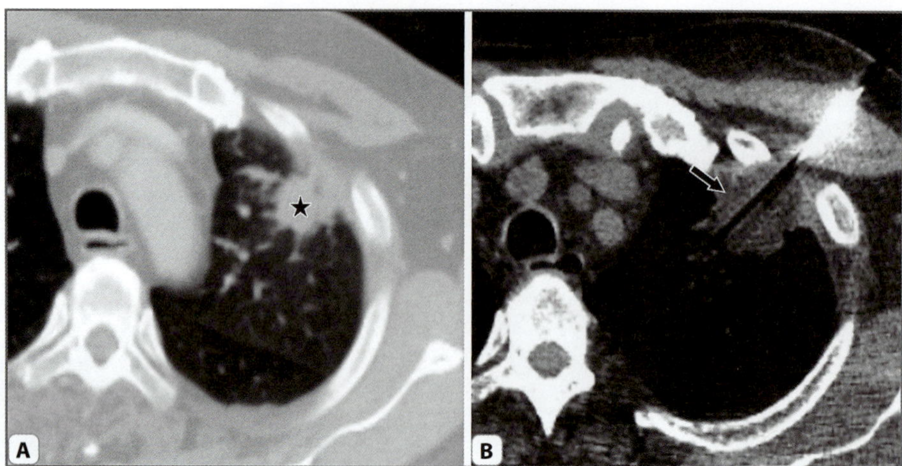

FIGS. 13A AND B: Axial CT images (A) lung window showing speculated nodule (asterix) in left upper lobe in 67-year-old male and (B) hypodense oval ice ball formation during cryoablation of same lung nodule.

reported cancer-specific 1-year survival is 83%, 2-year survival is 73% and 3-year survival is 61% for pulmonary tumors of mean size of 3.5 cm.[37]

Cryoablation works on the principle of freeze-thaw-freeze cycle. Pressurized argon gas is used to generate temperatures of less than –40°C and helium is used to increase the temperature to 20°C. There is cell rupture, protein denaturation and microvascular thrombosis-induced ischemia. One can accurately visualize the ablation zone as an "ice ball" on CT scan **(Fig. 13)**. Immunological modulation is a very well-known phenomenon with cryoablation which may help increase the efficacy of immunotherapy in cryoablation. Presently, cryoablation is considered safer than RFA and MWA for lung tumors near the chest wall or mediastinum. The newer cryoablation devices have the cautery option unlike the older equipment which decreases the risk of bleeding complications like pulmonary hemorrhage, hemoptysis and hemothorax.[38] However, the potential risk of a severe systemic adverse effect, i.e., cryoshock still remains.

VASCULAR INTERVENTIONS

The various vascular interventions are bronchial artery embolization, pulmonary artery embolization, superior vena cava (SVC) stenting and percutaneous vascular foreign body retrieval. Bronchial artery embolization will be discussed in another chapter.

Pulmonary Artery Embolization

Pulmonary artery embolization is done for pulmonary artery aneurysms and pulmonary arteriovenous malformations (PAVMs). Aneurysms and pseudoaneurysms of pulmonary arteries have several causes. The main pulmonary artery may be dilated by left-to-right shunts or pulmonary artery hypertension. Poststenotic dilatation following pulmonary valve disease may mimic an aneurysm. Central pulmonary artery aneurysms are caused by congenital disorders or vasculitis. Multiple aneurysms may be seen with infection (e.g., Rasmussen's aneurysms in tuberculosis, following septic emboli, necrotizing pneumonia, syphilis). Large pulmonary artery aneurysms present with hemoptysis, chest pain or dyspnea or may be seen as an incidental finding on CT or chest X-ray.

Pseudoaneurysms are usually seen in the right middle or lower lobe arteries. Distal arterial rupture with pseudoaneurysm formation is a rare complication of Swan–Ganz catheter placement. The patients present with hemoptysis or a lung mass on imaging studies. There is increase in incidence of *Mucor*-related pseudoaneurysms since COVID-19 pandemic. Transcatheter embolization of the parent artery with coils or vascular plugs is the treatment of choice and is usually successful **(Figs. 14 and 15)**.

PAVMs occur sporadically or in patients with hereditary hemorrhagic telangiectasia (HHT), also known as Osler-Weber-Rendu syndrome. PAVMs may also occur secondary to trauma. HHT is an autosomal dominant disorder in which there are telangiectasias of the mouth and telangiectasias or AVMs of the brain, gastrointestinal tract (GIT), liver, and lungs. Pulmonary AVMs are seen in 20–50% of patients with HHT and 60% have multiple lesions. Many patients are present with epistaxis.

The majority (90%) of AVMs are simple and have single segmental arterial supply. The rest are complex and have multiple segmental arterial supply. They are usually found in the lower lobes. The PAVMs are direct communications between pulmonary artery branches and veins and thus cause a right-to-left shunt. This results in dyspnea, fatigue, hemoptysis, stroke or brain abscess. The primary indication for embolization of PAVMs is prevention of neurologic complications.

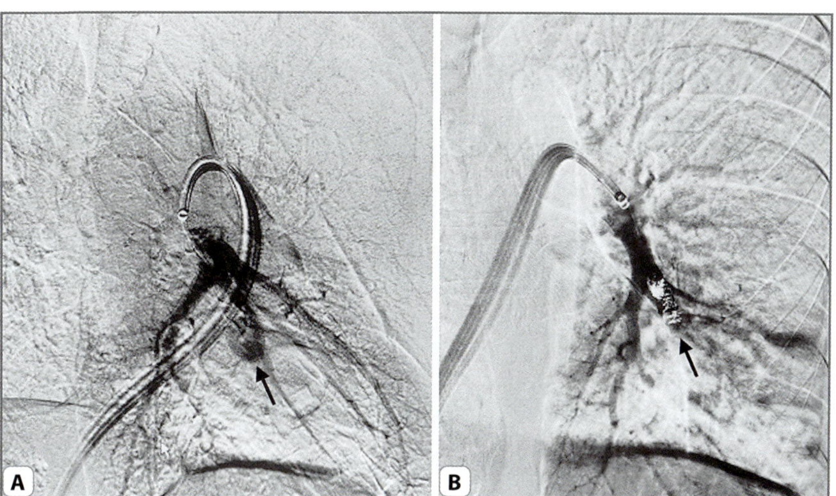

FIGS. 14A AND B: (A) Pulmonary angiogram showing contrast filled outpouching (arrow) arising from a branch of lower lobar pulmonary artery. (B) The branch supplying the pseudoaneurysm is embolized using microcoils (arrow).

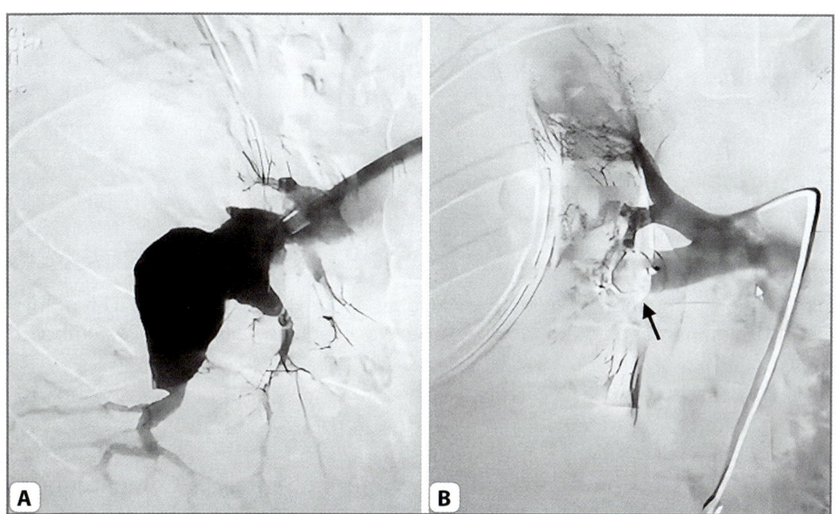

FIGS. 15A AND B: (A) Pulmonary angiogram in patient with *Mucor* infection showing large lobulated contrast-filled outpouching arising from a right descending pulmonary artery. (B) The branch supplying the pseudoaneurysm is embolized using vascular plug (arrow).

CT angiography is done to identify all feeding arteries. Pulmonary embolotherapy is the treatment of choice.[39] Many devices have been used for occlusion including coils and detachable balloons or vascular plugs **(Figs. 16A to D)**. Coils should be 1–2 mm larger than the artery being embolized and should be deployed near the nidus of the malformations. In small feeding arteries (<5 mm in diameter), detachable balloons may be preferred due to the precision of placement. Embolization is successful in more than 90% of patients. Postembolization syndrome with fever and chest pain is common. Complications occur in 10–20% of cases. Serious complications include paradoxical embolization of air or of the embolization device. All catheter and guide wire exchanges and coil introduction should be done "under water" to avoid air embolism to the brain.

Endovascular Therapy of SVC Obstruction

The superior vena cava (SVC) may be obstructed as a result of luminal disease (thrombus or tumor), extrinsic compression (tumor or lymph node) or mural disease (intimal hyperplasia or tumor invasion). Fibrosing mediastinitis is a localized or diffuse infiltrative disease that may be idiopathic or may be caused by chronic infection. The SVC is involved in one-third of cases. Significant SVC or bilateral brachiocephalic vein stenosis or obstruction

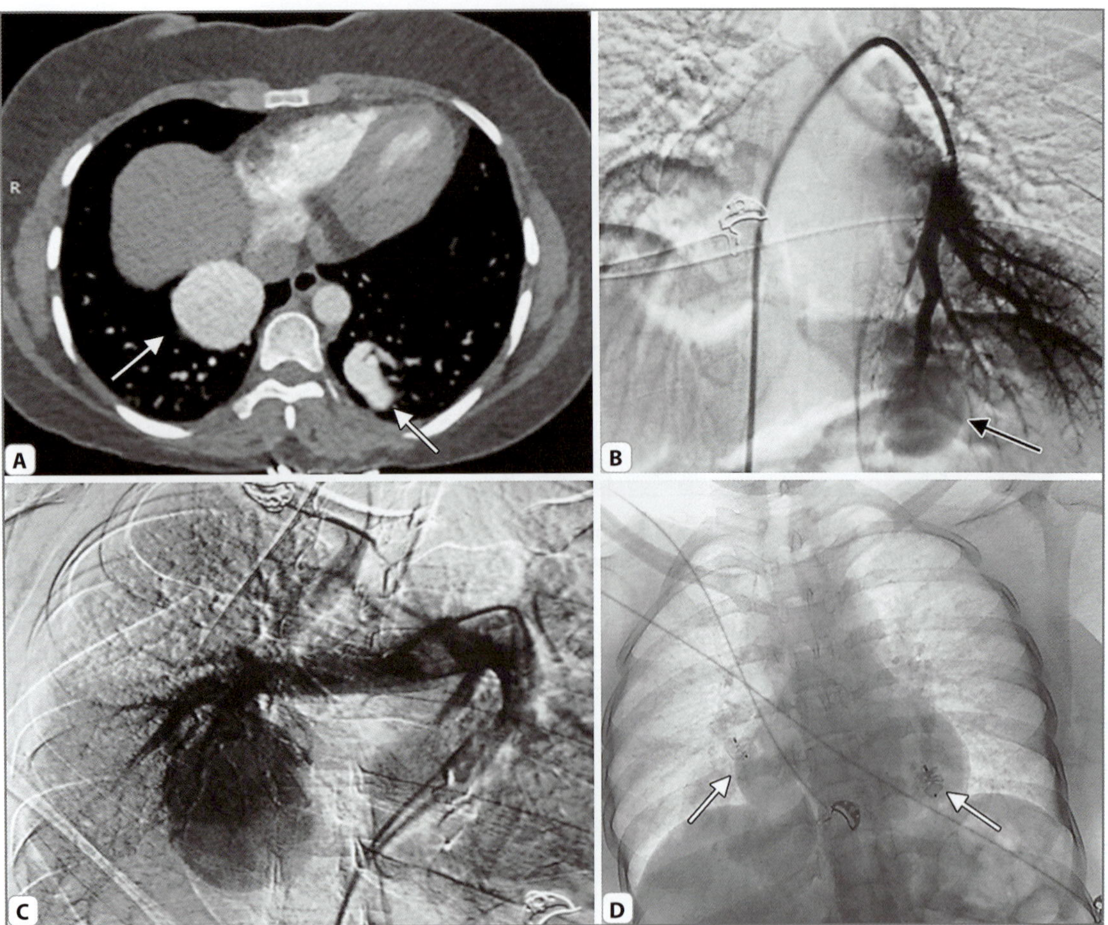

FIGS. 16A TO D: (A) Axial CECT showing pulmonary AVMs in lower lobes of both lungs (arrows). (B) Left pulmonary angiogram showing AVM in left lower lobe. (C) Right pulmonary angiogram showing large AVM in right lower lobe. (D) Postembolization radiograph showing both vascular plugs (arrows).

(AVM: arteriovenous malformation; CECT: contrast enhanced computerized tomography)

may lead to SVC syndrome. This is characterized by marked facial and neck swelling, bilateral arm swelling, cyanosis, shortness of breath, hoarseness and headache. Catheter directed therapy is considered only in patients with moderate to severe symptoms who fail to respond to less aggressive measures. SVC occlusion itself is rarely fatal, and most patients die due to the underlying malignant disease. Therefore, the aim of treatment is only short-term palliation of symptoms. Long-term patency is required in patients with benign SVC obstruction. Intravascular stents are effective in both benign and malignant SVC obstruction. In patients with benign obstruction, PTA is done before stenting. It probes the degree of stenosis and localizes the level of maximum resistance within the stenosed segment. PTA is not done prior to stenting in malignant disease but should be done after stenting to establish optimal venous return. Relative contraindications to the procedure are preterminal patients with malignant disease, extensive chronic venous thrombosis, endoluminal tumor growth and upper limb paralysis. Complications include stent migration or misplacement, formation of de novo thrombosis and pulmonary embolism.

Percutaneous Vascular Foreign Body Retrieval

The percutaneous method of retrieval avoids thoracotomy and open-heart surgery. The foreign bodies needing retrieval include lost central venous lines, Swan–Ganz catheters, ventriculoatrial shunts, port-a-cath, cardiac stimulator lines and pacemaker electrodes. Relative contraindications for retrieval are free-floating thrombus attached to the foreign body and chronic incorporation of the foreign body in a thrombus or vessel wall. The extraction is done by loop-snare technique, helical basket entrapment or the grasping forceps technique or a combination of the above **(Figs. 17A and B)**. The reported success rate of closed percutaneous retrieval is >90%.[40]

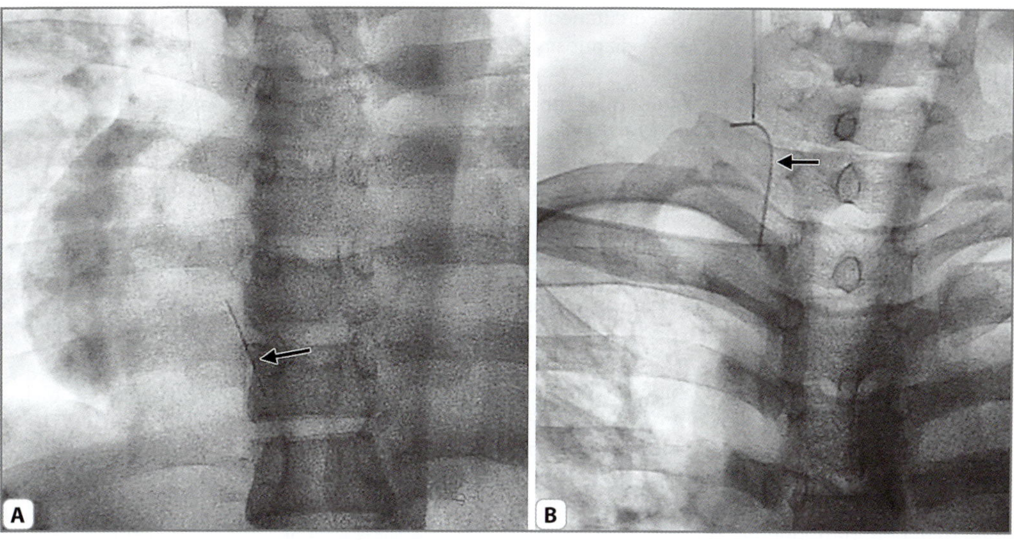

FIGS. 17A AND B: A piece of broken dialysis catheter guidewire (arrow in A) was successfully retrieved using snare (arrow in B).

Lung Chemoembolization/ Chemoinfusion

Chemoembolization in lung cancers can be performed from bronchial arteries, nonbronchial systemic arteries or pulmonary arteries depending upon the predominant supply to tumors. Chemoembolization is usually performed with chemotherapeutic agent (e.g., mitomycin) plus lipiodol solution. Recent phase I trial by Boas et al. showed that the chemoembolization in lung cancer is safe and technically successful.[41]

There are a few studies on safety and effectiveness of intra-arterial chemoinfusion using gemcitabine and cisplatin which showed promising results.[42] However, more studies are required to validate the efficacy of intraarterial therapies in unresectable lung cancers.

CONCLUSION

There is a myriad of procedures that can be performed by the interventional radiologist in the chest. However, there needs to be a close association between the radiologists, pulmonologists, oncologists, pathologists and thoracic surgeons to ensure the success of these procedures. The complication rate can also be kept low by following the prescribed guidelines for these interventions.

REFERENCES

1. Leyden OO. Uber infectiose pneumonie. Dtsch Med Wochenschr. 1883;9:52-5.
2. Hattori S, Matsuda M, Sugiyama T, Matsuda H. Cytologic diagnosis of early lung cancer: brushing method under X-ray television fluoroscopy. Dis Chest. 1964;45:129-42.
3. Ghaye B, Dondelinger RF. Imaging guided thoracic interventions. Eur Respir J. 2001;17:507-28.
4. Park B, Park J, Shin KM, Lim JK, Hong J, Cha JG, et al. Ultrasound-guided lung biopsy for small (≤2 cm) subpleural lung lesions: comparison of diagnostic yield and safety with larger lesions. J Thorac Dis. 2023;15(5):2485-96.
5. Ghaye B, Dondelinger RF, Dewe W. Percutaneous CT-guided lung biopsy: sequential versus spiral scanning. A randomized prospective study. Eur Radiol. 1999;9:1317-20.
6. Iguchi T, Matsui Y, Tomita K, Uka M, Umakoshi N, Munetomo K, et al. CT fluoroscopy-guided biopsy of pulmonary lesions contacting the interlobar fissure: An analysis of 72 biopsies. Diagn Interv Imaging. 2022;103(6):302-9.
7. Constantinescu A, Stoicescu ER, Iacob R, Chira CA, Cocolea DM, Nicola AC, et al. CT-Guided Transthoracic Core-Needle Biopsy of Pulmonary Nodules: Current Practices, Efficacy, and Safety Considerations. J Clin Med. 2024;13(23):7330.
8. Klein JS, Zarka MA. Transthoracic needle biopsy. Radiol Clin North Am. 2000;38:235-66.
9. Gupta S, Wallace MJ, Cardella JF, Kundu S, Miller DL, Rose SC, et al. Quality improvement guidelines for percutaneous needle biopsy. J Vasc Interv Radiol. 2010;21:969-75.
10. Cardella JF, Bakal CW, Bertino RE, Burke DR, Drooz A, Haskal Z, et al. Quality improvement guidelines for image-guided percutaneous biopsy in adults. J Vasc Interv Radiol. 2003;14:S227-30.
11. Saggiante L, Biondetti P, Lanza C, Carriero S, Ascenti V, Piacentino F, et al. Computed-Tomography-Guided Lung Biopsy: A Practice-Oriented Document on Techniques and Principles and a Review of the Literature. Diagnostics (Basel). 2024;14(11):1089.

12. Greif J, Marmor S, Schwarz Y, Staroselsky AN. Percutaneous core needle biopsy vs. fine needle aspiration in diagnosing benign lung lesions. Acta Cytol. 1999;43:756-60.
13. Protopapas Z, Westcott JL. Transthoracic hilar and mediastinal biopsy. Radiol Clin North Am. 2000;38:281-91.
14. Gupta S, Gulati M, Rajwanshi A, Gupta D, Suri S. Sonographically guided fine-needle aspiration biopsy of superior mediastinal lesions by the suprasternal route. Am J Roentgenol. 1998;171:1303-6.
15. Gupta S, Wallace MJ, Morello FA Jr, Ahrar K, Hicks ME. CT-guided percutaneous needle biopsy of intra-thoracic lesions by using the trans-sternal approach: Experience in 37 patients. Radiology. 2002;222:57-62.
16. Langen HJ, Klose KC, Keulers P, Adam G, Jochims M, Günther RW. Artificial widening of the mediastinum to gain access for extra pleural biopsy: Clinical results. Radiology. 1995;196: 703-06.
17. Bressler EL, Kirkham JA. Mediastinal masses: alternative approaches to CT-guided needle biopsy. Radiology. 1994;191:391-6.
18. Christopher DJ, Gupta R, Thangakunam B. Pleural effusion guidelines from ICS and NCCP Section 1: Basic principles, laboratory tests and pleural procedures. Lung India. 2024;41(3):230-48.
19. Klein JS, Schultz S, Heffner JE. Interventional radiology of the chest: Image-guided percutaneous drainage of pleural effusions, lung abscess, and pneumothorax. Am J Roentgenol. 1995;164:581-8.
20. Vetrugno L, Guadagnin GM, Orso D, Boero E, Bignami E, Bove T. An easier and safe affair, pleural drainage with ultra-sound in critical patient: a technical note. Crit Ultrasound J. 2018;10(1):18.
21. Collins TR, Sahn SA. Thoracocentesis: Clinical value, complications, technical problems, and patent experience. Chest. 1987;91:817-22.
22. Light RW. Parapneumonic effusions and empyema. Clin Chest Med. 1985;6:55-62.
23. Shankar S, Gulati M, Kang M, Gupta D, Suri S. Image-guided percutaneous drainage of thoracic empyema: Can sonography predict the outcome? Eur Radiol. 2000;10:495-9.
24. D'Agostino HB, Hurvitz D, Nall L, Toledo EG, Sangster GP. Transcatheter fluid drainage. In: Valji K (Eds). Vascular and Interventional Radiology, Elsevier, 2006; pp. 516-31.
25. Gobien RP, Stanley JH, Gobien BS, Vujic I, Pass HI. Percutaneous catheter aspiration and drainage of suspected mediastinal abscesses. Radiology. 1984;151:69-71.
26. Szapiro D, Ghaye B, Dondelinger RF. Pericardial tamponade: CT-guided percutaneous drainage. J Interv Radiol. 1996;11: 129-31.
27. Sewall LE. Franco AI, Wojtowycz MM, McDermott JC. Pneumatoceles causing respiratory compromise. Treatment by percutaneous decompression. Chest. 1993;103:1266-7.
28. Kalra N, Aiyappan SK, Jindal SL, Khandelwal N. Image-guided percutaneous drainage of an emphysematous bulla with a fluid level. Indian J Radiol Imaging. 2010;20:34-6.
29. Lang M, Lang AL, Chauhan N, Gill A. Non-surgical treatment options for pulmonary aspergilloma. Respir Med. 2020;164:105903.
30. Dupuy DE, Zagoria RJ, Akerley W, Mayo-Smith WW, Kavanagh PV, Safran H. Percutaneous radiofrequency ablation of malignancies in the lung. Am J Roentgenol. 2000;174:57-9.
31. Roy AM, Bent C, Fotheringham T. Radiofrequency ablation of lung lesions: Practical applications and tips. Curr Probl Diagn Radiol. 2009;38:44-52.
32. Akeboshi M, Yamakado K, Nakatsuka A, Hataji O, Taguchi O, Takao M, et al. Percutaneous radiofrequency ablation of lung neoplasms: Initial therapeutic response. J Vasc Interv Radiol. 2004;15:463-70.
33. Vogl TJ, Nour-Eldin NA, Albrecht MH, Kaltenbach B, Hohenforst-Schmidt W, Lin H, et al. Thermal ablation of lung tumors: Focus on microwave ablation. Rofo. 2017;189: 828-43.
34. Bonichon F, Palussiere, Godbert Y, Pulido M, Descat E, Devillers A, et al. Diagnostic accuracy of 18F-FDG PET/CT for assessing response to radiofrequency ablation treatment in lung metastases: a multicentric prospective study. Eur J Nucl Med Mol Imaging. 2013;40:1817-27.
35. Lencioni R, Crocetti L, Cioni R, Suh R, Glenn D, Regge D, et al. Response to radiofrequency ablation of pulmonary tumours: a prospective, intention-to-treat, multicentre clinical trial (the RAPTURE study). Lancet Oncol. 2008;9:621-8.
36. de Baere T, Auperin A, Deschamps F, Chevallier P, Gaubert Y, Boige V, et al. Radiofrequency ablation is a valid treatment option for lung metastases: experience in 566 patients with 1037 metastases. Ann Oncol. 2015;26:987-91.
37. Wolf FJ, Grand D, Machan JT, Dipetrillo TA, Mayo-Smith WW, Dupuy DE. Microwave ablation of lung malignancies: Effectiveness, CT findings, and safety in 50 patients. Radiology. 2008;247:871-9.
38. Lee KS, Erinjeri JP. Decision making in interventional oncology: Ablative options in the lung. Semin Intervent Radiol. 2017;34:176-81.
39. Mager JJ, Overtoom TT, Blauw H, Lammers JWJ, Westermann CJJ. Embolotherapy of pulmonary arteriovenous malformation: Long-term results in 112 patients. J Vasc Interv Radiol. 2004;15:451-6.
40. Leite TFO, Pazinato LV, Bortolini E, Pereira OI, Nomura CH, Filho JMDML. Endovascular Removal of Intravascular Foreign Bodies: A Single-Center Experience and Literature Review. Ann Vasc Surg. 2022;82:362-76.
41. Boas FE, Kemeny NE, Sofocleous CT, Yeh R, Thompson VR, Hsu M, et al. Bronchial or Pulmonary Artery Chemoembolization for Unresectable and Unablatable Lung Metastases: A Phase I Clinical Trial. Radiology. 2021; 301(2):474-84.
42. Yuan Z, Li WT, Ye XD, Dong S, Peng WJ. Intra-arterial infusion chemotherapy for advanced non-small-cell lung cancer: preliminary experience on the safety, efficacy, and clinical outcomes. J Vasc Interv Radiol. 2013;24(10):1521-8.e4.

Priya Jagia, Niraj Nirmal Pandey

CHAPTER

22 Chest Radiograph in Cardiac Disease

INTRODUCTION

Chest radiography is an important imaging technique used for assessment of heart disease.[1] A skilled interpretation of the chest radiograph may disclose important morphological changes and to some extent even indicate the functional status of the cardiovascular system. Despite the fact that it usually provides an indirect (inferential) information, and that other more specific imaging techniques for non-invasive cardiac imaging have now become available, the chest radiograph remains a widely available, economical and often the first examination performed in a patient with suspected cardiac disease. The size and shape of cardiac shadow can be determined and retained as a permanent record for future reference. A proper understanding of normal anatomy is essential for correct interpretation of pathological states.

The evaluation of the chest radiograph must begin with the assessment of the situs. Normally, in the upper abdomen, the liver and the inferior vena cava (IVC) lie on the right side, and the gastric fundus and the spleen lie on the left side. The systemic venous atrium lies on the right side and opposite the gastric fundus. This relationship is referred to as the "viscero-atrial situs" meaning that the atrial situs almost always conforms to the situs of the upper abdomen, irrespective of the situs or position of the remainder of the heart. The right-sided bronchus is shorter, wider, and more vertically oriented than the left bronchus. The right lung is tri-lobed whereas the left lung is bi-lobed. This is referred to as the "bronchial situs". In addition, the ascending aorta is generally on the same side as the systemic venous atrium and opposite the side of the gastric fundus.

Situs solitus implies that the liver, IVC, right atrium, and right-sided bronchus are on the right side, and the gastric fundus, spleen, and left-sided bronchus are on the left side. The position of the cardiac apex is not directly related to the visceroatrial situs and may not correspond with it. In addition, other issues to be considered include atrioventricular and ventriculoarterial connections, the loop of the aorta (dextro or levo), and the relation of cardiac chambers to each other.

CARDIAC SILHOUETTE

Cardiac Shape

Depending upon the build of the subjects, three types of shape may be encountered on a frontal radiograph. In hyposthenic individuals, it is long and narrow, in hypersthenic individuals, it is of transverse type, and in moderately built individuals, it is oblique or globular in shape. In adults, two-thirds of the heart lies on the left and one-third on the right side of mid-line. In infants, the heart is of transverse or globular type, and the right heart is almost equal in size to the left. In infants and young children, the thymic tissue often obscures the base of the heart and great vessels. By the age of 5–7 years, the globular infant heart attains the adult shape.

Cardiac Contours

Posteroanterior View

The right heart border consists of two segments. The upper segment is nearly vertical in normal young adults and is formed by the superior vena cava (SVC). The lower segment is usually convex and represents the lateral border of the right atrium (RA) separated by a notch. In old age, the upper border may become convex due to the tendency of the aorta to dilate and elongate. The convexity represents the right lateral aspect of the ascending aorta. In hyposthenic subjects with a vertical heart, it is sometimes possible to see a small segment of the IVC as a triangular shadow in the right cardiophrenic angle.

The left heart border can be divided into distinct segments. The uppermost is rounded and convex laterally and is formed by the posterior part of the transverse aortic arch and is called the aortic knuckle or knob. Immediately below this, a flat or concave border is represented by the trunk of pulmonary artery and is called the pulmonary conus. Prominence of the conus is a normal variation in young females and children. A small concavity along the left heart border below the region of the pulmonary conus represents the region of the left atrial appendage. The lowest and largest segment of the left border is formed by the left ventricle (LV). This segment may be relatively straight in asthenic individuals but is convex and rounded in hypersthenic individuals. Diaphragmatic or inferior border is often not defined, but it may be seen in tall, asthenic-built subjects and is represented by the right ventricle (RV) **(Fig. 1)**.

Right Anterior Oblique View

The anterior border from above downwards is formed by the transverse part of the arch of aorta, pulmonary trunk, RV and LV. The posterior border is formed by the left atrium (LA) above and RA below. The diaphragmatic surface is formed by the IVC, RA, and RV.

Left Anterior Oblique View

The anterior border from above downwards consists of the innominate vein, SVC, ascending aorta, RA appendage and RV. The posterior border from above downwards includes a small part of LA and LV.

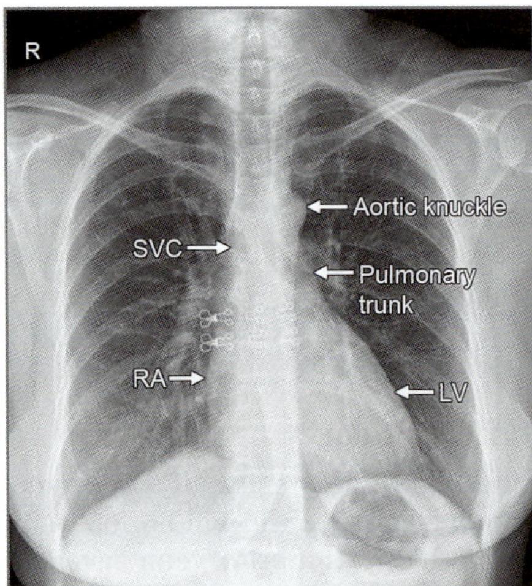

FIG. 1: Cardiac contours on a posteroanterior chest radiograph. The upper segment of the right heart border is formed by the superior vena cava (SVC) and the lower segment represents the lateral border of the right atrium (RA). The uppermost part of the left heart border is formed by the posterior part of the transverse aortic arch (aortic knuckle). The flat or concave border immediately below this, is represented by the pulmonary trunk while the lowest and largest segment of the left border is formed by the left ventricle (LV).

Lateral View

The anterior border is formed above by the RA appendage and below by the RV. The posterior border is formed above by LA and below by the LV.

Cardiac Size

The true size of the heart can only be assessed by orthodiagraphy with the help of an orthodiagraph. The method has now become obsolete. Conventional chest X-ray at a focus-film distance (FFD) of 6 feet provides some magnification and the size of the heart is more than 1 cm greater in width than the orthodiagraphic measurements. If the FFD is doubled to about 12 feet, the measurements on the film are equal to those made on orthodiagraph. But this is not practical. Therefore, radiographic size at 6 feet is taken as a true representative size of the heart although there is some magnification.

Mathematical numerical cardiac measurement on chest radiograph has many variables, including age, sex, height, weight, race, occupation, phase of respiration, pulmonary and abdominal disease, which elevate or depress the diaphragm, and pose mathematical problems so that prediction tables are seldom used. The easiest method of measurement of cardiac size is to assess the transverse cardiothoracic ratio (CTR). This is the most adopted practical method though it is a rough estimate. This represents the ratio between the transverse cardiac diameter and the widest internal diameter of the thorax in posteroanterior (PA) view **(Fig. 2)**. The adult heart that measures more than half of the widest internal diameter of the chest is considered enlarged. In neonates, a ratio of up to 60%, and in infants, a ratio of up to 55% is taken as normal. The CTR may increase in the elderly probably due to infolding of the ribs which reduces the transverse thoracic diameter. Cardiomegaly has been graded as mild,

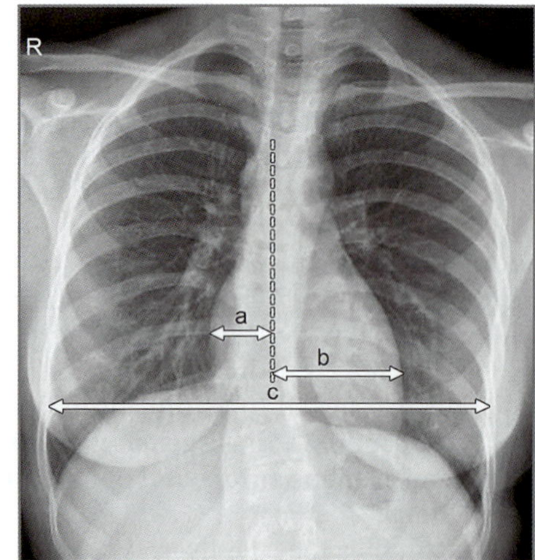

FIG. 2: Cardiothoracic ratio on a posteroanterior chest radiograph. It represents the ratio between the transverse cardiac diameter (a + b) and the widest internal diameter of the thorax (c) in the posteroanterior view.

moderate or severe by various authors based on the increase in the transverse diameter, but these classifications are not widely used.

Cardiac Volume

Volume measurement is not done as routine practice. It may be measured assuming the heart as an ellipsoid by the following formula:

$$V = l \times b \times d \times k \times m^3$$

where,

V = volume

l = long or oblique diameter. This is drawn from the lowermost point of the heart on left side to the notch separating RA and right vascular shadow.

b = broad diameter. It is obtained by joining the lower most point at the right cardiophrenic angle and uppermost point of the left vascular shadow.

d = AP diameter of the heart measured in lateral view. It is obtained by drawing a line from the point where the anterior border of the heart and sternum meet to the point of maximum convexity on the posterior surface of the heart.

m = magnification factor

k = 0.63

ASSESSMENT OF CHAMBER ENLARGEMENT

Right Atrium

When this is enlarged, the right heart border becomes more convex and also protrudes to the right, away from the midline. The maximum convexity of right cardiac border >3 cm beyond right lateral vertebral border suggests RA enlargement. In early stages, only RA appendage fills the space between front of the heart and back of the sternum. The most reliable sign for the enlargement of the right atrium in the frontal chest radiograph is the increase in its height. In normal individuals, the distance between the top of the arch and the junction of the SVC and the right atrium is more than the distance between the latter and the right cardiophrenic angle. When the reverse happens, the right atrium is said to be enlarged **(Fig. 3)**.

Left Atrium

This chamber does not take part in the formation of any part of the cardiac border in frontal projection in normal subjects. It lies in the mid-line and in a posterior location. It usually enlarges posteriorly and to the right causing indentation and displacement of the esophagus posteriorly. With further increase in size, enlargement is in all directions except anteriorly. The LA may project beyond the LV producing localized convexity of the left border of cardiac silhouette just below the PA segment. The earliest evidence of LA enlargement is seen as lifting up of the left main bronchus. However, this is difficult to appreciate on the chest radiograph. Subsequently, the carinal angle widens. The normal carinal angle ranges between 51–71 degrees. With LA enlargement, it becomes right angled or obtuse angled. When enlargement reaches this stage, the chamber is often large enough to produce an oval shaped, localized density on the right side and projecting outside the lower right cardiac border. This can be seen in frontal projection as a double density within the cardiac shadow on the right side **(Fig. 4)**. With massive enlargement, LA

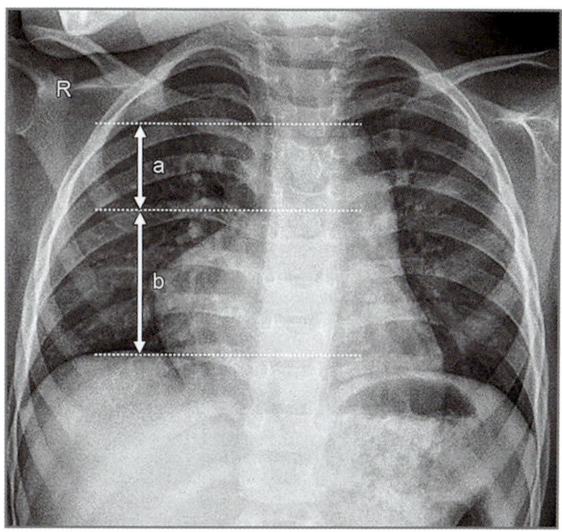

FIG. 3: Right atrial enlargement on a posteroanterior chest radiograph. The distance between the top of the arch and the superior vena cava—right atrium junction (a) is less than the distance between the latter and the right cardiophrenic angle (b) suggestive of right atrial enlargement.

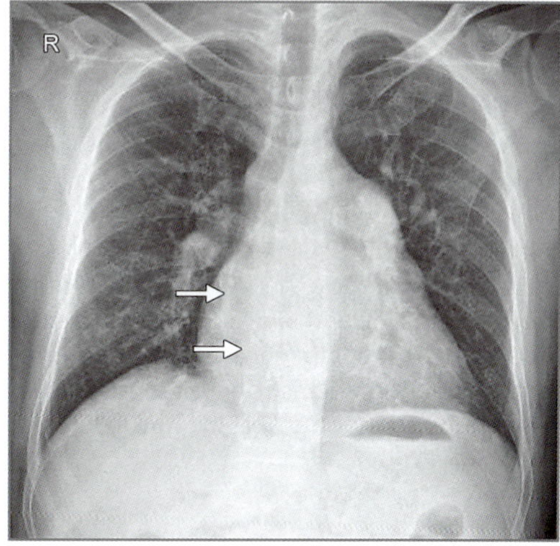

FIG. 4: Left atrial enlargement on a posteroanterior chest radiograph. In a patient with severe mitral stenosis, the left atrium (indicated by arrows) is producing an oval shaped, localized density on the right side and seen as a double density within the cardiac shadow on the right side suggestive of left atrial enlargement.

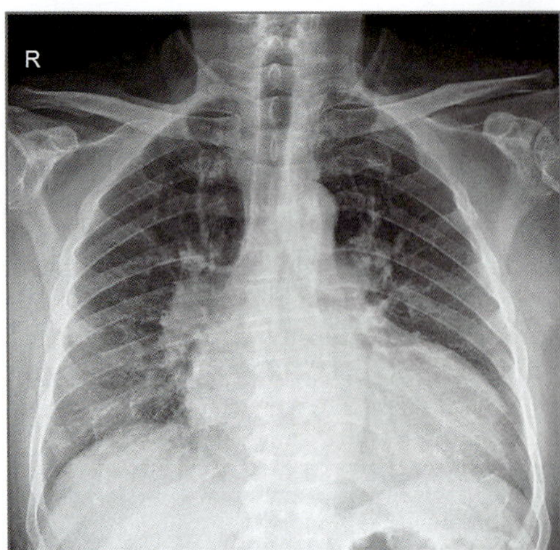

FIG. 5: Left ventricular enlargement on a posteroanterior chest radiograph. Left ventricular dilatation has resulted in cardiomegaly with shifting of the apex toward the left and downwards, combined with rounding of the apex.

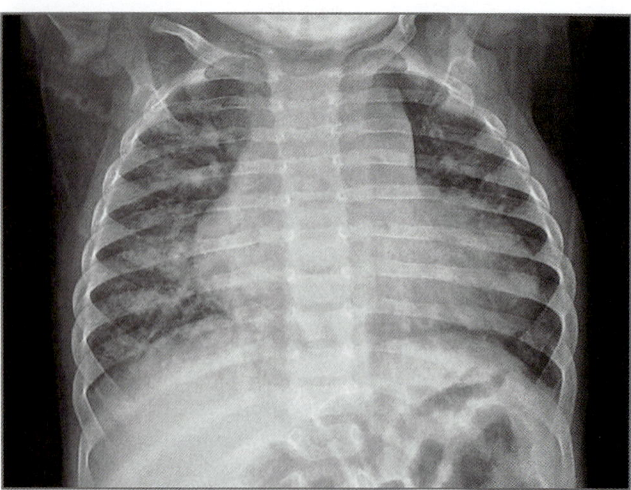

FIG. 6: Right ventricular enlargement on an anteroposterior chest radiograph. Right ventricular dilatation has resulted in elevation of the apex.

forms the right cardiac contour almost throughout except the upper part of SVC. The enlarged LA can compress the left or occasionally the right bronchus and cause collapse, obstructive emphysema or rarely recurrent infection distal to the compressed lower lobe bronchus.

Left Ventricle

It enlarges to the left and posteriorly and only slightly to the right and anteriorly. Hypertrophy produces rounding of the cardiac apex whereas dilatation causes elongation either to the left or to the left and downwards, often combined with rounding of the apex **(Fig. 5)**. Rounding may also affect the left cardiac border when the LV gradually encroaches upon the prevertebral space. Left ventricular enlargement is best assessed in PA, LAO and lateral views.

Right Ventricle

It enlarges chiefly to the left and anteriorly. The outflow tract enlarges first and this is best seen in RAO and lateral views. When enlargement is significant, pulmonary conus becomes prominent in PA view. In some cases, the left border may be formed by this ventricle and may cause rotation of LV to the left with elevation of the apex **(Fig. 6)**. In lateral view, there is encroachment upon the retrosternal space in the upper part. This rotation tends to swing the aorta to the right, so that the aortic knuckle becomes less prominent.

AORTA

The normal ascending aorta does not contribute to the cardiac silhouette in frontal projection. When dilated and elongated in old age, it bulges to the right beyond the SVC to form the right upper border. The posterior most part of the arch of the aorta forms the left upper cardiac border and is called the aortic knob or knuckle. In infants and young children, the aortic knob is not well seen. The aortic knuckle also becomes more prominent, somewhat enlarged and may show curvilinear calcification in old age. The descending aorta can usually be seen as a straight line passing downwards and toward mid-line to the left of spine. The following should be looked for during the assessment of the aortic shadow:

- Is it a D-loop or L-loop?
- Is the aortic knuckle right or left-sided?
- Is the aorta enlarged? If so, is there any disproportionate enlargement of the ascending or arch and descending aorta?
- Is there any calcification in the aorta? If so, its location (in the knuckle, descending thoracic or ascending aorta), pattern and extent.

Each of the above abnormalities has specific localizing value for the diagnosis.

PULMONARY VASCULATURE

A standard chest radiograph is a detailed record of the pulmonary vasculature. Pulmonary blood flow mirrors the pathophysiology of the heart since the pulmonary blood vessels are clearly visualized on a chest radiograph and abnormal patterns of blood flow can be identified.[2]

Normal Radiographic Anatomy

The analysis of pulmonary vascularity begins at the hilum. Pulmonary circulation begins at the pulmonary valve. The left border of the main pulmonary artery (MPA) forms the floor of pulmonary segment. The normal pulmonary segment (PAS) is concave or straight. The enlargement of MPA causes a convexity of the PAS. MPA bifurcates within the mediastinum into the right (RPA) and left (LPA) pulmonary arteries. The intrapulmonary branches parallel the bronchi, divide in an orderly manner, and gradually taper toward the periphery. The arteries and bronchial branches are approximately the same diameter at any particular level with the radio of 1:2:1. The LPA and left hilum are 1 cm above the RPA. The course of the pulmonary arteries is interlobular and inter-segmental. The veins are wider, less well defined and branch less often than the companion arteries. These are located medial to the companion artery in the upper zones, overlap each other in the mid-zone and are lateral to the artery in the lower zone. The pulmonary veins converge into the LA 2–3 cm below the hilum. The pulmonary arteries radiate from the hila above the pulmonary venous confluence. It is often difficult to differentiate the artery from the vein due to variable arterial supply and venous drainage. In normal individuals, the pulmonary arteries and veins in the outer one-third of the lung are too small to be seen in chest radiograph.

The right hilum is formed by the confluence of the shadows of the right upper lobe pulmonary vein and the right descending pulmonary artery (RDPA). These form a right angle. The width of the pulmonary vessels depends on the flow. Normal RDPA has a straight outer border. A convexity suggests an enlargement and concavity suggests a diminished size. In children, the ratio of RDPA to trachea is <1.0.[2] In adults, the normal transverse diameter of RDPA just above the origin of right middle lobe branch or 1.25 cm distal to the origin of right upper lobe branch is 10–16 mm in males and 9–15 mm in females in deep inspiration.[3] In erect position, blood flow is greater to the lower lobe because of gravity and differential intra-alveolar pressure. The lower lobe vessels are 2–3 times larger than the upper lobe vessels. In the erect chest radiograph, vessels in first intercostal space are <3 mm in diameter and those just above the diaphragm are up to 6 mm in diameter.

Increased Pulmonary Blood Flow (Pulmonary Plethora)

This is defined as an enlargement of vessels due to increased flow. The width of the pulmonary vessels depends on flow as long as the vascular reserve is not exceeded. Beyond this, the size depends on flow and pressure or pressure alone. Increased pulmonary flow can be caused by high output states, left to right (L-R) shunts, and admixture lesions. The pulmonary veins also enlarge as pulmonary arterial blood flow increases. Blood vessels become visible in the outer one-third of the lungs. In larger shunts, there is recruitment of upper lobe vessels, so that the differential flow between the upper and lower lobe vessels is lost **(Fig. 7)**. There is a fair correlation between vessel enlargement and shunt size. Shunts with QP:QS > 2:1 can be reliably detected. Very large volume shunts can also cause pulmonary venous hypertension (PVH).

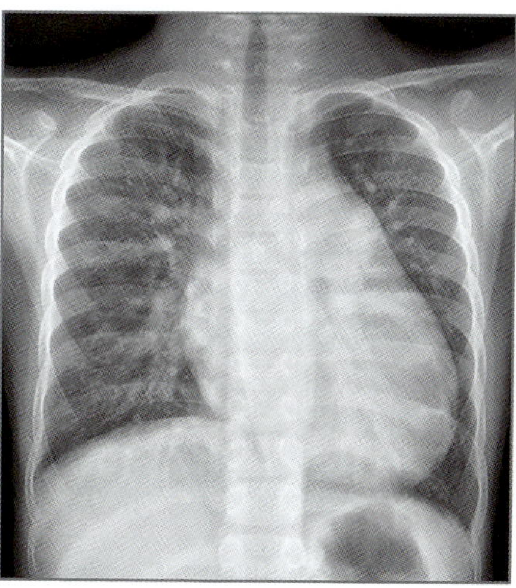

FIG. 7: Pulmonary plethora on a posteroanterior chest radiograph. The right descending pulmonary artery is dilated with prominent pulmonary conus along with visualization of dilated end-on vessels.

Gooding compared the diameter of the RDPA and trachea in children up to 14 years of age. The ratio in normal children at any age was close to one. 90% had diameters within 2 mm of each other, with one-third having diameters of the RDPA that was less than that of the trachea. When a L-R shunt was present, the diameter of the RDPA was never less than that of the trachea.[4,5]

Radiological signs of plethora are as follows:

- The presence of shunt vessels, end-on vessels more than two times the diameter of the accompanying bronchus
- Prominent upper and lower zone vessels
- En-face vessels below the tenth posterior rib
- Prominent vessels below the crest of the diaphragm
- RDPA diameter more than that of the trachea
- >6 vessels in peripheral one-third of the lungs
- RDPA > 16 mm in diameter
- Prominent hilar vessels on lateral view
- In infants and children, generalized mottling may be seen.

Plethora correlates with the size of L-R shunts better than the heart size.[6] With a normal or slightly increased heart size, QP:QS is >2:1 or 2:1 in 50%, with a larger heart, the shunt is >2:1 in at least 60% and with no plethora, the shunt is <2:1 in 100%. Assessment of plethora should not be based on measurements alone. However, measurements can be used in corroboration with a subjective impression.

Decreased Pulmonary Blood Flow (Pulmonary Oligemia)

It is difficult to diagnose pulmonary oligemia unless it is severe. Some normal people may have small pulmonary vessels. Oligemia can be caused by pulmonary outflow tract obstruction and intracardiac right-to-left (R-L) shunts.

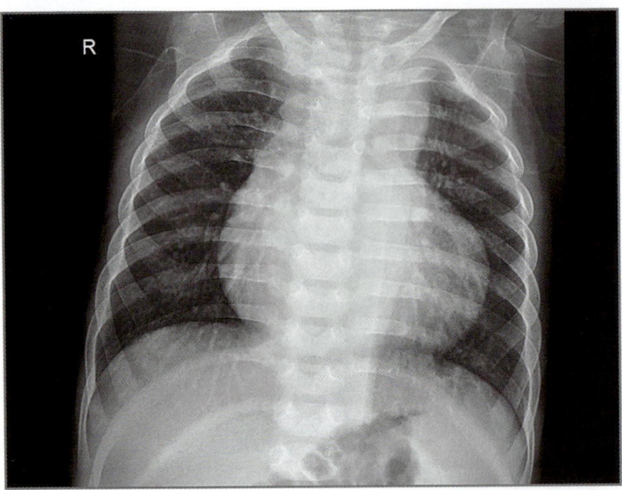

FIG. 8: Pulmonary oligemia on an anteroposterior chest radiograph. There is an overall appearance of an over-penetrated film with small hilar, lobar, segmental vessels.

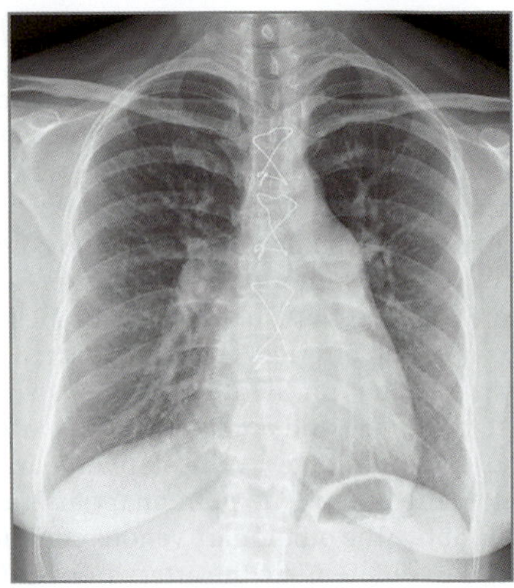

FIG. 9: Pulmonary arterial hypertension on a posteroanterior chest radiograph. There is an enlarged right descending pulmonary artery, convex pulmonary conus and dilated central pulmonary arteries with peripheral pruning.

The pulmonary arteries and veins are reduced in size, the central vessels become narrow, and peripheral arteries are not visible **(Fig. 8)**.

The radiological signs are as follows:

- Concave or absent MPA
- Overall appearance of an over-penetrated film
- <4 vessels in peripheral one-third of the lungs
- Small hilar, lobar, segmental vessels
- Decreased size and density of hilar vessels on lateral chest radiograph in the presence of cyanosis is suggestive of pulmonary oligemia.
- Enlarged bronchial and other systemic collateral arteries are seen in pulmonary atresia with ventricular septal defect (VSD) and in tetralogy of Fallot (TOF). These are seen as small, tortuous, nontapering and disorganized vascular markings not radiating from the hilum and also not conforming to known branching patterns of the pulmonary vessels. The hila are not enlarged.

Pulmonary Arterial Hypertension

This may be primary or secondary to PVH, long standing L-R shunts, pulmonary thromboembolic disease, respiratory disease, high altitude, drugs, and pulmonary arterial occlusion. It is said to be present if the mean pulmonary artery (PA) pressure is >20 mm Hg. The PAH is graded as mild, moderate and severe with the PA mean pressure ranging from 20–29, 30–49, and >50 mm Hg respectively. The central vessels from the MPA to the second order branching vessels dilate and peripheral (lobar) vessels constrict. The transition between centrally dilated and peripherally constricted vessels is more lateral in L-R shunts. The pruning of the pulmonary arteries is defined as more than a 50% loss of the vessel diameter at any degree branching and is suggestive of PAH **(Fig. 9)**. Chronic PAH leads to calcification of the MPA and proximal branches. The presence of calcification is pathognomonic of PAH. The severity of central dilatation has a rough correlation with the severity of PAH. In the lower pressure ranges, the ratio of the size of the hemithoracic diameter to the size of the MPA shows an approximate correlation with PA pressure.

Hyperkinetic PAH versus Eisenmenger PAH

In hyperkinetic PAH, peripheral vessels increase in size and number, and cardiac enlargement is proportional to the amount of L-R shunt. In Eisenmenger PAH, peripheral vessels decrease, central vessels increase further in size, heart size decreases, and the RV becomes more prominent.

Pulmonary Venous Hypertension

Pulmonary venous hypertension (PVH) is said to be present when the pulmonary capillary wedge pressure (PCWP) exceeds the normal range of 8–12 mm Hg. Progressive PVH produces changes reflecting the presence and severity of this disorder.

Stage 1: Redistribution/Cephalization of the Blood Flow

This may precede the clinical signs and symptoms. The PCWP ranges from 13–19 mm Hg. The changes are characterized by constriction, blurring of lower zone vessels, effacement of hilar angle, and dilatation of upper lobe vessels **(Fig. 10)**. With the increase in LA and PCW pressure, there is an increase in the capillary hydrostatic pressure. This results in an increase in the interstitial lung water and increased pulmonary lymphatic drainage, leading

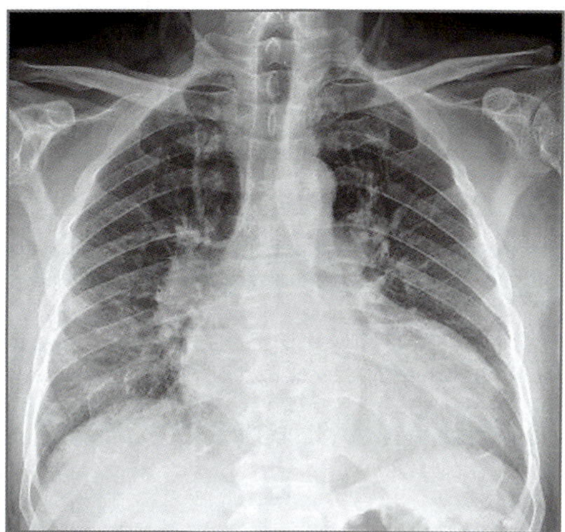

FIG. 10: Stage 1 pulmonary venous hypertension on a posteroanterior chest radiograph. There is presence of dilatation of upper lobe vessels (cephalization), blurring of lower zone vessels and effacement of hilar angle.

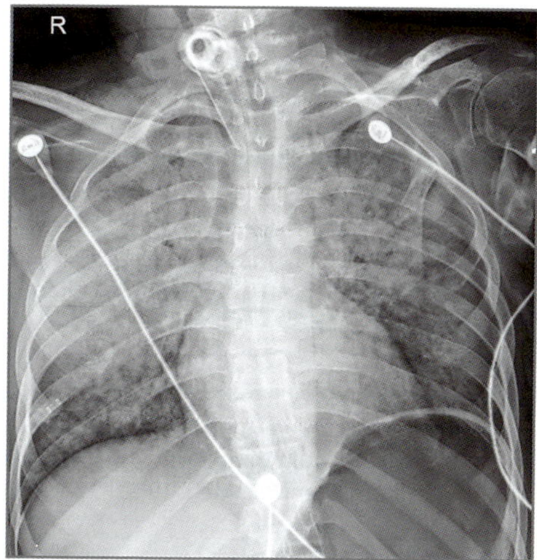

FIG. 12: Stage 3 pulmonary venous hypertension on an anteroposterior chest radiograph. There is presence of bilateral extensive pulmonary edema with relative sparing of the lung periphery.

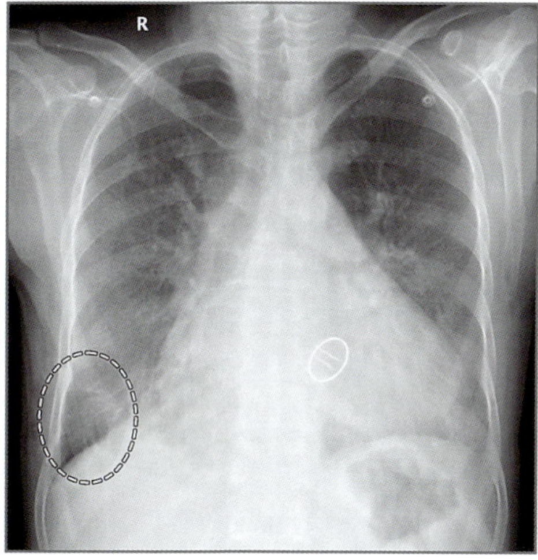

FIG. 11: Stage 2 pulmonary venous hypertension on a posteroanterior chest radiograph. There is presence of Kerley B lines (dotted circle), peribronchial cuffing, and a background haze.

to "cuffing" of fluid around small bronchi. The increased interstitial water gravitates to dependent areas, causing increased interstitial pressure and vascular resistance at lung bases. Thus, blood is diverted to upper lobes leading to vascular redistribution. Exceptions to this pattern of redistribution are basal emphysema and pulmonary parenchymal diseases of the upper lobe.

Stage 2: Interstitial Edema

It is characterized by the presence of Kerley lines, peribronchial cuffing, background haze, septal and interstitial edema, and pleural effusion **(Fig. 11)**. The PCWP ranges from 20–24 mm Hg.

Stage 3: Alveolar Edema

This occurs when the interstitial fluid accumulates at rates faster than can be removed by the lymphatics, The PCWP ranges from 25 mm Hg and above. Milking of edema fluid toward the hilum by the expanding lung imparts a "bat's wing appearance" **(Fig. 12)**. However, chronic lung disease and dependent posture may result in atypical patterns of edema. Pleural effusion occurs when pleural fluid formation by visceral pleura is faster than its absorption by the parietal pleura. This usually occurs when systemic venous pressure is also elevated, as in right heart failure. Several radiologic findings have been correlated with the level of PCWP in patients with acute and chronic heart failure.

Asymmetrical Pulmonary Blood Flow

This is due to the presence of vessels in one lung that are smaller than the other:

- *Localized decrease*: Pulmonary thromboembolism, chronic obstructive airway disease (COAD), arteritis, segmental stenosis.
- *Unilateral decrease*: Pulmonary artery branch atresia/stenosis, hemitruncus, TOF with unilateral pulmonary atresia.
- *Unilateral increase*: After shunt surgery (e.g., Blalock-Taussig shunt), Glenn shunt (on the side of shunt), PDA and anomalous origin of a pulmonary artery from the aorta.

CONCLUSION

It is obvious from the above description that the chest radiograph is a mathematical record of the events produced by cardiac disease. Its detailed and sequential interpretation provides important clues to the underlying heart disease and the functional impairment produced by it. The chest radiograph also serves as a useful method for follow-up after treatment in most cardiac conditions. Distinctive radiographic abnormalities in specific cardiac disorders will be dealt with in the following chapters.

REFERENCES

1. Radiology of the heart. In: Braunwald E (Ed). Heart Disease: A Textbook of Cardiovascular Medicine. Philadelphia: WB Saunders; 1992. pp. 204-324.
2. Coussement AM. Objective radiographic assessment of pulmonary vascularity in children. Radiology. 1973;109:649-54.
3. Chang CH. The normal roentgenographic measurement of the right descending pulmonary artery in 1085 cases. Am J Roentgenol Radium Ther Nucl Med. 1962;87:929-35.
4. Roberts WC. Radiologic differentiation of common anomalies. In: Adult Congenital Heart Disease; 1988. pp. 191-219.
5. Moes CAF. Analysis of the chest in the neonate with congenital heart disease. Radiol Clin North Am. 1975;13: 251-76.
6. Jefferson K, Rees R. Clinical Cardiac Radiology. London: Butterworth; 1980.

Arun Sharma, Manphool Singhal, Amarinder Singh Malhi

CHAPTER 23

Cardiac and Coronary Imaging on CT and MRI: Techniques and Anatomy

INTRODUCTION

Technical advancements in multidetector computed tomography (MDCT) and magnetic resonance imaging (MRI) have revolutionized the non-invasive assessment of almost every aspect of the cardiovascular system. Currently, it is now possible to evaluate the heart and the coronaries as a motion-free volume of data with acquisition of isotropic voxels. However, its application and interpretation require a thorough understanding of normal cardiac and coronary anatomy. Radiologists interpreting the scans should be aware of the normal anatomy and the variations for correct interpretation. Equally apt knowledge of imaging techniques is essential for data acquisition. The chapter describes normal cardiac and coronary anatomy along with precepts of imaging.

ANATOMY

This section describes normal anatomy pertinent to the cardiac chambers, coronary arterial and venous system and the pericardium.

Cardiac Anatomy

Heart is a pyramidal shaped structure enclosed within the pericardium. The right sided chambers are normally anterior and receive deoxygenated systemic venous blood via venae cavae with outflow to the pulmonary circulation.

The left sided chambers are posterior and receive oxygenated venous blood from the pulmonary circulation to pump into the systemic circulation.

Systematic anatomical approach is very important in elucidating exact anatomic cardiac details and include:

- Situs and cardiac orientation
- Systemic veins and right atrium
- Pulmonary veins and left atrium
- Right ventricle and tricuspid valve
- Left ventricle and mitral valve
- Great arteries and semilunar valves
- Coronary arteries
- Pericardium and pericardial recesses

Situs and Cardiac Orientation

Situs deciphers the position of the abdominal viscera, atria and the tracheobronchial tree.[1] Cardiac situs is defined by the atria as they maintain their laterality throughout the development. The thoracic situs is generally concordant with the cardiac situs and the tracheobronchial anatomy is more useful in situs anomalies as characteristic landmarks that differentiate the atria may not conform to the usual anatomy. The right main bronchus (eparterial) is shorter, vertically oriented and bifurcates early while the left bronchus (hyparterial) is longer, horizontal and placed below the left pulmonary artery or above the left atrium **(Fig. 1)**.[1,2] However, it should be noted that the configuration of the tracheobronchial tree does not predict the position of the ventricles, great arteries or the heart apex. Cardiac orientation or position describes the anatomic position of the cardiac apex in the chest and is left-sided or levocardia in situs solitus **(Fig. 2)**. In case of right-sided or midline heart, dextrocardia or mesocardia is used respectively.[2]

Systemic Veins and Right Atrium

Embryologically, right atrium (RA) (irregular ellipsoid shaped) is derived from the primitive atrium (trabeculated part) and the sinus venosus (smooth part) separated by the crista terminalis. It receives the deoxygenated blood from the two venae cavae, coronary sinus, and the thebesian veins. The RA appendage is triangular, broad based, larger than the left with a wide opening and have rough trabeculations or pectinate muscles **(Fig. 3)**.[3,4] The supradiaphragmatic inferior vena cava provides a reliable landmark for locating the anatomic RA.[5]

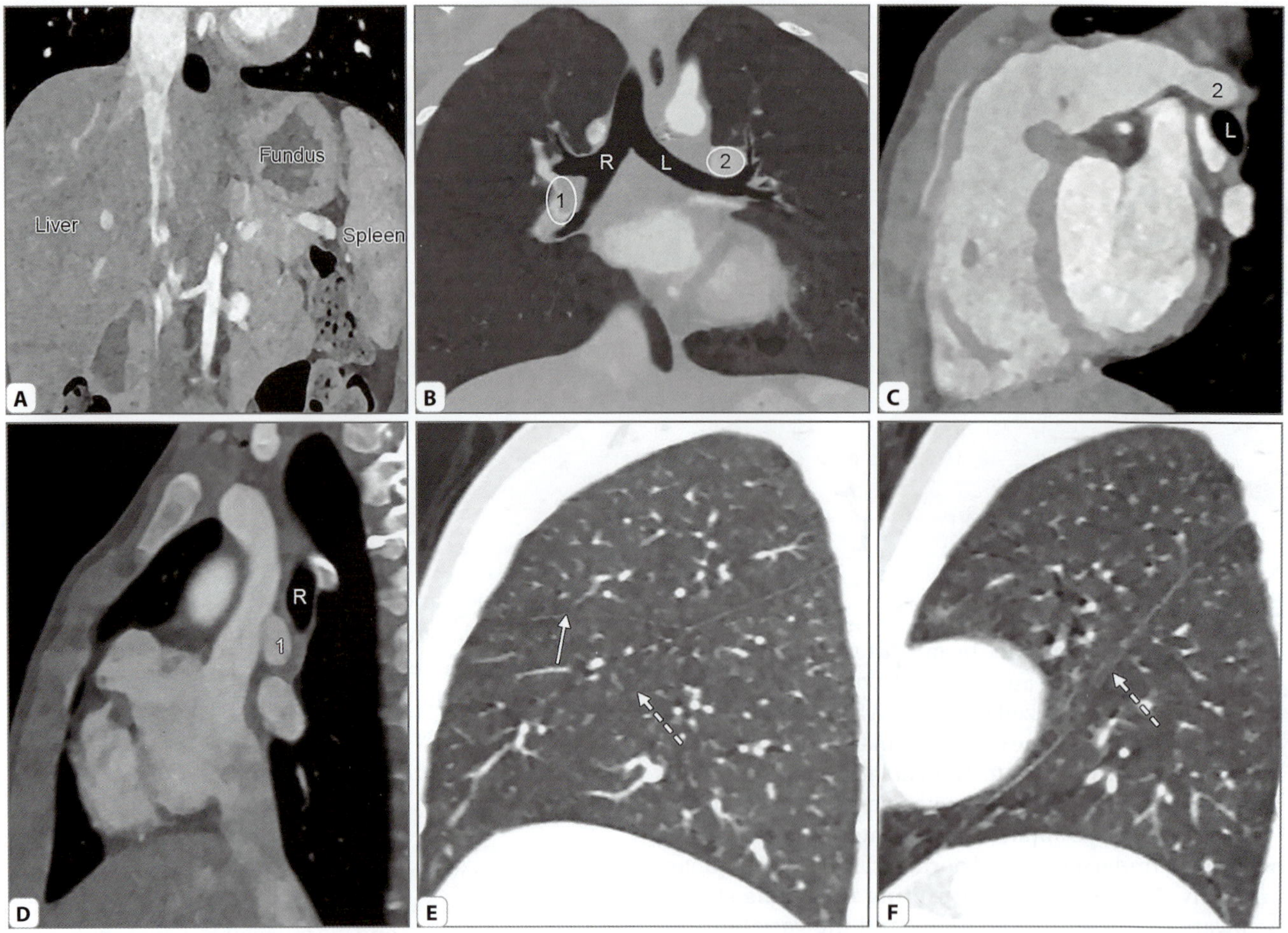

FIGS. 1A TO F: CT images (A to F) showing right sided liver with stomach fundus and spleen on left side (A) in situs solitus, shorter and more vertically oriented right (R) bronchus than left (L) bronchus (B). The right bronchus is positioned posterosuperior (eparterial) to the right (1) pulmonary artery (B and D) with the left bronchus is located below (hyparterial) the left (2) pulmonary artery (B and C). The right lung is trilobed with bilobed left lung. Dashed arrow (E and F) represents the oblique fissure while the arrow in (E) represents the horizontal fissure on right side.

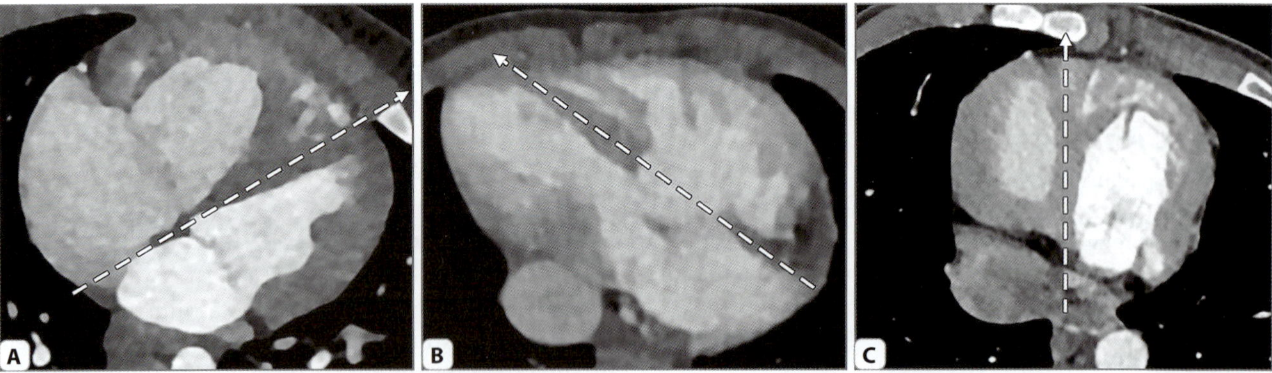

FIGS. 2A TO C: CT axial images (A to C) from different patients depicting the orientation of the cardiac apex toward the left (levocardia), right (dextrocardia) and the midline (mesocardia) respectively.

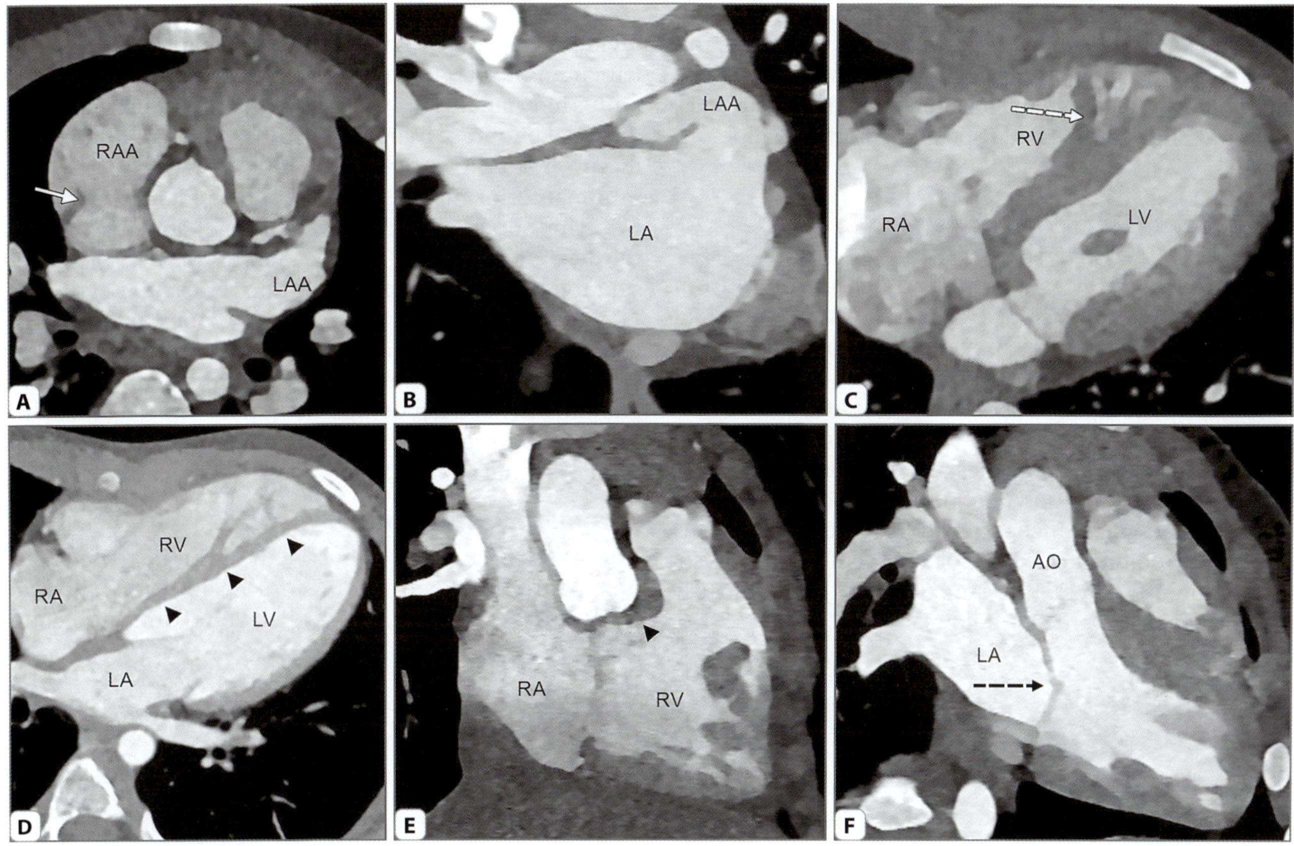

FIGS. 3A TO F: CT images (A to F) showing blunt, broad-based right (RAA) atrial appendage (A) with tubular and fingerlike left (LAA) atrial appendage (A and B). The right ventricle (RV) shows coarse trabeculations, moderator band (dashed arrow in C), well developed conus with lack of fibrous continuity (arrowhead in E) of the atrioventricular valve and the outflow tract while the left ventricle (LV) shows fine trabeculations with smooth septal surface (arrowheads in D) with aortomitral continuity (F). Dashed arrow in F represents the mitral valve.

Pulmonary Veins and Left Atrium

The left atrium (LA) is the most posterior chamber which normally receives the pulmonary venous return with its appendage being characteristically narrow, tubular, more elongated and fingerlike **(Fig. 3)**.[4] Both the atria are separated by the interatrial septum which features the fossa ovalis. The pulmonary veins should be evaluated for any anomalous drainage which can be partial or total and obstructive or nonobstructive in addition to the variant anatomy.[6,7]

Right Ventricle and Tricuspid Valve

The right ventricle (RV) consists of inlet, outlet (smooth), and apical (trabeculated) portions and receives blood from the RA with tricuspid valve (chordal attachments to the septum) across RA-RV. It is identified **(Fig. 3)** based on the presence of coarse trabeculae, characteristic moderator band (from apical portion of the septum to the anterior papillary muscle), well developed infundibulum, papillary muscle attachment to both the interventricular septum and the free wall. Also, it is characterized by the lack of the fibrous continuity of the atrioventricular (AV) valve and the outflow tract and can also be identified by the loop rule in complex cases.[4,8]

Left Ventricle and Mitral Valve

The left ventricle (LV) is conical and longer with thicker walls as compared to the RV with which it is separated through the interventricular septum. The septum normally bulges into the RV with rounded LV profile in the short axis view. It comprises of inlet, apical, and outlet portions with characteristic aorto-mitral continuity. It shows two papillary muscles (anterolateral and posteromedial), which are larger than those in RV with smooth septal surface and fine trabeculations **(Fig. 3)**. Moreover, it should also be noted that the tricuspid valve is positioned more apically than the mitral valve.[9]

Great Arteries and Semilunar Valves

Two great arteries, aorta and the pulmonary artery arise normally from the LV and the RV respectively with pulmonary valve being superior, anterior and to the left of aortic valve, presence of aortomitral continuity and well developed subpulmonic conus.[10,11] Variations can be observed with regard to the positions of the great arteries, including situs, inversus, transposition or malposition.

Coronary Anatomy

Coronary Arteries

The coronary arteries (right and left) originate from their respective aortic sinuses to run in the epicardial fat **(Figs. 4 and 5)** and carry oxygenated blood to the heart muscle. The right coronary artery (slightly inferior to the origin of the left coronary) runs in right atrioventricular groove and is dominant in 80–85% of the individuals.[12] It gives off the following branches; the conal branch (typical anterior course to supply the pulmonary outflow), right or acute marginal branches, posterior descending (PDA) artery (right dominance), posterolateral ventricular branch, and frequently (~55%) the sinoatrial (SA) nodal artery (typical course toward SVC inflow).

The left coronary artery is short (5–10 mm) and generally divides into the left anterior descending (LAD) and the left circumflex (LCX) coronary arteries. Trifurcation with ramus intermedius is seen in 15–30% cases which can have diagonal or obtuse marginal distribution depending upon its supply to the anterior or lateral LV wall.[13] LAD runs in the anterior interventricular sulcus (sometimes with overlying superficial myocardial bridge) and gives rise to the diagonal branches (supply anterior wall of LV) and the septal perforators (supply anterior ventricular septum). LCX runs in the left or posterior AV groove and gives off the obtuse marginal branches which supply the lateral LV wall. Moreover, it sometimes supplies the SA nodal artery and the PDA in a left dominant system. The diagonal and the obtuse marginal branches are numbered sequentially from proximal to distal.

Coronary Venous Anatomy

Coronary sinus is the largest vein of the heart, located posteriorly between the LA and LV to drain into the RA.[14] It receives the great cardiac vein (runs alongside

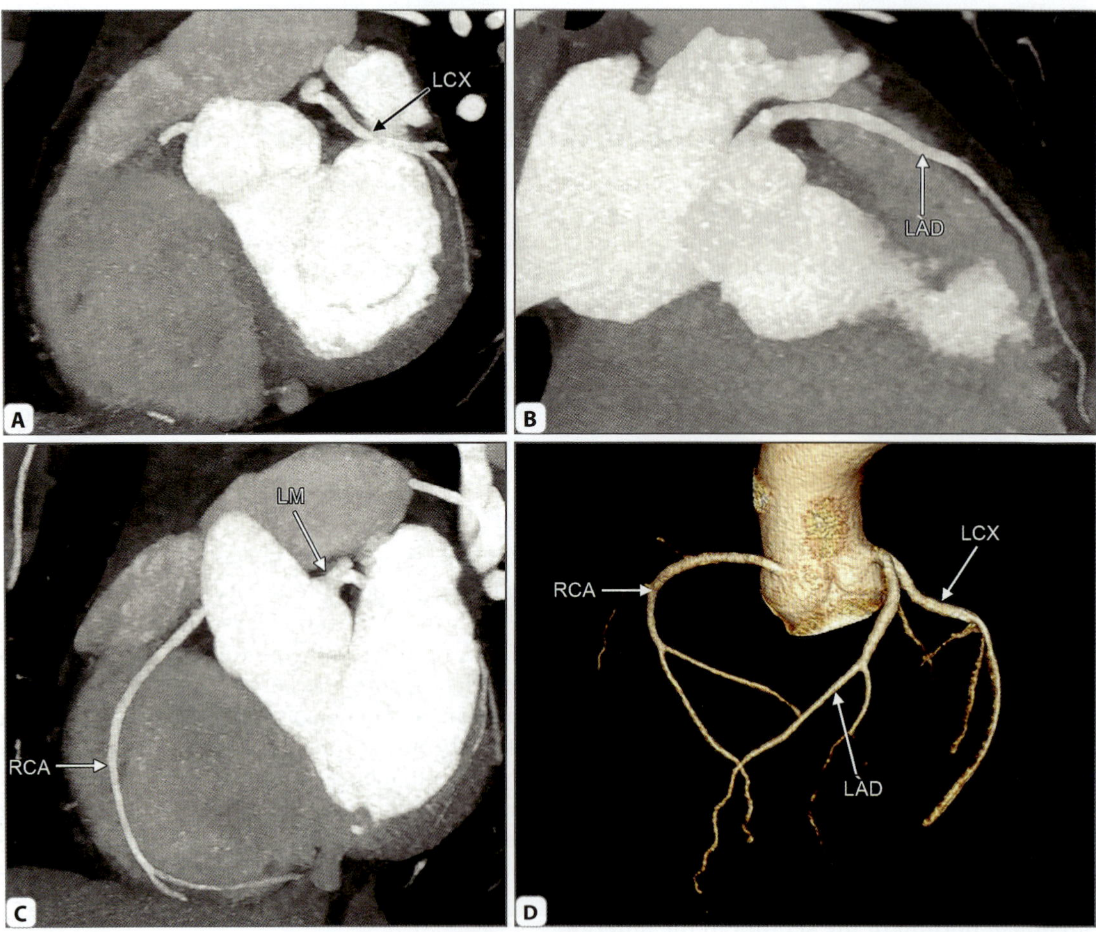

FIGS. 4A TO D: CT images (A to D) showing origin and the course of the coronary arteries using maximum intensity projection (A to C) and volume rendered (D) CT images is made of right coronary dominance in this patient with posterior descending artery from the RCA.
(LM: left main coronary artery; LAD: left anterior descending artery; LCX: left circumflex artery; RCA: right coronary artery)

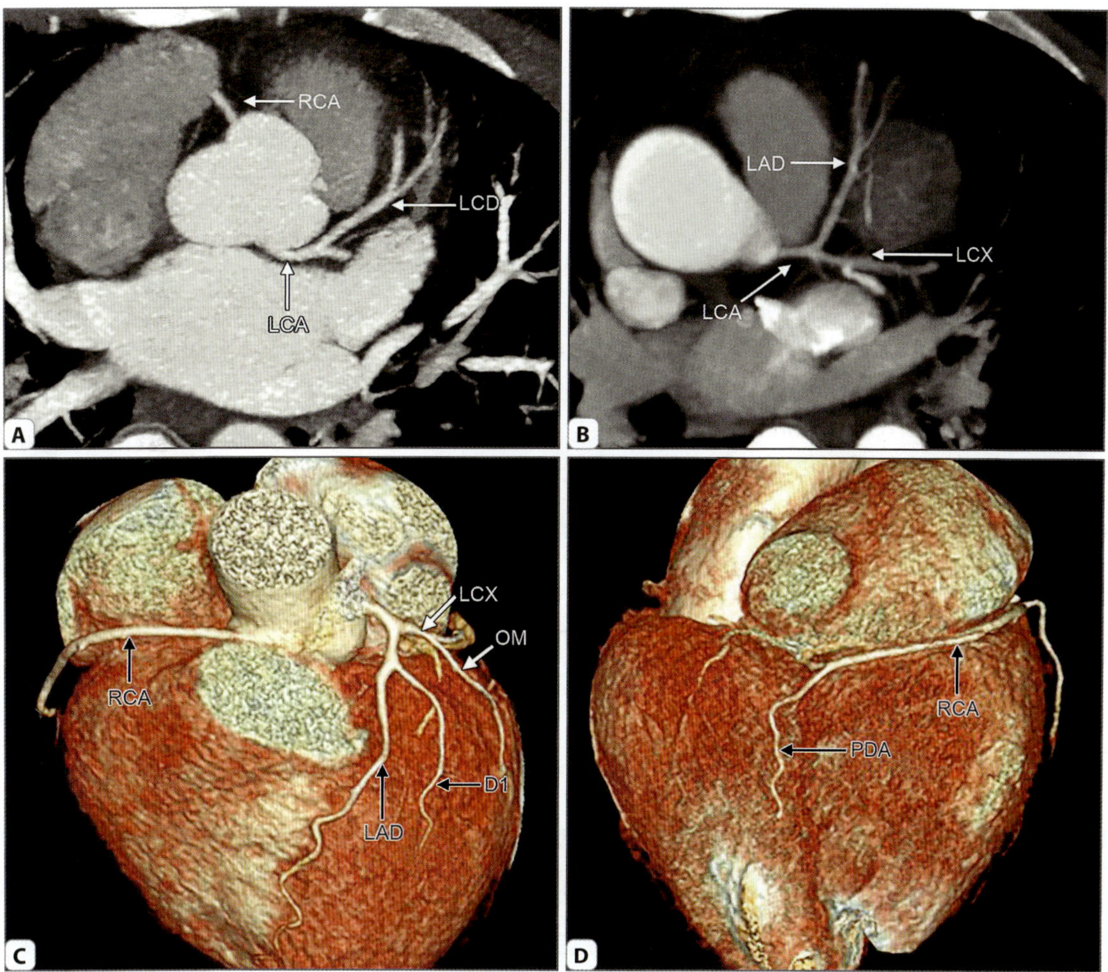

FIGS. 5A TO D: CT images (A to D) showing normal origin and the course of the coronary arteries with origin of right coronary artery (RCA) from the right or anterior sinus and origin of the left coronary (LCA) from the left or posterior sinus. LCA bifurcates into left anterior descending (LAD) and the left circumflex (LCX) artery. RCA and LCX runs in the right and the left atrioventricular groove respectively with LAD along anterior interventricular sulcus giving rise to the diagonal (D1) branches while LCX gives rise to obtuse marginal (OM) branches. Posterior descending artery (PDA) was seen arising from the RCA in this case with right coronary dominance.

LAD) proximally and the middle cardiac vein (runs alongside PDA) distally in addition to the other tributaries. Posterolateral vein which drains the lateral LV wall may be seen between these two larger tributaries. Additionally, veins draining the atria, RV and the thebesian veins constitute rest of the venous system. Knowledge of the venous anatomy is important for planning of ablation procedures, LV pacing and targeted drug therapy.[15]

Pericardial Anatomy

The pericardium is the protective covering which encloses the heart and the root of great vessels and is generally paper thin (<2 mm). It consists of outer fibrous and inner serous pericardium with visceral and parietal layers of serous pericardium being separated by the pericardial cavity containing approximately 15–50 mL of pericardial fluid.[16] Pericardial recesses are small pericardial spaces formed by the reflections of the pericardium which should not be misdiagnosed as abnormality such as lymph node, cyst or soft tissue.[17]

TECHNIQUES

MDCT in Cardiac and Coronary Imaging

Cardiac CT has now established its role in evaluation of all aspects of cardiovascular diseases, ranging from its role in screening, diagnosis, treatment optimization and follow-up. Current generation dual source CT scanners with sub-millimeter collimation and reduced gantry rotation times (up to 0.25 second) allow high temporal resolution (up to 66 ms) with acquisition of isotropic data (spatial resolution up to 0.24 mm) in a single breath hold.[18] ECG gating and special reconstruction algorithms are used to acquire motionless images of the heart.

ECG gated scans are primarily used for coronary assessment while the non-gated scans can be used in morphological evaluation of pulmonary arteries and veins, evaluation of congenital heart disease and pericardial assessment.

Coronary CT Angiography

Coronary CT angiography provides accurate atherosclerotic coronary plaque and stenosis assessment and prognostic utility in cardiovascular disease, receiving class 1, evidence level A recommendation supporting its use in both stable and acute chest pain settings.[19] Typical protocol has two components:

1. Coronary artery calcium (CAC) score
2. CT angiography after injection of IV contrast medium.

Coronary Artery Calcium Score

Coronary artery calcium is a surrogate marker of atherosclerosis and is assessed on the non-contrast phase (typical protocol includes axial MDCT acquisition with prospective ECG gating, from the level below the aortic arch to the base of the heart with a section thickness and section interval of 2.5 mm and 1 mm respectively) prior to coronary artery imaging with the use of IV contrast. CAC score using Agatston method (Agatston score) is then calculated with an automated software [calcification identified as high attenuation (>130 HU) with an area ≥ 1 mm^2] and is colour coded as per the coronary arteries **(Fig. 6)**.[20] It is an independent risk factor for coronary artery disease and is important in cardiovascular risk stratification, guiding preventive/statin therapy and predicting patient outcomes.

CT Coronary Angiography

CT coronary angiography (CTCA) is done after injecting contrast medium through a peripheral vein (usually right anterior cubital vein) and acquiring data in the peak aortic enhancement phase.

CTCA mandates optimal and uniform opacification of coronary arteries with minimal or no contrast in the right-sided cardiac chambers to avoid streak artifacts of the dense contrast. This is possible by using a high iodine concentration (320–400 mgI/mL) contrast and using dual power injector with saline chase.[21]

There are two techniques of determining the scan timing following contrast administration—bolus-tracking method and test-bolus method. Bolus tracking method is preferred as it is easy to use. This is done after placing region of interest in the ascending aorta with automatic triggering

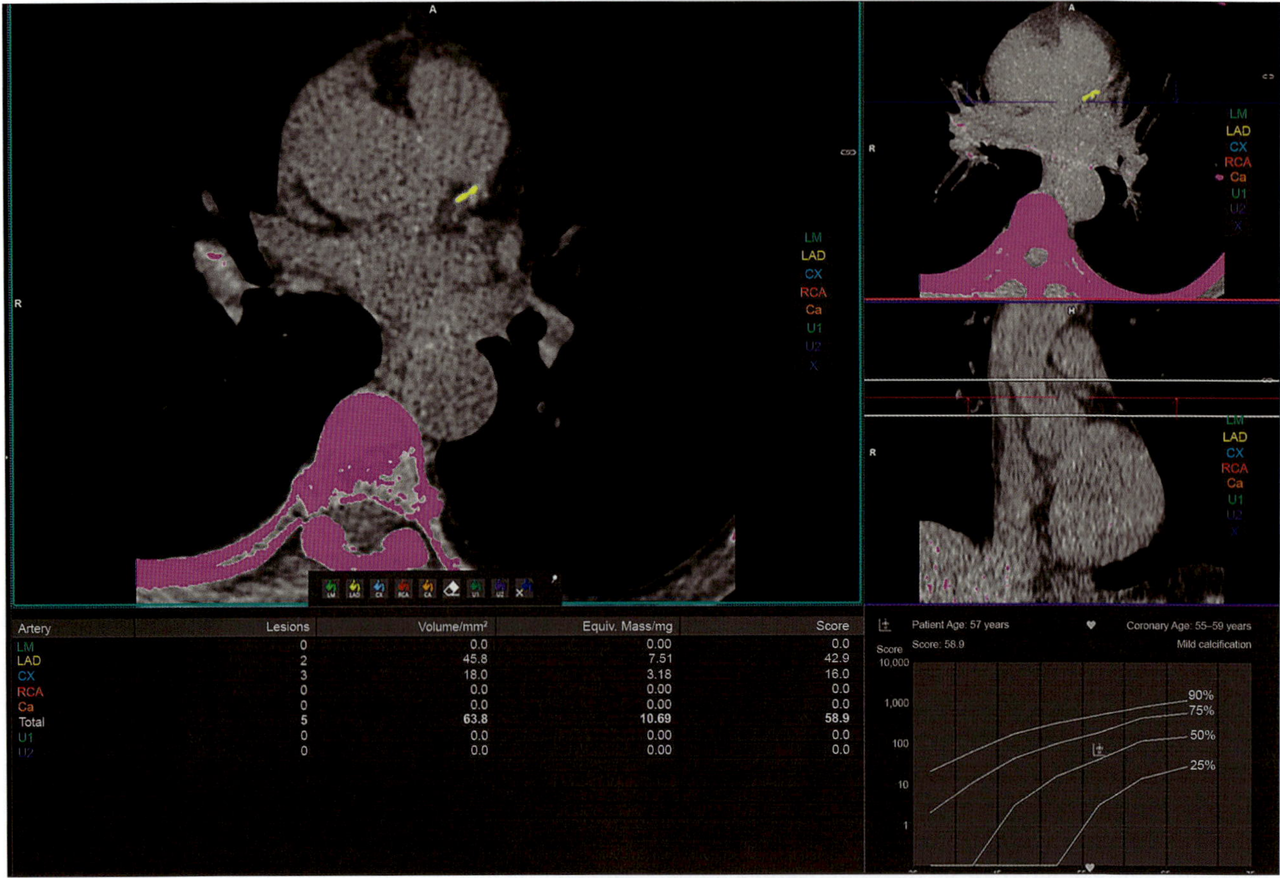

FIG. 6: CT images depicting the CT coronary calcium score using Agatston method using vendor specific software.

of scan, once a preset threshold (generally 100–125 HU) is achieved.[21]

CTCA can either be done using prospective or retrospective ECG gating.[22,23]

Prospective ECG Gating

This type of gating uses step and shoot sequential technique enabling data acquisition in certain phase of cardiac cycle, especially the mid-diastolic phase, when the cardiac motion is least. As optimal choosing of R-R interval is required, a regular heart rate is a prerequisite for prospective gating. It is associated with lower radiation exposure but does not allow functional analysis. Prospective high pitch helical scan is possible with latest dual source CT scanners.

Retrospective ECG Gating

Here the ECG information is simultaneously recorded with the attenuation data and is used only after the scan during image reconstruction to gate the CT data. It allows imaging of the entire cardiac cycle for functional analysis with fast continuous volume coverage and improved z-axis resolution at the expense of increased radiation dose. **Table 1** list the differences between prospective and retrospective ECG gated coronary artery acquisitions.

Postprocessing of Data

Many postprocessing techniques, including the maximum intensity projection (MIP), multiplanar reformation (MPR), curved reformation, volume rendering (VR), and the cine imaging are used for optimal assessment **(Figs. 4 and 7)**. Curved reformation is particularly helpful in coronary and bypass grafts assessment which allows the evaluation of the entire vessel along its centre line by sampling a given volume along a pre-defined curved anatomic plane **(Fig. 7)**. Automatic detection of the vascular centre line using existing software allows depiction of the whole length of the coronary artery in a single curved reformatted image. The data from all phases of the cardiac cycle can be displayed as cine loop and is useful for functional assessment, contractility, wall thickening and LV wall motion **(Fig. 8)**. 3D printing and virtual dissection techniques are particularly helpful in cases of complex congenital heart disease using acquired CT data.[24,25]

TABLE 1: Enumerates features of different types of ECG-gated CT acquisition of coronary arteries.

	Prospective ECG-gated CTCA	Retrospective ECG-gated CTCA
Technique	• "Step and shoot" • X-ray tube is switched on a pre-select short segment R-R interval of ECG (usually diastolic phase)	X-ray tube is switched on throughout the cardiac cycle
Temporal resolution	Low	High-provides functional information of ventricles and aortic valve
Heart rate consideration	Stable and low heart rate	Any heart rate (especially with current higher detectors and dual-source CT scanners)
Radiation exposure	Low radiation	High radiation

Cardiac CT beyond CTCA

Role of cardiac CT has now expanded to comprehensive cardiac evaluation beyond traditional CTCA including its use in electrophysiology applications, native and prosthetic heart valve assessment and transcatheter aortic valve implantation, etc. Further, incorporation of photon-counting CT, CT-derived fractional flow reserve, cardiac CT perfusion and the evolving artificial intelligence tools (plaque volume quantification and assessment of perivascular fat attenuation index reflecting coronary inflammation) may improve the diagnostic work up of cardiovascular disease.[26,27]

Magnetic Resonance in Cardiac and Coronary Imaging

Cardiac MRI is useful for evaluation of various cardiac diseases, including ischemic and non-ischemic cardiomyopathies, valvular heart disease, congenital anomalies, coronary artery disease and pericardial involvement.[28] It provides higher soft tissue contrast with lack of ionizing radiation. Contraindications to its use include intracranial aneurysm clips and the iron particles in the globe. Most patients with current generation pacemakers, prostheses and other implanted cardiac devices can safely undergo MRI evaluation at 1.5 T, keeping in view the implementation of standard appropriate precautions and manufacturer instructions.[29]

There are certain technical challenges unique to the cardiac MRI, particularly the rapid cardiac motion, pulsatility of great vessels and the respiratory motion which can be mitigated by the use of the ECG gating, navigator echo respiratory gating, improved field homogeneity, high-performance gradients and advanced pulse sequences.

On cardiac MR, three aspects are considered: (a) anatomy, (b) function, and (c) myocardial tissue characterization. Before these aspects are discussed, it is imperative to understand that heart lies in an oblique orientation in the chest cavity which is not in anatomical planes of the body. This demands creation of planes according to the position of the heart.

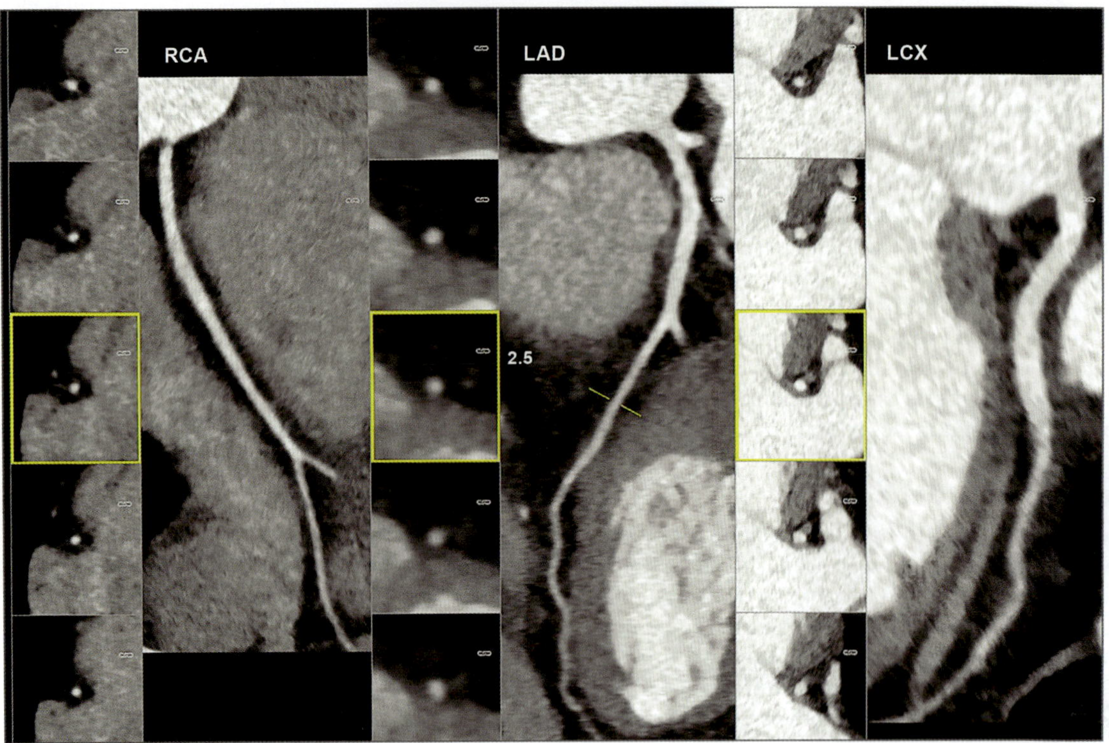

FIG. 7: Curved reformatted CT images depicting the coronary arteries.
(LAD: left anterior descending artery; LCX: left circumflex artery; RCA: right coronary artery)

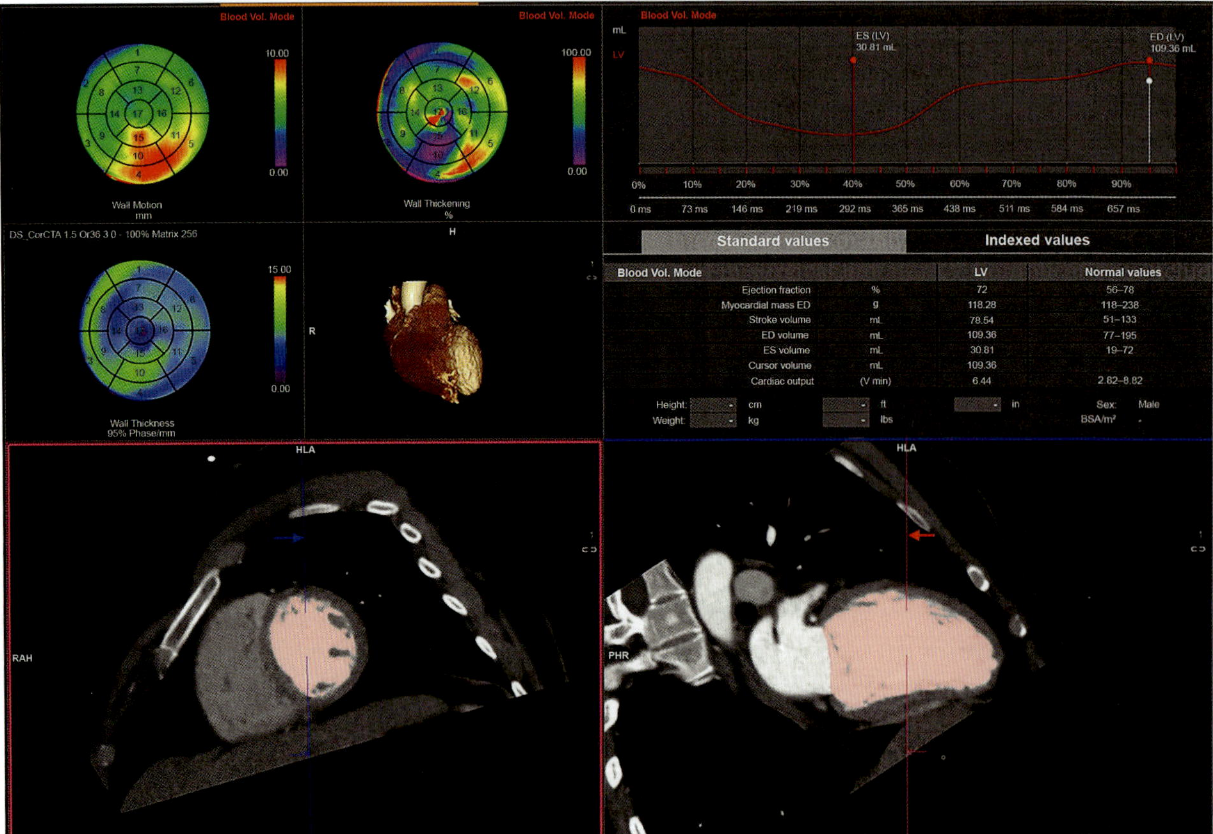

FIG. 8: CT image depicting the functional assessment using the cardiac CT data acquired using retrospective ECG gating showing normal systolic left ventricular function with normal ejection fraction in this patient with no coronary artery disease.

Cardiac Planes

The standard cardiac planes include horizontal long axis plane or four chamber view, short axis, and the vertical long axis or two chamber view **(Fig. 9)**.[30] These planes can be made along the long axis of the heart (line extending from the apex to the centre of the mitral valve) using the axial body plane images. The short axis plane extends perpendicular to this true long cardiac axis at the level of the mid portion of left ventricle. The vertical and the horizontal long axis planes can be generated by selecting the vertical or horizontal plane orthogonal to the short-axis plane. Depending upon the clinical indication, other planes such as right or left ventricular outflow, oblique sagittal plane (parallel to the axis of the aorta) can be used for optimal evaluation.

Pulse Sequences

Pulse sequences are software programs that describe the interplay of the magnetic field gradients and the RF pulses to produce requisite data with particular characteristics. These consist of sequences that provide both the static images (usually for anatomy and tissue characterization) and the cine images (for function).

Dark or black blood imaging **(Fig. 10)** is used to delineate the anatomical aspects.[30] In this sequence two inversion recovery (IR) pulses are used prior to the spin echo. This double inversion recovery (DIR) BB sequence attenuates the signal of flowing blood, and at the same time preserve signal from the surrounding stationary tissues.

Bright blood imaging can either be used for generation of the static images (for anatomy) or the cine imaging (for functional assessment). Previously GRE (gradient echo) sequences are used, but now steady-state free precession sequences (SSFP) are the work horse as it provides excellent images with great signal-to-noise ratio **(Fig. 10)**.[30,31]

Late gadolinium enhancement (LGE) imaging is the prime imaging sequence for myocardial tissue characterization and is used after setting an appropriate myocardial nulling time (on look-locker sequence) after

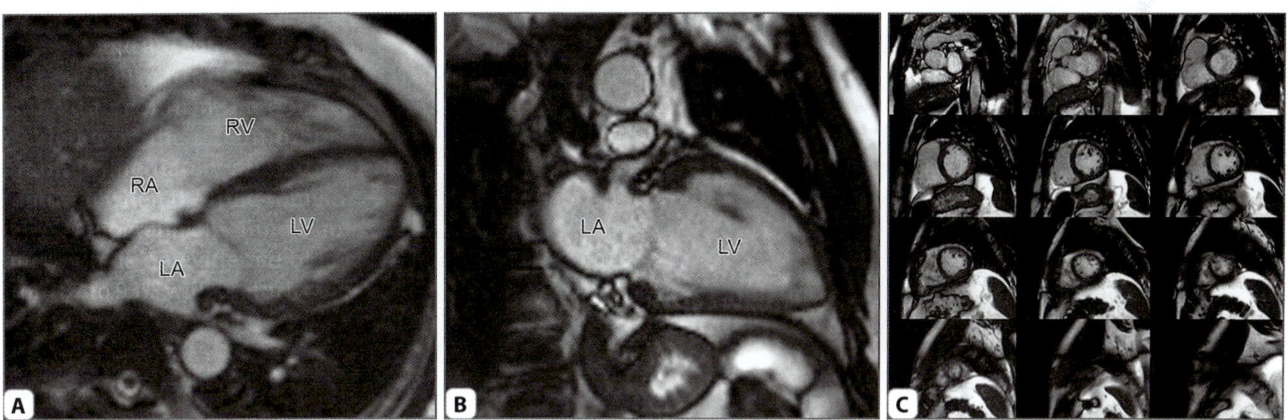

FIGS. 9A TO C: Cardiac imaging planes on SSFP cardiac MRI. Panel of images show (A) Horizontal long axis or four chamber view, (B) vertical long axis or two chamber view and (C) stack of short axis.

(LA: left atrium; LV: left ventricle; RA: right atrium; RV: right ventricle; SSFP: steady-state free precession sequences)

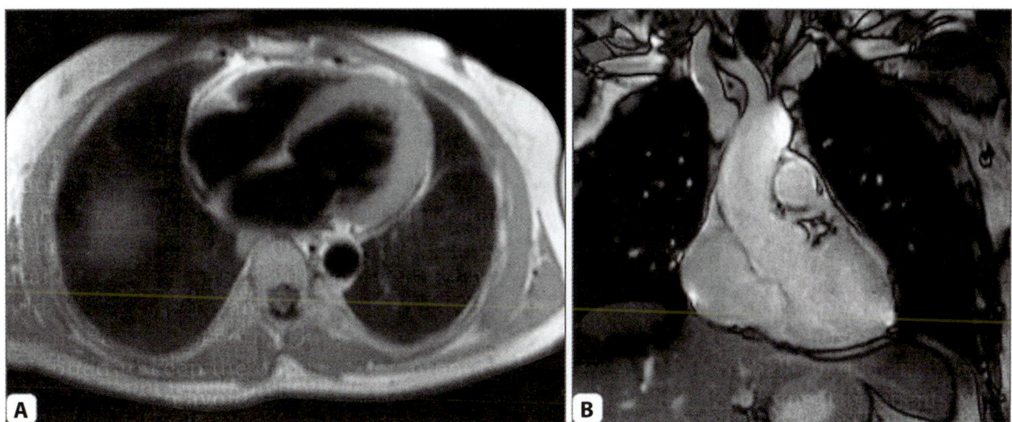

FIGS. 10A AND B: (A) Axial dark blood (double inverse recovery sequence); and (B) Coronal bright blood [still steady-state free precession sequences (SSFP)] image. These images are acquired for assessment of cardiac and extra-cardiac anatomy and further used for creation of cardiac imagining planes.

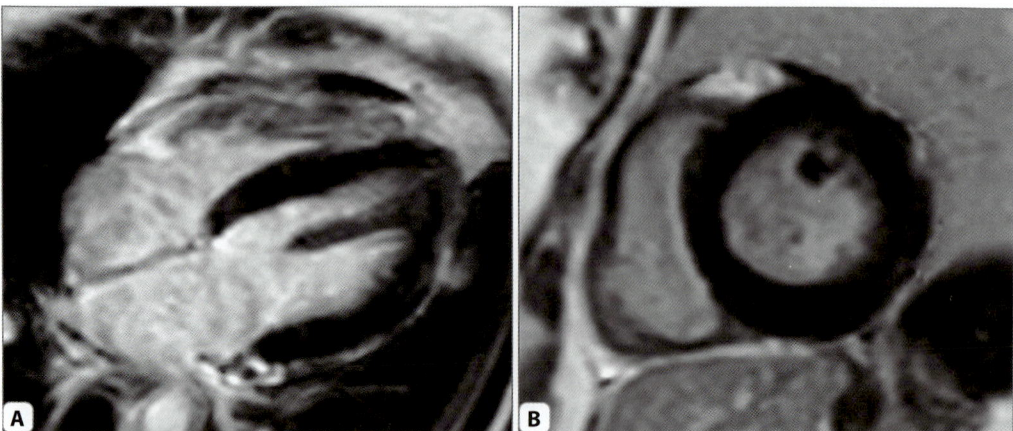

FIGS. 11A AND B: Late gadolinium enhancement (LGE) images in (A) four-chamber and (B) short axis-mid cavity planes. Note the myocardium is uniformly black in appearance.

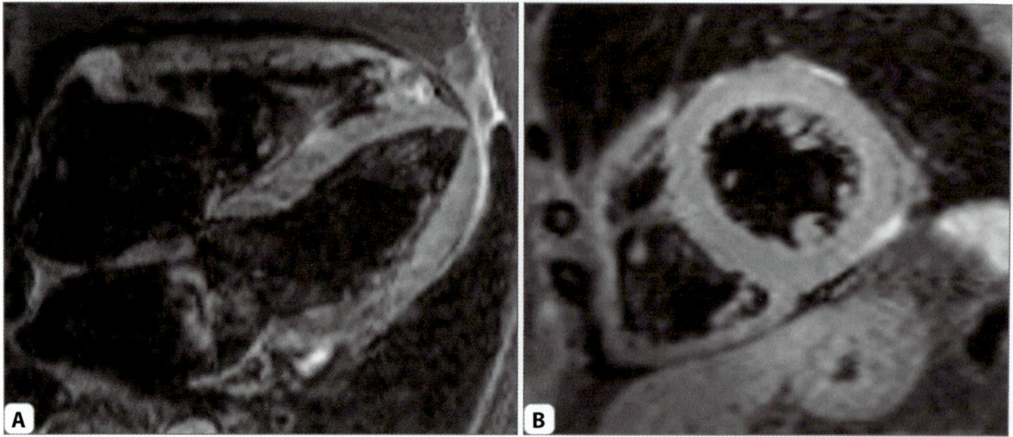

FIGS. 12A AND B: Short-tau-inverse-recovery (STIR) images in (A) four-chamber and (B) short axis-mid cavity planes. Note the myocardium is isointense in signal.

giving IV gadolinium. This sequence nulls the normal myocardium, that appears as uniformly dark/black and any pathology (edema or fibrosis—that expands extracellular space like amyloidosis) then strikingly appears bright **(Fig. 11)**.

Triple inversion recovery sequences (typically STIR—short-tau-inverse-recovery) uses a third inversion pulse in the previously described double inversion recovery (DIR) BB sequence that nulls the signal from fat and blood. This sequence is used for assessment of myocardial edema which manifests as bright signal in the region of abnormality **(Fig. 12)**.[30]

Phase-contrast imaging is a noncontrast technique that is frequently used to estimate the pulmonary and systemic blood flow to assess the shunt fraction and regurgitant fractions.[32,33]

Newer pulse sequences: Parametric mapping is the new addition that has capabilities of myocardial tissue characterization without the need of gadolinium. These are T1, T2 and T2*, which are useful in assessment of various diseases like amyloidosis, Anderson Fabry disease, myocarditis and iron overload in thalassemia patients.[34] Free breathing imaging, dark blood LGE and MR spectroscopy are some other sequences which are being integrated into the cardiac MR with encouraging results.[35-38] **Table 2** enumerates various types of pulse sequences used in cardiac MRI and the information provided by each of them.

Cardiac MRI needs skill, and every scan needs customization in respect to selection of various pulse sequences and imaging planes. Imaging data subsequently needs analysis on a dedicated workstation with suitable software for evaluation of ventricular functions and quantitative values.

TABLE 2: Enumerates various types of pulse sequences and their role in cardiac MRI.

Sequence	Role/Information provided
Basic	
Black blood (double inverse recovery sequence)—static images (usually T1 HASTE)	Anatomy—similar to CT scan
T2 STIR (short-tau-inversion recovery)—this is triple inversion recovery sequence that supress fat as well	Myocardial edema
Balanced-SSFP (steady-state free precession)—cine imaging: This provides high SNR (signal to noise ratio) where blood appear bright and myocardium appear gray. This is ECG- gated acquisition	Functional evaluation and morphology
Perfusion imaging	Myocardial ischemia
LGE: Delayed/Late enhancement—image contrast between scar/healthy myocardium is highest. It is usually SSFP sequence with a 180° inversion pulse given to null normal myocardium	Myocardial tissue characterization for scar and fibrosis
Additional	
T1 TSE/ T2 TSE FS	For assessment of myocardial thickening and characterization of masses
T1 TSE postcontrast	For assessment of pericardium/mass enhancement
Real time free breathing	For septal bounce—in constrictive pericarditis
Para-metric mapping	Myocardial tissue characterization
3D—whole heart fat supressed SSFP	Coronary arteries
Velocity-encoded phase contrast imaging	Flow quantification

CONCLUSION

With the advent of higher generation dual source CT and advanced MRI scanners, cardiac and coronary imaging have witnessed a considerable change. Apt knowledge of cross-sectional anatomy and post-processing tools are a must for optimal interpretation, so is the understanding of techniques for appropriate acquisition of data.

REFERENCES

1. Ghosh S, Yarmish G, Godelman A, Haramati LB, Spindola-Franco H. Anomalies of visceroatrial situs. AJR Am J Roentgenol. 2009;193(4):1107-17.
2. Pandey NN, Sinha M, Rajagopal R, Sharma A, Kumar S. Deciphering normal and anomalous viscero-atrial situs on multidetector CT angiography. Br J Radiol. 2019;92(1102):20190231.
3. Malouf JF, Edwards WD, Tajik AJ, Seward JB. Functional anatomy of the heart. In: Fuster V, Al- exander RW, O'Rourke RA, Roberts R, King SB, Wellens HJJ (Eds). Hurst's the heart. 11th ed. New York, NY: McGraw-Hill; 2005. pp. 45-82.
4. O'Brien JP, Srichai MB, Hecht EM, Kim DC, Jacobs JE. Anatomy of the heart at multidetector CT: what the radiologist needs to know. Radiographics. 2007;27(6):1569-82.
5. Jacobs JP, Anderson RH, Weinberg PM, Walters HL 3rd, Tchervenkov CI, Del Duca D, et al. The nomenclature, definition and classification of cardiac structures in the setting of heterotaxy. Cardiol Young. 2007;17 Suppl 2: 1-28.
6. Pandey NN, Sharma A, Jagia P. Imaging of anomalous pulmonary venous connections by multidetector CT angiography using third-generation dual source CT scanner. Br J Radiol. 2018;91(1092):20180298.
7. Pandey NN, Taxak A, Kumar S. Normal pulmonary venous anatomy and non-anomalous variations demonstrated on CT angiography: what the radiologist needs to know? Br J Radiol. 2020;93(1116):20200595.
8. Choe YH, Kim YM, Han BK, Park KG, Lee HJ. Morphologic diagnosis of congenital heart disease. RadioGraphics. 1997;17(2):403-22.
9. Yucel E, Bertrand PB, Churchill JL, Namasivayam M. The tricuspid valve in review: anatomy, pathophysiology and echocardiographic assessment with focus on functional tricuspid regurgitation. J Thorac Dis. 2020;12(5):2945-54.
10. Van Praagh R, Layton WM, Van Praagh S. The morphogenesis of normal and abnormal relationships between the great arteries and the ventricles: pathologic and experimental data. In: Van Praagh R, Takao A (Eds). Etiology and morphogenesis of congenital heart disease. Mount Kisco, NY: Futurama; 1980. pp. 271 316.
11. Lapierre C, Déry J, Guérin R, Viremouneix L, Dubois J, Garel L. Segmental approach to imaging of congenital heart disease. Radiographics. 2010;30(2):397-411.
12. Aricatt DP, Prabhu A, Avadhani R, Subramanyam K, Manzil AS, Ezhilan J, et al. A study of coronary dominance and its clinical significance. Folia Morphol (Warsz). 2023;82(1):102-7.

13. Khachatryan A, Chow RT, Srivastava MC, Cinar T, Alejandro J, Sargsyan M, et al. The Ramus Intermedius: A Bridge to Survival in the Setting of Triple-Vessel Total Occlusion. Cureus. 2024;16(5):e61288.
14. Van de Veire NR, Schuijf JD, De Sutter J, Devos D, Bleeker GB, de Roos A, et al. Non-invasive visualization of the cardiac venous system in coronary artery disease patients using 64-slice computed tomography. J Am Coll Cardiol. 2006;48(9):1832-8.
15. Bax JJ, Abraham T, Barold SS, Breithardt OA, Fung JWH, Garrigue S, et al. Cardiac re-synchronization therapy. Part 2–issues during and after device implantation and unresolved questions. J Am Coll Cardiol. 2005;46(12):2168-82.
16. Yamani N, Abbasi A, Almas T, Mookadam F, Unzek S. Diagnosis, treatment, and management of pericardial effusion- review. Ann Med Surg (Lond). 2022;80:104142.
17. Groell R, Schaffler GJ, Rienmueller R. Pericardial sinuses and recesses: findings at electrocardiographically triggered electron-beam CT. Radiology. 1999;212(1):69-73.
18. Ahmed Z, Campeau D, Gong H, Rajendran K, Rajiah P, McCollough C, et al. High-pitch, high temporal resolution, multi-energy cardiac imaging on a dual-source photon-counting-detector CT. Med Phys. 2023;50(3):1428-35.
19. Gulati M, Levy PD, Mukherjee D, Amsterdam E, Bhatt DL, Birtcher KK, et al. 2021 AHA/ACC/ASE/CHEST/SAEM/SCCT/ SCMR Guideline for the Evaluation and Diagnosis of Chest Pain: Executive Summary: A Report of the American College of Cardiology/American Heart Association Joint Committee on Clinical Practice Guidelines. J Am Coll Cardiol. 2021;78(22):2218-61.
20. Gupta A, Bera K, Kikano E, Pierce JD, Gan J, Rajdev M, et al. Coronary Artery Calcium Scoring: Current Status and Future Directions. Radiographics. 2022;42(4):947-67.
21. Singhal M, Subramanian P, Sharma A. Contrast Kinetics in CT Coronary Angiography. Indian J Radiol Imaging. 2024.
22. Desjardins B, Kazerooni EA. ECG-gated cardiac CT. AJR Am J Roentgenol. 2004;182(4):993-1010.
23. Liang CR, Ong CC, Chai P, Teo LLS. Comparison of radiation dose, contrast enhancement and image quality of prospective ECG-Gated CT coronary angiography: Single versus dual source CT. Radiography (Lond). 2021;27(3):831-9.
24. Yoo SJ, Hussein N, Peel B, Coles J, van Arsdell GS, Honjo O, et al. 3D Modeling and Printing in Congenital Heart Surgery: Entering the Stage of Maturation. Front Pediatr. 2021;9:621672.
25. Tretter JT, Gupta SK, Izawa Y, Nishii T, Mori S. Virtual Dissection: Emerging as the Gold Standard of Analyzing Living Heart Anatomy. J Cardiovasc Dev Dis. 2020;7(3):30.
26. Dodd JD, Leipsic JA. Evolving Developments in Cardiac CT. Radiology. 2023;307(3):e222827.
27. Jiang B, Guo N, Ge Y, Zhang L, Oudkerk M, Xie X. Development and application of artificial intelligence in cardiac imaging. Br J Radiol. 2020;93(1113):20190812.
28. Pennell DJ, Sechtem UP, Higgins CB, Manning WJ, Pohost GM, Rademakers FE, et al. European Society of Cardiology; Society for Cardiovascular Magnetic Resonance. Clinical indications for cardiovascular magnetic resonance (CMR): Consensus Panel report. J Cardiovasc Magn Reason. 2004;6:727-65.
29. Martin ET, Coman JA, Shellock FG, Pulling CC, Fair R, Jenkins K. Magnetic resonance imaging and cardiac pacemaker safety at 1.5-Tesla. J Am Coll Cardiol. 2004;43:1315-24.
30. Ginat DT, Fong MW, Tuttle DJ, Hobbs SK, Vyas RC. Cardiac imaging: Part 1, MR pulse sequences, imaging planes, and basic anatomy. AJR Am J Roentgenol. 2011;197(4):808-15.
31. Boxt LM. Cardiac MR imaging: a guide for the beginner. Radiographics 1999;19:1009-25; discussion, 1026-8.
32. Dunn TS 2nd, Patel P, Abazid B, Nagaraj HM, Desai RV, Gupta H, et al. Quantification of pulmonary/systemic shunt ratio by single-acquisition phase-contrast cardiovascular magnetic resonance. Echocardiography. 2019;36(6): 1181-90.
33. Colletti PM. Evaluation of intracardiac shunts with cardiac magnetic resonance. Curr Cardiol Rep. 2005;7(1):52-8.
34. Muser D, Chahal AA, Selvanayagam JB, Nucifora G. Clinical Applications of Cardiac Magnetic Resonance Parametric Mapping. Diagnostics (Basel). 2024;14(16):1816.
35. Tsampasian V, Cameron D, Sobhan R, Bazoukis G, Vassiliou VS. Phosphorus Magnetic Resonance Spectroscopy (31P MRS) and Cardiovascular Disease: The Importance of Energy. Medicina (Kaunas). 2023;59(1):174.
36. Longère B, Abassebay N, Gkizas C, Hennicaux J, Simeone A, Rodriguez Musso A, et al. A new compressed sensing cine cardiac MRI sequence with free-breathing real-time acquisition and fully automated motion-correction: A comprehensive evaluation. Diagn Interv Imaging. 2023;104(11): 538-46.
37. Holtackers RJ, Gommers S, Van De Heyning CM, Mihl C, Smink J, Higgins DM, et al. Steadily Increasing Inversion Time Improves Blood Suppression for Free-Breathing 3D Late Gadolinium Enhancement MRI With Optimized Dark-Blood Contrast. Invest Radiol. 2021;56(5):335-40.
38. Si D, Wu Y, Xiao J, Qin X, Guo R, Liu B, et al. Three-dimensional High-Resolution Dark-Blood Late Gadolinium Enhancement Imaging for Improved Atrial Scar Evaluation. Radiology. 2023;307(5):e222032.

Priya Jagia, Sanjeev Kumar, Akshit Kumar

CHAPTER 24

Imaging Approach in Children with Congenital Heart Disease

INTRODUCTION

Congenital heart diseases (CHDs) represent a spectrum of anomalies ranging from simple defects to complex structural malformations. The accurate diagnosis and effective management of these conditions heavily rely on imaging. The primary objectives of imaging have evolved from merely confirming a diagnosis to hemodynamic assessment (flow or shunt quantification) to strategically planning treatments (endovascular or surgical) and evaluating outcomes.

This chapter explores the role of imaging modalities such as chest radiographs, echocardiography, CT, and MRI in assessing patients with CHDs. We have incorporated diagnostic algorithms to assist in identifying CHDs, allowing for a systematic case-by-case approach.

Approximately seventy-five percent of cases of all CHDs either are not detected or do not have signs or symptoms warranting complete investigation in infants. Acyanotic CHDs including Left to right shunts, even large, rarely present with serious respiratory or cardiac difficulty in the first months of life, owing to high pulmonary vascular resistance. Cyanotic heart diseases, on the other hand, usually present early. Cyanotic CHDs can be severe pulmonary obstructive lesions (severe pulmonary stenosis with intact ventricular septum, pulmonary atresia), right to left shunts [tetralogy of Fallot (TOF)] or admixture lesions (total anomalous pulmonary venous return).[1]

These can further be classified as follows, based on pulmonary flow:

Group A: Lesions with decreased pulmonary blood flow—
- Pulmonary atresia (PA) or severe pulmonic stenosis (PS), with intact ventricular septum
- Tricuspid atresia
- Pulmonary atresia (or severe pulmonic stenosis) with VSD including TOF

Group B: Lesions with increased pulmonary blood flow—
- Transposition of great arteries (TGAs)
- Total anomalous pulmonary venous return with obstruction (TAPVR)

Group C: Lesions with severe pulmonary venous hypertension—
- Hypoplastic left heart (HLH)
- Severe coarctation of aorta with intact ventricular septum

PHYSICAL EXAMINATION

The conditions mentioned above might cause cyanosis, respiratory distress, or both in the first few days of life. Patients with TGA, pulmonary atresia (or stenosis) and tricuspid atresia have marked cyanosis with minimal or no respiratory distress in the neonatal period. On the other hand, respiratory distress is marked in TAPVC with obstruction and hypoplastic left heart syndrome, with little cyanosis. In Ebstein's, the child has cyanosis, tachypnea, systolic murmur and hepatomegaly which improves over the first weeks of life.

RADIOLOGICAL APPROACH

Chest Radiograph

A chest radiograph is the initial modality of choice in almost all cardiac diagnostic algorithms, particularly the CHDs. When systematically evaluated with relevant clinical information, it can help to categorise a patient into a specific CHD group with a certain degree of certitude, even if it does not specify the exact lesion.

General principles in the interpretation of chest radiographs in CHD include a sequential evaluation of

TABLE 1: Radiographic approach to acyanotic CHDs.

Normal aorta	Enlarged aortic knuckle	Enlarged aortic root
Left to right shunts:		
• Intracardiac shunts • *Pretricuspid*: ASD, PAPVD • *Post-tricuspid*: VSD	PDA	• RSOV • APW • CAF
Outflow lesions: • Aortic stenosis • CoA		

(APW: aortopulmonary window defect; ASD: atrial septal defect; CAF: coronary arteriovenous fistula; PAPVD: partial anomalous pulmonary venous drainage; PDA: patent ductus arteriosus; RSOV: ruptured aneurysm of sinus of Valsalva; VSD: ventricular septal defect)

TABLE 2: Radiographic approach to cyanotic CHDs.

Decreased pulmonary vascularity	Increased pulmonary vascularity
• *Enlarged aorta*: ○ TOF ○ VSD with pulmonary atresia ○ Tricuspid atresia ○ Single ventricle with PS ○ DORV with PS • *Normal aorta*: ○ Valvular PS ○ Ebstein's anomaly	• *Enlarged pedicle enlarged*: ○ Truncus arteriosus ○ TAPVC ○ Tricuspid atresia without PS • *Normal or narrow pedicle*: ○ D-TGA
Others: • Hypoplastic left heart syndrome • Severe coarctation of aorta with intact septum	

(DORV: double outlet right ventricle; PS: pulmonary stenosis; TOF: tetralogy of Fallot; TAPVC: total anomalous pulmonary venous connection; TGA: transposition of great vessels; VSD: ventricular septal defect)

the cardiac size, chamber enlargement, aorta, status of the pulmonary vasculature, assessment of the situs, and other associated abnormalities.

Traditionally, CHDs are classified as cyanotic or noncyanotic based on clinical presentation where noncyanotic patients typically present with symptoms of congestive cardiac failure like dyspnea, tachypnea or recurrent respiratory infections.

Using chest X-ray, these can be further classified by evaluating the pulmonary blood flow, the size of the heart, and the aorta, as described in **Tables 1 and 2**.

Left-to-right Shunt

A chest radiograph is useful in localizing the site of left-to-right (L-R) shunts in CHD. If the aortic knuckle is enlarged, the shunt is extracardiac and if the aorta is normal, the shunt is intracardiac.

Large Aorta

If the aortic knuckle is enlarged disproportionate to the ascending aorta, the L-R shunt is caused by patent ductus arteriosus (PDA). In PDA the heart is usually normal or mildly enlarged and lung vascularity is increased. In addition, pulmonary arterial hypertension (PAH) may be present.

If the ascending aorta is enlarged disproportionate to the aortic knuckle, the L-R shunt is at the aortic root level. The causes include a ruptured aneurysm of the sinus of Valsalva, aortopulmonary window, and coronary arteriovenous fistula.

- *Ruptured aneurysm of the sinus of Valsalva (RSOV)*: The heart size is usually enlarged with a biventricular or LV configuration. The aorta is enlarged with a disproportionate dilatation of the aortic root. The pulmonary conus is prominent, and lung vascularity is increased. There may be curvilinear calcification in it. In addition, in symptomatic patients, some evidence of PVH is also present. Usually, the right coronary sinus is involved and ruptures into the right ventricle.[2] The simultaneous presence of pulmonary plethora and PVH is characteristic of an RSOV.
- *Aortopulmonary window*: The heart size is usually enlarged with an LV configuration, there is disproportionate enlargement of the aortic root, pulmonary conus is prominent, lung vascularity is increased, and PAH is usually present.
- *Coronary arteriovenous fistula*: The heart size is usually normal and there may be LV configuration. There is disproportionate enlargement of the aortic root, pulmonary conus is prominent and lung vascularity is normal or increased. Chest radiograph may be normal because the shunt is usually small.

Normal Aorta

Normal or small aortic knuckle and inconspicuous ascending aortic shadow in a frontal chest radiograph in the presence of increased lung vascularity in a pink patient suggest an intracardiac L-R shunt. This shunt can be at a pre- or post-tricuspid level.

Pretricuspid Shunt

The pretricuspid shunt is produced by an atrial septal defect or a partial anomalous pulmonary venous drainage.

Atrial septal defect

The heart size is usually normal. There may be mild cardiomegaly in approximately 25% of the patients. There is right atrial enlargement with a right-sided configuration of the heart. Aortic shadows are normal in size with the ascending aortic shadow usually conspicuous by its absence in the upper right cardiac border. This sign is characteristic of an atrial septal defect (ASD). The heart appears to be shifted to the left and lung vascularity is increased. PAH may be present. The presence of associated anomalies may change this radiographic picture. Associated mitral valve disease should be suspected if LA/LA appendage is enlarged, PVH (especially if Kerley's lines) is present, or if the mitral valve is calcified. The association of ASD with mitral stenosis of rheumatic etiology is called "Lutembacher's syndrome".

Partial anomalous pulmonary venous drainage

This should be suspected if, in the presence of radiographic features of ASD, there is an abnormally enlarged shadow of the superior vena cava (SVC) or an abnormally directed pulmonary vein is seen.

Post-tricuspid L-R Shunt

This results from the presence of a VSD. This is the most common form of acyanotic CHD. The findings on chest radiograph in VSD depend on the shunt size and the direction of predominant flow. In a small <2:1 shunt, the chest radiograph may be normal. In the presence of a large >2:1 shunt, the heart size is usually enlarged with a left or a biventricular configuration, and there is evidence of LA enlargement, a normal aorta, and increased lung vascularity **(Figs. 1A to C)**. PAH may be present, in addition, there may be evidence of differential increase in lung vascularity in the right upper zone. In 3–5% of the patients, an associated right-sided aortic arch may be present.

Right-to-left (R-L) Shunt

Although chest radiographic features of most of the following conditions can be characteristic, it is important to remember that typical features are not usually seen in most patients. As with L-R shunts, the size of the aortic shadow is important in the localization of R-L shunts.

Large Aorta with Decreased Lung Vascularity

An enlarged aortic knuckle results from blood being shunted from the left to the right side of the heart, while reduced vascularity occurs due to limited blood flow to the pulmonary arteries. This is observed in conditions like TOF, pulmonary atresia with VSD, tricuspid atresia, double outlet right ventricle (DORV) with PS, and related disorders.

Tetralogy of Fallot: Etienne-Louis Fallot in 1888 described a tetralogy of defects, including pulmonary stenosis, a malaligned ventricular septal defect, overriding of the aorta and hypertrophy of the right ventricle. This is the most common form of cyanotic CHD in children. The pulmonic stenosis is usually infundibular in location. Additional valvular pulmonary stenosis and hypoplasia of the main pulmonary artery are also frequently present.

The chest radiograph shows a characteristic picture produced by a normal or mildly enlarged cardia, RV configuration with an uplifted apex (coeur-en sabot appearance), a large aortic knuckle, presence of pulmonary bay and pulmonary oligemia **(Fig. 2)**. A right-sided aortic arch is present in approximately 25% of the cases.[3]

Bronchial and nonbronchial aortopulmonary circulation is frequently present in case of severe pulmonary stenosis or pulmonary atresia.

The heart size may be enlarged in the presence of tricuspid or pulmonary regurgitation, absent pulmonary valve, severe anemia, bacterial endocarditis, pulmonary atresia, or bacterial infections.

In addition, a host of lung abnormalities largely due to defective bronchial cartilage and resultant tracheobronchomalacia may be associated. Occasionally, TOF may be associated with the congenital absence of a pulmonary artery, left more commonly than right. When this happens, parenchymal lung abnormalities are frequently associated.

Pulmonary atresia with VSD: There is mild cardiomegaly with RV configuration, a large aortic knuckle that frequently crosses the sternoclavicular joint into the neck, pulmonary bay, and peripheral oligemia. The aortic arch is right-sided

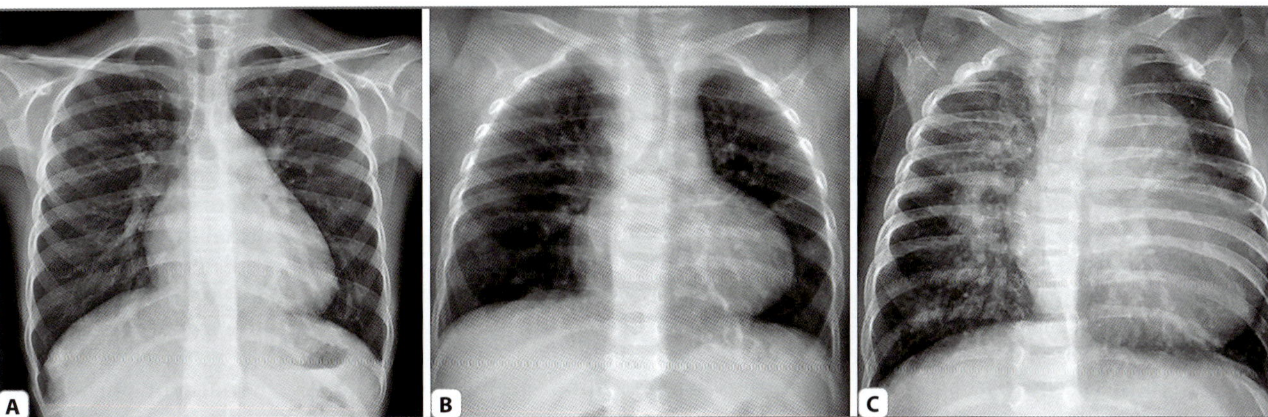

FIGS. 1A TO C: Left to right shunts: Radiographs of (A) ASD: Increased pulmonary vascularity with dilated right atrium. (B) VSD: Increased pulmonary vascularity with dilated right atrium, right ventricle. The main feature which differentiates from ASD is dilated left atrium (note increased carinal angle and double atrial shadow). (C) PDA: In addition to increased pulmonary vascularity, there is dilated aortic knuckle and dilated right and left ventricle in this case.

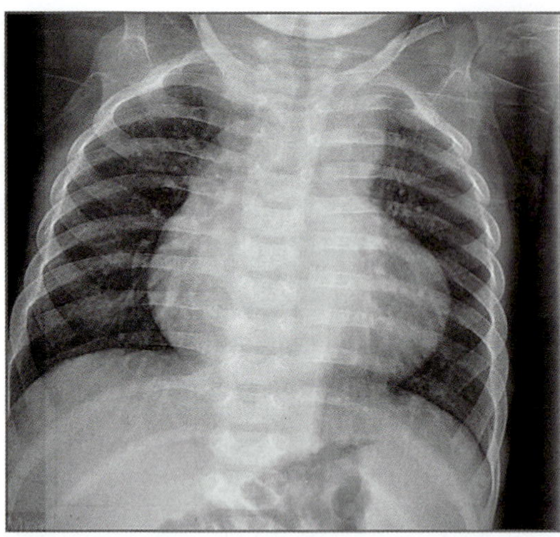

FIG. 2: Radiograph of tetralogy of Fallot: "Boot shaped" heart due to upturned cardiac apex (RV dilatation) and concave pulmonary arterial segment. Note should be made of reduced pulmonary vascularity.

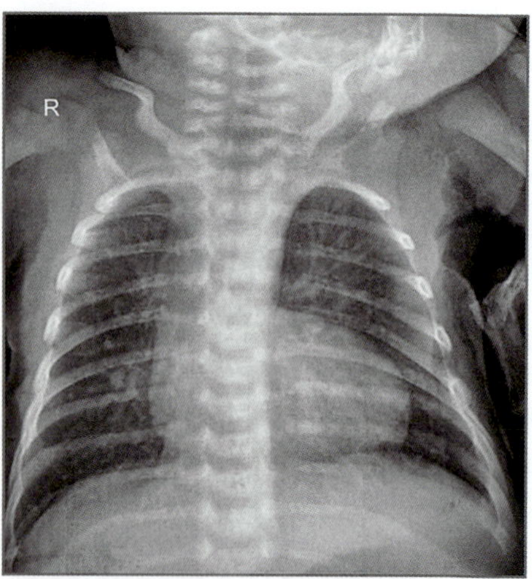

FIG. 3: Radiograph of transposition of great arteries (TGA): "Egg on side" appearance. This is due to the rightward displacement of the right ventricular outflow tract. Normally the right ventricular outflow tract is a left-sided structure and contributes to the mild convexity of the left mid cardiac contour.

in 30–40% patients. Collateral circulation by bronchial and nonbronchial aortopulmonary collaterals is frequently present.

Tricuspid atresia: The chest radiographic picture depends on the relationship of great vessels, the presence of PS, and the degree of RV hypoplasia.

A typical picture is seen in only 15–20% of the cases and consists of a normal-sized or mildly enlarged heart, LV configuration, straight right heart border, some evidence of LA enlargement, enlarged aorta, pulmonary bay, and decreased vascularity, provided that there is PS and the great vessels are normally related **(Fig. 3)**. The aortic arch is right-sided in one-third of the cases. If the pulmonary arteries are not located in their normal position, an abnormal relationship of great vessels should be suspected. In the absence of PS, there is evidence of increased lung vascularity.[4]

Normal or Narrow Pedicle with Increased Vascularity

D-TGA: This is the second most common cause of cyanotic heart disease in infancy. It is caused by a ventriculoarterial abnormality in which the aorta originates from RV and PA from LV.

The chest radiographic findings are characteristic, consisting of an enlarged heart, narrow pedicle, abnormally located pulmonary arteries, and increased lung vascularity. The shape of the heart is typical and resembles an "egg-on-side" **(Fig. 3)**. This pathognomonic picture is seen in patients in whom there is no evidence of pulmonary stenosis.[5]

Large Pedicle with Increased Vascularity

This combination is seen in truncus arteriosus, total anomalous pulmonary venous drainage (TAPVC), and tricuspid atresia without PS.

Truncus arteriosus: The heart is usually enlarged, there is LV configuration, the aorta is enlarged, pulmonary artery is not in its usual position, and lung vascularity is increased. The abnormal location of the PA may produce a characteristic picture described as "comma or water-fall" sign. This is more often seen on the left side. The aortic arch is right sided in about 50% of the cases.

TAPVC: This may be divided into four main groups according to the site or sites of connection, supracardiac, cardiac, infracardiac and mixed. The chest radiographic picture depends on the type of TAPVC.

In supracardiac type, which is also the most common, the heart is enlarged, the pedicle is wide with a classical "figure-of-8 or snowman's" appearance, produced by the dilated left vertical and left innominate veins and the right SVC. The left atrium is small and there is increased flow, as evidenced by pulmonary plethora **(Fig. 4)**.

In cardiac or mixed types, the picture may be nonspecific and consists of cardiomegaly, normal or enlarged aorta, and increased lung vascularity. A shadow of an enlarged abnormal pulmonary vein may be seen.

The scimitar sign is seen in the infradiaphragmatic type of TAPVC and is caused by the drainage of the right pulmonary vein into the IVC, hepatic or portal vein. This syndrome is often associated with hypoplasia or sequestration of the right lung.[6]

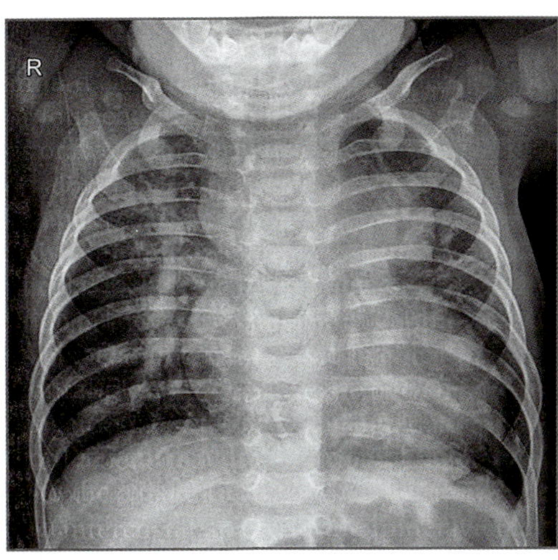

FIG. 4: Radiograph of supracardiac total anomalous pulmonary venous connection (TAPVC)—the upper part is formed by the vertical vein that drains the pulmonary venous return on the left and the dilated superior vena cava on the right. The lower part is formed by the enlarged heart.

Normal Aorta with Decreased Lung Vascularity

This combination can be seen in patients with Ebstein's anomaly, and valvular PS in failure.

Ebstein's anomaly: This produces a characteristic radiographic picture. There is severe cardiomegaly (reaching unto the ribs), evidence of RA enlargement, sharp, well-delineated cardiac margins as if drawn by a pencil, normal aorta and pulmonary oligemia.[7]

It can superficially resemble pericardial effusion, tricuspid regurgitation caused by chronic rheumatic heart disease (RHD), dilated cardiomyopathy (DCM), and Uhl's anomaly. Pulmonary vascularity is important in differentiating these conditions. In pericardial effusion, the lung vasculature is normal, and no specific chamber enlargement is present. In RHD, there is PVH and telltale signs of the underlying valvular disease are always present. In DCM, there is evidence of PVH. LA and LV may be enlarged.

Valvular PS: A chest radiograph may be normal except for a prominent pulmonary conus till there is severe PS with congestive failure. In such cases, there is cardiomegaly, RA enlargement, a normal aorta, prominent pulmonary conus produced by poststenotic dilatation of MPA and LPA, and peripheral pulmonary oligemia.

Other Conditions

Coarctation of aorta: This refers to a narrowing of the distal aortic arch and/or proximal descending aorta due to a discrete membrane or narrowing of the aortic isthmus. Findings on chest radiograph depend on the age of the patient, location of the coarct, ventricular function, competence of the aortic valve and associated abnormalities.

In an uncomplicated isolated coarctation, the heart size is usually normal. There may be left ventricular configuration. The classical feature of bilateral notching of the posterior and inferior margins of the 4th to 8th ribs is usually not seen in the first decade of life. The coarct segment is usually located in the juxtaductal region. Occasionally, it can be postductal and rarely preductal.

Postductal or juxtaductal coarctation produces typical radiographic features in the cardiac configuration, ribs and aorta. Rib notching is caused by the hypertrophied intercostal arteries that run along the posterior and inferior margins of the ribs. In juxtaductal coarct, the fourth to eight ribs are usually involved.

Coarctation proximal to the origin of the left subclavian artery results in unilateral right-sided rib notching. If the coarctation is proximal to an aberrant right subclavian artery, unilateral notching of the left ribs occurs.

Abnormal appearance of the aorta is seen in most patients. The ascending aorta is slightly dilated. "Figure-of-3" appearance of the descending aorta is characteristic but not commonly seen. The upper convexity is formed by the dilated subclavian artery and the lower convexity by the poststenotic dilatation of the descending aorta. Usually, a prominent or a flat knuckle is seen. If there is associated left ventricular decompensation, PVH may be present.

MULTISLICE CARDIAC CT

Echocardiography is the screening modality of choice for diagnosing and follow-up in CHDs. It is noninvasive, cost-effective, involves no radiation, and can be frequently repeated for follow-ups. It provides real-time imaging of the cardiac structures and functions, including the assessment of blood flow patterns with doppler techniques. However, echocardiography is operator-dependent and can be less effective for complex anatomies or postsurgical evaluations where metal or other structures might obscure imaging.

When echocardiography does not yield enough detail, cardiac CT or MRI should be used to clearly define the cardiac and vascular anatomy, particularly in complex CHDs, coronary anomalies, and postsurgical interventions. Cross-sectional imaging gives a superior view of the situs, central pulmonary arteries, pulmonary veins, AV-VA connections, and the aorta.

Multislice ECG-gated cardiac CT with its high resolution enables visualization of small, mobile heart structures. Although there's a concern of ionizing radiation, advanced techniques like fast low-dose accurate spiral helical (FLASH) CT scan image the heart in under a second, reducing radiation exposure by up to 80%. This method utilizes dual-source CT scanners for a higher temporal resolution (down to 66 milliseconds with third-generation scanners), and supports high-pitch scanning.[8] Additionally, scans can be prospectively gated, activating the X-ray beam only during the optimal cardiac phase, typically end-diastole.

Retrospective ECG-gated scan captures images at all phases of the cardiac cycle and images are reconstructed by selecting frames from different phases of the heart's motion, allowing for the creation of cine-like sequences. Retrospective ECG gating is reserved for cases where functional or valve motion assessment is required, in complex CHD cases and in patients with arrhythmias.

Some modern scanners allow for techniques like ECG dose modulation where retrospective data is collected but with reduced radiation during less critical phases of the cardiac cycle (systole), blending the benefits of both methods.[9]

Short-term sedation for CT is often necessary, especially in young children. At our institution, we ensure an anesthetist is present during the procedure, and the child remains admitted for a brief observation period post-scan. We use nonionic contrast at a dosage of 2–3 mL/kg of the child's body weight, administering it intravenously at a rate of 1.5–2 mL/s in infants.

We routinely use dual source CT scanner (Siemens Medical Solutions, Germany) for Cardiac CT. For children, a body weight based low dose protocol is used to limit the radiation exposure. Tube voltage of 80 kV has also been recommended for this purpose.

The scan delay is determined by bolus chase technique. In small children, the region of interest (ROI) is placed in right ventricle if pulmonary arteries need to be evaluated and in LV if aortic evaluation is required. Postprocessing involves reconstruction of multiplanar reformation (MPR), maximum intensity projection (MIP) and volume rendered (VRT) images on the dedicated workstation.

CARDIAC MRI

MRI provides outstanding anatomical detail without the need for ionizing radiation or contrast agents. However, it comes with challenges such as lengthy scan times, potential claustrophobia, and susceptibility to motion artifacts. Small children typically require anesthesia for the procedure, and to optimize image quality, a small coil is needed to cover the baby's chest, achieving the best signal-to-noise ratio.

The European Society of Cardiology (ESC) (2010) recommends cardiac MRI as an adjunct to echo when an echo study is suboptimal or when echo measurements are borderline or ambiguous, e.g., in the setting of volume overload.[10] The recommendations also include the following applications where cardiac MRI performs better than other modalities for the following:

- Quantification of RV volumes and ejection fraction, e.g., after repair of ToF.
- Evaluation of the right ventricular outflow tract (RVOT), RV–pulmonary artery (PA) conduits (site of stenosis or aneurysm), and the branch PA's.
- Quantification of pulmonary regurgitation (PR).
- Quantification of shunts.
- Detection and quantification of myocardial fibrosis.
- Tissue characterization (fibrosis, fat, iron loading, etc.).
- Evaluation of intra- and extracardiac masses.

For anatomic delineation, coronal, sagittal and axial nongated steady-state free precession images covering the entire chest are taken. Vascular anatomy is best delineated by doing a contrast-enhanced MR angiogram.

ECG-gated cine images in the short axis from the base of the ventricle to the apex help assess cardiac function and measure ventricular volume. Cine imaging across desired vascular planes can be done, e.g., along ventricular outflow tract, to rule out any stenosis or regurgitations.

Velocity-encoded phase-contrast MRI assess blood flow velocity and volume and thus helps in the quantification of shunts, stenoses and regurgitations; Systemic to pulmonary blood flow ratio (Qp/Qs) can be calculated by measuring flow in the pulmonary trunk and ascending aorta. Pressure gradient (ΔP) across a stenosis can be calculated by measuring maximum poststenotic velocity (V_{max}) by using Bernoulli's equation ($\Delta P = 4V^2_{max}$).

Newer techniques like 4D flow offer a detailed assessment of blood flow in CHDs by providing a 4D view (three spatial dimensions plus time) of cardiovascular hemodynamics. It's invaluable for visualizing complex, multidirectional flow patterns, allowing retrospective analysis of flow in any plane without extrascans, which helps understand anomalies like a bicuspid aortic valve or Fontan circulation. It quantifies flow metrics such as volume, velocity, and direction, aiding in evaluating shunts or valve regurgitation **(Figs. 5A to C)**. Additionally, it provides advanced hemodynamic data like kinetic energy and wall shear stress, which can guide clinical decisions by linking flow patterns to disease progression or cardiac changes.[11]

Myocardial parametric mapping and late gadolinium enhancement (LGE) help for detecting myocardial fibrosis in CHD patients, particularly postsurgery, aiding in assessing long-term myocardial effects.[12]

Sequential Segmental Approach of Analysing CT or MRI Images

Segmental approach in CHDs was developed independently in the 1960s by two groups: one headed by Richard Van Praagh and another by Maria Victoria de la Cruz. This system concentrated on the different topological arrangements of the three main components of heart—atria, ventricles, and great arteries.[13] Later, Robert H Anderson incorporated sequential analysis in it with a more detailed description of the AV-VA connections.[14] The sequential segmental approach is based on the three aspects of cardia—(1) Morphology of three components (atria, ventricles, and great vessels), (2) their interconnections, (3) Interrelationship between them.

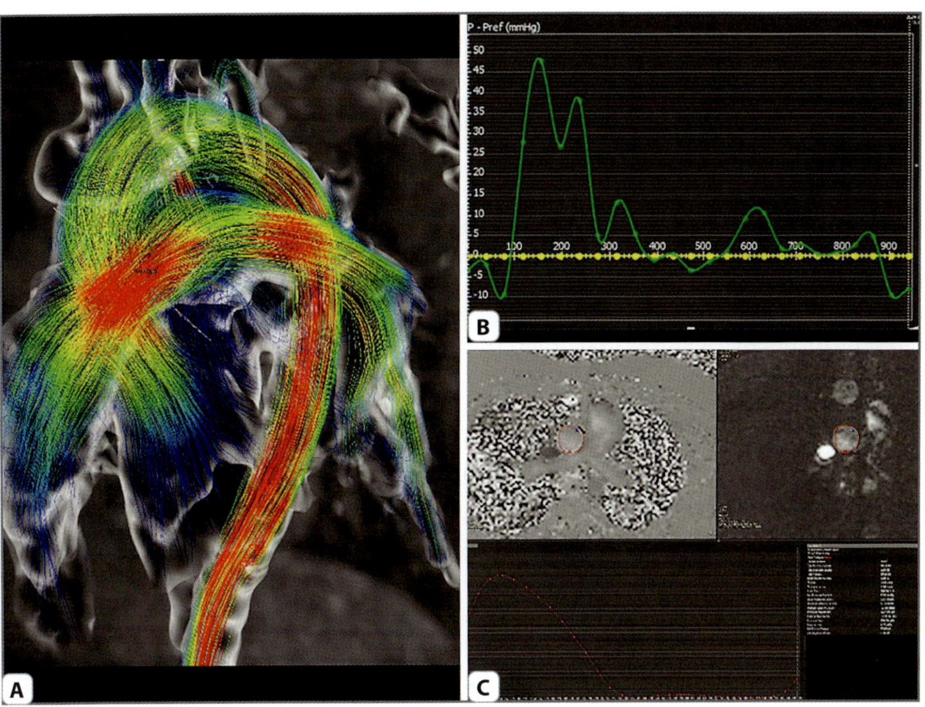

FIGS. 5A TO C: Phase contrast MRI techniques to calculate blood flow and pressure gradients. (A and B) 4D flow. (C) 2D flow showing the aortic flow and pressure measurements.

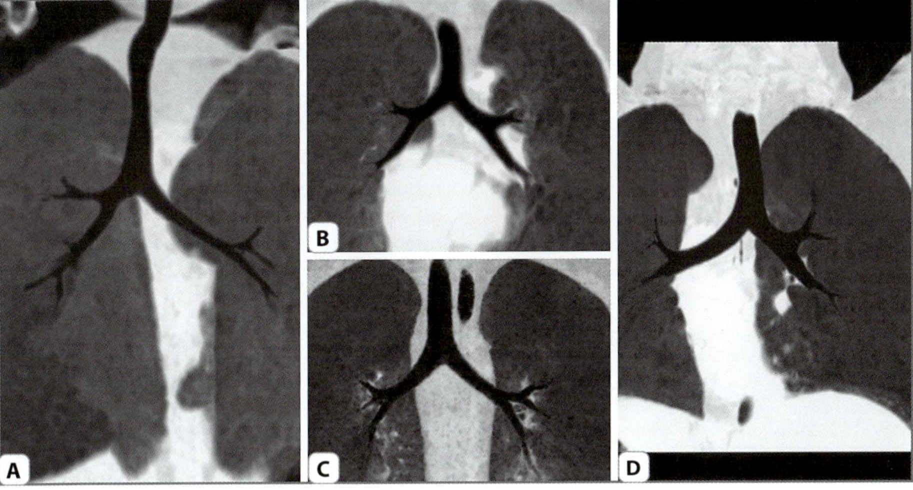

FIGS. 6A TO D: Possible thoracic situs. (A) Normal situs: Early right bronchus and long left bronchus. (B) Right isomerism. (C) Left isomerism. (D) Situs inversus.

Step 1: Identification of Visceroatrial Situs

Situs refers to the arrangement of organs in the body. Three arrangements may be possible: Normal arrangement—called situs solitus, a mirror image of normal—called situs inversus and when arrangement cannot be defined—called Situs ambiguous.

Visceral situs included identification of thoracic and abdominal situs.

Thoracic situs: Identified by bronchial anatomy, relationship of bronchi to the pulmonary arteries, and lobar pattern of the lungs. In a normal thoracic situs (solitus), the right bronchus is more vertical, wider, shorter, and more in line with the trachea than the left bronchus. The right upper lobe bronchus branches early and is positioned above the right pulmonary artery (eparterial bronchus), whereas the left bronchus is below the left pulmonary artery (hyparterial bronchus). The right lung is trilobed while the left lung is bilobed **(Figs. 6A to D)**.

Abdominal situs: In a normal abdominal situs (solitus), the liver and inferior vena cava are on the right side while the stomach, aorta, and spleen are on the left side. In an inversus arrangement, there is an exact mirror image of the normal arrangement. when the arrangement of abdominal organs does not fit into a clear category, it's referred to as situs ambiguous.

Atrial situs: It is defined by the position of the morphologically right and left atrium. The atria are identified by the morphology rather than the position of the chambers.

Table 3 illustrates the distinctive features that differentiate the right atrium from the left atrium **(Figs. 7 and 8)**.

Embryologically, suprahepatic IVC is closely related to the growth of the liver and right atrium and thus morphological right atrium and liver almost invariably develop on the right side. So, visceral situs is highly predictive of the atrial situs.

In a visceroatrial situs solitus, the morphologically RA and liver are positioned on the right side and the morphological LA, stomach and spleen are positioned on the left side. The right lung is trilobed whereas the left lung is bilobed. The situs inversus is an exact mirror image of the solitus. In an ambiguous situs, the position or assignment of RA and LA cannot be ascertained. The atrial situs ambiguity is usually seen with visceral organ ambiguity. This combination of visceral and atrial ambiguity can lead to "isomerism". Two forms of isomerism have been described: Right-sided isomerism with mid-line liver, asplenia, bilateral right bronchi and bilateral morphological right atria with abnormal pulmonary venous drainage; Left-sided isomerism with mid-line smaller liver, polysplenia, bilateral left bronchi and bilateral left morphological atria with abnormal systemic venous drainage **(Figs. 9 and 10)**.

TABLE 3: Features differentiating right and left atrium.

	Morphological RA	Morphological LA
Appendage	Large triangular with a broad base (tongue like) with wide orifice with RA	• Narrow and tubular (little finger like) • With narrow orifice with LA
Pectinate muscles	Extend up to AV junction	Confined to appendage
Crista terminalis	Present	Absent
IVC and hepatic veins	Usually drain into RA	–
Pulmonary veins	–	Usually drain into LA

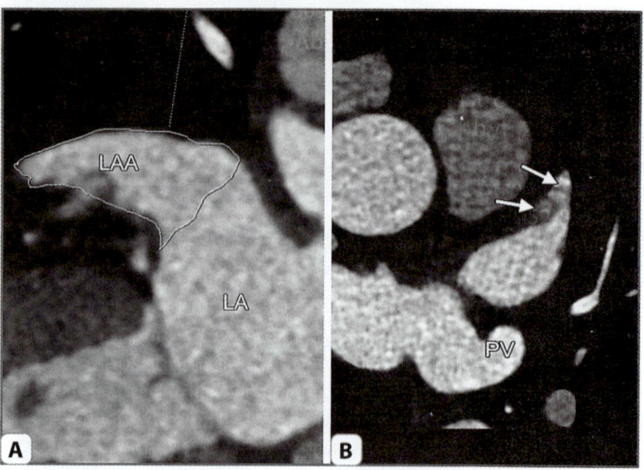

FIGS. 7A AND B: Features of morphological left atrium. (A) Long tubular auricle (LAA) with narrow opening into left atrium (LA). (B) Pectinate muscles within auricle and pulmonary veins (PV) opening into left atrium.

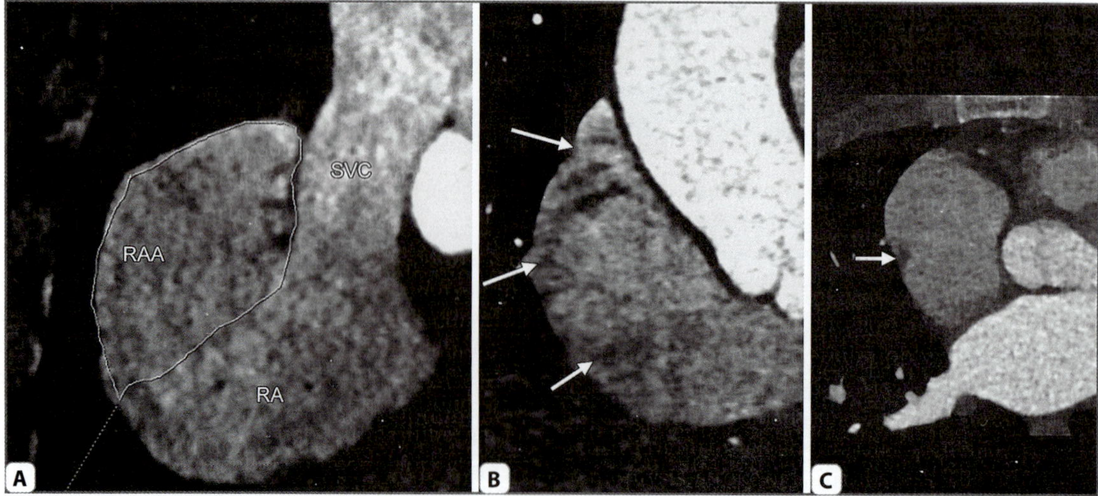

FIGS. 8A TO C: Features of morphological right atrium. (A) Pyramidal right auricle (RAA) with wide opening into right atrium (RA). (B) Pectinate muscle extending into right atrium (arrows). (C) Crista terminalis (arrow).

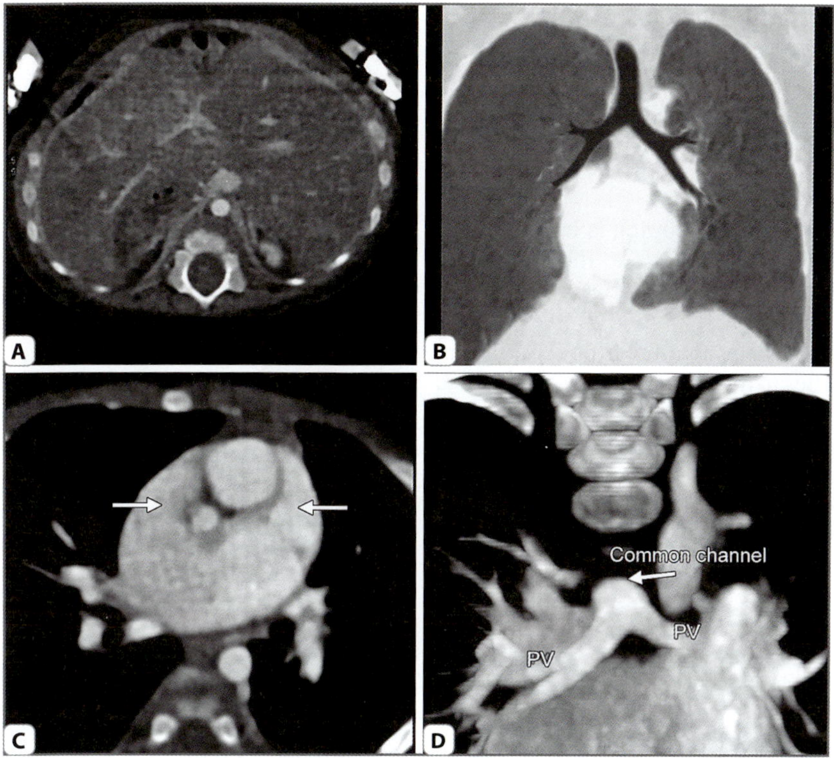

FIGS. 9A TO D: Right isomerism. (A) Large midline liver with asplenia. (B) Right-sided morphology of both bronchi. (C) Right-sided morphology both auricles (arrows). (D) Abnormal pulmonary venous drainage—TAPVC.

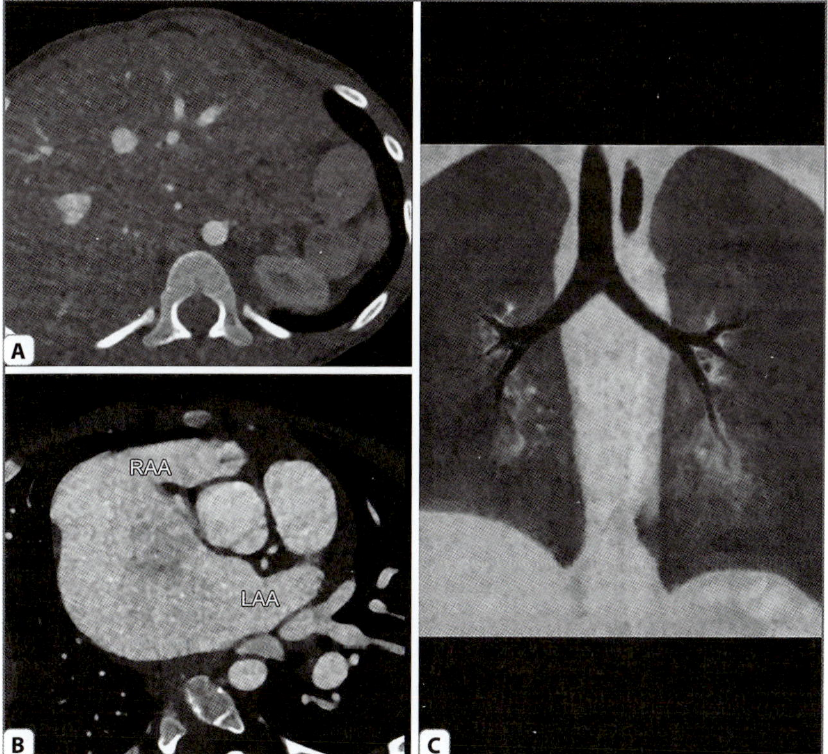

FIGS. 10A TO C: Left isomerism. (A) Polysplenia. (B) Left-sided morphology of bronchi. (C) Left-sided morphology of both auricles (RAA and LAA).

Step 2: Identification of Ventricles

Table 4 illustrates the distinctive features that differentiate the right atrium from the left atrium **(Figs. 11A to D)**.

Step 3: Ventricular Looping and Atrioventricular Connections

Embryologically, the ventricular looping is independent of the visceroatrial situs. This gives rise to the concept of concordance (RA-RV and LA-LV) and discordance (RA-LV and LA-RV).

A D-loop ventricle indicates that the inflow portion of the morphological RV lies to the right of the morphological LV and an L-loop ventricle suggests that the inflow portion of the morphological RV lies to the left of the morphological LV.

TABLE 4: Features differentiating right and left atrium.

	Morphological RV	Morphological LV
Moderator band	Present	Absent
Trabeculations	Coarse and irregular	Thin and fine
Septal surface	Coarse due to attachment of the septal papillary muscle	Smooth
AV valve	Tricuspid	Bicuspid
Continuity between AV valve and semilunar valve	Discontinuous by infundibulum	Fibrous continuity

The atrioventricular (AV) connection can be either univentricular or biventricular, depending on how the atria drain into the ventricles. Several types of AV connections have been identified in congenital heart diseases (CHDs) **(Figs. 12A to C)**.

- *Biventricular connection*:
  - Concordant: RA is connected to RV and LA to LV
  - Discordant: RA is connected to LV and LA to RV
  - Ambiguous: It can be associated with right or left atrial isomerism
- *Univentricular connection*:
  - Double-inlet ventricle: Both AV valves open into a single ventricle (e.g., DILV)
  - Atresia of one of the AV valve: Can be either tricuspid or mitral atresia

Step 4: Ventricular-arterial Connections

There can be four different forms of ventriculoarterial connections:

1. *Concordant*: When LV is connected to aorta and RV is connected to PA.
2. *Discordant*: When LV is connected to PA and RV to aorta (known as TGA).

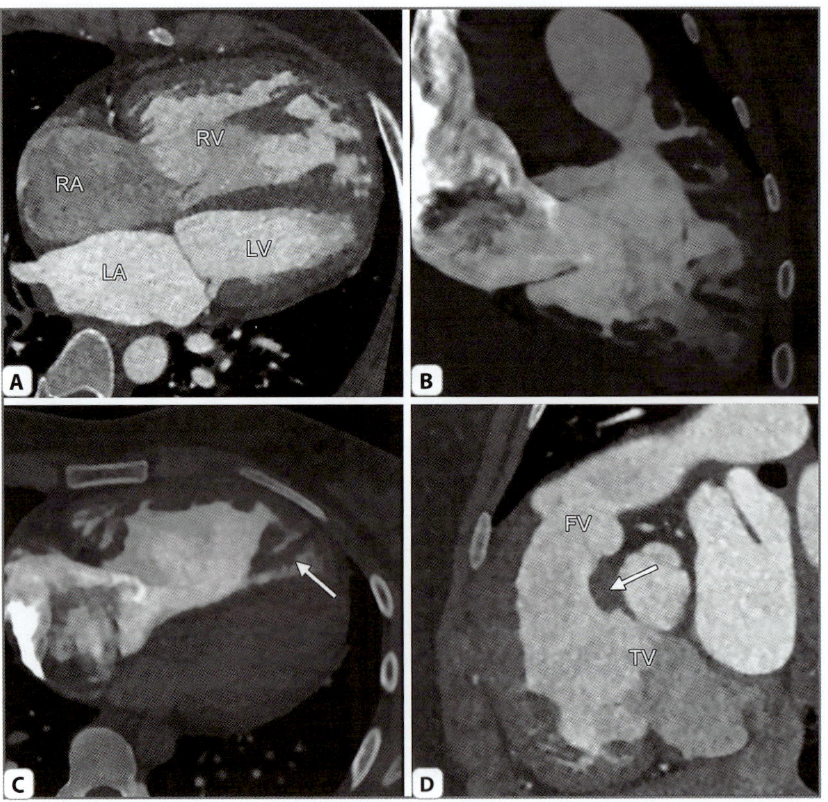

FIGS. 11A TO D: Features of morphological right ventricle. (A and B) Coarse trabeculations. (C) Moderator band (arrow). (D) Conus between pulmonary valve (PV) and tricuspid valve (TV).

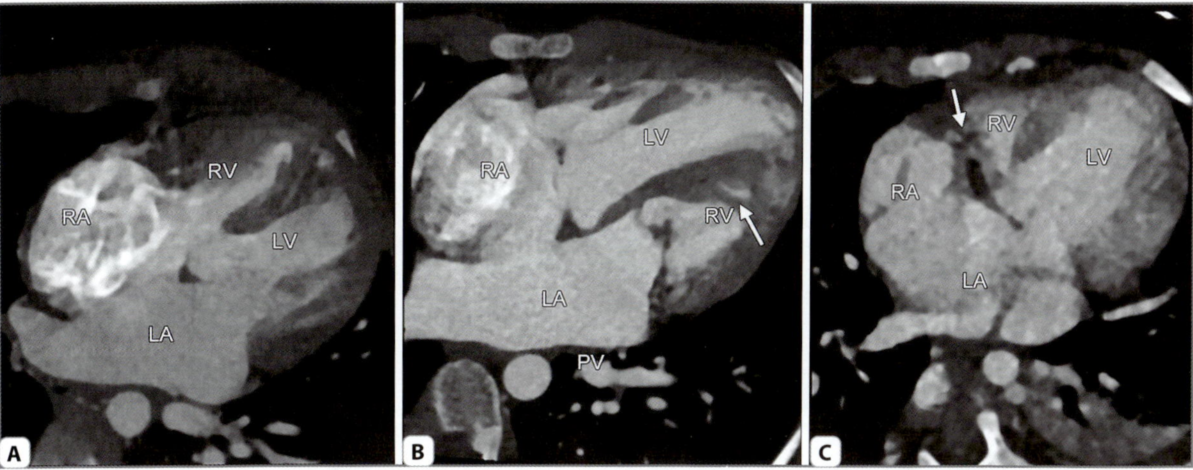

FIGS. 12A TO C: AV connections. (A) Biventricular concordant. (B) Biventricular discordant. (C) Univentricular in tricuspid atresia.

3. *Double outlet*: Both aorta and pulmonary artery arise predominantly (>50%) from one ventricle. This may be a double-outlet LV (DOLV) or a double-outlet RV (DORV).
4. *Single outlet*:
   - Only aorta connected, PA atresia
   - Only PA connected, aortic atresia
   - Truncus arteriosus.

Step 5: Spatial Relationship of Great Vessels

The position and relation of great arteries is defined at the level of ventriculoarterial valves; however, identification of the great arteries is based on the branching pattern. Normally, the ascending aorta is positioned posterior and to the right of the pulmonary artery (PA); it gives rise to at least one coronary artery and systemic branches. The main pulmonary artery (MPA) travels to the left and divides into the left (LPA) and right (RPA) pulmonary arteries **(Figs. 13A to D)**.

The following relationships of the great vessels may be possible:

- *Normal relation*: Aortic valve is rightward and posterior to the pulmonary valve
- *Inverse relation*: Aorta is leftward and posterior (e.g., situs inversus totalis)
- *D-transposition*: Aorta is anterior and to right of the MPA (e.g., D-TGA)
- *L-transposition*: Aorta is anterior and to left of the MPA (e.g., L-TGA)

Step 6: Assessment of Associated Abnormalities

After systematically evaluating the chambers and their connections, the associated intracardiac defects and anomalies should be identified.

- *Cardiac chambers*: Look for atrial and ventricular septal defects, chamber size, obstructions in ventricular outflow, etc.
- *Great vessels*: Check for variations in major vessel branching, the patency of the ductus arteriosus, significant aortopulmonary collaterals, hypoplasia of the aortic arch, the anatomy and size of the pulmonary arteries, and the coronary artery configuration.
- *Lung parenchyma and tracheobronchial tree*: Check for peripheral vasculature, mosaic attenuation, tracheobronchial compression or other lung lesions which may be present with CHDs.

CARDIAC CATHETERIZATION

With the advent of cardiac CT and MRI, diagnostic cardiac catheterization is now limited to a few conditions where hemodynamic information is required, e.g., a patient with combined aortic stenosis (AS) and pulmonary stenosis, or a patient with multiple levels of obstruction of both the systemic and pulmonary circulation, can be confusing when examined based on echocardiographic studies alone.[15]

Cardiac catheterization is vital for assessing pulmonary hypertension in CHD patients, determining pulmonary resistance for surgical and medical decisions, and evaluating responses to vasodilator therapy. It's particularly crucial before staged Fontan procedures for single-ventricle palliation, where it helps assess pulmonary resistance and detect venous obstructions, or high ventricular filling pressures, which could affect surgical outcomes.

In complex cases like pulmonary atresia, catheterization is key for mapping the pulmonary arterial and collateral supply, influencing surgical planning.

It's also essential for evaluating coronary artery anatomy in conditions like pulmonary atresia with an intact ventricular septum, especially for assessing RV-dependent coronary circulation.

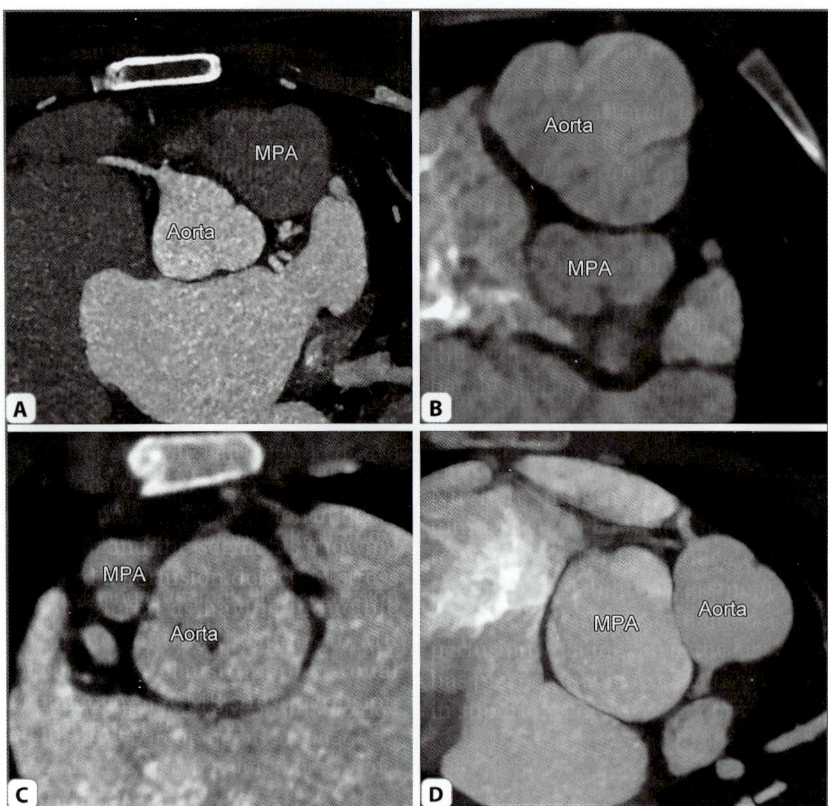

FIGS. 13A TO D: Spatial relationship of great vessels. (A) Normal; (B) D-TGA; (C) Inverse relation (L posed aorta); (D) L-TGA.

CONCLUSION

A multimodality approach individualized to each patient's clinical and safety profile is essential. With newer advances in imaging techniques, diagnostic algorithms are evolving with newer noninvasive techniques are taking centre stage. The initial focus of imaging in CHD relates to diagnosis and repair, this changes as patients age. These patients need extended follow-ups and repeated assessments, thus requiring a rational and methodical approach.

REFERENCES

1. Artman M, Mahony L, Teitel DF. Approach to the Cyanotic Infant. In: Neonatal Cardiology [Internet]. 3rd edition. New York, NY: McGraw-Hill Education; 2017 [cited 2024 Dec 25]. Available from: accesscardiology.mhmedical.com/content.aspx?aid=1140363192
2. Hoey ETD, Kanagasingam A, Sivananthan MU. Sinus of Valsalva Aneurysms: Assessment with Cardiovascular MRI. Am J Roentgenol. 2010;194(6):W495-504.
3. Apostolopoulou SC, Manginas A, Kelekis NL, Noutsias M. Cardiovascular imaging approach in pre and postoperative tetralogy of Fallot. BMC Cardiovasc Disord. 2019;19(1):7.
4. Park IS, Kim SJ, Goo HW. Tricuspid Atresia. In: Park IS (Ed). An Illustrated Guide to Congenital Heart Disease: From Diagnosis to Treatment—From Fetus to Adult [Internet]. Singapore: Springer; 2019 [cited 2024 Dec 25]. pp. 253-67. Available from: https://doi.org/10.1007/978-981-13-6978-0_12
5. Multimodality Imaging of Transposition of the Great Arteries | RadioGraphics [Internet]. [cited 2024 Dec 25]. Available from: https://pubs.rsna.org/doi/full/10.1148/rg.2021200069
6. Ferguson EC, Krishnamurthy R, Oldham SAA. Classic imaging signs of congenital cardiovascular abnormalities. Radiogr Rev Publ Radiol Soc N Am Inc. 2007;27(5):1323-34.
7. Jost CHA, Connolly HM, Dearani JA, Edwards WD, Danielson GK. Ebstein's Anomaly. Circulation. 2007;115(2):277-85.
8. Danad I, Fayad ZA, Willemink MJ, Min JK. New Applications of Cardiac Computed Tomography: Dual-Energy, Spectral, and Molecular CT Imaging. JACC Cardiovasc Imaging. 2015;8(6):710-23.
9. Tarkowski P, Czekajska-Chehab E. Dual-Energy Heart CT: Beyond Better Angiography—Review. J Clin Med. 2021;10(21):5193.
10. Kilner PJ, Geva T, Kaemmerer H, Trindade PT, Schwitter J, Webb GD. Recommendations for cardiovascular magnetic resonance in adults with congenital heart disease from the respective working groups of the European Society of Cardiology. Eur Heart J. 2010;31(7):794-805.

11. Rizk J. 4D flow MRI applications in congenital heart disease. Eur Radiol. 2021;31(2):1160-74.
12. DiLorenzo MP, Grosse-Wortmann L. Myocardial Fibrosis in Congenital Heart Disease and the Role of MRI. Radiol Cardiothorac Imaging. 2023;5(3):e220255.
13. Lapierre C, Déry J, Guérin R, Viremouneix L, Dubois J, Garel L. Segmental Approach to Imaging of Congenital Heart Disease. RadioGraphics. 2010;30(2):397-411.
14. Anderson RH, Shirali G. Sequential segmental analysis. Ann Pediatr Cardiol. 2009;2(1):24-35.
15. Feltes TF, Bacha E, Beekman RH, Cheatham JP, Feinstein JA, Gomes AS, et al. Indications for Cardiac Catheterization and Intervention in Pediatric Cardiac Disease. Circulation. 2011;123(22):2607-52.

Niraj Nirmal Pandey, Sanjeev Kumar

CHAPTER

25

Imaging in Ischemic Heart Disease

INTRODUCTION

Ischemic heart disease (IHD) continues to be one of the leading causes of mortality in developed countries. Even, in developing nations like India, the prevalence of IHD has risen markedly in the recent years.[1]

Ischemic heart disease is a complex entity with pathological changes noted in the coronary arteries as well as the myocardium. IHD includes different phases and clinical syndromes, and hence, imaging evaluation in IHD encompasses a wide gamut of indications which are highlighted in **Box 1**.

Conventionally, imaging modalities including transthoracic echocardiography, nuclear imaging and invasive catheter angiography have been used to evaluate various components of IHD. In recent times, computed tomography (CT) and cardiac magnetic resonance (CMR) have emerged as the diagnostic modalities of choice for almost all the aforementioned indications, with complementary roles depending on the phase of IHD. In general, CT can accurately detect coronary atherosclerosis in terms of the overall plaque burden, luminal stenosis caused by each plaque and presence of high-risk plaque features (HRPF), while CMR allows comprehensive evaluation of the function, perfusion, infarction and viability of the ventricular myocardium.[2] However, with recent technological advances, the scope of CT and CMR in IHD is increasingly overlapping.

The chapter focusses on the pathophysiological basis of IHD, their imaging correlates and evidence-based optimal CT/CMR imaging strategy depending on the phase and clinical syndromes of IHD.

BOX 1: Goals of imaging in ischemic heart disease.

- Assessment of presence, extent and characterization of coronary artery plaques
- Hemodynamic evaluation of blood flow obstruction caused by the coronary artery plaque
- Assessment of presence, extent and localization of myocardial ischemia
- Quantification of myocardial function
- Assessment of presence and extent of myocardial infarction (MI) and myocardium at risk
- Assessment of myocardial viability as a guide for revascularization
- Follow-up and imaging complications following MI

PATHOPHYSIOLOGICAL BASIS OF ISCHEMIC HEART DISEASE

Coronary atherosclerosis begins with the development of fatty streaks in the coronary artery walls which eventually progress to mature atherosclerotic plaques.[3] The plaque consists of a central lipid core with a fibrous cap and may progressively grow into the coronary artery lumen resulting in luminal blood flow obstruction. Subsequent to decrease in oxygenated blood flow to the working myocardium, myocardial ischemia may develop resulting in myocardial perfusion deficits, ECG changes, myocardial dysfunction and angina.[2] It is important to note that the hemodynamic significance of coronary artery stenosis may not relate directly to the degree of luminal stenosis.[4]

Also, it is well known that MI often arises from nonobstructive plaques.[5] Rupture of the thin fibrous cap exposing the thrombogenic core or surface endothelial erosions overlying the fibrous cap may trigger thrombus formation, which may lead to coronary artery occlusion and subsequently development of acute coronary syndrome (ACS).[6] Plaques precipitating these acute thrombotic events may demonstrate certain adverse characteristics or HRPFs such as presence of thin fibrous cap, positive remodeling, large necrotic core, microcalcifications, and intraplaque hemorrhage.[2]

Development of myocardial ischemia or MI affects the structure and function of the myocardium. Post MI, tissue necrosis and eventually irreversible scarring of the myocardium occurs which results in both systolic and diastolic myocardial dysfunction. Myocardial ischemia can result in areas of stunned myocardium which show dysfunction but are not infarcted and can potentially regain function. Severe myocardial ischemia can result in hibernating myocardium which shows dysfunction and can regain function if blood flow is improved. Eventually myocardial dysfunction can lead to the development of congestive heart failure and ischemic cardiomyopathy.

IMAGING MODALITIES

Multidetector Computed Tomography

Coronary Artery Calcium Scoring

The first step of a cardiac multidetector CT scan is usually a noncontrast electrocardiographically (ECG)-gated coronary artery calcium scoring scan, scanning the heart from the level of the carina to the caudal most extent of the heart. The quantified coronary artery calcium score (CACS) can be used in conjunction with reference databases that have stratified CACS by age, sex, and ethnicity to risk stratify patients on the basis of the likelihood of having a future coronary event **(Fig. 1)**.[7,8]

While the CACS can itself provide independent prognostic information in asymptomatic patients, it can also help in determining whether a symptomatic patient indicated for coronary CT angiography (CCTA) is a good candidate for the same. While there is no absolute threshold recommendation for a CACS that precludes a patient from undergoing CCTA, it may be difficult to interpret the CCTA images in the presence of dense calcification along the length of the coronary vessels and at branch points.

Coronary Computed Tomography Angiography

Following the CACS scan, an ECG-gated CCTA examination of the heart is performed including the same scan range as

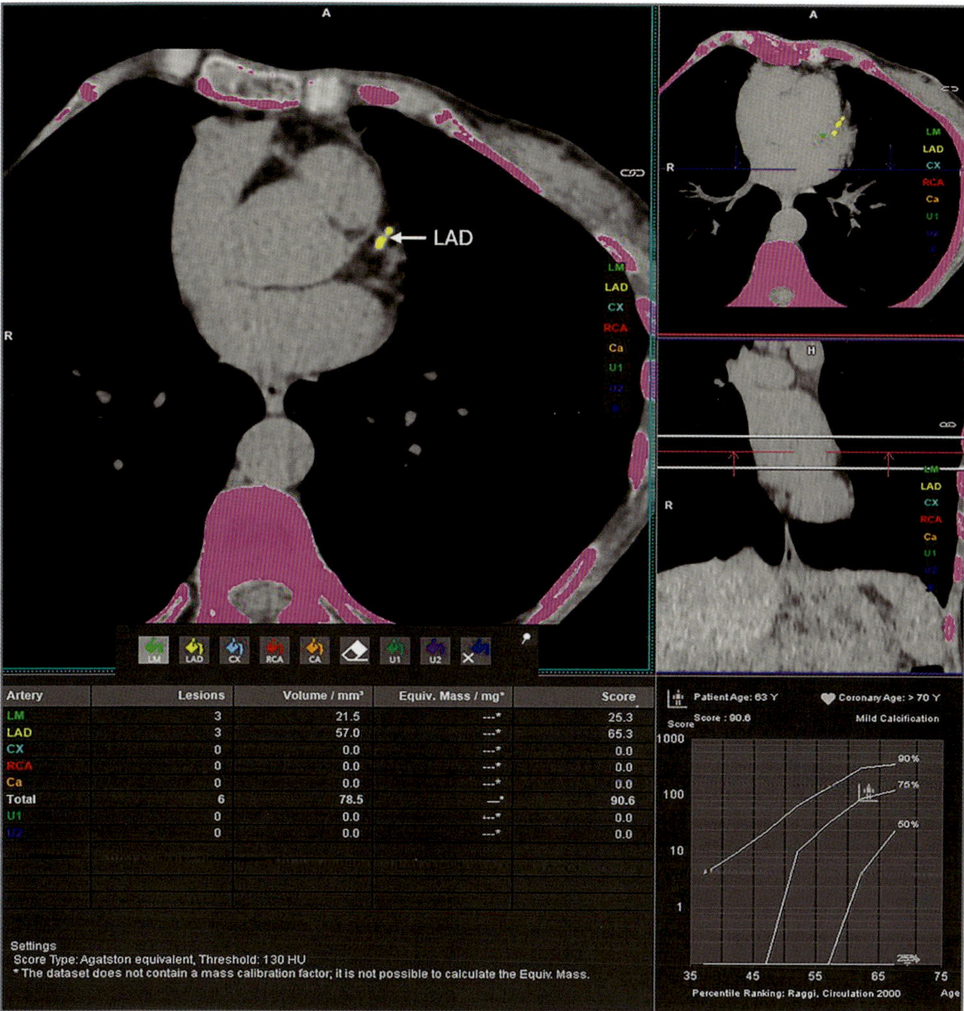

FIG. 1: Coronary artery calcium score assessment: Calcified plaques are noted in the left main coronary artery and the left anterior descending (LAD) artery with a total coronary artery calcium score of 90.6.

the CACS scan. The iodinated contrast agent, the volume and flow rate of the contrast, the method of contrast injection and scan triggering (using test bolus or automatic bolus tracking) and other scanner parameters like tube current and kilovoltage peak vary depending on operator preference and the technical considerations of the available CT scanner. The images are subsequently reconstructed with a small field of view to improve resolution **(Figs. 2 and 3)**.

A few crucial technical prerequisites for obtaining a CCTA of diagnostic quality are enumerated in **Table 1**.[9]

Electrocardiogram-gating during CCTA can be performed in two ways. A prospective ECG-gated CCTA (X-ray only turned on during part of the cardiac cycle) acquires images at predefined points in the cardiac cycle using a step-and-shoot sequential scanning method. Prospective ECG-gating requires presence of regular heart rate and rhythm. With an irregular heart rate, image acquisition can be triggered during the wrong phase of the cardiac cycle, causing mis-registration artifacts. The step-and-shoot sequential scanning produces individual trans-axial slices instead of volumetric data, with suboptimal z-axis resolution.

A retrospective ECG-gated CCTA (X-ray turned on during the entire cardiac cycle) obtains image sets along the entire cardiac cycle in the spiral mode. Using retrospective ECG-gated CCTA, data for all phases of the cardiac cycle can be reconstructed from the original volumetric dataset allowing for reconstruction of high-quality images along standard anatomic axis of the heart for the assessment of heart anatomy and for generation of dynamic cine sequences for assessment of ventricular function. It is advantageous for patients with arrhythmias or higher heart rates but also increases the radiation exposure to the patient compared to prospective ECG-gating.

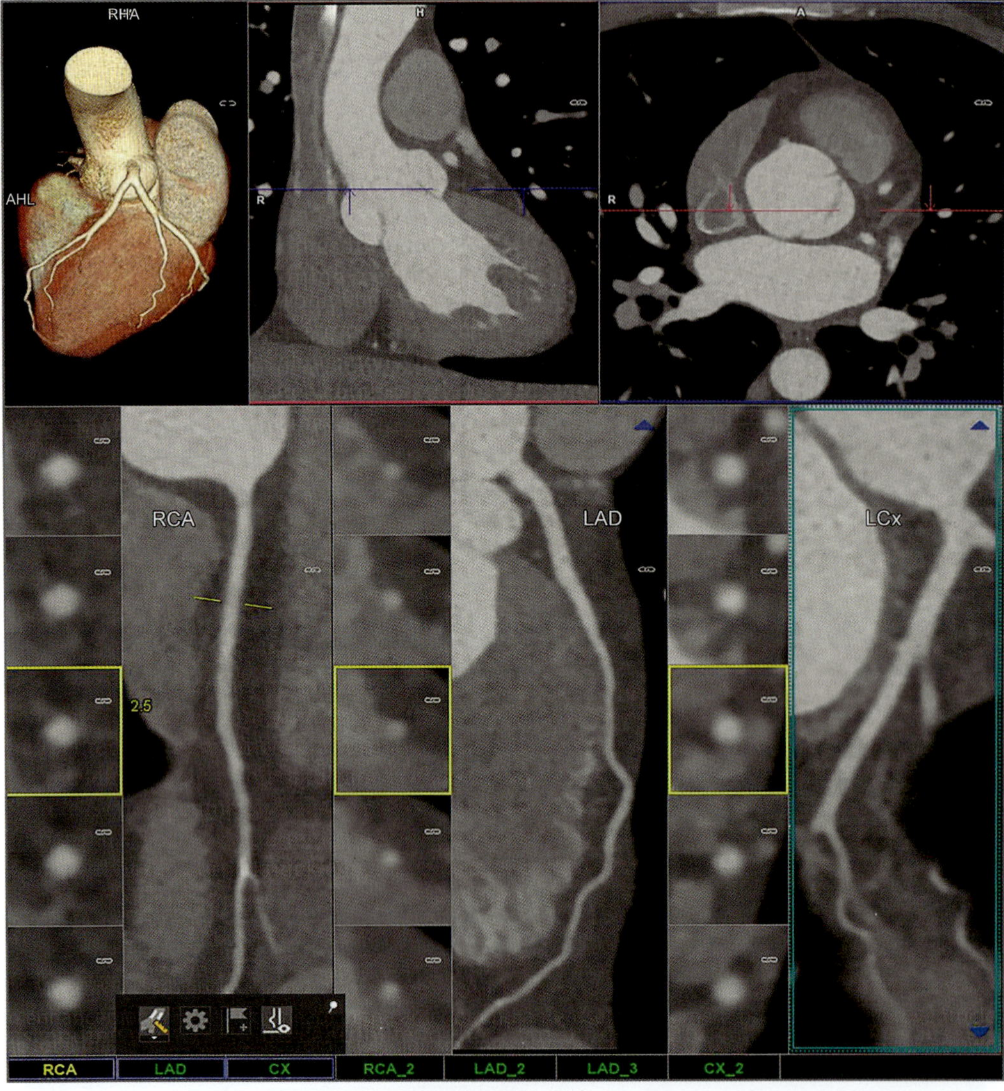

FIG. 2: Normal coronary CT angiography: Retrospective ECG gated CT coronary angiography shows normal opacification of the right coronary artery (RCA), left anterior descending (LAD) artery and left circumflex (LCx) artery on curved multiplanar reformatted images.

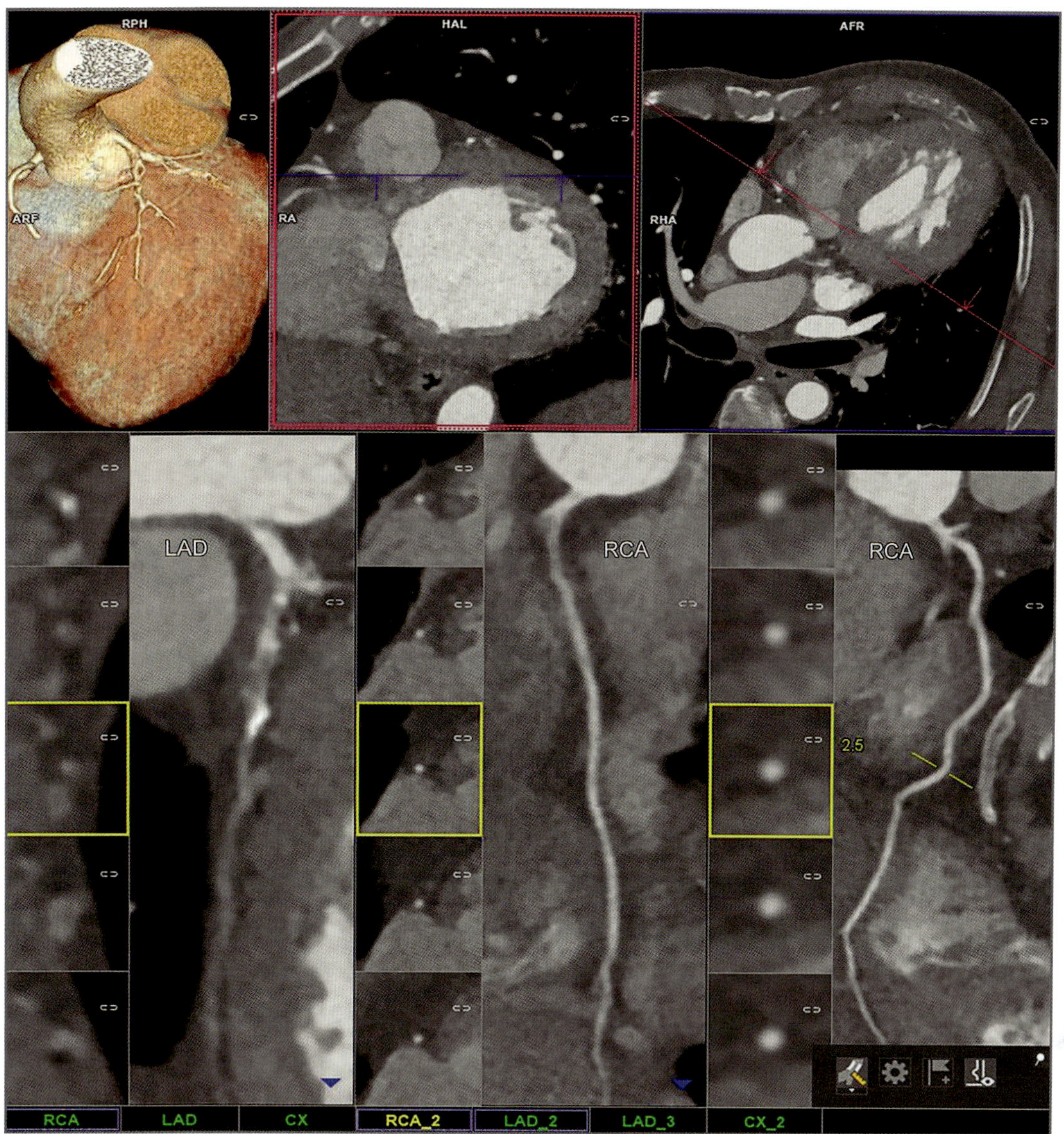

FIG. 3: Obstructive coronary artery disease on coronary CT angiography: Retrospective ECG gated CT coronary angiography shows near total occlusion of the proximal and mid left anterior descending (LAD) artery on curved multiplanar reformatted image. Note normal opacification of the right coronary artery (RCA).

TABLE 1: Technical prerequisites for obtaining a diagnostic quality CCTA.

Desirable characteristic	Function	Relevant technical parameter
High temporal resolution	Reduces motion artifacts	Rotation speed of the gantry tube
High spatial resolution	Allows detailed delineation of the coronary artery including the lumen and the walls	Detector properties, but also the reconstruction filter used, object contrast and image noise
Fast continuous coverage	Allows imaging of the whole heart in a single breath-hold	Detector size and pitch
Synchronization of scanning to the patient's heartbeat	Allows imaging during a consistent phase of the cardiac cycle	ECG gating

A major concern regarding CCTA is the exposure to ionizing radiation. Various radiation reduction strategies have been introduced to reduce radiation exposure to a level that is as low as reasonably achievable (the ALARA principle) **(Box 2)**.

Other challenges associated with CCTA have been highlighted in **Table 2**.[10]

The Society of Cardiovascular Computed Tomography has provided detailed guidelines for patient preparation before CCTA and the CT scanner requirements for performing CCTA which may be referred for guidance.[11]

Fractional Flow Reserve CT

Fractional flow reserve (FFR) CT is a novel postprocessing method that utilizes the CCTA imaging datasets and computational fluid dynamics to calculate FFR. FFR-CT involves the computation of coronary blood flow parameters like velocity and pressure, from the CCTA data. The computational steps are depicted in **Figure 4**.[10,12-14]

Fractional flow reserve CT utilizes the existing CCTA data and requires no additional imaging or radiation exposure. However, disadvantages of FFR-CT include the requirement of high-quality CCTA dataset as studies with artifacts may not be processed or may be incorrectly processed, limited availability and long processing times.[10]

Computed Tomography Stress Perfusion Imaging

Computed tomography stress perfusion imaging combines anatomic information obtained from CCTA and functional information obtained from the CT stress perfusion to anatomically detect coronary artery stenosis and

BOX 2: Radiation reduction strategies in coronary CT angiography.

- Limiting scan coverage to the area of the heart
- Retrospective ECG-gating with pulsed radiation delivering lower radiation dose outside the selected window in diastolic phase
- Lowering the tube voltage especially in patients with normal body habitus/body mass index
- Use of iterative reconstruction with lower tube current
- Using prospective ECG-gating wherever feasible

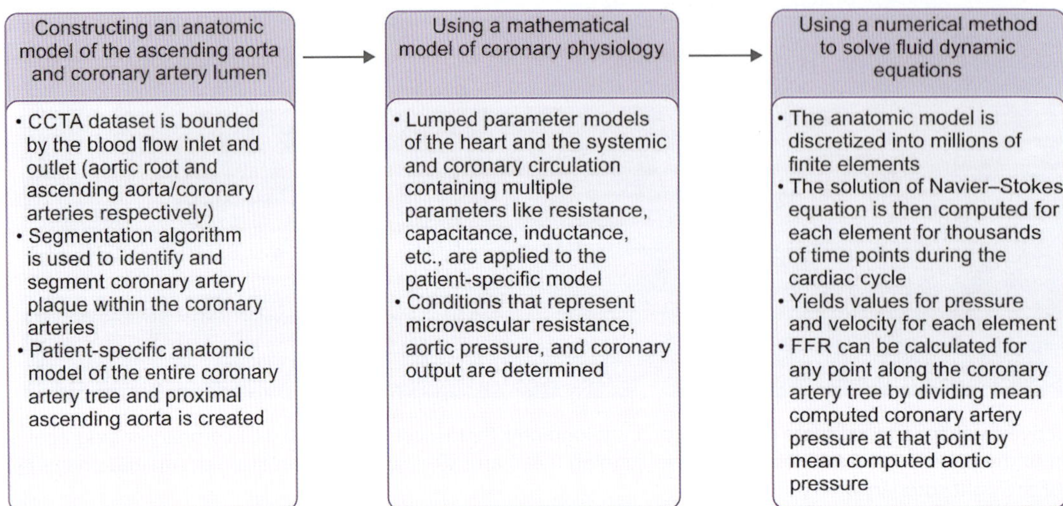

FIG. 4: Steps of computing fractional flow reserve (FFR) using coronary CT angiography (CCTA).

TABLE 2: Common challenges associated with CCTA.

Limitations	Cause	Problem solving strategies
Cardiac motion artifacts	High heart rate (>65 beats/min) and/or arrhythmia	• Heart rate control using oral and/or intravenous beta blockers • ECG-editing to remove data acquired during ectopic heartbeats • Using retrospective ECG-gating
Calcium blooming artifacts	Blooming of the dense calcified plaques leading to overestimation of stenosis severity	Using iterative reconstruction algorithms to reduce calcium blooming
Beam-hardening artifacts	Dark bands adjacent to areas of high attenuation such as dense contrast medium or metal	• Using a saline bolus chaser to clear contrast from the right heart • Using specific metal artifact reduction postprocessing softwares

subsequently establish its hemodynamic significance. It entails the performance of two CT examinations, at rest and at stress. The rest CT (the CCTA) is performed during the administration of iodinated contrast material while the stress CT perfusion is performed during the administration of a vasodilator agent (details included in the section under MR stress perfusion imaging) and iodinated contrast material. Either stress CT or rest CT may be performed first with a 10–20 minutes gap between the two examinations.

The stress CT technique can be static or dynamic.[15] In static CT perfusion, a single CT scan of the heart is obtained at peak myocardial perfusion during vasodilator stress; comparison of this scan with the rest CT scan allows for qualitative assessment of perfusion defects.[10,16] However, balanced ischemia may be missed.[10,17] In dynamic CT perfusion, multiple CT scans are obtained during the administration of the vasodilator and iodinated contrast which depict the wash-in and washout of contrast within the myocardium. While it results in a higher radiation dose to the patient, it allows both semiquantitative (using the upslope method) and fully quantitative (using indicator dilution theory) perfusion analyses.[10] Postprocessing involves extraction of time-attenuation curves of the arterial input function (from descending thoracic aorta) and the myocardium and quantification of the myocardial blood flow parameters using model-based deconvolution.[18] A major disadvantage is double exposure of the patients to both iodinated contrast and radiation.[10]

Cardiac Magnetic Resonance

Cine Sequences

Cine imaging involves image acquisition over several heart beats and results in a "segmented" acquisition of an individual cardiac plane. These sequences typically use a balanced steady-state free precession (bSSFP) or fast gradient echo technique.[19]

Usually a stack of ECG-gated cine images is acquired in the short-axis with a slice thickness of 6–8 mm covering both ventricles. These images provide a good contrast between the bright blood pool and the dark myocardium and have good spatial resolution. After drawing the endocardial contours, the modified Simpson's rule is used to calculate the volumetric and functional data including end-diastolic volume, end-systolic volume, stroke volume, cardiac output and ejection fractions for either ventricle. Drawing the epicardial contours as well allows for calculation of the ventricular mass and wall thickening.

Conventional T2-weighted Sequences

T2-weighted turbo spin echo sequences are used to detect increased water tissue content as an indirect measure of tissue edema or inflammation.

Cardiac Magnetic Resonance Stress Perfusion Imaging

In the resting state, blood flow to an ischemic myocardial segment may be compensated by various mechanisms. The aim of CMR stress perfusion imaging is to induce a high flow state (using vasodilators) or increased myocardial contractility (using inotropic agents), akin to physiological stress, which accentuates the difference between normally perfused myocardial segments which show increased perfusion owing to adequate myocardial reserve and the ischemic myocardium, which has a poor reserve.[2] Stress can be induced using various pharmacological agents, summarized in **Table 3.**[20]

After obtaining a written informed consent, where the entire procedure and expected side effects are clearly explained to the patient, two intravenous accesses are obtained in both upper limbs. Baseline cine images are performed, and perfusion images are planned with preferably three short axis slices (basal, mid, and apical LV myocardium). Adenosine is the most commonly used agent for CMR stress perfusion imaging and is administered as an infusion, at a dose starting at 140 µg/kg/min. The adequacy of response is assessed at 3 minutes following initiation. Adequate stress is defined as an increase in heart rate above 20 beats/min from baseline or a drop in systolic blood pressure of more than 10 mm Hg from baseline. If adequate response is not achieved, infusion rate can be increased (till a maximum of 210 µg/kg/min)

TABLE 3: Common pharmacological agents used in CMR stress perfusion imaging.

Agent	Route of administration	Principle	Contraindications
Adenosine (140 µg/kg/min)	Intravenous infusion	Vasodilator; nonspecific action on adenosine receptors (A2A, A2B)	Bronchospastic disease, hypotension (systolic blood pressure <90 mm Hg), atrioventricular block
Regadenoson (0.4 mg/5 mL) (not available in India)	Intravenous injection	Vasodilator; selective action on A2A receptors	Hypotension, atrioventricular block
Dipyridamole (0.56 mg/kg)	Intravenous infusion	Vasodilator; blocks adenosine reuptake into cells	Bronchospastic disease, hypotension (systolic blood pressure <90 mm Hg), atrioventricular block
Dobutamine (5 µg/kg/min)	Intravenous infusion	Inotropic stress	Severe hypertension, outflow obstruction, unstable angina, ventricular arrhythmias

and response assessed at 1-minute intervals. Whenever adequate response is achieved, gadolinium contrast (0.05 mmol/kg) is administered as a bolus from the opposite limb and the infusion of adenosine is continued at the same rate for one more minute. Stress perfusion images are obtained during this phase. Following the perfusion images, stress cine imaging can also be performed. After 15 minutes, gadolinium at the same dose and rate is administered again to obtain the resting perfusion images of the same slices. After 10 minutes of the second gadolinium administration, late gadolinium enhancement (LGE) images are obtained.[10]

Perfusion defects appear as hypoperfused (dark) areas, typically in a subendocardial location and last for several cardiac cycles (after initial peak enhancement in the ventricle, the first pass). Segments showing LGE are not evaluated (infarcted myocardium). Segments having a resting perfusion deficit (dark on resting perfusion images) are considered as artefactual, and the segments showing normal perfusion on rest and a perfusion defect on stress perfusion images are considered as having inducible ischemia. Apart from routine contraindications to MR imaging (patient on pacemakers/claustrophobia/renal failure), some specific challenges in CMR stress perfusion imaging are highlighted in **Table 4**.[21]

Delayed Enhancement MRI

Myocyte death (infarction) results in increased extracellular volume, which in turn results in slow wash in and delayed washout of the administered gadolinium-based contrast agent, compared to normal myocardial segments. When imaged 10–20 minutes postgadolinium administration, the infarcted myocardium appears bright (shortening of T1) due to this retention of contrast **(Fig. 5)**.[22] After an initial inversion scout sequence, the images are obtained during the time of inversion (TI) at which normal myocardium is nulled. The images are usually obtained at diastolic standstill, with the same slice thickness as used for cine imaging.

A subendocardial to transmural extent of LGE is usually seen with myocardial infarction. The extent of transmurality is graded according to the percentage of myocardium involved (<25%, 25–50%, 50–75%, and >75%), which indicate the severity of infarction and the possibility of viable myocardium being present. Areas of microvascular obstruction or intramyocardial hemorrhage appear as areas of low signal intensity within the bright infarct and denote a poor prognosis.

The conventional LGE sequences are susceptible to motion artefacts. Newer methods like single shot LGE (fast bSSFP readouts in a single cardiac cycle) or motion corrected LGE (MOCO) using motion correction algorithms can be used to tackle these.[23] The various types of LGE sequences commonly used are tabulated in **Table 5**. The presence of susceptibility artefacts is also challenging, especially in patients with pacemakers. In these situations, the wideband LGE can be employed, which uses a large bandwidth inversion recovery pulse, to eliminate artefacts.[24]

Nuclear Imaging

Nuclear imaging techniques like positron emission tomography (PET) and single positron emission computed tomography (SPECT) have well-established role in MI, myocardial viability assessment and myocardial perfusion imaging. SPECT has remained a workhorse for myocardial perfusion imaging but in the last two decades PET perfusion has picked up due to enhanced image quality that resulted in superior diagnostic accuracy over SPECT.

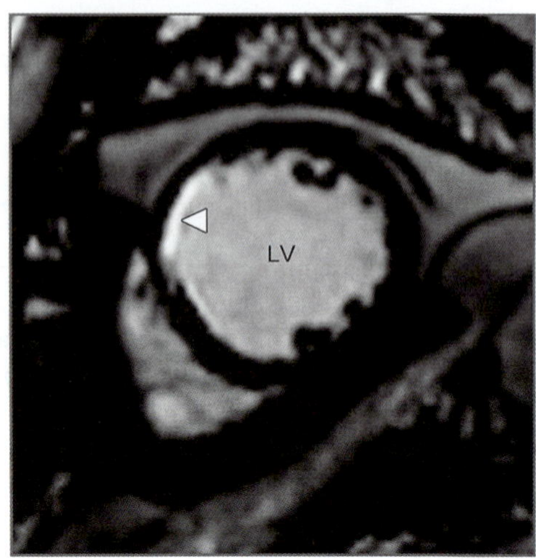

FIG. 5: Delayed enhancement MRI: Phase-sensitive inversion recovery images in the short axis view shows subendocardial late gadolinium enhancement (arrowhead) in the anterior segment of mid part of left ventricle (LV).

TABLE 4: Common challenges associated with CMR stress perfusion imaging.

	Challenge	Problem solving strategy
Gibb's artefact	Dark bands in subendocardial location mimicking perfusion defects	• Assess rest perfusion images—if present, consider as artefact • Usually one pixel wide, in the septum, does not persist for more than 3 cardiac cycles
Adequacy of stress response	May be difficult to ascertain based on vital parameters	Look for splenic switch off—spleen becomes dark, if stress response is adequate
Lack of response to stressors	Lack of adequate response even at maximal stress	Ensure patient is not on medications like theophylline or has taken caffeinated products in the last 24 hours

TABLE 5: Commonly used sequences for imaging late gadolinium enhancement.

Sequence	Underlying physics	Advantages	Disadvantages
FLASH/ GRE based PSIR	• Spoiled GRE sequence • Provides T1 weighted images	Better spatial resolution and image quality (in comparison to SSFP sequences)	• Requires breath-hold • Less SNR • Ghosting artifacts
SSFP based PSIR	• Steady state GRE sequence • Fully refocused steady state sequence • *Single shot*: All images acquired in 1 TR	• Very short TR, TE can be acquired with a breath-hold • High SNR • Less ghosting artifacts	• Less spatial resolution and image quality (as compared to FLASH GRE) • Less sensitive for detection of subtle LGE
Free breathing (FB) motion corrected (MOCO) PSIR	Eliminates pauses between FLASH slices and is therefore faster to acquire than a BH stack	• Single shot approach • Less ghosting artifacts due to poor breath-hold • Resolution and image quality of FLASH	
Dark blood LGE sequences	*Can be achieved by:* • *Nulling blood (manual)*: Gray rather than black blood • T2 prep (FIDDLE) • Magnetization transfer	• Higher contrast between infarcted myocardium and blood • Can detect subendocardial LGE better	Can miss thrombus
Fat water LGE sequences	• Dixon technique based PSIR • *Fat only image*: Fat is bright • *Water only image*: Fibrosis/ scar is bright	Differentiation between epicardial fat and subepicardial LGE	
Long TI sequence	TI ~ 600 ms at 1.5T and ~ 875 ms at 3T	• Nulls thrombus or regions of myocardium with MVO • Blood appears bright and myocardium appears gray	

(FIDDLE: flow-independent dark-blood delayed enhancement; FLASH: fast low-angle shot; GRE: gradient echo; LGE: late gadolinium enhancement; MVO: microvascular obstruction; PSIR: phase-sensitive inversion recovery; SNR: signal-to-noise ratio; SSFP: steady-state free precession; TE: echo time; TI: inversion time; TR: repetition time)

Single-photon emission computed tomography (SPECT) radioactive contrasts like Tc-99m tetrofosmin and Tc-99m sestamibi to generate 3-dimensional blood flow parameters. Tracers are taken up by myocardium in proportion to myocardial blood flow. Two sets of images are acquired after tracer injection at rest and other at stress (exercise or pharmacological stress). LV functions can also be evaluated using ECG gated SPECT.

Positron emission tomography has higher diagnostic accuracy owing to higher spatial resolution. PET with metabolic tracer like 18-FDG (Fludeoxyglucose F18) are regarded as gold standard for myocardial viability assessment. Fatty acids are the major substrate for non-ischemic heart. However, during ischemia, glucose becomes the major substrate. Hence, metabolic tracers like FDG are able to detect ischemic changes at cellular level. 18-FDG is usually combined with flow tracer like 13-N ammonia to assess myocardial perfusion. Hypoperfused/ dysfunctional myocardium (flow-metabolism mismatch) showing normal/increased 18-FDG uptake suggest viable myocardium. Decrease in both perfusion and 18-FDG uptake suggest infarction/scar.

EVALUATION OF VARIOUS COMPONENTS OF ISCHEMIC HEART DISEASE

Quantification of Coronary Plaque Burden

Coronary Artery Calcium Score

The Agatston method is the commonly used method for CACS assessment. In this method, weighted sum of coronary lesions having CT attenuation >130 HU are analysed. Plaque area is multiplied by a factor based on maximum plaque attenuation (factor 1: 130–199 HU; factor 2: 200–299 HU; factor 3: 300–399; and factor 4: >400).[25]

Coronary artery calcium score is used as an independent risk factor for atherosclerotic cardiovascular diseases, and it shows significant association with major cardiovascular events (all-cause mortality, cardiac mortality and nonfatal myocardial infarction) in medium- and long-term follow-up. Asymptomatic patients with CACS of zero and in the absence of additional risk factors is highly unlikely to have significant coronary obstruction with very low risk of adverse cardiovascular events. Patients can also be stratified for atherosclerotic cardiovascular disease risk based on their CAC score (no risk: 0; minimal risk: 1–10; mild:11–100; moderate: 101–400; high: >400).[26] CACS has also been incorporated in Coronary Artery Disease Reporting and Data System (CADRADS) for quantifying plaque burden in coronary arteries.[27]

Major global CACS guidelines recommend CACS screening for all asymptomatic individuals aged >40 years and having an intermediate level of risk. American College of Cardiology/American Heart Association (ACC/AHA) and Canadian Cardiovascular Society (CCS) also recommend use of CACS for decision making for appropriate use of statins. Multiple guidelines recommend withholding statins in individuals with CACS of zero and absence of other higher risk conditions like diabetes mellitus, smoking and family history of premature coronary heart disease followed by reassessment within 5 years for individuals > 40 years. Statin therapy is reasonable for CACS of 1–99 in individuals age ≥55 years. High intensity statin therapy is recommended for all age groups having CACS ≥100.[28]

Coronary Computed Tomography Angiography

In addition to locating and quantifying the stenosis, CCTA has an added advantage of direct visualization of the plaque which is not possible with catheter coronary angiography. Since CCTA has excellent spatial resolution, it can reliably distinguish between various types of plaques. It has high sensitivity (94%) and specificity (83%) for coronary plaque detection. It has an accuracy of 95% for detecting coronary artery stenosis when compared with invasive angiography.

Coronary plaques are described as calcified, partially calcified and noncalcified (soft) plaques. Noncalcified plaques can be further classified based upon their CT attenuation as lipid rich plaques (11–99 HU) and predominantly fibrous plaques (770û121 HU).[29] Imaging features of high risk/vulnerable plaques include low density (<30 HU) plaques, spotty calcification, positive remodeling and/or "napkin ring" sign. Positive remodeling is when the combined diameter of plaque and residual coronary lumen is more than the native artery diameter. "Napkin ring" sign refers to coronary plaque having central hypoattenuating area surrounded by high attenuation rim.[30]

The updated CADRADS with the intent to standardize CCTA reporting has graded coronary artery stenosis into no stenosis (0%), minimal (1–24%), mild (25–49%), moderate (50–69%), severe (70–99%) and occluded (100%). Similarly, CADRADS has also proposed a grading scale for coronary plaque burden based on CACS and the number and segments of coronary arteries involved.[27] CADRADS classifies patients with stable chest pain and acute chest pain into six categories (CADRADS 0 to 5) and suggests management based on severity.

Multiple large clinical trials including ACRIN-PA (American College of Radiology Imaging Network PA), ROMICAT II (Rule Out Myocardial Ischemia/Infarction by Computer Assisted Tomography), and CT-STAT (Coronary Computed Tomographic Angiography for Systematic Triage of Acute Chest Pain Patients to Treatment) have established the role of CCTA in low-to-intermediate risk patients presenting to emergency owing to its excellent negative predictive value of 99%.[31] CCTA also has prognostic significance with a 3-year risk for major adverse cardiovascular events (MACE) for a negative CCTA and a nonobstructive CCTA being 0.8% and 3.7% respectively.[32]

Cardiac Magnetic Resonance Angiography

Cardiac CMR is the gold standard imaging modality for assessment of cardiac structures, volume, functions and tissue characterization. However, as far as coronary artery angiography is concerned, CCTA still scores over MRA owing to its higher spatial resolution, shorter acquisition time, lower cost, wider availability and less artefacts. Owing to these shortcomings, CMRA has still not found a place among recommended/appropriate imaging modalities for coronary artery assessment.[33] However, recent advances in CMR techniques including motion correction, navigation techniques, reconstruction frameworks, higher field strength and use of nitrates have shown promising results. Multiple small validation studies have shown sensitivity, specificity, and negative predictive value of >80%.

Cardiac magnetic resonance has an added advantage in characterizing coronary plaques by analyzing T1 weighted (T1W), T2 weighted (T2W) and inversion recovery sequences. MRI can characterize plaque components like fibrous tissue, hemorrhagic tissue and calcification. However, sparse calcification may be masked by partial volume effect. Coronary plaques appearing hyperintense on noncontrast T1W images and are called high intensity plaque (HIP) and correlate with complicated plaques, lipid rich core and intraplaque hemorrhage.[34]

Noninvasive Functional Assessment of Coronary Artery Disease

Both CCTA and CCMRA provide anatomical details and have poor positive predictive value, hence, functional assessment of CAD is often required. Noninvasive functional assessment can be done using advanced CT and CMR techniques.

Fractional Flow Reserve Computed Tomography

Fractional flow reserve (FFR) is the ratio of maximum flow across a stenotic lesion to the maximum flow across a non-stenotic artery and hence it reflects the functional stenosis. Invasive FFR assessment is considered the gold standard for lesion specific ischemia. Only 49% of CCTA significant stenotic lesions are found significant on FFR assessment during invasive angiography resulting in lower positive predictive value of CCTA. Addition of CT derived FFR to CCTA results in increased specificity for lesion-specific ischemia. CT derived FFR value ranges between 0 and 1 with 0 reflecting complete occlusion and 1 reflecting no stenosis.

CT derived FFR values >0.8 are considered normal, values between 0.76 and 0.8 are considered borderline, and values ≤0.75 are considered abnormal. CT derived FFR values should be measured 1–2 cm distal to lesion as it correlates best with invasive FFR.

Fractional flow reserve CT is required only in patients having intermediate risk coronary anatomy. Low risk anatomy (stenosis <30%) can be managed with optimal medical therapy alone. High risk anatomy [≥50% stenosis of left main coronary artery (LMCA)/≥70% stenosis of left anterior descending (LAD) artery/triple vessel disease] can be referred for invasive coronary angiography. Significance of CT derived FFR lies in intermediate risk anatomy, i.e., 30–69% luminal stenosis or ≥70% stenosis of artery other than LMCA and LAD. If CT derived FFR comes out to be abnormal or borderline, then these patients are referred for ICA. However, in patients having normal CT derived FFR in intermediate risk anatomy, ICA and revascularization can be safely deferred with lower rate of MACE.[35]

Cardiac Magnetic Resonance Stress Perfusion Imaging

The temporal sequence of pathophysiological events which occur after onset of mismatch between myocardial oxygen demand and myocardial oxygen delivery is called the ischemic cascade **(Fig. 6)**. This ischemic cascade forms the basis of functional imaging. Functional significance of coronary stenosis can be assessed by demonstrating perfusion abnormality or wall motion abnormality on CMR stress perfusion imaging, CT stress perfusion imaging, positron emission tomography (PET) imaging and single photon emission computed tomography (SPECT) imaging.

Stress can be achieved with pharmacological vasodilatory stress or inotropic stress.[36] Administration of vasodilator agent causes dilation of nonstenotic coronary arteries resulting in increased blood flow. However, stenotic artery is already maximally dilated at rest to maintain myocardial oxygen demand and fails to respond to vasodilators. This results in maldistribution of blood flow with consequent hypoperfusion in segments supplied by the stenotic artery. Ischemia is predominantly diagnosed by perfusion deficit by using vasodilatory stress. However, wall motion abnormalities can also occur, particularly when stenosis is severe.

Inotropic stressor agent increases myocardial oxygen demand due to their inotropic and chronotropic effect. Vasodilation occurs secondary to increased myocardial oxygen demand but is not as vigorous as achieved with adenosine and dipyridamole. Therefore, ischemia is diagnosed primarily by inducible wall motion abnormality while perfusion deficits are less pronounced.

Cardiac magnetic resonance stress perfusion imaging is highly accurate for diagnosing CAD with sensitivity of 89% and specificity of 80%. Stress MR perfusion can be qualitative, semiquantitative and fully quantitative. Conventional qualitative cardiac stress MR perfusion is reported using 17 segment American Heart Association (AHA) model with exclusion of the apex (segment 17).

Qualitative CMR stress perfusion is reported based upon severity of defects (mild, moderate, and severity), transmural extent (subendocardial and transmural) and reversibility. Reversible perfusion defect is visible only on stress perfusion but not on rest perfusion. Semiquantitative CMR stress perfusion involves calculation of contrast enhancement ratio (CER) of myocardium [CER = (peak signal intensity of myocardial segment – baseline signal intensity of myocardial segment)/baseline signal intensity of myocardial segment] and myocardium-to-LV upslope ratio. However, semiquantitative CMR stress perfusion is currently not recommended as it does not significantly improve diagnostic accuracy over qualitative MR perfusion. Moreover, it underestimates perfusion deficits at high blood flow rates. Fully quantitative CMR stress perfusion maps are generated automatically using post processing software using arterial input function. It quantifies myocardial blood flow in milliliters per minute per gram tissue and is the most accurate method of MR stress perfusion.

Newer noncontrast techniques like arterial spin labelling (ASL) and blood oxygen dependent (BOLD) imaging are also being evaluated for myocardial perfusion imaging. ASL technique is based on the use of radiofrequency pulse to tag the protons in incoming arterial blood and has been conventionally used for noncontrast perfusion imaging of brain. BOLD perfusion technique makes use of deoxygenated hemoglobin as contrast material along with T2* oxygenation sensitive sequence.[10]

Computed Tomography Stress Perfusion

Computed tomography stress perfusion imaging is based on similar principles as CMR stress perfusion imaging. Dynamic CT stress perfusion imaging has high diagnostic accuracy (85%) when compared with invasive FFR as gold standard. The diagnostic accuracy of CT stress perfusion imaging is comparable to CMR stress perfusion imaging and PET and is superior to SPECT. Sequential addition of CCTA, FFR-CT and dynamic CT stress perfusion imaging further

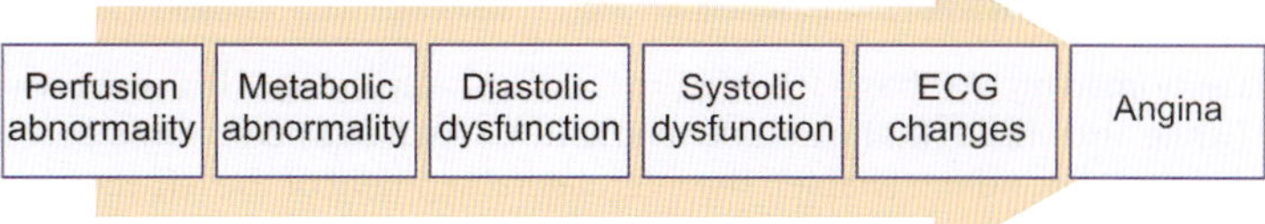

FIG. 6: Ischemic cascade: The temporal sequence of pathophysiological events which occur after onset of mismatch between myocardial oxygen demand and myocardial oxygen delivery.

increases diagnostic accuracy for detection of significant CAD. Dynamic CT stress perfusion imaging alone has the highest prognostic value for MACE when compared to CCTA and FFR-CT. Despite these promising results in various studies, dynamic CT perfusion is sparsely available and is not routinely used.[37]

Evaluation of Myocardial Infarction and Viability Assessment

Cardiac Magnetic Resonance

Prolonged myocardial ischemia results in MI which most commonly occurs due to coronary plaque rupture or erosion. Less common causes include coronary vasospasm, vasculitis, embolism, and coronary artery dissection.

Cardiac magnetic resonance is the imaging modality of choice for evaluation of evaluation of MI and viability assessment. MI results in increased extracellular volume with delayed wash-in and wash-out of gadolinium which is reflected as LGE. Most characteristically, LGE in MI occurs in the subendocardial region with variable degree of transmural extent. Transmural extent of LGE can be graded as 1–25%, 26–50%, 51–75%, 76–99%, and 100% **(Figs. 7A and B)**. LGE transmural extent of >50% is associated with lower likelihood of recovery after revascularization. Hence, reporting of cardiac magnetic resonance done for assessment of MI should include transmural extent of LGE in each AHA segment. Additional findings include wall motion abnormality, myocardial thinning, ventricular dilation, and reduced ejection fraction.

Cardiac magnetic resonance can be used to distinguish between hibernating and stunned myocardium. Stunned myocardium refers to prolonged regional dysfunction which persists for hours to weeks after transient stress induced ischemia, and it recovers without revascularization. Hibernating myocardium refers to chronic ischemia resulting in focal dysfunction which may recover after revascularization. Stunned myocardium shows normal perfusion while hibernating myocardium shows perfusion defect on CMR stress perfusion imaging.

Cardiac Computed Tomography

Computed tomography is not indicated for MI and viability assessment. However, several findings on CCTA which points toward MI include regional area of hypoperfusion, focal myocardial thinning, myocardial calcification and fatty metaplasia of myocardium. In dual energy CT, iodine maps can be generated for myocardium in which area of absent iodine uptake suggests MI. Regional wall motion abnormality and ventricular functions can be assessed in retrospectively gated cardiac CT. Recent studies have described delayed myocardial enhancement after iodinated contrast at 10–15 min in cardiac CT using a concept similar to CMR based LGE assessment. However, larger studies are required to validate results of CT delated myocardial enhancement.

Imaging of Complications

Complications of ischemic heart disease can be classified into electrical dysfunction (arrythmias), mechanical dysfunction (heart failure, myocardial rupture, dissection, aneurysm, papillary muscle dysfunction), thrombotic (mural thrombus, embolism) and inflammatory complications (pericarditis, postmyocardial infarction syndrome) **(Figs. 8A and B)**.

Figure 9 summarizes the imaging evaluation of various components of IHD.

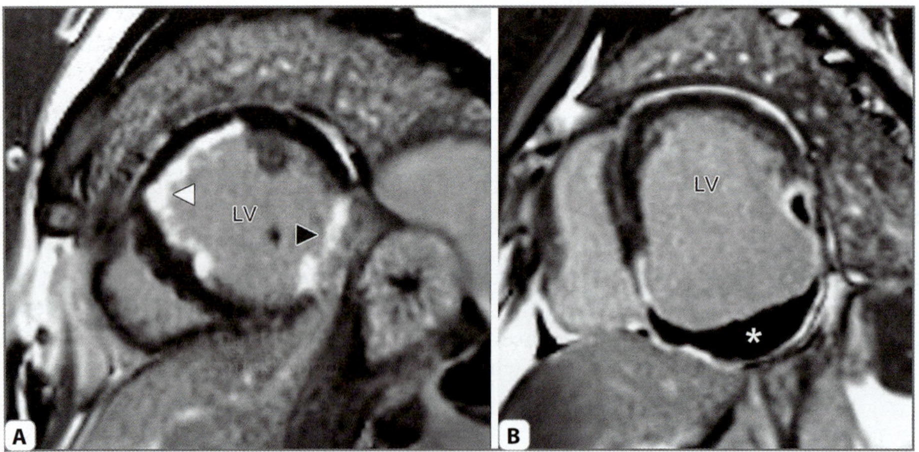

FIGS. 7A AND B: Myocardial viability imaging: (A) Phase-sensitive inversion recovery images in the short axis view shows subendocardial late gadolinium enhancement (white arrowhead) in the anterior and anteroseptal segment of mid part of left ventricle (LV) extending up to 50% of the total thickness of the myocardium (viable). The inferolateral segment of the left ventricle (black arrowhead) extending across the full thickness (100%) of the myocardium (nonviable). (B) In another patient, phase-sensitive inversion recovery images in the short axis view shows thinning, aneurysmal dilatation and transmural late gadolinium enhancement involving the inferoseptal, inferior and inferolateral segment (nonviable) of mid part of left ventricle. Note the peripheral thrombus (*) along the infarcted segment.

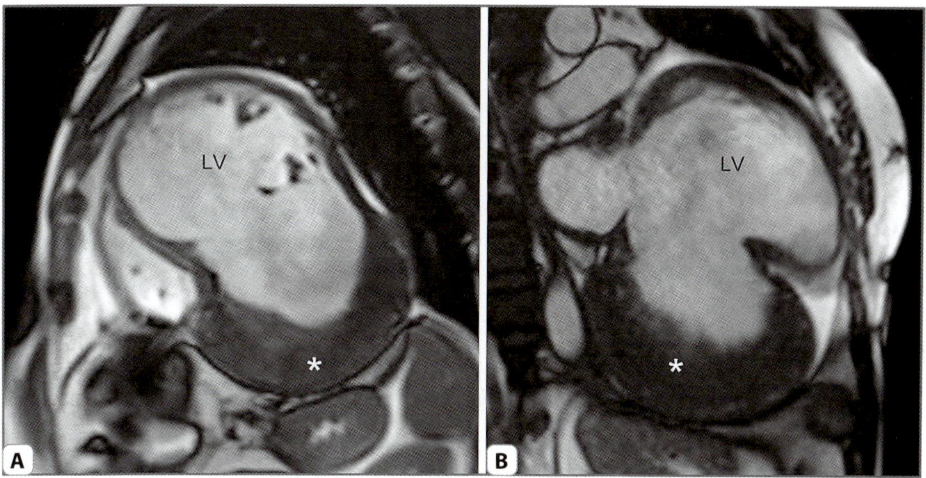

FIGS. 8A AND B: Left ventricular aneurysm after myocardial infarction: Steady-state free precession images in the short axis (A) and two-chamber (B) view shows aneurysm formation postmyocardial infarction involving the inferior and inferolateral segments of the basal and mid part of the left ventricle (LV) with peripheral thrombus (*).

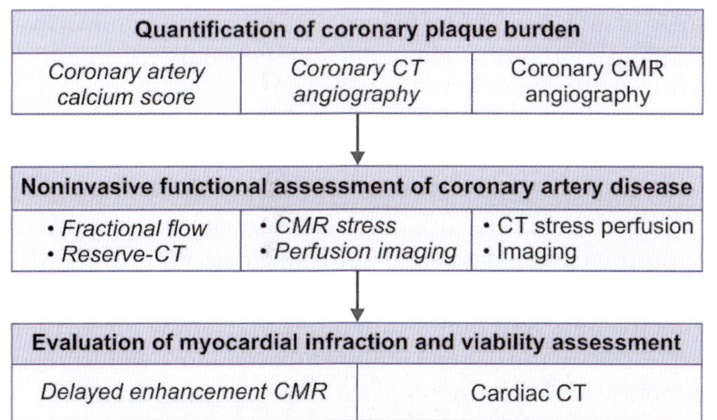

FIG. 9: Imaging evaluation of various components of ischemic heart disease. Italic indicates the imaging modalities of choice.

EVIDENCE-BASED GUIDELINES FOR THE USE OF IMAGING IN ISCHEMIC HEART DISEASE

Coronary Artery Calcium Scoring[38,39]

Class 2A recommendations:

- In asymptomatic adults at intermediate risk [≥7.5% to <20% 10-year atherosclerotic cardiovascular disease (ASCVD) risk] or selected adults at borderline risk (5% to <7.5% 10-year ASCVD risk), if risk based decisions for preventive interventions (statin therapy) remain uncertain
- In patients with stable chest pain, if the patient is low risk with no known CAD or if the patient is at intermediate-high risk with mildly positive stress test.

Coronary Computed Tomography Angiography[39,40]

Class 1A recommendations:

- In patient with acute chest pain, if the patient is at intermediate risk with no known CAD
- In patient with stable chest pain, if the patient is at intermediate-high risk with no known CAD

Class 1C recommendation: In patients with prior coronary artery bypass graft (CABG) with acute chest pain after acute coronary syndrome (ACS) ruled out.

Class 2A recommendations:

- In patient with acute chest pain, if the patient is at intermediate risk with mildly abnormal stress test within 1 year
- In patient with acute chest pain, if the patient is at intermediate risk with no known CAD and inconclusive prior stress test
- In patient with acute chest pain, if the patient is at intermediate risk with known nonobstructive CAD
- In patient with stable chest pain, if the patient is at intermediate-high risk with inconclusive or abnormal stress imaging
- In patients with chronic coronary syndrome, if there is change in symptoms or functional capacity persisting despite optimal medical management with prior revascularization (CABG/stents greater than 3 mm)

Class 2B recommendation: In patient with stable chest pain, if the patient is at intermediate-high risk with negative stress test and high clinical suspicion.

Fractional Flow Reserve Computed Tomography[39,40]

Class 2A recommendation: In patient with acute or stable chest pain, if the patient has an inconclusive CTCA or CTCA showing 40–90% in proximal or mid segment of coronary artery.

Cardiac Magnetic Resonance Stress Perfusion Imaging*[39,40]

*Stress echocardiography/SPECT/PET are alternatives

Class 1B recommendations:

- In patient with acute chest pain, if the patient is at intermediate risk with no known CAD
- In patient with stable chest pain, if the patient is at intermediate-high risk with no known CAD
- In patient with stable chest pain, if the patient has obstructive CAD and pain despite optimal medical therapy
- In patients with chronic coronary syndrome, if there is change in symptoms or functional capacity persisting despite optimal medical management

Class 2B recommendations:

- In patient with acute chest pain, if the patient is at intermediate risk with known CAD
- In patient with stable chest pain, if the patient is at intermediate-high risk with inconclusive imaging
- In patient with stable chest pain, if the patient has non-obstructive CAD with extensive plaques

Class 2C recommendations:

- In patient with acute chest pain, if the patient is at intermediate risk with no known CAD and inconclusive CCTA
- In patient with stable chest pain, if the patient is post-CABG with suspected ischemia

Viability Imaging Using Cardiac Magnetic Resonance*[41]

*Dobutamine stress echocardiography, SPECT, PET are alternatives.

Class 2A recommendation: In patient with stable coronary disease, for evaluation of viability in patients suitable for revascularization.

CONCLUSION

Assessment of the coronary vasculature and the ventricular myocardium using CT and CMR provides complementary information and thus a comprehensive evaluation of IHD across the various stages of the ischemic cascade up to the stage of advanced heart failure. CT is now the noninvasive imaging modality of choice for the coronary arterial tree while CMR plays a major role in the evaluation of the ventricular myocardium, including assessment of function, myocardial perfusion and tissue characterization. Advances in CT and CMR have allowed for functional assessment of CAD and therefore, have assumed a crucial role in guiding appropriate management. Future advances in CT and CMR technologies along with real world data demonstrating cost-effectiveness and better outcomes may allow for further expansion of the clinical utility and even more widespread adoption of these modalities in the evaluation of IHD.

REFERENCES

1. Kalra A, Jose AP, Prabhakaran P, Kumar A, Agrawal A, Roy A, et al. The burgeoning cardiovascular disease epidemic in Indians—perspectives on contextual factors and potential solutions. Lancet Reg Health Southeast Asia. 2023;12:100156.
2. Dweck MR, Williams MC, Moss AJ, Newby DE, Fayad ZA. Computed Tomography and Cardiac Magnetic Resonance in Ischemic Heart Disease. J Am Coll Cardiol. 2016;68(20):2201-16.
3. Ross R. Atherosclerosis—an inflammatory disease. N Engl J Med. 1999;340(2):115-26.
4. Kern MJ, Samady H. Current concepts of integrated coronary physiology in the catheterization laboratory. J Am Coll Cardiol. 2010;55(3):173-85.
5. Libby P. Mechanisms of acute coronary syndromes and their implications for therapy. N Engl J Med. 2013;368(21):2004-13.
6. Farb A, Burke AP, Tang AL, Liang TY, Mannan P, Smialek J, et al. Coronary plaque erosion without rupture into a lipid core. A frequent cause of coronary thrombosis in sudden coronary death. Circulation. 1996;93(7):1354-63.
7. Achenbach S, Raggi P. Imaging of coronary atherosclerosis by computed tomography. Eur Heart J. 2010;31(12):1442-8.
8. McClelland RL, Chung H, Detrano R, Post W, Kronmal RA. Distribution of coronary artery calcium by race, gender, and age: results from the Multi-Ethnic Study of Atherosclerosis (MESA). Circulation. 2006;113(1):30-7.
9. Ghekiere O, Salgado R, Buls N, Leiner T, Mancini I, Vanhoenacker P, et al. Image quality in coronary CT angiography: challenges and technical solutions. Br J Radiol. 2017;90(1072):20160567.
10. Sirajuddin A, Mirmomen SM, Kligerman SJ, Groves DW, Burke AP, Kureshi F, et al. Ischemic Heart Disease: Noninvasive Imaging Techniques and Findings. Radiographics. 2021;41(4):990-1021.
11. Abbara S, Blanke P, Maroules CD, Cheezum M, Choi AD, Han BK, et al. SCCT guidelines for the performance and acquisition of coronary computed tomographic angiography: A report of the society of Cardiovascular Computed Tomography Guidelines Committee: Endorsed by the North American Society for Cardiovascular Imaging (NASCI). J Cardiovasc Comput Tomogr. 2016;10(6):435-49.
12. Taylor CA, Fonte TA, Min JK. Computational fluid dynamics applied to cardiac computed tomography for noninvasive quantification of fractional flow reserve: scientific basis. J Am Coll Cardiol. 2013;61(22):2233-41.

13. Pantos I, Katritsis D. Fractional Flow Reserve Derived from Coronary Imaging and Computational Fluid Dynamics. Interv Cardiol. 2014;9(3):145-50.
14. Taylor CA, Figueroa CA. Patient-specific modeling of cardiovascular mechanics. Annu Rev Biomed Eng. 2009;11:109-34.
15. Patel AR, Bamberg F, Branch K, Carrascosa P, Chen M, Cury RC, et al. Society of cardiovascular computed tomography expert consensus document on myocardial computed tomography perfusion imaging. J Cardiovasc Comput Tomogr. 2020;14(1):87-100.
16. So A, Lee TY. Quantitative myocardial CT perfusion: a pictorial review and the current state of technology development. J Cardiovasc Comput Tomogr. 2011;5(6):467-81.
17. Rossi A, Merkus D, Klotz E, Mollet N, de Feyter PJ, Krestin GP. Stress myocardial perfusion: imaging with multidetector CT. Radiology. 2014;270(1):25-46
18. Rossi A, Uitterdijk A, Dijkshoorn M, Klotz E, Dharampal A, van Straten M, et al. Quantification of myocardial blood flow by adenosine-stress CT perfusion imaging in pigs during various degrees of stenosis correlates well with coronary artery blood flow and fractional flow reserve. Eur Heart J Cardiovasc Imaging. 2013;14(4):331-8.
19. Kramer CM, Barkhausen J, Bucciarelli-Ducci C, Flamm SD, Kim RJ, Nagel E. Standardized cardiovascular magnetic resonance imaging (CMR) protocols: 2020 update. J Cardiovasc Magn Reson. 2020;22(1):17.
20. Henzlova MJ, Duvall WL, Einstein AJ, Travin MI, Verberne HJ. ASNC imaging guidelines for SPECT nuclear cardiology procedures: Stress, protocols, and tracers. J Nucl Cardiol. 2016;23(3):606-39.
21. Ta AD, Hsu LY, Conn HM, Winkler S, Greve AM, Shanbhag SM, et al. Fully quantitative pixel-wise analysis of cardiovascular magnetic resonance perfusion improves discrimination of dark rim artifact from perfusion defects associated with epicardial coronary stenosis. J Cardiovasc Magn Reson. 2018;20(1):16.
22. Flavian A, Carta F, Thuny F, Bernard M, Kober F, Moulin G, et al. Cardiac MRI in the diagnosis of complications of myocardial infarction. Diagn Interv Imaging. 2012;93(7-8):578-85.
23. Wildgruber M, Settles M, Herrmann K, Beer AJ, Rummeny EJ, Huber AM. Inversion-recovery single-shot cardiac MRI for the assessment of myocardial infarction at 1.5 T with a dedicated cardiac coil. Br J Radiol. 2012;85(1017):e709-15.
24. Rashid S, Rapacchi S, Vaseghi M, Tung R, Shivkumar K, Finn JP, et al. Improved late gadolinium enhancement MR imaging for patients with implanted cardiac devices. Radiology. 2014;270(1):269-74.
25. Agatston AS, Janowitz WR, Hildner FJ, Zusmer NR, Viamonte M Jr, Detrano R. Quantification of coronary artery calcium using ultrafast computed tomography. J Am Coll Cardiol. 1990;15(4):827-32.
26. Shreya D, Zamora DI, Patel GS, Grossmann I, Rodriguez K, Soni M, et al. Coronary Artery Calcium Score: A Reliable Indicator of Coronary Artery Disease? Cureus. 2021;13(12):e20149.
27. Cury RC, Leipsic J, Abbara S, Achenbach S, Berman D, Bittencourt M, et al. CAD-RADS™ 2.0-2022 Coronary Artery Disease-Reporting and Data System. An Expert Consensus Document of the Society of Cardiovascular Computed Tomography (SCCT), the American College of Cardiology (ACC), the American College of Radiology (ACR), and the North America Society of Cardiovascular Imaging (NASCI). J Cardiovasc Comput Tomogr. 2022;16(6):536-57.
28. Golub IS, Termeie OG, Kristo S, Schroeder LP, Lakshmanan S, Shafter AM, et al. Major Global Coronary Artery Calcium Guidelines. JACC Cardiovasc Imaging. 2023;16(1):98-117.
29. Pohle K, Achenbach S, Macneill B, Ropers D, Ferencik M, Moselewski F, et al. Characterization of non-calcified coronary atherosclerotic plaque by multi-detector row CT: comparison to IVUS. Atherosclerosis. 2007;190(1):174-80.
30. Puchner SB, Liu T, Mayrhofer T, Truong QA, Lee H, Fleg JL, et al. High-risk plaque detected on coronary CT angiography predicts acute coronary syndromes independent of significant stenosis in acute chest pain: results from the ROMICAT-II trial. J Am Coll Cardiol. 2014;64(7):684-92.
31. Doris M, Newby DE. Coronary CT Angiography as a Diagnostic and Prognostic Tool: Perspectives from the SCOT-HEART Trial. Curr Cardiol Rep. 2016;18(2):18.
32. Hou ZH, Lu B, Gao Y, Jiang SL, Wang Y, Li W, et al. Prognostic value of coronary CT angiography and calcium score for major adverse cardiac events in outpatients. JACC Cardiovasc Imaging. 2012;5(10):990-9.
33. Hajhosseiny R, Bustin A, Munoz C, Rashid I, Cruz G, Manning WJ, et al. Coronary Magnetic Resonance Angiography: Technical Innovations Leading Us to the Promised Land? JACC Cardiovasc Imaging. 2020;13(12):2653-72.
34. Noguchi T, Nakao K, Asaumi Y, Morita Y, Otsuka F, Kataoka Y, et al. Noninvasive Coronary Plaque Imaging. J Atheroscler Thromb. 2018;25(4):281-93.
35. Rajiah P, Cummings KW, Williamson E, Young PM. CT Fractional Flow Reserve: A Practical Guide to Application, Interpretation, and Problem Solving. Radiographics. 2022;42(2):340-58.
36. Pakkal M, Raj V, McCann GP. Non-invasive imaging in coronary artery disease including anatomical and functional evaluation of ischaemia and viability assessment. Br J Radiol. 2011;84 Spec No 3(Spec Iss 3):S280-95.
37. Sliwicka O, Sechopoulos I, Baggiano A, Pontone G, Nijveldt R, Habets J. Dynamic myocardial CT perfusion imaging-state of the art. Eur Radiol. 2023;33(8):5509-25.
38. Arnett DK, Blumenthal RS, Albert MA, Buroker AB, Goldberger ZD, Hahn EJ, et al. 2019 ACC/AHA Guideline on the Primary Prevention of Cardiovascular Disease: A Report of the American College of Cardiology/American Heart Association Task Force on Clinical Practice Guidelines. Circulation. 2019;140(11):e596-e646.
39. Gulati M, Levy PD, Mukherjee D, Amsterdam E, Bhatt DL, Birtcher KK, et al. 2021 AHA/ACC/ASE/CHEST/SAEM/SCCT/SCMR Guideline for the Evaluation and Diagnosis of Chest Pain: A Report of the American College of Cardiology/American Heart Association Joint Committee on Clinical Practice Guidelines. Circulation. 2021;144(22):e368-e454.
40. Virani SS, Newby LK, Arnold SV, Bittner V, Brewer LC, Demeter SH, et al.; Peer Review Committee Members. 2023 AHA/ACC/ACCP/ASPC/NLA/PCNA Guideline for the Management of Patients with Chronic Coronary Disease: A Report of the American Heart Association/American College of Cardiology Joint Committee on Clinical Practice Guidelines. Circulation. 2023;148(9):e9-e119.
41. McDonagh TA, Metra M, Adamo M, Gardner RS, Baumbach A, Böhm M, et al.; ESC Scientific Document Group. 2021 ESC Guidelines for the diagnosis and treatment of acute and chronic heart failure. Eur Heart J. 2021;42(36):3599-3726.

Priya Jagia, Vineeta Ojha

CHAPTER

26

Imaging in Non-ischemic Cardiomyopathies

INTRODUCTION

Cardiomyopathies (CMPs) comprise a spectrum of chronic progressive heart muscle disorders which have distinct pattern of morphological, functional and electrophysiological characteristics. The European Society of Cardiology (ESC) position statement published in 2008 defined CMPs as myocardial disorders "in which the heart muscle is structurally and functionally abnormal, in the absence of coronary artery disease, hypertension, valvular disease and congenital heart disease sufficient to cause the observed myocardial abnormality".[1] CMPs are often confined to the heart but can be a part of systemic disorders, leading to chronic heart failure and cardiovascular death, if not diagnosed or managed timely.

CLASSIFICATION OF CARDIOMYOPATHIES

Cardiomyopathies are broadly classified into: (1) *Primary* CMPs (genetic/familial or non-genetic/acquired) comprise those few conditions that are either solely or predominantly confined to heart muscle. (2) *Secondary* CMPs are those group of conditions where the myocardial involvement occurs as part of a large number and heterogeneous variety of systemic disorders, usually affecting multiple organ systems. Overall, for imaging, it is helpful to categorize them into hypertrophic cardiomyopathy (HCM), dilated cardiomyopathy (DCM), restrictive cardiomyopathy (RCM), arrhythmogenic cardiomyopathy (ACM) as well as non-dilated LV cardiomyopathy (NDLVC). (3) This chapter will focus on these common CMP, but we will also describe certain miscellaneous forms of CMPs.

DIAGNOSTIC TECHNIQUES

It is important to determine the exact CMP phenotype and etiology as this determines the line of treatment and the patient survival.[2] Diagnostic work up in patients with suspected CMP includes clinical history and physical examination, a 12-lead ECG, laboratory studies, imaging and genetic testing as well as endomyocardial biopsy in certain patients. Endomyocardial biopsy, though is the gold standard technique, but has limitations in the form of sampling errors and poor sensitivity. Multimodality imaging forms the backbone of diagnosis and follow-up in patients with cardiomyopathies.[3]

The uses of the commonly used imaging modalities in the context of CMPs are given below **(Fig. 1)**:

- *Echocardiography*: It is recommended in all patients with cardiomyopathy and is usually the first line imaging modality.[3] It is safe, cheap and easily available and gives information about ventricular functions, chamber dilatations or myocardial hypertrophy, valve abnormalities as well as regional functional abnormalities. It is useful to categorize the patients into the primary phenotypes namely dilated type, hypertrophic pattern or restrictive phenotype. It is devoid of radiation or contrast administration, hence also allows for serial follow up for ventricular functions over time. The major disadvantage of echocardiography is that it does not allow for tissue characterization. It is also limited by availability of acoustic windows and is operator dependent. RV wall and KV apex may not be very well evaluable. Echocardiography also allows for the assessment of diastolic dysfunction (using transmitral flows), useful in diagnosis of restrictive CMP.
- *Computed tomography (CT) and CT angiography*: Cardiac CT angiography is useful to rule out congenital coronary anomalies or suspected coronary artery disease in a patient with CMP. Cardiac CT can demonstrate ventricular function and limited myocardial characterization. Although, its ability to do tissue characterization is limited, but CT may be used to do anatomical assessment in patients who have poor acoustic window for echocardiography or have contraindications to MRI.[3] Cardiac CT angiography

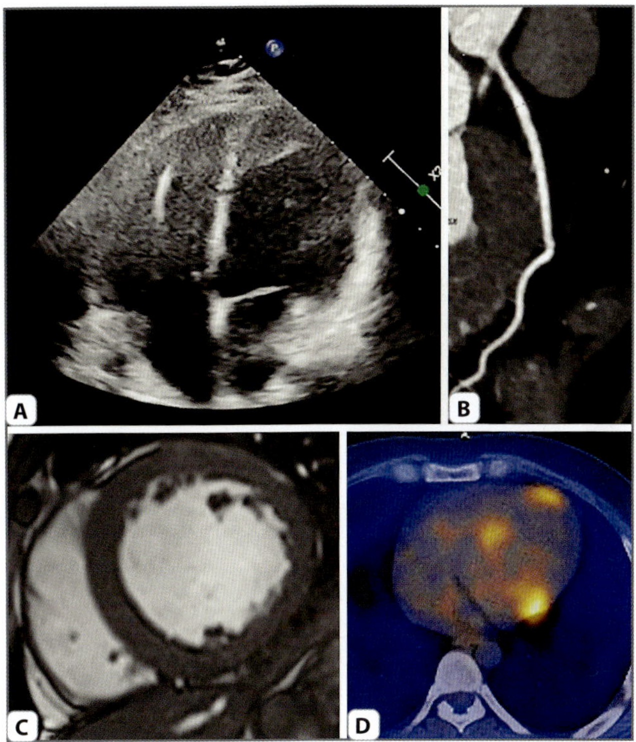

FIGS. 1A TO D: Common imaging modalities: (A) Echocardiography, (B) CT angiography showing a coronary artery in curvilinear reformat, (C) MRI cine snapshot in short axis view; and (D) PET image.

requires ECG gating and sometimes, administration of drugs (beta-blockers or vasodilators) to reduce heart rate or obtain good coronary visualization. Unlike MRI, it entails radiation exposure. CT is also useful to evaluate extracardiac structures like lung parenchymal changes and mediastinal lymphadenopathy, especially in sarcoidosis and other autoimmune disorders.

- *Cardiac magnetic resonance imaging (CMR)*: It is now considered the "in-vivo" gold standard imaging modality for the diagnosis and treatment monitoring of CMPs. The major advantage is the ability to do tissue characterization in addition to allowing for accurate functional evaluation.[4] Additionally, it allows for assessment of valve functions, perfusion, flows, shunts as well as the pericardium. It provides high-resolution images of the heart in any desired plane without any radiation. Contrast CMR is now recommended in patients with CMP at initial evaluation.[3] CMR is useful for diagnosis, prognosis, risk stratification, in guiding management, and for follow up in CMPs. It also helps in the assessment of therapeutic response in amyloidosis, Fabry, sarcoidosis, inflammatory CMP, and hemochromatosis.[3] The main sequences that are used are:
  - Spin echo (SE) T1- and T2-weighted imaging allows for tissue characterization like presence of fat (bright on T1 and suppresses on fat sat images) or edema (bright on T2).
  - Cine CMR helps assess cardiac morphology and function assessment.
  - Passage of gadolinium through the LV myocardium can be imaged during its first pass at rest and this provides important information about contrast kinetics of the myocardium. Stress perfusion CMR helps in assessment of inducible ischemia
  - Delayed enhanced CMR (DE-CMR) also known as late gadolinium enhancement (LGE) helps to differentiate ischemic from non-ischemic CMP based on the pattern of enhancement. LGE occurs in conditions where the extracellular volume increases due to myocardial fibrosis, inflammation or edema. The pattern of LGE is the backbone for etiological classification of CMPs.[5] Usually, subendocardial to transmural LGE pattern is suggestive of ischemic etiology, more so when conforming to coronary artery territory. Midwall or subepicardial LGE is likely suggestive of non-ischemic etiology **(Fig. 2)**.[5]
  - *Parametric mapping* for tissue characterization is newer CMR technique which is also part of the current ESC guidelines of CMP assessment.[3] Pre-contrast native T1 mapping reflects combined signal from myocytes and interstitial tissues and increases in diffuse fibrosis or infiltration of the heart. It reduces iron infiltration or lipid deposition (e.g., Fabry disease). Native T2 mapping is specific for the water content of the heart tissue and increases in myocardial edema (hence used to diagnose myocardial inflammation/myocarditis). Extracellular volume (ECV) mapping can be derived from the pre and post contrast T1 mapping values of the myocardium and blood and the patient's hematocrit values and is specific for the interstitium (extra cellular matrix). It increases in interstitial fibrosis or infiltrations like amyloid.[6] It is important to establish normal values of mapping techniques in each institute as these greatly vary depending on the scanner conditions and mapping techniques used. We have earlier published the values in our 1.5 Tesla scanner for native Indian population.[7] T2* mapping values decrease in iron overload and are the non-invasive gold standard for assessment of heart iron content in patients with Thalassemia.[8] **Table 1** summarizes the alterations in the values of tissue characterization parameters with disease states.
- *Nuclear medicine*: FDG-PET imaging is the technique of choice for the assessment of myocardial inflammation, useful for the detection of myocarditis or sarcoidosis. DPD/PYP scans are also part of the diagnostic algorithm in cardiac amyloidosis, especially ATTR amyloid. For assessment of inflammation, FDG-PET requires tougher dietary preparation of the patient using high-fat/low-carbohydrate diet, which may affect the imaging depending upon the quality of dietary preparation. PET/SPECT also suffer from poor spatial resolution

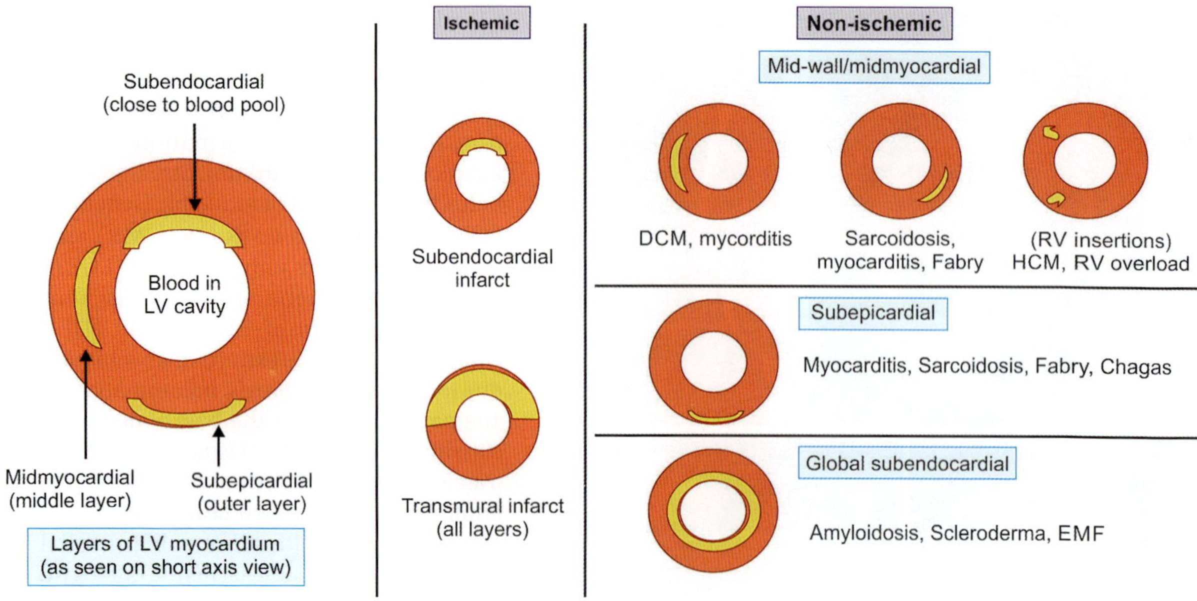

FIG. 2: Schematic diagram showing different patterns of late gadolinium enhancement (LGE) seen in various etiologies of cardiomyopathy.[5]

TABLE 1: Alterations in the values of tissue characterization (mapping) parameters with disease states.

Parameters	Increase	Decrease
Native T1	Inflammation, ischemia, infiltration (amyloid), diffuse fibrosis, scar	Iron, fat, hemorrhage, Anderson–Fabry
Native T2	Edema (inflammation), ischemia	Iron, hemorrhage
ECV	Amyloid, scar, diffuse fibrosis	Athlete's heart
T2*		Iron, hemorrhage
(ECV: extracellular volume)		

and radiation exposure. Newer innovations like hybrid PET-MRI have been developed to harness the potential of both MRI and PET with a case for offering higher diagnostic value.

- *Catheter angiography*: Catheter angiography assesses only the chamber lumen, with poor demonstration of myocardial changes. With the advancements in CT, the utility of catheter angiography in the diagnostic work-up of CMPs is to rule out CAD in patients who have high pretest probability of CAD.

The choice of imaging modality is usually guided by the yield of actionable results weighed against the costs, advantages, and limitations of each technique. Patient safety, ionizing radiation and the use of contrast media are important concerns guiding the imaging algorithm. The idea is to move from simpler and cheaper tests first to more complex and expensive tests as needed later. A few common cardiomyopathies in routine clinical practice are described below. All the various CMPs as described in this article henceforth, are appropriate indications for performing a CMR examination, according to the recently published societal document.[4]

NON-ISCHEMIC DILATED CARDIOMYOPATHY

Dilated cardiomyopathy (DCM) is defined by LV (or biventricular) systolic dysfunction and dilatation (increased LV end-diastolic volumes two or more standard deviations from normal corrected by age, gender, and body surface area) not attributed to loading conditions (e.g., hypertension or valvular heart disease) or coronary artery disease.[9] That said, sometimes DCM may coexist with CAD.[10] The anatomical abnormalities of DCM may include enlargement of other chambers as well **(Fig. 3A)**. There may be pleural or pericardial effusion or ventricular thrombi. The functional abnormalities are in the form of segmental wall motion abnormalities or global hypokinesia.

Echocardiography allows for the assessment of ventricular functions and anatomy. CMR is considered the imaging gold standard for evaluation of ejection fractions, especially for the RV. A low LVEF (< 35%) is a predictor for mortality and these patients may develop life-threatening arrythmias. Hence, such patients may be considered for prophylactic implantable cardiac defibrillator (ICD) placement.[3] Mitral or tricuspid regurgitation, if present, can be well demonstrated on both echocardiography and cine MR. Assessment of the RV size and systolic function is important in DCM patients since RV systolic dysfunction is a common and is a predictor of adverse outcome.

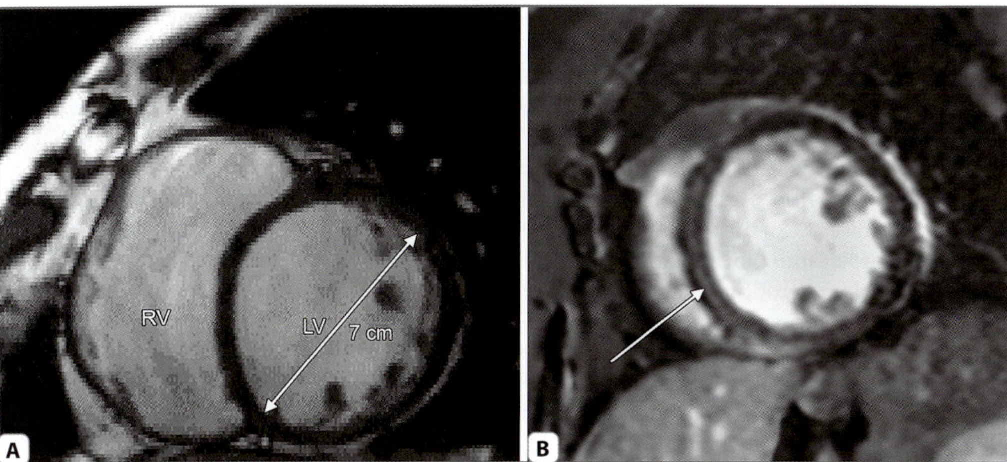

FIGS. 3A AND B: Cardiac MRI in patients with non-ischemic dilated cardiomyopathy (DCM): (A) Still from cine short-axis view showing dilated LV and RV with thin walls. (B) LGE (late gadolinium enhancement) image in short-axis view in a different patient shows the typical linear mid-myocardial LGE.

TABLE 2: Causes of non-ischemic dilated cardiomyopathy.

Broad classification	Causes of non-ischemic dilated cardiomyopathy
Genetic	Mutations in sarcomere proteins (e.g., Titin, myosin heavy chain, troponins), nuclear envelope, cytoskeleton elements (dystrophin, desmin), ion channels, mitochondrial or sarcoplasmic reticulum
Acquired	• Drugs and toxins (alcohol, recreational drugs) • Chemotherapeutic agents (anthracycline, monoclonal antibodies) • Endocrine (thyroid disorders) • Peripartum cardiomyopathy • Infectious and inflammatory (myocarditis) • Autoimmune diseases

BOX 1: Poor prognostic features for DCM on CMR.

- Poor prognostic features for DCM on imaging
- LVEF <35%
- RV systolic dysfunction
- Significant mitral regurgitation
- Presence and extent of LGE
- Increased T1/ECV mapping values
- Impaired strain values

(CMR: cardiac magnetic resonance imaging; DCM: dilated cardiomyopathy; ECV: extracellular volume; LVEF: left ventricular ejection fraction)

DCM can be genetic or acquired **(Table 2)**. The pattern of LGE helps in distinguishing the etiology of DCM **(Fig. 2)**.[5] The pattern of enhancement (LGE) in the myocardium can also help differentiate LV dysfunction related to DCM or CAD on CMR. LGE is seen in 35–40% of the patients with DCM, usually in the mid myocardial pattern in the interventricular septum **(Fig. 3B)**.[11,12] In DCM, LGE presence and increasing extent is a poor prognostic marker for arrythmia (ventricular tachycardia) and sudden cardiac death, regardless of the LV ejection fraction **(Box 1)**.[13] LGE picks up replacement fibrosis, but T1/ECV mapping detect the more diffuse interstitial fibrosis. Because of increased interstitial fibrosis in DCM, there is an increase in T1 mapping value as well, which can be a poor prognostic marker. Another novel imaging tool is strain imaging which analyses contractile properties of the myocardium and can be done using echocardiography and CMR. Impaired global longitudinal strain also predicts adverse outcomes in DCM and can also detect the disease earlier than actual contractile abnormalities. This becomes clinically important in patients on chemotherapeutic regimens.

HYPERTROPHIC CARDIOMYOPATHY

Hypertrophic cardiomyopathy (HCM) is characterized by significant myocardial hypertrophy which may be symmetric (concentric) or asymmetric, unexplained by other loading conditions like aortic stenosis or hypertension. It is usually caused by genetic mutations in sarcomeric genes like MYH7, etc., but may be caused due to non-sarcomeric genetic mutations as well.[3] Previous criteria have described HCM when septal thickness is more than 15 mm in end-diastole or when the ratio of thickness of septal wall to inferior wall at the midventricular level is >1.5, but recent research has highlighted the importance body surface area-based criteria of thickness rather than absolute values.[14,15] In HCM, the hypertrophy can be of many morphologic types like asymmetric septal (most common), mid-cavity predominant, apical or concentric. LV is usually hypercontractile. Diastolic dysfunction is common. Mitral regurgitation and left atrial dilatation may also be seen, which predisposes to the development of left atrial arrythmias.

Echocardiography allows for initial diagnosis but may not evaluate apical hypertrophy well. CMR accurately defines the site and extent of hypertrophy, especially at LV apex and echo-blind areas like RV. One-third of the patients can have systolic anterior motion of the anterior mitral leaflet and approximately 60–70% of the patients may have LV outflow obstruction. Cardiac function and flow dynamics of the outflow in cases of hypertrophic obstructive CMP (HOCM), including systolic anterior motion of mitral valve, are well seen on echocardiography and cine-CMR. Precise planimetric measurements of the LVOT area during systole can also be determined on CMR. LGE-CMR demonstrates a pattern of contrast uptake in the myocardium **(Fig. 4)**, particularly at the RV insertion points on the septum, usually seen in approximately 60% of the patients. Patients showing hyperenhancement are at increased risk of sudden cardiac death. Extensive LGE (≥15% of LV mass) associated with a two-fold greater risk of sudden death events.[3] **Box 2** describes the various poor prognostic features on CMR. CMR can help monitor the functional and anatomical outcome of surgical and pharmacological septal ablation. CMR is also useful to screen the relatives of probands. Sometimes, genotypic positive first-degree relatives who do not have phenotypic HCM may have soft markers on CMR like papillary muscle abnormalities (bifid/single papillary muscle), elongated mitral leaflet or myocardial crypts.[3]

BOX 2: Various poor prognostic features on CMR.

The imaging features on CMR which are poor prognostic factors for HCM:

- Thickness of LV wall > 30 mm
- LVOT gradient > 30 mm Hg
- *Increased left atrial size (> 45 mm)*: Consistent predictor for atrial fibrillation and stroke
- LVEF< 50% (burnt-out phase)
- *Apical HCM*: Apical aneurysm formation is predictor of adverse outcome
- *Perfusion abnormalities*: Early adverse marker
- *LGE representing fibrosis >15% of the LV myocardium*: Associated with adverse events like heart failure, angina, systolic dysfunction and sudden cardiac death

(CMR: cardiac magnetic resonance imaging; HCM: hypertrophic cardiomyopathy; LVEF: left ventricular ejection fraction; LVOT: left ventricular outflow tract)

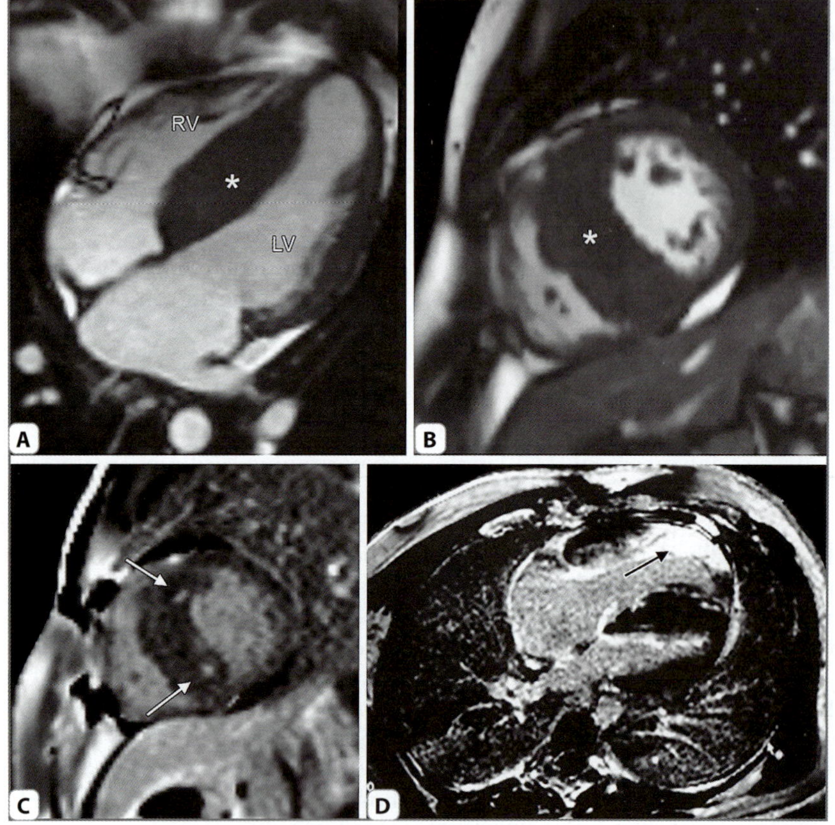

FIGS. 4A TO D: Cardiac MRI: A patient with hypertrophic cardiomyopathy (A to C) showing asymmetric thickening of interventricular septum, measuring 19 mm in end diastole (asterisk in cine four chamber image-A, and cine short axis view (B). LGE image in short axis (C) shows mid wall patchy LGE (white arrow, mainly along RV insertion points). LGE image in four chamber view in another patient (D) shows delayed dense enhancement in areas of hypertrophy in RV (black arrow), interventricular septum and LV.

TABLE 3: Differential diagnoses of hypertrophic cardiomyopathy (HCM) and differentiating points.

HCM	Athlete's heart	Hypertensive heart	Amyloid	Fabry disease
Asymmetric hypertrophy is common	Concentric hypertrophy (rarely > 16 mm)	Concentric hypertrophy (rarely > 16 mm)	Concentric hypertrophy	Concentric hypertrophy
Common LGE pattern: RV insertion points, patchy mid-wall	Not commonly seen	Not commonly seen	Diffuse subendocardial or transmural	Inferolateral wall of LV
LV cavity size reduced	LV cavity size increased	LV cavity size reduced	Unaffected/increased in late stage	Variable
Systolic anterior motion of the anterior mitral leaflet is typical; 1/3rd of the patients	Rare	Rare	Rare	Rare
Absent	Absent	Absent	Nulling abnormalities	Absent
Increased T1 mapping (diffuse fibrosis); ECV is increased but < 40%	ECV is reduced due to myocyte hypertrophy	T1 mapping may be increased	Gross increase in T1 mapping; ECV >40%	Low T1 mapping values (due to glycosphingolipid)

(CMR: cardiac magnetic resonance imaging; ECV: extracellular volume; HCM: hypertrophic cardiomyopathy; LVOT: left ventricular outflow tract)

Close differentials include amyloidosis, athlete's heart, Anderson–Fabry disease (AFD) or hypertensive heart disease. **Table 3** gives a few pointers to differentiate between the various etiologies.

RESTRICTIVE CARDIOMYOPATHY

The World Health Organization (WHO) defines RCM as a myocardial disease characterized by restrictive filling and reduced diastolic volume of either or both ventricles with normal or near-normal systolic function and wall thickness and it accounts for nearly 5% of all primary heart muscle disorders. **Table 4** summarizes the causes of RCM.

Restrictive cardiomyopathy is identified on CT and MRI by normal LV size and normal or mildly impaired systolic function, abnormal severe diastolic ventricular function and biatrial enlargement **(Fig. 5)**. CMR can characterize tissue, identify anatomic alterations and can quantify myocardial mass, ventricular volumes and ejection fraction, thus making it a useful modality for investigating infiltrative or restrictive CMPs. Common infiltrative disorders of the heart causing RCM include amyloidosis, endomyocardial fibrosis (EMF), sarcoidosis, hemochromatosis (or siderotic CMP).

Amyloidosis

Cardiac amyloidosis is characterized by infiltration of interstitium with misfolded amyloid protein. Cardiac involvement is seen with most forms of amyloidosis, although it is most common and most often clinically significant with type AL amyloidosis (primary amyloidosis), often associated with multiple myeloma or other monoclonal gammopathies. It is the most common cause of RCM outside the tropics. The other major type of cardiac amyloidosis is ATTR type, having a better prognosis than AL.

TABLE 4: Etiologies of restrictive cardiomyopathy (RCM).

Broad classification	Causes of restrictive cardiomyopathy
Genetic etiologies	Troponin, MYH7, filamin C mutations
Infiltrations	Amyloid, sarcoidosis, iron overload
Storage disorders	Anderson–Fabry disease, Gaucher's disease, glycogen storage disorders, mucopolysaccharidoses
Drug induced	Anthracyclines, methysergide, ergotamin, busulfan
Systemic diseases	EMF, scleroderma, diabetes, carcinoid, muscular dystrophy, malignancy
Radiation induced	

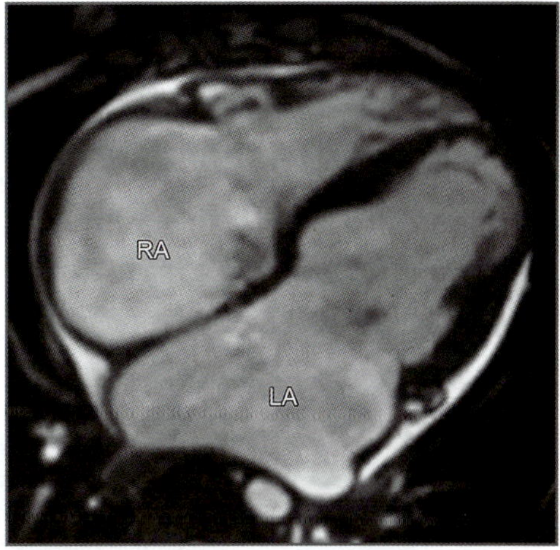

FIG. 5: Still from a cine cardiac MRI sequence in four chamber view in a patient with restrictive cardiomyopathy shows normal ventricular volumes and bi-atrial enlargement, characteristic appearance of this phenotype.

In the heart, amyloidosis leads to thickening of the left and right ventricular walls, sometimes associated with thickened right atrial walls, inter-atrial septum and the atrio-ventricular valves. On CT and CMR, the presence of these findings, in combination with pericardial and pleural effusions help to differentiate amyloidosis from other causes of hypertrophied myocardium. An increase in thickness of interatrial septum or posterior right atrial wall > 6 mm is quite specific for amyloid infiltration. There is a diffuse decrease in the myocardial signal intensity on both T1- and T2-weighted images. A ratio of myocardial to skeletal muscle signal intensity of < 1.0 at 20 ms TE is an important feature of cardiac amyloidosis.

On DE-CMR, diffuse contrast uptake is seen typically in the subendocardial or transmural pattern and does not match any specific coronary artery perfusion territory **(Fig. 6)**. Classic CMR LGE pattern has a sensitivity of 80% and specificity of 94% for the diagnosis of cardiac amyloidosis. Because the amyloid protein expands the extracellular space, there is preferential Gadolinium (extracellular agent) accumulation there causing shortening if inversion time, resulting in myocardial nulling abnormalities on TI scout images. Abnormal nulling pattern has sensitivity and specificity of 93% and 70% for the diagnosis of cardiac amyloidosis. Mahrholdt et al. reported that if > 50% of LV myocardium nulls earlier than LV cavity and if this region is not in a coronary artery distribution territory, then the diagnosis of cardiac amyloidosis is highly likely.[16] Advances in parametric mapping has revolutionized the diagnosis and management of cardiac amyloidosis. T1 mapping values increase, a value of >1164 ms at 1.5 Tesla has 98% positive predictive value for the diagnosis of cardiac amyloidosis, if clinically suspected **(Fig. 7)**.[17] ECV mapping values in amyloidosis are typically >40%. CMR, particularly T1 and ECV mapping values, can be used to follow up the patients on drug therapy in amyloidosis.

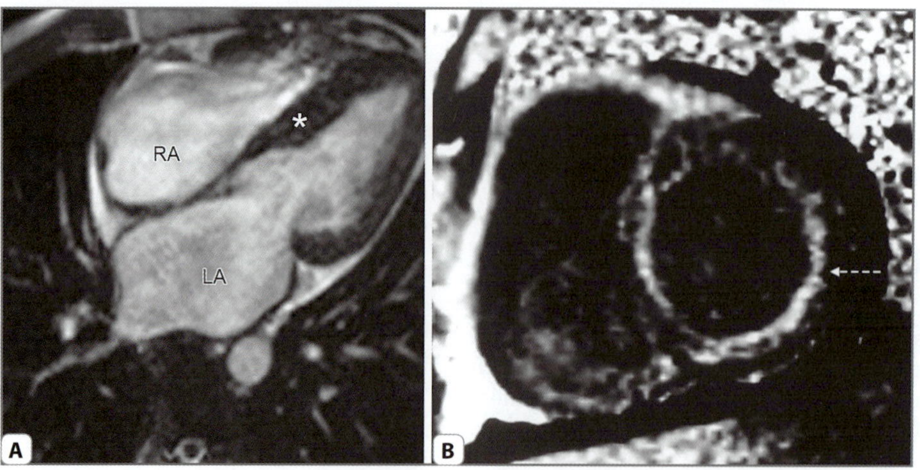

FIGS. 6A AND B: (A) Four chamber cine image on cardiac MRI shows diffuse thickening of LV walls (asterisk) and bi-atrial enlargement in a patient with amyloidosis. (B) Typical global subendocardial enhancement (dashed arrow) on LGE-MRI image in short-axis view, characteristic of amyloidosis.

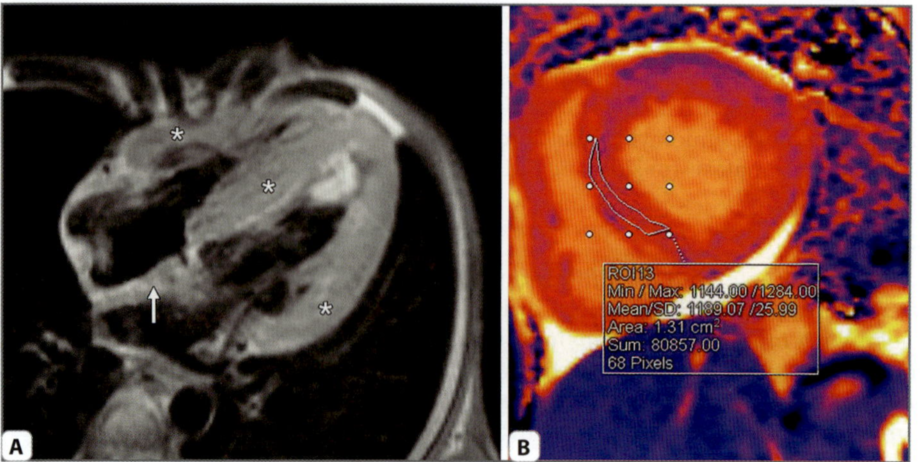

FIGS. 7A AND B: (A) Four chamber T2 sequence of cardiac MRI in patient with amyloidosis reveals diffuse thickening of myocardium of LV and RV (asterisks) and thickening of interatrial septum. (B) T1 color coded map shows diffusely increased T1 mapping values (~1189 ms), a feature of diffuse infiltration.

ECV is the earliest marker to track amyloid regression. T2 mapping also increases cardiac amyloidosis, particularly AL type, because of concomitant myocardial inflammation.[18] Nuclear medicine investigations like 99mTc-PYP or DPD scintigraphy are very useful for picking up ATTR amyloidosis. Grade 2/3 cardiac uptake has high specificity for ATTR.[19] **Table 5** summarizes typical findings and poor prognostic features of cardiac amyloidosis on imaging.

Endomyocardial Fibrosis

Endomyocardial fibrosis is characterized by extensive subendocardial fibrosis, apical thrombus formation and progressive diastolic dysfunction. This disease entity is a common cause of RCM in the tropics. EMF shows involvement of both ventricles, the LV, or RV in 50%, 40%, and 10% of cases, respectively. The etiology is unknown, though eosinophilia and immunopathological processes are thought to play a role in its pathogenesis.

Cardiac MR findings in EMF include high signal intensity along the endocardium of the apex on T2-weighted sequences, an overlying non-enhancing thrombus, with a distinct high signal intensity plane separating the thrombus from the underlying myocardium on gradient echo cine sequences. Cine-CMR shows mitral and tricuspid regurgitation and obliterated apices of the ventricles **(Fig. 5)**. DE-CMR shows a trilaminar appearance—non-enhancing clot in apex, followed subendocardial hyperenhancement of the underlying myocardium related to endocardial fibrosis, followed by a normal myocardium **(Fig. 8)**.[20] In advanced stages, there can be tethering of the AV valves or fibrosis of the papillary muscles, resulting in AV valve regurgitations.

Cardiac Sarcoidosis

Heart is involved in about 25% of patients with sarcoidosis but causes symptoms in only 5% of cases. An early diagnosis is important since early corticosteroid therapy can help in treating the myocardial inflammation, which, if persistent, may lead to malignant arrhythmias and sudden cardiac death. Echocardiography detects regional wall motion abnormalities, basal septal thinning, and ventricular dysfunction.

Cardiac MR has a sensitivity and specificity of 75–100% and 76.9–78% in diagnosing CS.[21] In the acute phase,

TABLE 5: Typical findings and poor prognostic features of cardiac amyloidosis on imaging.

Typical imaging findings in cardiac amyloidosis	Poor prognostic factors on imaging
Biventricular hypertrophy with bi-atrial dilatation (restrictive pattern)	RV, RA involvement
Thickening of valves, atrial septum	Increased myocardial mass
Normal function till end stage	Decreased LVEF
Diffuse subendocardial/transmural LGE	Transmural LGE
Increased native T1 and ECV mapping values, increased T2 mapping values in AL amyloidosis	ECV >40%
Abnormal nulling pattern, myocardial to skeletal muscle signal intensity ratio >1 at 20 ms TE	Cardiac thrombus
Reduced global longitudinal strain with apical sparing (Cherry on top pattern)	
Pericardial, pleural effusions, cardiac thrombi may be present	

(ECV: extracellular volume; LGE: late enhancement)

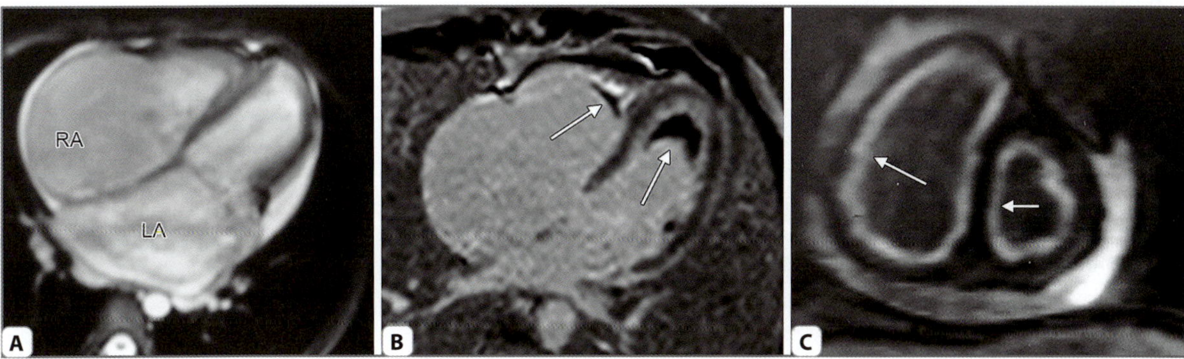

FIGS. 8A TO C: Cardiac MRI in a patient with endomyocardial fibrosis: Cine four chamber image (A) shows obliterated RV apex and biatrial dilatation. (B) LGE four chamber image shows a typical trilaminar appearance in both ventricles (white arrows)—non-enhancing clot in apex, followed subendocardial hyperenhancement of the underlying myocardium, related to endocardial fibrosis, followed by a normal myocardium. (C) LGE short-axis image in another patient showing diffuse subendocardial enhancement in both LV and RV (white arrows).

T2-weighted and early gadolinium enhanced images show focal areas of increased signal intensity and increased T2 mapping value suggesting inflammation. Confluent sarcoid granulomas show an increased peripheral T2 signal **(Fig. 9A)**. Focal myocardial thickening because of edema/ granuloma may be seen. Cine-CMR may show segmental wall motion abnormalities. On DE-CMR, patchy or focal enhancement is seen which is often mid wall rather than subendocardial or transmural **(Fig. 9B)**. The enhancement may be seen in the interventricular septum in the basal region and sometimes in the LV wall. Sometimes, papillary muscle and RV wall may be involved. In later burnt-out stages, features of DCM may be seen. Follow-up CMR can be done to see regression in T2 mapping values/edema or LGE. CMR may also show associated features such as pericardial effusion, mediastinal adenopathy, etc. Native T1 and T2 mapping may also be used in early detection of CS as seen in initial studies (Puntmann et al. JACC, 2016).

Nuclear imaging also helps in characterising CS. FDG-PET helps in diagnosing inflammation in the characteristic patchy distribution (usually with basal septal involvement), a feature typical for acute sarcoidosis. Abnormal perfusion is a sign of myocardial scarring and happens in subacute to chronic stages. The sensitivity and specificity of PET for CS is 89% and 78%, respectively.[22] Combined use of CMR and PET is useful in diagnosis with PET detecting inflammation (which guides initiation of steroid therapy) and CMR detecting LGE/scar (which guides placement of implantable defibrillator). **Table 6** summarizes the differential diagnosis of cardiac sarcoidosis. **Box 3** summarizes poor prognostic features of CS on CMR.

Iron Overload Cardiomyopathy

This is seen in patients with hemochromatosis or in those with hemolytic anemias like thalassemia where multiple and regular blood transfusions are required. Ferritin, commonly used for monitoring body iron overload, although correlates well with liver iron, does not correlate well with myocardial iron. CMR, using T2* MRI, is the current non-invasive gold standard method for detecting heart iron deposition **(Fig. 10, Table 7)**. Increasing iron causes decrease in T2*, which has been found to correlate with progressive LV dysfunction if untreated and has been validated through

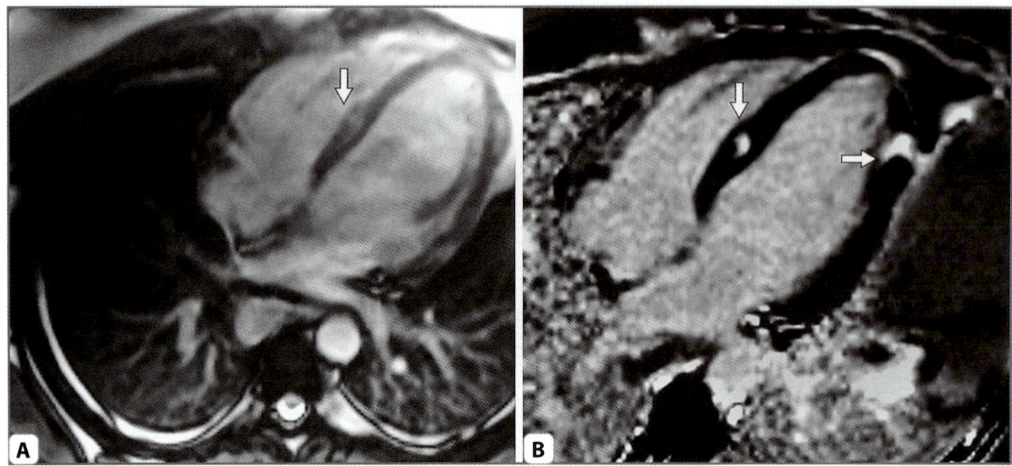

FIGS. 9A AND B: Cardiac MRI in a patient with sarcoidosis: (A) Cine four chamber image shows a hyperintense sarcoid granuloma in interventricular septum (block arrow). (B) The same granuloma shows enhancement on delayed contrast MRI (block arrows in LGE four chamber image). Another enhancing lesion in lateral wall of apical LV is also seen. Focal areas of enhancement like these are characteristic of sarcoid.

TABLE 6: The differential diagnosis of cardiac sarcoidosis and imaging features.

Differential diagnosis	Clinical features	Imaging findings
Sarcoidosis	High degree AV nodal blocks, ventricular arrythmias	Patchy LGE in subepicardial/mid-myocardial/transmural/subendocardial pattern, especially involving basal septum
Myocarditis	H/o viral fever, raised troponins	Subepicardial LGE, especially in inferolateral wall, myocardial edema on T2/T2 mapping
Non-ischemic DCM	Heart failure, may be familial	Dilated LV with global hypokinesia, linear mid wall LGE in septum
Asymmetric HCM	May be familial, syncopal episodes	Thick myocardium >15 mm in end diastole, patchy mid-wall LGE especially in RV insertion points

(ECV: extracellular volume; LGE: late enhancement)

various studies.[8] T2* MRI helps in planning chelation regimens in patients with thalassemia and is also useful in following up of treatment response in these patients. CMR also reveals an extensive myocardial signal loss on T1 and T2 weighted images. Restrictive patterns may be seen in earlier stages with late stages resulting in DCM.

Iron also decreases the T1 mapping values, and this can also be used to detect iron overload early. Our group found that the native T1 of <850 ms had high specificity (95.2%), sensitivity (94.2%) and negative predictive value (98.8%) for detecting T2* < 20 ms (significant iron overload). We use a rapid CMR protocol, including cine (for LV function, T2* mapping and T1 mapping), which takes about 9–10 minutes.[23] Strain abnormalities can also identify subclinical heart failure in patients with myocardial iron (T2* < 20 ms) but normal LV ejection fraction. We found global radial strain to be valuable in this regard.[24]

BOX 3: Poor prognostic features of cardiac sarcoidosis (CS) on CMR.

- Decreased LVEF <35%
- LV dilatation (increased LVEDV)
- RV, atrial involvement
- LGE presence and extent (>20%) – ventricular arrythmia and sudden cardiac death

(CMR: cardiac magnetic resonance imaging; ECV: extracellular volume; LGE: late enhancement)

ANDERSON–FABRY DISEASE

Anderson–Fabry disease is an X-linked disorder of lysosomal metabolism with lack of lysosomal α-galactosidase enzyme, resulting in the accumulation of glycosphingolipid in various tissues. In cardiac variants, myocardial hypertrophy is the main feature. This hypertrophy appears to be similar to that seen in HCM, but on DE-CMR helps it differentiate from HCM since the pattern of enhancement is different, with the basal inferolateral wall being the most common segment showing enhancement. Parametric mapping also helps in the detection of AFD, since most patients show low native T1 mapping (due to fat). Presence of myocardial scarring on LGE may imply that treatment with enzyme replacement therapy may be less effective at this stage, making a case for early initiation of this treatment, before fibrosis has developed.

ARRHYTHMOGENIC CARDIOMYOPATHY

Arrhythmogenic cardiomyopathy [earlier known as "arrhythmogenic right ventricular dysplasia" (ARVD)] is characterized by fibrosis and fatty replacement of the myocardium. It commonly involves the anterior wall of the right ventricle, in the so-called "triangle of dysplasia" (right ventricular subtricuspid area, the apex and the right ventricular infundibulum). It is more common in young males and has a familial occurrence.

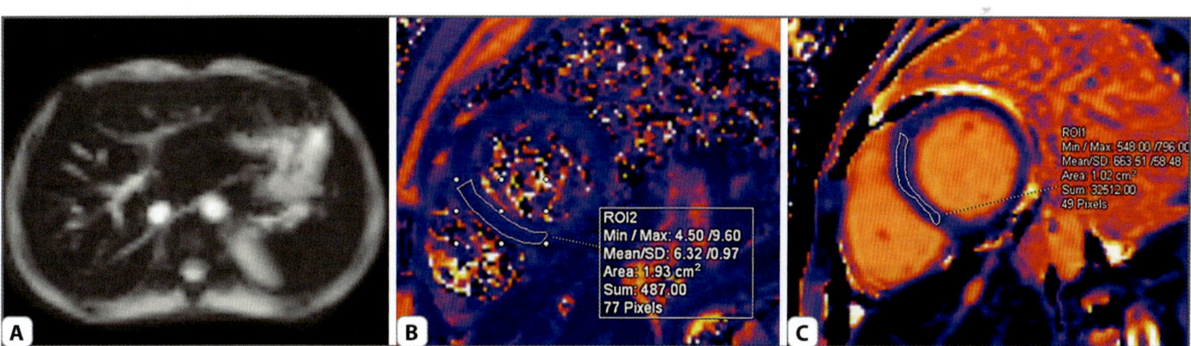

FIGS. 10A TO C: Cardiac MRI in patient with iron overload cardiomyopathy/siderosis: (A) TruFISP image shows dark liver and spleen; (B) T2* MRI of heart in short axis view shows T2* of ~6 ms (severe iron overload at 1.5 Tesla); and (C) T1 mapping of the heart shows reduced values (~663 ms).

TABLE 7: Reference values of T2* MRI of heart and liver.

Categories of iron overload	Myocardium		Liver	
	1.5 T	3 T	1.5 T	3 T
Normal	>20 ms	>12.6 ms	>15.4 ms	>8.4 ms
Mild–moderate	10–20 ms	5.8–12.6 ms	4.5–15.4 ms (moderate), 2.1–4.5 ms (mild)	2.3–8.4 ms (moderate); 1.05–2.3 ms (mild)
Severe	<10 ms	<5.8 ms	<2.1 ms	<1.05 ms

Biventricular involvement is common. It leads to progressive ventricular failure and dilatation and is an important cause of sudden cardiac death due to ventricular arrhythmias. The diagnostic criteria for ACM encompass genetic, electrocardiographic, pathophysiologic, and histopathologic factors and have evolved over time. **Table 8** summarizes the 2024 European Task Force consensus report which was refinement of the 2020 international Padua criteria. The major upgrade was the recognition of the LV involvement that may coexist ("biventricular") or exceed (arrhythmogenic left ventricular cardiomyopathy) the RV involvement.[25,26] The typical feature that is seen with the ALVC phenotypes is the subepicardial ring like LGE pattern in LV myocardium, which occurs in genetic mutations like desmoplakin or filamin C **(Fig. 11)**.[26]

The traditional imaging modalities used to evaluate right ventricular abnormalities include echocardiography and radionuclide angiography. However, all of them have low sensitivity and specificity for diagnosing ARVD, primarily because of their inability to accurately characterize structural and functional abnormalities of the right ventricle. Also, all these imaging modalities are limited by a lack of spatial resolution in diagnosing the typical fatty and fibrofatty changes of the right ventricular myocardium. Endomyocardial biopsy suffers from sampling errors, since involvement generally occurs in a segmental fashion. Due to its high resolution, large field of view and ability to quantify RV abnormalities, CMR has emerged as the imaging modality of choice in investigating ARVD. T1-weighted spin echo images show fatty infiltration as bright signal with thinning of the RV wall and RV dilatation **(Fig. 12)**. Cine-CMR shows decreased global function, regional wall motion abnormalities or aneurysms. Delayed enhancement CMR may show hyperenhancement in regions of fibrofatty replacement and thus may be useful to guide endomyocardial biopsy. Selection of patients who need implantable cardioverter defibrillator implantation is one of the most important issues in clinical management.

Cardiac MR can help measure intramyocardial fat and thus help monitor evolution of the disease. However, it should be remembered that significant fatty infiltration occurs in > 50% of normal hearts in elderly people. Also,

TABLE 8: Relevant simplified imaging-based criteria from the 2024 European consensus document for ACM diagnosis.[26]

Category	RV phenotype	LV phenotype
Morpho-functional ventricular abnormalities	*Major*: • RV Regional wall motion abnormality (RWMA), plus • Global RV dilatation, or • Dysfunction *Minor*: RV RWMA	*Minor*: Global LV systolic dysfunction
Structural	*Major:* Fibrous replacement +/– fatty tissue at histology *Minor*: RV LGE	*Major*: Ring like LV LGE (in ≥ 3 segments) *Minor:* LV LGE in 1–2 segments
Repolarization abnormalities		
Depolarization/conduction abnormalities		
Arrythmias		
Family history/genetics		

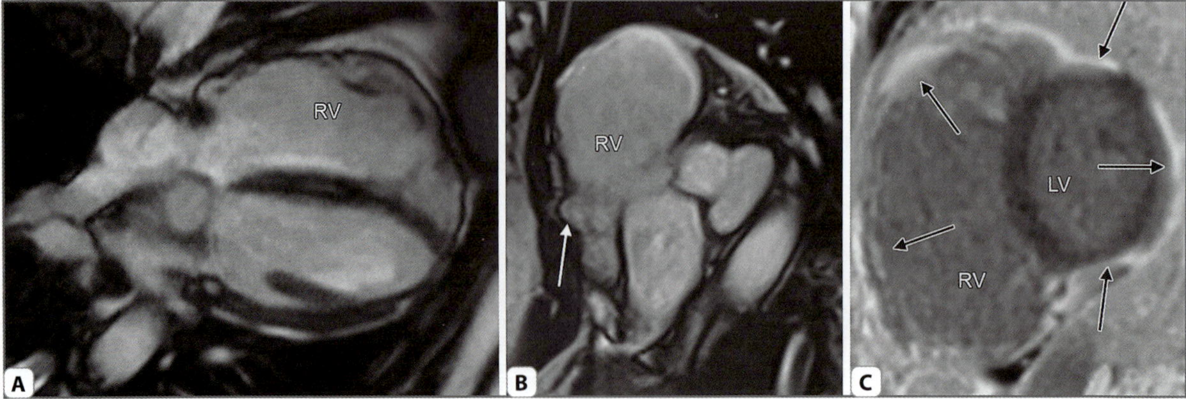

FIGS. 11A TO C: Cardiac MRI in a patient with genetic arrhythmogenic cardiomyopathy. (A) Cine four chamber image shows dilated RV; (B) Cine short axis image in systole shows small microaneurysms in RV free wall (white arrow); and (C) LGE image in short-axis view shows diffuse. RV free wall enhancement (black arrows) as well as subepicardial ring like LGE (black arrows) in LV. Findings confirm biventricular involvement.

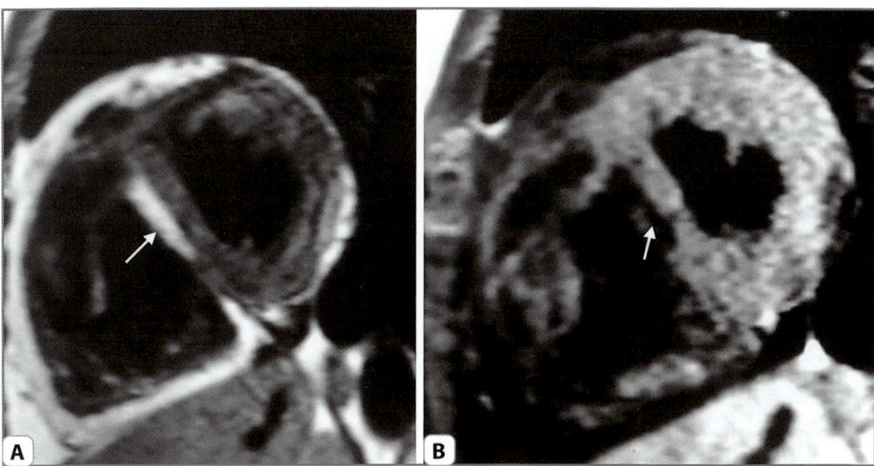

FIGS. 12A AND B: Cardiac MRI in a patient with genetic arrhythmogenic cardiomyopathy T1 weighted short axis image (A) showing bright signal along RV side in interventricular septum which nulls on fat saturated images (B) confirming fatty infiltration.

in 15% of control subjects, some degree of intramyocardial fat is seen in anterior apex of right ventricle. So, focal wall motion abnormalities are a more reliable indicator of ARVD than presence of isolated intramyocardial fat. Because first-degree relatives of individuals with ARVD have an increased chance of having the disease, with an increased risk of sudden death, CMR serves as an important tool for screening them for presence of pre-clinical disease.

LEFT VENTRICULAR NON-COMPACTION

In this CMP, there is the persistence of deep intertrabecular recesses in communication with the ventricular cavity. On imaging, the inner myocardial layer is spongy and less compacted compared to the outer compacted myocardium, giving a double layered appearance **(Fig. 13)**. Both CT and CMR image this differential compactness of the myocardium with superior spatial resolution, particularly in the ventricular apex whereas echocardiography has inherent diagnostic limitations. Lesser degrees of myocardial layering may also be seen in other CMPs. Peterson et al reported in 2005 that a non-compacted/compacted myocardium ratio of > 2.3 in diastole distinguished pathological non-compaction from other CMPs, with a specificity and negative predictive value of 99% each.[27] The same group has recently published a consensus which highlights that increased trabeculation may be frequently demonstrated on imaging in healthy individuals, as well as in physiological states like pregnancy, athletes, and with varied inherited or acquired cardiac diseases, and that the terminology non-compaction be replaced be excessive trabeculation of the left ventricle. They propose that the excessive trabeculation is a phenotype rather than a standalone CMP itself. The physiological variants (isolated trabeculations) do not need follow-up, but those with coexisting CMP should be treated for the primary CMP rather than the non-compaction. Clot formation is common due to stasis of the blood and the demonstration of the same should prompt anticoagulation.[28]

TAKOTSUBO CARDIOMYOPATHY

The condition is likely thought to be due to stress related catecholamine upsurge causing cardiac dysfunction .and is characterized by basal hypercontractile myocardium and a mid-apical LV ballooning **(Fig. 14)**. Patients usually present with all clinical manifestations of an ST elevation myocardial infarction including chest pain, ECG changes and enzyme elevation. However, coronary angiography is normal. CMR is useful to show the reversible functional abnormalities as well as absence of any enhancement on DE-CMR, confirming non-infarcted myocardium.[29] Recent literature suggests that although there is absence of major LGE (using +5 SD threshold criteria), there may be faint enhancement (on + 3SD threshold). T1 and T2 mapping values increase due to concomitant inflammation and edema. A follow-up at 3–6 months may demonstrate normalization of functional abnormalities, resolution of edema as well as LGE.[29]

MYOCARDITIS

It is usually viral in origin and characterized by inflammation of the myocardium. Although spontaneous recovery is common, active myocarditis may occasionally lead to sudden death, and 5–10% of cases may progress to chronic dilated CMP.

Patchy involvement limits the use of myocardial biopsy for the diagnostic purposes. Echocardiography is the initial screening modality, but CMR is more sensitive due to its ability of tissue characterization. CMR has high diagnostic value and may show focal areas of increased signal on T2-weighted images, representing active inflammation/

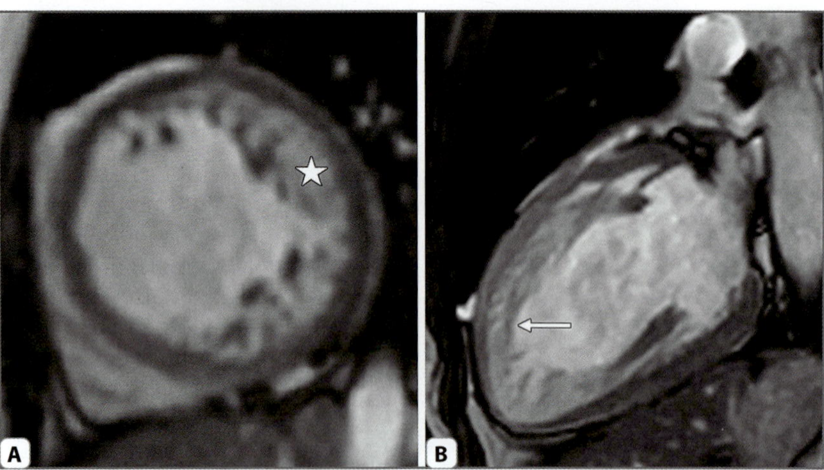

FIGS. 13A AND B: Cardiac MRI cine image in short axis (A) and two chamber view (B) shows double layered appearance of the LV myocardium with a non-compacted layer (star in A and arrow in B) alongside a compacted normal layer, in a patient with LV non-compaction.

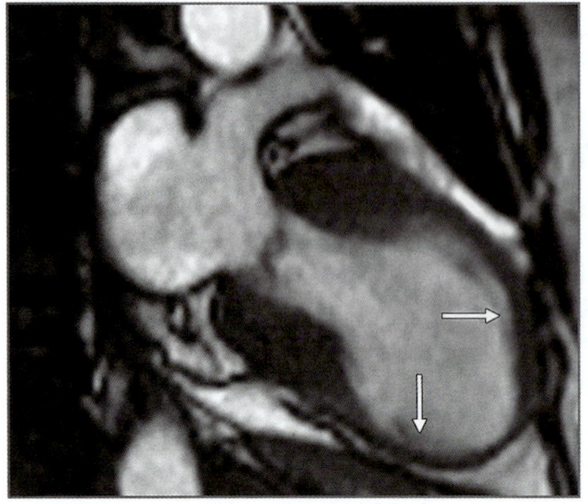

FIG. 14: Cardiac MRI cine image two-chamber view in end systolic frame shows mid-apical LV ballooning (arrows) in a patient with Takotsubo cardiomyopathy.

edema. Both early and late gadolinium enhancement may be seen in areas of myocardial necrosis on histology. Cine-CMR may show wall motion abnormalities. The late hyperenhancement is typically subepicardial and has "non-ischemic" pattern of distribution. It is known to occur predominantly in the lateral free wall. The previous Lake Louise criteria focused on the above findings of edema (T2), hyperemia (EGE) and necrosis (LGE).[30] However, the latest Lake Louise criteria has recognized the importance of parametric mapping, and these are summarized in **Table 9 (Fig. 15)**.[31] FDG-PET also shows areas of inflammation and shows good agreement with CMR.

MYOCARDIAL TUBERCULOSIS

Myocardial tuberculosis is very rare, the reported autopsy incidence being 0.14–0.3%. Tuberculosis of the heart

TABLE 9: Overview of the 2018 Lake Louise criteria for the CMR diagnosis of myocarditis.[31]

Type of criteria	Components of the criteria
Main criteria: Both criteria are needed to be present	• Myocardial edema (increased signal on T2 images, or increased T2 mapping values), and • Non-ischemic myocardial injury (increase of native T1 or ECV mapping values or non-ischemic pattern of LGE present)
Supportive criteria	• Pericarditis • Systolic LV dysfunction

generally involves the pericardium and may result in constrictive pericarditis. Myocardial tuberculosis is very unusual. CMR shows predominant involvement of right heart (tubercular myocarditis), especially right atrium, but may show diffuse myocardial thickening contiguous with the pericardial involvement (myopericarditis) more commonly. DE-CMR showed dense myocardial and pericardial enhancement. On histopathology, these may manifest as tubercular nodules with central caseation, miliary nodules, or a diffused infiltrative pattern with pericarditis. Definitive diagnosis requires demonstration of mycobacteria on biopsy specimens or caseating necrosis.

PERIPARTUM CARDIOMYOPATHY

Peripartum cardiomyopathy is heart failure that develops during the peripartum period in otherwise healthy women. Its causes are classified as inflammatory (e.g., viral) and noninflammatory (e.g., genetic etiology, malnutrition, hormonal). Diagnosis requires heart failure onset in late pregnancy or early postpartum, no prior heart disease, and no other obvious cause. CMR helps in diagnosis and

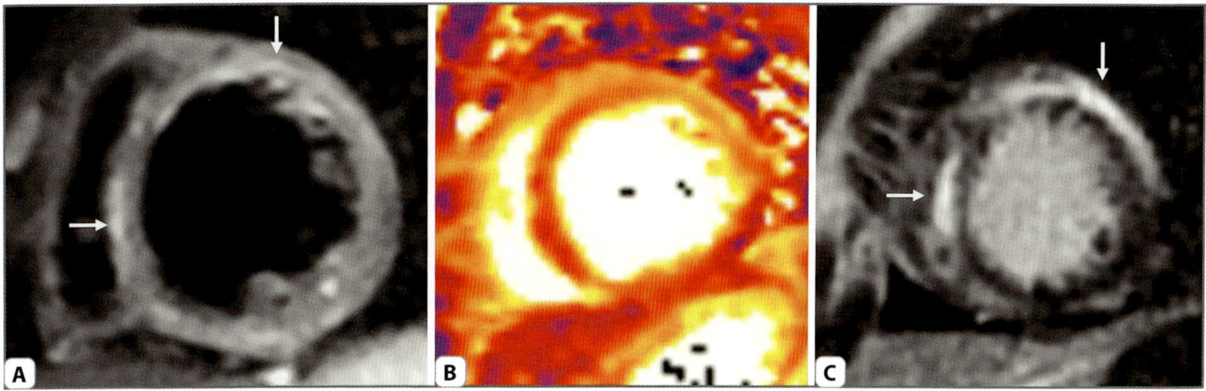

FIGS. 15A TO C: Cardiac MRI in a patient with acute myocarditis: T2/STIR short-axis image (A) show areas of myocardial edema (hyperintensity, arrows) confirmed on T2 mapping image (B) which showed increased values (63 ms). (C) LGE image in short-axis view shows areas of subepicardial LGE (arrows), characteristic of myocarditis.

follow-up, and shows findings like myocardial edema and midmyocardial LGE in anterior and lateral segments. T1 and ECV mapping may show raised values.

CONCLUSION

Cardiomyopathies are a heterogeneous group of myocardial disorders associated with distinct anatomical, functional and electrophysiological alterations of the heart. Traditional imaging techniques are limited in their assessment of the myocardium. Echocardiography is usually the first line investigation. Cardiac CT is useful to rule out coronary artery disease (ischemic etiology). CMR has emerged as the investigation of choice for imaging in CMPs, primarily because of its ability to allow for accurate functional assessment and tissue characterization. FDG-PET plays a role in detecting myocardial inflammation and in diagnosis of ATTR amyloidosis.

REFERENCES

1. Elliott P, Andersson B, Arbustini E, Bilinska Z, Cecchi F, Charron P, et al. Classification of the cardiomyopathies: a position statement from the European Society of Cardiology Working Group on Myocardial and Pericardial Diseases. Eur Heart J. 2008;29:270-6.
2. Felker GM, Thompson RE, Hare JM, Hruban RH, Clemetson DE, Howard DL, et al. Underlying causes and long-term survival in patients with initially unexplained cardiomyopathy. N Engl J Med. 2000;342:1077-84.
3. Arbelo E, Protonotarios A, Gimeno JR, Arbustini E, Barriales-Villa R, Basso C, et al. 2023 ESC Guidelines for the management of cardiomyopathies. Eur Heart J. 2023;44(37):3503-26.
4. Leiner T, Bogaert J, Friedrich, MG. et al. SCMR Position Paper on clinical indications for cardiovascular magnetic resonance. J Cardiovasc Magn Reason. 2020;22:76.
5. Shah DJ, Judd RM, Kim RJ. Myocardial viability. In: Edelman RR, Hesselink JR, Zlatkin MB, Crues JV, (Eds). Clinical Magnetic Resonance Imaging. 3rd edition. New York, NY: Elsevier, 2006.
6. Messroghli DR, Moon JC, Ferreira VM, Grosse-Wortmann L, He T, Kellman P, et al. Clinical recommendations for cardiovascular magnetic resonance mapping of T1, T2, T2* and extracellular volume: A consensus statement by the Society for Cardiovascular Magnetic Resonance (SCMR) endorsed by the European Association for Cardiovascular Imaging (EACVI) [published correction appears in J Cardiovasc Magn Reson. 2018;20(1):9.
7. Shaw M, Ojha V, Jagia KP, Malhi AS, Chandrashekhara SH, Kumar S, et al. Reference values of myocardial native T1 and T2 mapping values in normal Indian population at 1.5 Tesla scanner. Int J Cardiovasc Imaging. 2022;38(11):2403-11.
8. Anderson LJ, Holden S, Davis B, Charrier CC, Bunce NH, Firmin DN, et al. Cardiovascular T2-star (T2*) magnetic resonance for the early diagnosis of myocardial iron overload. Eur Heart J. 2001;22(23):2171-9.
9. Pinto YM, Elliott PM, Arbustini E, Adler Y, Anastasakis A, Böhm M, et al. Proposal for a revised definition of dilated cardiomyopathy, hypokinetic non-dilated cardiomyopathy, and its implications for clinical practice: a position statement of the ESC working group on myocardial and pericardial diseases. Eur Heart J. 2016;37(23):1850-8.
10. Assomull RG, Shakespeare C, Kalra PR, Lloyd G, Gulati A, Strange J, et al. Role of cardiovascular magnetic resonance as a gatekeeper to invasive coronary angiography in patients presenting with heart failure of unknown etiology. Circulation. 2011;124:1351-60.
11. Assomull RG, Prasad SK, Lyne J, Smith G, Elizabeth D Burman ED, Khan M, et al. Cardiovascular magnetic resonance,

fibrosis, and prognosis in dilated cardiomyopathy. J Am Coll Cardiol. 2006;48(10):1977-85.

12. Wu KC, Weiss RG, Thiemann DR, Kitagawa K, Schmidt A, Dalal D, et al. Late gadolinium enhancement by cardiovascular magnetic resonance heralds an adverse prognosis in nonischemic cardiomyopathy. J Am Coll Cardiol. 2008;51(25):2414-21.
13. Klem I, Klein M, Khan M, Yang EY, Faisal Nabi F, Ivanov A, et al. Relationship of LVEF and Myocardial Scar to Long-term Mortality Risk and Mode of Death in Patients with Nonischemic Cardiomyopathy. Circulation. 2021;143(14):1343-58.
14. Elliott PM, Anastasakis A, Borger MA, Martin Borggrefe M, Cecchi F, et al. 2014 ESC Guidelines on diagnosis and management of hypertrophic cardiomyopathy: the Task Force for the Diagnosis and Management of Hypertrophic Cardiomyopathy of the European Society of Cardiology (ESC). Eur Heart J. 2014;35(39):2733-9.
15. Hughes RK, Shiwani H, Rosmini S, Augusto JB, Burke L, Jiang Y, et al. Improved Diagnostic Criteria for Apical Hypertrophic Cardiomyopathy. JACC Cardiovasc Imaging. 2024;17(5):501-12.
16. Mahrholdt H, Wagner A, Judd RM, Sechtem U, Kim RJ. Delayed enhancement cardiovascular magnetic resonance assessment of non-ischemic cardiomyopathies. Eur Heart J. 2005;26:1461-74.
17. Baggiano A, Boldrini M, Martinez-Naharro A, et al. Noncontrast Magnetic Resonance for the Diagnosis of Cardiac Amyloidosis. JACC Cardiovasc Imaging. 2020; 13(1 Pt 1):69-80.
18. Ridouani F, Damy T, Tacher V, Derbel H, Legou F, Sifaoui I, et al. Myocardial native T2 measurement to differentiate light-chain and transthyretin cardiac amyloidosis and assess prognosis. J Cardiovasc Magn Reson. 2018;20(1):58.
19. Garcia-Pavia P, Rapezzi C, Adler Y, Arad M, Cristina Basso C, Brucato A, et al. Diagnosis and treatment of cardiac amyloidosis: a position statement of the ESC Working Group on Myocardial and Pericardial Diseases. Eur Heart J. 2021;42(16):1554-68.
20. de Carvalho FP, Azevedo CF. Comprehensive Assessment of Endomyocardial Fibrosis with Cardiac MRI: Morphology, Function, and Tissue Characterization. Radiographics. 2020;40(2):336-53.
21. Jeudy J, Burke AP, White CS, Kramer GB, Frazier AA. Cardiac sarcoidosis: the challenge of radiologic-pathologic correlation: from the radiologic pathology archives. Radiographics. 2015;35(4):1316.
22. Youssef G, Leung E, Mylonas I, Nery P, Kathryn Williams K, Wisenberg G, et al. The use of 18F-FDG PET in the diagnosis of cardiac sarcoidosis: a systematic review and meta-analysis including the Ontario experience. J Nucl Med. 2012;53(2):241-8.
23. Singh SP, Jagia P, Ojha V, Seth T, Naik N, Ganga KP, et al. Diagnostic Value of T1 Mapping in Detecting Iron Overload in Indian Patients with Thalassemia Major: A Comparison with T2* Mapping. Indian J Radiol Imaging. 2023;34(1):54-9.
24. Ojha V, Ganga KP, Jagia P, Seth T, Roy A, Naik N, et al. Role of CMR feature-tracking derived left ventricular strain in predicting myocardial iron overload and assessing myocardial contractile dysfunction in patients with thalassemia major. Eur Radiol. 2021;31(8):6184-92.
25. Corrado D, Perazzolo Marra M, Zorzi A, Beffagna G, Cipriani A, Lazzari MD, et al. Diagnosis of arrhythmogenic cardiomyopathy: The Padua criteria. Int J Cardiol. 2020;319:106-14.
26. Corrado D, Anastasakis A, Basso C, Bauce B, Blomström-Lundqvist C, Bucciarelli-Ducci C, et al. Proposed diagnostic criteria for arrhythmogenic cardiomyopathy: European Task Force consensus report. Int J Cardiol. 2024;395:131447.
27. Petersen SE, Selvanayagam JB, Wiesmann F, Robson MD, Francis JM, Anderson RH, et al. Left ventricular non-compaction: insights from cardiovascular magnetic resonance imaging. J Am Coll Cardiol. 2005;46(1):101-5.
28. Petersen SE, Jensen B, Aung N, Friedrich MG, Colin J McMahon CJ, Mohiddin SA, et al. Excessive Trabeculation of the Left Ventricle: JACC: Cardiovascular Imaging Expert Panel Paper. JACC Cardiovasc Imaging. 2023;16(3):408-25.
29. Ojha V, Khurana R, Ganga KP, Kumar S. Advanced cardiac magnetic resonance imaging in takotsubo cardiomyopathy. Br J Radiol. 2020;93(1115):20200514.
30. Friedrich MG, Sechtem U, Schulz-Menger J, Holmvang G, Alakija P, Cooper LT, et al. Cardiovascular magnetic resonance in myocarditis: a JACC white paper. J Am Coll Cardiol. 2009;53(17):1475-87.
31. Ferreira VM, Schulz-Menger J, Holmvang G, Kramer CM, Carbone I, Sechtem U, et al. Cardiovascular magnetic resonance in nonischemic myocardial inflammation: expert recommendations. J Am Coll Cardiol. 2018;72(24):3158-76.

Sanjeev Kumar, Aprateem Mukherjee

CHAPTER

27

Imaging Evaluation of Cardiac Masses

INTRODUCTION

Cardiac masses, despite being rare, are now being more frequently encountered. This may be attributed to increase in availability and access to multimodality imaging techniques such as echocardiography, CT and MRI. Cardiac masses encompass both neoplastic and non-neoplastic lesions involving the heart. The identification of any cardiac as benign or malignant is important from prognostic point of view. Reaching an accurate diagnosis is important, as management strategies vary depending upon the etiology. Additionally, it is necessary not to misinterpret normal cardiac structures and variants as cardiac masses. Therefore, radiologists need to be familiar with the imaging appearances of various cardiac masses as well as normal structures and variants.

The advent and evolution of multidetector CT (MDCT) and MRI technology over the last two decades has markedly improved our ability to evaluate and plan the optimal management of various pathological conditions that may affect the heart. Prior to the availability of these modalities, the diagnosis of cardiac masses was difficult to make and often not possible ante-mortem. In this review, we discuss the clinical presentation, classification, and modalities utilized for imaging along with the imaging features of various cardiac mass lesions.

CLINICAL FEATURES

Cardiac masses may be symptomatic or found incidentally as part of some other evaluation). Hence, a high degree of clinical suspicion is needed to make a reliable diagnosis.

Symptomatic masses may present as:

- Constitutional symptoms (fever, weight loss, arthralgias), paraneoplastic syndrome
- Symptoms related to location within the heart (valvular dysfunction such as regurgitation, arrhythmias, mass effect causing obstruction to blood flow, pericardial effusion)
- Systemic or pulmonary thromboembolic effects from the tumor.

Multimodality Imaging in Cardiac Masses

The goal of imaging in cardiac masses is, firstly, to localize the mass within the cardiac chambers; to ascertain whether the mass is benign or malignant in nature and to provide a reasonable diagnosis/narrow list of differentials for the lesion. Imaging in paramount to establish the accurate site of the mass as biopsy may then be planned for final histological diagnosis. Till date however, there is no single modality that possesses all the above characteristics. This, therefore, necessitates a multimodality approach in order to make an accurate and complete diagnosis.

Echocardiography

Transthoracic echocardiography (TTE) is usually the first imaging modality for assessment of cardiac masses. The mass maybe pickup up incidentally, in asymptomatic cases where echocardiography is being performed for another purpose, or workup for a suspected cardiac pathology. Echocardiography is most cases, can localize the mass within the cardiac chambers. It is capable of providing most of the required information regarding the lesion location, extent, mobility and hemodynamic consequences.

Advantages

- Noninvasive, relatively cheap and easily available modality.
- No use of ionizing radiation or iodinated contrast media.

- Portable (can be performed bedside).
- Can localize the site, size of the lesion.
- Allows for evaluation of cardiac function, cardiac valves (if involved by the mass).
- Hemodynamic evaluation (whether mass causing valvular obstruction).

Disadvantages

- Needs operator experience and expertise.
- Visualization of mass maybe limited by poor echo windows, (e.g., obese patients, mass at right ventricle apex, masses in left atrium, small valvular masses)
- Poor tissue characterization of the mass.
- Extent of large masses and extracardiac involvement cannot be adequately evaluated.

Transesophageal Echocardiography

Transesophageal echocardiography is an advanced echocardiographic technique where the ultrasound transducer is introduced via the esophagus to get better images of the cardiac structures. TEE provides higher resolution images because the ultrasound transducer is closer to the heart and gives better assessment of masses involving the cardiac valves—their size, mobility and hemodynamic parameters. Newer techniques such as 3D-TEE provides better visualization real time assessment of cardiac valves and it's relationship with cardiac masses, if any. However, TEE is an invasive procedure and may not be suitable for everyone, such as those with esophageal diseases or strictures.

Cardiac Magnetic Resonance Imaging

After a cardiac mass is picked up on echocardiography or any other imaging modality, the next step in imaging is usually a cardiac MRI. Cardiac MRI allows a comprehensive, noninvasive assessment for the diagnosis as well as follow-up of cardiac masses.

Advantages

- *Detection and tissue characterization*: CMR allows high-resolution imaging of cardiac masses with the added advantage of using various sequences for tissue characterization of masses such as T1, T2-weighted imaging and postcontrast sequences (perfusion, early and late gadolinium enhancement). Newer techniques such as parametric mapping (T1 and T2 mapping) also allow quantitative assessment beyond the conventional tissue characterization.
- The multiplanar capabilities of MRI allows accurate localization of the site of the mass, size of the lesion and it's relation to surrounding cardiac structures-this is crucial for surgical planning. Extracardiac involvement can also be accurately assessment with cardiac MRI which can potentially change the management approach.
- MRI does not involve use of ionizing radiation or potentially nephrotoxic contrast (except for a small risk of causing nephrogenic systemic fibrosis with use of gadolinium in underlying severe renal insufficiency).

Disadvantages

- Limited availability of expertise, scanner and software.
- Longer scanning time.
- Susceptibility to motion artifacts with requirement of a stable heart rate.

Cardiac CT

The development of MDCT technology has dramatically improved the spatial and temporal resolution for cardiac imaging. Gating the cardiac images to the electrocardiogram (ECG) can be accomplished either by scanning or reconstructing raw data at the point of least cardiac motion.

Advantages

- Generates three-dimensional images with isotropic resolution. This allows for multiplanar reconstructions in any oblique planes.
- Short acquisition time. This is helpful in scanning unstable or pediatric patients. The latter often require deep sedation or even general anesthesia for doing MRI.
- Volume rendered reconstructions provide a useful roadmap to the surgeon for tumor resection.
- Excellent for detection of calcifications within mass/calcified masses.
- Allows assessment of coronary artery disease in elderly patients/evaluation of involvement of coronary artery by masses.
- Assessment of any lung abnormalities.

Disadvantages

- Entails use of ionizing radiation.
- Uses iodinated contrast agents (maybe contraindicated in patients with renal failure, contrast allergy).
- Poorer tissue contrast compared to cardiac MRI.

Angiocardiography

Prior to the advent of noninvasive modalities, angiocardiography was the only modality available for detecting cardiac masses. Besides being invasive, this is an indirect assessment based on the presence of a filling defect or a change in the luminal outline. Angiography is imprecise, often misleading, and can easily miss small lesions and intramurally located masses. Further, there is a real risk of embolization of dislodged tumor fragments during catheterization.

With the availability of noninvasive modalities that directly image the myocardium and the lesion and can also allow for tissue characterization, angiography is rarely indicated at present for demonstration of cardiac masses. The only situations where it is still performed include:

- Suspicion of valvular or outflow tract obstruction by the mass, where catheterization may demonstrate a hemodynamically significant pressure gradient.
- *In vascular lesions*: For example sinus of Valsalva (SOV) aneurysm or ventricular pseudoaneurysm
- Demonstration of coronary artery anatomy and tumor vascularity prior to surgery **(Fig. 1)**
- Performing endomyocardial biopsy for indeterminate lesions.

It is important to note that MRI and ECHO are capable of quantifying obstruction, MDCT can demonstrate coronary anatomy, while both MRI and MDCT can equally assess vascular lesions. Therefore, angiography can easily be avoided for these indications.

MRI SEQUENCES FOR EVALUATION OF CARDIAC MASSES

A cardiac MRI acquisition should be tailored to location and type of suspected cardiac masses. A protocol for MR acquisition in cardiac masses is shown in **Table 1**.

CLASSIFICATION OF CARDIAC MASSES

Cardiac tumors have a cumulative prevalence of 0.002–0.3% as determined in autopsy series.[1] Primary cardiac neoplasms include both benign and malignant histological types **(Flowchart 1)**.

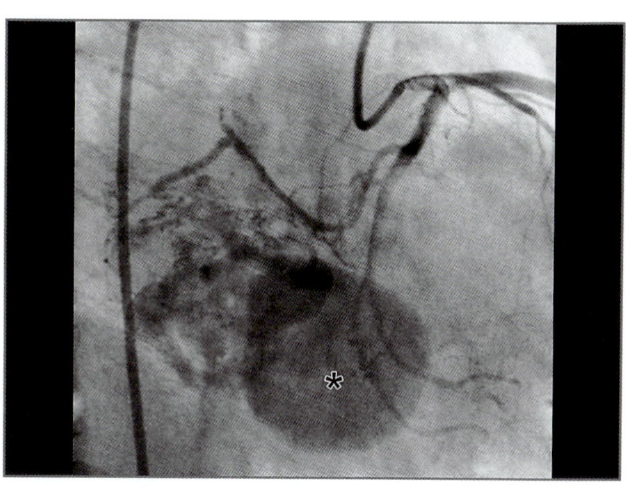

FIG. 1: Left coronary angiogram in a known case of right atrial myxoma. The atrial branches of the left circumflex artery are seen to supply a vascularized area within interatrial septum (representing the stalk) with an oval mobile mass (asterisk) that enhances immediately afterwards.

TABLE 1: Basic cardiac MRI protocol for evaluation of cardiac masses.

Sequence	Localizers
Balanced steady-state free precession (bSSFP) sequences covering the entire thorax	Localization of mass within the thoracic cavity and extrathoracic involvement, if any
T1/T2/STIR covering the mass	Tissue characteristics of the lesion
Cine-SSFP sequences	• Standard cardiac planes – short axis, four-chamber and two-chamber planes for cardiac functions. Chamber containing the cardiac mass should be included to assess mobility of the mass • Additional views maybe planned depending on the location of the mass
Postcontrast perfusion sequences	To be planned in orthogonal planes encompassing the mass for assessment of perfusion. Perfusion imaging can be useful to demonstrate increased tumor vascularity typical of malignant lesions such as angiosarcomas
Early gadolinium (EGE) and late gadolinium enhancement (LGE) including high TI	• Delayed enhanced imaging is useful to detect intramurally located lesions, distinguish tumors from thrombi, differentiate benign from malignant masses and identify areas of tissue necrosis • High TI PSIR sequences to differentiate mass from thrombus
• Other sequences (maybe optional depending on availability) • Parametric mapping T1/T2 mapping • Tagging • DWI/ADC	Allows quantitative assessment of tissue characteristics: • Myocardial tagging methods create a grid pattern on the myocardium and can thus help to differentiate contracting myocardial tissue from noncontractile tumor. This may help detect tumors of muscle consistency, such as rhabdomyomas • Maybe performed to assess for diffusion restriction (e.g., Lymphomas may show diffusion restriction)

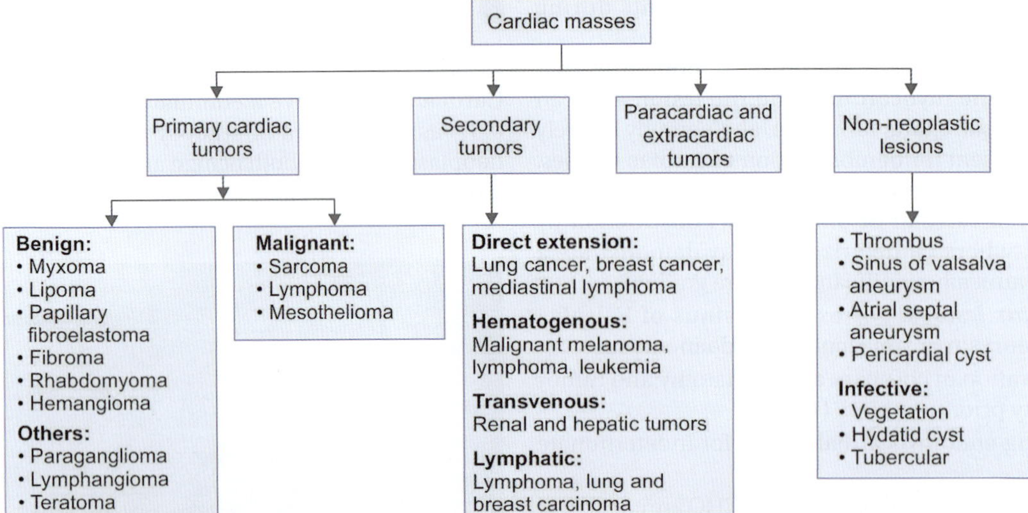

FLOWCHART 1: Overview of classification of cardiac masses.

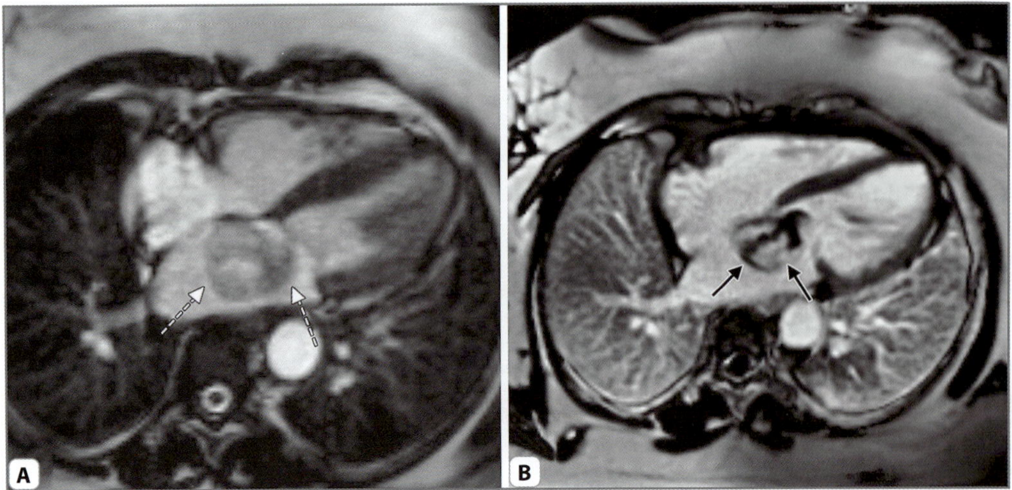

FIGS. 2A AND B: Four-chamber cine image (A) shows left atrial mass with narrow stalk attached to the interatrial septum. Late gadolinium enhances images (B) shows the heterogeneous enhancement of the mass. This was surgically removed and histopathologically confirmed as a myxoma.

Primary Cardiac Tumors

Benign Tumors

Myxoma: Myxomas are the most common benign tumor (50%) found in adults. They arise from embryologic rests that get entrapped during the septation phase of cardiac embryogenesis.

These tumors usually present between the fourth and seventh decades of life with mean age of diagnosis of about 50 years. They are more common in women (around 70% occur in women). Clinically, they may present in three ways:

1. Clinically silent (20%).
2. Classic triad—constitutional symptoms (fever, malaise), mitral valve obstruction (mimicking mitral stenosis), and embolic phenomenon
3. Nonspecific in presentation.

Thromboembolic events occur in 35% of left-sided myxomas to the brain, kidney, spleen and extremities and 10% of right-sided myxomas to the lung. Friable and gelatinous myxomas are more likely to embolize than firm and fibrous lesions.[2]

Location: Approximately 75% of myxomas are found in the left atrium, typically, in the interatrial septum in the region of the fossa ovalis; 20% of myxomas are located in the right atrium, and rare cases are found in the ventricles.

Imaging appearance ***(Fig. 2)***: On echocardiography, myxomas appear as homogeneous or heterogeneous mass, with echogenic foci owing to calcification and hypoechoic areas from hemorrhage, necrosis or cysts. Well defined, smooth, lobular, or oval and often pedunculated. Myxomas are typically solitary, varying in size from 1–15 cm appearing as a well-defined spherical or ovoid intracavitary mass, which typically has lobular contours and frequently calcified. On MRI, they are isointense on T1-weighted images, higher signal intensity on T2-weighted images owing to the high extracellular water content.

Regions of acute hemorrhage within myxomas appear as hypointense on both T1- and T2-weighted images, and older regions appear hyperintense as the hemoglobin becomes oxidized to methemoglobin, varying amounts of myxoid, hemorrhagic, ossific, and necrotic tissue. Cine imaging shows highly mobile, occasionally prolapsing through the mitral valve and causing obstruction. On SSFP sequences, they appear as hyperintense relative to the myocardium but hypointense relative to the blood pool. LGE usually shows patchy enhancement. Many myxomas have a layer of surface thrombus which appear as low signal intensity on LGE images.

Most lesions are sporadic. Carney's complex is an autosomal dominant disorder consisting of cardiac myxomas, hyperpigmented skin lesions and various extracardiac tumors.

Lipoma: Second most common primary benign cardiac neoplasm (8–12%) and are composed of mature adipose tissue.[3] They occur across a wide age range commonly seen in middle-age and older adults.

Nearly 50% of lipomas arise subendocardially and the rest are epicardial or endomyocardial in location. The left ventricle (LV) and RA are the most frequently involved.

Lipomas are usually detected incidentally. However, they may cause arrhythmias or valvular dysfunction. Subepicardial lipomas can compress the coronary arteries, which leads to ischemic chest pain.

Imaging appearance: Both CT and MRI are highly specific and sensitive in the detection of lipomas. They appear as well defined, homogeneous, encapsulated tumors homogeneous high signal intensity (relative to myocardium) on T1-weighted images that markedly suppresses with the application of additional fat-saturation prepulses. Similar signal intensity of surrounding chest wall fat on T1- and T2-weighted images **(Fig. 3)**. They do not enhance with contrast material. As with soft-tissue lipomas, cardiac lipomas do not show enhancement with the administration of a contrast material.

CT characteristically shows a homogeneous, non-enhancing masses with fat attenuation.

Lipomatous hypertrophy of the interatrial septum (IAS), although not a true neoplasm, has been included in various reports of cardiac lipomas. This is defined as any fatty thickening of the IAS at the level of the fossa ovalis that exceed 2 cm in transverse dimension. It is seen in older, obese patients and is frequently associated with increased epicardial fat. It has a typical "dumbbell" shape on imaging.

Papillary fibroelastoma: They are benign endocardial papillomas composed of avascular fronds of connective tissue lined by endothelium. They comprise nearly 10% of all primary cardiac tumors and 75% of all valvular neoplasms.[4] They are usually found on downstream side of the cardiac valves (ventricular side of mitral and aortic side of aortic valves). Despite this predilection, these tumors are not known to cause valvular dysfunction. The tumor usually has a narrow stalk and is mobile.

Patients are typically middle-aged and present with embolic complications, particularly cerebral, related to the predilection for left-sided valves.

Imaging features: Small, highly mobile homogeneous valvular mass (usually attached to the downstream side with a small pedicle). Papillary fibroelastomas are usually not observed on CT or MR images as they are small (<1.5 cm in diameter) and are attached to the moving valves.[4] MRI typically demonstrates the presence of a mass on a valve leaflet or on the endocardial surface. These tumors can create turbulence in the blood flow, which might be demonstrated with the use of cine MRI.

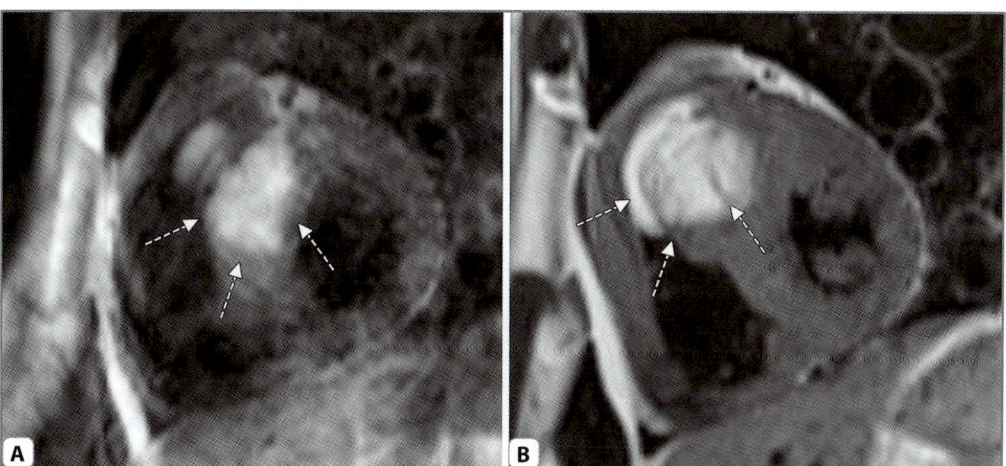

FIGS. 3A AND B: Short-axis T1W (A) and T2W (B) images show a T1/T2 hyperintense mass which suppressed on fat-sat images (not shown) within interventricular septum—a case of intracardiac lipoma.

Rhabdomyoma: They are the most common primary cardiac tumors in infants and children. About 75% of neonatal primary tumors are rhabdomyomas. These tumors are often associated with tuberous sclerosis in up to 50% of cases.[5]

Location: Usually intramurally in the ventricular myocardium with equal distribution on the right and left side of the heart and multiple lesions may be present in up to 90% of cases.

They typically present during the first year of life and can be asymptomatic or can protrude into the ventricular chambers, causing obstruction.

- *Imaging appearance*: On echocardiography: Small, well-circumscribed (multiple) nodules or a pedunculated mass in a cardiac cavity.
- MRI: Isointense to normal myocardium on T1-weighted images, hyperintense on T2-weighted image with minimal or no enhancement **(Fig. 4)**.

Majority remain asymptomatic and spontaneously regress before the age of 4 years.

Fibroma: Fibromas are neoplasms that mainly affect infants and children, being the second most common tumors found in this age group after rhabdomyomas. They are usually solitary tumors and are most often located intramurally in the ventricles involving the interventricular septum. These occur with increased frequency in patients with Gorlin syndrome and familial adenomatous polyposis.

Clinical presentation: Typically present in pediatric or young adult life.

Patients may present with ventricular arrhythmias and sudden death secondary to interference with conduction pathways. Large tumors can also cause dyspnea.

Imaging appearance:

- MRI: Isointense relative to normal myocardium on T1-weighted images and are characteristically hypointense on T2-weighted images. No contrast enhancement during perfusion imaging due to their avascularity and intense hyperenhancement on LGE image as gadolinium diffuses into interstitial spaces **(Fig. 5)**. The use of CT shows fibromas as homogeneous masses with soft-tissue attenuation, which may be either sharply marginated or infiltrative. Calcification is often observed.[6]

  In a child, the presence of a solitary, calcified, ventricular mass favors a fibroma whereas multiple tumors located in both atria and ventricles with other features of tuberous sclerosis favor rhabdomyomas.
- *Hemangioma:* These are tumors of vascular origin composed of either capillaries (capillary hemangiomas) or cavernous spaces (cavernous hemangiomas). They comprise 10% of primary benign tumors of the heart. The tumors are typically solitary and found in either ventricle but can be located in any chamber.
- *Imaging characteristics*: Cardiac hemangiomas are heterogeneous as depicted on precontrast CT images and are intensely enhanced as seen on CT images obtained after the administration of a contrast material. On MR, they are typically heterogenous and hyperintense on T1- and T2-weighted images owing to slow blood flow.

  During and after contrast agent administration they are intensely hyperintense due to their vascular content **(Fig. 6)**[7]—but there may be regions of inhomogeneity owing to calcification or fibrous septa.
- *Paraganglioma*: Cardiac paragangliomas make up 2% of all paragangliomas. Their most common location is in the left atrium (55%), followed by the interatrial septum (16%) and the anterior surface of the heart (10%). On echocardiography, they are typically seen as large, echogenic left atrial masses with broad base of attachment and occasionally may show infiltration. CT usually shows a circumscribed, heterogenous, low attenuation mass that enhances strongly with contrast **(Fig. 7)**. On MRI, the tumor is iso- to hypointense on T1W images. Increased SI on T1W images may be due to hemorrhage. It is markedly hyperintense on

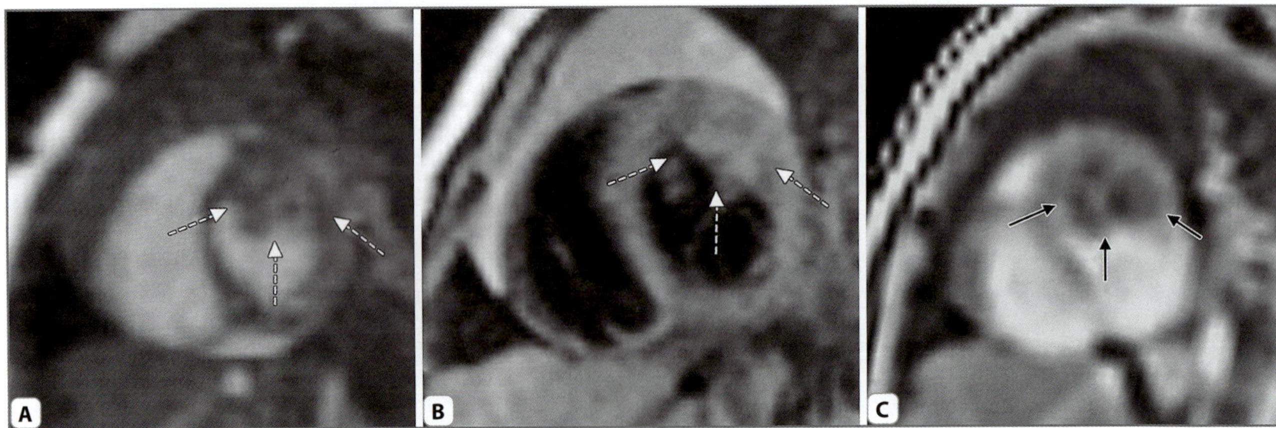

FIGS. 4A TO C: Rhabdomyoma: Short-axis TRUFI (True Fast Imaging with steady-state-free precession) image (A) T2W image, (B) shows a mass in the anterior LV myocardium which is slightly hyperintense on T2 and showing minimal to mild contrast enhancement (C).

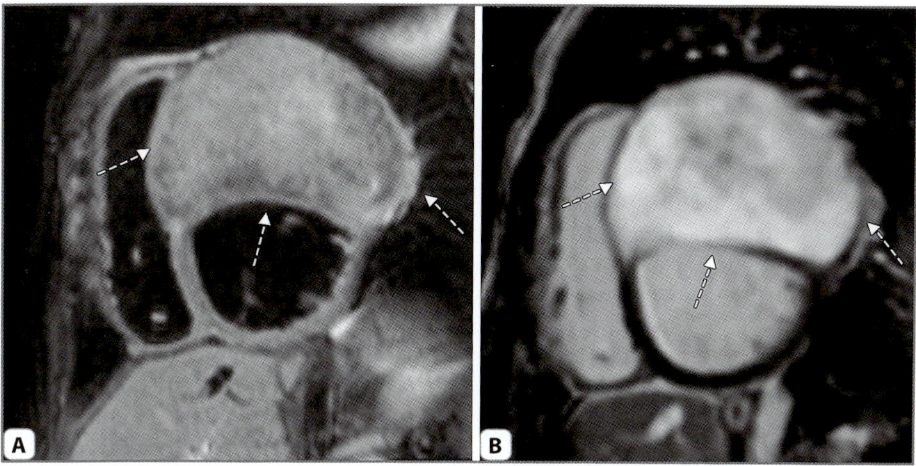

FIGS. 5A AND B: Dark blood STIR (Short Tau Inversion Recovery) image (A) shows a large isointense mass with areas of hypointensity in the anterior LV wall. The mass showed intense homogenous enhancement on postcontrast LGE images (B) characteristic of fibroma.

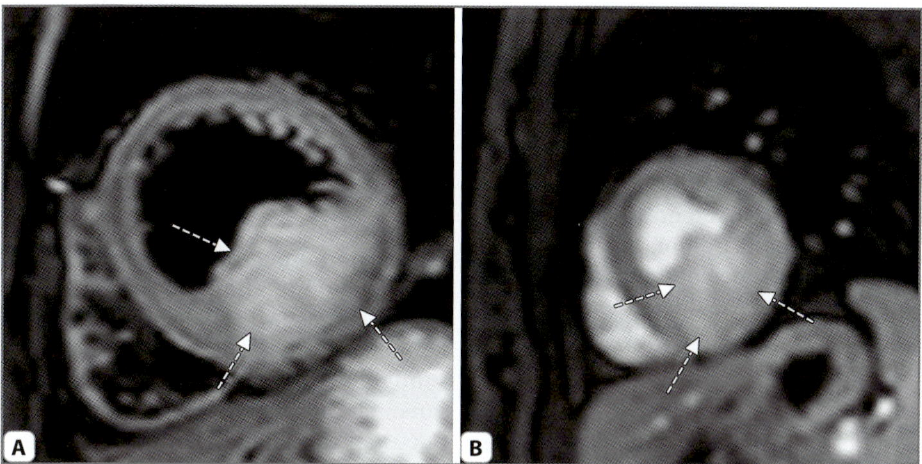

FIGS. 6A AND B: Dark blood STIR (Short Tau Inversion Recovery) image (A) shows a T2 hyperintense lesion in inferior LV wall which shows peripheral filling of contrast on perfusion images (B) characteristic of hemangioma.

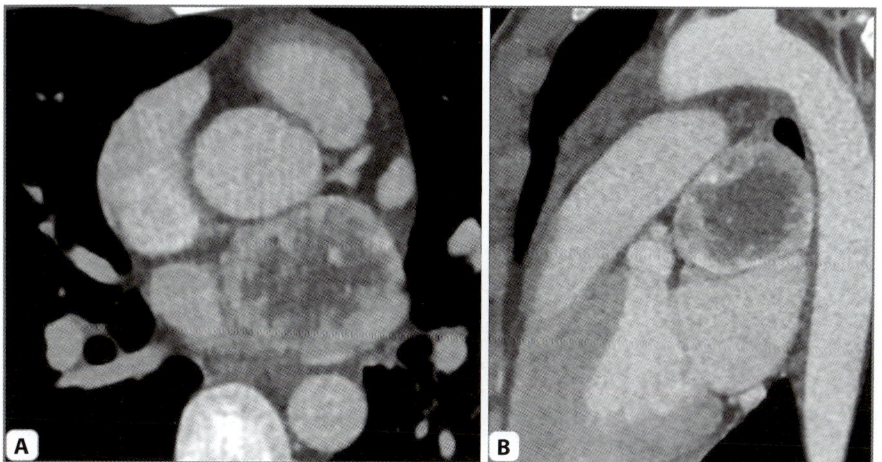

FIGS. 7A AND B: Postcontrast cardiac CT images in axial (A) and sagittal reformat (B) shows an enhancing lesion with central hypodense areas just superior to the left atrium—case of paraganglioma.

T2W images. Intense enhancement is usually noted with gadolinium. Nonenhancing areas may represent necrosis within the lesion.

- *Lymphangioma*: These are benign lymph containing neoplasms. Most lesions occur in children. They may be associated with other lymphovascular masses of the neck or the mediastinum. The most common location is in the pericardial spaces. These tumors may present with cardiac tamponade. CT features have not been described. MRI demonstrates an increased SI mass on T1W and T2W images.

Primary Malignant Tumors

Malignant primary cardiac tumors are extremely rare and represent only 5–6% of primary cardiac tumors. Among them, the majority are represented by sarcomas, followed by lymphomas and mesotheliomas.

Sarcoma: The most common cardiac sarcomas are angiosarcomas that comprise 37% of all cases.[6] These are highly aggressive tumors that arises from endothelial cells lining the lymphatics or blood vessels.

The most common location is right atrium (~75% of cases) and infiltrates into the pericardium, tricuspid valve, right ventricle, and right coronary artery.

Clinically, they usually present with right-sided heart failure or tamponade as the tumors tend to occur in the right atrium and involve the pericardium. Presentation is late, and there is often the presence of metastases at the time of diagnosis, particularly to the lung. The tumor has been reported to occur over a wide age range. They have a poor prognosis, with a mean survival of 6 months following presentation.

Imaging features: There are two morphological subtypes of the tumor: a well circumscribed intracavitary mass, or a diffusely infiltrative lesion of the myocardium.

- *Echocardiography*: Echogenic nodular or lobulated mass in the right atrium, with pericardial effusion or direct pericardial extension. Transesophageal echo (TEE) provides superior image resolution and better visualization about the valves, the site of tumor implantation and wall infiltration, especially those located in the posterior cardiac structure.
- *Cardiac CT*: Low-attenuated mass in the right atrium, which might be irregular or nodular. There may be pericardial effusion or thickening. Involvement of right coronary artery can be demonstrated well on cardiac CT angiography.
- *CMR*: Appears as a large heterogenous mass, with areas of high signal intensity as seen on T2-weighted images representing the blood-filled spaces within the neoplasm. A papillary or "cauliflower" appearance can be observed as a specific MR feature of angiosarcoma, with a nodular area of high signal intensity interspersed within areas of intermediate signal intensity as seen on T1- and T2-weighted images. In cases with diffuse pericardial infiltration, some investigators have described linear enhancement along the vascular spaces as a "sunray" appearance.[8] Perfusion MRI shows early and increased contrast uptake within the tumor **(Fig. 8)**. Delayed contrast enhancement is heterogenous on both CT and MRI.

Hemangiopericytomas are rare cardiac sarcomas that are indistinguishable from angiosarcomas on imaging.

Other cardiac sarcomas: Although angiosarcomas are the most common cardiac sarcomas, all types of sarcomas, including undifferentiated sarcomas, malignant fibrous histiocytomas (MFHs), leiomyosarcomas, osteosarcomas, lymphosarcomas, myxosarcomas, neurogenic sarcomas, synovial sarcomas, neurofibrosarcomas, and Kaposi's sarcomas can affect the heart. Although most angiosarcomas occur in the right atrium, the other sarcomas affect the left atrium more frequently, which is an important differentiating feature.[6]

- *Leiomyosarcomas* are malignant tumors of smooth muscle origin. They are rare and highly aggressive.

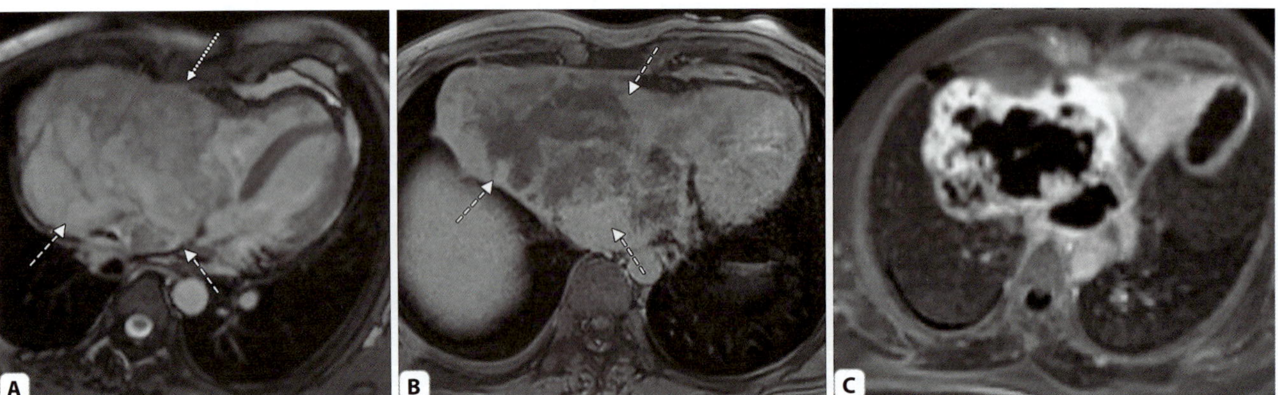

FIGS. 8A TO C: Four-chamber image (A) shows a large bulky heterogeneous lesion completely filling the right atrium. Postcontrast image (B) and LGE image (C) shows the heterogeneous enhancement of the lesion. Hypointense areas in (C) likely represent areas of hemorrhage/thrombus.

Most lesions (75%) arise in the superior vena cava (SVC) or the IVC and extend to the heart. Intracardiac lesions are usually seen in the posterior left atrium and present as sessile masses that can have a mucoid appearance. LA masses usually invade mitral valve and pulmonary veins. Mean survival time without treatment is reported to be 6 months from the time of diagnosis.

- *Rhabdomyosarcomas* are more frequent in infants and children. They present as bulky, invasive masses (usually more than 10 cm). They can occur at multiple sites within the heart, including the valves—unlike other sarcomas.
- *Malignant fibrous histiocytomas* consist of primitive mesenchymal, fibroblastic, and histiocytic cells arranged in a storiform pattern.[9] The most common location of MFHs is the left atrium where the tumors are usually attached to the posterior wall.[9] Distinguishing MFHs from a benign cardiac tumor might be difficult on a clinical and imaging basis, but MFH is far more aggressive and has a greater propensity for recurrence and infiltration. MRI demonstrates the presence of MFH as a mass with a nonspecific signal intensity as seen on T1- and T2-weighted images. A MFH arises from the posterior wall of the left atrium and can extend into the pulmonary veins. This finding would not normally be expected with a myxoma.
- *Lymphoma:* Primary cardiac lymphoma refers to the one involving only the heart or pericardium.[10] These tumors are extremely rare, with a reported incidence of 0.15–1%. When they occur, they are usually aggressive B-cell lymphomas seen more commonly in immunocompromised individuals. It most commonly arises in the RA but may involve any chamber. Sometimes, large pericardial effusion or thickening may be the only finding. Cardiac mass may be a polypoidal or an infiltrative intramural lesion. The latter may be diffuse form of infiltration of lymphoma cells in the myocardium, mimicking classic hypertrophic cardiomyopathy.

Imaging characteristics: CT images show cardiac lymphomas as hypo- or iso-attenuated infiltrative soft tissue masses as compared with the myocardium, and the masses demonstrate heterogeneous enhancement after the administration of a contrast agent. On MRI, they usually appear as iso- to hypo-intense to cardiac muscle on both T1W and T2W images. They may be bright on T2W images. Contrast enhancement may be homogenous, heterogenous or minimal, with areas of low enhancement seen in the center of the lesion as compared with the periphery.

Angiosarcoma versus lymphoma:

- Angiosarcomas are usually much more aggressive than lymphomas, involve larger areas of the heart, and even penetrate the valves and great vessels, an atypical finding in cardiac lymphoma.
- Central necrosis is another common feature of angiosarcoma and is less likely seen with lymphoma.
- Additionally, angiosarcomas tend to show prominent enhancement after contrast material administration at both CT and MRI, whereas, lymphoma typically does not have such strong enhancement patterns.
- *Pericardial mesothelioma*: This most common primary pericardial neoplasm constitutes 15% of all malignant cardiac tumors. Unlike metastatic tumors to the pericardium, mesotheliomas are generally restricted to involvement of the pericardium without actually spreading to the cardiac chambers. There is no association with asbestos exposure. Cross-sectional imaging helps to define the extent of the lesion and optimize the surgical approach. Contrast enhancement helps to differentiate the tumor from adjacent, normal myocardium. SI characteristics on MRI are nonspecific.

Secondary Neoplasm

Metastases to the heart are 30 times more common than primary cardiac tumors.[11] The tumors that most frequently metastasize to the heart are lung and breast cancers, melanomas and lymphomas.[12]

Metastasis may involve the heart through direct extension or through hematogenous, venous or lymphatic spread. Although imaging findings are not characteristic of any particular type of tumor, CT and particularly MRI is helpful in delineating the site and extent of cardiac and paracardiac involvement. The extent of involvement revealed by imaging may lead to a modification of the radiotherapy planning or the addition of chemotherapy.

The epicardium is the site most often affected by metastases.[11,12] Spread is mainly via a retrograde route through the mediastinal lymphatics, leading to implantation in the epicardial surface of the heart. Other tumors such as melanomas and sarcomas usually spread hematogenously to the myocardium and epicardium through the coronary arteries, or less commonly, by the implantation of cancer cells through the vena cava.[12]

Direct extension can occur with thymic, bronchial, breast and esophageal malignancies due to the proximity of the primary lesions to the heart. Invasion of the pericardium may be seen as interruption of the normal pericardial outline with nodular or diffuse pericardial thickening, hemorrhage, or effusion. Myocardial involvement is suspected when there is irregularity of the outline. Delayed enhanced MRI helps to demonstrate the extent of the cardiac invasion **(Fig. 9)**.

Paracardiac and Extracardiac Tumors

These are mediastinal lesions that may extrinsically compress the cardiac structure or invade it. Anterior mediastinal masses include thymoma, thymo-lipoma, lymphoma, teratoma, teratocarcinoma and thyroid masses. Masses of neurogenic, airway (bronchogenic cyst or bronchial malignancy) or esophageal (carcinoma, duplication, leiomyoma) origin are the most common middle or posterior mediastinal lesions about the heart.

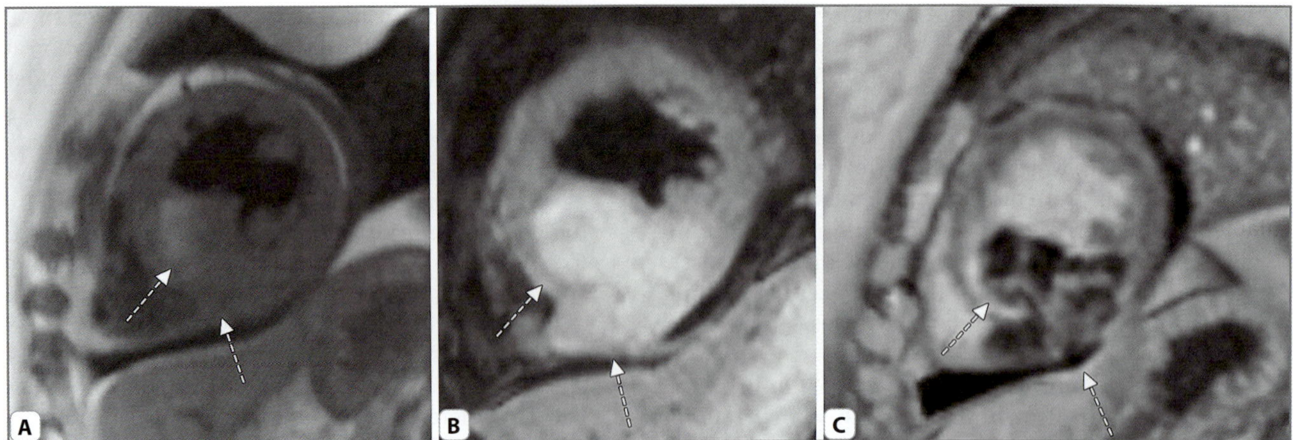

FIGS. 9A TO C: An adult patient with known malignancy elsewhere showing a mass in the inferoseptal LV myocardium (white arrows) which is isointense on T1 (A), hyperintense on T2 (B) and showing heterogenous enhancement on postgadolinium images (C). Metastatic deposit from known primary.

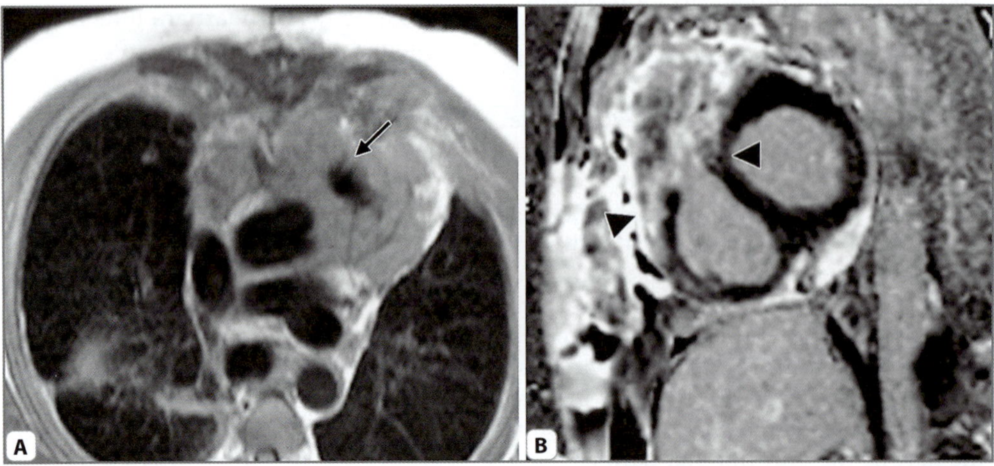

FIGS. 10A AND B: Axial SE T1W (left) and short-axis delayed enhanced (right) MRI images in a patient with anterior mediastinal tumor. The mass is seen to encase and infiltrate the right ventricular outflow tract (irregular outline, arrow) and extends up to the ascending aorta. Delayed enhanced image shows the heterogeneous mass also involves the RV myocardium and the upper IVS (arrowheads).

The direct orthogonal imaging capability of MRI makes it ideally suited to delineate the site of origin, extent and involvement of the heart by these tumors **(Fig. 10)**. CT and particularly MRI may localize the etiology by their ability to characterize tissue components. CT shows the presence of calcium and fat in germ cell tumors. On MRI, cystic lesions typically have a very high SI on the T2W images. High SI on T1W images may suggest high protein content, fat or hemorrhage within the lesion. Fat suppression techniques will distinguish fat, and GRE sequences will demonstrate hemosiderin deposits in chronic hemorrhage. Thymolipomas are anterior mediastinal lesions that usually conform to the shape of surrounding structures. CT and MRI characteristically display a mixture of fat and soft tissue within the lesion. Benign and invasive thymomas can, to some extent, be differentiated on MRI. The invasive thymomas tend to be more inhomogeneous, multinodular in appearance and less well defined in outline.

Non-neoplastic Lesions

Thrombus: Thrombus are the most common cardiac "masses" and require prompt recognition and institution of appropriate treatment. Prior infarct (particularly in apical and interventricular septal location) and markedly depressed left ventricular systolic function predispose to thrombus formation in the left ventricular apical regions. Atrial fibrillation predisposes to thrombus formation in the LA appendage, whereas, factors causing diastolic dysfunction (e.g., restrictive cardiomyopathy) or presence of mechanical valves, interatrial septal devices, and appendage occluder devices are other common factors leading to atrial thrombus formation.

Imaging characteristics: Thrombus are most commonly and best diagnosed by transthoracic Echo. Presence of predisposing conditions along with a soft-tissue mass located in expected regions is the hallmark of echocardiographic diagnosis of intracardiac thrombi. Finding of a mass in the absence of predisposing conditions outlined above as well as of systemic hypercoagulable state make etiologic classification of a cardiac mass challenging by echo.

- *MRI*: The signal intensity characteristics of a thrombus vary with MRI and are dependent on the age of the thrombus. An acute thrombus will appear bright as seen on both T1- and T2-weighted MR images, whereas a subacute thrombus will appear bright as seen on T1-weighted images with hypointense areas seen on T2-weighted images due to the paramagnetic effects of methemoglobin and shortening of the T2 relaxation times. A chronic organized thrombus will exhibit hypointensity as seen on both T1- and T2-weighted images **(Fig. 11)** due to a depleted water content.[13] Contrast enhanced MRI can be utilized to detect thrombus by increasing the inversion time to longer intervals—a long T1 of approximately 600 ms (at 1.5T). This helps in nulling avascular tissue (such as thrombus) which is appear as homogenously black on the high T1 images.[14]
- *Aneurysm of sinus of Valsalva (SOV)*: SOV aneurysm is most commonly congenital in origin and caused by a deficiency of elastic tissue in the tunica media.[15] Rarely it may be acquired secondary to aortic valve endocarditis or trauma. Most SOV aneurysms arise from the right and noncoronary sinuses. Unruptured SOV aneurysms are usually clinically silent and discovered serendipitously on ECHO as a vascular mass. Rupture most often occurs into the right atrium or right ventricular outflow tract and may be a catastrophic event or present with rapid onset of heart failure caused by pronounced left to right shunting.

  Although transesophageal ECHO is better for demonstration of site of communication of the aneurysm with a coronary sinus and its extension into a chamber wall (in case of unruptured aneurysms), it is an invasive technique and may be uncomfortable for the patient.

  On CT, SOV aneurysm appears as a thin-walled crescent shaped outpouching that is contiguous with the aortic root **(Fig. 12A)**. Occasionally, they are partially or completely thrombosed. MRI is very useful to confirm its vascular nature, by showing a signal void on SE sequences **(Fig. 12B)**. Both modalities are particularly useful for demonstrating extension into the adjacent cardiac chambers, valves and septum which can be difficult to fully evaluate with echo.
- *Atrial septal aneurysm*: This is a localized protrusion of the primary component of the interatrial septum (IAS) through the fossa ovalis region, or a diffuse bulging of the entire septum into either of the atria. It may be associated with other congenital cardiac anomalies, or with acquired lesions that result in unequal pressures in the two atria. Due to thrombus formation in the concavity of the aneurysm, pulmonary or systemic embolic events may occur. The presence of an associated atrial septal defect may result in paradoxical embolism. Although the diagnosis is usually made on ECHO, stagnant blood within aneurysm concavity may simulate a cystic tumor. Similar problems may result on SE MRI. Hence cine-SSFP MRI should be done and this shows blood flow within the aneurysm, as well as the mobility of the aneurysmal IAS.
- *Pleuro-pericardial cyst*: Though the most common pericardial mass lesion, these are very rare, the reported incidence being 1:100,000 of the general population. They are thought to be congenital in origin. The most common location is in the right cardiophrenic angle, although they may also be seen in left cardiophrenic angle and posterior mediastinum. Patients are usually asymptomatic; the lesion often

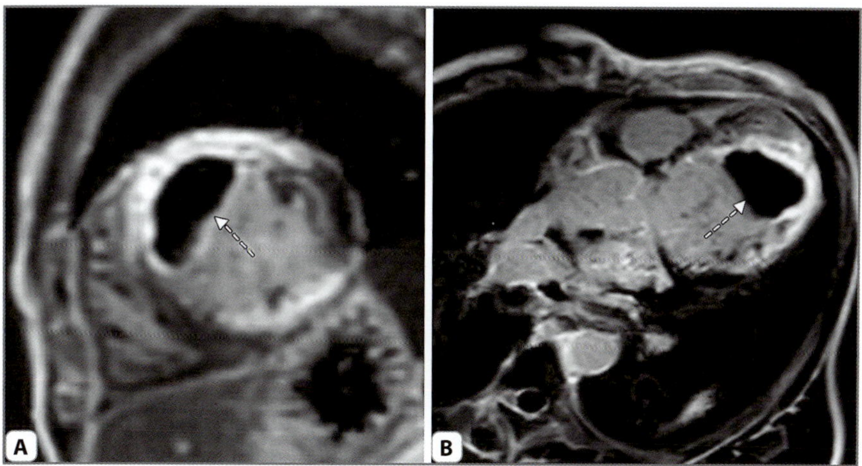

FIGS. 11A AND B: Short axis (A) and four chamber (B) LGE images in an elderly patient with poor cardiac function shows a nonenhancing hypointense mass (arrows) adhered to the wall of LV cavity—typical appearance of left ventricular thrombus.

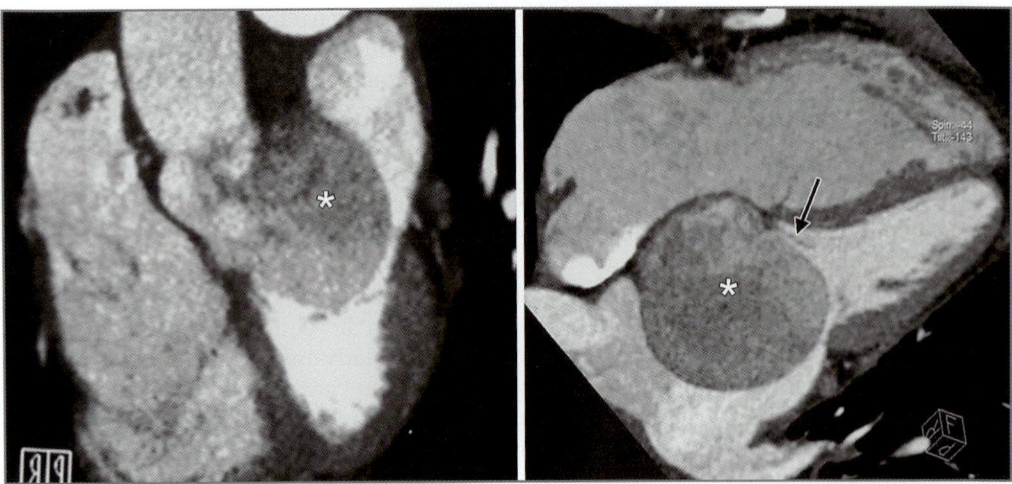

FIG. 12A: MDCT in a case of SOV aneurysm, sagittal (left) and 4-chamber (right) images. A round lesion (asterisk) with heterogeneous enhancement in this early arterial phase (due to turbulent flow) arises from the aortic root and projects leftwards, posteriorly and inferiorly into LA. It also impinges on the mitral valve (arrow in figure on right)

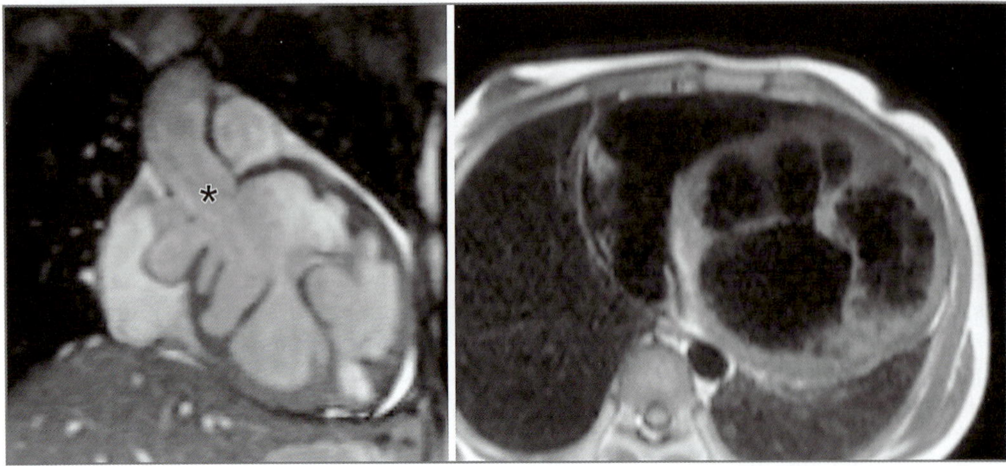

FIG. 12B: Coronal oblique SSFP (left) and axial SE T1W (right) MRI in a case of SOV aneurysm. The lesion arises from the aortic root (asterisk), is multilobulated, and burrows into the interventricular septum. The lesion shows multiple large signal voids, consistent with its vascular nature.

being detected incidentally on imaging. Lesions are typically stable, and surgical excision is rarely required. CT typically shows a well marginated cyst of fluid attenuation. There may or may not be a perceptible wall. MRI characteristically shows a well circumscribed, homogenous paracardiac mass with iso- to hypo-intensity on T1W and hyperintensity on T2W images. Intracystic septae may be observed following paramagnetic contrast agent administration. The major role of MRI is in differentiating pericardial cysts from other mediastinal masses and thus avoiding an inadvertent surgery.

Infective Lesions

- *Vegetation*: Valvular vegetations may appear as a mass lesion related to the valvular apparatus. Small vegetations are usually not visible on cardiac CT or cardiac MRI. These modalities are mainly indicated for detection of the extent of perivalvular invasion, including abscess and/or fistula formation. Cine-SSFP MRI is useful to detect small lesions.
- *Hydatid cyst*: Cardiac hydatid is rare, constituting constitute 0.5–2% of all hydatid locations in the human body. The most common location is the LV (60%), followed by RV (10%), pericardium (7%), pulmonary artery (6%) and IVS (4%). Right-sided lesions are seen to expand into the chamber cavity and subendocardially, while the left sided lesions more often grow subepicardially. The heart also can be secondarily affected by direct contact with hydatid cysts originating from the liver or the lung. They are usually asymptomatic but larger lesions can rarely

cause coronary compression and chest pain.[16] They may also rupture leading to anaphylaxis, tamponade or pericardial constriction. Echocardiography, CT, and MRI can show the cystic nature of the mass and its relation to the cardiac chambers. The cysts may be single or multiple, uniloculated or multiloculated, and thin or thick walled. MRI depicts the exact anatomic location and nature of the internal and external structures and is the technique used for post-treatment follow-up. The appearance of a hydatid cyst on MRI is usually a characteristic oval lesion that is hypointense on T1-weighted images and hyperintense on T2-weighted images **(Fig. 13)**. MRI also demonstrates a thin low intensity peripheral rim on T2W images, reported to be a characteristic sign of a hydatid cyst. This is thought to represent dense fibrous capsule from reactive host tissue.[17]

- *Tuberculoma*: Cardiac involvement in tuberculosis is usually tuberculous involvement of the pericardium leading to pericarditis and subsequently calcific pericardium leading to constriction. Myocardial involvement of tuberculosis is exceedingly rare, with reported overall autopsy incidence of myocardial involvement ranging from 0.14–0.3%.[18,19] A mass like tuberculoma is described in isolated case reports[19] commonly involving the right atrium, close to SVC-RA junction or the right ventricle **(Fig. 14)**. However, extensive infiltration of the myocardium, inseparable from pericardium and with the heart appearing literally "boxed in" has also been described. MRI appearance

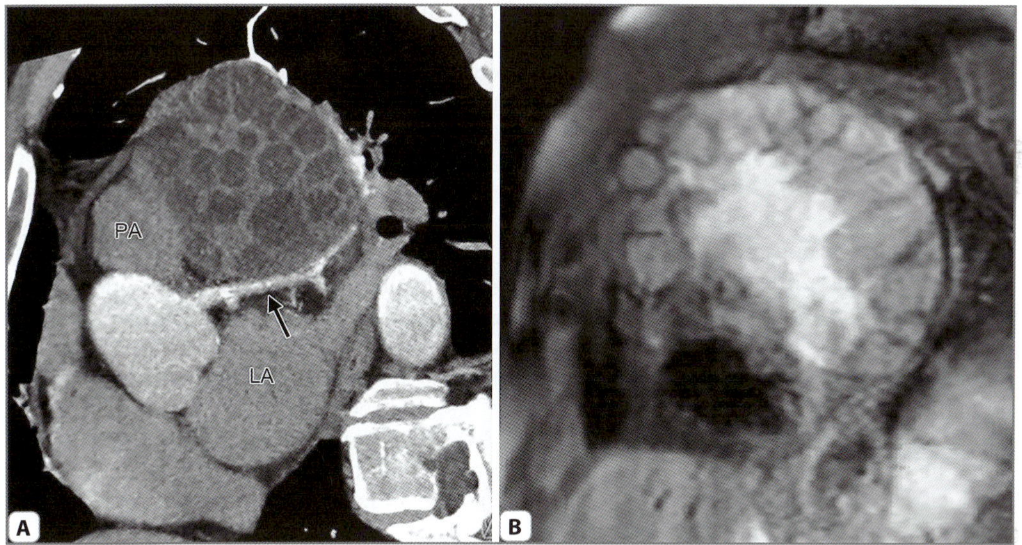

FIGS. 13A AND B: Short-axis cardiac CT (A) and short-axis SE T2W (fat-suppressed) MRI (B) images in a patient with hydatid cyst. The lesion shows multiple daughter cysts and abuts the PA, LA and the left circumflex artery (arrow). In (B) the typical hypointense rim to the lesion is seen.

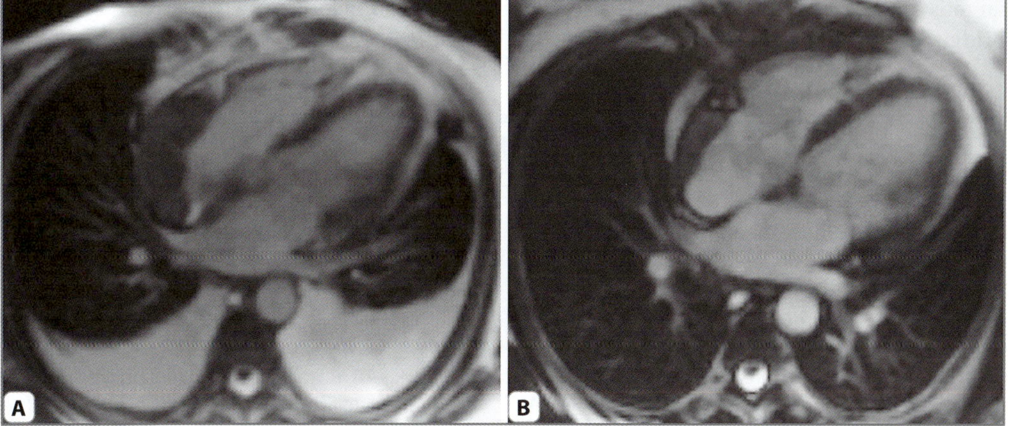

FIGS. 14A AND B: SSFP MRI in 4-chamber view in a case of RA tuberculoma, pre anti-tubercular therapy (A) and 8 months post anti-tubercular therapy (B) There is a homogeneous, well-marginated right atrial mass that has significantly reduced in size following treatment. Pleural effusions have also disappeared.

is usually that of a mass with a central isointense core (central caseation), a hypointense rim (fibrous capsule) and a thin hyperintense line (inflammatory cellular infiltrate). Contrast images demonstrate ring enhancement around a central nonenhancing core.

VARIANT AND NORMAL ANATOMICAL STRUCTURES SIMULATING A CARDIAC MASS

- *Pericardium*: Extension of the normal pericardial space into its various recesses and presence of small amounts of normally occurring pericardial fluid within them may lead to a false diagnosis of a pericardial or a vascular tumor. A typical example is a high extending superior pericardial recess that may simulate an enlarged lymph node, vascular tumor or an aortic dissection.
- *Left atrium*: The left atrial appendage is lined with thin, pectinate ridges, compared to the body of the LA that has a smooth endocardial outline. These ridges may be confused with thrombi. Also, other posterior mediastinal lesions such as cysts, esophageal tumors, and even a tortuous descending aorta may, at times, be misinterpreted as a LA mass. The multiplanar imaging capability of MDCT and MRI is useful in this regard to avoid a false-positive diagnosis.
- *Left ventricle*: False chordae and tendons are accessory structures that may appear as linear strands extending through the LV cavity, particularly on echo.
- *Right atrium*: The Chiari network consists of fibrous strand-like structures arising from the region near the Eustachian valve and extending into the RA cavity. On MRI, these have a SI similar to that of the myocardium and should not be misdiagnosed as a tumor or a thrombus. The crista terminalis is a prominent muscular ridge that runs along the posterior wall of the RA from the orifice of the SVC to that of the IVC. It may present as a nodular mass on axial MDCT or MRI but is resolved as a linear ridge on oblique coronal reconstructions.
- *Right ventricle*: The moderator band is a thin muscular band extending from the mid-portion of the IVS to the free wall of the RV across the cavity. It may enlarge and simulate a RV mass, particularly in patients with enlargement or hypertrophy. MDCT or MRI help to delineate its points of attachment, with an attenuation/SI similar to that of the adjacent myocardium.

CONCLUSION

A high index of clinical suspicion, supported by reliable noninvasive imaging, is necessary to make a definite diagnosis of a cardiac mass lesion. Although echocardiography is universally accepted as the initial modality for evaluation of a suspected intracardiac mass, it has significant limitations. Echo is the best modality however, for valvular lesions.

MDCT is useful for vascular lesions, calcification and fat content, and for demonstration of coronary anatomy prior to surgery. It is also useful for staging malignant lesions. MDCT is distinctly superior to MRI in pediatric patients due to a significantly less scanning time. Overall, MDCT has significantly limited ability to characterize tissues compared to MRI.

Due to its superior contrast resolution and availability of multiple sequences (including perfusion and delayed enhancement), MRI is the ideal modality for complete evaluation of cardiac masses. It is capable of simultaneously assessing their nature, extent and hemodynamic consequences. The most common cardiac "mass" is a thrombus. Among the neoplastic lesions, metastasis are almost thirty times more common than primary cardiac tumors. Within the primary cardiac tumors, benign masses are much more common than primary malignant tumors, the most common primary cardiac tumor being a myxoma. The most common malignant primary cardiac tumor is angiosarcoma. Knowledge of various cardiac masses is imperative to differentiate between neoplastic, non-neoplastic and nonpathologic entities mimicking a mass, in order to avoid an inadvertent surgery.

REFERENCES

1. Sutsch G, Jenni R, von Segesser L, Schneider J. Heart tumors: incidence, distribution, diagnosis. Exemplified by 20,305 echocardiographies. Schweiz Med Wochenschr. 1991;121:621-9.
2. Moriyama Y, Saigenji H, Shimokawa S, Toyohira H, Taira A. The surgical treatment of 30 patients with cardiac myxomas: a comparison of clinical features according to morphological classification. Surg Today. 1994;24:596-8.
3. Burke A, Virmani R. Atlas of tumor pathology. 3rd ed. Washington, DC: Armed Forces Institute of Pathology; 1996. Tumors of the heart and great vessels; pp. 79-90.
4. Edwards FH, Hale D, Cohen A, Thompson L, Pezzella AT, Virmani R. Primary cardiac valve tumors. Ann Thorac Surg. 1991;52:1127-31.
5. Webb DW, Thomas RD, Osborne JP. Cardiac rhabdomyomas and their association with tuberous sclerosis. Arch Dis Child. 1993;68:367-70.
6. Burke AP, Rosado-de-Christenson M, Templeton PA, Virmani R. Cardiac fibroma: clinicopathologic correlates and surgical treatment. J Thorac Cardiovasc Surg. 1994;108:862-70.
7. Newell JD, Eckel C, Davis M, Tadros NB. MR appearance of an arteriovenous hemangioma of the interventricular septum. Cardiovasc Intervent Radiol. 1988;11:319-21.

8. Yahata S, Endo T, Honma H, Ino T, Hayakawa H, Ogawa M, et al. Sunray appearance on enhanced magnetic resonance image of cardiac angiosarcoma with pericardial obliteration. Am Heart J. 1994;127:468-71.
9. Okamoto K, Kato S, Katsuki S, Wada Y, Toyozumi Y, Morimatsu M, et al. Malignant fibrous histiocytoma of the heart: case report and review of 46 cases in the literature. Intern Med. 2001;40:1222-6.
10. Cuotinsinger CR, Wilson J, Yoneda K. Primary cardiac lymphoma. Cancer. 1989; 64:521-5.
11. Lam KY, Dickens P, Chan AC. Tumors of the heart. A 20-year experience with a review of 12,485 consecutive autopsies. Arch Pathol Lab Med. 1993;117:1027-103.
12. Klatt EC, Heitz DR. Cardiac metastases. Cancer. 1990;65: 1456-9.
13. Sparrow PJ, Kurian JB, Jones TR, Sivananthan MU. MR imaging of cardiac tumors. Radiographics. 2005;25: 1255-76.
14. Pazos-López P, Pozo E, Siqueira ME, García-Lunar I, Cham M, Jacobi A, et al. Value of CMR for the differential diagnosis of cardiac masses. JACC Cardiovasc Imaging. 2014;7:896-905.
15. Sasson L, Katz MG, Ezri T, Tamir A, Rozenman Y, Geva Y, et al. Ruptured sinus of Valsalva aneurysm complicated by myocardial ischemia: pathogenetic mechanisms. Cardiovasc Pathol. 2006;15:291-3.
16. Girish NK, Singh D, Pandey NN, Mukherjee A, Yadav R, Jagia P. Cardiac hydatid cyst causing coronary arterial compression. J Cardiovasc Comput Tomogr. 2024:S1934-5925(24)00440-4.
17. Dursun M, Terzibasioglu E, Yilmaz R, Cekrezi R, Olgar S, Nisli K, et al. Cardiac hydatid disease: CT and MRI findings. AJR Am J Roentgenol. 2008;190(1):226-32.
18. Rose AG. Cardiac tuberculosis: a study of 19 patients. Arch Pathol Lab Med. 1987;11:422-26.
19. Gulati GS, Singh S, Arepalli CD, Sharma S, Kothari SS, Airan B, et al. Superior vena caval obstruction after complete resolution of cardiac tuberculoma. Clin Radiol. 2008;63:605-9.

Vineeta Ojha, Niraj Nirmal Pandey

CHAPTER

28

Imaging of Valvular Heart Disease

INTRODUCTION AND EPIDEMIOLOGY

Valvular heart disease (VHD) is among the most common cardiac disorders, primarily due to the high prevalence of rheumatic fever in India. Rheumatic heart disease (RHD) remains the leading cause of valvular heart disease in regions such as the Middle East, the Indian subcontinent, and Africa.[1] It most often affects the mitral valve, followed by the aortic, tricuspid, and pulmonary valves. The resulting lesions can cause stenosis, incompetence, or a combination of both in the affected valve. Other common causes of VHD include calcific degeneration of the valves, bicuspid aortic valve, myxomatous valvular disease, congenital, infective or neoplastic causes. Of the total number of cardiac surgeries worldwide, VHD accounts for 10–20% and becomes more prevalent with increasing age.[2] Advances in medical science have improved life expectancy for VHD patients. According to the OxVALVE study, 31% of individuals over 65 years had valve disease, though only 10% had moderate-to-severe involvement. Mild mitral or aortic regurgitation was the most frequently observed finding.[3]

CLINICAL PRESENTATION AND MANAGEMENT

Mild to moderate VHD may remain asymptomatic for a long time. Difficulty in breathing is the most common symptom. Conditions like mitral stenosis which cause atrial dilatation may lead to atrial fibrillation. Chronic left sided lesions may further lead to pulmonary hypertension. Symptomatic patients with ventricular dysfunction often need surgical replacement of the diseased valve. In asymptomatic patients, exercise testing to unmask the symptoms is recommended. Sometimes, severe regurgitant lesions may be offered repair on case to case basis. Recent times have seen drastic improvement in percutaneous valve replacement technologies like transcatheter aortic and pulmonary valve interventions, mitraClip, etc., and hence these are gaining popularity.

IMAGING TECHNIQUES

The primary objectives of imaging in valvular heart disease, regardless of its cause are enumerated in the **Box 1** and **Figure 1**.

Advancements in noninvasive imaging techniques have significantly improved the ability to determine the anatomical location of valvular abnormalities and their hemodynamic and functional consequences. These developments have also enhanced the understanding of the natural history of valvular diseases and enabled accurate diagnosis using noninvasive methods. The various imaging modalities are detailed below.[4-6]

- *Chest radiography*: Useful for initial evaluation, it provides insights into cardiac size, pulmonary

BOX 1: Goals of imaging in valvular heart disease (VHD).

- To confirm the diagnosis of VHD through qualitative and quantitative assessment of all valves
- Confirm the etiology
- To grade the severity (qualitative and quantification)—mild/moderate/severe disease
- Evaluating the hemodynamic impact of valvular disease on pulmonary vasculature and ventricular function
- Assessment of ventricular function (ejection fractions and volumes)
- To evaluate associated abnormalities—e.g., associated aortic coarctation in bicuspid aortic valve, myocardial fibrosis (on MRI), pulmonary vascular pathologies, etc.
- Guide treatment
- To follow-up after treatment

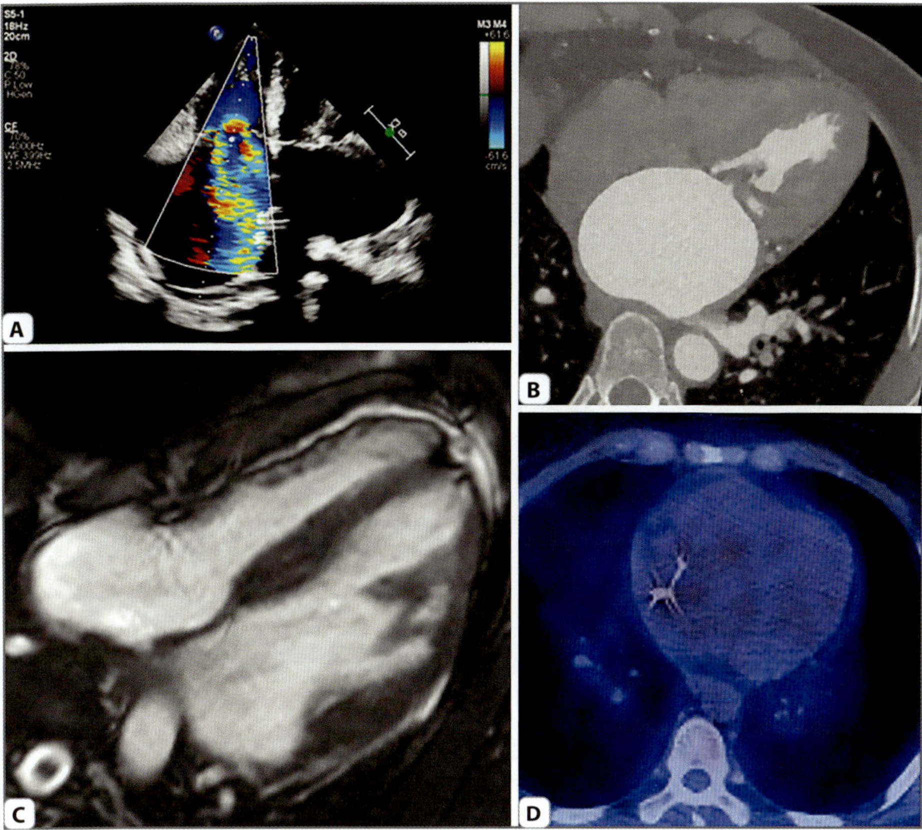

FIGS. 1A TO D: Imaging modalities for assessment of valvular heart disease: (A) Echocardiography (B) CT (C) MRI (D) PET scan.

vasculature, arterial and venous hypertension, and secondary lung changes. This widely accessible, simple-to-use technique provides a repeatable, reproducible, and permanent patient record. Imaging features such as calcification location, chamber enlargement patterns, poststenotic dilatations, pulmonary venous and arterial hypertension, and lung changes can assist in identifying the type of VHD. Additionally, chest radiographs are useful for follow-up, allowing comparisons of heart size and pulmonary vasculature over time.

- *Echocardiography*: A widely available, noninvasive, real-time imaging tool that allows visualization of cardiac chambers and valves in multiple planes. It is the first line imaging technique and enables reliable quantification of stenosis, regurgitation, ventricular function, chamber size, wall thickness, valvular orifice size, transstenotic pressure gradients, and regurgitant volume. Its findings are often comparable to cardiac catheterization and angiography. It also aids in identifying any associated pathologies. Assessment of ventricular function and volumes forms an integral part of the examination. However, its limitations include operator dependency and the need for an adequate acoustic window. Also, assessment of the right ventricle function is a challenge and CMR is often preferred for the same.

  If transthoracic echocardiography (TTE) yields suboptimal results or there is concern for complications such as thrombosis, prosthetic valve dysfunction, or infective endocarditis, transesophageal echocardiography (TEE) may be utilized. TEE is also commonly used during percutaneous valve repair procedures.[5,6]
- *Multi-slice computed tomography (MSCT)*: It plays a crucial role in evaluating valvular heart disease (VHD). It is particularly effective in assessing valve calcification, analyzing coronary and great vessels, planning for transcatheter aortic valve implantation (TAVI), and diagnosing prosthetic heart valve dysfunction **(Fig. 2)**. It has a high spatial and temporal resolution, strong signal to noise ratio, multiplanar reconstruction capabilities, volume rendering and endoluminal viewing capabilities. CT provides detailed information on chamber sizes, volumes, valve morphology, cardiac output, stroke volume, and ventricular mass. It allows for rapid evaluation, useful in children by avoiding general anesthesia . However, it's use requires consideration of contrast administration and radiation exposure, which must be weighed against the diagnostic benefits.[5,6]

  Typical protocol for CT for VSD at our institute includes ECG gated (retrospective) scan (after administering nonionic iodinated contrast medium) to evaluate

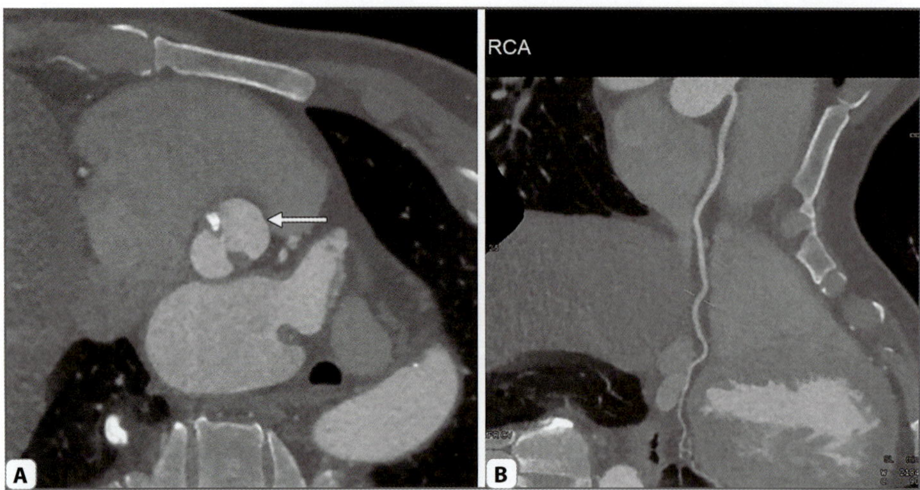

FIGS. 2A AND B: CT angiography multiplanar reconstructed view at the level of aortic valve (A) shows bicuspid aortic valve in a patient with aortic stenosis. (B) Curvilinear reconstruction shows right coronary artery (RCA) with no significant disease.

valve motion, ventricular function with automated kV and tube current modulation. The field of view ranges from the arch of aorta to diaphragm.

- *Cardiac magnetic resonance imaging (CMR)*: It is being increasingly utilized in selected cases for detailed evaluation of valvular disease and its hemodynamic effects. Magnetic resonance imaging (MRI) offers valuable insights in specific cases, particularly in regurgitant lesions. It is particularly useful for assessing valve anatomy in challenging scenarios, such as postcardiac surgery or complex congenital heart conditions. MRI allows precise quantification of stenosis and regurgitation through phase-contrast sequences, while also providing detailed evaluation of ventricular function and volumes. Furthermore, MRI is instrumental in detecting myocardial scars and characterizing tissue, aiding in patient prognosis. Magnetic resonance angiography (MRA) enhances the role of MRI in valvular heart disease by delivering detailed visualization of great vessel anatomy. CMR is noninvasive, devoid of radiation and has excellent resolution. **Table 1** describes the utility of CMR in preoperative evaluation and the sequences used for the same.[4]
- *Invasive catheter angiography*: It is not routinely used for diagnosis solely. It may be useful in selected cases for hemodynamic assessment, coronary arterial assessment and during percutaneous interventions of the valves. It enables the measurement of pressures and oxygen saturation within cardiac chambers and great vessels, facilitating a detailed hemodynamic assessment.
- *Nuclear medicine/PET scan*: It is useful in assessment of perivalvular and systemic complications in prosthetic heart valve infections as well as inflammatory valvular pathologies. In calcific AS, it helps in detecting inflammation and osteoblastic activity.[5]

TABLE 1: Utility of CMR in preoperative evaluation and the sequences used during scanning.

Characteristics of VHD	Importance of CMR	Sequences used for the same
Valve morphology	Bicuspid/tricuspid leaflet morphology, valvar/supravalvar/subvalvar stenoses, aortic root diameters-functional MR	Cine SSFP imaging
Etiology	Rheumatic/degenerative/neoplastic/infective/congenital	Cine SSFP imaging, T1 TSE
Functions	Ventricular functions and volumes, atrial sizes, strain, regional wall motion	Cine SSFP imaging
Severity	Regurgitation volumes and fractions, stenosis (gradient) quantification, flow volume, peak velocity, valve area	Phase contrast, volumetry on cine
Myocardial characterization	Myocardial scar	LGE, T1 mapping, perfusion

- *Fluoroscopy*: It is a valuable tool for evaluating valvular calcification and is frequently utilized in assessing valve dysfunction as well as monitoring patients undergoing treatment for such conditions. It allows visualization of leaflet motion in most prosthetic valves, except for bioprosthetic valves, making it particularly useful in detecting mechanical abnormalities.

Multimodality imaging facilitates better disease management and improves patient outcomes by providing a comprehensive understanding of valvular pathology. **Table 2** summarizes the major imaging modalities and **Table 3** provides the appropriate imaging technique as per the indications.[7]

With this background, let us have a look at the common pathologies affecting the heart valves.

MITRAL VALVE

The mitral valve apparatus consists of the mitral annulus and two leaflets, supported by chordae tendineae, which are anchored to the anterolateral and posteromedial papillary muscles. The mitral annulus has a distinctive D-shaped configuration, with the anterior portion forming the straight edge and the posterior portion forming the curved edge **(Fig. 3)**. The anterior annulus is in fibrous continuity with the aortic annulus, while the posterior annulus is attached to the endocardium.[8]

Mitral Regurgitation

Mitral regurgitation (MR) results form a fraction of blood being shunted from the LV into the LA during ventricular

TABLE 2: Summary of common imaging modalities.

Modality	Information
Chest radiography	• *Cardiac size*: Enlarged chambers suggest chronic volume or pressure overload • *Pulmonary vasculature*: Signs of pulmonary venous hypertension or edema • *Calcifications*: Visible in advanced valvular disease, particularly in the aortic or mitral valves • *Postoperative evaluation*: Changes following valve replacement or repair
Transthoracic echocardiography (TTE)	• *First-line investigation*: Noninvasive, portable, and widely available • *Key assessments*: Valve morphology, gradient measurement, effective orifice area, regurgitant volume, and ventricular function • *Real-time imaging*: Enables dynamic evaluation
Transesophageal echocardiography (TEE)	• *Higher resolution*: Provides detailed views of posterior structures • *Indications*: Prosthetic valve assessment, infective endocarditis, or suboptimal TTE results • *Intraprocedural utility*: Used during valve repair or replacement
Cardiac magnetic resonance (CMR)	*CMR is the gold standard for ventricular volume and function assessment. Its role in VHD includes*: • *Quantification*: Accurate measurement of regurgitant volume and fraction • *Fibrosis detection*: Late gadolinium enhancement (LGE) helps in risk stratification • *Anatomy*: Evaluation of valve morphology and associated vascular abnormalities • *Pre-TAVI planning*: Assessment of annular dimensions and aortic root anatomy. *Limitations*: • Underestimation of transvalvular gradients • Longer acquisition times and contraindications in patients with certain implants
Cardiac computed tomography (CT)	*Multislice CT (MSCT)*: • *Valve calcification*: Superior to other modalities for detecting and quantifying calcification • *Pre-TAVI evaluation*: Annular dimensions, coronary artery anatomy, and vascular access • *Prosthetic valve assessment*: Identifies structural abnormalities or pannus formation *CT angiography (CTA)*: • Provides detailed vascular anatomy • Useful for planning complex surgeries or interventions *Limitations*: • Radiation exposure and iodinated contrast risks
Fluoroscopy	• *Dynamic assessment*: Visualizes prosthetic valve motion, especially mechanical valves • *Adjunct tool*: Used intraoperatively or during catheter-based interventions

Cardiac catheterization	• Invasive but provides definitive hemodynamic data
	• *Indicated for*:
	  ○ *Coronary evaluation*: In older patients or those at risk for atherosclerosis
	  ○ *Presurgical planning*: When noninvasive imaging is inconclusive

PET CT	• Inflammation (native valve or within calcium) • Infection

TABLE 3: Appropriate imaging tools for VHD as per indications.[7]

Broad indication	Specific indication	Appropriate modality
Initial evaluation of VHD in a asymptomatic patient	• Clinically suspected VHD in an asymptomatic patient (unexplained murmur) or • High risk for VHD (E.g., history of RHD or known disease associated with VHD or a family history of bicuspid aortic valve)	Transthoracic echocardiography (TTE) is appropriate (CT, MRI or TEE are not considered appropriate)
Initial evaluation in a symptomatic patient	Most of the symptomatic patients	TTE is the preferred initial imaging option
	Respiratory failure or hypoxemia	Cardiac CT after TTE
Subsequent/ additional testing for VHD for clarification of diagnosis	Inadequate TTE due to patient characteristics	Transesophageal echocardiography (TEE) *Alternative*: CMR>CT
	Native or prosthetic heart valves assessment in symptomatic patients	TEE *Alternative*: Cardiac CT >valve fluoroscopy
	Suspected infective endocarditis with negative TTE	TEE *Alternative*: ^{18}FDG-PET/CT
	Chronic secondary mitral regurgitation (to rule out ischemia and assess viability)	CMR *Alternative*: FDG-PET or viability
	RV function and volume (in tricuspid/pulmonary valve lesions), quantify PR/TR (right sided)	CMR
	Stenotic lesions(in AS and MS) to assess and quantify calcification	CT
Follow-up testing	VHD after surgical valve replacement/ endocarditis	TTE
	Bicuspid aortic valve and ascending aortic dilatation of more than 4 cm	CT = CMR
	Suspected valve dysfunction postsurgical valve replacement	TTE = fluoroscopy → CT if needed
Transcatheter intervention for VHD	Pre-TAVR evaluation	CT
	Intraprocedural evaluation during TAVR	TTE, TEE or fluoroscopy
	Postprocedural evaluation after TAVR	TTE

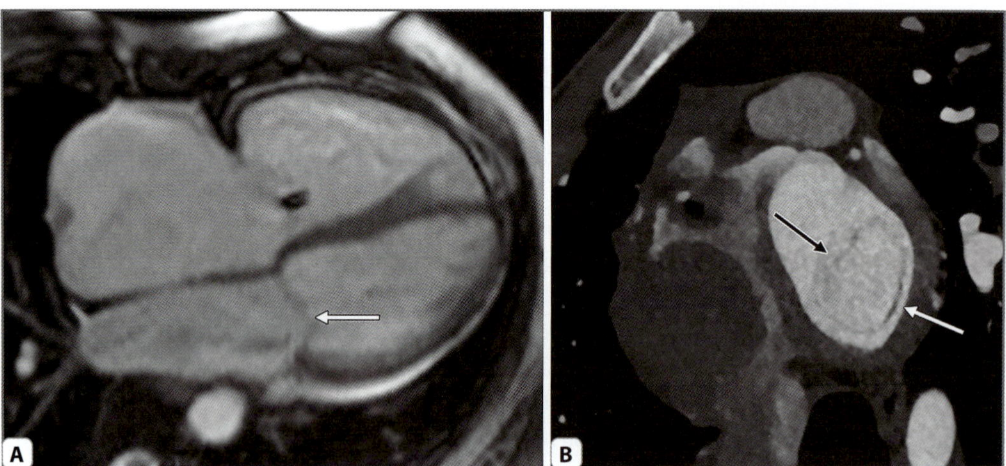

FIGS. 3A AND B: (A) MRI SSFP (TruFISP) image in four chamber view shows closed mitral valve leaflet (white arrow). (B) CT angiography multiplanar reconstructed image at the plane of mitral valve shows the D-shaped appearance of the mitral valve with black arrow pointing toward anterior leaflet and white arrow pointing toward posterior leaflet.

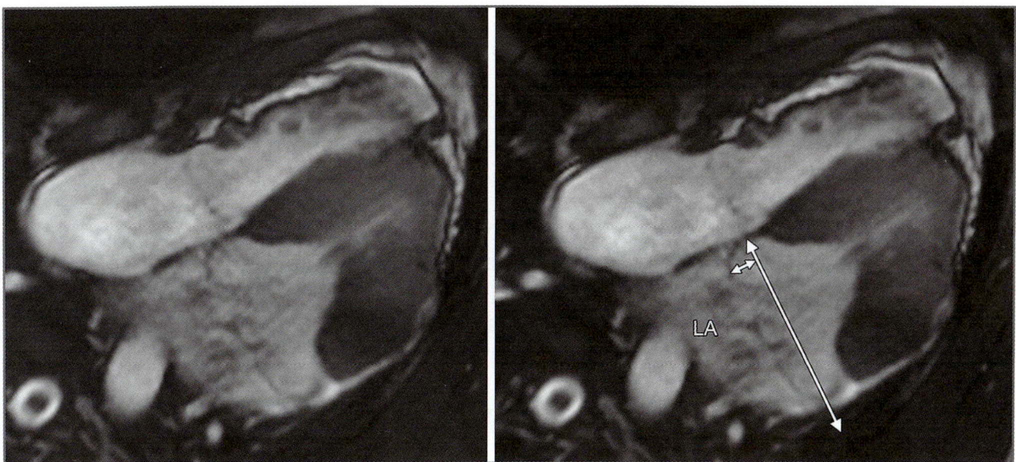

FIG. 4: Cardiac MRI cine end systolic frame in a patient with mitral regurgitation shows upward displacement of the mitral valve leaflet into the left atrium (LA) (4 mm in this case), suggestive of mitral valve prolapse (cut off >2 mm displacement).

systole, this volume further adding up to the LV volume causing volume overload. Primary MR occurs due to dysfunctional mitral valve apparatus.

Mitral valve prolapse (MVP) is a common cause of MR and is characterized by the systolic displacement of one or both mitral valve leaflets into the left atrium due to elongation or redundancy of the leaflets and chordae tendineae **(Fig. 4)**. It is often associated with myxomatous degeneration of the mitral valve, leading to leaflet thickening and billowing. MVP can be asymptomatic or present with symptoms such as palpitations, chest pain, or fatigue. Secondary MR results due to dilatation of mitral annulus due to LV dilatation **(Table 4)**. Left ventricular dysfunction, whether due to an acute myocardial infarction or ischemic and nonischemic cardiomyopathies, can impair papillary muscle function, increasing the risk of mitral valve dysfunction (secondary MR).[8]

TABLE 4: Etiologies of mitral regurgitation (MR).

Primary MR	Secondary MR	Based on acuity
Mitral valve prolapse (with/without mitral annular disjunction)	*Dilated cardiomyopathy*: • Ischemic • Nonischemic • Sarcoid • Toxic	*Acute MR*: • Myocardial infarction • Infective endocarditis • Acute myocarditis
Flail leaflets	Hypertrophic cardiomyopathy	*Chronic MR*: • Mitral valve prolapse • Rheumatic heart disease • Cardiomyopathy

Chest X-ray usually shows cardiomegaly with LV configuration **(Fig. 5)**. The hallmark of mitral valve disease is selective LA enlargement. Enlargement of the LA appendage (LAA) is pathognomonic of rheumatic etiology and can vary from a simple straightening of the left heart border to a large bulge in the typical site, immediately below the left main bronchus **(Fig. 5)**. Rarely, LA or LAA may show calcification either in its wall or in the clot lining the wall. Valvular calcification, generally seen on fluoroscopy, strongly suggests a rheumatic etiology. In contrast, mitral annular calcification is often seen in age-related degenerative disease and in the postoperative patient after closed mitral valvotomy **(Fig. 6)**. In MR, LA enlargement is usually gross or aneurysmal and may also lead to clot formation in LA appendage due to stasis of blood.

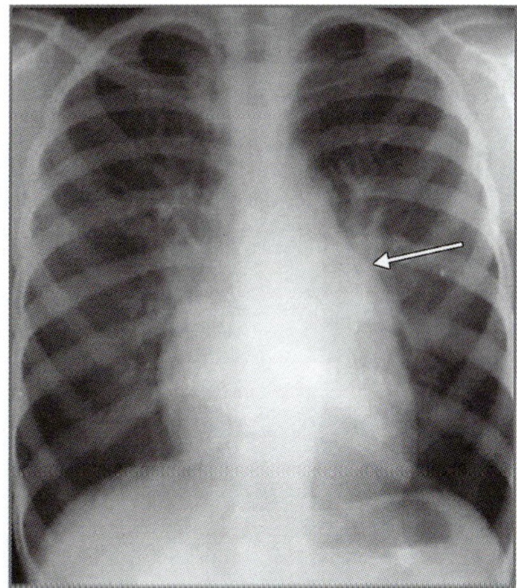

FIG. 5: Chest radiograph in a patient with MR shows a large heart, LV and LA enlargement, and mild PVH. White arrow shows enlargement of the LA appendage.

Echocardiography is the mainstay for evaluation of MR. It allows for assessment of MV anatomy, severity of MR as well as LV cavity size and function **(Fig. 7)**. Short-axis view at the level of the mitral valve orifice is crucial for performing direct planimetry and estimating the effective regurgitant orifice area (EROA), an EROA exceeding 40 mm^2 or a regurgitant volume ≥60 mL/beat indicates severe primary MR is generally recommended as a threshold for surgical intervention, as it is associated with higher rates of cardiac events.[9] CT angiography is useful to rule out coronary artery disease in selected patients. It may also be used to rule out clot formation in LA appendage which has propensity to embolize.

Cardiac magnetic resonance (cine SSFP) is useful in assessment of the valve morphology. Diagnosis is typically made using echocardiography, which shows leaflet prolapse of more than 2 mm beyond the annular plane **(Fig. 4)**. It plays a role in quantifying MR volume as it is more reproducible than echocardiography, especially when combined with other valvular abnormalities, and to evaluate ventricular functions (Class I recommendation as per ACC).[7]

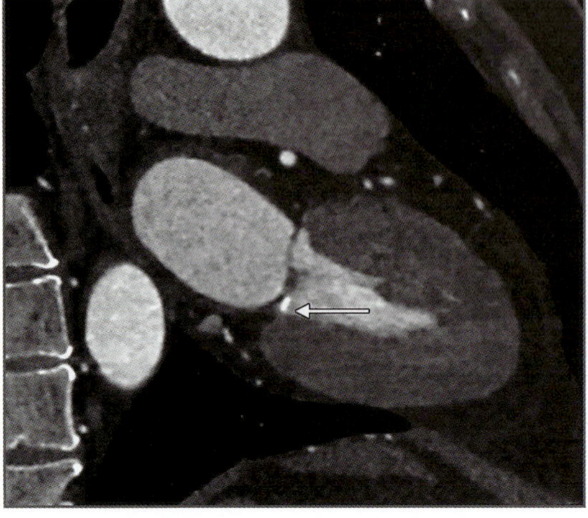

FIG. 6: CT angiography image in two chamber view shows speck of mitral annular calcification (white arrow) in a patient who presented with aortic stenosis and resultant LV hypertrophy.

MR volume is calculated on CMR using the formula below **(Fig. 8)**:

In isolated MR and without any cardiac shunts, LV stroke volume = MR volume + forward flow in aorta (Aorta).

Hence, MR volume = LV stroke volume – Aorta forward flow

Mild, moderate and severe MR is graded on the basis of regurgitant fraction as follows: Mild (<30%), moderate (30–49%) and severe (>50%). The presence of LV myocardial scar on CMR is one of the prognostic factors for adverse LV remodeling.[9,10]

Mitral Annular Disjunction and Arrhythmogenic Mitral Valve Prolapse

Mitral annular disjunction (MAD) is a structural abnormality characterized by the separation of the mitral annulus from the left ventricular myocardium, typically involving the posterior annulus. It is increasingly recognized as a marker of arrhythmic risk, particularly in patients with MVP. Arrhythmogenic mitral valve prolapse (AMVP) refers to a subset of MVP associated with malignant ventricular arrhythmias, including sudden cardiac arrest. The mechanism underlying AMVP is believed to involve mechanical stress from the prolapsing leaflets, myocardial fibrosis near the mitral annulus, and papillary muscle

MR volume = LV stroke volume – Aorta forward flow

TR volume = RV stroke volume – PA forward flow

AR or PR volume = Directly quantified form phase contrast sequence above the level of the valve annulus

FIG. 8: Formulae for calculating the regurgitant volumes [mitral, tricuspid, aortic and pulmonary regurgitation: MR, TR, AR, PR; Pulmonary artery (PA)].

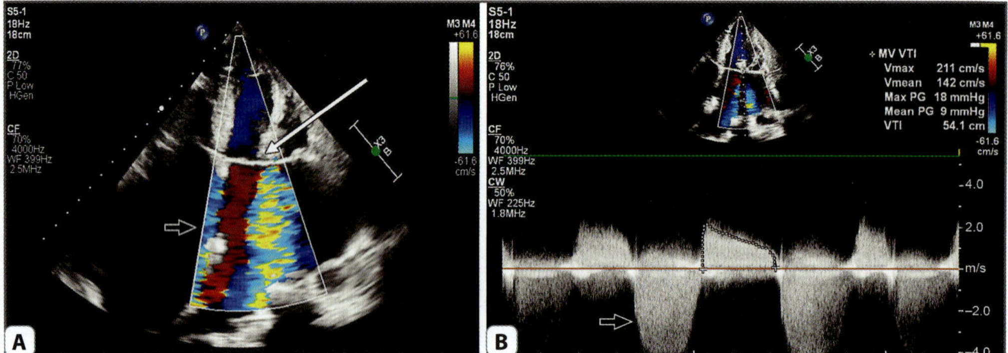

FIGS. 7A AND B: Transthoracic echocardiography with color doppler (A) shows thickened mitral valve leaflets (white thick arrow) in a patient with MS as well as MR (postmitraClip). The thick black arrow is pointing toward the regurgitant jet in LA (suggesting MR). (B) shows tracing of doppler showing regurgitant flow below the baseline. The tracing of MS jet is showing mean pressure gradient of 9 mm Hg.

Courtesy: Dr Avinash Mani, Consultant Cardiology, Fortis Escorts Heart Institute, Delhi.

FIGS. 9A TO C: Cine SSFP image in end diastolic (A) and end-systolic (B) frames in the same patient as in **Figure 4** (with MVP) shows mitral annular disjunction (MAD) (black arrow). (C) LGE image shows mild thinning and thin subendocardial enhancement in inferolateral segment (white arrow).

traction, which together create a substrate for ventricular arrhythmias. Cardiac MRI plays a pivotal role in diagnosing MAD and detecting fibrosis using LGE, helping stratify arrhythmic risk in these patients **(Fig. 9)**.[11]

Mitral Stenosis

It is most commonly caused by rheumatic heart disease. Connective tissue disorders, carcinoid disease, radiation and congenital causes are other etiologies implicated.

Characteristic findings are seen on chest X-ray. In MS, the heart size can be normal if assessed only by frontal projection **(Fig. 10)**. However, by volumetry, it is found to be enlarged in a majority of cases. Still a completely normal heart size can be seen in approximately 10% of the patients with critical MS. In MS, enlargement of LA may be mild or moderate but is rarely gross. In both MR as well as MS, the size of LA bears no correlation with the severity of the lesion as it is more dependent on the pliability of the atrial wall because of inflammation in rheumatic disease. The hemodynamic changes in the pulmonary circulation are sensitive indicators of the severity of disease in MS. Frequently, the mitral valve has a combined lesion. In such situations, it is usually not possible to assess the severity of each lesion by chest radiography alone. However, a dominant MS can be suggested by small heart and LA relative to the severity of PVH. A large heart and LA with relatively mild PVH changes suggests a dominant MR. Similarly, a concomitant involvement of aortic valve and tricuspid valve can be suggested if there is prominence of ascending aorta or right atrium, respectively.

Echocardiography is the mainstay for evaluation **(Fig. 7)**. **Table 5** gives the ACC criteria for evaluation of severity of MS based on valve planimetry (valve area) and mean diastolic pressure gradient. A valve area of <1 cm^2 is suggestive of severe MS.[9] CMR can offer the same information as well, with the phase contrast sequence [with velocity encoding (VENC)] used to measure gradient across the valve. Phase contrast method is principally based on the phase shifts of moving spins in the magnetic field gradient.

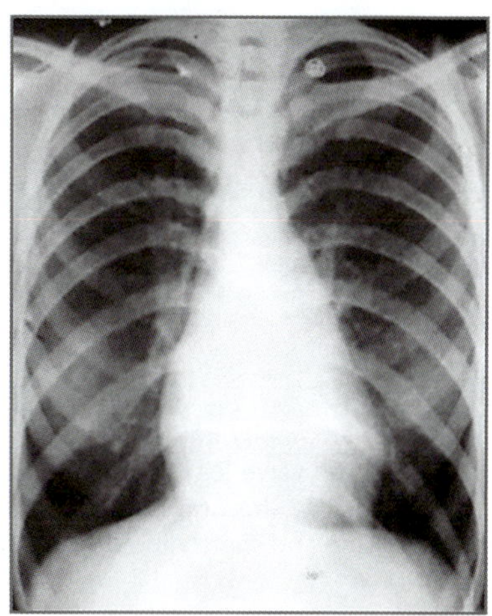

FIG. 10: Chest radiograph in a patient with MS shows normal heart size, LA enlargement and mild PVH.

TABLE 5: ACC (2008) criteria for severity of MS.

Grade	Mean gradient (mm Hg)	Valve area (cm^2)
Normal	0	4–6
Mild	<5	1.6–3.9
Moderate	5-10	1–1.5
Severe	>10	<1

The extent of phase shifts of moving spins is proportional to the velocity along the velocity-encoding direction. Velocity-encoding is performed by using bipolar gradient pulses. Its direction can be selected in any orthogonal or oblique axis of the body. Velocity-encoding of blood flow in each pixel provides 2D quantitative velocity mapping of the vascular system. Once velocity across a vessel is obtained, gradient can be derived using formula gradient = $4\,(V_{max})^2$. However, this technique is fraught with challenges. The jet of MS is seen as a dephasing dark jet across the mitral valve in cine SSFP image.

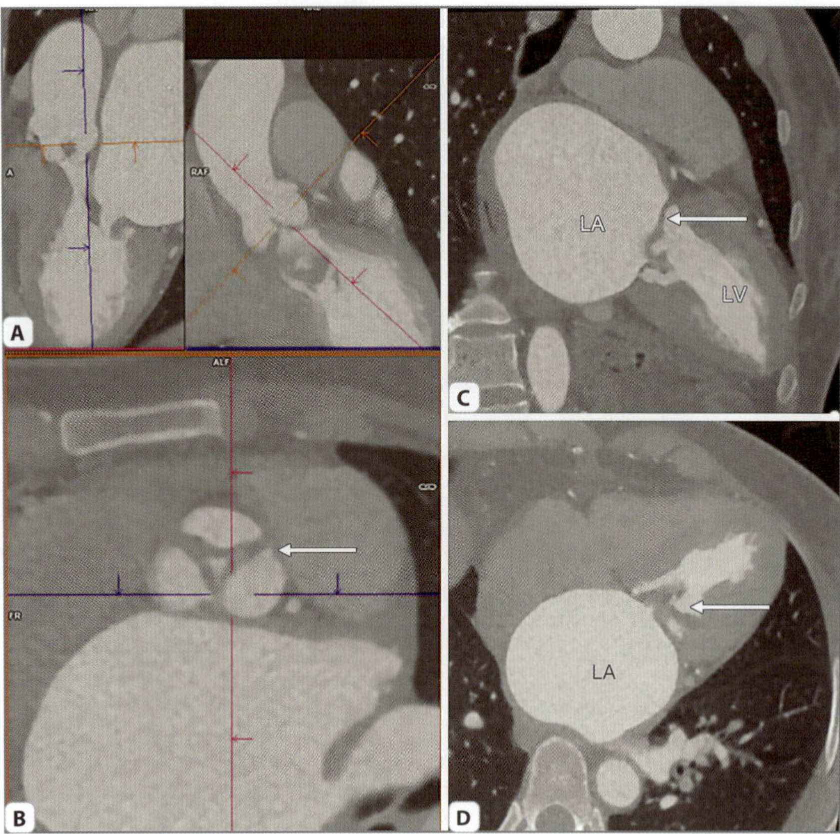

FIGS. 11A TO D: CT angiography images in a patient with rheumatic aortic stenosis and mitral stenosis. (A) shows the planning of the plane across the aortic valve leaflets in two orthogonal views. (B) shows thickened tricuspid aortic valve leaflets (white arrow). (C) shows two chamber view showing thickened mitral valve leaflets (white arrow). (D) Four chamber view shows mitral subvalvular deformity (with thickening and shortening of subvalvular apparatus) in the same patient.

MS leads to stasis of blood in LA and LA appendage and may cause clot formation in the appendage, which can further embolize. CT is useful in the assessment of mitral annular calcification and any coexisting coronary artery disease **(Figs. 2 and 6)**. CT and MRI both help in assessment of valve thickening and subvalvular deformity **(Fig. 11)**. CT also helps in ruling out left atrial appendage clot **(Fig. 12)**. Symptomatic patients moderate to severe MS need surgical or percutaneous management.[10]

TRICUSPID VALVE

Tricuspid Regurgitation

Tricuspid regurgitation (TR) is categorized as either primary, resulting from intrinsic tricuspid valve dysfunction, or secondary, caused by annular dilation. The most common involvement of tricuspid valve is in the form of a functional regurgitation secondary to RV dilatation. Primary TR occurs because of rheumatic process, Ebstein anomaly, infective endocarditis, carcinoid disease or connective tissue disorders.

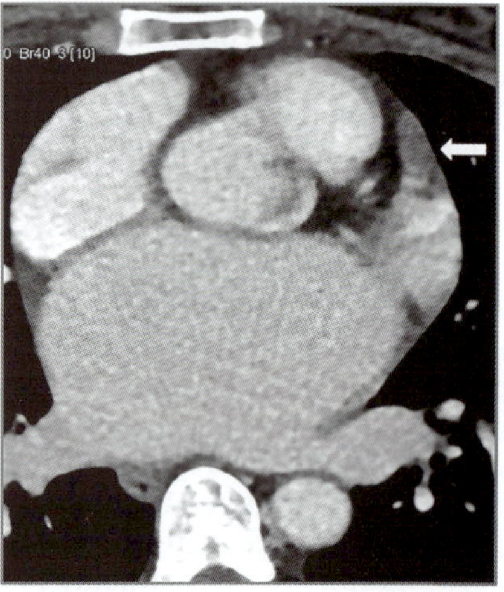

FIG. 12: CT delayed phase image in the same patient as **Figure 10** (with mitral and aortic stenosis), showing a small nonopacified clot at the tip of the left atrial appendage (white block arrow).

The characteristic chest X-ray radiological feature is a large RA **(Fig. 13)**. The increase in the height of the RA relative to that of the vascular pedicle provides

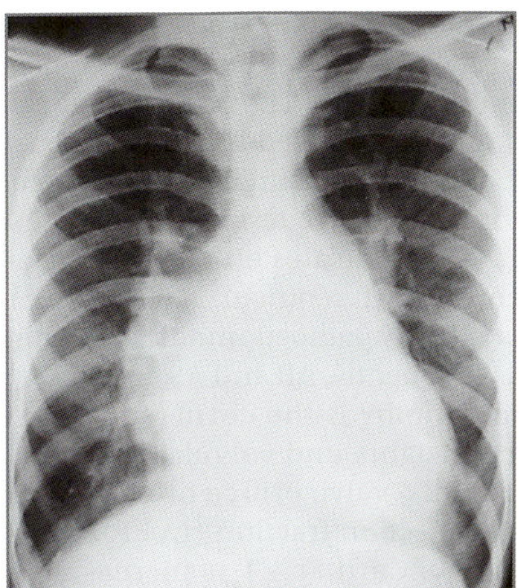

FIG. 13: Chest radiograph in a patient with MS and TR shows mild cardiomegaly, LA and RA enlargement and PVH.

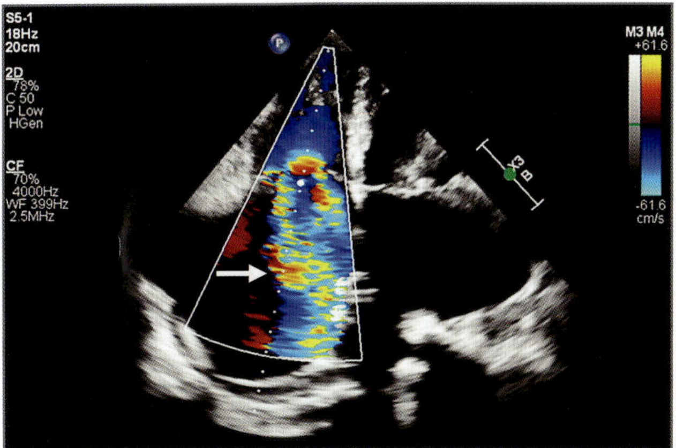

FIG. 14: Transthoracic echocardiography shows regurgitant jet of TR (white arrow).

Courtesy: Dr Avinash Mani, Consultant Cardiology, Fortis Escorts Heart Institute, Delhi.

the most specific index of its enlargement. Although echocardiography (TEE) is the first line investigation, it offers limited evaluation of the RV itself **(Fig. 14)**. CMR is preferred for quantitative and qualitative evaluation in TR and RV volumetry. TR is seen as a dephasing black jet on cine/SSFP sequences **(Fig. 15)**.

TR volume is calculated in the same way as MR volume on CMR **(Fig. 7)**.

RV stroke volume = TR volume + forward flow in pulmonary artery (PA)

TR volume = RV stroke volume – PA forward flow

ESC defines severe TR as regurgitant volume of >45 mL/beat or effective regurgitant orifice area >40 mm^2.[9,12] Severe TR resulting in right heart failure requires corrective surgery. Percutaneous repair/replacement may be considered in suitable cases who cannot undergo surgical repair/replacement. Development of pulmonary hypertension in TR is a poor prognostic feature.

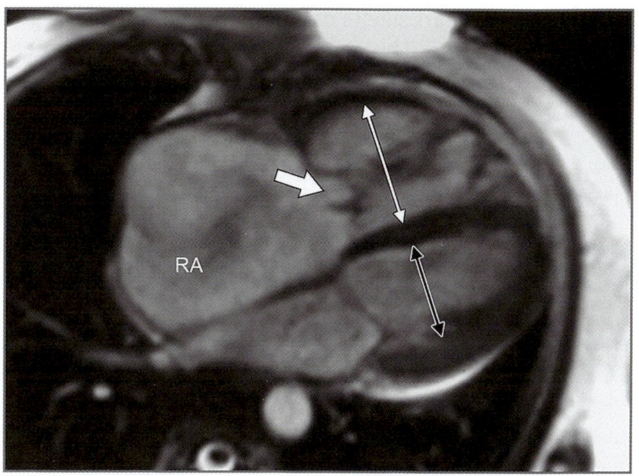

FIG. 15: Cine SSFP frame in four chamber view in systole shows the dephasing jet of tricuspid regurgitation (TR, white block arrow). RA is dilated. RV is also dilated (white arrow) compared to LV (black arrow). RV function was 45%.

Tricuspid Stenosis

Tricuspid stenosis (TS) is rare. Rheumatic etiology is the most common cause in India. Congenital causes, endocarditis and carcinoid syndrome are other important etiologies. Echocardiography (TEE) is the mainstay; however, CMR is useful for RV assessment, to assess valve anatomy and to calculate gradient across the valve. Valve area <1 cm^2 or mean gradient of >5 mm Hg is considered significant enough to cause systemic venous congestion.[9] Surgical repair of severe TS is considered in symptomatic patients and those undergoing left sided corrective surgeries. Percutaneous transcatheter treatment may also be considered in suitable cases.

AORTIC VALVE

Aortic valve is usually tricuspid. Aortic annulus is the plane where the cusps insert. The cusps attach at the annulus and to each other at "commissures". Although less commonly seen , but bicuspid morphology is an important cause of congenital aortic stenosis (AS).

Aortic Stenosis

Calcific AS is present in 1 – 2% of individuals aged 65 years or older and 12% of those aged 75 years or older. The primary causes of valvular AS include congenital bicuspid valve, calcific degeneration of a tricuspid valve, rheumatic heart disease, congenital valve stenosis, severe atherosclerosis, and hypercholesterolemia. Fixed left ventricular (LV) outflow obstruction can occur above (supravalvular AS) or below (subvalvular AS) the valve, while dynamic obstruction may result from hypertrophic cardiomyopathy.

AS is characterized by LV hypertrophy. On radiograph, the heart shows characteristic LV configuration in the form of rounding of cardiac apex, low apex and elongation of left border. Heart size is normal or minimally enlarged in stenotic lesions. The ascending aorta shows a typical poststenotic dilatation in AS **(Fig. 16)**. Aortic valve calcification is more frequently seen in AS with a bicuspid valve than in AS of rheumatic etiology. Calcification is also seen on fluoroscopy. The presence of calcification in the aortic valve is localized based on its characteristic location and movement. Minimal LA enlargement and PVH can be seen in aortic valve lesions. However, significant enlargement of LA indicates either an associated mitral valve involvement or left ventricular failure. A prominent LA appendage is virtually pathognomonic of rheumatic mitral valve disease. Frequently, AR and AS coexist.

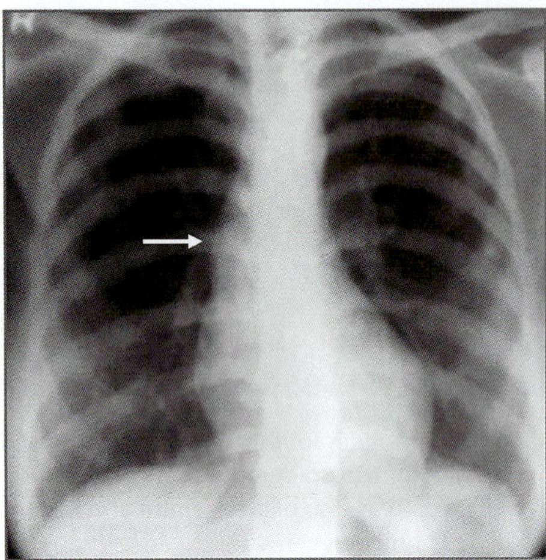

FIG. 16: Chest radiograph in a patient with valvular AS shows normal heart size, LV configuration, poststenotic dilatation (white arrow) of the ascending aorta and normal lung vasculature.

Echocardiography is the cornerstone for assessing AS, providing insights into valvular anatomy, severity, pressure gradients, valve orifice area, LV hypertrophy, left ventricular ejection fraction (LVEF), and coexisting mitral pathology. Cardiac CT is increasingly used for evaluating AS, particularly in assessing aortic root and valve calcification, coronary artery disease, and aortic dimensions **(Figs. 17 and 18A)**. CT angiography plays a crucial role in preprocedural planning for surgical AV replacement or transcatheter aortic valve implantation (TAVI), offering precise measurements of the annulus, sinus of Valsalva, sinotubular junction, and ascending aorta, along with evaluation of the aorta and its branches.

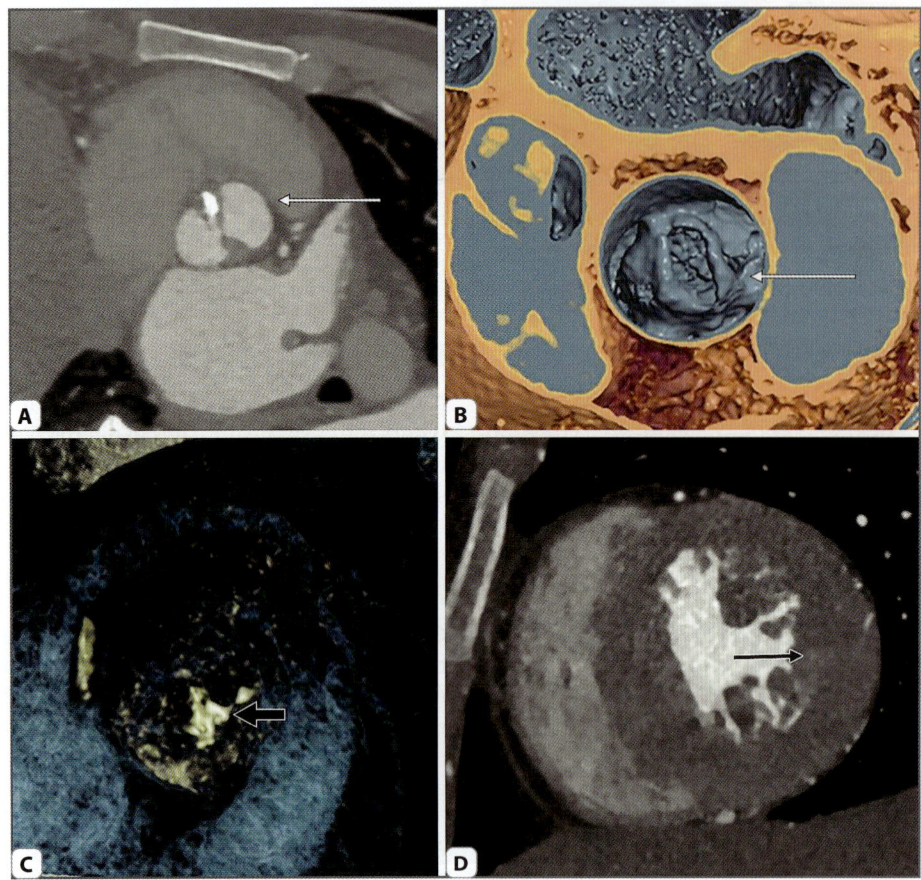

FIGS. 17A TO D: CT angiography images. (A) Multiplanar reconstructed image at the level of the valve shows bicuspid aortic valve (white arrow) with thickened and calcified leaflets in a patient with AS. (B) Volume rendered image also shows the bicuspid morphology. (C) Volume rendered image (calcium view) shows speck of calcification (black arrow) in the valve. (D) short axis view shows myocardial hypertrophy (thick LV wall).

CMR is valuable for functional assessment and monitoring aortic dimensions in patients with bicuspid valves, requiring serial imaging over several years. LGE detected on CMR serves as a prognostic tool, as the presence of myocardial fibrosis is linked to worse outcomes in patients with AS. CMR is also effective for evaluating valve morphology, aortic anatomy, and annular dimensions, particularly during preprocedural planning for TAVI **(Fig. 18B)**. However, CMR is not recommended for assessing stenosis severity, as it tends to underestimate transvalvular velocities. The advancement sin CR like 4D flow MRI helps in assessment of complex flow patterns in ascending aorta in the patients with bicuspid aortic valves and are being investigated **(Fig. 19)**. It can also allow for the assessment of aortic wall shear stress.[4,13]

AS can be graded as shown in **Table 6**.[9] AV replacement is advised for patients with severe AS and a left ventricular ejection fraction below 50%, as well as for those with severe asymptomatic AS undergoing coronary artery bypass grafting (CABG) or other cardiac surgeries. In patients not suitable for surgical repair, TAVI may be offered.

Aortic Regurgitation

Aortic regurgitation may result from congenital malformations of the aortic valve, rheumatic heart disease, connective tissue disorders (like Marfan's) or hypertension. It may also result from conditions causing dilatation of aortic root and ascending aorta (functional regurgitation), e.g., age-related aortic dilatation and aortic cystic medial necrosis.

Radiograph shows LV dilatation. The heart shows a moderate or severe enlargement in regurgitant lesions. Ascending aortic dilatation is more diffuse and also involves the aortic knuckle in aortic regurgitation **(Fig. 20)**. In presence of AR, the size of the heart roughly parallels the severity of regurgitation. Echocardiography is usually the initial investigation of choice for AR quantification and LV volumetry and functional evaluation. It may show bicuspid or thickened valves. Vena contracta width of >0.6 cm and holo-diastolic reversal of flow in descending aorta are characteristics of severe AR.[9] Transesophageal echocardiography may sometimes provide more detailed assessment. Invasive angiogram can also demonstrate aortic regurgitation, although not used solely for this purpose **(Fig. 21)**.

The CT allows for assessment of the maximum diameter of the dilated aorta, which is an important determinant for surgery. Although CMR, being radiation free, can be used for serial evaluation of the same. CMR provides precise quantification the AR volume and fraction, with

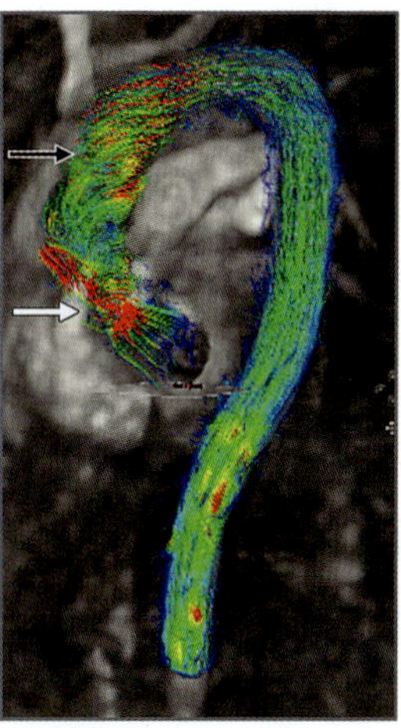

FIG. 19: 4D flow MRI image showing increased velocity (red lines, white arrow) of blood streamlines in a patient with bicuspid aortic valve and AS and vortices of swirling flow (black arrow) in ascending aorta.

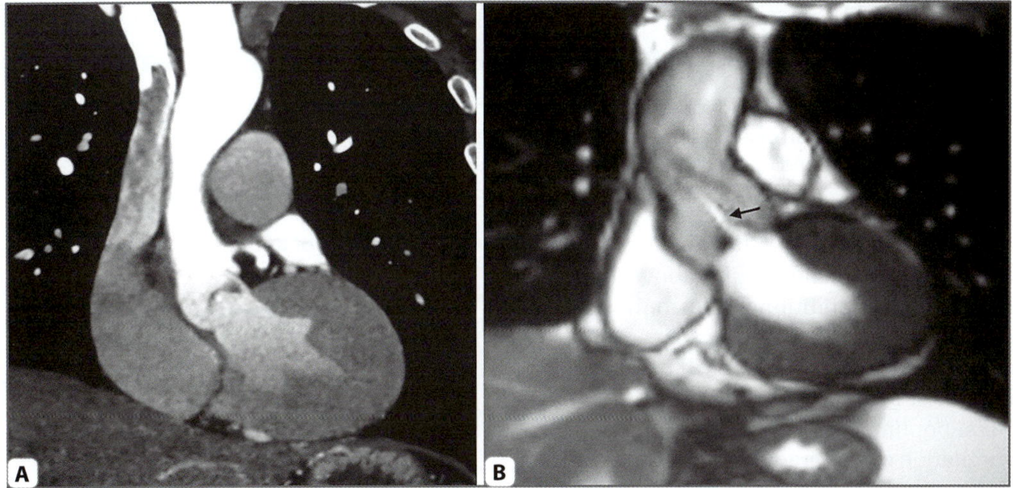

FIGS. 18A AND B: (A) Cine coronal image reconstructed from ECG-gated CT images shows doming of the bicuspid aortic valve in systole. (B) Oblique coronal view on cine bright blood MRI image showing poststenotic jet in ascending aorta in a patient with aortic valvular stenosis.

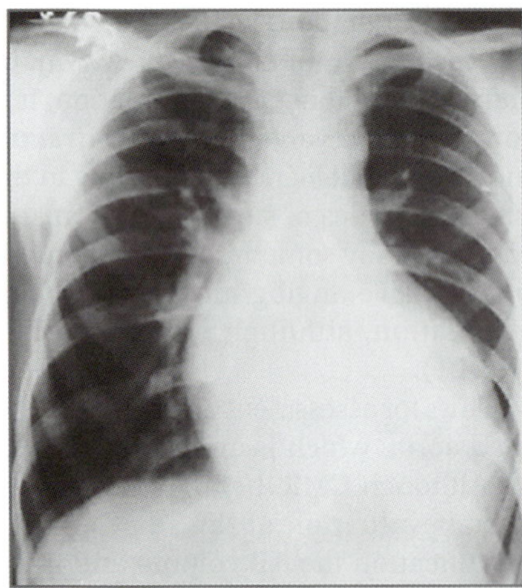

FIG. 20: Chest radiograph in a patient with AR shows a large heart, LV configuration, dilated aorta and mild PVH.

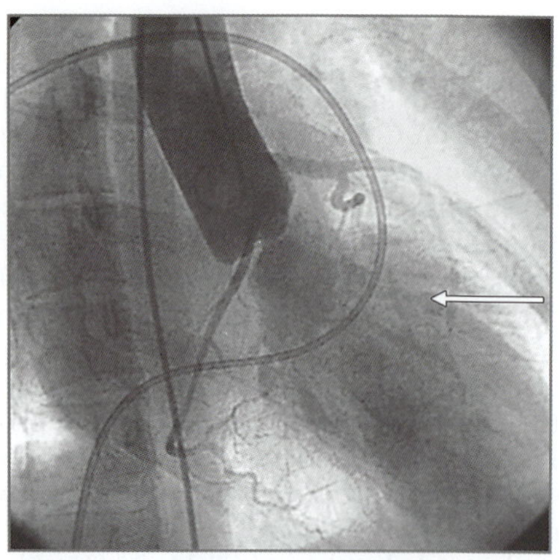

FIG. 21: Aortic root angiogram in the RAO view in a patient with severe AR shows opacification of the entire LV.

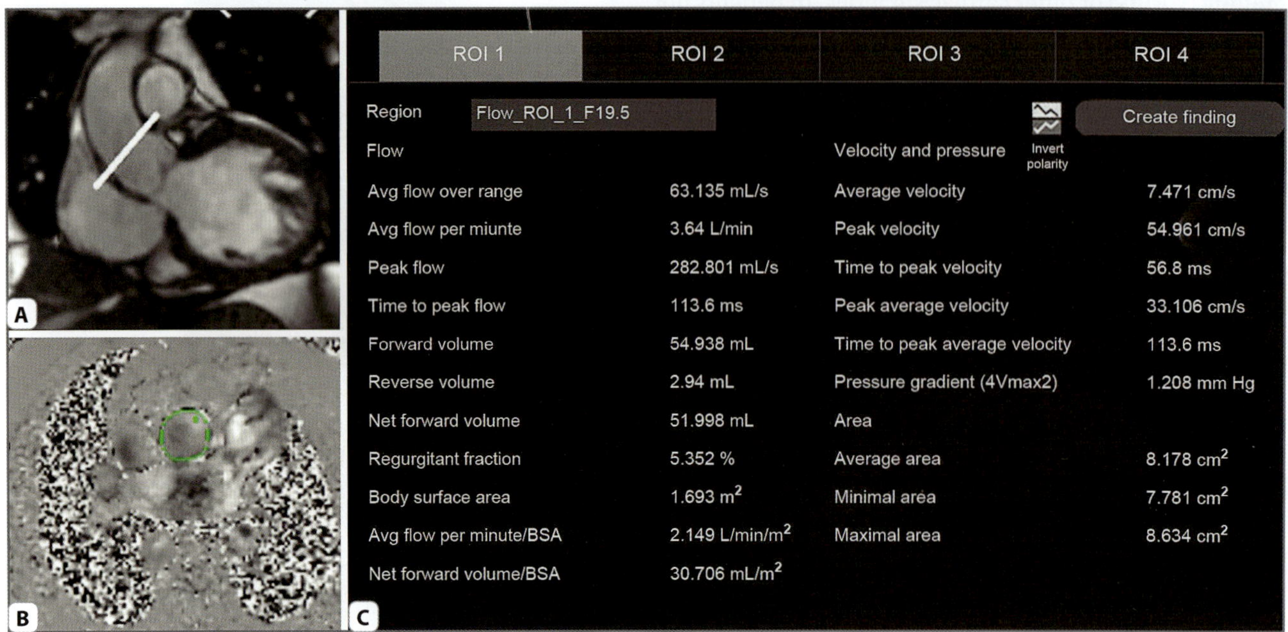

FIGS. 22A TO C: 2D phase contrast flow MRI for aorta: (A) shows planning of aortic flow above the valve level (white line), (B) phase image acquired at the slice with region of interest along the aorta (green circle). (C) shows the measurements that can be obtained flow quantification, regurgitant volume and fraction (here 5.3%) as well as pressure gradient.

phase contrast (PC) method being the most accurate. It involves planning a through plane slice just above the aortic root **(Fig. 22)**. CMR offers additional information about LV functions, volumes and myocardial scar, especially important in asymptomatic severe AR. CMR is particularly recommended when echocardiographic assessment is inconclusive or suboptimal.[9,10]

Aortic regurgitation can be graded as shown in **Table 6**. Surgery is recommended for symptomatic patients or asymptomatic patients with low LV function (<50%). In addition, simultaneous repair of the aortic sinuses or replacement of the ascending aorta is indicated if aortic diameter is >45 mm.[9]

TABLE 6: Grading of aortic stenosis and aortic regurgitation.

Grading	AS	AR
Mild	Mean gradient <20 mm Hg or valve area >1.5 cm^2	Regurgitant fraction (RF) <30% or vena contracta width of <0.3 cm
Moderate	Mean gradient 20–40 mm Hg or valve area 1–1.5 cm^2	RF 30–49% or vena contracta width of 0.3–0.6 cm
Severe	Mean gradient >40 mm Hg and valve area <1 cm^2	RF >50% or vena contracta width of >0.6 cm

PULMONARY VALVE

Pulmonary Stenosis

Congenital PS is the most frequent cause and is often associated with syndromes such as tetralogy of Fallot (TOF), Noonan syndrome and Williams syndrome. Rheumatic heart disease may rarely cause PS, usually in conjunction with the involvement of other valves. Differentiating valvular PS from subvalvular (infundibular) or supravalvular stenosis is critical for determining appropriate management. Echocardiography allows limited assessment of the pulmonary valve. Cardiac MRI is highly effective in distinguishing these conditions and is the gold standard for assessing RV function and volume. Velocity-encoded phase-contrast (VENC-PC) imaging can be used to measure the gradient across the pulmonary valve, aiding in severity assessment. While specific gradient thresholds for intervention are not universally defined, a gradient exceeding 64 mm Hg typically warrants repair. Management options for PS include percutaneous balloon valvuloplasty, transcatheter pulmonary valve replacement, or surgical valve replacement, depending on the severity and underlying anatomy.[9,10]

Pulmonary Regurgitation

Pulmonary regurgitation most commonly results from annular dilatation secondary to pulmonary artery hypertension or infective endocarditis. It is also frequently seen as a residual finding after the surgical correction of TOF or following balloon dilatation for PS. Other causes include congenital abnormalities of the valve leaflets, such as fenestrations, malformations, or supernumerary leaflets, and carcinoid syndrome. As with other regurgitant valvular diseases, cardiac MRI plays a pivotal role in evaluating PR. It provides quantitative assessment of the PR fraction and qualitative evaluation of valve leaflets **(Figs. 23 and 24)**. Additionally, RV volume and functional analysis are critical in planning surgical interventions. Symptomatic severe PR warrants treatment, whereas, replacement is considered in asymptomatic patients with PR >25% and increased indexed volumes of the right ventricle (dilated dysfunctional RV).[9,10]

PROSTHETIC HEART VALVE

The available prosthetic valves, for replacement of diseased native valves, are broadly categorized into mechanical valves and bioprosthetic valves, TTE is typically the first-line investigation for evaluating PHVs. However, its sensitivity can be limited due to acoustic shadowing from metallic components. Cine fluoroscopy is particularly useful for assessing leaflet motion in cases where echocardiography suggests increased transvalvular gradients. However, fluoroscopy alone cannot provide comprehensive details such as flow dynamics or the presence of leaks, making it a complementary rather than standalone modality. CT imaging is effective for evaluating valvular morphology, identifying structural abnormalities, and detecting complications such as paravalvular leaks, calcifications, thrombus, and pseudoaneurysms or abscesses. It provides detailed anatomical information critical for comprehensive assessment. MRI can be performed when TTE results are suboptimal or when CT is contraindicated. MRI is safe in patients with metallic heart valves, allowing for additional functional and anatomical insights when needed. Patients with PHVs require continuous clinical and imaging follow-up to ensure early detection and management of potential complications, which can significantly improve outcomes. Common complications of PHVs are summarized in **Table 7**.[14,15]

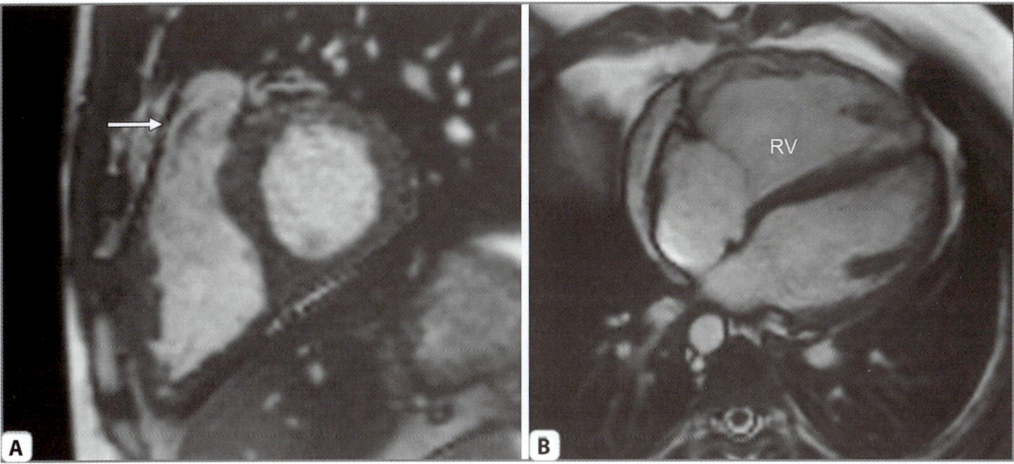

FIGS. 23A AND B: Cardiac MRI cine SSFP image in short axis (A) view shows dephasing jet of PR in a patient after repair of tetralogy of Fallot. (B) Four chamber cine SSFP image shows dilated RV.

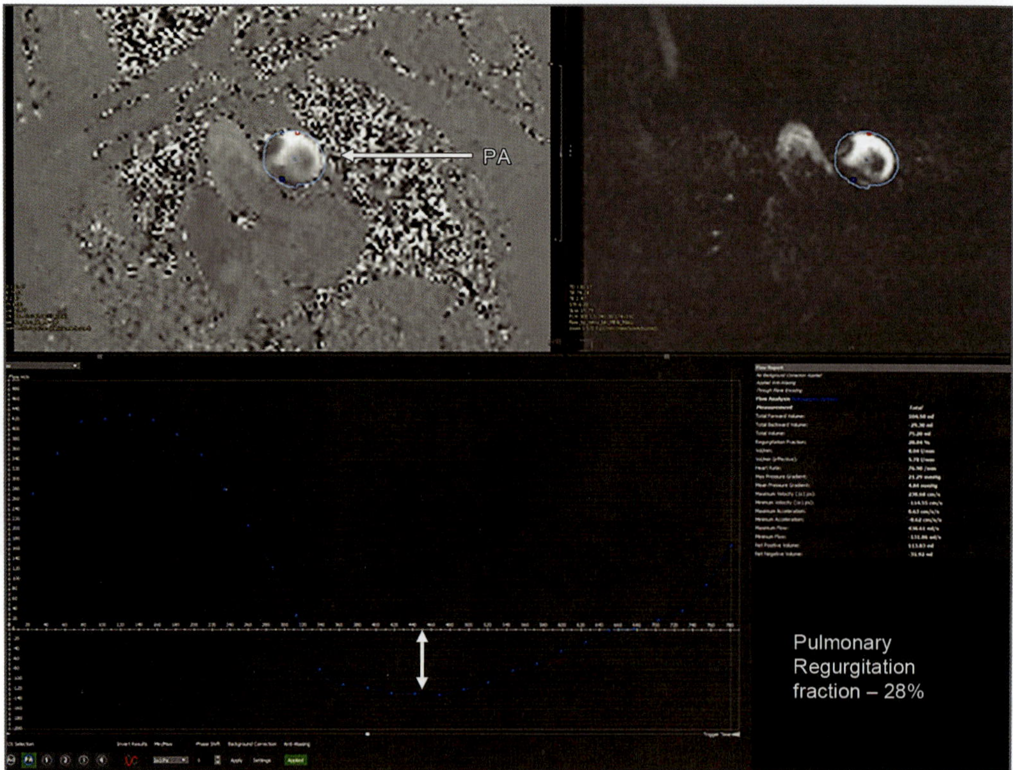

FIG. 24: Flow assessment of main pulmonary artery on phase contrast MRI in the same patient as **Figure 23** shows pulmonary regurgitant volume of 29 mL, PR fraction of 28% (also depicted in the curve).

TABLE 7: Complications of prosthetic heart valves.

Functional and hemodynamic complications	• Stenosis, • Regurgitation, and • Leaflet dysfunction (e.g., a stuck leaflet). A stuck leaflet may result from restricted or absent mobility of the valve leaflet due to structural failure or a space-occupying lesion such as thrombus or pannus. Leaflet angles, measured relative to the orifice plane, should be compared with manufacturer-provided opening and closing angles to diagnose valve dysfunction accurately
Structural complications	• *Thrombus or pannus formation*: Differentiating these is essential as they require distinct management approaches. CT is useful for the same • *Hypoattenuating leaflet thickening (HALT)*: Subtle changes detectable on CT imaging • *Paravalvular leaks*: Gaps between the valve and the surrounding tissue • *Infective endocarditis*: Infections leading to abscesses, pseudoaneurysms, or fistula formation • *Patient–prosthesis mismatch*: Inadequate size of the prosthetic valve relative to the patient's needs • *Structural valve failure*: Degeneration or dysfunction of the valve • *Valve dehiscence*: Loosening or separation of the valve from its attachment site

CONCLUSION

A thorough evaluation of VHD involves not only assessing the severity of lesions but also understanding their etiology, conducting functional assessments, performing risk stratification, and planning appropriate interventions. Effective clinical decision-making relies on combining clinical evaluation with multimodality imaging to meet these objectives. Echocardiography remains the cornerstone and first-line imaging tool. However, advancements in 3D imaging have expanded the roles of cardiac CT and CMR in managing VHD. CMR offers distinct advantages by providing detailed assessments of valve pathology, ventricular function, and myocardial fibrosis.

REFERENCES

1. Manjunath CN, Srinivas P, Ravindranath KS, Dhanalakshmi C. Incidence and patterns of valvular heart disease in a tertiary care high-volume cardiac center: a single center experience, Indian Heart J. 2014;66(3):320-6,
2. Nkomo VT, Gardin JM, Skelton TN, Gottdiener JS, Scott CG, Enriquez-Sarano M. Burden of valvular heart diseases: a population-based study. Lancet. 2006;368(9540):1005-11.
3. d'Arcy JL, Coffey S, Loudon MA, Kennedy A, Pearson-Stuttard J, Birks J, et al. Large- scale community echocardiographic screening reveals a major burden of undiagnosed valvular heart disease in older people: the OxVALVE Population Cohort Study. Eur. Heart J. 2016;37(47):3515-22
4. Myerson SG. CMR in Evaluating Valvular Heart Disease: Diagnosis, Severity, and Outcomes. JACC Cardiovasc Imaging. 2021;14(10):2020-32.
5. Bax J, Delgado V. Advanced imaging in valvular heart disease. Nat Rev Cardiol. 2017;14:209-23.
6. John B Chambers, Saul G Myerson, Ronak Rajani, Gareth J Morgan-Hughes, Marc R Dweck. Multimodality imaging in heart valve disease. Open Heart. 2016;3:e000330.
7. Doherty JU, Kort S, Mehran R, Schoenhagen P, Soman P. ACC/AATS/AHA/ASE/ASNC/HRS/SCAI/SCCT/SCMR/STS 2017 Appropriate Use Criteria for Multimodality Imaging in Valvular Heart Disease: A Report of the American College of Cardiology Appropriate Use Criteria Task Force, American Association for Thoracic Surgery, American Heart Association, American Society of Echocardiography, American Society of Nuclear Cardiology, Heart Rhythm Society, Society for Cardiovascular Angiography and Interventions, Society of Cardiovascular Computed Tomography, Society for Cardiovascular Magnetic Resonance, and Society of Thoracic Surgeons. J Am Coll Cardiol. 2017;70(13):1647-72.
8. Morris MF, Maleszewski JJ, Suri RM, Burkhart HM, Foley TA, Bonnichsen CR, et al. CT and MR imaging of the mitral valve: radiologic-pathologic correlation. Radiographics. 2010;30(6):1603-20.
9. Nishimura RA, Otto CM, Bonow RO, Carabello BA, Erwin JP 3rd, Guyton RA, et al. 2014 AHA/ACC Guideline for the Management of Patients With Valvular Heart Disease: executive summary: a report of the American College of Cardiology/American Heart Association Task Force on Practice Guidelines. Circulation. 2014;129(23):2440-92.
10. Otto CM, Nishimura RA, Bonow RO, Carabello BA, Erwin JP 3rd, Gentile F, et al. 2020 ACC/AHA Guideline for the Management of Patients With Valvular Heart Disease: Executive Summary: A Report of the American College of Cardiology/American Heart Association Joint Committee on Clinical Practice Guidelines. Circulation. 2021;143(5):e35-71.
11. Van der Bijl P, Stassen J, Haugaa KH, et al. Mitral Annular Disjunction in the Context of Mitral Valve Prolapse: Identifying the At-Risk Patient. JACC Cardiovasc Imaging. 2024;17(10):1229-45.
12. Vahanian A, Alfieri O, Andreotti F, Antunes MJ, Barón-Esquivias G, Baumgartner H, et al. Guidelines on the management of valvular heart disease (version 2012) The Joint Task Force on the Management of Valvular Heart Disease of the European Society of Cardiology (ESC) and the European Association for Cardio Thoracic Surgery (EACTS), Eur. Heart J. 2012;33(19):2451-96.
13. Sträter A, Huber A, Rudolph J, Berndt M, Rasper M, Rummeny EJ, et al. 4D-flow MRI: technique and applications. Rofo. 2018;190(11):1025-35.
14. Gulsin GS, Singh A, McCann GP. Cardiovascular magnetic resonance in the evaluation of heart valve disease. BMC Med. Imaging. 2017;17:67.
15. Rajiah P, Moore A, Saboo S, Goerne H, Ranganath P, MacNamara J. et al. Multimodality imaging of complications of cardiac valve surgeries. Radiographics. 2019;39(4):932-56.

Jyoti Kumar, Sapna Singh, Gaurav Shanker Pradhan

CHAPTER

29

Imaging of the Pericardium

INTRODUCTION

Pericardial diseases could be a variety of benign and malignant disorders.[1] The initial approach to the evaluation of pericardial disease is usually performed with echocardiography and chest radiography. While echocardiography has its own advantages, namely high temporal and spatial resolution, easy availability, no involvement of ionizing radiation, it is usually limited by poor acoustic window, poor soft tissue characterization and operator variability. In addition, it can be very difficult to detect pericardial thickening or calcification.[2,3] Plain radiography, on the other hand, may not be able to differentiate various pericardial disorders.[4]

Computed tomography (CT) and magnetic resonance imaging (MRI) techniques are complementary to echocardiography and used as second line modality. They provide excellent anatomic details, help in localizing pericardial pathology as well as depicting associated abnormalities of the lung and mediastinum. The advent of multidetector CT with its excellent temporal resolution helps us to image pericardium devoid of cardiac motion artifacts. Multiplanar reformats allow better visualization of pericardial pathology with easy communication to the referring physician.[5] A cinematic display of cardiac motion is now possible on CT with electrocardiography (ECG) gating and high-resolution thin section images can be obtained. Increased sensitivity to detect calcification is another advantage of CT. MRI provides superior soft tissue characterization than CT and echocardiography. MRI can provide excellent display of cardiac motion in patients with regular heart rhythm.[5-8] The role of various imaging modalities based on European Society of Cardiology (ESC) guidelines[9] and American Society of Echocardiography (ASE) consensus[10] is depicted in **Table 1**.

TABLE 1: Various imaging modalities to evaluate pericardial pathology as per ESC guidelines and ASE consensus.

	Echocardiography	Computed Tomography	Cardiac Magnetic Resonance
Role	First modality of choice	Second modality of choice	Second modality of choice
Advantages	• Can be used bedside • Functional evaluation possible • Hemodynamic assessment can be done on Doppler	• Short acquisition time • Calcification diagnosed reliably • Extracardiac findings assessed	• Superior tissue characterization compared with Echo and CT • Excellent temporal resolution for hemodynamic evaluation • Late gadolinium imaging (LGE) with MRI can delineate ongoing pericardial inflammation
Disadvantages	• Limited evaluation in case of poor acoustic window, in obesity • Operator dependent • Less soft tissue characterization	Ventricular function not assessed (in case of prospective gating)	Time-consuming examination

(ESC: European Society of Cardiology; ASE: American Society of Echocardiography)

ANATOMY

The pericardium has an outer fibrous layer and an inner serous layer. The inner serosal layer is further composed of outer parietal and inner visceral layers. The outer parietal layer lines the inner surface of the fibrous pericardium, and the inner visceral layer forms the epicardium.[11-13] The pericardial cavity lies between the parietal and visceral layers. Normally, up to 50 mL fluid may be present in this potential space created by two opposing serosal surfaces.

Ligaments attach the outer pericardium to sternum and diaphragm. The serosal layer forms two complex sleeves as it reflects around major vessels. One of these sleeves encloses the aorta and pulmonary trunk, and the other encloses the superior and inferior vena cava and the four pulmonary veins. These reflections form the sinuses and recesses **(Fig. 1)**. The transverse sinus is the channel in between these two sleeves around the arteries and veins and the oblique sinus is the channel behind the left atrium. The recesses are the blind ends of these sinuses **(Box 1)**. These sinuses and recesses can collect fluid within them in case of pericardial effusion. With the advent of MDCT, visualization of pericardial recesses without fluid accumulation is also possible.[13]

The normal pericardium can be seen as a thin line <2 mm in thickness.[14] On CT, it appears as a thin linear density surrounding the heart better visualized over the right ventricle **(Fig. 2A)**. It appears as a hypointense line on MR surrounded by epicardial fat on one side and pericardial fat on the other side on T1, T2 weighted and gradient images **(Fig. 2B)**.[15-17] Pericardial fat is the anterior meditational fat seen anterior to the pericardium while the epicardial fat lies between the visceral layer of pericardium and the outer wall of myocardium.[1] The volume of epicardial fat has been linked with the risk of coronary artery disease.

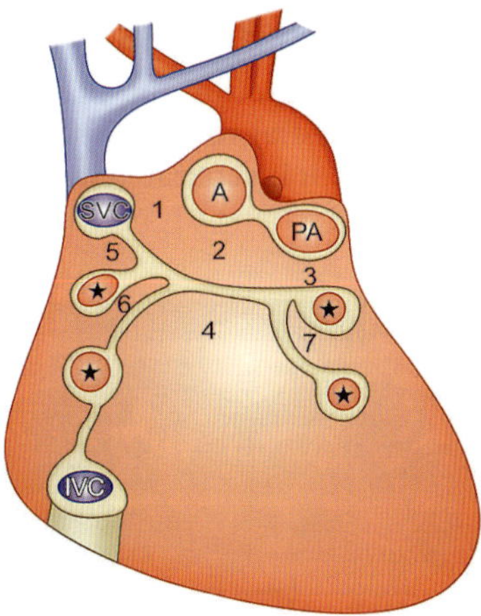

FIG. 1: Schematic representation of pericardium. Transverse sinus (2) with right and left pulmonic recesses (1 and 3). Oblique sinus (4), postcaval recess (5) and right and left pulmonary venous recesses (6 and 7).

(A: aorta; PA: pulmonary artery; SVC: superior vena cava; IVC: inferior vena cava; H: pulmonary veins)

BOX 1: Sinuses and recesses of pericardium.

- *Transverse sinus*:
  - Superior aortic sinus
    - Anterior triangular extension
    - Posterior crescentic extension
    - Right lateral extension
  - Inferior aortic recess
  - Right and left pulmonic recesses
- *Oblique sinus*:
  - Posterior pericardial recess
- *Recesses of pericardial cavity proper*:
  - Right and left pulmonary venous recesses
  - Postcaval recess

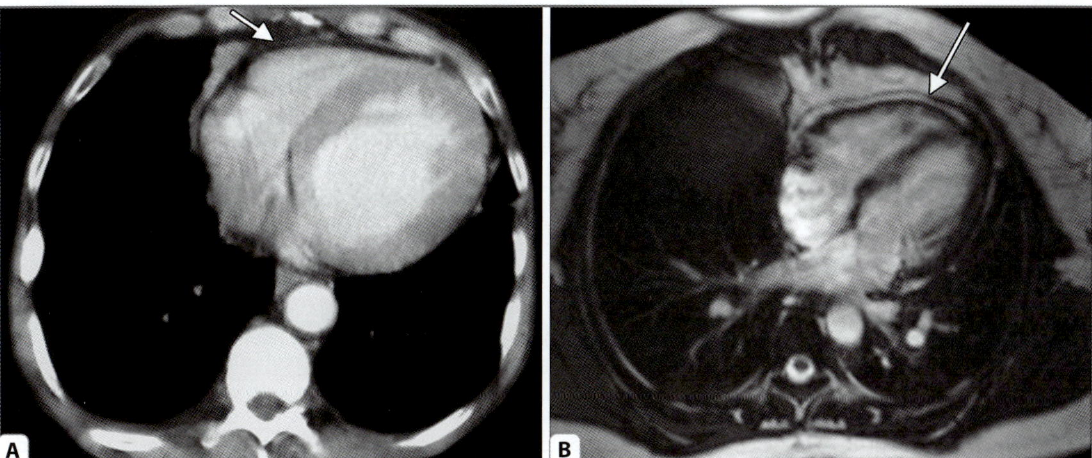

FIGS. 2A AND B: (A) Axial contrast enhanced CT scan shows normal pericardium (arrow) outlined by epicardial fat and mediastinal fat on either side. Note made of subsegmental atelectasis in right lung; (B) Short axis cine gradient echo MR image shows normal pericardium as a thin curved line (arrow) surrounded by bright epicardial and pericardial fat on either side.

TRANSVERSE SINUS AND RECESSES

The transverse sinus lies behind the aorta and the main pulmonary artery and superior to the left atrium.

Superior Aortic Recess

The cranial most extent of this sinus is the superior aortic or superior pericardial recess. It can further be divided into posterior, right, and anterior portions depending on relationship with aorta. The posterior portion is seen as a crescentic fluid collection just posterior to the ascending aorta. It can be mistaken for a lymph node. The fluid in this posterior portion lies directly posterior to the aorta with no intervening fat. The crescent shape and fluid attenuation are other distinguishing features from lymph nodes. Multiplanar reformats aid in depicting continuity of the pericardial recesses with the fluid in the pericardial sac. The anterior portion passes between the aorta and pulmonary artery, resulting in a triangular shape between them **(Fig. 3A)**.[13]

Inferior Aortic Recess

Inferiorly, the transverse sinus extends between the ascending aorta and the right atrium and forms the inferior aortic recess. This extends caudally till the level of the aortic valve annulus and lies anterior to the left atrium **(Figs. 4A and B)**.

Right and Left Pulmonic Recesses

Laterally, the transverse sinus ends in right and left pulmonic recesses **(Figs. 3B to D)**. The former lies inferior to the right pulmonary artery. The left pulmonic recess lies below the left pulmonary artery. Below this lies the left superior pulmonary vein. Fluid within these recesses can sometimes simulate lymph nodes.[18]

Oblique Sinus and Recess

The oblique sinus lies superior and posterior to the left atrium and posteromedial to the superior pulmonary veins **(Figs. 5A and B)**. It is separated from the transverse

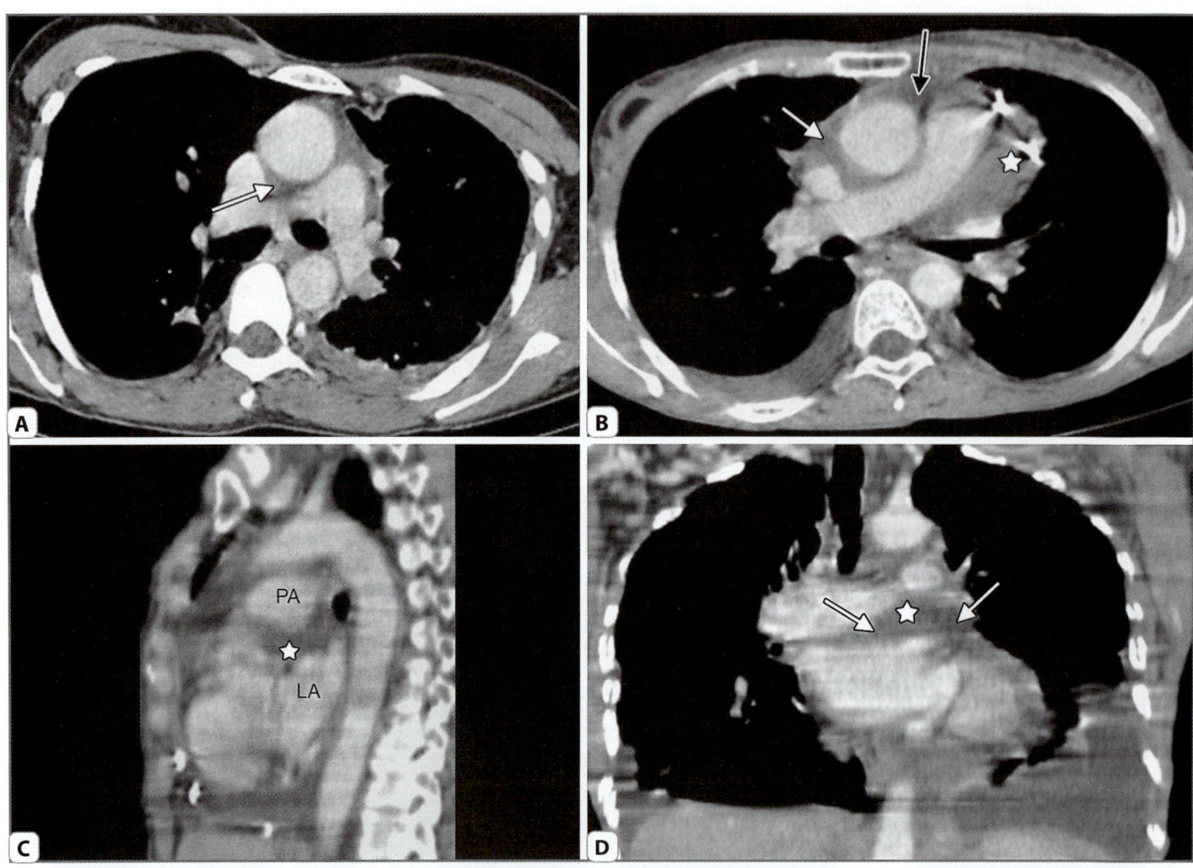

FIGS. 3A TO D: (A) Axial CECT shows the posterior extension of the superior aortic recess posterior to the ascending aorta, as a crescentic fluid collection (arrow); (B) Axial CECT shows left pulmonic recess of the transverse sinus (asterisk). Pericardial fluid is also seen in the anterior (black arrow) and right (white arrow) portions of the superior aortic recess. Note made of pericardial drainage catheter in situ; (C) Sagittal reformation shows the transverse sinus (asterisk) between pulmonary artery (PA) and left atrium (LA). Note made of pericardial drainage catheter in situ; (D) Coronal reformation shows transverse sinus (asterisk) along with right and left pulmonic recesses (arrows) at its right and left ends.

FIGS. 4A AND B: (A) Axial contrast enhanced CT scan shows inferior aortic recess between the right atrium and aortic root (asterisk). Note made of pericardial drainage catheter in situ; (B) Coronal reformation shows the vertical extent of the transverse sinus with its superior and inferior aortic recesses (asterisk). Note made of pericardial drainage catheter in situ.

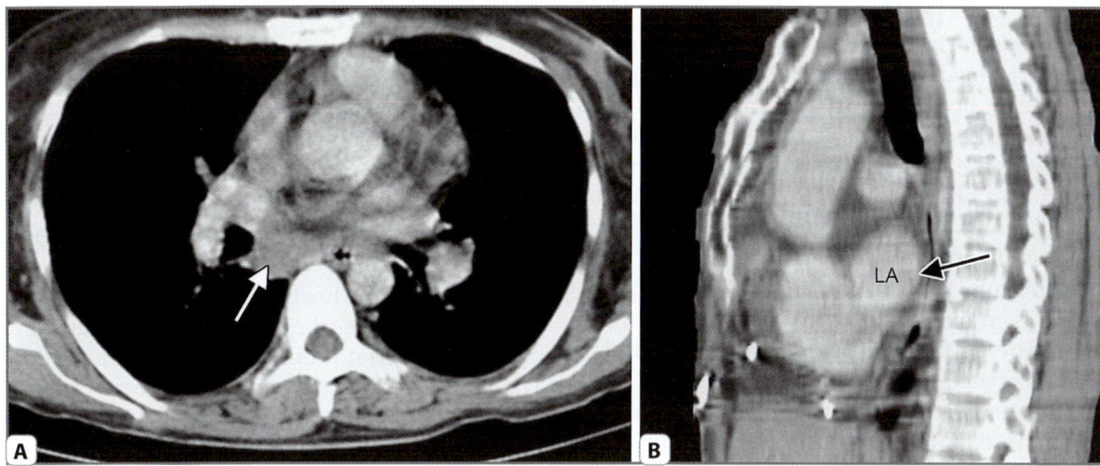

FIGS. 5A AND B: (A) Axial contrast enhanced CT scan shows posterior pericardial recess of the oblique sinus (arrow) superior to the left atrium, medial to bronchus intermedius and posteromedial to the superior pulmonary veins; (B) Sagittal reformation shows the oblique sinus (arrow) between the left atrium anteriorly and the esophagus posteriorly.

sinus by a pericardial reflection between the right and left superior pulmonary veins. Since this lies just anterior to the esophagus, fluid here may be mistaken for esophageal lesions and sometimes even as bronchogenic cysts.

The cranial reflection is the posterior pericardial recess. This extends behind the right pulmonary artery and medial to the bronchus intermedius **(Fig. 5A)**. Fluid within this recess can mimic peribronchial or subcarinal lymph nodes.[11]

Recesses of the Pericardial Cavity Proper

Right and Left Pulmonary Venous Recesses

The right and left pulmonary venous recesses are recesses of the pericardial cavity proper, located between the superior and inferior pulmonary veins on either side.

Fluid in these pulmonary venous recesses can be mistaken for bronchopulmonary lymph nodes. These may be distinguished by the fact that fluid lies both anterior and posterior to the veins whereas, lymph nodes lie only on one side and may narrow the vein.[11]

Postcaval Recess

The postcaval recess is another small recess from the pericardial cavity proper, lying posterior to the superior vena cava (SVC) and to its right.[11]

PHYSIOLOGY

The pericardium supports the heart and cardiac function in the following major ways:[19]

- It fixes the heart within the anterior mediastinum protecting it from surrounding organs
- Its elasticity limits excessive dilatation of cardiac chambers in response to increased preload

- It equalizes compliance between right and left ventricle. When stroke volume of left ventricle is altered due to elevated systemic vascular resistance, it helps in adaptation of stroke volume of the right ventricle accordingly (ventricular coupling).
- The respiratory changes in intrathoracic pressure are directly transmitted to the pericardial cavity and then to the cardiac chambers. The effect is greater on the right ventricle than on the left because of its thinner wall.

CONGENITAL PERICARDIAL ANOMALIES

Congenital pericardial abnormalities include pericardial cyst, pericardial diverticula and congenital absence of pericardium.

Pericardial Cyst (Box 2)

Pericardial cyst is a rare lesion which results from pinching off of parietal pericardial recess. It can be found throughout the mediastinum, but the most common location is the right anterior cardiophrenic angle. A pericardial cyst elsewhere in the mediastinum may be difficult to differentiate from a bronchogenic or thymic cyst.[8] When a pericardial cyst has a residual communication with the pericardial space, it is called a pericardial diverticula.[4] This communication may however be difficult to delineate. Owing to this communication, there may be changes in size and shape of the diverticula when evaluated at different points of time.

Although usually asymptomatic, few patients may have chest pain, dyspnea, cough, pneumothorax, or fever. Another rarer presentation may be due to bronchial compression.

The pericardial cyst is usually sharply demarcated round or ovoid mass in the region of right cardiophrenic angle silhouetting the cardiac border. The cyst may have a pointed upper border as it droops down into the cardiophrenic region from higher up. On cross-sectional imaging, it is a well-defined unilocular, thin walled homogenous nonenhancing mass contiguous with the pericardium. Ultrasound can depict the cystic lesion adjacent to pericardium. On CT, it has fluid attenuation and on MRI, it matches the signal characteristics of water. Presence of proteinaceous contents within the cyst can result in occasional high signal on T1 weighted images. There is no restriction on diffusion imaging. Additionally, a pericardial cyst does not normally cause mass effect on the heart. The cysts may get infected and then show peripheral enhancement and mass effect. Internal enhancement, soft tissue or fat component, thickened wall or septae or mass effect raise the suspicion of a cystic tumor. Symptomatic and complicated cysts may need to be resected.[11]

BOX 2: Pericardial cyst.

- Rare congenital lesion
- Most common location is right cardiophrenic angle
- Typical imaging features—well-defined cyst with thin wall, no internal septations, low signal on T1 weighted MR and high signal on T2 weighted MR images
- Mass effect and enhancement not seen unless infected

CONGENITAL ABSENCE OF THE PERICARDIUM (BOX 3)

Congenital absence of the pericardium is an uncommon abnormality which may be partial or complete. Apart from congenital etiology, pericardial defect may also be acquired after surgery or trauma.[20]

Absence of left pericardium is more common than complete absence.[3] Bilateral and isolated right sided defects are very rare. There may be other congenital anomalies along with pericardial defect which include cardiac anomalies (atrial septal defect, patent ductus arteriosus), and anomalies of the lung (bronchogenic cysts, pulmonary sequestration), chest wall (pectus excavatum) and diaphragm.[21] Patients are generally asymptomatic although vague chest pain can occur due to lack of fixation.[20,21] A focally deficient pericardium may allow a part of the heart to herniate through the defect. It most often involves the left atrial appendage. Rarely, there may be left atrial infarction resulting in sudden death. The left coronary artery may also be compressed by the herniation through this defect. This can rarely result in ischemia, especially during activity. In such situations, surgical closure or enlargement of the defect may be performed.[19]

In complete absence of left pericardium, heart is displaced to the left side on plain radiographs. The segments of the heart that make up the left heart border can be seen more distinctly. The aorta and main pulmonary artery are

BOX 3: Congenital absence of pericardium.

- Rare anomaly
- Left-sided absence commoner than complete absence
- *Radiographic findings*:
  - Left ventricle and pulmonary artery displaced to left
  - Main pulmonary artery borders distinctly seen
  - Pulmonary artery/left atrial appendage may be prominent in partial absence
- *CT/MR findings*:
  - Leftward shift of cardiac axis
  - Prominent atrial appendage
  - Lung seen interposed between aorta and main pulmonary artery

seen more clearly due to the interposition of lung between them. In partial absence of the left pericardium, pulmonary artery or left atrial appendage may be prominent depending upon the location of pericardial defect.[4,22]

Normally, CT and MR may not depict the pericardium along its entirety. The pericardium may not be normally seen over the left atrial appendage and the left ventricle and should not be misinterpreted as pericardial defect. Secondary signs, which include posterior and leftward shift of the cardiac axis, prominent atrial appendage and separation of the aorta and main pulmonary artery due to lung tissue interposition become more important features. Occasionally, lung tissue can be seen inferior to the heart, interposed between the heart and the diaphragm. The herniation may be intermittent; hence left lateral decubitus position of the patient can assist in diagnosing pericardial defects. Also, functional examination can pick up greater mobility of the cardiac apex which is otherwise essentially stationary in a normal cardiac cycle.[23]

PERICARDIAL EFFUSION

The various causes of pericardial effusion include heart failure, renal insufficiency, infection (bacterial, viral, tubercular), neoplasm (carcinoma of the lung, breast, lymphoma, melanoma) and injury (trauma, myocardial infarction). Other causes may be hypothyroidism, connective tissue disorder, acquired immune deficiency syndrome (AIDS) or radiation pericarditis.[24]

The role of imaging is to confirm the presence and extent of fluid, to characterize the nature of fluid, to rule out pericardial inflammation, to determine its hemodynamic impact and to guide pericardiocentesis. Echocardiography is generally the first imaging modality used because of high sensitivity, specificity, easy availability and low cost **(Fig. 6A)**. Limited acoustic window may impair the utility of this modality in many cases. With the exception of transesophageal echocardiography, it is not a reliable technique for estimating pericardial thickness and in assessment of loculated pericardial effusions. CT and MR provide a wider field of view and are superior in detecting the amount, nature and distribution of the fluid. Focal fluid accumulation may be seen posterolateral to the left ventricle and along the inferolateral wall of the right ventricle owing to their dependent locations. Superior pericardial recess is another common location of focal fluid accumulation.[19]

The size of a pericardial effusion may be semi-quantitatively assessed by the thickness of fluid anterior to the right ventricle. Pericardial width of >4 mm may be regarded as abnormal. Using criteria established by echocardiography, a pericardial effusion may be quantified as small (<5 mm); moderate (5–10 mm); or large (>10 mm).[24,25] On a chest radiograph, pericardial effusion is suspected when there is diffuse cardiac silhouette enlargement without specific chamber enlargement. Filling of the retrosternal space, enlargement of normal cardiac borders, development of "flask" configuration and bilateral hilar overlay may be seen in larger effusions **(Fig. 6B)**. On the lateral projection, "epicardial fat pad" sign is diagnostic of pericardial disease. This is positive when the anterior pericardial stripe, bordered by the epicardial fat and mediastinal fat on either side, is seen to be thicker than 2 mm. It may also be seen in the frontal view because of the presence of abundant fat between the pericardium and pleura at the cardiac apex. This is seen as a radiolucent stripe internal to and parallel to the left lower cardiac border.[19] Rapid increase in cardiac size also suggests presence of pericardial effusion. On a chest radiograph, pan chamber cardiac enlargement and large anterior mediastinal tumor may simulate pericardial effusion.

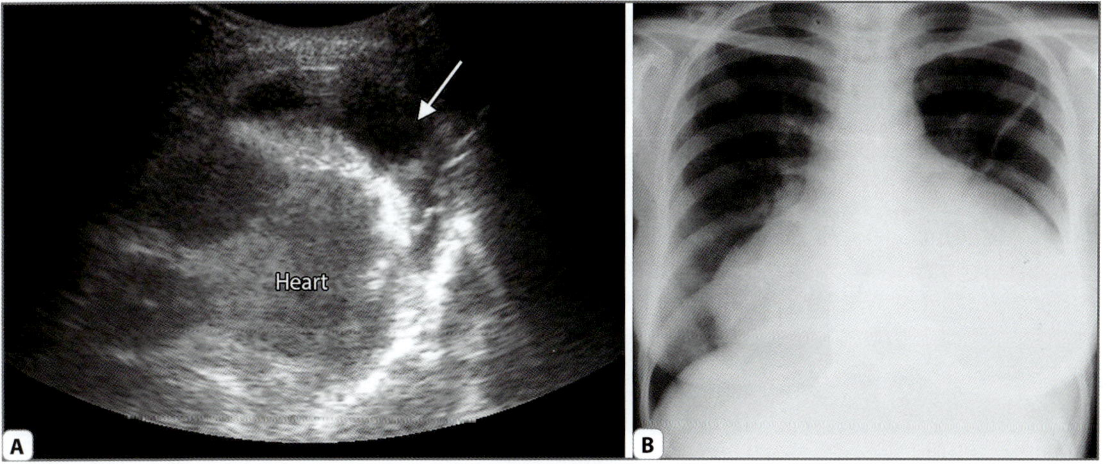

FIGS. 6A AND B: (A) Pericardial effusion. Ultrasound chest depicts fluid in the pericardial cavity (arrow); (B) Frontal chest radiograph shows enlarged "flask" shaped cardiac silhouette without specific chamber enlargement with bilateral hilum overlay sign.

On CT, the attenuation values of pericardial fluid are only of limited value. Serous effusions tend to have near-water attenuation values (<10 HU) **(Figs. 7A and B)**, while exudative effusions can range from 20 to 60 HU **(Figs. 7C and D)**. Chylopericardium can also present with low attenuation values but may be difficult to distinguish from transudative effusions. Acute hemopericardium can have attenuation values in the range of 60–80 HU, but if blood represents only a portion of the fluid, the attenuation values can then be similar to that of exudative effusions. High attenuation suggests hemopericardium in the history of trauma, surgery or aortic dissection. Generally, 30 HU is a useful cut off between simple effusions and bloody or proteinaceous effusions.[12] Pericardial enhancement can be seen in case of pericardial inflammation. It may sometimes be difficult to distinguish between pericardial effusion and thickening on CT which is better appreciated on echocardiography or MRI. Echocardiography is limited by poor acoustic window, location of effusion and characterization of pericardial effusion.

MRI may be performed to further characterize pericardial effusions. Transudates have a low signal intensity on T1-weighted images and high signal intensity on T2-weighted images and GRE cine images **(Figs. 8A and B)**. Exudates have a higher signal intensity on T1-weighted images and low signal intensity on T2-weighted images due to high cellularity and protein content within **(Figs. 9A and B)**. Hemopericardium is characterized by high signal on T1-weighted images and may be low signal on T2-weighted images and GRE cine images. Hemorrhage or infection should be suspected on cine imaging when the effusion fluid is clearly complex and inhomogeneous, containing regions of different signal intensity.[26,27] The gradient images may better characterize a hemopericardium as they facilitate the visualization of fibrinous strands and presence of coagulated blood. The T1 and T2 signal intensity of a hemorrhagic pericardial effusion is dependent on the duration of the hematoma. However, certain artifacts like non-linear motion of pericardial fluid during cardiac motion may falsely cause high signal on T1-weighted

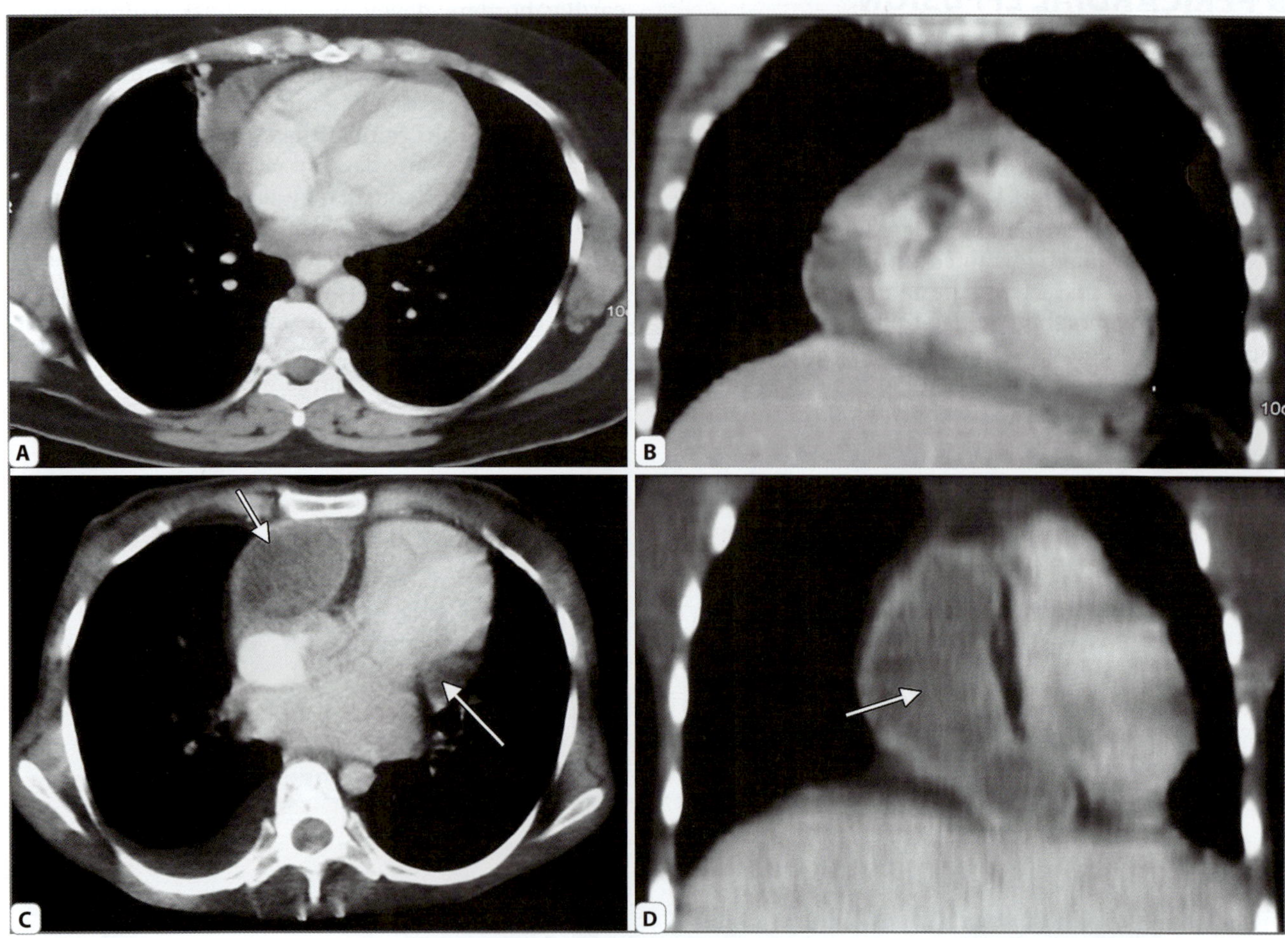

FIGS. 7A TO D: (A and B) Pericardial effusion. Axial CECT (A) and coronal reformatted (B) images show small simple pericardial effusion (HU = 10); (C and D) Exudative pericardial effusion. Axial CECT (C) and coronal reformatted (D) images show high attenuation loculated effusion (HU = 45) (arrows) in atrioventricular groove in a case of tubercular pericarditis.

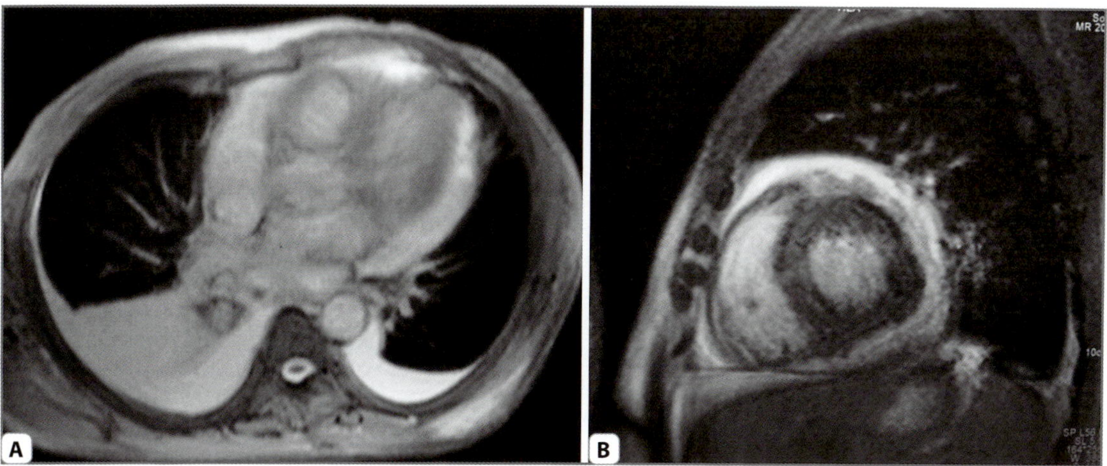

FIGS. 8A AND B: Pericardial effusion. Moderate simple effusion is seen on four chamber (A) and short axis; (B) cine SSFP images. Bilateral pleural effusions are also seen.

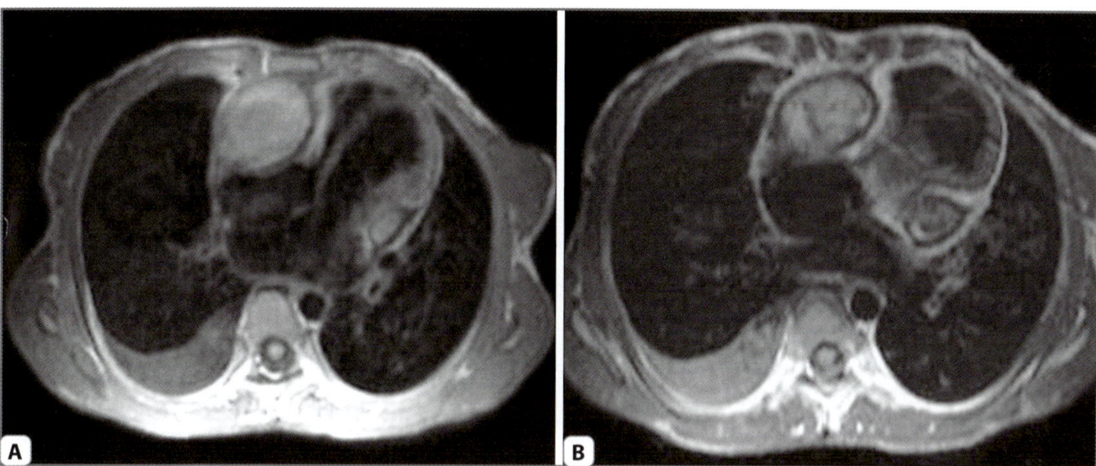

FIGS. 9A AND B: Exudative pericardial effusion. Axial dark blood T1 and T2-weighted images show exudative effusion in the atrioventricular groove and associated pericardial thickening. It is seen as high signal intensity on T1-weighted images (A) with complex and inhomogeneous signal intensity on T2-weighted images (B). Note made of right pleural effusion.

spin-echo CMR even within a transudative effusion.[12] Effusion secondary to malignancy may have associated pericardial thickening and nodularity. MR is superior to CT in differentiating pericardial effusion from thickening. The high signal intensity on cine and T2-weighted images allows to clearly distinguish between pericardial effusion and thickened pericardium which is low signal intensity on these sequences. Phase sensitive inversion recovery (PSIR) delayed enhancement imaging not only aids in assessing pericardial and myocardial inflammation but can also help in distinguishing dark appearing pericardial fluid from bright epicardial fat on this sequence.

CARDIAC TAMPONADE (BOX 4)

Slow accumulation of pericardial fluid may cause adaptive expansion of the pericardium with accumulation of up to 3 L of fluid without significant hemodynamic consequence.[28] However, in cases of rapid accumulation, as little as 100–200 mL of fluid may result in an effusion under tension or cardiac tamponade, especially if the pericardium has limited compliance owing to pericardial inflammation/scarring.[20] The resultant increased pericardial pressure is then transmitted to the cardiac chambers. Cardiac

BOX 4: Cardiac tamponade.

- Life-threatening condition requiring urgent intervention
- Causes include trauma, cardiac surgery, inflammation, pericardial neoplasm, aortic dissection
- Speed of fluid accumulation key determinant of symptoms
- Primarily a Clinical diagnosis, in combination with findings on echocardiography
- Role of CT and MR limited to atypical/chronic cases

tamponade is a low cardiac output state due to excessive fluid in the pericardial space that compresses the heart, especially the right ventricle. Owing to decreased filling of the right ventricle, tamponade can result in life-threatening hemodynamic compromise. Diagnosis is primarily clinical. It is based on clinical criteria in combination with hemodynamic findings on echocardiography that can depict collapse of right ventricular free wall during diastolic phase, right atrial collapse during late diastole/ systole, paradoxic motion of the interventricular septum, greater respiratory variations and distended hepatic veins and inferior vena cava due to back flow. "Flow velocity paradoxus" refers to increased flow across tricuspid and pulmonic valves and decreased flow across mitral and aortic valves during inspiration.

CT and MR have a limited role in the evaluation of acute cardiac tamponade; only long standing or less severe forms may sometimes be seen. CT and MRI may be helpful in nonemergent situations when echocardiographic findings are equivocal. The heart size, excluding the pericardial space is normal or decreased. This is contrary to restrictive cardiomyopathy and pericardial constriction in which the atria are typically enlarged.[3,5] The cavae and hepatic veins which are exterior to the pericardium dilate to accommodate back pooling of blood. Eventually, if pericardial pressure exceeds the ability of the circulation to fill the heart, the right sided cardiac chambers collapse.[5] Leftward bowing of the interventricular septum is a nonspecific finding that may be seen in any condition with right side volume or pressure overload.

Cine CT and MRI can show the dynamic features suggestive of tamponade. There is collapse of the right ventricular free wall in early diastole and collapse of the right atrial free wall in early systole. This is because in early diastole less blood is present in the right ventricle than in the right atrium, and so, the right ventricle has the least pressure to counteract the pressure of the pericardial effusion. In early systole, the right atrium has less blood than the right ventricle, so the right atrium has less pressure. This collapse is especially evident during expiration which decreases the right heart filling. Throughout the cardiac cycle there is enhanced ventricular coupling from the taut pericardial space. This most often manifests as abnormal motion of the intraventricular septum. This is seen on cine images as septal rocking or sigmoid septum configuration. The diastolic dysfunction characteristic of tamponade is also well-evaluated on cine images.[5]

When cardiac tamponade is atypical, CT and MR may be better than echocardiography. In these unusual situations, the effusions tend to be loculated and exert mass effect on a part of the heart not well-visualized by transthoracic echocardiography, including the right atrium and left atrium. Oftentimes, these effusions are malignant, postradiation, or postinfectious.

PERICARDITIS

Nonconstrictive Pericarditis (Box 5)

Pericarditis is an inflammatory response of the pericardium which may be a result of various conditions, which include infectious, noninfectious and idiopathic causes **(Table 2)**. Most of the idiopathic causes may be viral in etiology, occurring weeks after the viral infection, secondary to an immune response to the infection. After myocardial infarction, pericarditis may occur in the first few days or less commonly a few weeks later secondary to inflammatory response to cardiac proteins. The latter is known as Dressler syndrome and can present with fever and pericardial friction rub.

In acute pericarditis, the pericardium may develop a small effusion and become slightly thickened. On contrast enhanced CT and MRI, acute pericarditis shows enhancement of the pericardium, which can show smooth thickening (>4 mm) **(Fig. 10)**. Enhancement is better appreciated in the venous phase than in the arterial phase of contrast administration. Associated small effusion may or may not be seen. There are accompanying inflammatory changes in the pericardial fat which may be increased or stranded. The absence of these findings does not exclude the diagnosis. On CT imaging, it may sometimes be

BOX 5: Nonconstrictive pericarditis.

- Inflammatory response of pericardium involving pericardial thickening and effusion
- Enhancement of pericardium can be seen
- Findings may be localized to part of pericardium
- No features of constriction

TABLE 2: Causes of pericarditis.

Infectious	• Viral • Bacterial (*Mycobacterium tuberculosis* most common) • Fungal • Parasitic
Noninfectious	• Post cardiac injury • Systemic inflammatory disorders (systemic lupus erythematosus, rheumatoid arthritis, scleroderma) • Drug reaction • Radiation • Metabolic conditions (chronic renal disease) • Pericardial trauma • Surgery • Malignancy

difficult to differentiate a small effusion from pericardial thickening which may be resolved on echocardiography. Also, care needs to be taken for assessment of pericardium in its entirety as the findings may only be localized. The presence of myopericarditis on imaging increases the risk of complications. On follow-up, the findings may resolve or progress to scarring.

Pericarditis secondary to tuberculosis, radiation, chronic renal failure, systemic inflammatory disorders, trauma and surgery is more likely to become chronic than viral or drug related pericarditis.

In chronic inflammatory pericarditis, there is development of fibrosis, adhesions and calcification. The effusion may increase or pericardium can get more thickened. The thickened pericardium may show calcification and irregular contour. On MRI, the pericardium is thickened, irregular with variable early enhancement. Delayed enhancement is seen owing to fibrosis. Tagging sequence in MRI can be used to detect adhesions, in which case the grid lines remain intact **(Figs. 11A to C)**. MRI cannot show calcification as well as seen on CT. Fibrous/calcific pericarditis may be asymptomatic or can lead to constrictive pericarditis.[1,29]

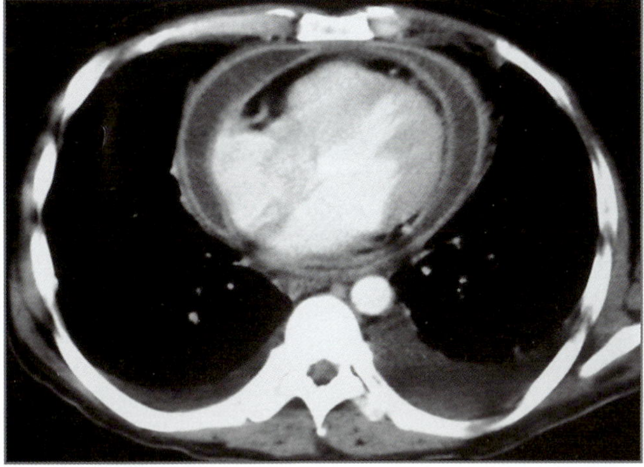

FIG. 10: Nonconstrictive pericarditis. Axial CECT shows enhancing thickened smooth pericardium with associated effusion in a known case of tuberculosis. Bilateral pleural effusions are also seen.

Constrictive Pericarditis (Box 6)

Constrictive pericarditis is a condition in which cardiac function is impaired by a thickened, rigid and often calcified pericardium. This results in diastolic dysfunction of the heart and subsequent right heart failure. Clinical symptoms and radiological concordance are required to make this diagnosis. It can clinically mimic restrictive cardiomyopathy, hepatic disease, and congestive heart failure. The distinction between constrictive pericarditis and restrictive cardiomyopathy is very important, since the former would benefit from pericardial stripping and the latter would not. Constrictive pericarditis may be secondary to prior surgery, infection, trauma, radiation, uremia, connective tissue disorder, neoplasm or may be

BOX 6: Constrictive pericarditis.

- Reduced pericardial compliance leading to diastolic dysfunction
- Causes include infection, radiation exposure, prior surgery, trauma and postoperative setting
- *Morphological findings*:
  - Pericardial thickening, calcification, enhancement
  - Tubular shape of ventricles
  - Compression of right sided chambers
  - Sigmoid shaped ventricular septum
  - Atrial enlargement
  - Dilated hepatic veins/IVC
  - Pleural effusion, ascites
- *Findings on functional evaluation*:
  - Septal bounce on cine MRI
  - MR tagging technique—tag lines remain unbroken in case of pericardial adhesions
- Dynamic MRI findings help distinguish constrictive pericarditis from restrictive cardiomyopathy

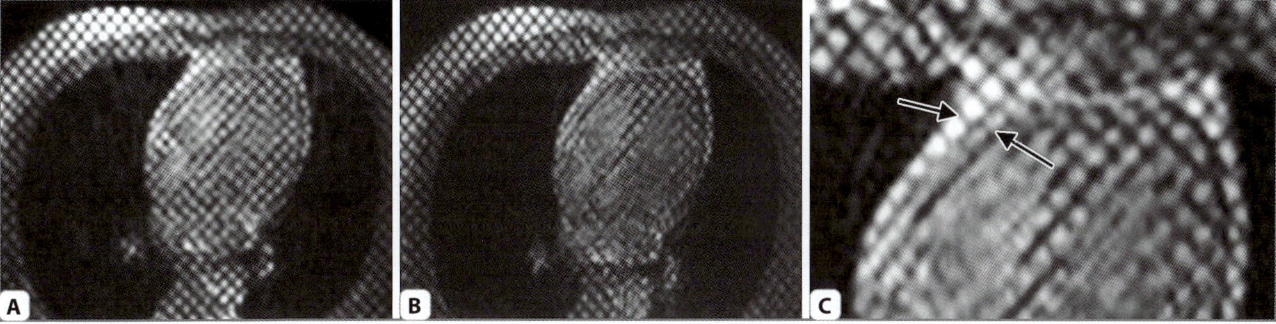

FIGS. 11A TO C: GRE tagging MRI in a healthy volunteer in axial plane. The continuity of the tags is lost during cardiac contraction because of shear motion between visceral and parietal layer of the pericardium [seen on the enlarged view (C)].

idiopathic. It is more often a sequel to purulent and tubercular pericarditis than viral amongst infectious causes.[30] In addition to diastolic dysfunction, there is ventricular interdependence where volume increase in one ventricle results in decrease in volume in the other ventricle.

Echocardiography is the initial modality used. However, if findings are equivocal, additional imaging may then be required using CT and MRI. Both morphological and functional hemodynamic aspects aid in the diagnosis. CT and MRI findings center on the demonstration of global or focal thickened or calcified pericardium which is usually greater over the right ventricle, along with secondary morphologic signs of constriction. These include a conical or tubular shape of the ventricles, compression of the right-sided cardiac chambers, sigmoid-shaped interventricular septum, enlargement of the atria, narrowing of the atrioventricular grooves and large inferior and superior vena cava in comparison with descending aorta[30-32] **(Fig. 12)**. The absence of pericardial thickening does not rule out pericardial constriction.

Delayed pericardial enhancement is usually seen owing to presence of fibrosis (>70 seconds postcontrast imaging). A small amount of pericardial effusion may also be seen. Calcification of the pericardium is better visualized on CT and strongly suggests constriction of tubercular etiology.[13] Other causes of pericardial calcification include viral, uremic pericarditis, collagen vascular disease, postoperative setting, radiation exposure and asbestosis. However, the presence of constriction and calcification are not always related. Atrial dilatation may or may not be seen depending on whether the entire pericardium is abnormal or just the anterior part. This is an insensitive finding as patients with restrictive cardiomyopathy may also demonstrate atrial dilatation. Pleural effusions, hepatic congestion, and ascites are the other non-specific findings. It should be remembered that the diagnosis of pericardial constriction is made only in the appropriate clinical setting.[33,34]

Since the diagnosis of constriction is ultimately that of altered physiology, cine imaging is a more direct means of confirming the diagnosis. The most sensitive and specific

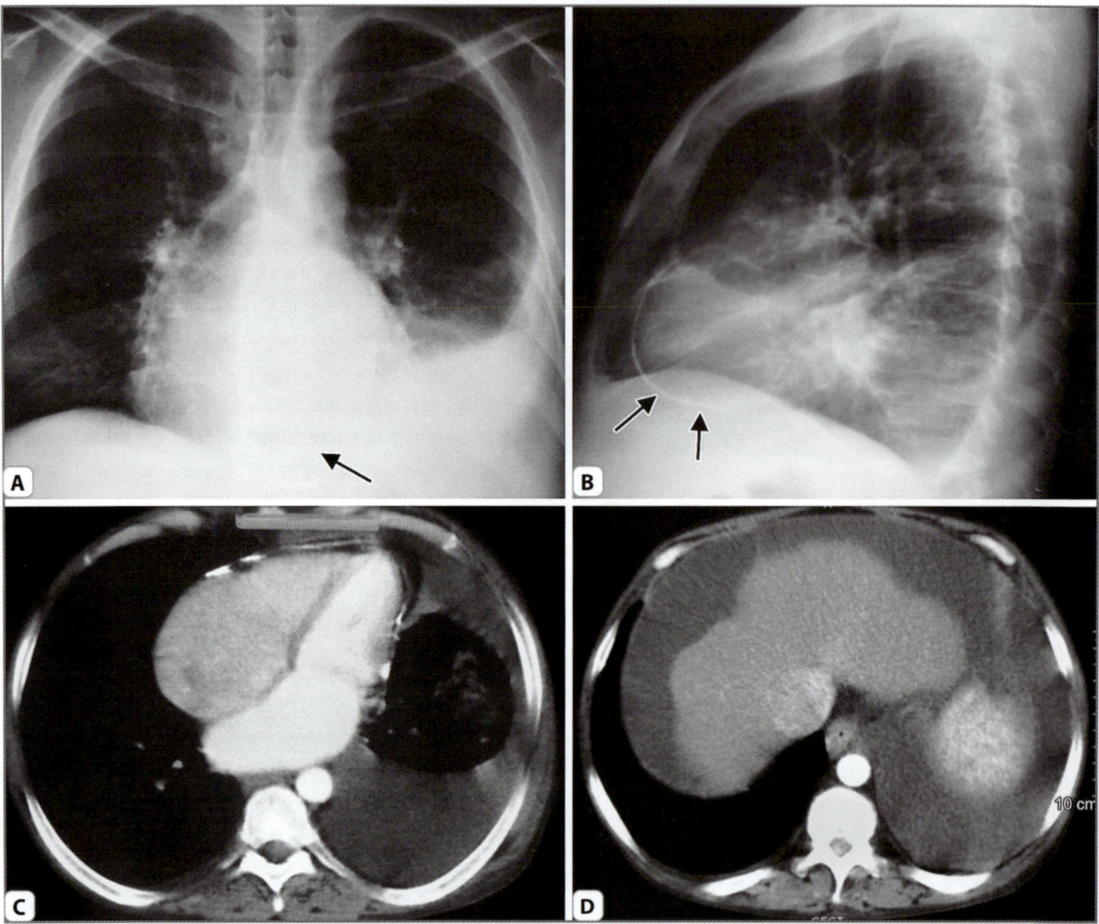

FIGS. 12A TO D: Calcific constrictive pericarditis. In a patient with distant history of tuberculosis, posteroanterior (A) and lateral (B) chest radiographs demonstrate curvilinear calcification (arrows) along the lower left and diaphragmatic cardiac border; (C and D) Axial CECT shows global pericardial thickening with calcification. The ventricles are tubular shaped with dilated atria and IVC. Associated left pleural effusion and ascites noted. Liver appears congested with irregular outline suggestive of cardiac cirrhosis.

finding is the septal bounce, seen on retrospectively gated cine MRI or cardiac CT angiography. In early diastole, the pressure in the right ventricle is transiently higher than the left, causing the septum to bow leftward due to ventricular interdependence **(Fig. 13)**. When the left ventricular pressure once again becomes higher, it pushes the septum rightward; the result is shivering of the ventricular septum or septal bounce.[1] Although septal bounce may be seen in other conditions, it is highly pronounced in constrictive pericarditis.

Septal bounce is most pronounced during inspiration, as the negative intrathoracic pressure results in more rapid right heart filling than the left. On expiration, there is increased pulmonary venous return as the intrathoracic pressure increases, septum appears relatively normal. Respiratory variations of the diastolic septal bounce can be assessed using non-gated free breathing on MRI. This technique aids in differentiating constrictive pericarditis from restrictive cardiomyopathy.[4,33-35]

Underlying myocardium also needs to be evaluated in cases of constrictive pericarditis as the presence of the myocardial factor (myocardial atrophy or fibrosis) is a contraindication to pericardiectomy, because of the risk of acute dilatation or rupture of one or both cardiac chambers following surgery.[28] Imaging also aids in planning surgery. The presence of a fat plane between the myocardium and pericardium indicates easier dissection.[36]

There are atypical forms of constrictive pericarditis. *Effusive constrictive pericarditis* is a rare variant that represents a combination of pericardial tamponade and constrictive pericarditis. Large pericardial effusion is seen along with features of noncompliant pericardium. This is seen most often following radiation therapy. The typical clinical setting is that pericardial effusion is identified in a patient with symptoms of heart failure and despite drainage of the effusion, the patient continues to have abnormal pericardial dynamics. *Transient or inflammatory constrictive pericarditis* results often secondary to viral insult which may result in transient constrictive physiology.[16] There is accompanying active inflammation of the pericardium. Increased T2 signal with prominent late gadolinium enhancement suggests actively inflamed pericardium. Normal T2 signal with increased late gadolinium enhancement is suggestive of subacute form while normal T2 signal and no late gadolinium enhancement represents chronic phase.

Focal pericarditis may result in constriction if present in strategic location. *Occult constrictive pericarditis* refers to presence of constriction only when there is volume overload and not on routine examination **(Fig. 13)**.

PNEUMOPERICARDIUM

Pneumopericardium may result from blunt or penetrating trauma. Other rarer causes may be infectious pericarditis or from a gastrointestinal fistula, increased intrathoracic pressure as in asthma or barotrauma in intubated patients, with adjacent lung infection/cancer, esophageal rupture, cocaine abuse or liver abscess rupture. Pneumopericardium following pneumothorax or pneumomediastinum usually indicates a disruption of the pericardium. On erect chest radiographs, it is seen as a radiolucent band around the heart ("halo sign") limited superiorly by the pericardial reflection at the root of great vessels **(Fig. 14)**. Air may be seen in the transverse pericardial sinus giving the "transverse band of air" sign. Lateral radiographs may show lucency of air behind the sternum and anterior to the base of heart and root of aorta ("triangle of air" sign).[37,38] In the setting of penetrating trauma, the presence of pneumopericardium should prompt investigation for potential cardiac laceration. Rarely, tension pneumopericardium may result in tamponade. This may be seen as a progressively decreasing cardiothoracic ratio. CT shows distension of SVC, IVC, hepatic veins, renal veins and periportal lymphedema.

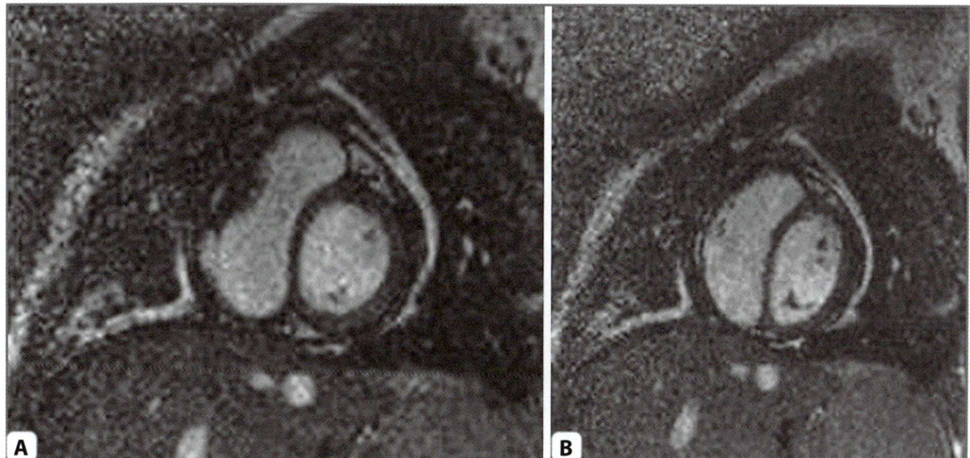

FIGS. 13A AND B: Short axis cine MR images in a patient with constrictive pericarditis in systole (A) and diastole (B) show straightening of the interventricular septum in diastole indicative of impaired right ventricular filling. Pericardium is focally thickened posterior to the left ventricle.

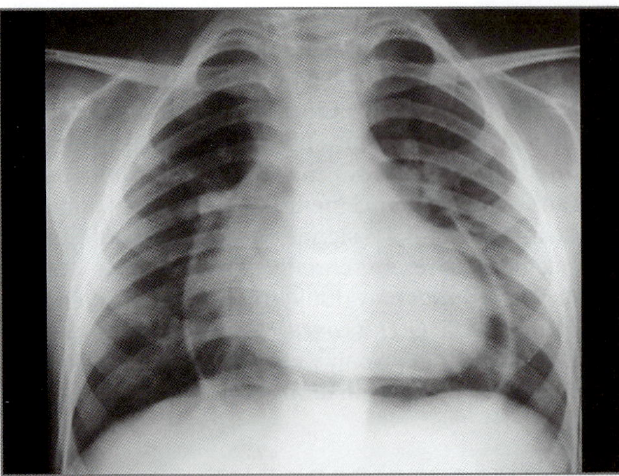

FIG. 14: Pneumopericardium. Posteroanterior chest radiograph shows radiolucent band of air surrounding the heart giving the "halo sign".

PERICARDIAL TUMORS

Metastases (Box 7)

Metastases to the pericardium are more common than involvement of pericardium by primary tumors.

Metastases to the heart and pericardium have been reported at autopsy in 10–12% of patients with known primary malignancies.[4,11] Pericardial metastases may result from contiguous spread from lung or mediastinum. Other modes may be lymphatic, hematogenous or transvenous route. The common sources of pericardial metastases are lung and breast cancer. Leukemias, lymphomas and melanomas are the other malignancies that can spread to the pericardium. Pericardial metastases when seen are a negative prognostic factor.

An effusion is the most common manifestation of metastatic pericardial disease. Pericardium can get irregularly thickened, and nodularity or tumor deposits may be seen. To distinguish between inflammatory etiology and metastases (when effusion and thickening are the only findings), follow-up may be required. With metastatic involvement, pericardium may be diffusely involved encasing the heart or there may be enhancement of portions of pericardium. Direct pericardial invasion may be suggested when the pericardial line is not seen between the adjacent primary mass and the pericardium and there is pericardial effusion. However, pericardium may remain intact adjacent to a primary lung mass. In these cases, hemorrhagic effusion, seen as high-signal on spin echo MR images confirms the extension of the mass to the pericardium **(Figs. 15A and B)**.[39] On MRI, most deposits show low-signal on T1 and high-signal on T2-weighted images. Metastatic melanoma is an exception; high-signal intensity on T1-weighted images is virtually pathognomonic of this diagnosis. The malignant tumor usually enhances significantly after the administration of contrast material. In a patient with a known primary tumor and pericardial effusion, other differential diagnoses are drug-induced and radiation-induced effusions.

BOX 7: Pericardial metastases.

- Metastases are commoner than primary pericardial tumors
- *Mode of spread to pericardium*:
  - Direct spread
  - Lymphatic
  - Hematogenous
  - Transvenous
- *Imaging findings include*:
  - Pericardial effusion
  - Pericardial thickening
  - Pericardial mass
- Hemorrhagic pericardial effusion adjacent to a lung/mediastinal mass is suggestive of pericardial invasion

Primary Pericardial Tumors

Primary pericardial tumors are rare and are more likely to be malignant than primary cardiac tumors. Pericardial tumors include benign tumors (lipoma, benign teratoma, fibroma, and hemangioma) and malignant tumors (mesothelioma, lymphoma, sarcoma and liposarcoma, malignant teratoma). Although pericardial mesotheliomas are rare tumors accounting for less than 1% of all malignant mesotheliomas, they account for nearly half of primary pericardial tumors.[39]

Chest radiography in patients with pericardial mesothelioma typically demonstrates cardiac enlargement, evidence of pericardial effusion, an irregular cardiac contour or diffuse mediastinal enlargement. In the early stage of disease, CT and MR may only show pericardial thickening and complex effusion which can mimic chronic pericarditis. Later in the disease, enhancing masses may be seen. Pericardial mesothelioma carries a very poor prognosis.

Lymphoma and sarcoma typically present with large masses accompanied by effusion. Most lymphomas occur secondary to systemic disease. Primary pericardial lymphoma may also be encountered, presenting as diffuse infiltration or a solitary mass. Rarely, there may be effusion without soft tissue mass in primary effusion lymphoma.

Most intrapericardial germ cell tumors are benign tumors, although malignant teratomas may be encountered in the pediatric population as a heterogeneous mass.

Histopathology is usually necessary to achieve a definitive diagnosis of most pericardial tumors. The diagnosis of few tumors can be aided by specific signal and attenuation characteristics. Lipoma has low attenuation on CT images and high signal intensity on T1-weighted SE images. Presence of calcium or fat in a pericardial mass on CT suggests the diagnosis of a teratoma. Fibroma characteristically has low signal intensity on T2-weighted images with poor enhancement characteristics.[40,41]

Other entities that may simulate a pericardial mass are pericardial hematoma, lymphatic malformation, coronary artery aneurysm and pericardial gossypiboma.[5,19] The signal

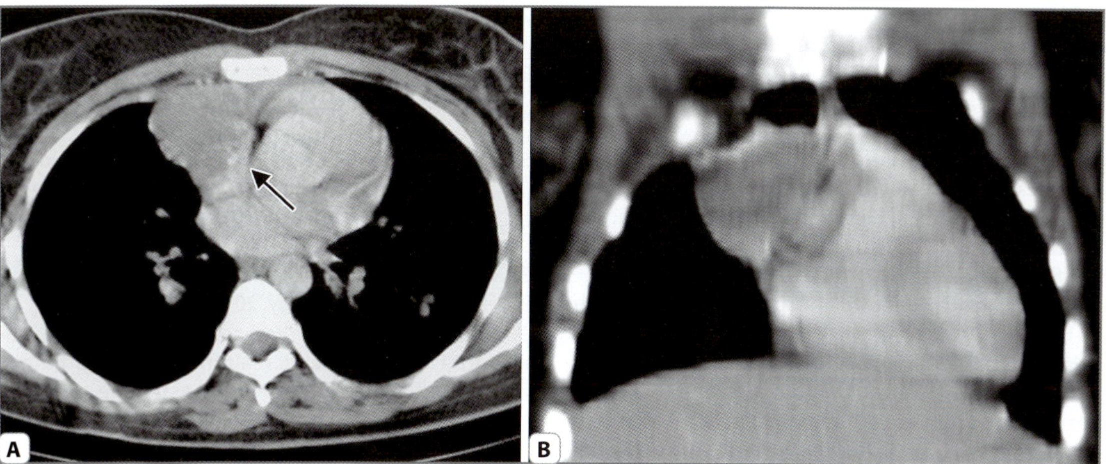

FIGS. 15A AND B: Axial CECT (A) and coronal reformation (arrow); (B) shows thymic carcinoma with direct invasion of the pericardium.

characteristics of pericardial hematoma are age related. Lymphatic malformation is seen as a nonenhancing fluid attenuation serpiginous lesion with internal septations (septations are usually absent in a pericardial cyst). There is no surrounding invasion. A coronary artery aneurysm should be suspected when a smooth enhancing mass is seen along the expected course of a coronary artery. Pericardial gossypiboma should be considered in a patient with previous cardiac surgery.

CONCLUSION

Congenital disease, infection, injury, neoplasm may all affect the pericardium. Although echocardiography is often initially used to evaluate the pericardium, CT and MR are useful for further evaluation of the disease processes. Integrated role of multiple imaging modalities helps establish the diagnosis in the appropriate clinical setting and facilitates management decisions.

REFERENCES

1. Fadl SA, Nasrullah A, Harris A, Edwards R, Kicska G. Comprehensive review of pericardial diseases using different imaging modalities. Int J Cardiovasc Imaging. 2020;36(5):947-69.
2. Gulati G, Sharma S, Kothari SS, et al. Comparison of echo and MRI in the imaging evaluation of intracardiac masses. Cardiovasc Intervent Radiol. 2004;27(5):459-69.
3. Grizzard JG, Ang GB. Magnetic resonance imaging of pericardial disease and cardiac masses. Magn Reson Imaging Clin N Am. 2007;15:579-607.
4. Ünal E, Karcaaltincaba M, Akpinar E, Ariyurek OM. The imaging appearances of various pericardial disorders. Insights Imaging. 2019;10(1):42.
5. Misselt AJ, Harris SR, Glockner J, Feng D, Syed IS, Araoz PA. MR imaging of the pericardium. Magn Reson Imaging Clin N Am. 2008;16:185-99.
6. Budoff MJ, Achenbach S, Blumenthal RS, et al. Assessment of coronary artery disease by cardiac computed tomography: A scientific statement from the American Heart Association Committee on Cardiovascular Imaging and Intervention, Council on Cardiovascular Radiology and Intervention, and Committee on Cardiac Imaging, Council on Clinical Cardiology. Circulation. 2006;114(16):1761-91.
7. Coles DR, Smail MA, Negus IS, et al. Comparison of radiation doses from multislice computed tomography coronary angiography and conventional diagnostic angiography. J Am Coll Cardiol. 2006;47(9):1840-5.
8. Wang ZJ, Reddy GP, Gotway MB, Yeh BM, Hetts SW, Higgins CB. CT and MR imaging of pericardial disease. Radiographics. 2003;23:S167-80.
9. Adler Y, Charron P, Imazio M, Badano L, Barón-Esquivias G, Bogaert J, et al. 2015 ESC Guidelines for the diagnosis and management of pericardial diseases: The Task Force for the Diagnosis and Management of Pericardial Diseases of the European Society of Cardiology (ESC) Endorsed by: The European Association for Cardio-Thoracic Surgery (EACTS). Eur Heart J. 2015;36(42):2921-64.
10. Klein AL, Abbara S, Agler DA, Appleton CP, Asher CR, Hoit B, et al. American Society of Echocardiography clinical recommendations for multimodality cardiovascular imaging of patients with pericardial disease: endorsed by the Society for Cardiovascular Magnetic Resonance and Society of Cardiovascular Computed Tomography. J Am Soc Echocardiogr. 2013;26(9):965-1012.
11. Rajiah P, Canan A, Saboo SS, Restrepo CS, Bolen MA. MRI of the Pericardium. Radiographics. 2019;39(7):1921-2.
12. Lopez Costa I, Bhalla S. Computed tomography and magnetic resonance imaging of the pericardium. Semin Roentgenol. 2008;43(3):234-45.
13. Truong MT, Erasmus JJ, Gladish GW, Sabloff BS, Marom EM, et al. Anatomy of pericardial recesses on multidetector CT: Implications for oncologic imaging. AJR Am J Roentgenol. 2003;181:1109-13.

14. Delille JP, Hernigou A, Sene V, et al. Maximal thickness of the normal human pericardium assessed by electron-beam computed tomography. Eur J Radiol. 1999;9:1183-89.
15. Oyama N, Oyama N, Komuro K, Nambu T, Manning W, Miyasaka K. Computed tomography and magnetic resonance imaging of the pericardium: anatomy and pathology. Magnetic Resonance in Medical Sciences. 2004;3(3):145-52.
16. Chetrit M, Xu B, Verma BR, Klein AL. Multimodality Imaging for the Assessment of Pericardial Diseases. Curr Cardiol Rep. 2019;21(5):41.
17. Kligerman S. Imaging of Pericardial Disease. Radiol Clin North Am. 2019;57(1):179-99.
18. Broderick LS, Brooks GN, Kuhlman JE. Anatomic pitfalls of the heart and pericardium. Radiographics. 2005;25:441-53.
19. Bogaert J, Francone M. Cardiovascular Magnetic resonance in pericardial diseases. J Cardiovasc Magn Reson. 2009;11(1):14.
20. O' Leary SM, Williams PL, Williams MP. et al. Imaging the pericardium: appearances on ECG – gated 64 detector row cardiac computed tomography. BJR. 2010;83:194-205.
21. Van Son JA, Danielson GK, Schaff HV, et al. Congenital partial and complete absence of the pericardium. Mayo Clin Proc. 1993;68(8):743-47.
22. Ellis K, Leeds NE, Himmelstein A. Congenital deficiencies in partial pericardium: Review with two new cases including successful diagnosis by plain roentgenography. AJR Am J Roentgenol. 1959;82:125-37.
23. Psychidis-Papakyritsis P, de Roos A, Kroft LJM. Functional MRI of congenital absence of the pericardium. Am J Roentgenol. 2007;189:W312-4.
24. Rajiah P. Cardiac MRI: Part 2, Pericardial disease. AJR. 2011;197:W621-34.
25. Czum Jm, Silas AM, Althoen MC. Evaluation of the pericardium with CT and MR. ISRN cardiology 2014 :2014:174908.
26. Glockner JF. Imaging of pericardial disease. Magn Reson Imaging Clin N Am. 2003;11(1):149-62, vii.
27. Yared K, Baggish AL, Picard MH, Hoffmann U, Hang J. Multimodality imaging of pericardial disease. JACC Cardiovasc Imaging. 2010;3(6):650-60.
28. Rienmuller R, Groll R, Lipton MJ. CT and MR imaging of pericardial disease. Radiol Clin North Am. 2004;42(3):587-601.
29. Kim JS, Kim HH, Yoon Y. Imaging of pericardial diseases. Clinical Radiol. 2007;62:626-31.
30. Imazio M, Brucato A, Maestroni S, et al. Risk of constrictive pericarditis after acute pericardiectomy. Circulation. 2011;124(11):1270-5.
31. Suh SY, Rha SW, Kim JW, et al. The usefulness of three-dimensional multidetector computed tomography to delineate pericardial calcification in constrictive pericarditis. Int J Cardiol. 2006;113:414-16.
32. Bogaert J, Francone M. Pericardial disease: Value of CT and MR imaging. Radiology. 2012;267(2):340-56.
33. Thavendiranathan P, Verhaert D, Wall MC, et al. Simultaneous right and left heart realtime, free-breathing CMR flow quantification indentifies constrictive physiology. JACC Cardiovasc Imaging. 2012;(1):15-24.
34. Verheart D, Gabriel RS, Johnston D, Lytle BW, Desai, MY Klein AL. The role of multimodality imaging in the management of pericardial disease. Circ Cardiovasc Imaging. 2010;3(3): 333-43.
35. Francone M, Dymarkowski S, Kalantzi M, et al. Realtime cine MRI of ventricular septal motion: A novel approach to assess ventricular coupling. J Magn Reson Imaging. 2005;21(3): 305-9.
36. Westwood MA, Moon JC. Cardiovascular magnetic resonance for pericardial disease. Indian J Radiol Imaging. 2007;17(2):133-6.
37. Ho ML, Gutierrez FR. Chest radiography in thoracic polytrauma. AJR Am J Roentgenol. 2009;192:599-612.
38. Mirvis SE. Imaging of acute thoarcic injury: The advent of MDCT screening. Semin Ultrasound CT MRI. 2005;26:305-31.
39. Grebenc ML, Christenson MLR, Burke AP, et al. Primary cardiac and pericardial neoplasms: radiologic-pathologic correlation. Radiographics. 2000;20:1073.
40. Fussen S, De Boeck BW, Zellweger MJ, et al. Cardiovascular magnetic resonance imaging for diagnosis and clinical management of suspected cardiac masses and tumours. Eur Heart J. 2011;32(12):1551-60.
41. Hoffmann U, Globits S, Frank H. Cardiac and paracardiac masses: Current opinion on diagnostic evaluation by magnetic resonance imaging. Eur Heart J. 1998;19:553-63.

Manphool Singhal, Arun Sharma, Sanjeev Kumar

CHAPTER

30

Imaging and Interventions of Aorta

INTRODUCTION

The word "Aorta" is derived from *Latin* word: aorta, and *Greek*: aorte which means "a strap to hang (something by)". This term was first used by Aristotle while describing the aorta: how it seems to be "suspended" above the heart.[1] The function of the aorta has been documented since the ancient times of Bible and Talmud, where it was noted as one of three major vessels entering or leaving the heart, and how its perforation was linked to death.[2]

The aorta is the largest artery in the body which carries oxygenated blood from the left ventricle to various organs of the body. It also functions both as a conduit and a reservoir. Its viscoelastic and compliance properties are responsible for the laminar blood flow during systole and modulate continued forward flow during diastole.[3]

Aorta is an elastic artery and its wall consists of:

- *Intima*: A thin endothelial layer
- *Media*: The thickest layer consisting of smooth muscles, collagen and elastic fibers.
- *Adventitia*: The outermost layer of collagen and elastic fibers also containing vasa vasorum, nerves and lymphatics.

SEGMENTATION ANATOMY OF AORTA

Aorta is divided into the following parts **(Figs. 1A and B)**:

- *Root*: Comprises of three aortic sinuses and extending from aortic valve to sinotubular junction where it becomes the ascending aorta.
- *Ascending aorta*: Extends from sinotubular junction to the origin of brachiocephalic artery.
- *Arch of aorta*: Extends from the origin of brachiocephalic artery to the origin of left subclavian artery.
- *Descending aorta*: Extends beyond the origin of left subclavian artery till aortic bifurcation at L4 level into common iliac arteries. It is further divided into thoracic

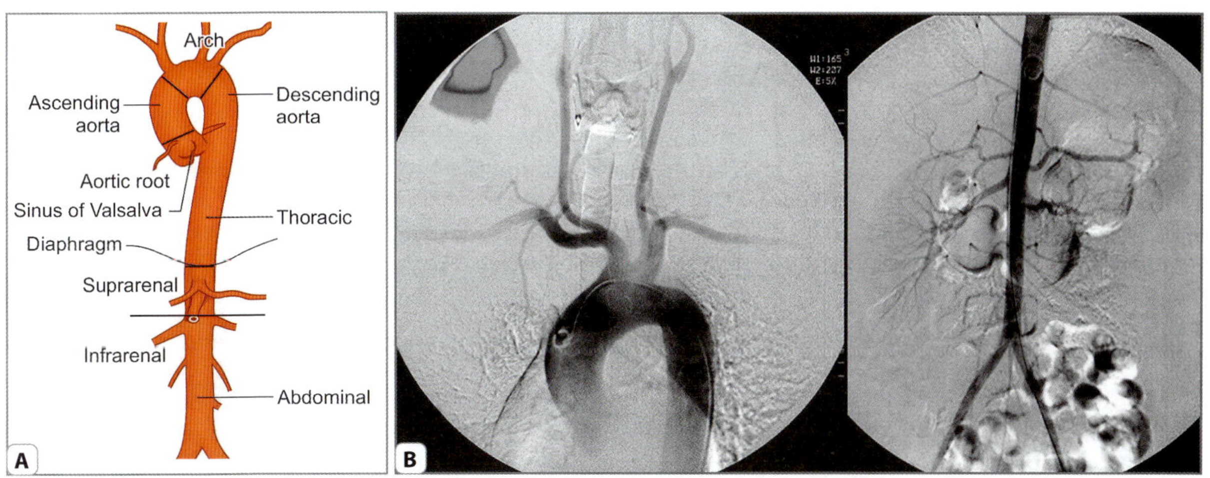

FIGS.1A AND B: (A) Segmentation anatomy of aorta. (B) Normal angiographic anatomy: Arch and abdominal aortogram (DSA) shows normal branches.

and abdominal portions by the diaphragm, where the aorta passes through the aortic hiatus at D12 level.

A normal narrowing may be present just distal to the left subclavian artery and proximal to ligamentum arteriosum called *isthmus*. Just beyond it, there may be a focal dilatation of the aorta, known as *aortic spindle*.

IMAGING OF AORTA: BASICS

Radiological evaluation of the anatomy and the pathology involving the aorta has undergone considerable refinement in recent years, which has been possible largely due to availability of multidetector CT (MDCT), dual source CT (DSCT) scanners and higher strength newer magnetic resonance imaging (MRI) and advanced software's. These modalities have largely replaced traditional contrast aortography.[4] Technological advances such as isotropic data acquisition with three-dimensional reconstruction capabilities, shorter acquisition times, improvement in processing and volume rendering have made it possible to visualize the aorta and its branches precisely. As a result, the role of catheter angiography is being restricted to special indications and to patients who may require catheter-based interventions.[5]

Angiographic Anatomy

The aorta is broadly divided into thoracic and abdominal aorta **(Fig. 1)**. The thoracic aorta begins at the aortic root just cranial to the aortic valve as the ascending aorta. It courses superiorly and to the left until the origin of the right brachiocephalic trunk where the aortic arch begins. The aortic arch continues cranially and posteriorly and gives rise to the left common carotid and left subclavian arteries. At this point, the aorta turns caudally and posterior to form the descending thoracic aorta. A normal narrowing called the *isthmus* may be present just distal to the left subclavian artery and proximal to the ligamentum arteriosum. The isthmus is commonly present in younger individuals and may be focal or extended over a long distance with a mild dilatation beyond it. It may form a small diverticulum called the *ductus diverticulum* **(Fig. 2)**. The descending thoracic aorta continues caudally in the posterior mediastinum slightly on the left side, anterolateral to the spine and posterolateral to the esophagus. It passes through the diaphragmatic hiatus at D12 level where it continues in the retroperitoneum on the left side as the abdominal aorta up to the iliac bifurcation. With age, the aorta shows enlargement of its diameter and tends to follow a more tortuous course.

The major branches which arise from the aorta are as follows:

- *Ascending aorta*: Right and left coronary arteries
- *Aortic arch*: Right brachiocephalic trunk (right subclavian and right common carotid artery), left common carotid artery and left subclavian artery

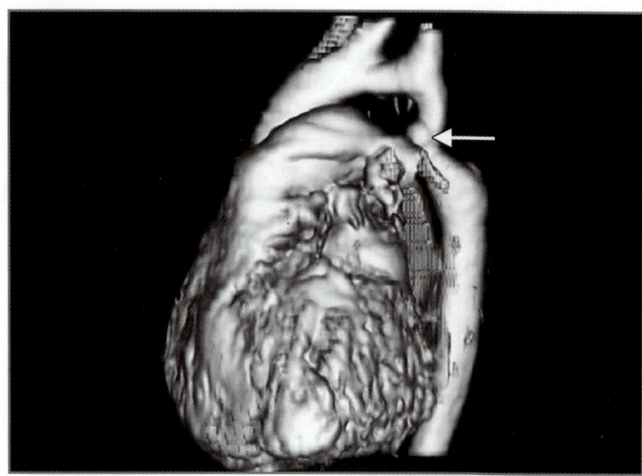

FIG. 2: Ductus diverticulum: CT angiogram (CTA) (volume rendered—VR) shows isthmus and diverticulum (arrow).

- *Descending thoracic aorta*:
  - Visceral branches: Pericardial branches, bronchial arteries (one on the right and two on the left side), mediastinal branches and phrenic branches.
  - Parietal branches: Intercostal arteries and subcostal arteries
- *Abdominal aorta*:
  - Ventral: Unpaired—celiac axis, superior mesenteric artery and inferior mesenteric artery
  - Lateral: Paired—inferior phrenic artery, middle suprarenal artery, renal artery, testicular or ovarian arteries
  - Dorsal: Lumbar (5-paired), median sacral (unpaired)
  - Terminal: Common iliac arteries (paired).

The Measurement (Diameter) of Aorta

The aortic diameter varies with body size, sex and ageing. The average mean diameter is as follows:[6]

- *Aortic root*: 3.6 cm
- *Aortic arch*: 3.5 cm
- *Proximal descending aorta*: 2.6 cm
- *Distal descending aorta*: 2.4 cm
- *Abdominal aorta*: 2.0 cm

In adults, the aortic diameter increases by approximately 0.1 cm per decade.

Normal Anatomic Variations

There are various normal anatomic variations involving the arch, brachiocephalic vessels and visceral branching patterns of the abdominal aorta. The most common variation is the common origin of brachiocephalic trunk and left common carotid artery which is seen in approximately 20% of the population **(Fig. 3)**. In about 5% of the population, the left vertebral artery arises directly from

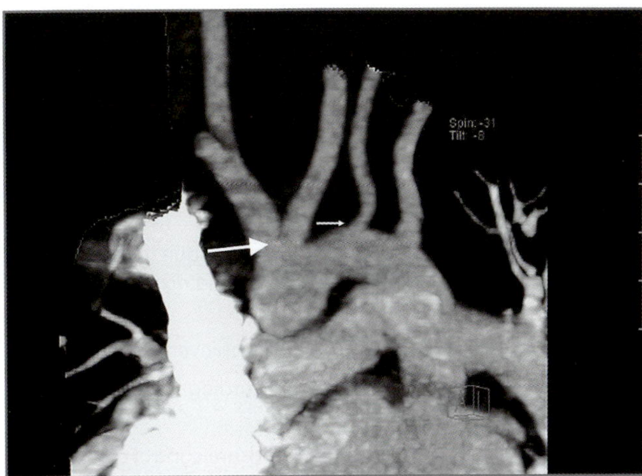

FIG. 3: MIP image of CTA showing common origin of right brachiocephalic and left common carotid arteries (thick arrow). Also seen is the direct origin of the left vertebral artery from arch of aorta (thin arrow).

the aorta **(Fig. 3)**. In 1%, there is a common origin of both common carotid arteries and a paired brachiocephalic trunk. Aortic arch anomalies include an aberrant origin of the right subclavian artery as the last branch of the thoracic aorta just distal to left subclavian artery (1%), right-sided aortic arch (1%), and aberrant origin of left subclavian artery (1%), etc.[7]

The most common variant of the abdominal aorta involves the origin of the hepatic artery. The left lobe of the liver may be supplied completely or partially by the left hepatic artery originating from the left gastric artery (25%). The "replaced origin" of the right hepatic artery from the superior mesenteric artery (SMA) may be seen in 10% of the population. Rarely, the common hepatic artery may take origin directly from the SMA or the aorta or the celiac axis and SMA may have a common origin.[7]

IMAGING MODALITIES

- *Noninvasive*:
  - Ultrasound (US): Transthoracic echocardiography (TTE), duplex scanning, color Doppler (CD), transesophageal echocardiography (TEE) and intravascular ultrasound (IVUS).
  - Computed tomography (CT): MDCT or DSCT
  - MRI: Three-dimensional contrast enhanced MR angiography (3D CE-MRA), bright blood (steady state free precession-SSFP) imaging, various black blood inversion sequences, a short tau inverse recovery (STIR) and phase contrast (PC) sequences for flow quantifications
  - Nuclear fusion imaging: Nuclear fusion imaging (PET) with 18-flurorodeoxyglucose (18F-FDG) with either CT or MRI has an increasing role now in the evaluation of systemic vasculitis, in the detection of vascular inflammation, delineating disease extent as well as treatment response evaluation
- *Invasive*: Catheter angiography—conventional or digital.

In addition, plain radiographs of the chest and/or abdomen, barium swallow, etc., may suggest aortic disease and may provide some clues for further imaging.

Ultrasound

Ultrasound, whether TTE or abdominal duplex scanning is the first noninvasive imaging modality for evaluation of aortic diseases and has sufficient accuracy for the purpose of diagnosis as well as surveillance. Technological improvement including combination of B-mode with pulsed wave Doppler and color flow mapping have increased the utility of US in the diagnosis as well as follow-up of aortic diseases. It is cost effective and portable with no hazards of ionizing radiation. However, the quality of the examination may be affected by patient factors such as bowel gas, obesity and it is highly operator dependent.

Transesophageal echocardiography and IVUS are two major advances in US that have modified preoperative aortic imaging.

Transesophageal echocardiography: It has overcome many of the limitations of TTE and has a high degree of accuracy in skilled hands. One of the main advantages of TEE, especially in unstable patients, is that the examination can be performed safely and quickly at the bed side.

High resolution imaging of the thoracic aorta is possible with TEE. A 5 MHz one or two phased array transducer is mounted on the top of a gastroscope which is manipulated in the esophagus to get high resolution images of the thoracic aorta. The high image quality is possible because of close proximity to the heart and great vessels, absence of interposed air/bone and excellent acoustic coupling of the transducer face with the esophageal mucosa. In thoracic aorta imaging, TEE provides excellent information except for a 1–3 cm segment of the distal ascending aorta or proximal arch which cannot be imaged because of tracheal air; this is known as the "blind-spot".[8]

The limitations are that it requires a great deal of the physician's skill, and it is not possible in patients suffering from esophageal stricture/tumors.

Intravascular ultrasound: It is a relatively new imaging modality, used mainly during coronary and peripheral interventions. It provides 2D, cross-sectional images of the vessel lumen with good resolution. It allows evaluation of plaque morphology, vessel walls, and perivascular structures. It has not been used widely in aortic evaluation, but it has the potential to provide useful information.[9]

Computed Tomography

The advances in CT technology have broadened its use for screening, diagnosis, endovascular treatment planning or preoperative evaluation and post-treatment follow-up of aortic diseases. It is more commonly used than MRI because of fast acquisition, high temporal and spatial resolution, and provision for ECG-gating especially for assessment of ascending aorta.[10-12]

Computed Tomography Angiography Technique

With the advent of MDCT and DSCT scanners, entire aorta and its branches can be imaged in a single breath hold with excellent image quality without venous contamination.[10]

Present scanners allow acquisition with radiation optimization with high temporal resolution (66 milliseconds-192 DSCT). Newer techniques like prospective triggering, ECG-based tube current modulation, body adaptive automatic dose calculation (exposure), excellent image quality with lower tube kilovoltage (kVp) setting by iterative images reconstruction algorithms have revolutionized the vascular imaging like never before.[10,13-15]

Recent CT advancement of photon-counting detector CT offers many advantages compared with energy-integrating detector CT, including better detector efficiency, higher image contrast, lower image noise with availability of spectral information.

For ascending aorta evaluation ECG gating is usually desirable especially when imaging Standford type A dissection and aneurysm for simultaneous evaluation of coronary arteries, and for planning transcatheter aortic valve implantation (TAVI).

A typical protocol for image acquisition of entire aorta on a 64-MDCT/128-DSCT (which we routinely use at our institution) is given below, which can be customized according to the area of interest (thoracic or abdominal aorta).

Area coverage: The scan should cover area 3 cm above the aortic arch till the level of femoral heads, to include the entire aorta and the origins of its major branches. The imaging till proximal femoral arteries is essential for planning of endovascular treatment.

Contrast injection protocol: Since the aorta is a large artery, dilution of contrast occurs rapidly thus a high rate of injection is required. If possible, dual head pressure injector with saline chase is recommended to minimize/avoid artifacts caused by the high-density contrast in the superior vena cava. Flow rate should be 3–4 mL/s and volume should be calculated as follows:

$$\text{Flow rate} \times (\text{scan time} + \text{scan delay})$$

This should be followed by saline chase with the same flow rate for 5–6 seconds.

Acquisition of data: Since, imaging is to be done when the contrast density is maximum in the lumen, "bolus chase" technique is preferred over fixed time delay, with threshold of contrast density kept between 100–200 HU (at level of ascending aorta) to trigger the acquisition with delay of 4–5 seconds to achieve maximum luminal enhancement **(Table 1)**.[16,17]

TABLE 1: Scan protocol for 128 DSCT angiography of the entire aorta.

CT coronary angiography scan parameters	Details of parameters
Scan area	3 cm above the aortic arch till the level of femoral heads
Data acquisition technique	Bolus tracking technique (region of interest in the ascending aorta with preset of 100 HU)
Scan delay	5 seconds after achievement of 100 HU
Kilovoltage	100–120 KV according to body habitus, sex, and age
Tube current	Automatic exposure control system-based tube current modulation
Detector collimation	2 × 64 × 0.6 mm
Slice acquisition	2 × 128 × 0.6 mm by means of a z-flying focal spot
Gantry rotation time	280 milliseconds
Temporal resolution	75 milliseconds
Reconstructed slice thickness	0.75 mm with a reconstruction increment of 0.5 mm
Image window	Soft-tissue convolution kernel (B26f)
ECG gating (for ascending aorta only)	Retrospective ECG gating with tube current modulation
Image post-processing	Images construction in multiplanar, maximum intensity projection and volume rendering along with axial data set

Data analysis: Data thus acquired can be reconstructed in axial or 3D images [maximum intensity projections (MIP), shaded surface display (SSD) or volume rendered technique (VRT)]. The 3D depiction of the entire aorta depicts the entire extent of the pathology in a single image and any number of desired projections can be made. This can be done with either VRT or MIP technique **(Figs. 4A to C)**. When detailed evaluation of pathology is required thin MIP up to 0.5 mm can be made and evaluated.

The major advantages of computed tomography angiography (CTA) over a digital subtraction angiography of the aorta are visualization of the wall and its surrounding changes. Pathologies like intramural hematoma can be easily overlooked on digital subtraction angiography (DSA). The other advantages being rapid imaging time, uniform arterial enhancement, lack of motion artifacts, identification of branch vessels, ease of use and it being less expensive. The major limitation includes lack of "flow quantification".

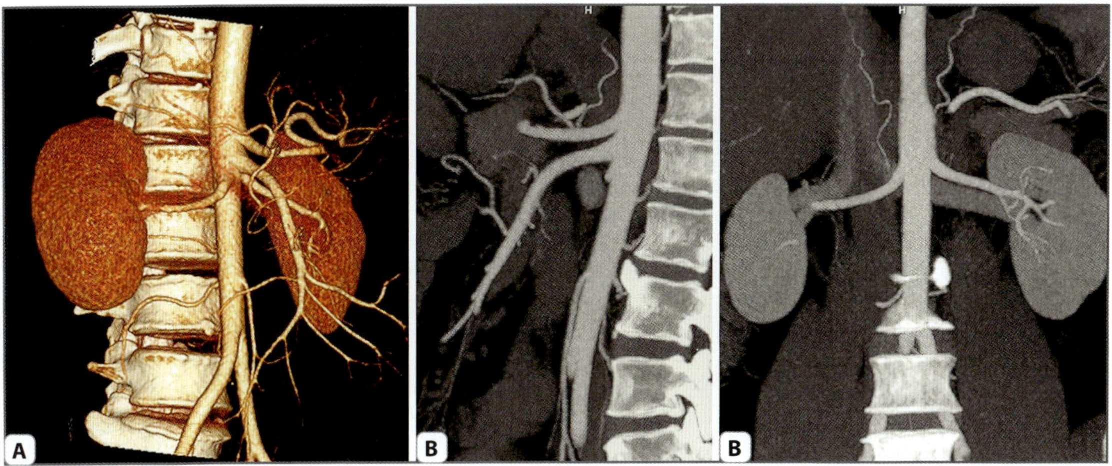

FIGS. 4A TO C: Normal abdominal CTA acquired on 128 DSCT: Volume rendering (A) and maximum intensity projection (B and C) projections showing major branches of aorta.

Magnetic Resonance Imaging and Magnetic Resonance Angiography

Magnetic resonance angiography (MRA) of the aorta offers certain advantages over CTA. Most important is that since it does not involve radiation, repeated examination can be done as required for follow-up, safely without any radiation concern.

One major advantage of MRI is that flow quantification and direction of flow can now be determined with advanced MR applications and MR angiography techniques.

Several techniques are available to image the aorta and can be broadly classified into:[11,12,18-22]

- 3D-contrast enhanced MR angiography (3D CE MRA)
- White blood imaging—static and cine imaging
- Black blood imaging—static imaging
- Phase contrast (PC) sequences—for flow quantification

3D Contrast-enhanced Magnetic Resonance Angiography

3D contrast-enhanced magnetic resonance angiography (3D CE-MRA) is gadolinium-enhanced 3D gradient echo (3D-GRE) where thin contiguous image partitions are obtained in a single breath-hold. It uses heavily T1-weighted 3D-GRE technique and is the work horse for evaluation of vascular abnormalities of primarily thoracic aorta **(Fig. 5)**. It allows post-processing just like CTA and techniques like MIP reformation, volume rendering and multiplanar reformation of the images can be generated for analysis.[11,12,23]

It is done with injection of gadolinium-based contrast agents (0.1 mmol/kg body weight) with a flow rate of 2–5 mL/s, followed by a saline flush of 20 mL injected at the same flow rate immediately after contrast administration. Scan can be started after a fixed time interval as determined by doing a test scan using a small amount of contrast or by MR fluoroscopy method when contrast reaches left ventricle.

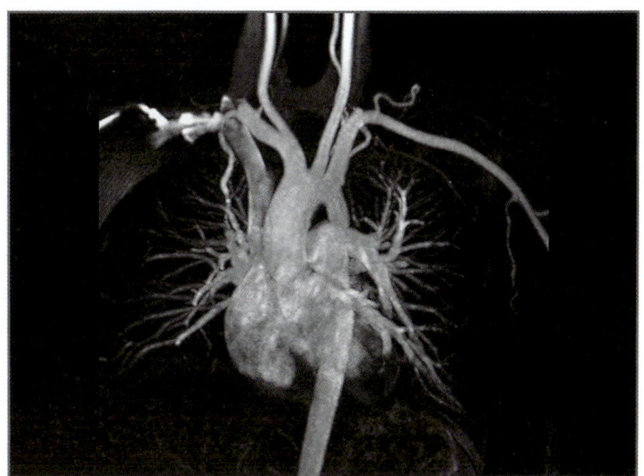

FIG. 5: 3D MIP image at 3T of contrast enhanced MRA showing aortic arch, ascending and descending thoracic aorta and its major branches with high spatial resolution and without any artifacts.

Bright Blood Imaging

Bright blood imaging provides images with blood having hyperintense signal that works on steady-state free-precession (SSFP) sequence (FIESTA, TrueFISP). It is a short TE and TR sequence, which provides very high and homogenous intraluminal signals even in cases of turbulent flow because this sequence depends mainly on the function of the T2/T1 ratio **(Figs. 6A to D)**.

Steady-state free-precession images can be acquired in both breath-hold and free-breathing manners, either with or without ECG-gating and navigator/respiratory trigger. SSFP can provide rapid bright-blood images with high-contrast resolution. SSFP sequences can also be

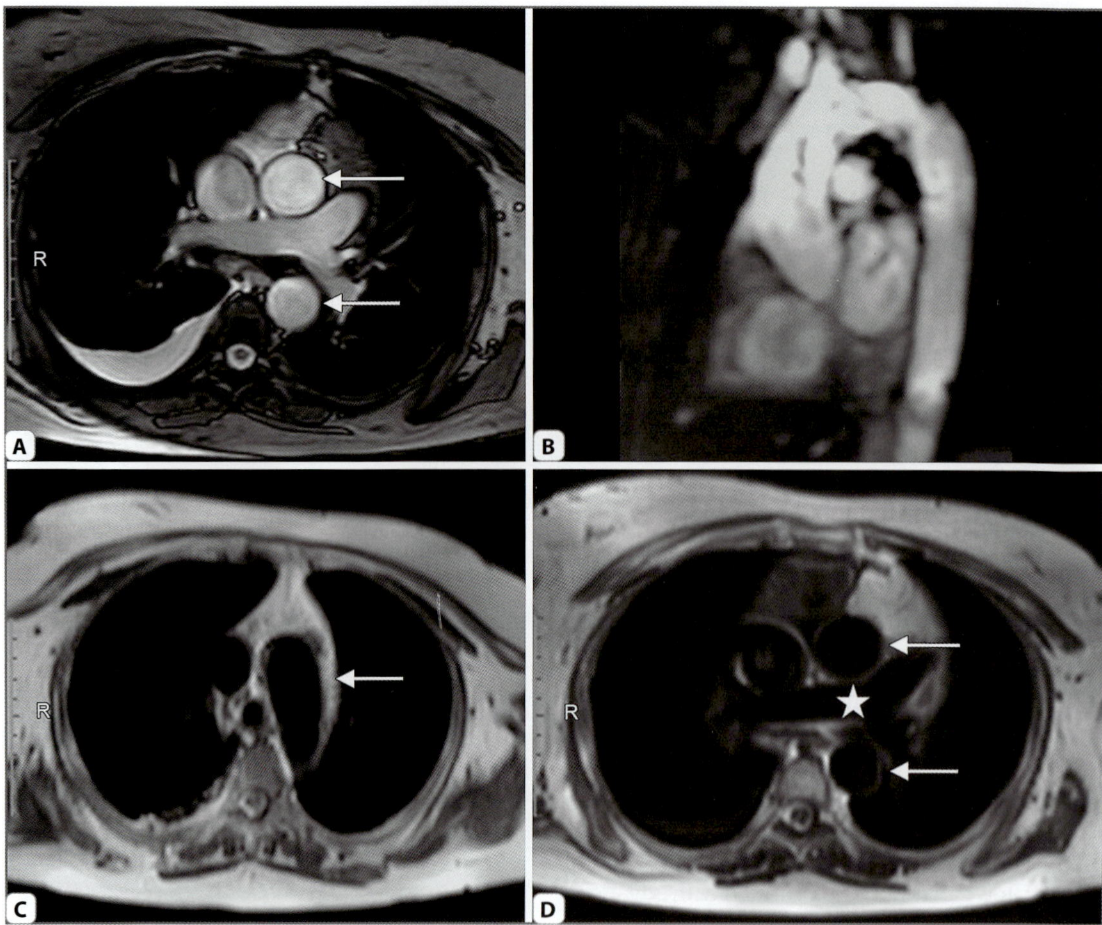

FIGS. 6A TO D: Top row-Axial (A) and "candy cane" view (B) SSFP images (bright blood images) at 3T through the thoracic aorta showing bright aortic lumen (arrows in A) due to sensitivity of the method to flowing blood. (C and D) Axial black blood double inversion recovery sequence images at 3T through the thoracic aorta showing aortic dark aortic lumen with well-delineated arch (arrow in C), ascending and descending thoracic aorta (arrows in D) and pulmonary arteries (asterisk in D)

acquired in a cine mode, and have become the foundation for cine imaging. Advantages are the higher signal-to-noise ratio (SNR), shorter imaging duration, and freedom from the reliance on inflow effects for signal generation. This sequence has benefited from the application of parallel imaging techniques, allowing high temporal resolution, large field of view (FOV) imaging of the thoracic aorta, and left ventricular outflow during acceptable breath-holds as low as 5–6 seconds. The inherently high blood signal achieved using SSFP throughout a cine acquisition period has been shown to aid evaluation of aortic mural and valvular characteristics and allowing exclusion of aortic dissection. SSFP is the most promising of the "bright-blood" non-contrast enhanced MR angiography techniques.[20-22]

Black Blood Imaging

Black blood employs the inherent contrast between the rapidly flowing blood (flow void) and aortic wall to generate images so that aortic wall is well depicted. It can be obtained either with spin echo (either conventional or echo-train spin-echo techniques) or double inversion recovery sequences. Short tau inversion recovery (STIR) sequence is restricted for demonstration of wall edema.[11,20,21] Usually image acquisition is with ECG-gating, exploiting the contrast between rapidly flowing blood and the aortic wall **(Figs. 6A to D)**.

Black blood imaging is recommended when analysis of aortic wall pathology is desirable such as mural hematoma and aortoarteritis. It may also be useful for the depiction of intraluminal abnormalities, such as dissection flaps and tumor thrombus.

Luminal signal void occurs because intravascular protons only produce signal if they are exposed to both a 90° excitation pulse and subsequent refocusing pulse while traveling through the image slice.[11,12] Therefore, low flow and entry/exit slice phenomena may produce high signal in the aortic lumen, artificially simulating wall disease, so before any conclusion is drawn all sequences and imaging planes need careful inspection and interpretation.

Phase Contrast Sequences

Quantification of aortic flow, especially in aortic regurgitation, stenosis, congenital heart diseases and coarctation of aorta is required for management which is possible with PC sequences. It is based upon the principle that protons passing through a magnetic field gradient undergo a phase change in proportion to velocity, and this is utilized to measure the flow velocities within the aortic lumen during the entire cardiac cycle for measurement of forward flow, regurgitation and stenosis.[24-26]

18-flurorodeoxyglucose with either CT or MRI

Fusion imaging of fluorine-18-fluorodeoxyglucose (18F-FDG) PET with CT/MRI is now emerging as the modality of choice as it not only provides the anatomical imaging with high spatial resolution also specific information about disease activity as 18F-FDG is a surrogate marker of increased activity of inflammatory cells.

In specific it delineates extent of vascular inflammation and response to treatment in cases of aortitis. It also helps in selection of appropriate sites for biopsy—histopathologic confirmation of diagnosis.[27-29]

Catheter Angiography

It is the most definitive study in the evaluation of aortic disease. Both conventional angiography and DSA provide detailed anatomic information including the aberrant origin of vessels. But DSA saves time, expenses on films and on contrast. The overlying bowel gas or osseous structures that obscure the area of interest are avoided. Contrast related complications may be avoided by using CO_2 gas as contrast agent. Intravenous DSA, once the preferred noninvasive technique, has largely been discarded because of technical difficulties and poor contrast resolution. Nonetheless, it can be used in a limited way in acute settings like trauma. There has been progressive decrease in the size of catheter used from 6–7 French to 4–5 French, low flow rates and smaller arterial punctures with overall reduction in mortality and morbidity rate. All these factors have pushed the most invasive investigation into an outpatient procedure.[5]

Technique

A 5 or 6F arterial sheath is placed in the femoral or brachial artery by puncturing it with 18G puncture needle under strict aseptic precautions under local anesthesia: 2,500 U of heparin is used normally for diagnostic studies. A 5F pigtail catheter is introduced over a 0.035"/0.032" guide wire in the ascending aorta (for arch study) 2.5 inches above the aortic valve or in the abdominal aorta (around T12) just above the origin of celiac axis. 25–30 cc of non-ionic contrast is injected at a flow rate of 12–14 cc/s through a power injector. A 45° LAO projection is taken for arch study and a straight AP and lateral views are taken for the abdominal aorta. Further studies like selective injection into branch vessels, lateral or oblique projection may be done depending upon the initial aortographic findings. After reviewing the entire study, the catheter and the arterial sheath are removed and pressure compression is applied at puncture site for 12–15 minutes till the bleeding stops.

Complications of Angiography

These are divided into three major categories: Reactions to contrast media, complications related to arterial puncture site and systemic complications related to arterial catheterization. A proper and carefully applied technique may reduce the complications rate to less than 0.1%.[30]

The contraindications of angiography include:

- Previous anaphylactic contrast reaction
- Low cardiac output, and
- Anuria and bleeding diathesis.

INDICATIONS FOR IMAGING THE AORTA

Various diseases afflicting the aorta may warrant either noninvasive or invasive aortic imaging. The diseases can be classified as:

- *Congenital*:
  - Aortic arch anomalies
  - Coarctation
  - Aortic atresia
  - Aortic stenosis
- *Acquired*:
  - Aneurysms
  - Dissection
  - Aortitis
  - Trauma
  - Atherosclerosis

CONGENITAL AORTIC ANOMALIES

Aortic Arch Anomalies

- Left aortic arch with aberrant origin of right subclavian artery **(Figs. 7A and B)**
- *Right aortic arch*:
  - With mirror image branching
  - With aberrant origin of the left subclavian artery
- Cervical arch
- Double aortic arch **(Figs. 8A and B)**

The detailed description and imaging findings are discussed in relevant chapters in this book.

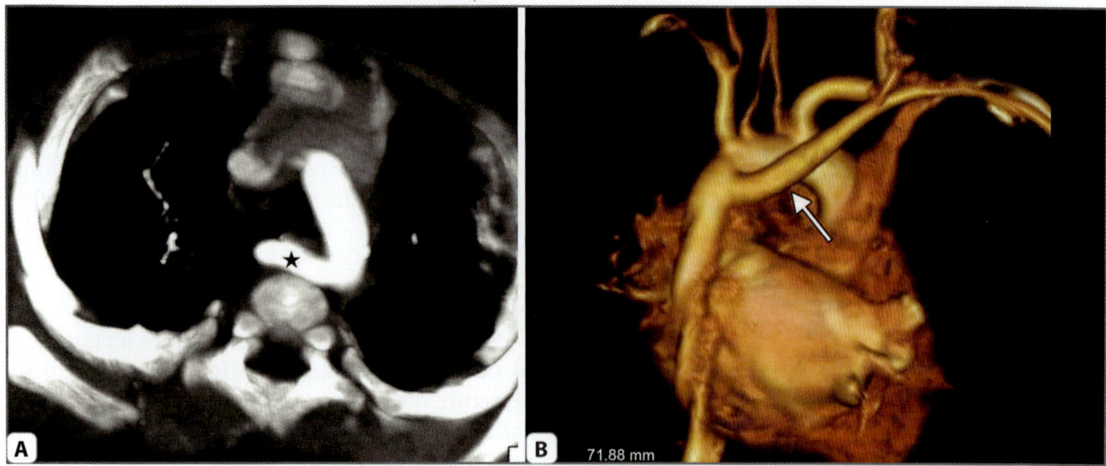

FIGS. 7A AND B: (A) MIP axial and (B) VR (posterior projection shows aberrant origin of right subclavian artery (asterisk and arrow) with retroesophageal course (asterisk) from left-sided arch.

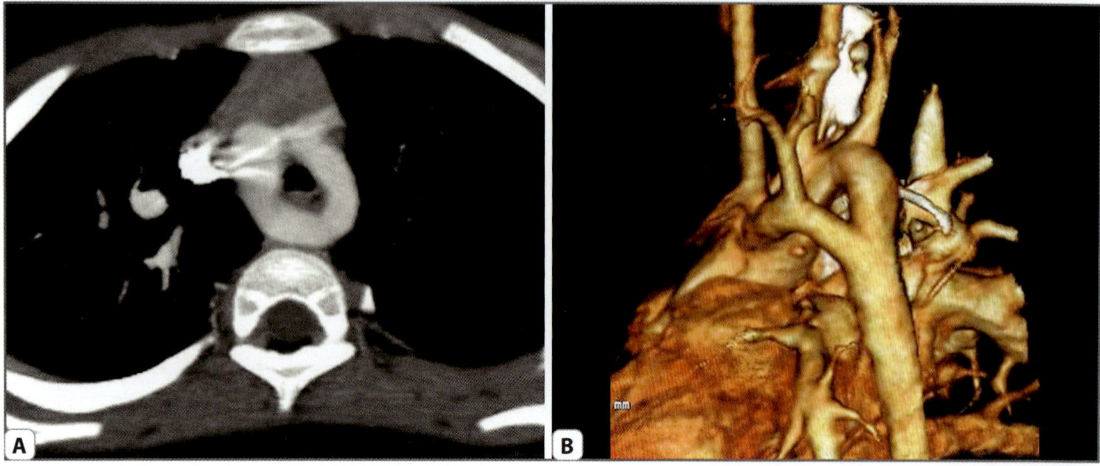

FIGS. 8A AND B: (A) MIP axial and (B) VR image (posterior projection) shows double aortic arch encircling trachea.

Coarctation of Aorta

It is a congenital aortic narrowing in the region of the isthmus. It is more common in males (M:F = 4:1) and is rare in blacks. It is of two types:

1. *Localized or adult or postductal or juxta-ductal type*: It is the most common type where there is a short segment narrowing close to the ligamentum arteriosum. Coexistent cardiac anomalies are uncommon.
2. *Tubular hypoplasia or infantile or preductal or diffuse type*: There is hypoplasia of a long segment of the aortic arch after the origin of the brachiocephalic trunk. Coexistent cardiac anomalies are common.

Associated Anomalies

- Bicuspid aortic valve (25–50%)
- *Cardiac shunts*:
  - Patent ductus arteriosus (PDA) (33%)
  - Ventricular septal defect (VSD) (15%)
- Turner's syndrome (13–15%)
- Cerebral berry aneurysms (5–7%)

A review of the natural history of coarctation revealed that of those patients who survived infancy, 20% were dead before the age of 20 years, 50% by 32 years and 90% by 58 years.[31] Most common causes of death are due to cardiac failure, aortic rupture, infective endocarditis, intracerebral hemorrhage, etc.

Hemodynamics in Adults

The collateral circulation distal to the coarctation is through the subclavian arteries and its branches like internal mammary artery to intercostal arteries, scapular artery to anterior spinal artery and transverse cervical artery to lateral thoracic artery.

Radiological Findings

Conventional X-ray of Chest

- *Rib notching* **(*Table 2*)**: It usually takes several years to develop. It is due to pressure erosion by the enlarged and tortuous intercostal arteries. It is typically bilateral but asymmetrical and is best seen on the inferior aspects of

TABLE 2: Causes of rib notching.

Aortic obstruction	Pulmonary oligemia
Coarctation	Fallot's tetralogy
Takayasu's arteritis	Pulmonary artery atresia
Thrombosis of abdominal aorta	*Miscellaneous*:
Subclavian artery obstruction	• Chronic SVC or IVC obstruction
Blalock–Taussig shunt	• Intercostal AV fistula
Takayasu's arteritis	• Fallot's tetralogy
Coarctation	• Pulmonary artery atresia

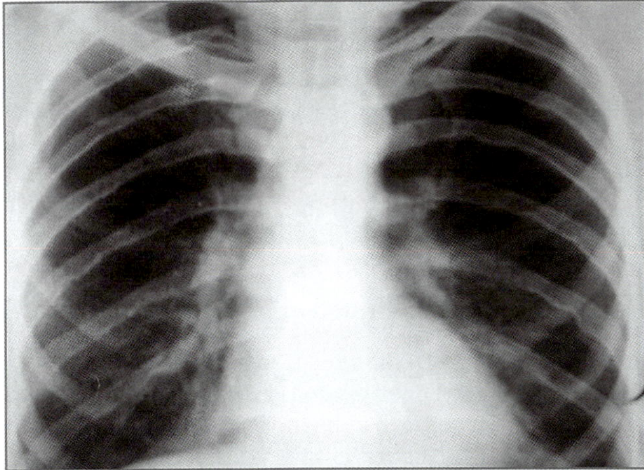

FIG. 9: Chest X-ray showing notching of posterior ribs bilaterally most prominent along inferior borders in a case of aortic coarctation.

the posterior thirds of 4th to 9th ribs **(Fig. 9)**. It will be seen only on the left side if there is an aberrant origin of the right subclavian artery below the coarctation and only on the right side if there is involvement of the left subclavian artery in the coarctation.

- Left ventricular hypertrophy.
- "Figure-of-3" appearance—it is due to dilated left subclavian artery above the coarctation (CoA), a pinching at the site of CoA and the post-stenotic dilatation below.
- Small and flat aortic knuckle.

Angiography: It has been used for long to image CoA. Cardiac catheterization is also required to evaluate cardiac abnormalities and for the measurement of pressure gradient across the lesion. CoA can usually be crossed from the femoral route but may require brachial artery catheterization in extreme stenosis. Multiple views are required in asymmetric lesions. The angiograms reveal the site, degree and size of the stenosis as well as the collateral circulation **(Figs. 10A to F)**.

Noninvasive Imaging

Computed tomography angiography, MRA and USG are often used in conjunction with angiography in the evaluation of coarctation. CTA can depict the morphology of the coarcted segment with good spatial resolution as well as status of aortic arch vessels and collaterals. However, it is not able to measure the gradient across the lesion, nor the direction of the flow. Still, it is an important investigation for planning stent graft implantation and follow-up imaging after surgery **(Figs. 10A to F)**.

Magnetic resonance angiography now in addition to the anatomic details can give the information of the dynamics involved in the coarctation of aorta, noninvasively **(Fig. 11)**.

Phase-contrast velocity-encoded cine MR can give reliable information regarding flow velocity, flow volume and the pressure gradient across the stenosed segment. Also, it can give information regarding the collaterals and direction of flow in them. Though this technique is promising, its use in routine clinical practice is limited because it also suffers from certain drawbacks like underestimation of flow volume and velocity and is also poor in small vessel assessment.

Management of Aortic Coarctation

Societal guidelines recommend that coarctation correction should be performed as early as possible (ideally as early as possible in childhood) to reduce the long-term morbidity and enhance survival.[32,33] The indications for corrective treatment are listed in **Box 1**. Percutaneous interventions and surgical correction are both acceptable options for coarctation repair. A multidisciplinary team (i.e., cardiologist, interventionists, and surgeons) with experience in treating patients with congenital heart disease should be involved in deciding the management protocol and is dependent on the morphology, age, associated cardiac lesions as well as the availability of either an experienced interventionist or surgeon. A suggested algorithmic approach to manage coarctation is given in **Flowchart 1**.

Balloon angioplasty may also be performed as a palliative procedure in very sick patients as part of a staged protocol for initial stabilization of the patient.

Pseudocoarctation is a condition that results from an elongation of the distal aortic arch which, as it is fixed at the arterial ligament, bulges backwards above and below this point causing a "double aortic" bulge. There is no hemodynamic obstruction. It may present as a mediastinal mass and the true nature can be demonstrated on CT or MRI.

Interrupted aortic arch is a rare condition in which a localized atresia of the arch occurs distal to the left subclavian artery (Type A: 42%), **(Figs. 12A to C)** distal to the left common carotid artery (Type B: 53%) or distal to the brachiocephalic trunk (Type C: 5%). It is usually associated with various cardiac anomalies like PDA and VSD.

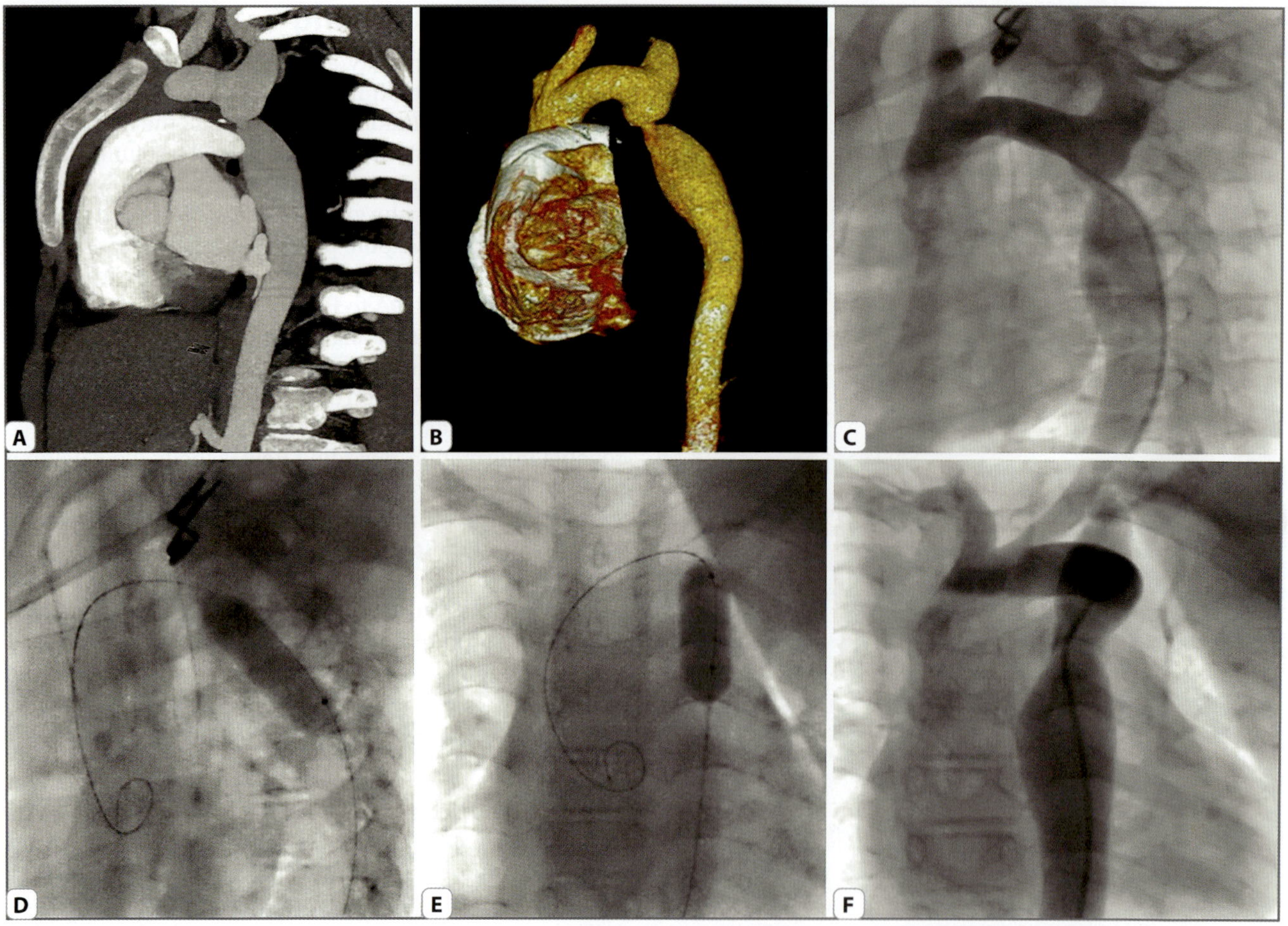

FIGS. 10A TO F: Balloon angioplasty of aortic coarctation. (A to C) Computed tomography and angiography showing coarctation of aorta; (D and E) balloon angioplasty of the coarctation; (F) Post balloon angioplasty angiography showing significant reduction in severity of stenosis.

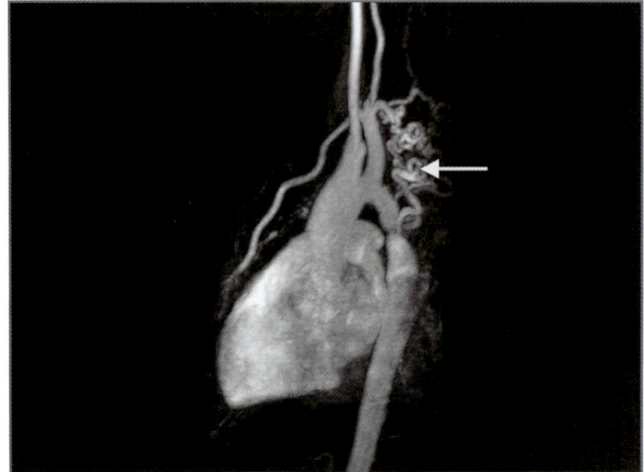

FIG. 11: MRA-MIP image lateral projection shows the coarctation, its length and the status of the aorta proximal and distal to it. Also note presence of collaterals seen on this MRA image (arrow).

BOX 1: Indications for corrective treatment.

- Peak to peak (or maximum instantaneous) coarctation gradient ≥20 mm Hg
- Peak to peak coarctation gradient <20 mm Hg in the presence of significant coarctation with imaging evidence of significant collateral flow

ACQUIRED AORTIC DISEASES

In this section, imaging in particular reference to endovascular and surgical management of aortic aneurysms, pathologies causing acute aortic syndrome, surveillance of aortic aneurysms is discussed in detail.

Imaging of common inflammatory aortitis like Takayasu and IgG4 related aortitis are also described. Infective or mycotic inflammatory pathologies have been included in the aneurysm section.

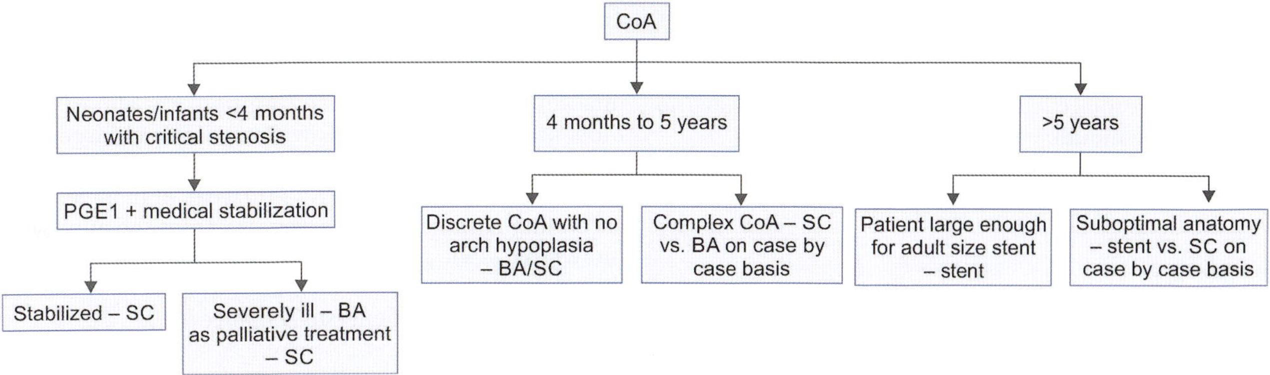

FLOWCHART 1: Approach to treatment of coarctation of aorta.
(CoA: coarctation; BA: balloon angioplasty; PGE1: prostaglandin E1; SC: surgical correction)

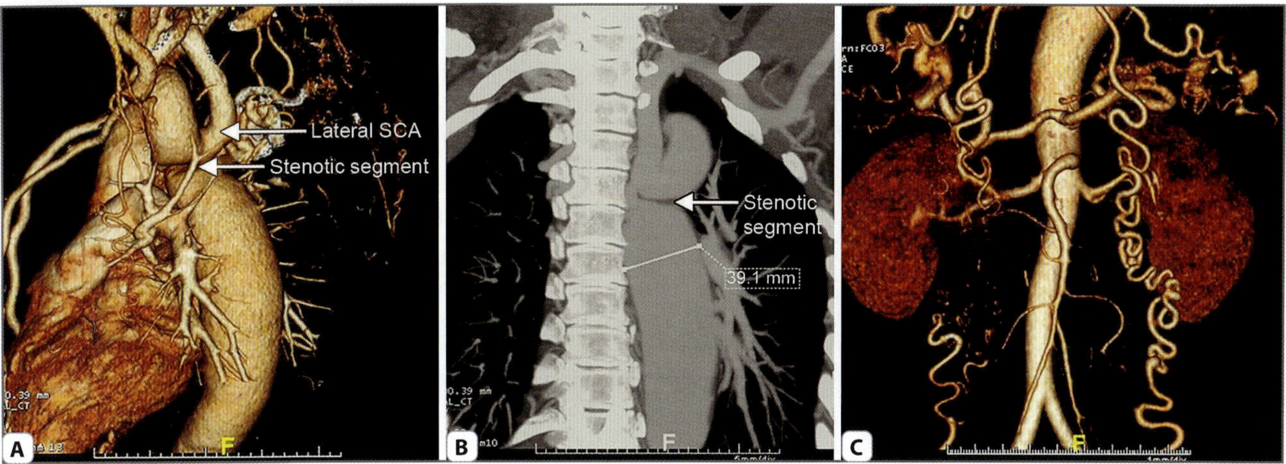

FIGS. 12A TO C: (A) CTA MIP image sagittal projection and (B) VR image show discontinuity of descending thoracic aorta just distal to origin of left subclavian artery. (C) Note extensive collaterals.

AORTIC ANEURYSMS

An aneurysm is a localized or diffuse dilatation of an artery. Aneurysm is defined as a permanent focal dilatation of the artery having ≥ 50% increase in diameter compared with the expected normal diameter of the artery in question. Ectasia is arterial dilatation <150% of normal arterial diameter. Arteriomegaly is diffuse arterial dilatation involving several arterial segments, with an increase in diameter > 50% in comparison with the expected normal arterial diameter.[34]

Incidence

The incidence of aortic aneurysm varies from 4% (60–70 years) to 11% (70 years and above) and is probably increasing. Patients with hypertension, coronary artery disease, peripheral vascular disease and those whose immediate family have aneurysms are at a higher risk of developing aortic aneurysms.

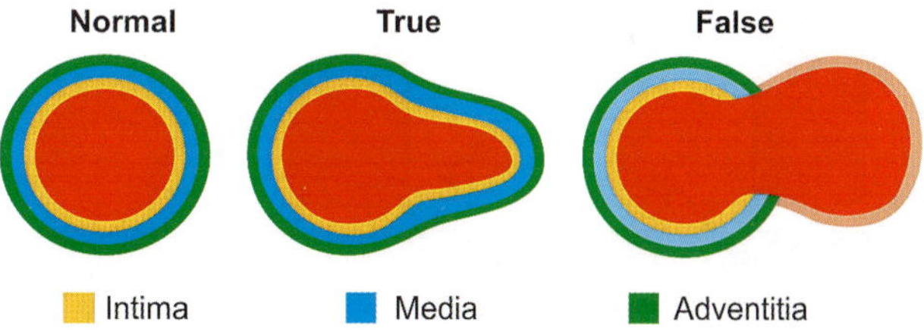

FIG. 13: Diagram showing differentiation of true (covered by all layers) from false/pseudoaneurysm (arterialized periarterial hematoma).

Classification

An aneurysm can be classified as:

- *True or false* ***(Fig. 13)***: True aneurysms consist of all three layers of the arterial wall (intima, media, and adventitia) whereas false aneurysms are due to focal perforation of the aortic wall limited externally by the adventitia, perivascular connective tissue, or by hematoma.

- *Saccular or fusiform* **(*Figs. 14A to D*)**: Saccular aneurysms usually arise from a distinct portion of the aortic wall and have a mouth, while fusiform aneurysms involve the total circumference of an artery and have no distinctive mouth.
- *Congenital or acquired*: Acquired aneurysms are more frequent than congenital aneurysms.

Etiology

- Atherosclerosis (70–80%)
- Cystic medial necrosis (Marfan syndrome, Ehlers-Danlos syndrome.)
- Mycotic/Infective (2–2.5%)—usually saccular
  - Tuberculosis (typically affects thoracic aorta),
  - Syphilis (90% affects ascending or arch of aorta)
  - Other infections (*Staphylococcus, Streptococcus, Salmonella* infection)
- Vasculitis (Takayasu's and Giant cell arteritis)
- Spondyloarthropathies [Ankylosing spondylitis, rheumatoid arthritis (RA), psoriasis, Behçet's syndrome, Reiter's syndrome, relapsing polychondritis]
- Post-traumatic (5–8%)—90% involving the isthmus and 8% in ascending aorta.

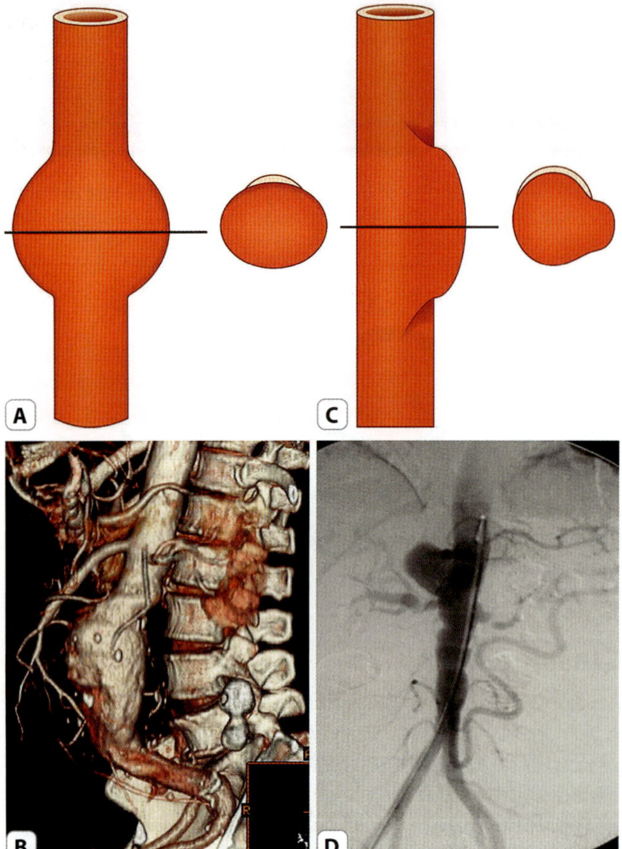

FIGS. 14A TO D: Images showing fusiform (A and B) saccular (C and D) aneurysms.

Growth Rates of Aneurysm

The mortality rate of untreated aortic aneurysms is unacceptably high and, once ruptured, it is almost 100%. Most aneurysms (80%) show progressive enlargement. The rate of growth is significantly greater for aneurysms of the descending aorta, at 1.9 mm/year, than those of the ascending aorta, at 0.7 mm/year.[35] Larger the aneurysm, more rapid is the growth. As the size (radius) of aneurysm increases, the wall tension increases, which tends to further increase the size of aneurysm *(Laplace law)*.

Risk of Rupture

Diameter of the aneurysm is the best predictor of rupture risk. Other parameters associated with increased risk are type of aneurysm (Saccular > Fusiform), wall stress, rate of expansion, family history, hypertension, smoking and gender (more common among females). Estimated annular rupture risk of abdominal aortic aneurysm (AAA) is tabulated in **Table 3**.[35,36]

Diagnostic Imaging

Physical examination, plain radiography and ultrasound are usually sufficient to establish a diagnosis of aneurysm, but these are inadequate in planning and implementing endovascular or surgical treatment. The preoperative imaging must provide the following information:[10,11,37]

- Location, size, angulations, craniocaudal extension and type of aneurysm.
- The maximum diameter of any dilatation, measured from the external wall of the aorta, perpendicular to the true axis of flow, and the length of the abnormally dilated aorta.
- Integrity of the wall, presence of intramural hematoma, penetrating ulcers and associated thrombus.
- Involvement of visceral arteries or adjacent structures.
- Associated anatomic variations.
- Unrecognized intra-abdominal/intrathoracic conditions, e.g., cholelithiasis.
- Complications of aneurysm, e.g., rupture, infection, thromboembolism.

TABLE 3: Rupture risk per year of AAA in relation to diameter of aneurysm.

AAA diameter (cm)	Rupture risk (%/years)
<4	0
4–5	0.5–5
5–6	3–15
6–7	10–20
7–8	20–40
>8	30–50

- Measurements of aortic valve, sinuses of Valsalva, sinotubular junction, and ascending aorta in patients with presumed or documented genetic syndromes who are at risk for aortic root disease.
- Comments on coronary arteries for ascending aorta aneurysms.
- Comment on vascular access site for endovascular treatment.

Plain Radiography

Plain radiography may suggest a diagnosis of aortic aneurysm but information essential for preoperative planning cannot be obtained. Findings include:

- Widening of mediastinum; in a standard supine chest radiography, if the mediastinum measures >8 cm, it is highly suggestive of thoracic aortic aneurysm **(Fig. 15)**
- Localized dilatation of ascending aorta/knuckle/descending aorta with or without curvilinear calcification **(Figs. 16A and B)**
- Depressed left main bronchus, tracheal displacement, obliteration of aorto-pulmonary window, cardiomegaly (thoracic aortic aneurysm) **(Figs. 17A to C)**
- Mural calcification, displacement of adjacent organs of gastrointestinal tract (GIT), vertebral erosion (abdominal aortic aneurysm) **(Figs. 18A and B)**.

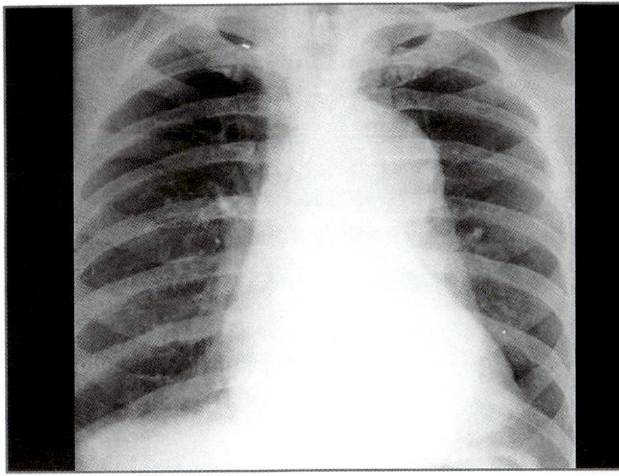

FIG. 15: Chest radiograph in a case of large thoracic aortic aneurysm showing mediastinal widening.

Ultrasound

Ultrasound has sufficient accuracy to size aortic aneurysms for the purpose of diagnosis as well as surveillance to detect expansion **(Figs. 19A and B)**. It has the following advantages:

- It confirms the clinical diagnosis of an aneurysm.
- It serves as a screening modality for follow-up of patients with aortic aneurysms, especially abdominal aortic aneurysms.
- It has a detection rate of 100% with size measurement within 4 mm of that obtained at surgery
- It is cost effective and portable.

The limitations of ultrasound are:

- It fails to provide reliable information regarding visceral artery involvement and craniocaudal extension.
- Obesity and intestinal gas hinder adequate evaluation
- Expertise and experience are required for providing other essential morphological information.

Transesophageal echocardiography and IVUS have limited role in the diagnosis, however, it may further modify the preoperative planning in aortic aneurysms. IVUS helps in accurate measurement of the aneurysm for selection of stent grafts during endovascular repair and helps in prevention of type I endoleaks.

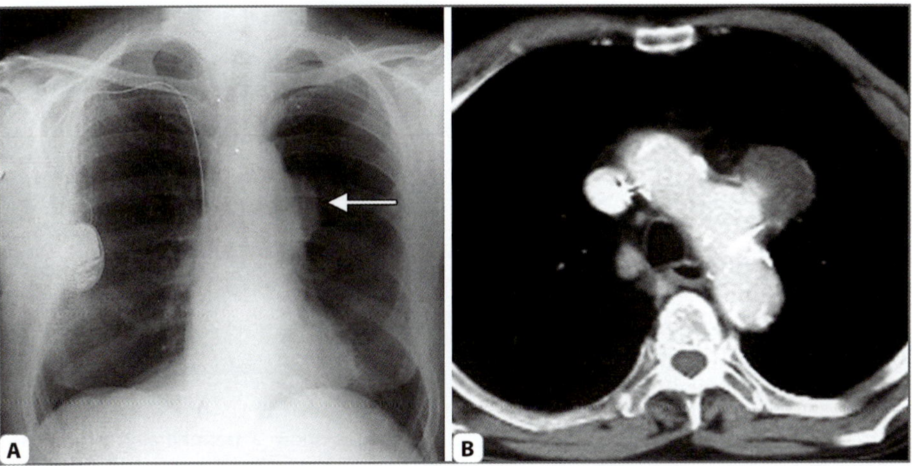

FIGS. 16A AND B: Chest radiograph in PA view shows prominent aortic knuckle (A), which on CTA (B) showed a peripherally thrombosed arch aneurysm with a penetrating ulcer.

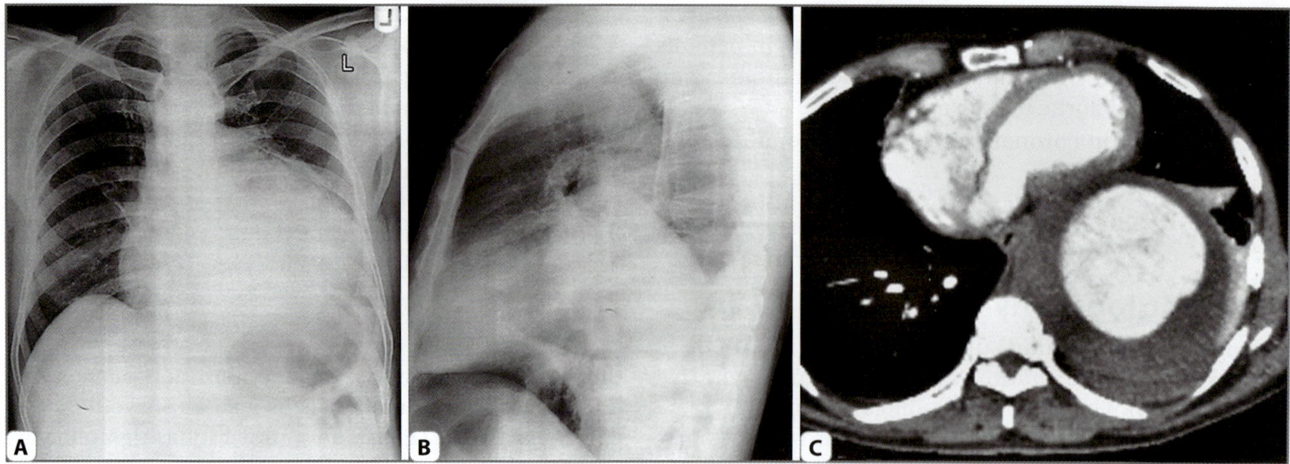

FIGS. 17A TO C: Chest radiograph in PA view shows cardiomegaly (A), which on lateral projection (B) shows a radio-opaque opacity overlying lower thoracic vertebra with loss of normal radiolucency. Subsequently on CTA (C) it was a large peripherally thrombosed DTA aneurysm.

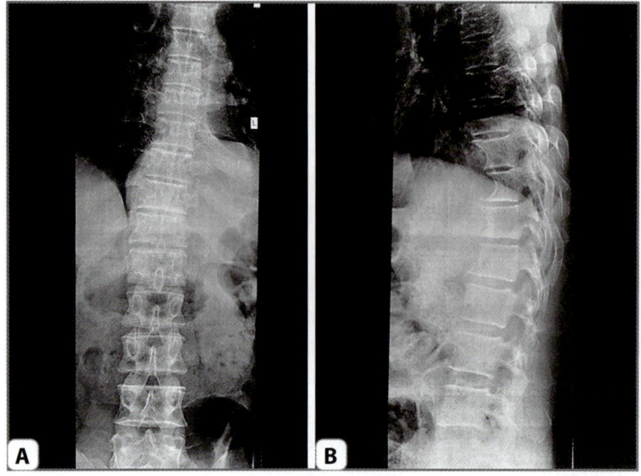

FIGS. 18A AND B: Front (A) and lateral thoracolumbar (B) spine radiograph shows a thoraco-abdominal mass like lesion with well-defined lateral margins on both sides of spine. On lateral view anterior scalloping of lower dorsal vertebral bodies is prominently seen. On CTA it turned out to be a large mycotic aneurysm (refer **Fig. 23**).

Computed Tomography and Magnetic Resonance Imaging

Computed tomography and MRI are the modalities of choice for imaging of aorta, however, CT is preferred over MRI because of shorter scanning time and high temporal and spatial resolution. MR angiography is usually recommended for post-treatment evaluation. Computed tomography permits one to choose an imaging plane in any arbitrary space orientation, measure the tortuous aorta in true cross-section and obtain an accurate diameter. Breath-held dynamic contrast-enhanced MRI also allows rapid acquisition of images in any plane, independent of

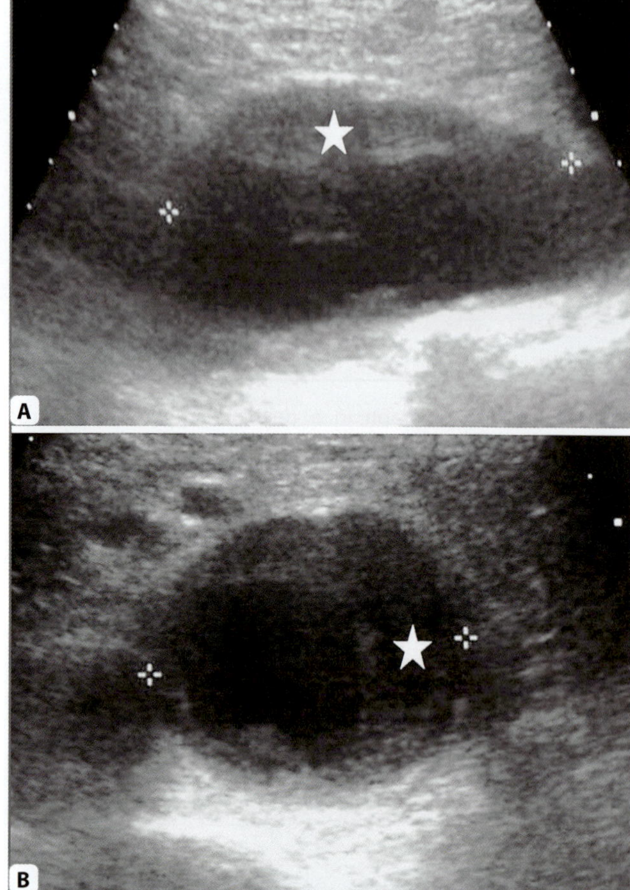

FIGS. 19A AND B: US abdomen longitudinal (A) and transverse (B) images show a peripherally thrombosed (along left lateral wall—asterisk) fusiform aneurysm of abdominal aorta.

flow, however disadvantages include non-visualization of calcifications and contraindications for MRI.[10-12,21,22,38]

In specific cases of ascending arch aneurysm, ECG gated study should be considered for simultaneous evaluation of coronary arteries as significant CAD may be treated with bypass grafts in one sitting.

Important Aneurysmal Features to be Assessed with Computed Tomography or Magnetic Resonance Imaging[22,38,39]

- Proximal extent of the aneurysm whether it involves major vessels or aortic root. The surgical approach differs if there is involvement of major vessels **(Fig. 20)**.

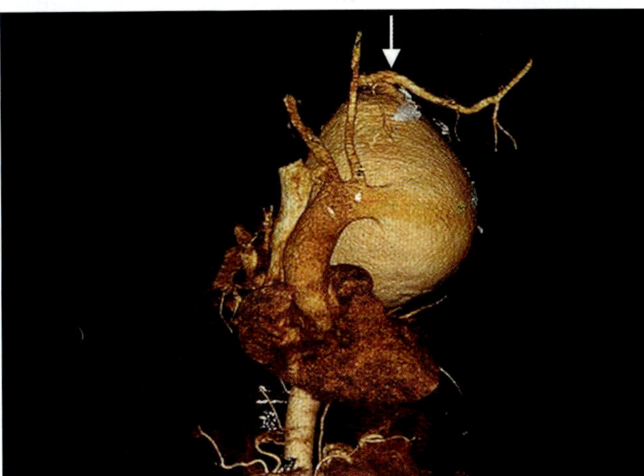

FIG. 20: Aortic aneurysm: CTA–VR projection shows large saccular aneurysm arising from distal aortic arch and descending thoracic aorta. Note that this 64-slice VR projection clearly shows the origin of left subclavian artery from the aneurismal sac (arrow) and sparing of right brachiocephalic and left common carotid.

- Distal extent of the aneurysm. Choice of the graft type depends on whether the aneurysm involves the common iliac vessels **(Figs. 21A to C)**.
- Congenital anomalies. The incidental anomalies like accessory renal artery or retroaortic/circumaortic left renal vein may warn an interventionist/surgeon to take due care during repair.
- *Etiology*: Based on imaging characteristics as whether it's inflammatory, mycotic or atherosclerotic (discussed in detail later).

Inflammatory aneurysm: It is a variant of atherosclerotic aneurysm characterized by inflammatory and/or fibrotic changes in the periaortic regions **(Fig. 22)**. These changes are probably due to local autoallergic reaction to certain atherosclerotic plaque components. Aneurysmal repair is difficult for these patients because of fibrosis and involvement of important structures, e.g., ureter, GIT, vena cava, etc. CT or MRI demonstrates well-defined soft tissue mass with sharply defined margins surrounding the aneurysm in the anterolateral aspect with sparing of the posterior aspect. The contrast enhancement is variable. CT may rarely demonstrate infiltrative soft tissue mass with poorly defined margins or lobulated mass mimicking a pseudotumor. More details are enumerated in the aortitis section.

CT or MRI findings of mycotic aneurysm include **(Figs. 23A to C)**:

- Saccular or irregular contour
- Little or no mural calcification
- Is adjacent to normal appearing adjacent aorta
- Perianeurysmal fibrosis with or without air
- *Ruptured aneurysm*. CT or MRI demonstrates freshly hemorrhaged blood in the mediastinum/retroperitoneum and focal area of indistinctness in the aortic wall **(Figs. 24 to 26)**. The overall accuracy varies from 87–97%. Distinction between acute or chronic

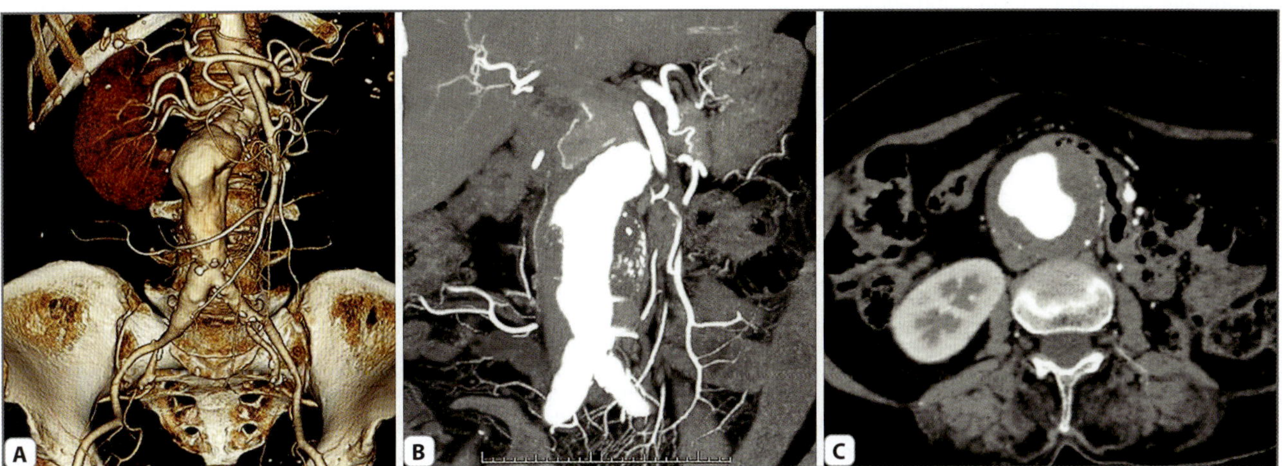

FIGS. 21A TO C: CTA-VR (A), MIP coronal (B) and axial (C) images demonstrate peripherally thrombosed fusiform infrarenal abdominal aortic aneurysm extending into both common iliac arteries.

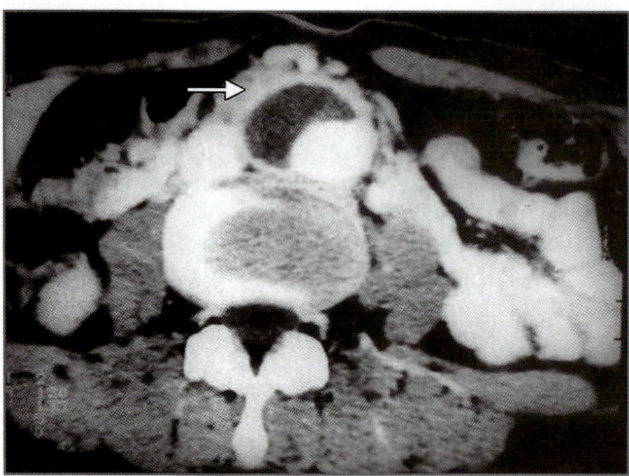

FIG. 22: Inflammatory aortic aneurysm: CECT shows a rind of soft tissue in right anterolateral aspect (arrow) of a partially thrombosed aneurysm (perianeurysmal fibrosis).

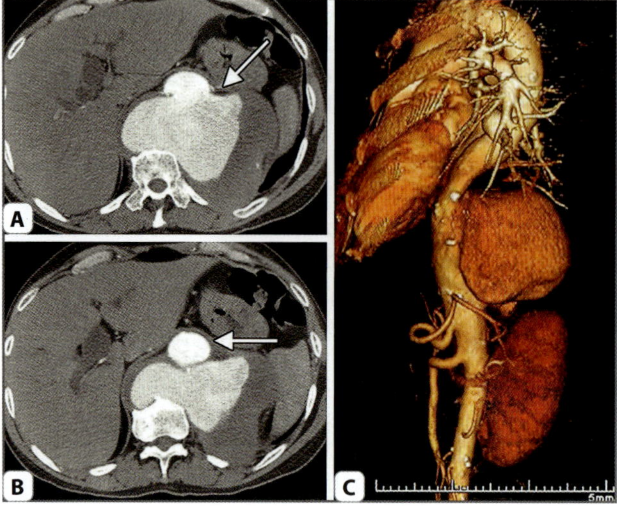

FIGS. 23A TO C: (A and B) CTA axial and (C) VR images show a large peripherally thrombosed juxta-diaphragmatic pseudoaneurysm (mycotic aneurysm) having lobulated outline with normal appearing anteriorly displaced aorta (thick arrow in B). Rent is posterior wall of aorta (thin arrow in A) is well seen. Note anterior scalloping of vertebral bodies (B). CTA pictures are of patients shown in **Figure 18**.

contained rupture is based on duration and severity of symptoms, the hematocrit and hemodynamic stability rather than on anatomic features demonstrated on CT/MRI.

Catheter Angiography

Catheter angiography has a limited role in diagnosis and follow-up aneurysms. However, with the advent of newer endovascular treatment methods, it has a definitive role in preoperative evaluation and treatment planning of aortic aneurysms. It provides detailed arterial anatomy including aberrant origins, the location of the aneurysm relative to branch vessels and demonstrates occlusive lesions.

Surveillance of Small Abdominal Aortic Aneurysms

The risk of rupture of small (5 cm) AAA is low, and hence careful surveillance up to a diameter of 5.5 cm is safe, unless there is rapid expansion (1 cm/year) or patient becomes symptomatic. Since the benefits of early surgery over surveillance with later surgery are comparable, patient preference is important, especially for AAA 4.5- 5.5 cm in diameter. The diameter of 5.5-cm appears to be an appropriate threshold for repair in an "average" patient based on the current evidence. For women, or AAA with greater than average rupture risk, elective repair at 4.5–5.0 cm is an appropriate threshold for repair.[40] Based on a recent individual-based meta-analysis of trials and observational studies with repeated AAA measurements over time, intervals of 3, 2, and 1 year(s) can be safely proposed for AAAs of 30–39, 40–44 and 45–54 mm diameter, respectively, with a rupture risk of 1% in men. Women with 45 mm AAA had a risk of rupture equivalent to men with a 55 mm AAA, so a lower intervention threshold, rather than shorter intervals of follow-up, may be considered.[41]

Management of Aortic Aneurysms

Ascending Aortic and Arch Aneurysms

The treatment of ascending aortic and arch aneurysms remains a surgical replacement. The extent of surgery depends on the status of the aortic valve, coronary arteries, and great vessels. Aortic valve replacement and complete arch replacement with reimplantation of the arch vessels may be required if the aortic valve is diseased or if the origins of the great vessels are involved. Hybrid debranching procedures as described in the section on dissection may be used in arch aneurysms where surgical grafts are placed to the great vessels from the ascending aorta followed by stent-graft placement across the arch from the ascending to the descending aorta.

Aneurysms of the Descending Thoracic Aorta

The relationship of the aneurysm to the arch vessels and the abdominal aortic visceral arteries determines the treatment. Involvement of these major aortic branches in the aneurysm increases the difficulty and morbidity of intervention. Complications of operative repair include a mortality rate of 5–10%, paraplegia due to spinal cord ischemia, renal failure, stroke and respiratory failure.[42]

An attractive alternative to open surgical repair is endovascular repair where the anatomy is suited for stent graft placement. Stent-grafts function by depressurizing the aneurysm sac. Anatomical prerequisites and the procedure itself are similar to those described in the section on aortic dissection.

FIGS. 24A TO G: Non-contrast axial CT images (A and B), axial CTA (C to F) and VR (G) images shows fusiform infrarenal abdominal aortic aneurysm (black asterisk in C, D and G) with active contrast leak (block black arrow in D) associated hyperdense hematoma (black arrow in E and F) and associated significant periaortic stranding (white arrow in A and B). Patient expired on day 2 of admission and a diagnosis of IgG4 periaortitis was made on autopsy.

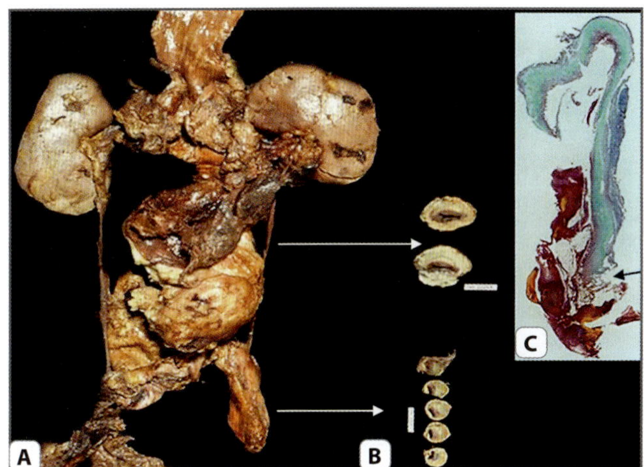

FIGS. 25A TO C: Autopsy specimen shows (A) gross specimen with evidence of blood collection in the area of aortic rupture confirmed (B and C) by cross-sections at the site of rupture and histopathology (arrow in C).

Courtesy: Professor Ritambra Nada, Department of Histopathology, PGIMER, Chandigarh, India.

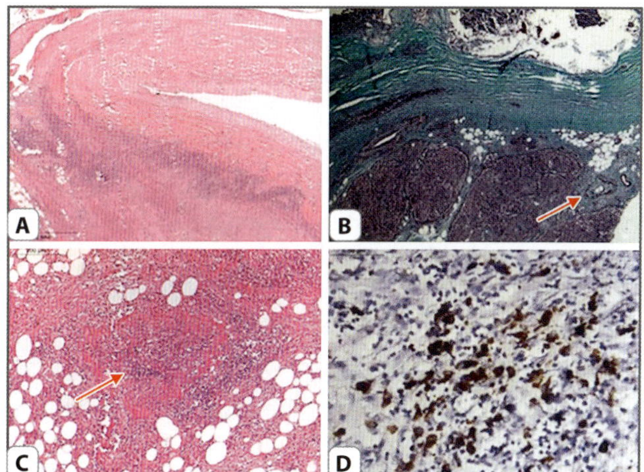

FIGS. 26A TO D: Photomicrograph shows (A) inflammatory periaortitis which had (B) evidence of fibrosis and venulitis (arrow). (C) shows obliterative venulitis (arrow) with immunohistochemistry (IHC) showing (D) IgG4 positive cells. Stains for CD3 CD20 were negative (which are positive in aortoarteritis—not shown here).

Courtesy: Professor Ritambra Nada, Department of Histopathology, PGIMER, Chandigarh, India.

Stent-graft repair of thoracoabdominal aneurysms requires either a hybrid procedure with surgical debranching of the abdominal aortic branches followed by stent-graft placement, or branched stent-grafts **(Figs. 27A to D)**. Debranching procedures are major surgical interventions, which increases the morbidity and mortality of the procedure. Branched stent-grafts are less invasive for the patient but are complex time-consuming procedures with the expertise for such procedures being available in only certain tertiary care centers in India.

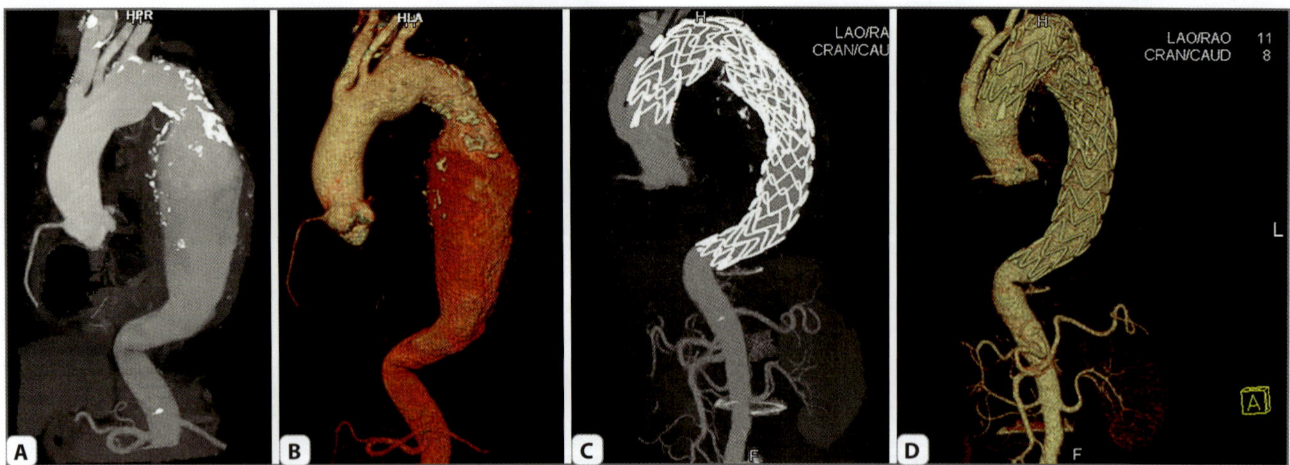

FIGS. 27A TO D: Descending thoracic aortic aneurysm treated with a stent graft after debranching to extend the proximal landing zone. (A and B) Oblique MIP and VRT computed tomography (CT) image showing the extent of the aneurysm. (C and D), CT of same patient 1 month after placement of a stent graft. The stent graft extends proximal and distal to the aneurysm with exclusion of the aneurysm sac. Transposed innominate artery to the ascending aorta is also noted.

BOX 2: Indications for treatment of abdominal aortic aneurysms (AAA).

- AAA ≥5 cm diameter
- Symptomatic aneurysms regardless of size:
    - Contained-rupture AAA
    - Inflammatory AAA
- Rapidly expanding (>5 mm/year) AAA
- High-risk for complication with open repair

Multilayered flow modulator devices and stents are currently being developed for treatment of true fusiform aneurysm and hold promise for future application.[43]

Aneurysms of the Infrarenal Abdominal Aorta

Infrarenal AAA which fulfils the criteria for treatment **(Box 2)** may be treated by placement of a stent-graft or surgery. The mortality rate is 3–6% for elective surgery and 25–50% for emergent repair of a ruptured aneurysm making endovascular treatment attractive. Careful pre-procedural planning **(Table 4)** is paramount as up to 37% of all patients may not be suitable candidate for endovascular aortic repair (EVAR).[44]

Patients must meet several anatomic criteria to be eligible for a stent graft **(see Table 4)**. Three types of stent graft configurations can be used to treat infrarenal AAA depending on the anatomic suitability. Most patients treated with current devices receive bifurcated stent-grafts as shown in **Figures 28A to F**. Other alternatives include aortounilateral iliac graft with surgical femoral-femoral bypass.[45] This type is used when the patient's anatomy is not suitable for a bifurcated graft. A single stent graft (similar to DTA stent graft) may also be used in rare situations where the proximal and distal landing zones are adequate.

TABLE 4: Eligibility criteria for interventional management of abdominal aortic aneurysm.

Criteria	Favorable	Unfavorable
Proximal aneurysm neck		
• Diameter	<32 mm	>32 mm
• Length	>1.5 cm	<1.5 cm
• Angulation	< 60°	>60°
• Morphological configuration	Cylindrical; Tapered	Reverse taper
• Calcification/ thrombus	< 90% circumference involved	>90% circumference involved
Aneurysm sac		
• Residual lumen	>18 mm	>18 mm
• Distal aortic diameter	>20 mm	<20 mm
• Extension	CIA not involved	CIA involved
Ileofemoral vessels		
• CIA diameter	<25 mm	>25 mm
• Landing zone length	>10 mm	>10 mm
• EIA diameter	>6 mm	>6 mm
• Tortuosity	<90°	<90°
• Calcification/ Thrombus	< 50% circumference involved	> 50% circumference involved

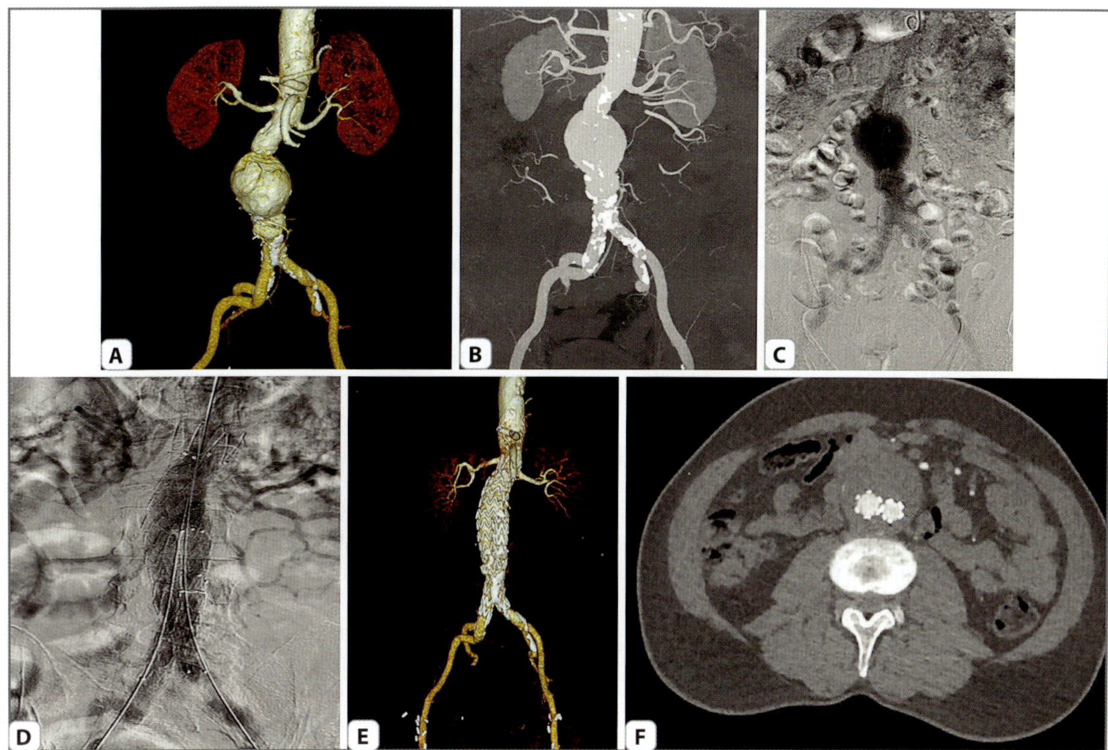

FIGS. 28A TO F: Infrarenal abdominal aortic aneurysm treated with a branched stent-graft. (A to C) VRT and MIP computed tomography images and aortogram showing an infrarenal abdominal aortic aneurysm. (D) Aortogram after deployment of stent graft shows exclusion of the aneurysm. (E) VRT computed tomography images of the same patient on 1 month follow-up; (F) Axial image showing good opacification of both limbs of the stent graft with aneurysm sac thrombosed.

ACUTE AORTIC SYNDROME

Acute aortic syndromes (AAS) constitute a spectrum of conditions characterized by disruptions in the integrity of the aortic wall presenting with acute pain as the leading symptom in most cases. They include classic aortic dissection, intramural hematoma, penetrating aortic ulcer, and aortic aneurysm rupture **(Fig. 29)**. Because of the life-threatening nature of these conditions, prompt and accurate diagnosis is paramount. Misdiagnosis of these conditions, usually because of confusion with myocardial ischemia, can lead to undue mortality. Benign conditions or findings that can mimic AAS on imaging studies are aortitis, atheromatous plaque, prior surgery of aorta, pericardial recess, remnant of a non-patent PDA, streak and motion artifacts on CT, and periaortic fat and hemiazygos sheath.[38]

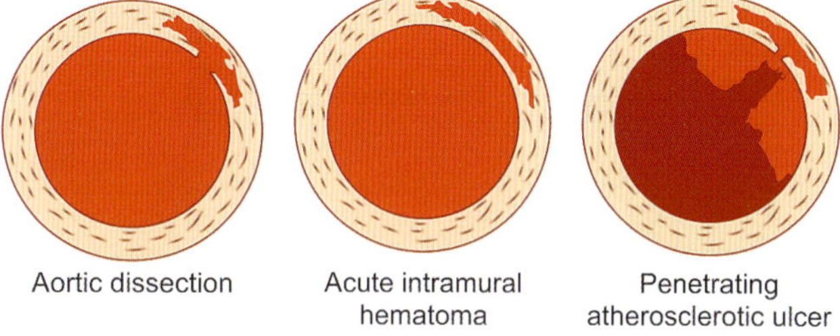

FIG. 29: Schematic diagrams demonstrating dissection, penetrating ulcer and intramural hematoma.

AORTIC DISSECTION

Aortic dissection is the most common acute emergency affecting aorta, occurring 2–3 times more frequently than acute rupture of an aortic aneurysm. The peak incidence is in the sixth and seventh decades of life, men are affected more than women. The clinical presentation is with acute onset of chest pain, congestive heart failure, abdominal pain, or stroke. Approximately 15–20% may be asymptomatic and incidentally diagnosed. The predisposing conditions are hypertension (70–90%), pre-existing aortic diseases (Marfan syndrome, coarctation) or aortic valve disease, aortitis, family history of aortic diseases, history of cardiac surgery, cigarette smoking, direct blunt chest trauma and use of intravenous drugs. Though the exact pathogenesis is somewhat controversial, the most accepted theory for long is that the initial event is a tear in the intima which allows blood to enter the aortic wall creating a true and false lumen. Demonstration of intimal flaps is thus essential to make the diagnosis. It is now recognized that degeneration of the media leads to rupture of the vasa vasorum of the aortic wall which leads to dissecting hematoma between the media and adventitia which may or may not rupture through the intima into the aortic lumen. This explains the fact that no intimal tear is found at autopsy in a small number of cases of aortic dissection.[46]

Classification

The DeBakey classification categorized aortic dissections into:

- *Type I (29–34%)*: Originates in the ascending aorta and extends to a variable distance beyond the aortic arch
- *Type II (12–21%)*: Confined to ascending aorta
- *Type III (50%)*: Originates distal to the left subclavian artery. It is subclassified into type IIIA up to diaphragm and type IIIB: below diaphragm.

This classification has been replaced by "Stanford classification" which takes into account of extent of dissection rather than location of entry site and divided into type A (involving the ascending aorta) and type B (not involving the ascending aorta) **(Fig. 30)**. Approximately 70% of dissections are type A and 30% are type B. Type A carries high mortality and morbidity and requires urgent intervention as compared to type B dissection, which is usually managed conservatively **(Table 5)**.[47]

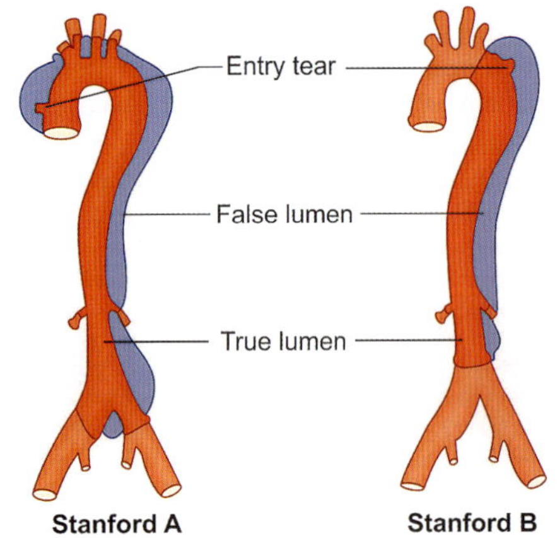

FIG. 30: Diagram showing Stanford types of dissections.

TABLE 5: Characteristics of Standford type A and type B aortic dissections.

Feature	Type A	Type B
Frequency (%)	65–70	30–35
Male: Female ratio	2:1	3:1
Average age (years)	50–55	60–70
Hypertension (%)	50	80
Atherosclerosis	+/-	+ +
Aortic insufficiency (%)	50	10
Intimal tear	Always present	Absent in 5–10%
Treatment	Urgent surgery	Usually, conservative
Acute mortality (%)	90–95	35–50

IMAGING

The goal of imaging is not merely to detect presence and extent of AD but to define other important features:[38]

- Differentiation of true and false lumen
- Location of intimal tears
- Coronary artery ostia integrity (in type A)
- Aortic valve function
- +/– pleural or pericardial effusion.

There is no consensus as to which examination(s) should be used in the diagnosis of aortic dissections. The initial imaging should consist of a chest radiograph (CXR) and a TTE. Plain film findings include widening of the mediastinum and aortic contour, changes in aortic contour from prior examination(s), and displaced intimal calcification. However, a normal CXR does not exclude the diagnosis. TTE may show a pericardial effusion, adequately images the aortic valve and the aortic root but does not show the arch and descending aorta with confidence (blind spot). Transesophageal echocardiography (TEE) has overcome many of the limitations of TTE and has a high degree of accuracy in skilled hands. One of the main advantages of TEE, especially in unstable patients, is that the examination can be performed safely and quickly at the bed side and can be used to monitor changes in-theater and in post-operative intensive care.

Computed tomography: CT angiographic protocols typically begin with low-dose non-contrast CT to exclude the possibility of intramural hematoma (IMH), followed by contrast-enhanced ECG gated CTA. The coverage includes the entire thorax, abdomen, and pelvis to allow delineation of the extent of a flap and its extension into branch vessels and to evaluate for end-organ ischemia (e.g., bowel or kidneys), and possible extravasation **(Figs. 31 and 32)**.

The CT findings in aortic dissection include the following:

- *Precontrast images*:
  - Internal displacement of intimal calcification.
  - Visible intimal flap as a linear structure slightly higher in attenuation than surrounding blood.
  - High attenuation thrombosed false lumen, if acutely thrombosed.
  - Enlargement of long segment of the aorta
  - Pericardial, mediastinal and/or pleural hemorrhage, secondary to rupture.
- *Postcontrast images **(Figs. 31 and 32)***:
  - Contrast filled true and false lumen separated by intimal flap; false lumen typically seen in outer curvature of aorta.
  - Delayed enhancement of the false lumen because of slower flow.
  - Thrombosis of false lumen, with enhancement of only the true lumen.
  - Compression of true lumen by thrombosed false lumen.

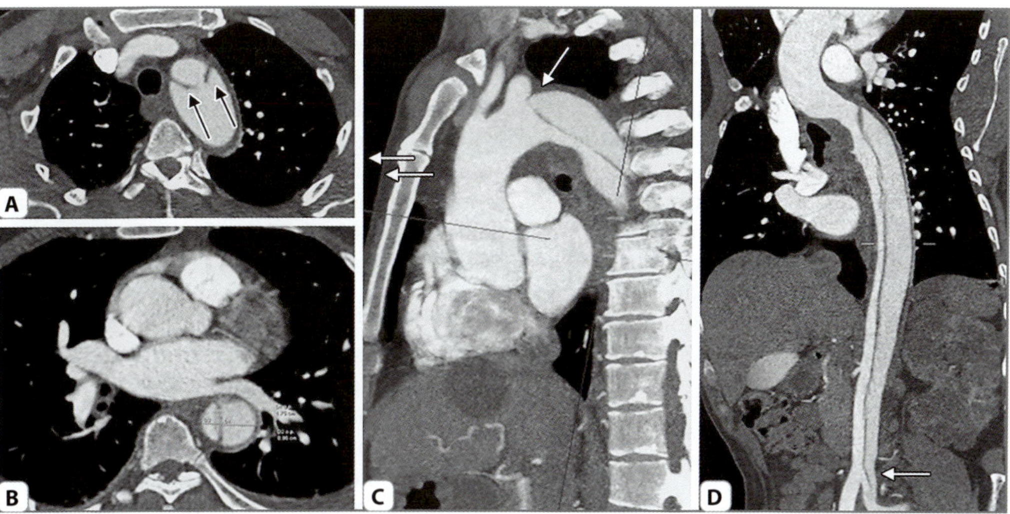

FIGS. 31A TO D: (A and B) CTA axial and (C) reconstructed sagittal and (D) stretched images show type B dissection with entry point juxta-posed to the origin of left subclavian artery (arrows in A and C). Note "beak sign" with convex flap toward posterior false lumen (A). (D) Note extension of flap into the left common iliac artery.

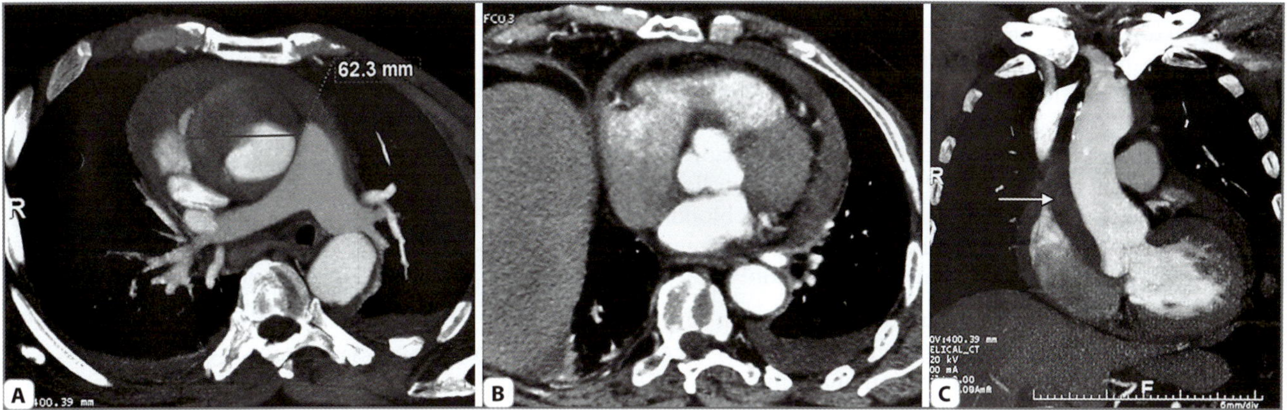

FIGS. 32A TO C: (A and B) CTA axial and oblique coronal images showing type A dissection with thrombosis of false lumen (A and C) with rupture into pericardial and right pleural cavities (A to C).

- Extension of dissection into branch vessels.
- Ischemia/infarction of organs supplied by branch vessels from false lumen.

Computed Tomography Signs of Aortic Dissection

Differentiation between true and false lumens of AD is important in planning of treatment with percutaneous endovascular grafts or surgical repair. It is critical to identify the lumen of origin of major branches such as coronary, carotid, renal and mesenteric arteries before treatment, as viscera supplied by false lumen are at risk when false lumen is spontaneously or surgically occluded **(Table 6)**.

The convex face of the intimal flap is usually toward the FL that surrounds the TL **(Figs. 31A to D)**. The FL usually has slower flow and a larger diameter and may contain thrombi. In type A AD, the FL is usually located along the

TABLE 6: CT features for differentiating true from false lumen.

Features	True lumen	False lumen
Continuity of lumen with lumen of uninvolved portion of aorta (most reliable)	+	–
Direction of free edges of the dissection flap at entrance tear	–	+
Aortic Cobweb	–	+
Outer wall calcification	+	–
Beak sign	–	+
Thrombosis	–/+	++
Peak flow	Faster	Slower
Size	Smaller and compressed	Larger and toward intimal concavity

right anterolateral wall of the ascending aorta and extends distally, in a spiral fashion, along the left posterolateral wall of the descending aorta **(Figs. 32A to C)**. Slender linear areas of low attenuation may be observed in the FL, corresponding to incompletely dissected media, known as the "Cobweb sign", a specific finding for identifying the FL. Discrimination between the FL and TL is utmost important to identify collaterals perfused exclusively by the FL, as well as when endovascular therapy is considered.[48]

If possible, ECG-triggered CTA should be done for type A dissection for simultaneous evaluation of coronary arteries so that bypass grafts can be placed in one-sitting **(Figs. 33A and B)**.

Magnetic resonance imaging: It has been shown to be an effective alternative technique to CT for evaluation of aortic dissection with a reported sensitivity and specificity of 98%. MRI not only gives anatomical but also functional information required for treatment planning, however because of ease of CT and its wider availability, CT is often the modality of investigation and MR is reserved for follow-up **(Figs. 34A and B)**.

Black blood imaging shows the intimal flap as thin linear structure in the aortic flow void. True lumen shows preservation of the flow void whereas the false lumen is seen as an area of increased signal intensity because of turbulent flow.

Phase contrast images can be done to identify aortic insufficiency, intimal tear sites and to differentiate slow flow from thrombus in the false lumen. Combining black blood, bright blood with gadolinium-enhanced 3D MRA images can comprehensively give the required information.[19,24,38,49]

Aortography: It is highly accurate in the detection and evaluation of aortic dissection with diagnostic accuracy over 95%. The direct signs are identification of an intimal flap, and a contrast filled with true and false lumen. Indirect signs are aortic wall thickening, aortic regurgitation, compression of the true lumen, nonvisualization of branch vessels and abnormal catheter position. False negative study may be seen when the false lumen is thrombosed, intimal flap not tangential to the X-ray beam, intimal tear proximal to the catheter and absence of intimal flap in some cases. Noninvasive imaging is more accurate in providing the diagnosis and therefore aortography is no longer used for the diagnosis of AD, except during coronary angiography or endovascular intervention.

Management of Aortic Dissection

Current classifications systems are not comprehensive at describing all the information pertinent to a surgeon/interventionist about the dissection. Information regarding chronicity of symptoms, location of primary entry tears, direction of flap extension (antegrade, retrograde, mixed), complications and patency of the false lumen are vital.

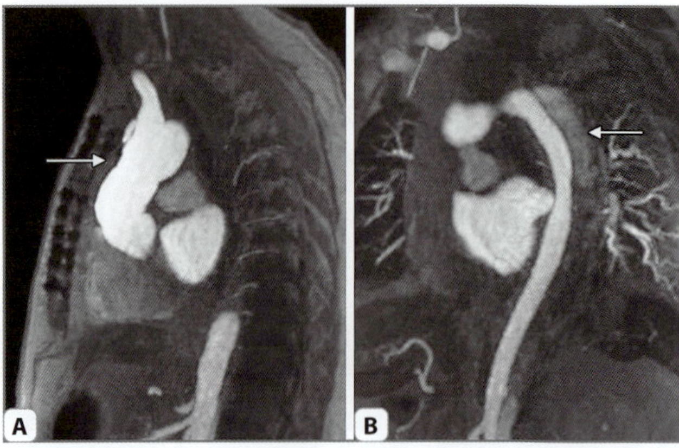

FIGS. 34A AND B: 3D-CE-MRA oblique coronal views in a post operative patient of type A dissection (post Bentall) show normally opacified ascending aorta (arrow in A) and faintly opacified false lumen (usually due to slow flow) in descending thoracic (arrow in B) and normally opacified true lumen.

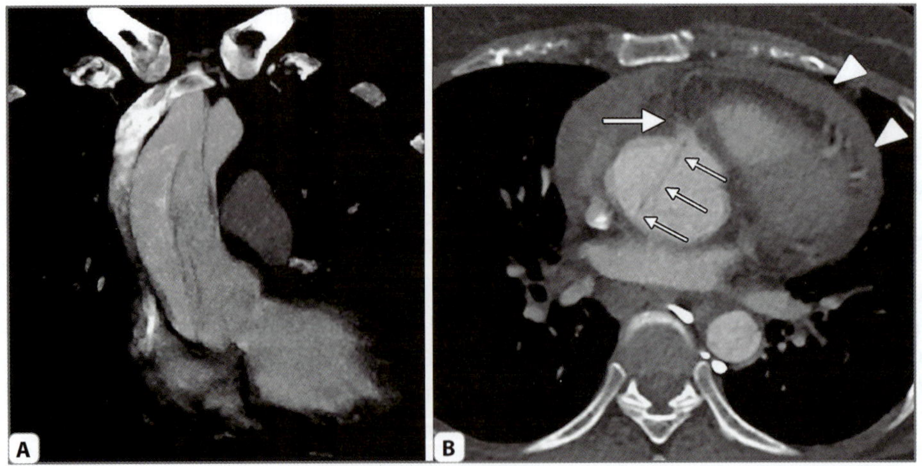

FIGS. 33A AND B: ECG-triggered CTA of ascending aorta oblique coronal and axial images show type A dissection (A and B) with intimal flap (thin arrows) extending into the ostia of right coronary artery (thick arrow). Note hemopericardium (arrowheads).

A mnemonic-based approach to the evaluation of aortic dissection was proposed by Dake et al.[50] The DISSECT classification system guides the radiologist through an assessment of six critical characteristics that facilitate a complete description of the most salient details that currently influence the selection of a treatment. The features of aortic dissection that are to be mentioned in the report are enumerated in **Table 7**.

Acute type A aortic dissection constitutes a surgical emergency since these patients are at high risk for a life-threatening complication such as aortic regurgitation, cardiac tamponade, stroke, frank rupture and myocardial infarction. Medical management has a mortality of up to 50% as compared to the operative mortality of 7–36% in experienced centers.[51,52]

At certain advanced centers, a hybrid approach to the repair of type A aortic dissection, referred to as the "frozen elephant trunk repair", may be attempted. This involves combination of an open approach to surgically repair the ascending aorta, while deploying a stent-graft to manage the descending aorta.

Type B dissection is generally managed initially with the best medical therapy as given in **Box 3**.

TABLE 7: DISSECT classification.

D: Duration of symptoms	• *Acute*: <2 weeks from onset of symptoms • *Subacute*: 2 weeks to 3 months after symptom onset • *Chronic*: >3 months from initial symptoms
I: Intimal tear location	Ascending aorta, aortic arch, descending aorta, abdominal aorta, unknown
S: Sizes	Maximum aortic diameter at any level
SE: Segmental extent	Proximal entry and distal re-entry tear locations

C: Complications	• Cardiac tamponade
	• Rupture
	• Branch vessel malperfusion
	• Static and/or dynamic branch involvement with accompanying stroke, paraplegia, coronary, mesenteric, visceral, renal, and/or extremity symptoms
	• Progression of aortic involvement with proximal or distal extension of dissection Involvement of aortic valve in case of type A dissection
	• *Other*:
	  ○ Uncontrollable hypertension
	  ○ Uncontrollable clinical symptoms
	  ○ Rapid false lumen dilation
	  ○ Overall trans-aortic enlargement of >10 mm within the first 2 weeks of initial diagnosis

T: Thrombosis of false lumen	Patent, completely or partially thrombosed

Intervention (surgical or endovascular) for descending thoracic aortic dissection is reserved for patients who develop complications as described in **Table 7**.

Type B aortic dissection with such complications is associated with mortality rates that can exceed 60%. Interventional management consists of placing a stent graft over the proximal entry tear which has been shown to acutely depressurize the false lumen and restore normal flow in the true lumen **(Figs. 35A to F)**.

The endograft should be sized to the estimated diameter of the true lumen, not the overall diameter of the dissected aorta. Successful stent-graft exclusion in the thoracic aorta, or any other aortic segment, necessitates at least 15-mm proximal and distal "landing zones" of non-diseased aorta to achieve fixation and seal. However, in case the proximal landing zones are inadequate, there are strategies and techniques designed to "extend the landing zone". These techniques may be endovascular (use of branched stent graft, chimney, or snorkel technique) or surgical debranching techniques to extend the landing zones. These techniques are known as debranching techniques. Using the classification proposed by Criado et al.[53] landing zones can be classified into five types **(Fig. 36)**. The complexity of procedures required to lengthen the landing zones increases as the landing zone of stent graft extends more proximally.

An endovascular procedure with proximal landing zones at Zone 3 and 4 is an optimal situation and requires no extra step for aortic interventions. A proximal landing zone involving Zone 2 would require either coverage (and occlusion) or transposition of the left subclavian artery (LSA). If the left common carotid artery (CCA) origin (Zone 1) is involved, transposition to the right CCA via a carotid-carotid bypass can be performed. If the disease involves the full entire aortic arch, coverage of the innominate artery (IA) would be required along with transposition of the IA and left CCA to the ascending aorta **(Figs. 37A to E)**. Alternatively, branched stent graft or chimney techniques can be used in these cases in centers where expertise is available.

When critical organ ischemia is not relieved by occlusion of the proximal entry tear with a stent graft, bare stents can be placed from the true lumen of the aorta into the true lumen of the branch vessel to restore flow.[54] Another

BOX 3: Best medical management for aortic dissection.

Four main management goals for type B dissection patients either with or without surgical/interventional management

1. Antihypertensive drugs to minimize the aortic wall shear stress caused by increased blood pressure
2. Continued monitoring for high-risk clinical conditions/presence of complications which would require immediate treatment
3. Serial imaging to detect signs of progression, re-dissection, or aneurysm formation
4. Optimal pain management

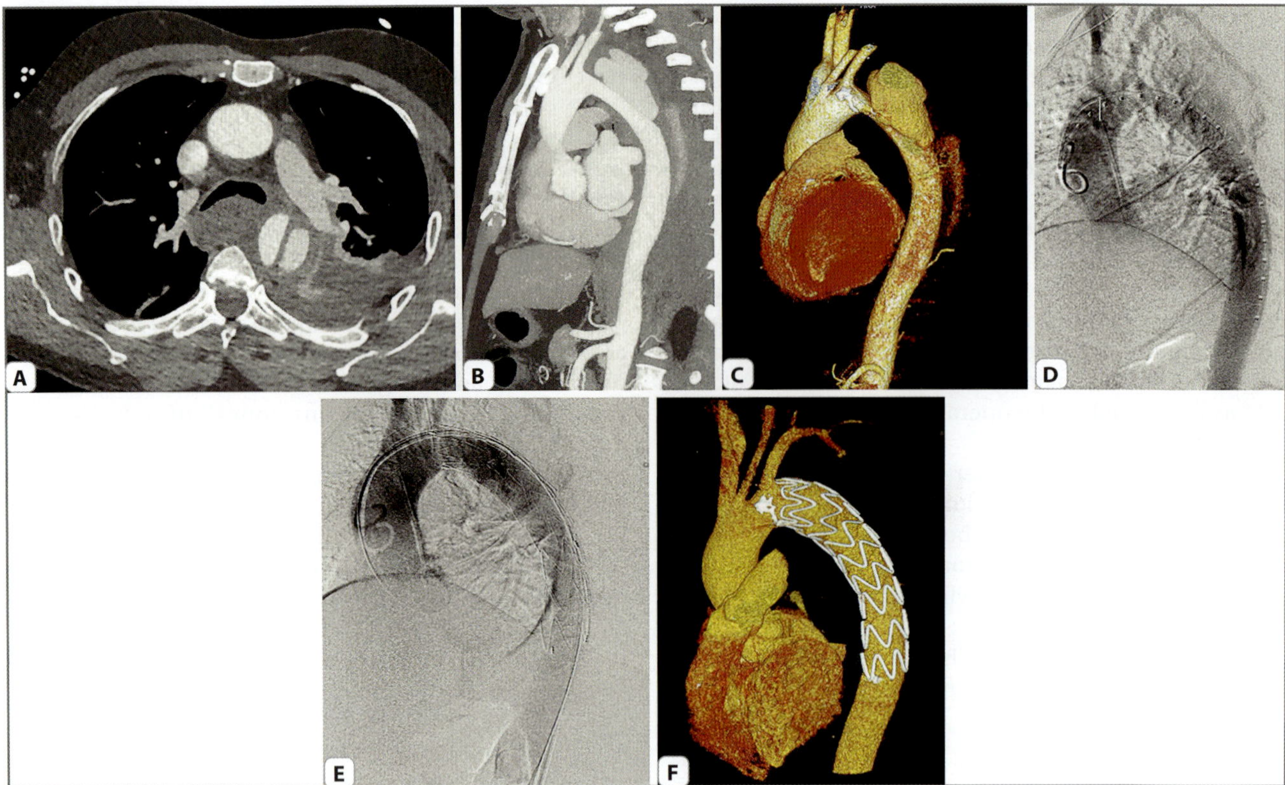

FIGS. 35A TO F: Stent-graft treatment of ruptured type B aortic dissection. (A and B) Axial, sagittal MIP and VRT images showing type B dissection with proximal tear distal to left subclavian artery. (C) aortogram in the left anterior oblique projection with faint opacification of the false lumen as it fills more slowly than the true lumen. (D) Angiogram after a stent-graft placement over the entry tear in the true lumen of the descending thoracic aorta. The true lumen has a normal diameter, and the false lumen is no longer opacified. (E and F) 1 month follow-up CT image showing stent in situ.

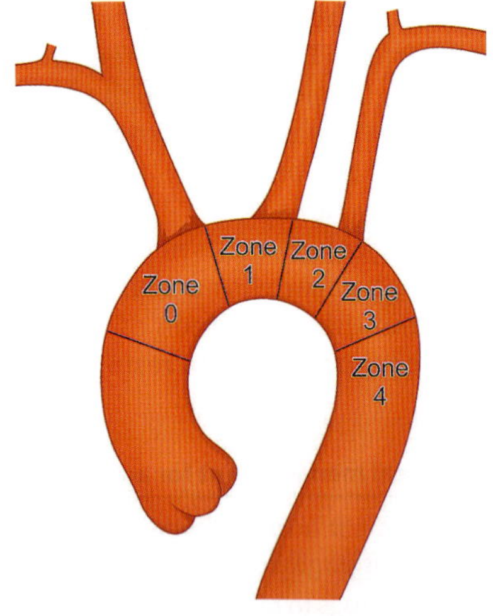

FIG. 36: Criado classification of aortic landing zones.

minimally invasive option is percutaneous fenestration of the aortic flap. This intentionally causes creation of a large distal exit tear, which decompresses the false lumen and relieves the dynamic obstruction of the true lumen. This is usually done as a lifesaving or as an adjunctive procedure as mortality with fenestration alone can be high. One of the ways to create a fenestration is to cross the intimal flap with an intravascular ultrasound to guide the puncture. This fenestration may then be enlarged using angioplasty balloons.

Delivery systems for thoracic stent-grafts tend to be large, so assessment of the femoral arteries, iliac arteries and abdominal aorta is necessary when evaluating a patient for one of these procedures. Surgical placement of a temporary graft to the common iliac artery or distal aorta (termed a *conduit*) may be required to deliver the endograft in patients with small or diseased pelvic arteries.

Although type B complicated aortic dissection can be handled by stent graft placement, with various adjunctive techniques, total surgical repair may be needed for those whose anatomy cannot support a stent-graft.

A summary of the prerequisites and challenges for interventional management is given in **Table 8**.

Endovascular intervention in patients with uncomplicated dissection may improve long-term outcomes by favorably influencing the dynamic relationship of the true and false lumen however, the results of multiple studies support a complication and patient-specific approach to type B dissection as the best treatment paradigm.

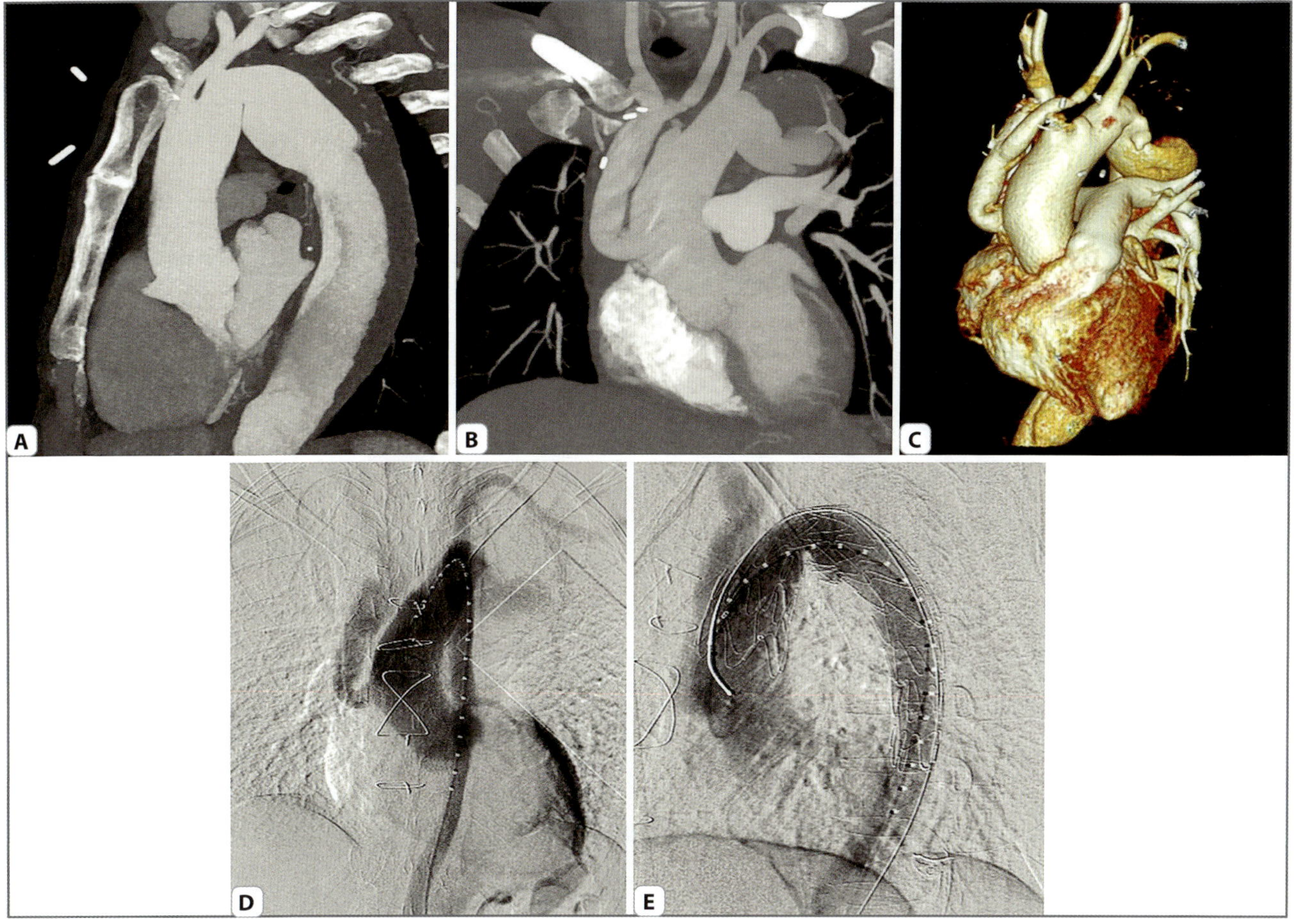

FIGS. 37A TO E: Stent-graft treatment with debranching technique of ruptured type B aortic dissection with unfavorable proximal landing zone anatomy. (A) Oblique sagittal image showing acute angulation of arch with proximal tear at the root of the left subclavian artery (not shown in image); (B to D) Oblique coronal, VRT images and aortogram showing innominate artery transposed to ascending aorta effectively "elongating the proximal landing zone". The left common carotid was transposed to the innominate artery. (E) Angiogram after a stent-graft placement over the entry tear in the true lumen of the descending thoracic aorta. The true lumen has a normal diameter and the false lumen is no longer opacified.

TABLE 8: Prerequisites for interventional management of dissection.

Proximal landing zone	• Atleast 1.5 cm normal aorta distal to left subclavian artery • If unavailable debranching procedures to extend the proximal landing zone
Distal landing zone	1.5–2 cm normal aorta above celiac artery
Landing zone diameters	Varies with device
Severe angulation of proximal or distal aorta	Longer landing zones needed which may necessitate debranching
Patency and caliber of pelvic arteries	• Minimal external iliac/common femoral artery diameter required 7 mm • Smaller vessels may require direct access to the common iliac artery or abdominal aorta via surgical conduit

A suggested algorithmic approach to management of AD is given in **Flowchart 2**.

INTRAMURAL HEMATOMA

Intramural hematoma is diagnosed by the presence of a circular or crescent-shaped thickening of >5 mm of the aortic wall in the absence of detectable blood flow. It accounts for approximately 10–25% of AAS. IMH was first believed to be result of rupture of the vasa vasorum, allowing bleeding between the elastic lamina of the aortic media. However, recent findings suggest that at least some IMHs may be initiated by small intimal tears that are undetectable by current aortic imaging modalities and are often overlooked on gross inspection of the aorta at the time of surgery or autopsy.[55-58] IMH can be associated with several conditions, including spontaneous ("typical") aortic dissection, penetrating ulcer, aortic trauma, and iatrogenic dissection (cardiac catheterization, cardiac surgery).

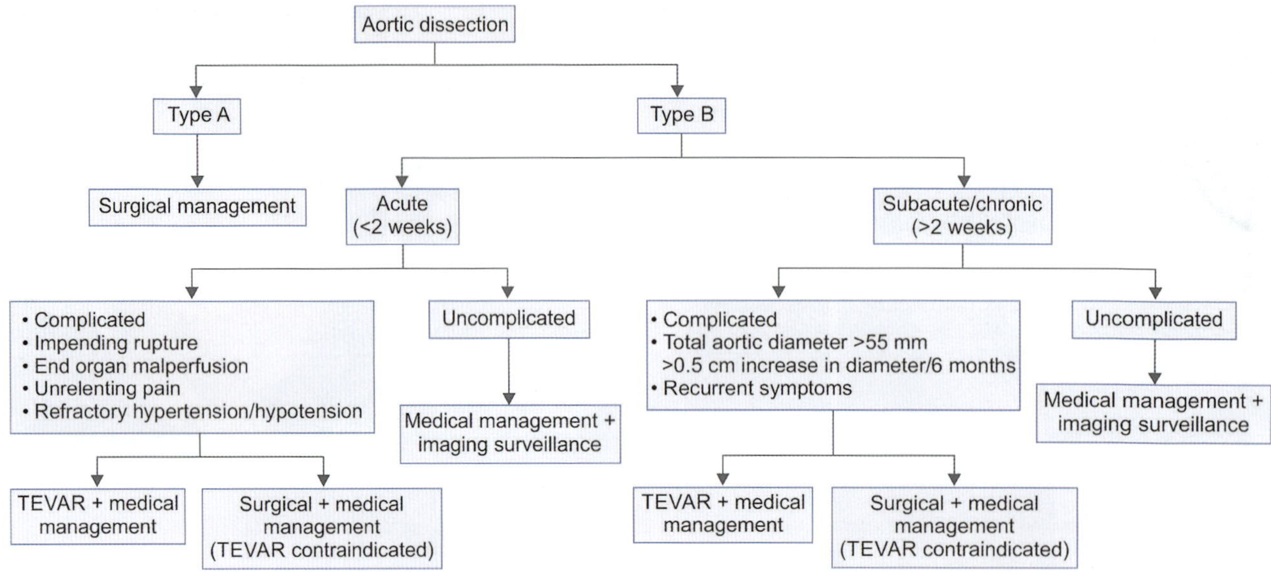

FLOWCHART 2: Treatment strategy for dissection of aorta.
(TEVAR: thoracic endovascular aortic repair)

Imaging features of IMH are **(Figs. 38A and B)**:

- Focal aortic wall thickening (crescentic > concentric)
- Preserved luminal shape with smooth luminal border
- Absence of dissection flap and false lumen
- Echolucent regions may be present in the aortic wall
- Central displacement of intimal calcium.

Predictors of complication and surveillance: Maximum aortic diameter (>40 to 50 mm), wall thickness (>10–12 mm) and associated periaortic hemorrhage or pleural effusion has been described as a predictor of progression. IMH may weaken the aortic wall and either progress outward with aortic expansion and/or rupture **(Figs. 39A to C)** or inward with disruption of the intima-media, resulting in typical aortic dissection. Therefore, serial imaging is necessary to rule out progression in patients who receive only medical treatment. Although there are no established guidelines for the optimal frequency and longitudinal duration for surveillance imaging of patients with IMH, Evangelista et al. on the basis of the significant dynamic evolution of IMH, recommended imaging at 1, 3, 6, 9, and 12 months from the time of diagnosis. Once stability has been documented, surveillance imaging may be annual.[59]

PENETRATING AORTIC ULCER

Penetrating aortic ulcer (PAU) is defined as ulceration of an aortic atherosclerotic plaque penetrating through the internal elastic lamina into the media.[60] These lesions represent 2–7% of all AAS. Most common location of PAU is the middle and lower descending thoracic aorta, and less frequently noted in the aortic arch or abdominal aorta. Propagation of the ulcerative process may either lead to IMH, pseudoaneurysm, or even aortic rupture or an acute AD, and hence requires close follow-up.[61]

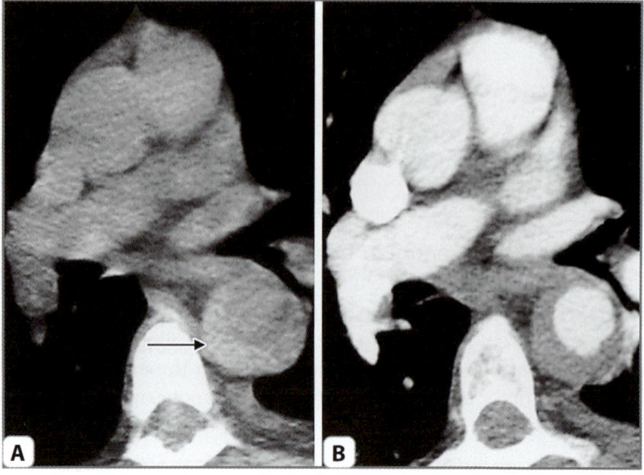

FIGS. 38A AND B: Non-contrast (A) axial and post-contrast CTA (B) images show high density crescentic thickening along right posterolateral wall of distal descending thoracic aorta.

On non-contrast CT, PAU resembles an IMH. Contrast-enhanced CT is the technique of choice for diagnosis of PAU, which shows characteristic finding of localized ulceration, penetrating through the aortic intima into the aortic wall **(Figs. 39A to C)**. Focal thickening or high attenuation of the adjacent aortic wall suggests associated IMH. The limitation of MRI is that it is unable to detect displacement of intimal calcification, which frequently accompanies PAU.

Management of Intramural Hematoma and Penetrating Aortic Ulcer

The management goals and treatment protocol for IMH and PAU are similar to type A and B AD. Surgery is advocated in

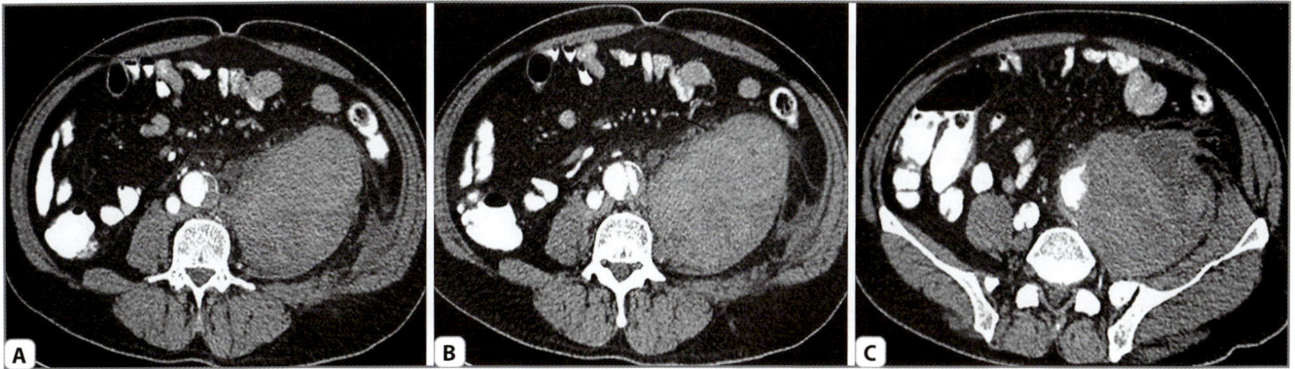

FIGS. 39A TO C: Serial CTA axial sections (craniocaudal) of distal abdominal aorta near bifurcation shows intramural hematoma along left lateral wall (A) penetrating ulcer (B) and rupture (C) leading to a large retroperitoneal hematoma (A to C).

patients with type A IMH and ascending aortic ulcerations. Initial medical therapy is advocated in patients with type B IMH and descending thoracic aortic PAU. Some authors suggest that a symptomatic ulceration that is 20 mm in diameter or greater, or 10 mm in depth, should be managed aggressively.[62]

Complicated type B IMH with expansion of the hematoma, continued pain, development of hemorrhagic pleural effusion, or rupture requires more aggressive management with stent graft placement or surgery. The endovascular procedure is similar to that described for aortic dissection.

AORTITIS

Aortitis is an inflammatory condition of the aortic wall which can be infectious or noninfectious in origin. Imaging is required for assessment of aortitis and is crucial in establishing the diagnosis. CT, MRI, and nuclear fusion imaging (PET CT/MRI) are the main imaging modalities for initial diagnosis and follow-up.[63,64]

Takayasu's Arteritis

Takayasu's arteritis (TA) is a necrotizing, obliterative and segmental primary large vessel panarteritis of unknown etiology that affects the aorta and its major branches including the pulmonary artery. It is most common in young Asian women and occurs about 10 times more commonly in women than in men. The etiologically factors implicated are previous tubercular infection, genetic factors and autoimmune mechanisms. The diagnosis of Takayasu's arteritis is often delayed because of a nonspecific clinical presentation. Ishikawa's criteria (sensitivity 60.4% and specificity 95%) and American College of Rheumatology criteria (sensitivity 77.4% and specificity 95%) have been widely used for diagnosis of this disease. Modified diagnostic criteria for Takayasu's arteritis by Sharma et al. have led to an early diagnosis of this condition thereby preventing high morbidity and mortality **(Table 9)**.[65,66]

The sensitivity and specificity using this modified diagnostic criteria is 92.5 and 95% respectively.

Incidence:
- 2.6 new cases/million/year
- 2.2% at autopsy

Pathology: TA is a T-cell-mediated panarteritis which begins in adventitial vasa vasorum with inward progression. Destructive perivascular cuffing of vasa vasorum is followed by fibrosis and calcifications and leads to aneurysmal dilatations followed by stenosis of aorta and its branches. Arterial wall inflammation with adventitial mononuclear infiltration, multiple granulomas and perivascular cuffing of the vasa vasorum observed in early stages, followed by chronic fibrosis and wall calcification in later stages. Chronic necrotizing wall inflammation causes destruction of the media with resultant stenosis and/or aneurysm formations.[63,66-68]

Types (Fig. 40)[69]

- *Type I* involves only the branches of the aortic arch.
- *Type IIa* involves the aorta only at its ascending portion and/or at the aortic arch. The branches of the aortic arch may be involved as well. The rest of the aorta is not affected.
- *Type IIb* affects the descending thoracic aorta with or without involvement of the ascending aorta or the aortic arch with its branches. The abdominal aorta is not involved.
- *Type III* is concomitant involvement of the descending thoracic aorta, the abdominal aorta, and/or the renal arteries. The ascending aorta and the aortic arch and its branches are not involved.
- *Type IV* involves only the abdominal aorta and/or the renal arteries.
- *Type V* is a generalized type, with combined features of the other types.

Note: Involvement of the coronary and pulmonary arteries should be indicated as C(+) or P(+), respectively.

TABLE 9: Modified diagnostic criteria for Takayasu's arteritis, Sharma et al.[65]

Three major criteria	
1. Left mid subclavian artery lesion	The most severe stenosis or occlusion present in the mid portion from the point 1 cm proximal to the vertebral artery orifice up to 3 cm distal to the orifice determined by angiography
2. Right mid subclavian artery lesion	The most severe stenosis or occlusion present in the mid portion from the right vertebral artery orifice to the point 3 cm distal to orifice determined by angiography
3. Characteristic signs and symptoms of at least 1 month duration	These include limb claudication, pulselessness or pulse differences in limbs, an unobtainable or significant blood pressure difference (>10 mm Hg systolic blood pressure difference in limb), fever, neck, pain, transient amaurosis, blurred vision, syncope, dyspnea or palplitations
Ten minor criteria	
1. High ESR	Unexplained persistent high ESR >20 mm/h (Westergren) at diagnosis or presence of the evidence in patients' history
2. Carotid artery tenderness	Unilateral or bilateral tenderness of common carotid on palpation. Neck muscle tenderness is unacceptable
3. Hypertension	Persistent blood pressure >140/90 mm Hg brachial or >160/90 mm Hg popliteal
4. Aortic regurgitation or annuloaortic ectasia	• By auscultation or Doppler echocardiology or angiography • By angiography or two-dimensional echocardiography
5. Pulmonary artery lesion	Lobar or segmental arterial occlusion or equivalent determined by angiography or perfusion scintigraphy, or presence of Stenosis, aneurysm, luminal irregularity or any combination in pulmonary trunk or in unilateral or bilateral pulmonary arteries determined by angiography
6. Left mid common carotid lesion	Presence of the most severe stenosis or occlusion in the mid portion of 5 cm in length from the point 2 cm distal to its orifice determined by angiography
7. Distal brachiocephalic trunk lesion	Presence of the most severe stenosis or occlusion in the distal third determined by angiography
8. Descending thoracic aorta lesion	Narrowing, dilatation or aneurysm, luminal irregularity or any combination determined by angiography: tortuosity alone is unacceptable
9. Abdominal aorta lesion	Narrowing, dilatation or aneurysm, luminal irregularity or aneurysm combination
10. Coronary artery lesion	Documented on angiography below the age of 30 years in the absence of risk factors like hyperlipidemia or diabetes mellitus

Note: Presence of two major or one major and two minor criteria or four minor criteria suggests a high probability of Takayasu's arteritis.

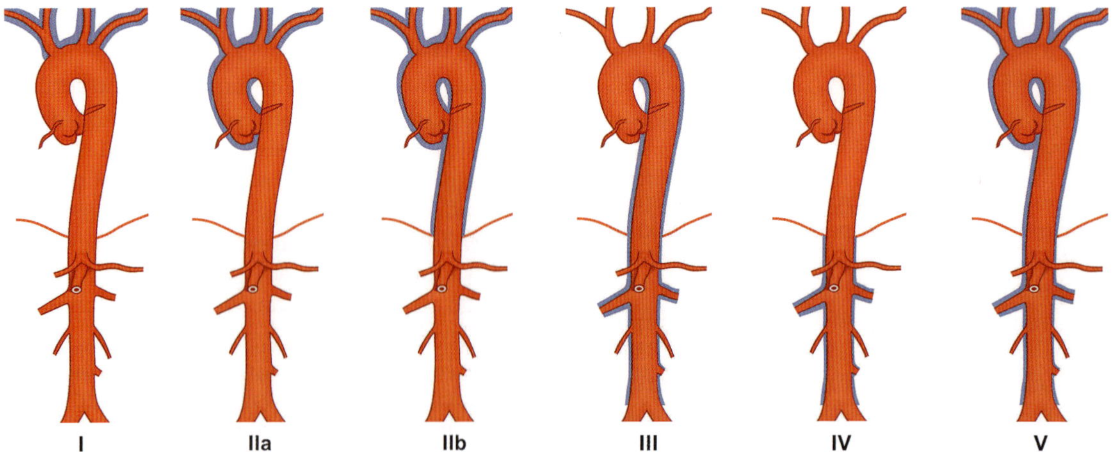

FIG. 40: Schematic diagrams show types of Takayasu's arteritis.

The commonly involved arteries are left subclavian artery (50%), left common carotid (20%), brachiocephalic, renal arteries, celiac trunk, SMA and pulmonary arteries (50%).

Imaging Findings

Almost all the available imaging modalities have some role in diagnosis and follow-up of TA, however currently CT, MRI and/or PET CT/MRI are the main imaging modalities. Role of conventional angiography in diagnosis of TA is almost obsolete and restricted for interventional procedures.[70]

Early/acute stage: The arterial wall thickening **(Fig. 41)** can be detected on CT or MRI (fat suppressed T1-weighted postcontrast MR images) as soft tissue thickening encircling the aorta (swollen intima) with circumferential peripheral contrast enhancement (inflamed media and adventitia. On T2-weighted sequences mural edema is depicted as high signal. Nuclear fusion imaging (PET) with 18-flurorodeoxyglucose (18F-FDG) with either CT or MRI is now emerging as the initial diagnosis and assessment of disease activity with high sensitivity of 60–90% and specificity of 88–100% as 18F-FDG is a surrogate marker of increased activity of inflammatory cells.[70-73]

Chronic stage: The disease is characterized by development of aneurysm and linear stenosis of descending and abdominal aorta. There may be long diffuse or short segmental irregular stenosis with occlusion of the major branches of the aorta near its origin **(Fig. 42)**. There may be skip lesions, abundant collateralization, saccular or fusiform aortic aneurysm (10–15%) **(Fig. 43)**.[74,75] These findings can be seen on conventional angiography, CTA or MRA. Cross-sectional imaging, in addition, shows arterial wall thickening, mural calcium deposition and full thickness calcification which is very suggestive of chronic phase of disease.[76,77]

FIG. 41: Takayasu arteritis: CTA source image showing circumferential mural thickening of the lateral common carotid and subclavian arteries.

Management of Takayasu Arteritis

Active TA is treated with steroids or immunosuppressants before revascularization as revascularization during the active phase can increase the risk of procedure-related complications, including restenosis and dissection.[78] Occlusion/restenosis rate of transluminal angioplasty with or without stent implantation in active disease is reported to be as high as 71.4% after a follow-up of 1.3 years.

Symptomatic TA is treated with revascularization of the affected vessels. In general, surgical bypass or endovascular intervention should be avoided during the active phase of TA, unless the presence of an acute life-threatening condition outweighs the risk any intervention including restenosis and dissection.[78-80]

Even in life-threatening situations (hypertensive encephalopathy, flash pulmonary edema and congestive

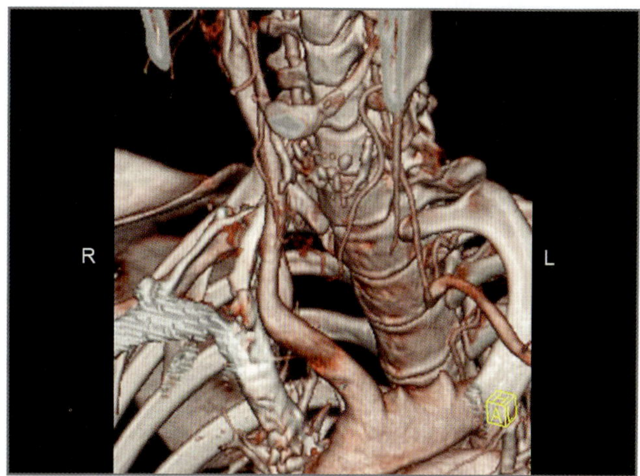

FIG. 42: Takayasu arteritis: CTA VR image showing total occlusion of left common carotid and subclavian arteries just beyond their origins.

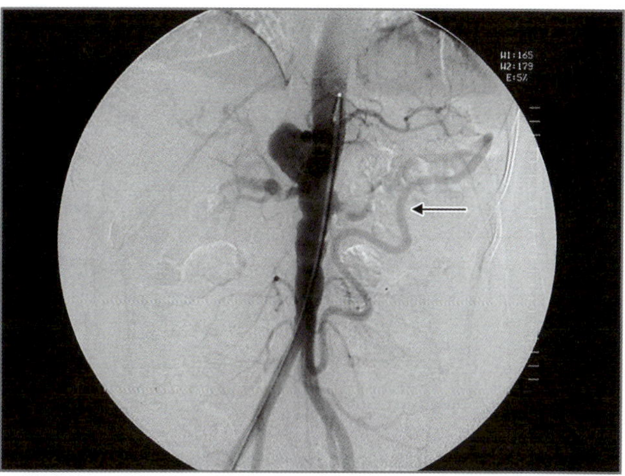

FIG. 43: Takayasu arteritis: DSA shows aneurysmal dilatation of the abdominal aorta above renal arteries, irregular aortic contour, collaterals from IMA (arrow).

heart failure), endovascular treatment is the treatment modality that carries the lowest risk of morbidity and mortality to the patient and should be considered before open surgical therapy. This is due to the fact that, surgical procedures are complicated by graft reocclusion, anastomotic site aneurysm and increased morbidity. The progressive inflammatory nature of TA has also a widespread problem limiting use of reconstructive surgery.

In the chronic fibrotic stage, the principle of treatment is revascularization either by surgery or balloon angioplasty. Balloon angioplasty is a relatively simple and cost-effective method for relief of stenotic lesions in patients with TA **(Figs. 44A to D)**. It avoids the risks of anesthesia and shortens the hospital stay. Percutaneous angioplasty yielded excellent results with success rates ranging from 81 to 100% and low morbidity and mortality.[78]

The problem with balloon angioplasty is recurrence of the stenosis, which is however, easily tackled by a secondary reintervention. Studies also reported improved results with primary stenting; however, stenting is better reserved for flow limiting dissections or persisting stenoses after balloon angioplasty. Moreover, the presence of long segment juxta diaphragmatic stenosis involving the origin of visceral arteries, often in a young child precludes the use of a stent. The risk of stent occlusion is also higher due to protracted nature of the disease with waxing and waning of disease activity.

Immunoglobulin G4-related Aortitis

Immunoglobulin G4 (IgG4) related diseases are of unknown etiology which can affect any organ from head to toe. It is characterized by diffuse or focal tumor like lesions with lymphoplasmacytic infiltrate enriched with IgG4 positive plasma cells and fibrosis. They are often associated with elevated serum IgG4 levels. It predominantly affects males in their fourth to sixth decades, however exact incidence is unknown. It is a great mimicker with varying differential diagnosis on imaging, ranging from inflammatory lesions to malignancy.[81]

Recognition of imaging findings can suggest a diagnosis, which can be confirmed on serology, and histopathology. This is of paramount importance as the disease responds to immunosuppressive therapy. On pathology the lymphoplasmacytic cells are IgG4 positive with negative CD3 and CD20 staining which are markers for T-cell and B-cell related inflammation respectively and are positive in aortoarteritis.

On imaging a soft tissue like mass is seen encasing aorta and its branches, typically without any luminal compromise unlike aortoarteritis. The soft tissue is hypodense on CT **(Figs. 45A and B)** and demonstrates varying signal intensity on MR depending on degree and stage of fibrosis.[82] Contrast enhancement can be variable depending upon degree of fibrosis.

In long-standing cases aneurysmal dilatation of abdominal aorta and extensive wall thickening with or without periaortic inflammatory extension can be seen.[83] Rupture though uncommon with IgG4-related disease may be seen **(refer Figs. 24 to 26)**.

18F-FDG PET-CT and CT are useful in detecting inflammatory activity in the aneurysmal wall **(Figs. 46A to D)** and assessing treatment response.[84]

AORTIC TRAUMA

Traumatic injuries to the aorta may result from either blunt (nonpenetrating, indirect) or sharp (penetrating, direct) trauma. Penetrating trauma is usually caused by stab or bullet wounds that puncture the aortic wall. Rare causes include misplacement of spinal fixation screws and lacerations from spinal fractures. Blunt aortic injuries (BAIs) are far more common, and the aortic wall

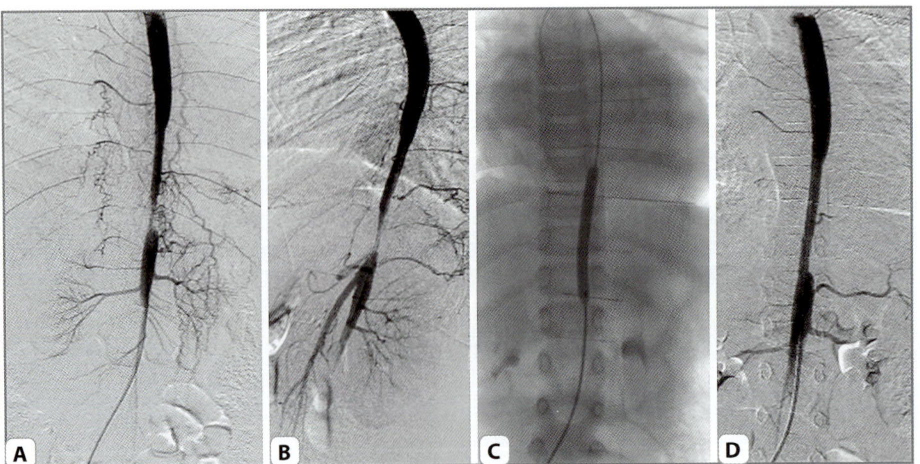

FIGS. 44A TO D: Balloon angioplasty in a patient of Takayasu arteritis with heart failure. (A and B) aortogram showing long segment tight stenosis of the juxta-diaphragmatic thoracic aorta. (C) Balloon angioplasty of the stenosed segment. (D) Postangioplasty aortogram showing significant reduction of degree of stenosis with reduction of the trans-stenotic gradient from 65 to 15 mm Hg.

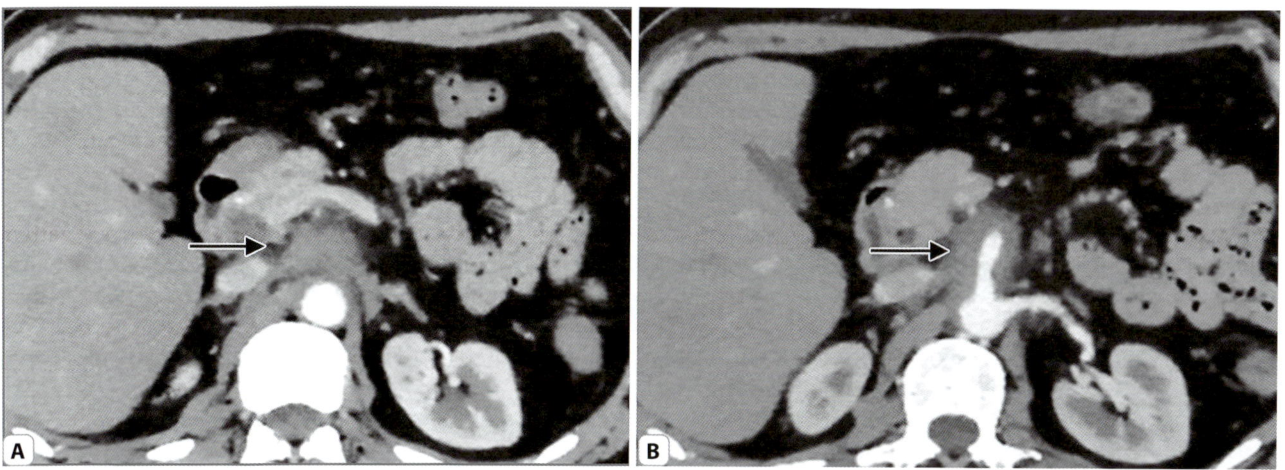

FIGS. 45A AND B: CTA axial images an ill-defined soft tissue is seen in preaortic location (black arrow in A) which is encasing the celiac artery from its origin (black arrow in B) without any luminal compromise.

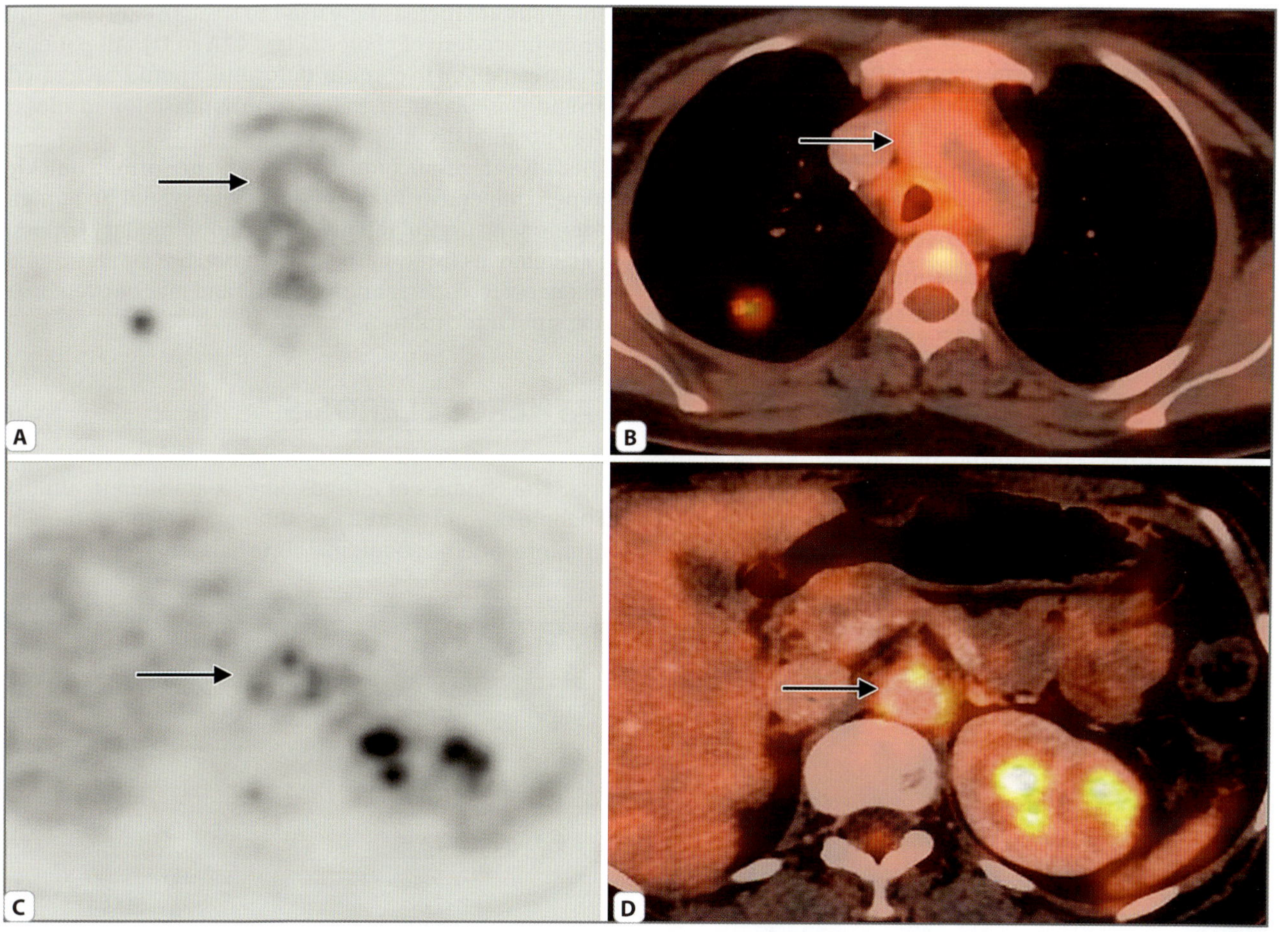

FIGS. 46A TO D: 18F-FDG PET and fused PET-CT images show increased activity in arch of aorta and abdominal aorta at the level of origin of celiac axis.

Courtesy: Dr Rajender Basher, Assistant Professor, Department of Nuclear Medicine, PGIMER, Chandigarh, India.

is damaged from the inside to the outside, from the intima to the adventitia.

Traumatic transaction of the aorta is a common cause of death in high-speed accidents. Sudden deceleration causes torsion and a shearing stress at the isthmus where the aorta is relatively fixed. "Osseous pinch" effect is due to pinching of the aorta between the manubrium and medial end of clavicle anteriorly and spine posteriorly. It is due to this pinch that there is posterior displacement of the heart which generates aortic torsion.[85] About 90% of traumatic tears occur around the isthmus. The other sites include aortic arch with avulsion of brachiocephalic trunk (4.5%), ascending aorta (1%), and descending aorta (2.5%). These patients often have multiple injuries and pose a considerable challenge for early and rapid imaging.

Grading of Aortic Injuries[86]

- *Grade 0*: Normal mediastinum and normal aorta
- *Grade I*: Abnormal mediastinum and normal aorta. 5–10% of blunt trauma of chest may have isolated mediastinal hematoma
- *Grade II*: Minimal aortic injury (differential diagnosis of ductus arteriosus remnant or atherosclerosis)
- *Grade III*: Confined aortic injury
- *Grade IV*: Aortic disruption

Imaging

The chest X-ray is a good screening tool for detection of mediastinal hemorrhage but affords little as far as definitive diagnosis is concerned. An AP erect chest film with the patient leaning forward is ideal rather than a supine film with 90% sensitivity, 95% specificity and 95% negative predictive value.

The plain X-ray findings include widening of the superior mediastinum, an abnormal aortic contour, shift of the trachea to the right, inferior displacement of the left main bronchus, widening of left paravertebral stripe, etc.

CT: Plain CT may demonstrate mediastinal hematoma. CECT may show an abrupt change in aortic contour, intimal flap, pseudoaneurysm, pseudocoarctation and extravasation of contrast. CTA shows 96.2% sensitivity, 99.8% specificity and 99.7% accuracy for the diagnosis of aortic injury.

MRI: In an acute setting of multiple injuries, MR is not recommended.

Aortography: It is the definitive mode of diagnosis but in view of the high sensitivity of CT, aortography is indicated only in selected cases of chronic aortic trauma.

Management of Thoracic Aortic Injury

The initial management of the patient with a contained aortic transection is stabilization of vitals. Patients with multiple injuries can be managed medically for several days or weeks until an intervention can be performed. The conventional therapy of aortic transection was surgery, but stent-grafts are increasingly used to treat TAI and now the current procedure of choice **(Figs. 47A to D)**. All patients with external aortic contour deformity should be treated with endovascular stent graft as soon as possible and atleast before hospital discharge.

Its advantages include that it can be performed quickly and percutaneously in the patients who would be at high risk for open surgical repair and cardiopulmonary bypass. The challenges faced in this population are similar to the challenges faced in treating type B AD and may be overcome using similar techniques.

ATHEROSCLEROSIS

Atherosclerosis is the most common disease involving aorta. The changes of atherosclerosis are seen in almost all people beyond middle age although they often remain asymptomatic. The abdominal aorta below the renal arteries

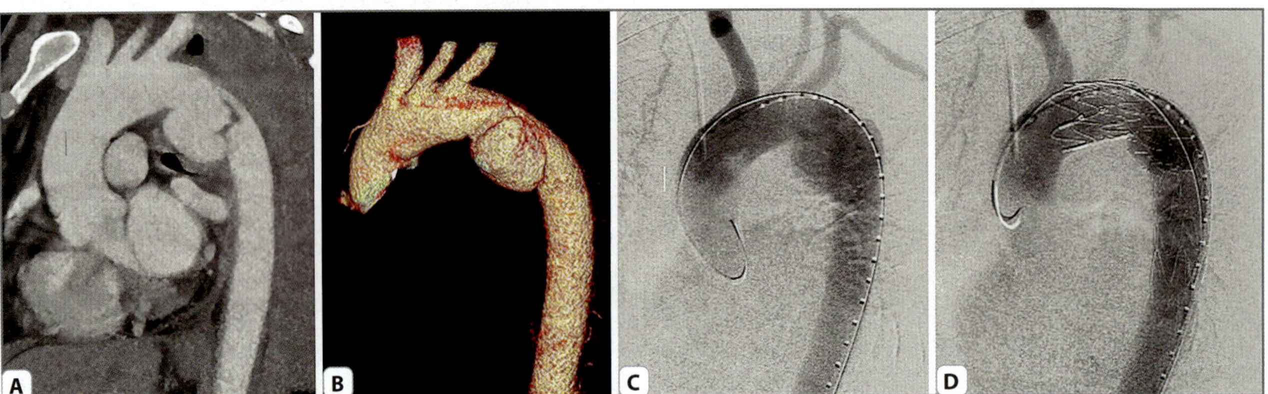

FIGS. 47A TO D: Stent-graft repair of traumatic aortic transection. (A and B) Computed tomography images showing transection with (A) pseudoaneurysm of the proximal descending thoracic aorta; (C) Angiogram prior to stent-graft placement shows in (A). (D) Angiogram following stent-graft placement. The pseudoaneurysm is excluded. Note that the left subclavian artery was sacrificed with its ostia covered by the stent graft.

is the most common site of atherosclerosis and most patients with aortoiliac occlusive disease also have associated femoral and distal arterial occlusions. Reconstruction of the aorta and the iliac arteries by thromboendarterectomy, shunts, stents or angioplasties is an extremely satisfactory therapy for disabling arteriosclerosis obliterans of the aortoiliac system. CTA and DSA are the most effective imaging modalities for the demonstration of aorto iliac obstruction sites, distal run off vessels or collateral vessels and associated stenosis or occlusions of the major visceral arteries.

Pathology

Variable combination of changes of the intima of arteries with focal accumulation of lipids, complex carbohydrates, blood and blood products, fibrous tissue and calcium are the hallmark of atherosclerosis. The disease is divided into:

- *Early changes*: Fatty streak and gelatinous elevation reflected on imaging as "smooth plaque".
- *Fibroatheromatous plaque*: It is seen on imaging as irregular plaque, plaque ulceration, etc. **(Fig. 48)**.
- *The complicated lesion*: Hemorrhage in the plaque, fibrogenesis leading to irregularity and tortousity, weakening of the wall leading to aneurysm formation and calcification **(Fig. 49)**. Stenosis and occlusion may be due to combinations of plaque, fibrosis and calcification.

Imaging

The gross morphological changes can be seen on all imaging modalities. These signs are:[87]

- Diffuse narrowing of the vessels
- Irregular vascular contours and diameters
- Nicks, filling defects and calcifications along the vessel wall
- Spotty or ragged density of the opaque contrast column
- Vessels that are generally large or tortuous or both.
- Saccular dilatations and aneurysm
- Stenosis and or frank occlusion of a vessel (obliterative arteriosclerosis)

Cross-sectional imaging may show a greater degree of luminal compromise, intimal atherosclerosis, mural thrombus and the surgeons may palpate a greater hardening of vessel wall than is seen on catheter angiograms.

Occlusion of the aorto-iliac system: It may be the terminal event in slowly progressive arteriosclerotic stenosis and may be tolerated without medical attention. The blood flow through a vessel may be relatively adequate until the vessel diameter is reduced to about 70%. Acute occlusion may occur following emboli from the heart, atherosclerotic plaques or aneurysms.

Complete occlusion of aorta: It rarely extends upwards to involve the renal arteries but at surgery, the renal and other visceral arteries are frequently found to be partially involved **(Figs. 50A to D)**. Syphilis, aortic dissection and atherosclerosis have been reported to cause complete aortic occlusion. "Leriche syndrome" is due to complete occlusion of the terminal part of abdominal aorta and bilateral common iliac arteries.

Collateral pathways: In stenotic or occlusive disease extensive collateral pathways open up.

- *Visceral collateral network*: The SMA and IMA form the major visceral collateral circulation.
  - Aortic occlusion above IMA: The SMA acts as the main affluent vessel through the left branch of middle colic artery into left colic branch of the IMA (effluent vessel). The "meandering mesenteric artery" or "central anastomotic artery" represents this communication **(Fig. 51)**.

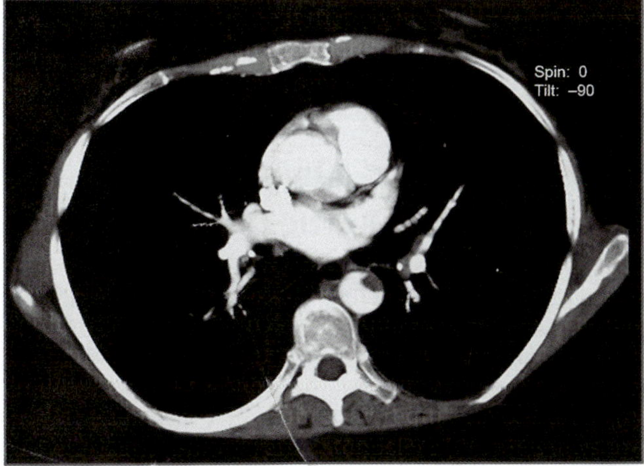

FIG. 48: Atheromatous aortic disease: CTA source image shows atheromatous plaque along anterolateral wall of aorta and projecting into the lumen.

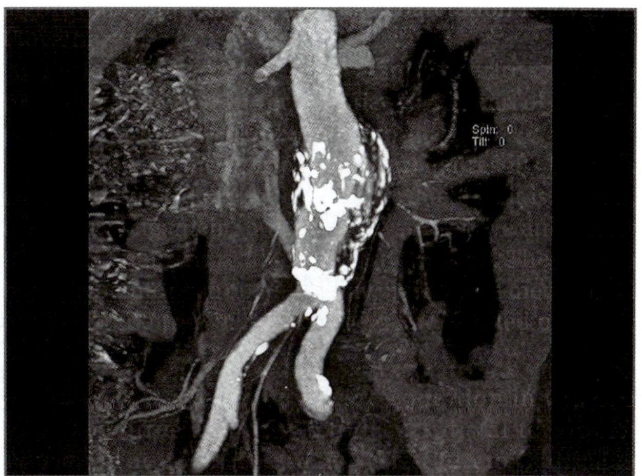

FIG. 49: Atheromatous aortic disease: Large plaque with circumferential calcifications, aortic dilatation, and mural thickening.

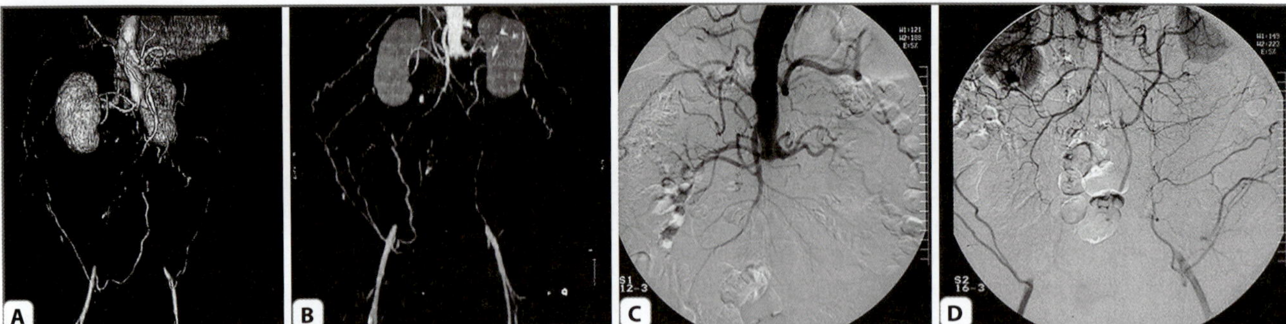

FIGS. 50A TO D: Atherosclerotic complete occlusion of aorta: CTA – (A) VR; (B) MIP projections show complete block of abdominal aorta just distal to renal arteries with collaterals and run off to distal external iliac arteries. DSA (C and D) confirms the findings of CTA.

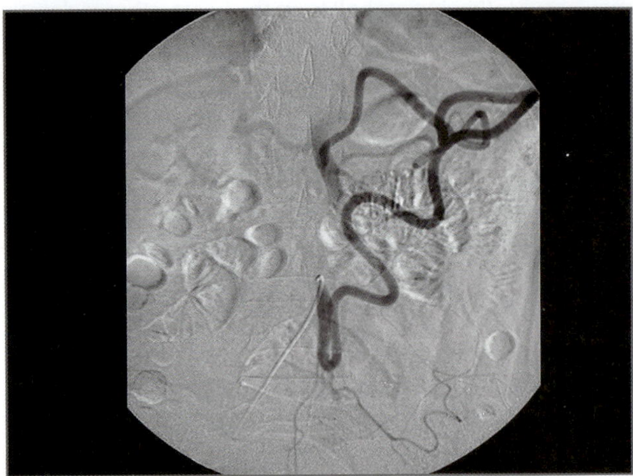

FIG. 51: Visceral collateral network: DSA shows IMA-SMA collateral network.

- Aortic occlusion below IMA: The IMA acts as a key source of collateral circulation via retiform anastomosis between superior hemorrhoidal branches and middle and inferior hemorrhoidal branches of the internal iliac arteries which may reconstitute the external iliac artery.

- *Parietal collateral network*: The parietal vessels that may be seen to bridge aortic occlusions are the intercostals, subcostal, lumbar and median sacral branches of the aorta with iliolumbar, lateral sacral, superior gluteal and obturator branches of the internal iliac arteries, and deep iliac circumflex and medial and lateral circumflex branches of the external iliac and deep femoral arteries. Lumbar branches have anastomotic connections with iliolumbar and gluteal branches of the internal iliac artery. The epigastric arteries may form an important collateral circulation (Winslow's pathway), i.e., from the intercostals and internal mammary artery to the external iliac arteries through the epigastric arteries.

The indications for intervention in patients with occlusive disease of aorta are moderate to severe claudication, rest pain, acutely threatened limb and hemodynamically significant lesion proximal to a distal lesion for which revascularization is being attempted. Patients with mild claudication should undergo medical management with exercise therapy first. Surgical options including aorto-femoral bypass, axillofemoral bypass, femoral–femoral bypass, and aortic endarterectomy are effective treatments but more morbid compared to endovascular approaches. Endovascular management includes balloon angioplasty with or without stenting. Stent placement is indicated for patients with obstructive dissection during balloon angioplasty, recanalization of total occlusions, or lesions that are likely to cause distal embolization. Stent-grafts may be used to exclude symptomatic ulcerated plaque, but otherwise currently have little role for aortic occlusive disease.

Postoperative Aorta

Computed tomography angiography or MRA is the preferred modality for evaluating postoperative aorta for demonstration of perigraft fluid collection and acute hemorrhage. It is also more informative in the diagnosis of graft infection, aortoenteric fistula, anastomotic pseudoaneurysm. These modalities are also very helpful in evaluating the efficacy of endovascular treatment in aortic diseases.[88]

Recent Societal Guidelines for Management of Aortic Diseases

The 2022 American College of Cardiology/American Heart Association Guideline and 2024 European Society Guidelines for aortic diseases has recommended endovascular treatment option as class 1 indication in management of type B aortic dissection, intramural hematoma and penetrating aortic ulcer. Endovascular approach as first approach even in atherosclerotic aortic occlusive lesion if it does not compromise the result of surgery later on.[89,90]

CONCLUSION

Noninvasive imaging of the aorta has almost replaced invasive aortography. US is a good screening modality to confirm or exclude aneurysm, dissection, atherosclerosis etc., but additional anatomic information needs to be obtained prior to an elective repair or endovascular treatment. TEE provides additional information for the thoracic aorta except in the area of the proximal arch (blind spot). Contrast enhanced CT should be used routinely both for preoperative and postoperative assessment of aortic diseases. At a reasonable cost and low-risk to patients, CT and CTA can provide the diagnosis, operability, and anatomic definition including concomitant intra-thoracic or intra-abdominal abnormalities. The recent advances in MR hardware, sequences and computational ability pose a real challenge to all imaging techniques. MR can now provide all the information needed for evaluating aortic diseases, anatomic as well as functional and gadolinium enhanced 3D MRA may replace catheter angiography for both preoperative and postoperative evaluation. Angiography is indicated to answer specific questions posed by the results of clinical examination and/or CT or MRI or as a prerequisite to endovascular intervention. Knowledge of indication of treatment (medical vs. interventional) of different aortic pathologies is of paramount importance. Surgery has been traditionally used in management of these patients. However, with increasing expertise and development of hardware, endovascular techniques have become the first line of management in many of these aortic pathologies.

ACKNOWLEDGMENTS

Dr Sreedhar BC, Department of Radiodiagnosis, PGIMER, Chandigarh for his active support in literature search and preparation of manuscript, Dr Chirag Jain, Department of Radiodiagnosis, PGIMER, Chandigarh for his contribution to art work, Professor Ritambra Nada, Department of Histopathology, PGIMER, Chandigarh for pathology specimens and slides, and Dr Rajender Basher, Additional Professor, Department of Nuclear Medicine, PGIMER, Chandigarh for providing PET-CT images.

REFERENCES

1. Douglas H. "Aorta". Online Etymology Dictionary. Retrieved 9 October; 2017.
2. Rosner F. Medicine in the Bible and the Talmud: selections from classical Jewish sources (Augm. ed.). Hoboken, NJ: KTAV Pub. House;1995. pp. 87-96.
3. Goldstein SA, Evangelista A, Abbara S. Multimodality imaging of diseases of the thoracic aorta in adults: from the American Society of Echocardiography and the European Association of Cardiovascular Imaging: endorsed by the Society of Cardiovascular Computed Tomography and Society for Cardiovascular Magnetic Resonance. J Am Soc Echocardiogr. 2015;28:119-82.
4. Wolf YG, Zarins CK. Noninvasive aortic imaging. In: Bruce L Gewetz (Ed.) Philadelphia: WB Saunders; 2000;1:34-40.
5. Rosenblum JD, Leef JA. Aortography. In: Bruce L Gewetz (Ed.) Philadelphia: WB Saunders; 2000;1:41-50.
6. Lucarotti ME, Shaw E, Heather BP. Distribution of aortic diameter in a screened population. Br J Surg. 1992;79:641-2.
7. Jaffee RB. Radiographic manifestations of congenital anomalies of the aortic arch. RCNA. 1991;29:319-34.
8. Shinley BR. Transesophageal echocardiography in the diagnosis of aortic disease. Seminars in US, CT and MRI. 1993;14:106-16.
9. Benenati JF. Intravasclar ultrasound: the role in diagnostic and therapeutic procedures. RCNA. 1995;33:31-50.
10. Kumamaru KK, Hoppe BF, Richard T, et al. CT Angiography: Current technology and clinical use. Radiol Clin North Am. 2010;48:213-35.
11. Rajiah P. CT and MRI in the Evaluation of Thoracic Aortic Diseases. International Journal of Vascular Medicine. 2013. p. 16.
12. Litmanovich D, Bankier AA, Cantin L, et al. CT and MRI in diseases of the aorta. AJR Am J Roentgenol. 2009;193:928-40.
13. Gutstein A, Wolak A, Lee C, et al. Predicting success of prospective and retrospective gating with dual-source coronary computed tomography angiography: development of selection criteria and initial experience. J Cardiovasc Comput Tomogr. 2008;2:81-90.
14. Gies M, Kalender W A, Wolf H, et al. Dose reduction in CT by anatomically adapted tube current modulation. I. Simulation studies. Med Phys. 1999:26;2235-47.
15. Leschka S, Stolzmann P, Schmid F T, et al. Low kilovoltage cardiac dual-source CT: attenuation, noise, and radiation dose. Eur Radiol. 2008;18:1809-17.
16. Macari M, Israel GM, Berman P, et al. Infrarenal abdominal aortic aneurysms at multi-detector row CT angiography: intravascular enhancement without a timing acquisition. Radiology. 2001;220:519-23.
17. Cademaritiri F, Mollet N, van der Lugt A, et al. Noninvasive 16-row multislice coronary angiography: usefulness of saline chaser. Eur Radiol. 2004;14:178-83.
18. Czum JM, Corse WR, Ho VB. MR angiography of the thoracic aorta. Magn Reson Imaging Clin N Am. 2005;13:41-64.
19. Sakamoto I, Sueyoshi E, Uetani M. MR Imaging of the Aorta. Radiol Clin N Am. 2007;45:485-97.
20. Amano Y, Takahama K, Kumita S. Non-contrast-enhanced MR angiography of the thoracic aorta using cardiac and navigatorgated magnetization-prepared three-dimensional steady-state free precession. J Magn Reson Imaging. 2008;27:504-9.
21. Gebker R, Gomaa O, Schnackenburg B, et al. Comparison of different MRI techniques for the assessment of thoracic aortic pathology: 3D contrast enhanced MR angiography, turbo spin echo and balanced steady state free precession. Int J Cardiovasc Imaging. 2007;23:747-56.

22. Galizia MS, Bolen MA, Flamm SD. MRI of the thoracic aorta. Applied Radiology. 2015:22-6 (www.appliedradiology.com).
23. Prince MR, Yucel EK, Kaufman JA, et al. Dynamic gadolinium-enhanced three-dimensional abdominal MR arteriography. J Magn Reson Imaging.1993;3:877-81.
24. Russo V, Renzulli M, Buttazzi K, et al. Acquired diseases of the thoracic aorta: role of MRI and MRA. Eur Radiol. 2006;16:852-65.
25. Russo V, Renzulli M, Palombara CL, et al. Congenital diseases of the thoracic aorta: role of MRI and MRA. Eur Radiol. 2006;16:676-84.
26. Hom JJ, Ordovas K, Reddy GP. Velocity-encoded Cine MR Imaging in Aortic Coarctation: functional assessment of hemodynamic events1. MPH. Radiographics. 2008;28:407-16.
27. Lee YH, Choi SJ, Ji JD, et al. Diagnostic accuracy of 18F-FDG PET or PET/CT for large vessel vasculitis. Für Rheumatologie. 2016;75:924.
28. Danve A, O'Dell J. The role of 18F fluorodeoxyglucose positron emission tomography scanning in the diagnosis and management of systemic vasculitis. Int J Rheum Dis. 2015;18:714-24.
29. Glaudemans AWJM, de Vries EFJ, Galli F, Dierckx RAJO, Slart RHJA, Signore A. The Use of F-FDG-PET/CT for Diagnosis and Treatment Monitoring of Inflammatory and Infectious Diseases. Clin Dev Immunol. 2013:2013:623036.
30. Khandelwal N, Gupta S. Current concepts in imaging aortic aneurysms. In Sanjiv Sharma (Ed). Recent advances in imaging and intervention in cardiovascular diseases. Singapore Springer. 1996;58-62.
31. Campbell M. Natural history of coarctation of aorta. Br Heart J. 1970;32:633-40.
32. Silversides CK, Marelli A, Beauchesne L, et al. Canadian Cardiovascular Society 2009 Consensus Conference on the management of adults with congenital heart disease: executive summary. Can J Cardiol. 2010;26:143-50.
33. Feltes TF, Bacha E, Beekman RH 3rd, et al. Indications for cardiac catheterization and intervention in pediatric cardiac disease: a scientific statement from the American Heart Association. Circulation. 2011;123:2607-52.
34. Hiratzka LF, Bakris GL, Beckman JA, et al. 2010 ACCF/AHA/ AATS/ ACR/ASA/SCA/SCAI/SIR/STS/ SVM Guidelines for the diagnosis and management of patients with thoracic aortic disease. A report of the American College of Cardiology Foundation/ American Heart Association Task Force on Practice Guidelines, American Association for Thoracic Surgery, American College of Radiology, American Stroke Association, Society of Cardiovascular Anesthesiologists, Society for Cardiovascular Angiography and Interventions, Society of Interventional Radiology, Society of Thoracic Surgeons, and Society for Vascular Medicine. J Am Coll Cardiol. 2010;55:e27-e129.
35. Davies RR, Goldstein LJ, Coady MA, et al. Yearly rupture or dissection rates for thoracic aortic aneurysms: simple prediction based on size. Ann Thorac Surg. 2002;73:17-27.
36. Brewster DC, Cronenwett JL, Hallett JW Jr, et al. Guidelines for the treatment of abdominal aortic aneurysms. Report of a subcommittee of the Joint Council of the American Association for Vascular Surgery and Society for Vascular Surgery. J Vasc Surg. 2003;37:1106.
37. LaRoy LL, Cormier PJ, Matalon TAS, et al. Imaging of abdominal aortic aneurysms. AJR. 1989;152:785-92.
38. Goldstein SA, Evangelista A, Abbara S, et al. Multimodality imaging of diseases of the thoracic aorta in adults: from the American Society of Echocardiography and the European Association of Cardiovascular Imaging: endorsed by the Society of Cardiovascular Computed Tomography and Society for Cardiovascular Magnetic Resonance. J Am Soc Echocardiogr. 2015;28:119-82.
39. Prince MR, Yucel EK, Kaufman JA, et al. Dynamic gadolinium-enhanced three-dimensional abdominal MR arteriography. J Magn Reson Imaging.1993;3:877-81.
40. Brewster DC, Cronenwett JL, Hallett JW Jr, et al. Guidelines for the treatment of abdominal aortic aneurysms. Report of a subcommittee of the Joint Council of the American Association for Vascular Surgery and Society for Vascular Surgery. J Vasc Surg. 2003;37:1106.
41. Bown MJ, Sweeting MJ, Brown LC, et al. Surveillance intervals for small abdominal aortic aneurysms: a meta-analysis. JAMA. 2013;309:806-13.
42. Walsh SR, Tang TY, Sadat U, et al. Endovascular stenting versus open surgery for thoracic aortic disease: systematic review and meta-analysis of perioperative results. J Vasc Surg. 2008;47:1094-8.
43. Zhang Y, Teng Z, Lu Q, et al. Management of complicated aortic aneurysms using multiple overlapping uncovered stents: mid-term outcome from a cohort study. Medicine (Baltimore). 2014;93:e209.
44. Sadat U, Boyle JR, Walsh SR, et al. Endovascular vs open repair of acute abdominal aortic aneurysms: a systematic review and meta-analysis. J Vasc Surg. 2008;48:227-36.
45. Kaufman JA, Geller SC, Brewster DC, et al. Endovascular repair of abdominal aortic aneurysms: current status and future directions. AJR Am J Roentgenol. 2000;175:289-302.
46. William DM, Joshi A, Dake MD, et al. Aortic cobwebs: An anatomic marker identifying the false lumen in aortic dissection–imaging and pathologic correlation. Radiology. 1994;190:167-74.
47. Nienaber CA, vonKodolitsch Y, Nicholas V, et al. The diagnosis of thoracic aortic dissection by non invasive imaging procedures. N Engl J Med. 1993;328:1-14.
48. LePage MA, Quint LE, Sonnad SS, et al. Aortic dissection: CT features that distinguish true lumen from false lumen. AJR Am J Roentgenol. 2001;177:207-11.
49. Pereles FS, McCarthy RM, Baskaran V, et al. Thoracic aortic dissection and aneurysm: evaluation with nonenhanced true FISP MR angiography in less than 4 minutes. Radiology. 2002;223:270-4.
50. Dake MD, Thompson M, van Sambeek M, et al. DISSECT: a new mnemonic-based approach to the categorization of aortic dissection. Eur J Vasc Endovasc Surg. 2013;46:175-90.
51. Nienaber CA, Eagle KA. Aortic dissection: new frontiers in diagnosis and management: Part I: from etiology to diagnostic strategies. Circulation. 2003;108:628-35.
52. Hagan PG, Nienaber CA, Isselbacher EM, et al. The International Registry of Acute Aortic Dissection (IRAD): new insights into an old disease. JAMA. 2000;283:897-903.
53. Criado FJ, Barnatan MF, Rizk Y, et al. Technical strategies to expand stent-graft applicability in the aortic arch and

proximal descending thoracic aorta. J Endovasc Ther. 2002;9(Suppl 2):II32-8.

54. Midulla M, Renaud A, Martinelli T, et al. Endovascular fenestration in aortic dissection with acute malperfusion syndrome: immediate and late follow-up. J Thorac Cardiovasc Surg. 2011;142:66-72.
55. Banning AP. Aortic intramural hematoma. N Engl J Med. 1997;337:1476-7.
56. Chao CP, Walker TG, Kalva SP. Natural history and CT appearances of aortic intramural hematoma. Radiographics. 2009;29:791-804.
57. O'Gara PT, DeSanctis RW. Acute aortic dissection and its variants. Toward a common diagnostic and therapeutic approach. Circulation. 1995;92:1376-8.
58. Park KH, Lim C, Choi JH, et al. Prevalence of aortic intimal defect in surgically treated acute type A intramural hematoma. Ann Thorac Surg. 2008;86:1494-500.
59. Evangelista A, Garcia-del-Castillo H, Gonzalez-Alujas T, et al. Diagnosis of ascending aortic dissection by transesophageal echocardiography: utility of Mmode in recognizing artifacts. J Am Coll Cardiol. 1996;27:102-7.
60. Bolger AF. Aortic intramural haematoma. Heart. 2008;94:1670-4.
61. Nathan DP, Boonn W, Lai E, et al. Presentation, complications, and natural history of penetrating atherosclerotic ulcer disease. J Vasc Surg. 2012;55:10-5.
62. Eggebrecht H, Plicht B, Kahlert P, et al. Intramural hematoma and penetrating ulcers: indications to endovascular treatment. Eur J Vasc Endovasc Surg. 2009;38:659-65.
63. Litmanovich DE, Yıldırım A, Bankier AA. Insights into imaging of aortitis. Insights Imaging. 2012;3:545-60.
64. Moyano JC, Magarolas MA, González EC, et al. Nonurgent aortic disease: clinical-radiological diagnosis of aortitis. Radiology. 2013;55:469-82.
65. Sharma BK, Siveski-Iliskovic N, Singal PK. Takayasu arteritis may be underdiagnosed in North America. Can J Cardiol. 1995;11:311-6.
66. Sharma BR, Jain S, Suri S, et al. Diagnostic criteria for Takayasu arteritis. International Journal of Cardiology. 1996:54 Suppl:S141-7.
67. Restrepo CS, Ocazionez D, Suri R, et al. Aortitis: imaging spectrum of the infectious and inflammatory conditions of the aorta. Radiographics. 2011;31:435-51.
68. Kerr GS, Hallahan CW, Giordano J, et al. Takayasu arteritis. Ann Intern Med. 1994;120:919-29.
69. Gotway MB, Araoz PA, Macedo TA, et al. Imaging findings in Takayasu's arteritis. AJR Am J Roentgenol. 2005;184:1945-50.
70. Matsunaga N, Hayashi R, Sakamoto I, et al. Takayasu's arteritis. Protean radiologic manifestations and diagnosis. Radiographics. 1997;17:579-91.
71. Gornik HL, Creager MA. Aortitis. Circulation. 2008;117: 3039-305.
72. Kobayashi Y, Ishii K, Oda K, et al. Aortic wall inflammation due to Takayasu arteritis imaged with 18F-FDG PET coregistered with enhanced CT. J Nucl Med. 2005;46:917-22.
73. Meller J, Grabbe E, Becker W, et al. Value of F-18 FDG hybrid camera PET and MRI in early Takayasu aortitis. Eur Radiol. 2003;13:400-5.
74. Webb M, Chambers A, AL-N A, et al. The role of 18F-FDG PET in characterising disease activity in Takayasu arteritis. Eur J Nucl Med Mol Imaging. 2004;31:627-34.
75. Sharma S, Rajani M. Aortic occlusion in nonspecific aortoarteritis (Takayasu disease): incidence and spectrum of involvement. Australas Radiol. 1993;37:57-9.
76. Sharma S, Rajani M, Talwar KK. Angiographic morphology in nonspecific aortoarteritis (Takayasu's arteritis): a study of 126 patients from north India. Cardiovasc Intervent Radiol. 1992;15:160-5.
77. Sharma S, Sharma S, Taneja K, et al. Morphological mural changes in the aorta in non specific aortoarteritis (Takayasu's arteritis): assessment by intravascular ultrasound imaging. Clin Radiol. 1998;53:37-43.
78. Sharma S, Sharma S, Taneja K, et al. Morphologic mural changes in the aorta revealed by CT in patients with nonspecific aortoarteritis (Takayasu's arteritis). AJR. 1996;167:1321-5.
79. Keser G, Direskeneli H, Aksu K. Management of Takayasu arteritis: a systematic review. Rheumatology (Oxford). 2014;53:793-801.
80. Liang P, Tan-Ong M, Hoffman GS. Takayasu's arteritis: vascular interventions and outcomes. J Rheumatol. 2004;31:102-6
81. Hedgire SS, McDermott S, Borczuk D, et al. The spectrum of IgG4-related disease in the abdomen and pelvis. AJR Am J Roentgenol. 2013;201:14-22.
82. Stone JH, Zen Y, Deshpande V. IgG4-related disease. N Engl J Med. 2012;366:539-51.
83. Kasashima S, Zen Y, Kawashima A, et al. Inflammatory abdominal aortic aneurysm: close relationship to IgG4-related periaortitis. Am J Surg Pathol. 2008;32:197-204.
84. Kasashima S, Zen Y. IgG4. IgG4-related inflammatory abdominal aortic aneurysm. Curr Opin Rheumatol. 2011;23:18-23.
85. Wintermark M, Wicky S, Schnyder P. Imaging of acute traumatic injuries of thoracic aorta. Eur Radiol. 2002;12:431-42.
86. Gavant ML. Helical CT grading of traumatic aortic injuries. RCNA. 1999;37:553-70.
87. Lipchick EO, Rogoff SM. The abnormal abdominal aorta: Arteriosclerosis and other diseases. In: Abrahams HL Little (Ed). Brown and Company, Boston. 1983;2:1057-78.
88. Sawhney R, Kerlan RR, Wall SD. Analysis of initial CT findings after endovascular repair of abdominal aortic aneurysms. Radiology. 2001;220:157-60.
89. Erwin III JP, ACC Solution Set Oversight Committee, Cibotti-Sun M, Elma M. 2022 Aortic Disease Guideline-at-a-Glance. JACC. 2022;80:2348-352.
90. Mazzolai L, Teixido-Tura G, Lanzi S, Boc V, et al. ESC Scientific Document Group. 2024 ESC Guidelines for the management of peripheral arterial and aortic diseases. Eur Heart J. 2024;45:3538-700.

Manphool Singhal, Arun Sharma,
Ujjwal Gorsi, Mandeep Garg

CHAPTER

31

Imaging in Pulmonary Thromboembolism

INTRODUCTION

Pulmonary embolism (PE) is the third most common acute cardiovascular event disease following coronary artery disease and stroke.[1] Most commonly it's a consequence of migration of thrombus from lower limb veins thrombus.[2,3] Acute pulmonary thromboembolism (APE) is an emergent condition, if not diagnosed and treated in time is almost always fatal. This, thus mandates timely and accurate diagnosis. After the advent of multidetector CT (MDCT) scanners, the conventional ventilation-perfusion scan (VP scan) has been replaced with MDCT derived pulmonary angiography (CTPA) with better clinical outcomes.[4-6]

Chronic thromboembolic disease (CTED) on the other hand results due to incomplete resolution and recanalization of acute emboli and often results in pulmonary hypertension.

This chapter describes the role of various imaging modalities in diagnosis of PE with focus on MDCT pulmonary angiography.

ACUTE PULMONARY EMBOLISM

Acute pulmonary thromboembolism most of the time is a consequence of migration of deep vein thrombus (DVT) from the lower limb veins.[2,3] For both DVT and APE an annual incidence of 100–200/100,000 inhabitants has been reported.[4]

Clinical features of APE are often nonspecific and deceptive, however, the commonest symptom in appropriate clinical setting is sudden onset of severe breathlessness. If diagnosed and treated in time, outcomes are rewarding. Hence imaging plays a leading role in evaluation of patients suspected of having APE.

When embolic burden is high enough to cause sustained systemic hypotension (systolic arterial pressure <90 mm Hg) for at least 15 minutes which is not due to cause other than PE with symptoms and signs of shock and chest pain its termed as massive PE.[7] Clinical scores such as Wells[8] and Geneva scores[9] are important scores which allows assessment of clinical pre-test probability of APE. Electrocardiography (ECG), D-dimer, chest radiograph and compression ultrasound of lower limbs are the initial investigations.

D-dimer levels are raised in APE and therefore a most important laboratory screening test for APE that has a high sensitivity and very high negative predictive. As 90% of APE originate from DVT in a lower limb,[10] for symptomatic DVT, compression ultrasound of veins of lower limb has a high sensitivity (>90%) and specificity (95%).[11]

Imaging Techniques

Chest Radiography

Chest radiography is useful to exclude other causes of acute chest pain when APE is suspected. It is important to exclude pneumonia, pneumothorax, pericardial effusion aortic dissection, and free intraperitoneal air as symptoms because of these entities may mimic those due to APE. In addition, ventilation perfusion scan interpretation is dependent on whether the chest radiograph is normal or abnormal.[12]

Although chest radiograph is the first investigation performed in patients of suspected pulmonary embolism, unfortunately the radiographic features of acute pulmonary embolism are rather nonspecific. Findings which may be seen are Hampton hump (peripheral, wedge-shaped consolidation with a rounded medial margin representing infarct), Westermark sign (oligemia of lung beyond the occluded vessel), Fleischner sign (prominent central pulmonary artery) plate like atelectasis, small pleural effusion and elevated ipsilateral hemidiaphragm **(Fig. 1)**.[13] Not all patients with APE have positive finding on chest X-ray. Normal chest skiagrams have been reported in the presence of APE in 12–30% of patients.

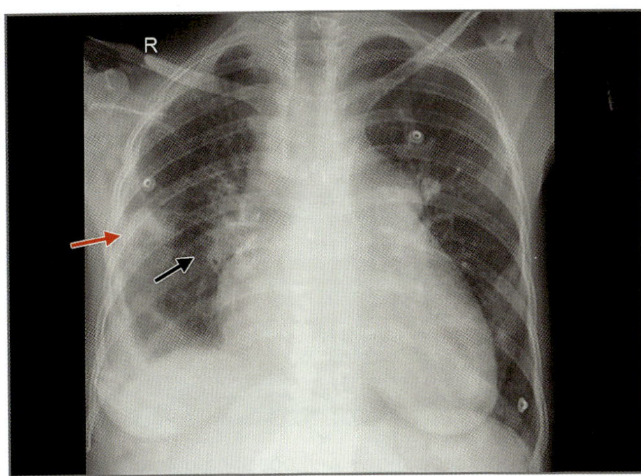

FIG. 1: Acute pulmonary embolism (APE). Dilated central pulmonary artery with dilated right descending pulmonary artery proximally and acute cut-off (black arrow). Note right-sided pleural effusion with peripheral wedge-shaped opacity in right middle zone suggestive of infarct (red arrow).

Transthoracic Echocardiography

The role of transthoracic echocardiography (TTE) for diagnosis of APE is limited however, is essential for assessment of right ventricular dysfunction at presentation and on follow-up after initiation of therapy. In addition, associated right atrial and right ventricular thrombus may also be diagnosed with TTE.

CT Angiography

CT pulmonary angiography (CTPA) is standard for diagnosis of APE as it is accurate, safe and can be performed rapidly. It has replaced catheter angiography for diagnosing PE.[14] It is considered the best imaging modality for those with intermediate or high clinical risk for APE and those with abnormal D-dimer values. PIOPED II (Prospective Investigation of Pulmonary Embolism Diagnosis) studied the accuracy of CTPA with V/Q and conventional pulmonary angiography. Sensitivity of 83% and specificity of 96% were shown in patients with a high pretest probability of PE.[14] However, scanners used in the PIOPED II study were 4, 8 or 16-row scanners, with rapid evolution of multidetector computed tomography (MDCT) with higher detectors with large area coverage, even greater accuracy is achieved.[15-18] Another advantage of CTPA is ability to detect alternative causes for clinical symptoms mimicking APE[19] unlike ventilation/perfusion scan (V/Q scan) and catheter angiography.

For CTPA 80–100 mL (less with higher detector CT scanners) of nonionic iodinated contrast is injected intravenously at a rate of 4 mL/s from an antecubital vein. To time optimal contrast delivery to the pulmonary vessels at the time of imaging, test bolus and automated bolus tracking techniques are very helpful. Test bolus technique is especially useful in patients who have delayed opacification of the pulmonary arteries due to poor cardiac function. Although caudal to cranial scanning is often used to reduce effect of respiratory motion at the lung bases where more emboli are seen and more diaphragmatic motion occurs, the availability of ultrafast MDCT scanners usually obviates this modification.

Recently with the availability of higher detector and dual source CT scanners with sub-millimetric detectors the diagnosis of sub-segmental PE is possible. Studies with ECG-gating acquisition have reported improved diagnosis of PE.[20,21]

Dual-energy CT

With the implementation of MDCT scanners with two X-ray tubes (dual-source CT) and a single tube with two focal spots (dual-energy), both iodinated contrast material-enhanced and soft-tissue images from a single imaging examination can be obtained. This feature is useful in APE imaging as the area of perfused lung can be directly assessed and quantified in addition to the standard documentation of clot burden and presence of right heart strain.[22]

Dual-energy CT (DECT) derived CTPA provide vascular images along with lung perfusion [iodine distribution maps/lung perfusion blood volume (PBV) images] **(Figs. 2A and B)**. This permits quantitative assessment of regional iodine density, a marker for pulmonary perfusion which is akin to V/Q scan or single photon-emission computed tomography (SPECT) V/Q scan.[4,23] The diagnostic accuracy of iodine maps along with vascular maps for occlusive acute PE is high even for the detection of subsegmental thrombi.[23-25] The negative predictive value of DECT-CPA for exclusion of PE is virtually 100%.[26] In addition, DECT techniques have the potential to reduce contrast dose without compromising diagnostic capabilities.[27]

Spectral CT, which is now a reality, has reported further reduction in both the iodine load and radiation dose to the patient. As shown by Szucs-Farkas et al. using a contrast injection of 75 mL (300 mg iodine/mL) and 80 kVp, images which were obtained were found to be equivalent to the standard dose of 100 mL (300 mg iodine/mL) and standard 100 kVp for diagnosing PE. The radiation dose was significantly less with this protocol (6.8 mSv for 100 kVp and 4.8 mSv for 80kVp).[28]

Ventilation/Perfusion Scan

A V/Q scan analyzes both the pulmonary blood flow and alveolar ventilation and is interpreted in correlation with a chest radiograph. It is an alternative test for patients who cannot undergo CTPA. The ability to detect pulmonary embolism (PE) on a V/Q scan can be improved by the addition of SPECT imaging, which provides cross-sectional imaging of the lungs.[29] V/Q scans assess for perfusion defects without matched ventilation defects, the combination of which is suggestive of PE. V/Q scans are

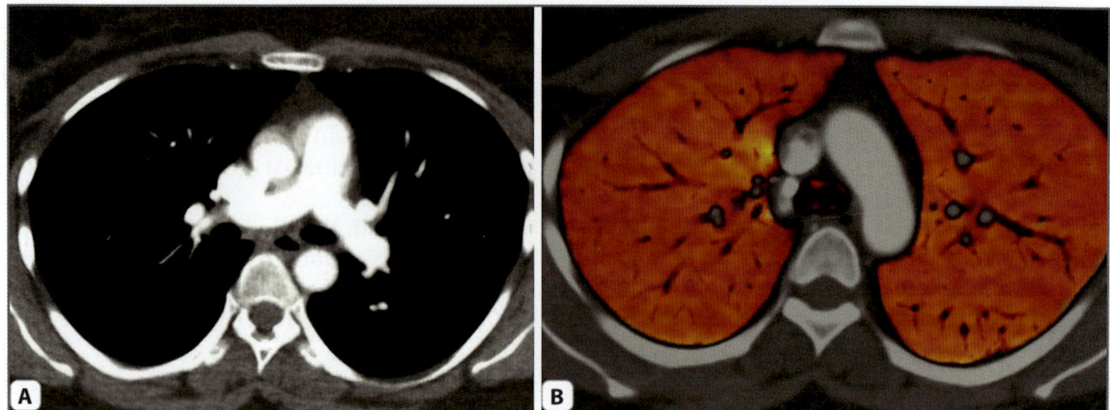

FIGS. 2A AND B: Dual energy CT pulmonary angiography (CTPA): (A) Axial vascular image shows well opacified pulmonary arteries. (B) Axial image of iodine maps shows homogenous and uniform distribution of iodine in the lung parenchyma.

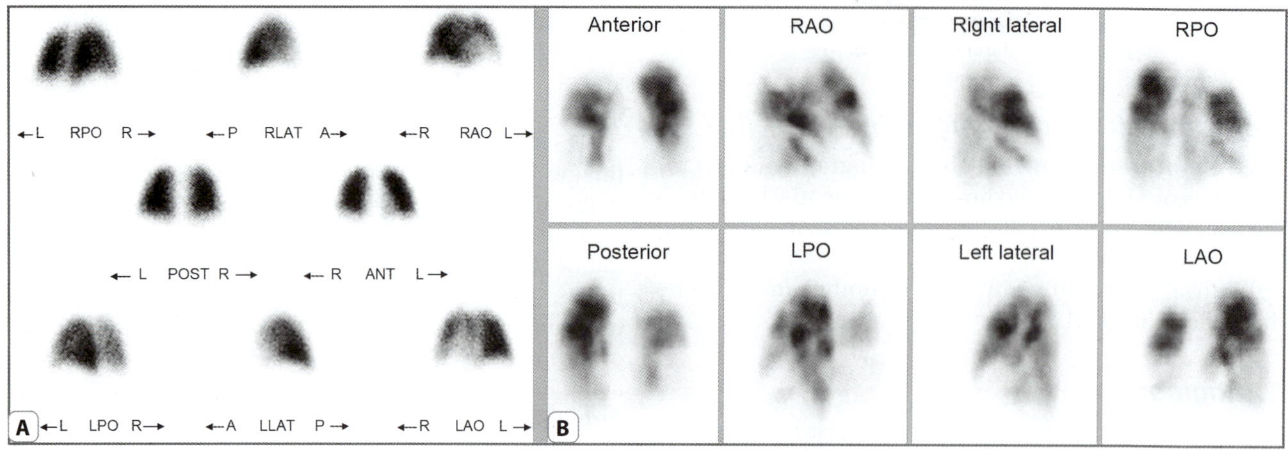

FIGS. 3A AND B: (A) Lung perfusion scan shows normal perfusion pattern. (B) Lung perfusion scan in another patient shows multiple large perfusion defects in both lungs, suggesting a high probability for pulmonary embolism.

reported as normal, very low probability, low probability, intermediate probability, and high probability, on the basis of the number and sizes of unmatched defects as well as in correlation with the chest radiograph **(Figs. 3A and B)**. A normal V/Q scan indicates that the chances of PE are <5% whereas high-probability V/Q scan indicates that chance of PE is >90%.[30] In pregnant women, V/Q scan may be preferred rather than CTPA. The American Thoracic Society and the Society of Thoracic Radiology recommends that for pregnant women in whom PE is suspected but whose chest radiograph is normal, the V/Q scan should be performed. However, CTPA is to be carried out rather than a V/Q scan if abnormality is detected on chest radiograph.[31]

Magnetic Resonance Imaging

Role of MR pulmonary angiography (MRPA) in management is limited due to long acquisition times, which limits its widespread use in diagnosis of APE. Needless, it is useful in certain clinical conditions where CTA is contraindicated.

MRPA consists of a three-dimensional (3D) heavily weighted-T1 gradient echo MRI sequences acquired during first-pass perfusion following intravenous injection of gadolinium via pressure injector to visualize the pulmonary arteries. Non-contrast enhanced MRPA can be performed using steady-state free precession (SSFP) free-breathing real-time imaging technique with additional navigator-gating, which is used to obtain the images in the same phase without the need for breath-hold **(Figs. 4A to D)**.[32]

Digital Subtraction Angiography

For the diagnosis of APE, CTPA has largely replaced catheter angiography, that provides similar results without the complications of invasive catheter angiography. Filling defects within main pulmonary arteries or their branches arteries or cut-off of a pulmonary artery branch is most

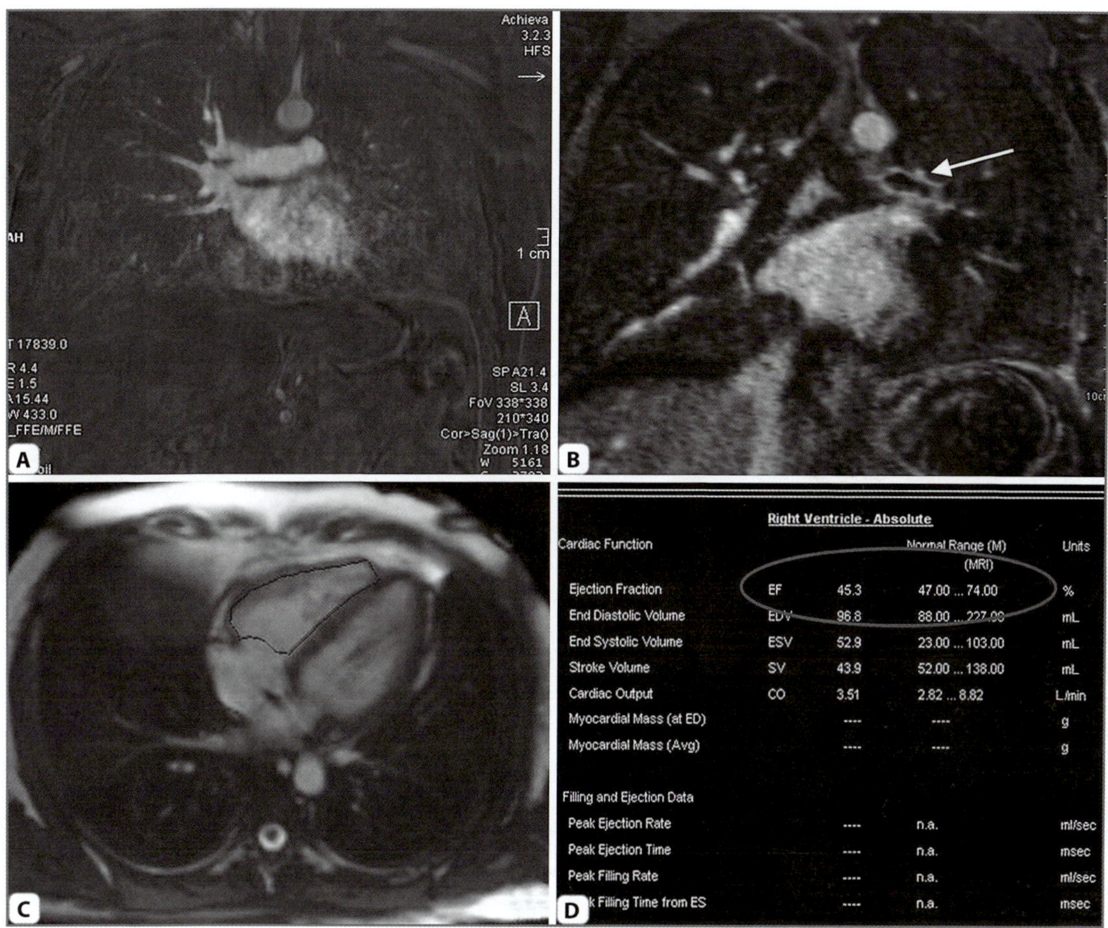

FIGS. 4A TO D: Acute pulmonary embolism. Coronal MRA images (A and B) show acute thrombus in left pulmonary artery (arrow in B) with normal right pulmonary artery. (C) Cine steady-state free precession (SSFP) static image—calculation of right ventricle (RV) function. (D) Volumetry showing RV dysfunction with decreased ejection fraction (EF) (EF-45.3%).

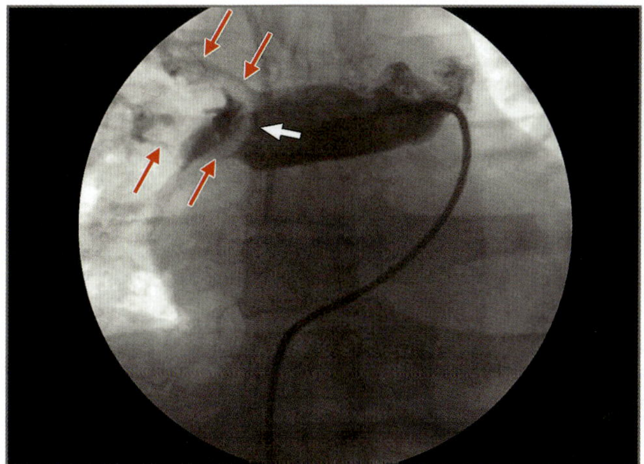

FIG. 5: Acute pulmonary embolism (APE). Catheter angiography of pulmonary artery confirming the filling defects in the right pulmonary artery (red arrows) typically forming concave margin (white arrow) suggestive of acute pulmonary embolism.

accepted diagnostic sign of APE **(Fig. 5)**.[12] Currently role of catheter angiography is limited for catheter-directed thrombolysis.

Imaging Features of Acute PE on CTPA

CTPA unambiguously, is now the standard of care imaging modality for diagnosis of acute PE. Findings of APE on CTPA are described below though imaging features are similar in all angiographic studies.

Vascular Features

CTPA shows hypodense filling defects in the pulmonary vasculature and radiological features depend upon the degree of obstruction: complete or partial.[9,33]

Complete obstruction: The lumen is entirely occupied by thromboembolic material which is completely obstructed and amputated ("arterial cut-off sign") **(Fig. 6)**. Acute thrombus usually has acute margins and concave filling defect or "trailing edge" within the opacified pulmonary arteries. The diameter of the pulmonary artery may be increased because of impaction of the thrombus by pulsatile flow **(Fig. 7)**. CTPA in this setting scores over the conventional catheter angiography as it demonstrates the status of distal circulation and thrombus burden **(Figs. 8A and B)**. If the thrombi are in the segmental or sub-segmental arteries caliber of the vessel at the level of obstruction is either normal or enlarged as compared to chronic PTE **(Fig. 9)**.

In partial obstruction intraluminal central or eccentric filling defects are seen surrounded by contrast **(Fig. 10)**. The morphology of emboli varies according to whether the vessel is imaged in short axis ("rim" or "polo mint" sign) or long axis ("railway track" sign) **(Figs. 8 and 10)**.[5] When analyzing small segmental branches for presence of emboli, appropriate window and level values should be chosen to avoid false negative due to presence of dense contrast media.

Recently ECG gated high pitch acquisition of CPTA has been studied in APE to address motion (both respiratory and cardiac) related artifacts for accuracy and results are encouraging **(Fig. 11)**.[20,21]

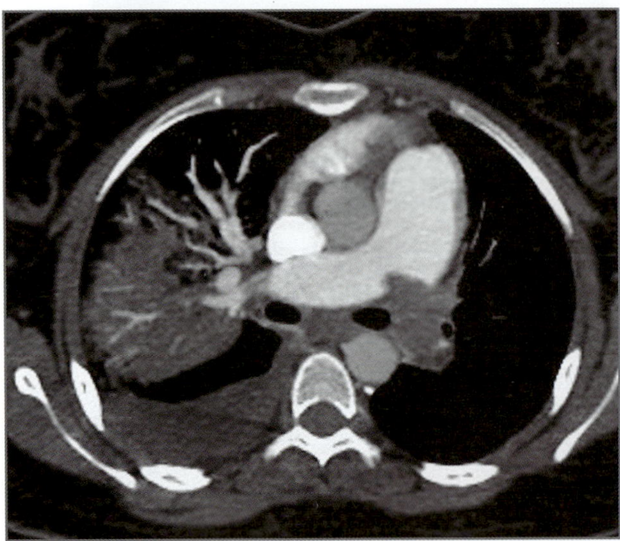

FIG. 6: Acute pulmonary embolism (APE) with complete obstruction. CT pulmonary angiography (CTPA) shows complete luminal occlusion of the left main pulmonary artery by hypodense thrombus expanding the artery ("arterial cut-off sign"). Note paucity of pulmonary arteries in the left lung. A patch of consolidation with pleural effusion is seen on right side.

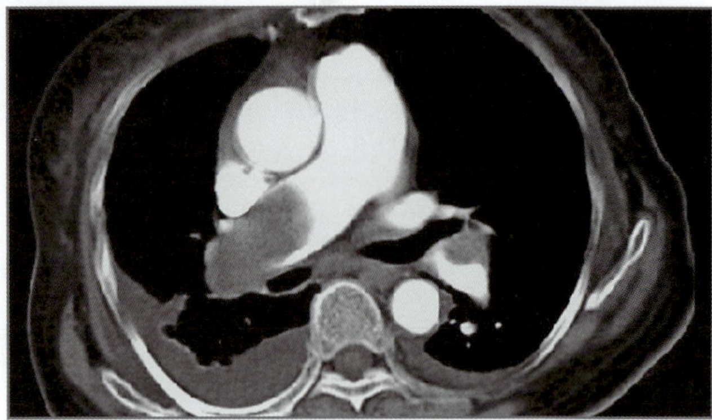

FIG. 7: Acute pulmonary embolism (APE). CT pulmonary angiography (CTPA) revealing hypodense filling defect with acute margins and concave filling defect or "trailing edge" in the right main pulmonary artery and left lower pulmonary artery branch with expansion of lumen, as well as bilateral pleural effusions.

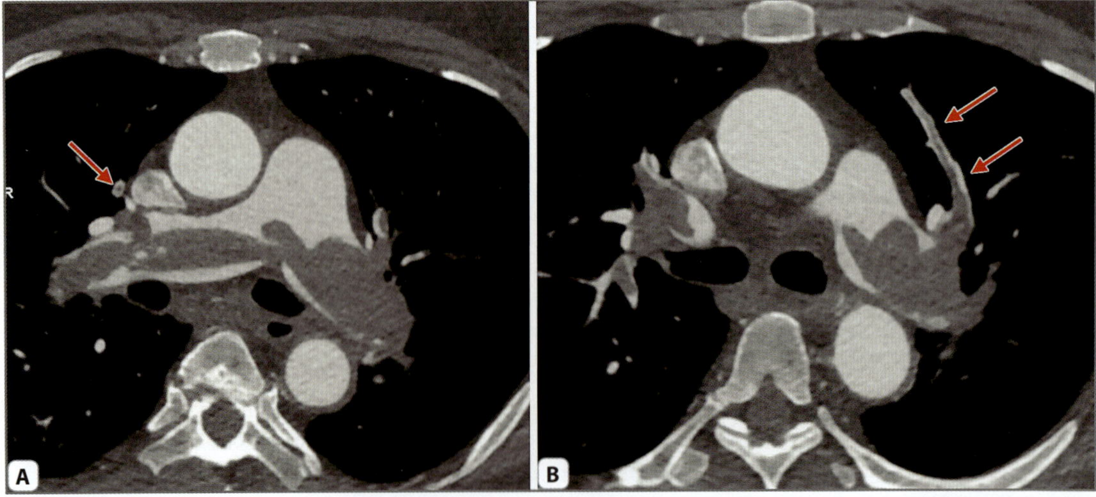

FIGS. 8A AND B: Acute saddle pulmonary embolism. CT pulmonary angiography (CTPA) revealing a large volume pulmonary embolism that straddles the bifurcation of the pulmonary trunk extending into left and right pulmonary arteries. Note concave margins of the thrombus with the opacified lumen. The thrombus is extending into the segmental branches with partial filling defects giving rise to a typical "tram-track appearance" in left superior pulmonary artery (B) (arrows) and "rim" or "polo mint" sign in the sub-segmental branch of the right upper pulmonary artery (A) (arrow).

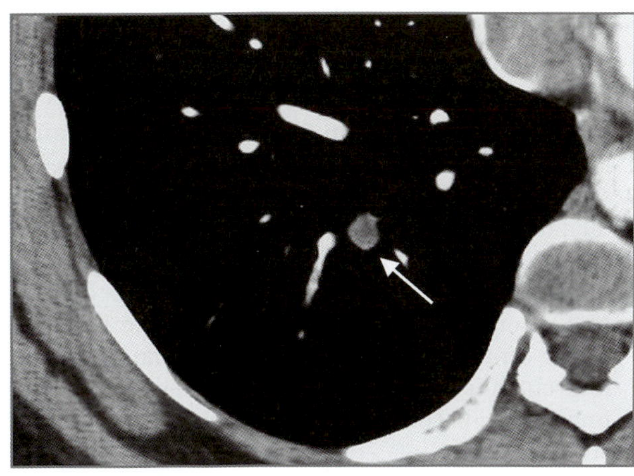

FIG. 9: Acute pulmonary embolism (APE) with complete obstruction. CT pulmonary angiography (CTPA) shows complete luminal occlusion with an expanded segmental artery (arrow).

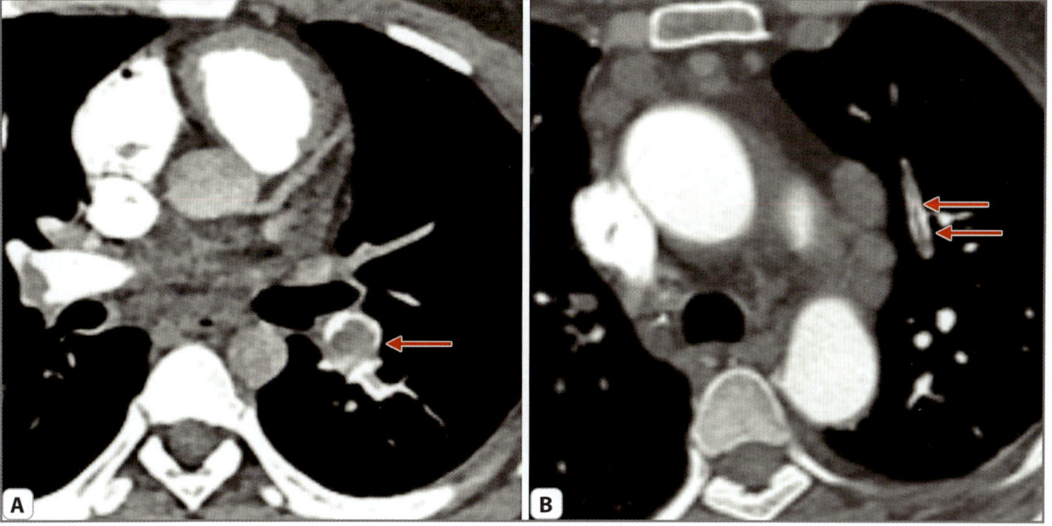

FIGS. 10A AND B: Acute pulmonary embolism (APE) with partial obstruction. (A) Axial CT pulmonary angiography (CTPA) image shows an eccentric filling defect in the left lower pulmonary artery forming acute angles with respect to the vessel wall (arrow). (B) Axial CTPA image in another patient demonstrate central hypodense filling defect surrounded by peripheral contrast in sub-segmental branch of left upper lobe pulmonary artery giving rise to typical "tram-track appearance (arrows)". Same image in perpendicular plane will appear as "polo mint sign" (refer **Fig. 8A**).

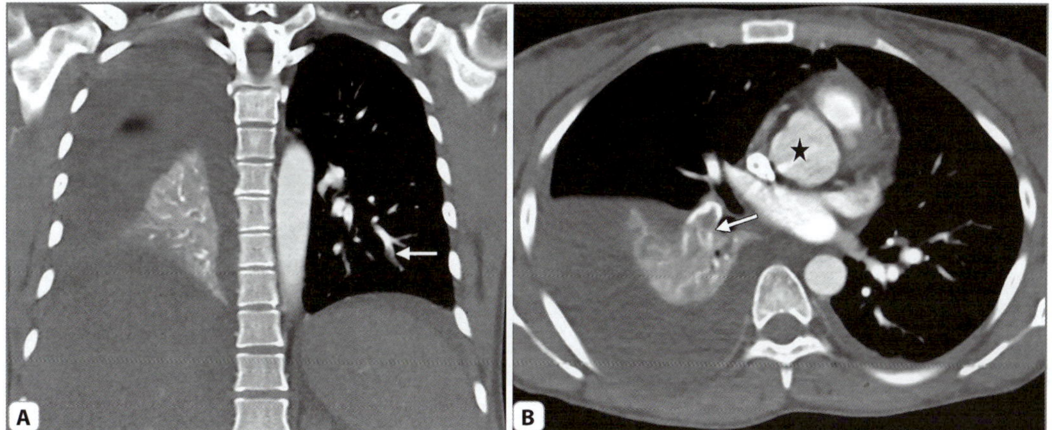

FIGS. 11A AND B: High-pitch ECG-gated CT pulmonary angiography (CTPA). Coronal (A) image shows hypodense filling defect in one of the subsegmental branches of the left inferior pulmonary artery (arrow). Axial (B) image show hypodense filling defect in a segmental branch of the right inferior pulmonary artery (arrow). Note clearly discernible segmental and subsegmental branches of pulmonary arteries and aortic sinus (asterisk) devoid of motion artifacts.

Parenchymal Features

Complete occlusion of the artery causes the complete loss of perfusion with distal infarct which manifests triangular subpleural consolidation or ground-glass opacity with fine reticular areas **(Fig. 12)**. When obstruction is partial, there is a reduced flow rate (oligemia) which causes nonuniform arterial perfusion of the lung parenchyma with reduced vessel diameter and patchy areas of low attenuation on CT or low signal on MRI (mosaic attenuation pattern). Atelectasis and pleural effusion may also be seen.

On DE-CTPA the perfusion defects are seen as typical wedge shapes areas of iodine defects.[25,26] This along with presence of filling defects in pulmonary vasculature adds accuracy and helps in diagnosis of sub-segmental PE which otherwise may be missed if only vascular images are analyzed **(Fig. 13)**.

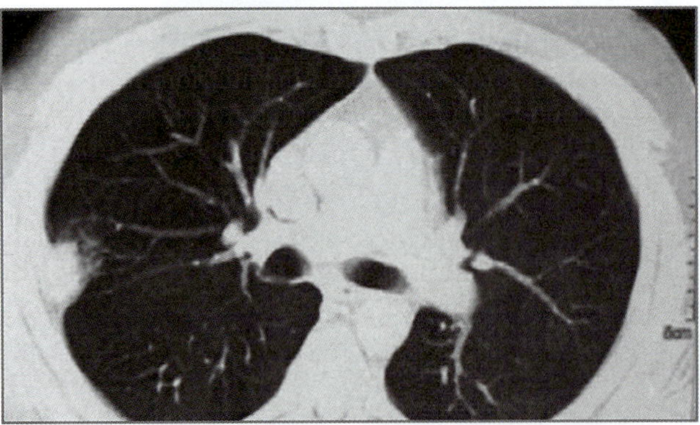

FIG. 12: Pulmonary infarct. Axial CPTA image (lung window) in a patient of acute PE shows characteristic peripheral wedge-shaped infarct in right middle lobe.

Cardiac Features

In acute PE, right ventricle (RV) after load is rapidly increased as a result of obstruction to pulmonary arterial flow and the increase in PVR. Features of RV after load include dilatation of the RV, bowing of the interventricular septum, dilatation of superior and inferior vena cava, dilatation of azygos vein, dilatation and reflux of contrast in the inferior vena cava and hepatic veins may also be present. Right ventricle dilatation is assessed commonly by RV/left ventricle (LV) ratio which can be calculated either on axial images or on a multiplanar reformatted four-chamber view. If the RV/LV ratio is >1.0 (on axial CT images) or >0.9 (on four-chamber view), RV dysfunction is suggested.[34]

CHRONIC THROMBOEMBOLIC DISEASE

Chronic thromboembolic disease (CTED) results due to incomplete resolution and recanalization of acute emboli. There occurs organization and endothelialization of thromboembolic material which may appear as laminated thrombi, single bands parallel to the vessel (shelves) or complex web-like network as well as complete vascular occlusions. The pathophysiological basis explaining transition from acute to chronic thromboembolism is uncertain; however, failed thrombolysis, a localized inflammatory response and localized endothelial dysfunction are thought to be responsible.[35] The CTPA findings of chronic thromboembolic pulmonary embolism include parenchymal and vascular signs.[9,33]

- *Vascular findings* include complete obstruction, indicated by a tapered occluded vessel, eccentric

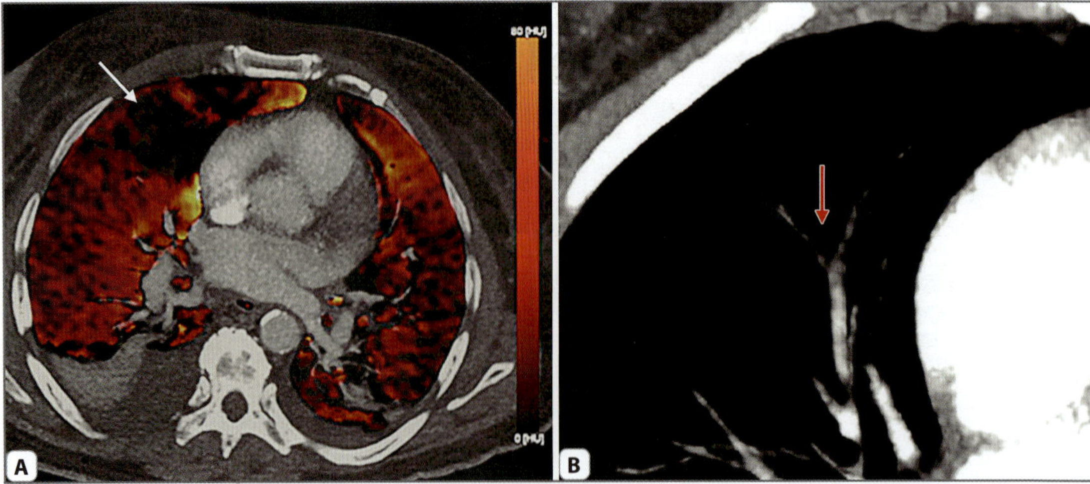

FIGS. 13A AND B: Dual energy-computed tomographic pulmonary angiography (DE-CTPA). Axial DE-CTPA iodine (perfusion) image (A) shows a peripheral wedge-shaped area of perfusion defect (white arrow) is seen in right middle lobe. Axial maximum intensity projection (MIP) vascular image (B) shows occlusion of corresponding subsegmental artery (red arrow) supplying the area. This was missed on solo evaluation of vascular maps.

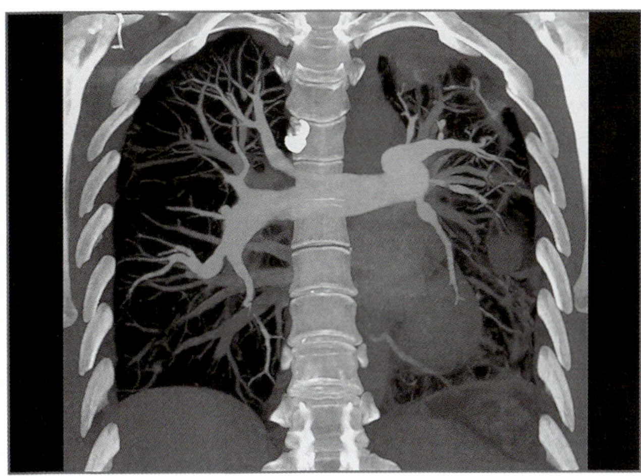

FIG. 14: Chronic thromboembolism with pulmonary hypertension. CT pulmonary angiogram coronal reformatted image showing dilated central pulmonary arteries with eccentric narrowing of proximal right upper lobar pulmonary artery, posterior segmental branch of right lower, and left descending pulmonary artery with segment of post-stenotic dilatation (typical of chronic pulmonary thromboembolism), with relative oligemia in right middle and bilateral lower lobes.

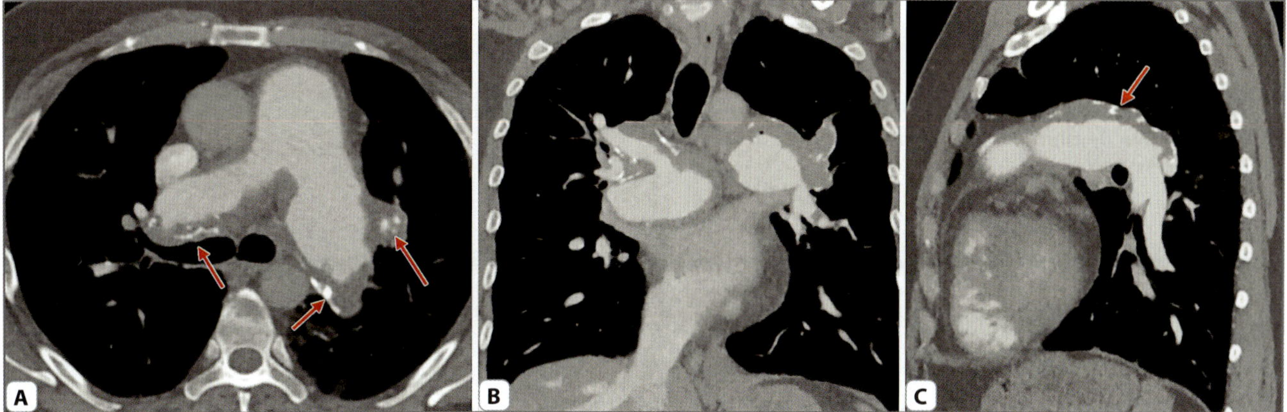

FIGS. 15A TO C: Chronic thromboembolic pulmonary embolism. Axial (A), coronal (B) and sagittal (C) CT pulmonary angiography (CTPA) images show eccentric hypodense filling defects with specks of calcifications in the right and left pulmonary arteries. Note the irregular lumen with obtuse margins of thrombus with the opacified arteries.

narrowing of pulmonary arteries with segments of post-stenotic dilatation **(Fig. 14)**, partial filling defects, indicated by obtuse mural margins with the vessel wall **(Fig. 15)** with or without calcifications. Partial filling defects are also indicated by the presence of webs or bands and collateral systemic supply **(Fig. 16)**.

- *Parenchymal findings* include scars from prior pulmonary infarction mosaic pattern of perfusion **(Fig. 17)**, cylindrical bronchial airway dilatation and systemic perfusion of the peripheral pulmonary arterial bed.[36]

CTPA is also a useful modality in assessing whether patients can be candidates for surgery or not. If the main, lobar, or proximal segmental arteries are involved, patients are considered for resection whereas if distal segments are involved medical treatment is considered.

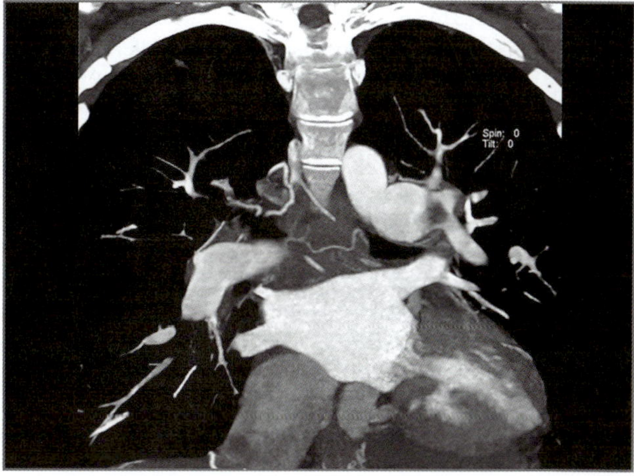

FIG. 16: Chronic pulmonary embolism. Multidetector CT (MDCT) coronal reformation showing hypertrophied bronchial arteries.

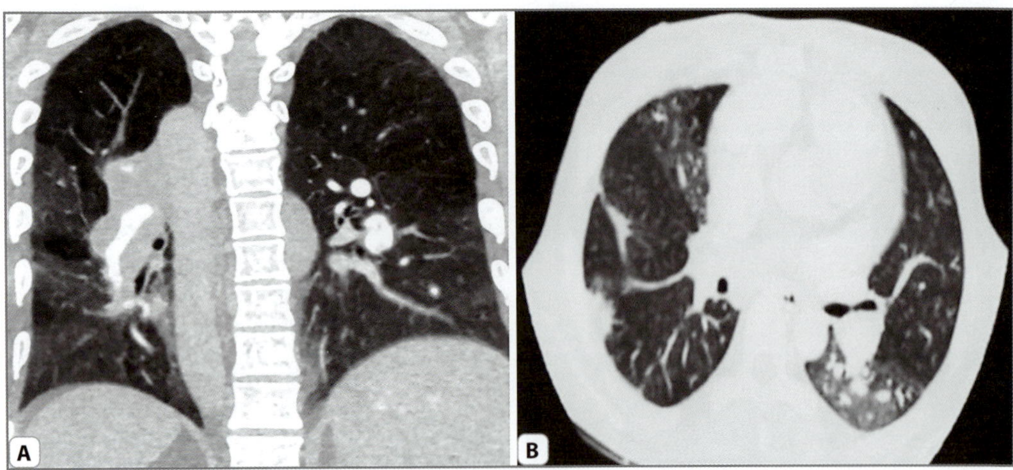

FIGS. 17A AND B: CT scan coronal reformatted image (lung window) in a case of chronic pulmonary thromboembolism shows (A) a mosaic perfusion pattern with wide regional variations in attenuation of the lung parenchyma and disparity in size of the segmental vessels. Axial CT scan image (B) in another patient shows mosaic attenuation with a peripheral parenchymal infarct and scar in right lower lobe.

CONCLUSION

Diagnosis of PE demands and accurate diagnosis as timely diagnosis and treatment significantly reduces morbidity and mortality. MDCT derived CTPA is the diagnostic imaging modality of choice for diagnosis of acute and chronic PE. Recently, ECG-gated and dual energy CTPA has been tried with success for detection of even subsegmental PE.

REFERENCES

1. Goldhaber SZ, Bounameaux H. Pulmonary embolism and deep vein thrombosis. Lancet. 2012;379(9828):1835-46.
2. Agarwal R, Varma S. Acute pulmonary embolism. Eastern J Med. 2013;14:57-68.
3. Sevitt S, Gallagher N. Venous thrombosis and pulmonary embolism. A clinico-pathological study in injured and burned patients. Br J Surg. 1961;48:475-89.
4. Konstantinides SV. ESC guidelines on the diagnosis and management of acute pulmonary embolism. Eur Heart J. 2014;35(45):3145-6.
5. Stein PD, Fowler SE, Goodman LR, Gottschalk A, Hales CA, Hull RD, et al. Multidetector computed tomography for acute pulmonary embolism. N Engl J Med. 2006;354(22):2317-27.
6. Remy-Jardin M, Pistolesi M, Goodman LR, Gefter WB, Gottschalk A, Mayo JR, et al. Management of suspected acute pulmonary embolism in the era of CT angiography: a statement from the Fleischner Society. Radiology. 2007;245: 315-29.
7. Ruggiero A, Screaton NJ. Imaging of acute and chronic thromboembolic disease: state of the art. Clin Radiol. 2017;72(5):375-88.
8. Wells PS, Anderson DR, Rodger M, Ginsberg JS, Kearon C, Gent M, et al. Derivation of a simple clinical model to categorize patients probability of pulmonary embolism: increasing the models utility with the SimpliRED D-dimer. Thromb Haemost. 2000;83(3):416-20.
9. Wicki J, Perneger TV, Junod AF, Bounameaux H, Perrier A. Assessing clinical probability of pulmonary embolism in the emergency ward: a simple score. Arch Intern Med. 2001;161(1):92-7.
10. Sevitt S, Gallagher N. Venous thrombosis and pulmonary embolism. A clinico-pathological study in injured and burned patients. Br J Surg. 1961;48:475-89.
11. Le Gal G, Righini M, Sanchez O, Roy PM, Baba-Ahmed M, Perrier A, et al. A positive compression ultrasonography of the lower limb veins is highly predictive of pulmonary embolism on computed tomography in suspected patients. Thromb Haemost. 2006;95(6):963-6.
12. Sista AK, Kuo WT, Schiebler M, Madoff DC. Stratification, imaging, and management of acute massive and submassive pulmonary embolism. Radiology. 2017;284(1):5-24.
13. Abdelaziz MM, Wali SO, Hamad M, Krayem A, Samman YS. Pulmonary embolism: a diagnostic approach. Annals of Thorac Medicine. 2006;(1):31-40.
14. Stein PD, Fowler SE, Goodman LR, Gottschalk A, Hales CA, Hull RD, et al. Multidetector computed tomography for acute pulmonary embolism. N Engl J Med. 2006;354(22): 2317-27.
15. Bunch PM, Fulwadhva UP, Wortman JR, Primak AN, Madan R, Steigner ML, et al. Motion artifact reduction from high-pitch dual-source computed tomography pulmonary angiography. J Comput Assist Tomogr. 2018;42:623-9.
16. Bauer RW, Schell B, Beeres M, Wichmann JL, Bodelle B, Vogl TJ,et al. High-pitch dual-source computed tomography pulmonary angiography in freely breathing patients. J Thorac Imaging. 2012;27:376-81.

17. Hou DJ, Tso DK, Davison C, Inacio J, Louis LJ, Nicolaou S, et al. Clinical utility of ultra-high pitch dual source thoracic CT imaging of acute pulmonary embolism in the emergency department: are we one step closer towards a non-gated triple rule out? Eur J Radiol. 2013;82:1793-8.
18. Lu GM, Luo S, Meinel FG, McQuiston AD, Zhou CS, Kong X, et al. High-pitch computed tomography pulmonary angiography with iterative reconstruction at 80 kVp and 20 mL contrast agent volume. Eur Radiol. 2014;24:3260-8.
19. Cummings KW, Bhalla S. Pulmonary vascular diseases. Clin Chest Med. 2015;36:235-48.
20. Bolen MA, Renapurkar RD, Popovic ZB, Heresi GA, Flamm SD, Lau CT, et al. High-pitch ECG-synchronized pulmonary CT angiography versus standard CT pulmonary angiography: a prospective randomized study. AJR American journal of roentgenology. 2013;201:971-21.
21. Thakur R, Singhal M, Aggrawal AN, Gorsi U, Sharma N, Bhalla A, et al. Comparison of high-pitch prospective electrocardiogram-gated pulmonary CT angiography with standard CT pulmonary angiography on dual-source CT for detection of subsegmental pulmonary embolism in patients suspected of acute pulmonary embolism. Pol J Radiol. 2022;87:e296-e303.
22. Fink C, Johnson TR, Michaely HJ, Morhard D, Becker C, Reiser M, et al. Dual-energy CT angiography of the lung in patients with suspected pulmonary embolism: initial results. Rofo. 2008;180(10):879-83.
23. Thieme SF, Becker CR, Hacker M, Nikolaou K, Reiser MF, Johnson TRC. Dual energy CT for the assessment of lung perfusion-correlation to scintigraphy. Eur J Radiol. 2008;68(3):369-74.
24. Pontana F, Faivre JB, Remy-Jardin M, Flohr T, Schmidt B, Tacelli N, et al. Lung perfusion with dual-energy multidetector-row CT (MDCT): feasibility for the evaluation of acute pulmonary embolism in 117 consecutive patients. Acad Radiol. 2008;15(12):1494-504.
25. Weidman EK, Plodkowski AJ, Halpenny DF, Hayes SA, Perez-Johnston R, Zheng J, et al. Dual-Energy CT Angiography for Detection of Pulmonary Emboli: Incremental Benefit of Iodine Maps. Radiology. 2018;289(2):546-53.
26. Yadav V, Singhal M, Maralakunte M, Sharma N, Sharma A, Lal A. Comparison of Dual-Energy Computed Tomography Pulmonary Angiography-Derived Contrast Enhancement with Standard Dual-Energy Pulmonary Angiography in Diagnosing Subsegmental Pulmonary Embolism: A Prospective Study. Indian J Radiol Imaging. 2023;33(4): 456-62.
27. Delesalle MA, Pontana F, Duhamel A, Faivre JB, FlohrT, Tacelli N, et al. Spectral optimization of chest CT angiography with reduced iodine load: experience in 80 patients evaluated with dual-source, dual-energy CT. Radiology. 2013;267(1): 25666.
28. Szucs-Farkas Z, Christe A, Megyeri B, Rohacek M, Vock P, Nagy EV, et al. Diagnostic accuracy of computed tomography pulmonary angiography with reduced radiation and contrast material dose: a prospective randomized clinical trial. Invest Radiol. 2014;49(4):201-8.
29. Sirajuddin A, François CJ, Kanne JP. Imaging studies for pulmonary vascular disease. Clinical Pulmonary Medicine. 2015;22(6):307-21.
30. Bajc M, Albrechtsson U, Olsson CG, Olsson B, Jonson B. Comparison of ventilation/perfusion scintigraphy and helical CT for diagnosis of pulmonary embolism; strategy using clinical data and ancillary findings. Clin Physiol Funct Imaging. 2002;22:392-7.
31. Leung AN, Bull TM, Jaeschke R, Lockwood CJ, Boiselle PM, Hurwitz LM, et al. American Thoracic Society documents: an official American Thoracic Society/Society of Thoracic Radiology Clinical Practice Guideline—evaluation of suspected pulmonary embolism in pregnancy. Radiology. 2012;262:63546.
32. Kluge A, Luboldt W, Bachmann G. Acute pulmonary embolism to the subsegmental level: diagnostic accuracy of three MRI techniques compared with 16-MDCT. Am J Roentgenol. 2006;187(1):W7-14.
33. Wittram C, Kalra MK, Maher MM, Greenfield A, McLoud TC, Shepard JA. Acute and chronic pulmonary emboli: angiography-CT correlation. AJR Am J Roentgenol. 2006;186(6 Suppl 2):S421-9
34. Furlan A, Aghayev A, Chang CC, Patil A, Jeon KN, Park B, et al. Short-term mortality in acute pulmonary embolism: clot burden and signs of right heart dysfunction at CT pulmonary angiography. Radiology. 2012;265(1):283-93.
35. Lang IM, Pesavento R, Bonderman D, Yuan JX-J. Risk factors and basic mechanisms of chronic thromboembolic pulmonary hypertension: a current understanding. Eur Respir J. 2013;41(2):462-8.
36. Pena E, Dennie C, Veinot J, Muñiz SH. Pulmonary hypertension: how the radioglogist can help. Radiographics. 2012;32:9-32.

Devasenathipathy Kandasamy, Shivanand Gamanagatti, Chandrashekhara SH

CHAPTER 32

Peripheral Vascular Diseases: Imaging and Interventions

INTRODUCTION

Peripheral vascular disease (PVD) encompasses a wide spectrum of disorders that affect the blood vessels of the upper and lower extremities. The prevalence of PVD increases with age, rising from approximately 2.5% in individuals aged 50–59 years to 14.5% in those over 70 years of age.[1] Imaging plays a pivotal role in the management of PVD, enabling detailed assessment of the arterial anatomy, the extent and severity of vascular disease, and guiding therapeutic decision-making.[2] Endovascular therapies have emerged as a lower-risk alternative to traditional surgical bypass procedures, particularly in patients with multiple comorbidities. Also, interventional treatments are increasingly being recognized as the first-line management strategy for PVD, whenever clinically feasible.[3,4]

Causes and Risk factors for Peripheral Vascular Disease

- *Atherosclerosis*:
  - Most common cause of PVD, particularly affecting the lower limbs.
  - Typically, a disease of the elderly, commonly seen in individuals over 50 years of age.
  - Risk factors for developing atherosclerosis include[1,5]:
    - Smoking
    - Diabetes mellitus
    - Hyperlipidemia
    - Hypertension
  - Atherosclerosis leads to plaque buildup in the arteries, which narrows the vessels and reduces blood flow, especially in the lower extremities.
- Non-atherosclerotic causes:[1,5,6]
  - *Takayasu arteritis*:
    - Primarily affects the aortoiliac segment (aorta and its branches).
    - Inflammatory condition that causes narrowing of large arteries.
  - Buerger's disease:
    - Commonly affects the femoropopliteal and tibioperoneal circulation (blood vessels in the legs).
    - Strongly associated with smoking and affects small and medium-sized arteries, leading to inflammation and clot formation.
- *PVD in younger patients*:
  - Less common in younger individuals.
  - Common causes of PVD in this group include:
    - Trauma: Physical injury leading to vascular damage.
    - Thromboembolism: Blood clots that block blood flow.
    - Arteritis: Inflammation of arteries, which can cause vessel narrowing or blockage.
    - Popliteal artery entrapment syndrome and cystic adventitial disease

This emphasizes that while atherosclerosis is predominant, other conditions like Takayasu arteritis, Buerger's disease, and specific causes in younger patients (e.g., trauma, arteritis) are also important contributors to PVD.

Anatomic Subsets for Localizing Disease in the Lower Extremity[1,2]

Refer to **Table 1**.

Anatomic Subsets for Localizing Disease in the Upper Extremity (Table 2)[1,2]

- Upper extremity peripheral arterial disease (PAD) is less common than lower extremity PAD, but it can occur due to atherosclerosis, trauma, embolism, or vasculitis.[1]
- Subclavian steal syndrome is a unique condition in upper extremity PAD where blood is "stolen" from the vertebrobasilar circulation, causing neurological symptoms alongside arm claudication.

Key Terms Used in Peripheral Arterial Disease[7]

Refer to **Table 3**.

TABLE 1: Anatomic subsets for localizing disease in the lower extremity.

Anatomic subset	Arteries involved	Typical symptoms
Aortoiliac segment	Infrarenal aorta, common and external iliac internal iliac arteries	Buttock, hip, thigh claudication; erectile dysfunction
Femoropopliteal segment	Common and superficial femoral artery, popliteal artery	Thigh and calf claudication
Infrapopliteal segment	Tibial-peroneal trunk, anterior tibial artery, posterior tibial artery, peroneal artery, plantar pedal loop, and pedal vessels (common plantar, medial plantar, and lateral plantar arteries)	Calf, ankle, foot claudication; rest pain, ulcers
Multilevel disease	*Multiple segments*: Aortoiliac, femoropopliteal, infrapopliteal	Diffuse leg pain; rest pain, ulcers

TABLE 2: Anatomic subsets for localizing disease in the upper extremity.

Anatomic subset	Arteries involved	Typical symptoms
Subclavian artery	Subclavian artery	Arm claudication, subclavian steal syndrome
Axillary artery	Axillary artery and branches	Arm fatigue, coldness, numbness
Brachial artery	Brachial artery, deep brachial artery	Forearm claudication, weak pulse
Radial and ulnar arteries	Radial and ulnar arteries	Hand claudication, coldness, ulcers
Palmar arch	Superficial and deep palmar arches	Digital ischemia, ulcers, reduced grip strength
Digital arteries	Proper digital arteries supplying fingers	Digital ulcers, gangrene, Raynaud's phenomenon

TABLE 3: Key terms used in PAD.

Term	Description
Acute limb ischemia (ALI)	Sudden (<2 weeks) reduction of blood flow to a limb, often marked by pain, pallor, pulselessness, poikilothermia (coolness), paresthesias, or paralysis. Classified by the Rutherford system
Angiosome-based blood flow	Refers to continuous arterial flow to a specific anatomical region of skin and deep tissues. In peripheral arterial disease (PAD), this is the area supplied by an infrapopliteal artery, often associated with wounds
Claudication	Muscle pain, cramping, or discomfort in the lower extremities triggered by walking and relieved by rest (within 10 minutes). Severe cases are known as functionally limiting claudication, a sign of chronic PAD
Chronic limb-threatening ischemia (CLTI)	A chronic condition (>2 weeks) involving rest pain, nonhealing wounds, ulcers, or gangrene due to arterial blockage, posing a risk for limb loss. CLTI reflects the chronic and dangerous nature of the condition
Endovascular revascularization	Minimally invasive procedures for restoring blood flow, using methods like balloon angioplasty, stenting (bare-metal, drug-coated, or covered), or atherectomy
Hybrid revascularization	A treatment strategy that combines both endovascular and surgical revascularization methods, performed either simultaneously or in stages
Inflow vs. outflow	Inflow refers to arteries located above the superficial femoral artery (aortoiliac and common femoral arteries), while outflow pertains to arteries below it (popliteal and infrapopliteal arteries)
Multispecialty care team for PAD	A team of experts from various fields working together to assess and treat PAD, especially CLTI. The team typically includes specialists in endovascular and surgical interventions, wound care, and foot surgery
Regions of the foot	• *Forefoot*: Contains phalanges, metatarsals, and sesamoid bones, located from the tarsometatarsal joint forward • *Midfoot*: Encompasses the navicular, cuboid, and cuneiform bones, located between the transverse tarsal and tarsometatarsal joints • *Hindfoot*: Includes the calcaneus and talus bones, spanning from the ankle joint to the transverse tarsal joint

Continued

Continued

Term	Description
Surgical revascularization	Procedures that restore blood flow surgically, such as endarterectomy (plaque removal), thrombectomy, or bypass surgery
Thrombolysis	The use of thrombolytic drugs, often delivered via a catheter to dissolve blood clots in an artery
Tissue loss	• *Minor*: Involves nonhealing ulcers or localized gangrene • *Major*: Significant tissue damage above the transmetatarsal level, making foot salvage unlikely

TABLE 4: Clinical subsets of PAD.

Term	Description
Asymptomatic peripheral arterial disease (PAD)	Around 20–59% of individuals with diagnosed PAD may not exhibit leg symptoms. These patients may limit their activity to avoid ischemic pain, staying below their threshold. Some asymptomatic patients may still develop symptoms during objective walking tests
Chronic symptomatic PAD	• This is the most common symptomatic form of PAD, where patients experience claudication or other non-joint-related leg symptoms that can hinder walking ability • Claudication is typically described as pain, cramping, or fatigue in the buttocks, thighs, calves, or feet during walking, which resolves within about 10 minutes of resting
Chronic limb-threatening ischemia (CTLI)	• A severe subset of PAD, with an estimated incidence of 11–20% in PAD patients • Symptoms include ischemic rest pain, nonhealing wounds, ulcers, or gangrene lasting more than 2 weeks. CLTI is responsible for most PAD-related limb amputations
Acute limb ischemia (ALI)	• A sudden reduction in leg blood flow that endangers limb viability • Symptoms appear acutely (within less than 2 weeks) and include pain, pallor, pulselessness, coolness (poikilothermia), and possible paralysis • Causes include embolism, thrombosis in a native artery or at a previous revascularization site, trauma, or peripheral aneurysms with embolization
Rutherford classification of ALI	ALI is categorized as follows: • *Class I (viable)*: No sensory or motor loss, with audible arterial and venous Doppler signals • *Class IIa (marginally threatened)*: Mild to moderate sensory loss (limited to toes) without motor loss. Arterial Doppler signal may be inaudible, while venous signal remains audible • *Class IIb (immediately threatened)*: Sensory loss beyond the toes with mild to moderate motor weakness. Arterial Doppler signal is absent, but venous signal is audible • *Class III (irreversible)*: Complete sensory and motor loss, with absent arterial and venous Doppler signals, making major tissue loss or nerve damage inevitable

CLINICAL ASSESSMENT FOR PERIPHERAL ARTERIAL DISEASE

Clinical assessment is a central component of evaluation for PAD. Recognition of patterns (clinical subsets) of clinical presentation of PAD will direct clinical evaluation, diagnostic testing, and treatment, as well as determine the urgency of care.[8]

Clinical Subsets of Peripheral Arterial Disease

The clinical presentation of patients with objectively confirmed PAD can be categorized into four clinical subsets **(Table 4)**.[8]

Direct Clinical Evaluation

- Clinical assessment for PAD begins with recognition of risk factors for PAD **(Table 5)** to assist in identification of patients at risk.[8]
- The history and physical examination **(Table 5)** are important to identify patients at increased risk of PAD, assess for lower extremity symptoms, and assess for pulse deficits and other signs of PAD, including lower extremity wounds.
- Suggestive clinical history or the presence of any abnormal physical examination finding concerning for PAD requires prompt evaluation with the ankle-brachial index (ABI) to establish the diagnosis of PAD.

TABLE 5: Patients at increased risk for PAD.

Risk group	Description
Age ≥ 65 years	Individuals aged 65 years or older.
Age 50–64 years with risk factors	Individuals aged 50–64 years who have risk factors for atherosclerosis, such as diabetes, a history of smoking, dyslipidemia, hypertension, chronic kidney disease, or a family history of PAD
Age < 50 years with diabetes and another risk factor	Individuals under 50 years of age who have diabetes in addition to at least one other atherosclerosis risk factor
Individuals with known atherosclerotic disease	People diagnosed with atherosclerosis in other vascular regions, such as coronary, carotid, subclavian, renal, mesenteric arteries, or abdominal aortic aneurysm (AAA)

(PAD: peripheral arterial disease)

- For patients in whom the diagnosis of PAD has been established, further imaging workup is needed to determine the treatment strategy (surgical, endovascular, medical therapy, and preventive foot care)

History and Physical Examination Findings Suggestive of Peripheral Arterial Disease[8]

History

- Claudication
- *Pain types*: Aching, burning, cramping, discomfort, or fatigue
- *Location*: Buttock, thigh, calf, or ankle
- *Onset/Offset*: Factors like distance, exercise, uphill walking, and time taken to relieve symptoms after rest (typically less than 10 minutes for typical claudication)
- Non-joint-related symptoms in the lower limbs during activity, or symptoms that limit walking ability but are not characteristic of typical claudication
- Muscular discomfort in the lower extremities during walking, requiring more than 10 minutes of rest to alleviate
- Leg weakness, numbness, or fatigue during walking without associated pain
- Ischemic rest pain
- History of slow or nonhealing wounds in the lower limbs
- Erectile dysfunction

Physical Examination[8]

- Abnormal pulse detection in the lower extremities (femoral, popliteal, dorsalis pedis, or posterior tibial arteries)
- Presence of vascular bruits (e.g., in the epigastric, periumbilical, or groin areas)
- Nonhealing wounds on the lower limbs
- Gangrene in the lower extremities
- Other signs of ischemia, such as uneven hair growth, nail changes, calf muscle wasting, or color changes (pallor when elevated, rubor when dependent)

DIAGNOSTIC TESTING FOR PERIPHERAL ARTERIAL DISEASE[4,8,9]

Diagnostic testing for suspected PAD requires a multifaceted approach that incorporates history and physical examination, ankle-brachial index, and additional physiological testing, as well as noninvasive and potentially invasive (angiography) imaging.

Physiological Testing

Refer to **Box 1**.

Imaging Testing (Table 6 and Fig. 1)

In patients with functionally limiting claudication with inadequate response to medical therapy (including structured exercise) and patients with CLTI for whom revascularization is being considered, imaging tests should be done for assessment of anatomy and severity of disease and to determine potential revascularization strategy.[8,10,11]

BOX 1: Physiological testing.

- Resting ankle-brachial index (ABI)
- *Resting ABI interpretation*:
  - Abnormal (ABI ≤ 0.90)
  - Borderline (ABI 0.91–0.99)—go for exercise ABI
  - Normal (ABI 1.00–1.40)
  - Noncompressible (ABI > 1.40)—go for toe-brachial index (TBI)
- Exercise (treadmill) ABI
- *Toe pressure/TBI with waveforms*: TBI >0.7 normal, TBI < 0.7 abnormal
- Transcutaneous oxygen pressure ($TcPO_2$)
- *Skin perfusion pressure (SPP)*:
  - $TcPO_2$ and SPP are testing modalities that can be used for perfusion assessment
  - A $TcPO_2$ of >30 mm Hg or an SPP of >40 mm Hg can predict wound healing
  - $TcPO_2$ < 30 associated with major amputation

TABLE 6: Imaging testing.

Duplex ultrasound	Screening modality in patients with inconclusive physiological testing and in patients with claudication, where in diagnosis of PAD to be made
CT angiography	Equivocal or positive doppler findings, First modality in patients with CLTI, ALI and in patients with claudication with failed medical therapy
MR angiography	wherever CT angiography is contraindicated or inconclusive
Catheter angiography	Problem solving modality, mainly for interventional purpose
(ALI: acute limb ischemia; CTLI: chronic limb-threatening ischemia)	

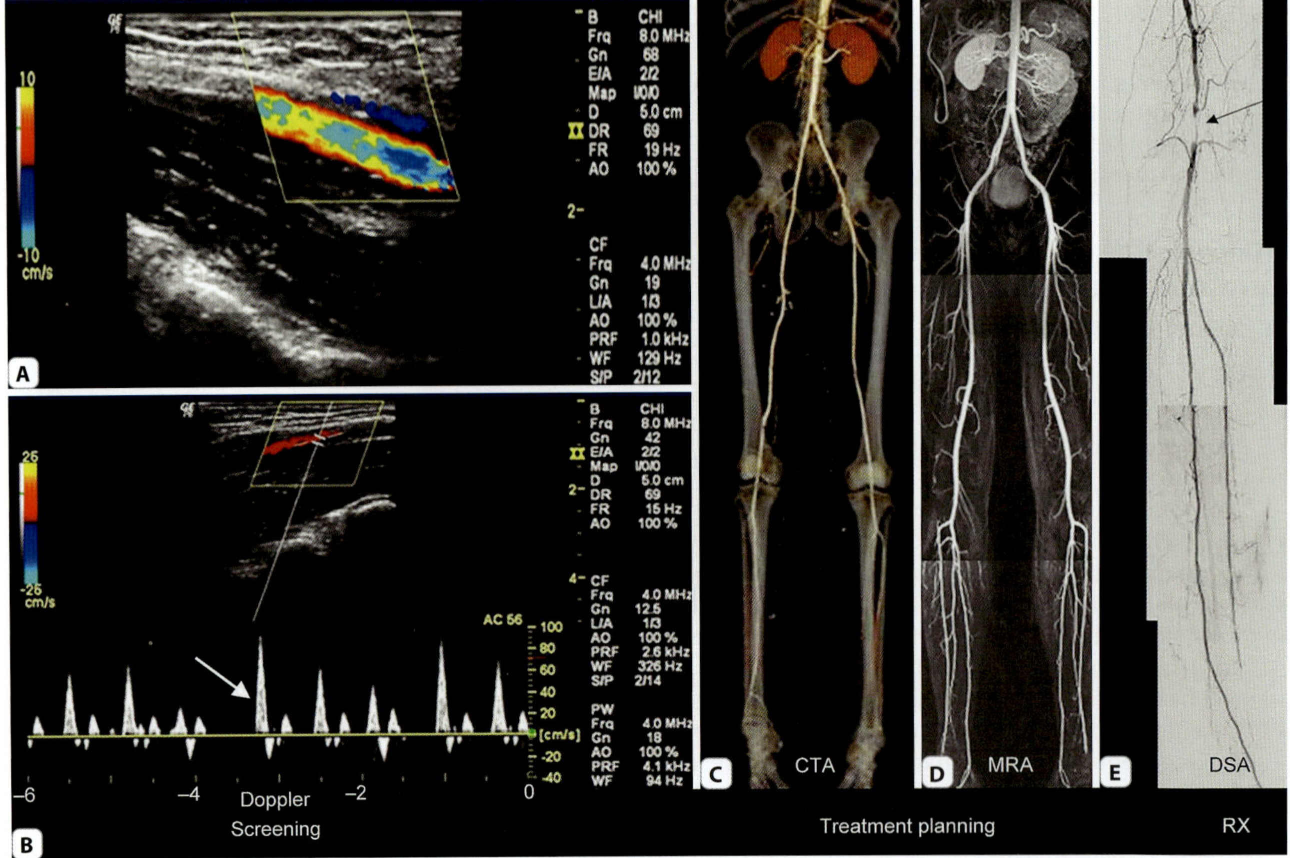

FIGS. 1A TO E: Normal lower extremity arteries on imaging. Color Doppler (A) with spectral tracing (B) of superficial femoral artery showing an uniform calibre artery which is showing typical triphasic flow pattern. Volume rendered technique (VRT) image (C) showing normal appearance of abdominal aorta and bilateral lower limb arteries. The course, calibre and relationship of vessels with the bones are shown on the VRT image. Maximum intensity projection (MIP) image (D) acquired in three stations showing normal abdominal and lower extremity arteries. Digital subtraction angiography (DSA) image (E) performed as part of interventional treatment showing occlusion in mid superficial femoral artery (arrow).

Goals of Imaging and Special Challenges of Imaging

Refer to **Box 2**.

Duplex Ultrasound[12-15]

Role:

- As a screening modality, in patients with inconclusive physiological testing and in patients with claudication, where in diagnosis of PAD to be made
- To locate and grade the stenosis
- For surveillance after bypass/endovascular treatment
- To identify puncture site complications such as hematoma, pseudoaneurysm, AV fistula after arterial access

Advantages:[10]

- Noninvasive, nonionizing, easily available, inexpensive, does not require nephrotoxic contrast
- Provides information about vessel walls and plaque morphology **(Fig. 2)**

- Spectral analysis provides hemodynamic information
- *In comparison to catheter angiography*: Pooled sensitivity of 87% and pooled specificity of 94%

Disadvantages:
- Operator dependent, time-consuming
- Not suitable for treatment planning
- Difficult visualization of aortoiliac segment, adductor and calf regions
- Detection of collaterals is low
- Presence of gas and calcification degrade images
- Infrapopliteal arteries challenging to image in their entirety
- Insufficient documentation

BOX 2: Goals of Imaging and Special Challenges of Imaging.

Goals of imaging:
- Identify arterial inflow and outflow lesions suitable for treatment
- *Assess their morphology and anatomical location*:
  - Therapeutic strategy (endovascular/surgery/combined)
  - Endovascular: Access route (antegrade, retrograde, cross-over, transbrachial)
  - Surgery: Possible origins and landing zones of bypass grafting

Special challenges: Critical limb ischemia—
- Imaging of the crural arteries
- Early venous overlay due to AV-shunting/cellulitis
- Calcified vessels (diabetics)
- High rate of patients with chronic renal failure/relevant co-morbidities

Technique of Doppler Ultrasound[13-15]

- The full length of the arterial segment(s) of interest should be evaluated with color Doppler
  - Curvilinear probe (2–5 MHz) for aortoiliac segments
  - Linear (7–12 MHz) probe for femoropopliteal imaging and calf arteries
- Acquire spectral Doppler waveforms with velocity measurements with the angle between the direction of moving blood and the direction of the ultrasound beam kept at less than or equal to 60°
- Suspected abnormalities should also be imaged with gray scale ultrasound and spectral Doppler waveforms with velocity measurements should be obtained and documented along the length of the arterial segment(s) and at any area of color or gray scale abnormality.
- The location and the length of any diseased or non-visualized segment(s) should be documented.

Parameters and Optimization of Doppler[14,15]

Optimization of Color Doppler

- *Color box*:
  - Refers to the square area within a gray scale ultrasound image where color Doppler data is displayed.
  - The size and depth of the box influence image resolution and quality.
  - To maximize frame rate, the box should be minimized and positioned as superficially as possible.
  - The "steer" function should be used to tilt the color box according to the arterial axis in longitudinal scans.
- *Color gain*:
  - Refers to the adjustment of flow data amplification to enhance flow visualization.

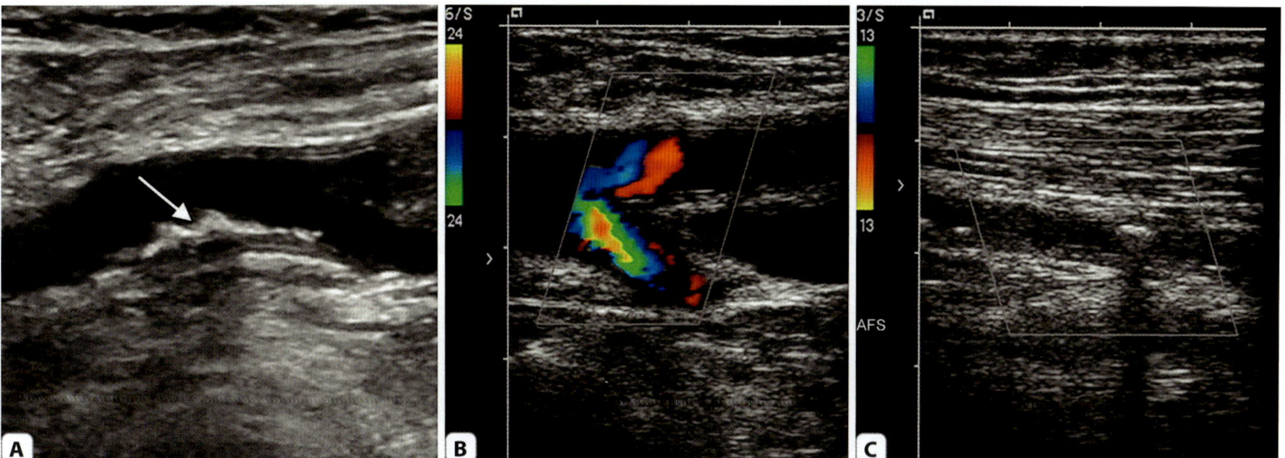

FIGS. 2A TO C: Arterial narrowing on color Doppler. B mode USG image (A) at the level of bifurcation of common femoral artery showing calcified plaques (arrow). Color Doppler image at the same level (B) and at the level of superficial femoral artery (C) showing no flow due to narrowing of the vessel.

- Color gain should be set as high as possible without introducing background color noise.
- *Color velocity scale*:
  - Indicates the range of flow velocities shown in the color Doppler image.
  - If the pulse repetition frequency (PRF) is set lower than the arterial flow velocity, color aliasing will occur.
  - Uniform color flow within an artery can be achieved by adjusting the gain or scale.
  - Color flow artifacts outside the artery can be minimized by decreasing the gain or increasing the scale.
- *Inversion*:
  - Refers to electronically reversing the flow direction, which may complicate interpretation.
  - Flow direction should be assessed using the color bar settings.
- *Wall filter (WF)*:
  - Eliminates low-frequency noise resulting from vessel wall motion below a specified frequency threshold.
  - WF settings are typically predefined by the manufacturer.

Optimization of Spectral Doppler[13-15]

- *Sample volume or gate*:
  - The sample volume cursor consists of parallel lines on either side of the arterial axis.
  - The sample volume should be positioned in the centre of the arterial lumen.
  - Its size generally ranges between 1/3 and 1/2 of the lumen's diameter.
- *Doppler angle*:
  - The angle formed by the Doppler line and the arterial axis should be between 45° and 60° for optimal accuracy.
  - The central line within the artery on Doppler ultrasound represents the axis of blood flow.
- *Doppler spectrum and baseline*:
  - The Doppler spectrum is a graphical representation of frequency variations over a short time and is displayed against a baseline.
  - The direction of flow relative to the transducer is indicated by its position above or below the baseline.
  - Flow toward the transducer is shown as positive velocity above the baseline.
  - To correct aliasing artifacts in the Doppler spectrum, the baseline can be lowered or the velocity scale increased.

Interpretation of Findings (Fig. 3)[14,15]

- Normal extremity artery shows a triphasic high resistance flow pattern with a preserved spectral window and PSV ranging from 120 to 60 cm/s from iliac artery to dorsalis pedis artery
- At the level of stenosis, the systolic flow rate across the stenosis increases and the flow changes from streamlined to turbulent, leads to increase in peak systolic velocity (PSV) and spectral broadening causing obliteration of spectral window.

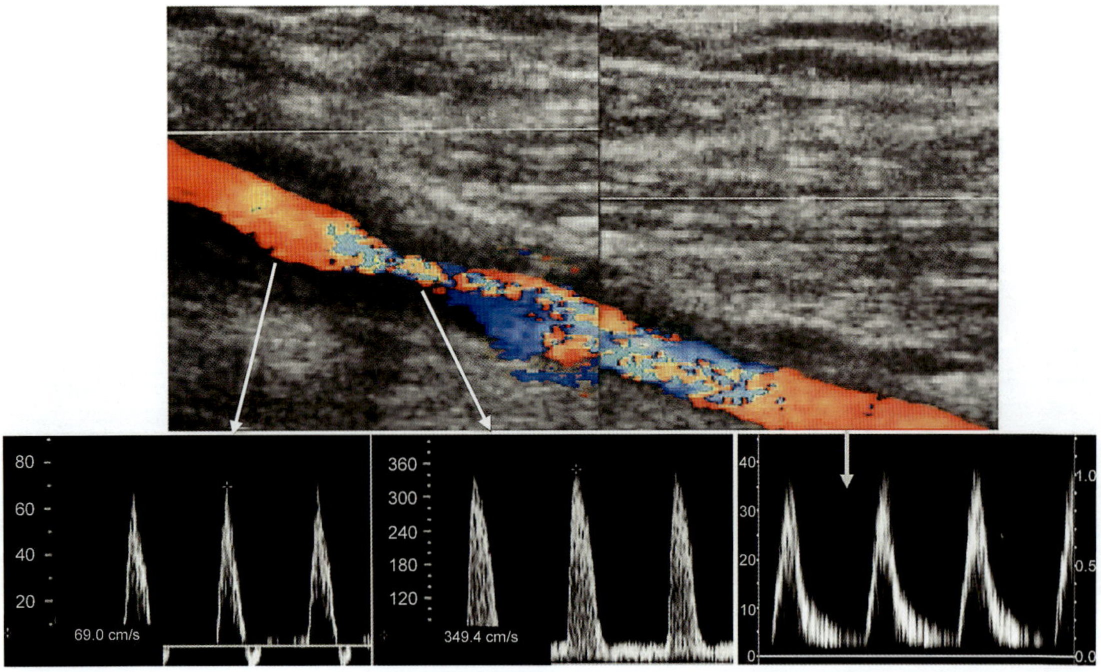

FIG. 3: Color Doppler with spectral wave patterns at normal part of artery, at the level of stenosis and distal to stenosis.

- To eliminate the variations in the PSV between vessel segments and patients, a ratio of PSV at the site of abnormality and at the normal proximal vessel is taken. The commonly used criteria to diagnose >50% stenosis is PSV ratio >2, PSV >200 cm/s, color aliasing and spectral broadening
- Monophasic flow used to describe abnormal waveforms with a single phase found distal to a hemodynamically significant arterial obstruction

Computed Tomography[10,16-18]

Computed tomography is the modality of choice to evaluate patients with peripheral vascular disease extremity **(Fig. 4)**. The advent of multidetector CT has revolutionized CT angiography (CTA) leading to faster and high-quality acquisition of images. Higher resolution compared to MRI and capability of 3D image generation are additional highlights.

Indications:
- Equivocal or positive doppler findings
- Patients with CLTI and ALI
- Patients with claudication after failed medical therapy

Advantages:
- Fast scanning, high spatial resolution, isotropic imaging, imaging of surrounding tissues
- Less invasive
- *Greater scan coverage*: Fast depiction of the whole vascular tree within one breath hold, including inflow and outflow vessels
- Accuracy comparable to catheter angiography
- Easily interpretable by the surgeon

Disadvantages:
- Higher radiation dose
- With significant and dense calcifications, interpretation becomes difficult. Hence, less valuable in CLI because of extensive crural artery calcifications **(Fig. 5)**
- Inconsistent/poor pedal vessel visualization
- Nephrotoxicity of iodinated contrast agents
- Risk of severe reaction to contrast medium

Technique of Computed Tomography Angiography[18-20]

- Recent multidetector CT (MDCT) technology (64-MDCT and more) allows submillimeter resolution, more coverage per rotation of tube and decrease in amount of contrast volume required for angiography.
- With the increasing speed of acquisition, the entire arterial tree from abdominal aorta and the arterial system of the lower limbs can be acquired within seconds in the first pass of contrast.
- With the current available scanning speed, CT systems may "outrun" the physiologic progress of the contrast medium bolus, and it is critical to capture the peak enhancement of the arterial tree to obtain good quality images.
- If the acquisition time is too long, venous contamination (return) may spoil the quality of the examination.
- Hence, it is mandatory to tailor the acquisition to the type of CT system used, the pathology, and the patients' condition.
  - For example, the presence of stenosis, occlusion or aneurysm may slow the arterial flow down.
  - Elderly patients, as well as patients with cardiac disease, may also have a slow flow

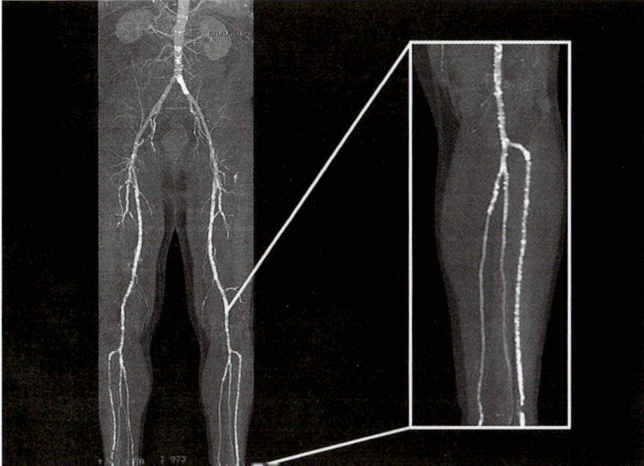

FIG. 4: Vessel wall calcification on computed tomography angiography (CTA). Maximum intensity projection (MIP) image of a CTA data set showing extensive vessel wall calcification involving the entire arterial tree. This is considered as a limitation of CTA in which the evaluation of vessel wall narrowing is known to be hampered by extensive calcifications.

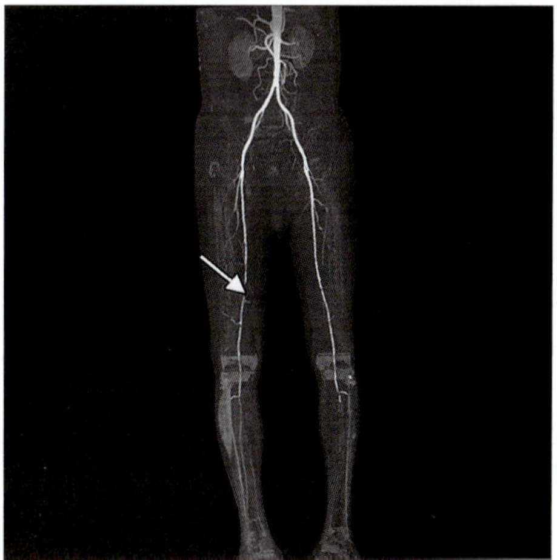

FIG. 5: Arterial narrowing on computed tomography angiography (CTA). Maximum intensity projection (MIP) image with bone removal of CTA data set showing short segment narrowing at the level of distal superficial femoral artery and good distal run-off. MIP image can provide an overview of the entire arterial tree on a single image based on the CTA data set which is otherwise huge.

- The timing, rate of injection, contrast volume and the scanning speed of the scanner should be adjusted meticulously to avoid poor opacification of arteries

Injection Protocols (Table 7)[19]

If there is suspected severe disease with slow flow, then a slower contrast injection bolus and longer scan time may be preferred. This can be achieved by reducing the table speed, through the scanner, i.e., the pitch, and by slowing the gantry rotation time.

Advantages of Dual-energy CT in Peripheral Vascular Disease[10,20,21]

Refer to **Table 8**.

Image Processing (Table 9)[10]

With the above post-processing methods especially the CPR along with axial images, stenosis can be easily categorized into mild (0–50%), moderate (50–70%) and severe (>70%).[7,8]

TABLE 7: Injection protocols.

Parameters and technique	Standard antegrade acquisition	Retrograde acquisition
Direction of acquisition	Craniocaudal	Caudocranial
Amount contrast injection	100 mL followed by 40 mL saline	100 mL followed by 40 mL saline
Rate of injection	4 mL saline	4 mL saline
Trigger point	Abdominal aorta T12 level, 150–200 HU	Popliteal artery, 100 HU
Rotation time and pitch	0.5 second or less, pitch < 1	0.5 second, pitch > 1

TABLE 8: Advantages of dual-energy CT in peripheral vascular disease.

Advantage	Explanation
Improved material differentiation	DECT can differentiate between materials such as calcium, iodine, and soft tissue, enhancing diagnostic accuracy
Reduced beam-hardening artifacts	Helps minimize artifacts caused by dense materials like calcium, improving image quality and vessel visualization
Enhanced plaque characterization	Automatic plaque characterization and removal which can give accurate stenosis measurements
Perfusion assessment	Provides additional information on tissue perfusion, helping assess the extent of ischemia in PAD
Reduced contrast use	Low kVp images enhances the better visualization of contrast, allows better visualization of arterial tree at lower iodinated contrast doses and less radiation dose
Virtual non-contrast imaging	Can create virtual non-contrast images from contrast-enhanced scans, reducing the need for multiple scans
Accurate vessel imaging	Improves visualization of small vessels and detection of stenosis, benefiting treatment planning
Bone removal	Accurate bone removal to generate high quality 3D images

(DECT: dual-energy CT; PAD: peripheral arterial disease)

TABLE 9: Image processing.

Feature	Description
Isotropic submillimeter resolution	Allows reconstruction of the computed tomography angiography (CTA) 3D dataset in any anatomic orientation. Axial images are very important
Reconstruction algorithms	3D data is reconstructed using multiplanar reformatted (MPR), maximum intensity projection (MIP), and volume rendered (VR) algorithms and cinematic rendering technique • MIP generate angiographic maps close to digital subtraction angiography (DSA) images • Volume rendering technique (VRT) provides 3D relationship of vessels to adjacent bones • Cinematic rendering shows facilitates 3D and depth perception
Automatic reconstruction	Basic axial, coronal, and sagittal MPR images are automatically reconstructed immediately after CT acquisition

Continued

Continued

Feature	Description
Postprocessing	Image data is transferred to dedicated software to generate intuitive and clinically useful images
MIP **(Fig. 5)**	MIP is a type of rendering in which the voxel with maximum value will be displayed from any point of view. The wall calcification and vessel contour are well-delineated on MIP and give an overview of the entire arterial tree. It can be used in two modes full-volume (thick) mode and sub-volume (thin) mode. Thin MIP is useful in depicting the inflow circulation (aortoiliac) so that the overlying abdominal visceral arteries are not visualized. Thick MIP is useful in showing the outflow circulation (femoropopliteal and tibioperoneal)
Curved MPR images	Curved planar reconstruction (CPR) is a specialized form of MPR in which the image can be reformatted in any curved plane. CPR is useful to visualize the entire length of artery in one image. It can also be used to create orthogonal axial images perpendicular to the axis of the artery so that the stenosis measurements can be done accurately even in the presence of calcified plaques
VRT **(Fig. 6)**	VRT is a postprocessing technique which can give 3D perspective of the entire volume. It is useful to provide spatial relationships with the adjacent structures such as collaterals and bone which is immensely helpful for interventional radiologists and surgeons. However, the distinction between the calcified plaque and vessel wall contour is not that well-visualized on VRT

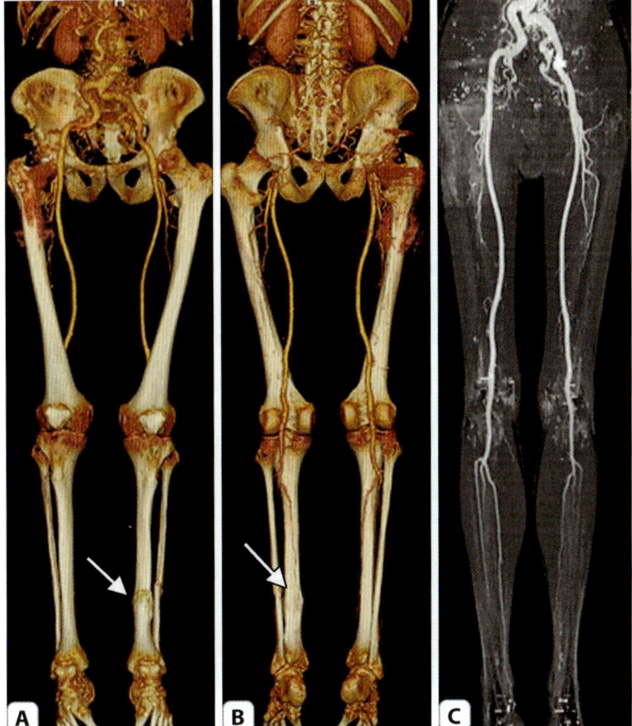

FIGS. 6A TO C: Computed tomography angiography (CTA)—one stop shop technique in skeletal trauma. Volume rendered technique (VRT) images of CTA in front (A) and back (B) views showing fracture of both bones in the left leg (arrow). Maximum intensity projection (MIP) image with bone removal (C) of the same patient showing attenuated arteries in the left leg. CTA in this situation can provide information about the skeletal and soft tissue injuries apart from showing the detailed anatomy of the lower limb arterial tree.

Magnetic Resonance Angiography[10,21]

Magnetic resonance imaging has undergone several technological improvements over decades and with the current scanners it is possible to scan the entire arterial tree in a single injection of contrast. MRA provided detailed visualization of blood vessels, aiding in the diagnosis and treatment planning of PAD **(Fig. 7)**. MRA techniques can be performed with or without the use of intravenous contrast agents, contrast enhanced MRA (CE-MRA) and non-contrast enhanced MRA (non CE-MRA).

Advantages:[10]

- Fast, non-invasive technique, out-patient procedure as compared to DSA
- No ionizing radiation as compared to CT
- No risk of contrast nephropathy as compared to CT
- Highest diagnostic accuracy compared with DSA
- Treatment planning possible/superior than with color doppler
- Not affected by arterial calcification
- Superior depiction of infrapopliteal arteries
- Compared to CTA is that it can generate images without overlapping bones
- Unique capability of MRI is that it can generate angiographic images without contrast media which comes handy in patients with chronic renal disease and patients with contraindication to iodinated contrast media

Disadvantages:

- Cost intensive, high-tech examination of limited availability
- Time consuming compared to CT angiography

- High magnetic field strength (contraindicated in patients with pacemaker, cochlear implants, metallic foreign bodies)
- Risk of nephrogenic systemic fibrosis for certain contrast agents
- Contraindicated in patients with claustrophobia
- Potential signal loss in presence of stents (bare metal more than nitinol)
- Image interpretation is affected by venous contamination with CE-MRA as compared to CTA and DSA **(Fig. 8)**

Advantages and Disadvantages of Magnetic Resonance Angiography in Tabular Form[10]

Refer to **Table 10**.

Key Components of CE-MRA Technique for Lower Limbs[10,11]

- *Basic concept of MRA*:
  - Fast and robust MRA technique depends on the T1 shortening effect of gadolinium-based contrast agents.

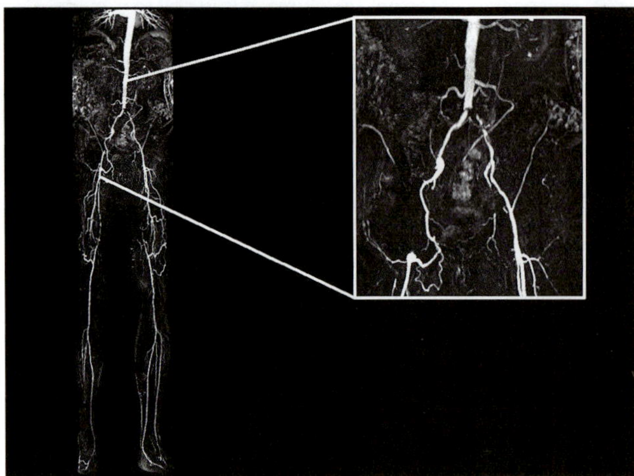

FIG. 7: Arterial narrowing on magnetic resonance angiography (MRA). Maximum intensity projection (MIP) image of MRA data set showing extensive atherosclerotic involvement of aorta and lower limb arteries. There is complete occlusion of bilateral common iliac arteries till superficial femoral arteries with good distal run-off. Extensive vessel wall calcifications do not hamper the vessel assessment on MRA which is an advantage over computed tomography angiography (CTA).

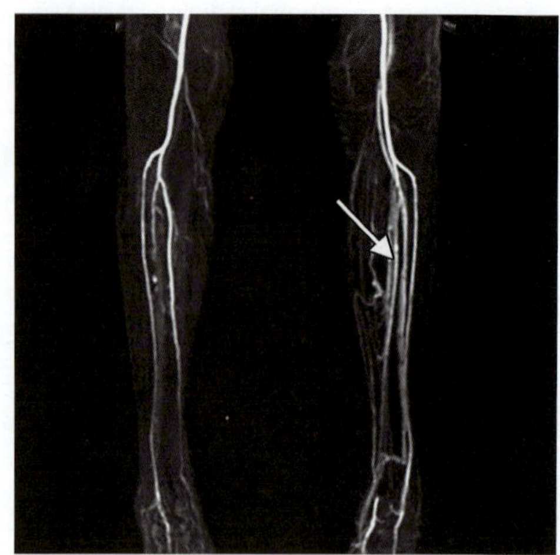

FIG. 8: Venous contamination in magnetic resonance angiography (MRA). Maximum intensity projection (MIP) image of MRA data set of bilateral legs showing venous contamination (arrow) in the left side. Venous contamination which usually occurs in the last station of data acquisition due to time delay can degrade the diagnostic quality of MRA.

TABLE 10: Advantages and disadvantages of magnetic resonance angiography.

Aspect	Advantages	Disadvantages
Non-invasive	MRA is non-invasive and does not require arterial puncture or catheterization	Compared to traditional angiography, MRA is slightly less precise in small vessel imaging
No ionizing radiation	MRA avoids the risks associated with radiation exposure, making it safer for repeat imaging	Some sequences, particularly non-contrast MRA, may take longer, which can cause discomfort for the patient
Excellent soft tissue contrast	MRA provides high-resolution imaging of blood vessels and surrounding tissues, allowing detailed analysis of both arterial stenosis and plaques	Can produce motion artifacts if the patient is unable to remain still during the scan
Assessment of blood flow	Time-resolved imaging sequences allow for evaluation of blood flow dynamics and identification of hemodynamically significant lesions	In non-contrast MRA, slow or turbulent blood flow can cause artifacts or reduced image quality
Contrast-enhanced MRA	Provides high spatial resolution and fast acquisition times with excellent visualization of the arterial tree	Requires gadolinium-based contrast agents, which carry risks for patients with renal insufficiency (nephrogenic systemic fibrosis)
Non-contrast MRA	Suitable for patients with renal insufficiency as it avoids gadolinium contrast	Non-contrast techniques generally have lower spatial resolution and longer acquisition times

Continued

Continued

Aspect	Advantages	Disadvantages
Wide field of view	Can image large portions of the vascular tree (e.g., whole limb imaging) in a single acquisition	The presence of metal implants (e.g., stents, pace-makers) can produce artifacts that affect image quality
Detection of arterial stenosis	Highly accurate in detecting stenosis and occlusions in peripheral arteries, making it an important tool in PAD management	In small, tortuous, or distal vessels, it may be less accurate compared to conventional angiography
Follow-up	Ideal for follow-up evaluations due to the absence of radiation and repeated contrast exposure, especially for chronic PAD patients	Non-contrast methods can be less accurate for subtle lesions or in areas with complex anatomy
Tissue characterization	Provides insight into plaque composition and vessel wall integrity, which is useful for PAD prognosis and treatment planning	Interpretation of MRA requires expertise, and technical challenges in specific cases can limit diagnostic accuracy
Interpretation	Image interpretation is not affected by calcified plaques as compared to CTA	Affected by venous contamination with CE MRA as compared to CTA

(CTA: computed tomography angiography; MRA: magnetic resonance angiography; PAD: peripheral arterial disease)

- CE-MRA sequence is a fast sequence with preferential filling of central k space which determines the contrast resolution of the image.
- Usually precontrast as well as post contrast volume sets are acquired and subtracted to obtain the MRA image. Subtraction using precontrast mask provides good background tissue suppression and showing only the vessels.

- *Patient positioning*:
  - The patient is positioned supine in the MRI scanner, with the lower limbs positioned within the field of view.
  - Comfortable positioning is important to minimize patient movement during the scan, which could cause motion artifacts.
- *Coil selection*:
  - Multichannel body and peripheral vascular coils are used to achieve high signal-to-noise ratio and spatial resolution.
  - A phased-array surface coil or dedicated vascular coil may be used to cover the entire lower limb arterial tree.
- *Field of view (FOV) and stations*:
  - The FOV with overlapping areas typically includes the abdominal aorta, iliac arteries, and the entire length of the lower limb arteries down to the feet.
  - MRA usually done in three stations namely aortoiliac, thigh and calf region and between the acquisitions the table has to move quickly to next station.
  - This technique is called three stations, moving table technique in which the contrast bolus is followed from aortoiliac to calf in the same order.
  - The aortoiliac station is usually done with breath holding to minimize motion blurring.
  - However, this three-station method can sometimes lead to venous contamination in the third station resulting in nondiagnostic studies
- *Methods to overcome the venous contamination*:
  - Thigh compression cuffs and pillow under the knee to slow down the venous return
  - Use of non-contrast MRA for the calf station
  - Acquiring calf station in a separate contrast injection.
  - Time resolved MRA of calf region which generates images in every 1–2 seconds to differentiate arteries from veins.
- *Contrast agent*:
  - A gadolinium-based contrast agent is injected intravenously to enhance the blood vessels.
  - The contrast is administered through a power injector typically at a dose of 0.1–0.2 mmol/kg body weight, followed by a saline flush.
  - Single bolus technique: We typically use 0.2 mmol/kg of an extracellular gadolinium agent injected at a rate of 1.5–2 mL/s.
  - Split bolus technique: A split dose delivery of 2 mL/s for 10 seconds followed by 0.5–1.0 mL/s for the remaining contrast agent can be used for long scanning times when proper sharing of the bolus is problematic.
- *Timing of contrast administration*:
  - CE-MRA relies on optimal timing of contrast injection to capture the arterial phase (before venous contamination).
  - If the data is acquired during the inflow of contrast, ringing artifacts will degrade the image quality. Thus, the image acquisition should be performed during the plateau phase of the arterial enhancement. Hence the timing of contrast injection and start of scanning are of paramount importance.
  - Bolus triggering technique in which rapid real time images are taken and once the contrast arrival is ascertained, the MRA sequence is triggered manually

- In bolus tracking, a test bolus or real-time monitoring helps determine the correct scan initiation time based on the arrival of the contrast in the abdominal aorta or common femoral artery.
- *Imaging sequences*:
  - CE-MRA typically uses 3D fast gradient-echo sequences (e.g., FLASH or SPGR) with short TR (repetition time) and TE (echo time).
  - This allows for rapid acquisition of high-resolution images with excellent depiction of vascular anatomy.
  - Parallel imaging techniques (such as GRAPPA or SENSE) and compressed sensing may be applied to accelerate the scan and reduce breath-hold time.
- *Breath-hold and scan duration*:
  - For imaging the abdominal and pelvic vessels, patients may be asked to hold their breath to reduce motion artifacts.
  - Lower limb segments, where breath-hold is not required, can be scanned continuously as the patient remains still.
  - The total imaging time is generally a few minutes, but with multi-station approaches, scanning may be done in stages with automatic table movement.
  - 1–3 min/station/segment
- *Postprocessing*:
  - After the acquisition, images are post-processed using maximum intensity projection (MIP) techniques to create 3D visualizations of the arteries.
  - MIP reconstructions are particularly useful for detecting stenoses, occlusions, and aneurysms.
  - Multiplanar reformations (MPR) and curved planar reconstructions (CPR) may be used to further evaluate the vessels.

Noncontrast Enhanced Magnetic Resonance Angiography Technique[22-24]

Advantages:
- *No risk of nephrotoxicity*: Especially suitable for patients with chronic kidney disease or those at risk of contrast-induced nephropathy.
- No need for contrast agents, making it safer in patients allergic to gadolinium.
- Can be used repeatedly in patients for follow-up examinations without concerns over cumulative contrast exposure.

Techniques:
- *Time-of-flight (TOF) MRA*:
  - Relies on the flow of unsaturated blood into an imaging slice, producing high signal in arteries.
  - Suitable for detecting stenosis or occlusion in the aortoiliac and femoro-popliteal segments
  - Long scanning time
  - Poor image quality from patient motion, poor SNR, loss of signal when flow is complex, turbulent or oriented parallel to the slice plane
- *Fresh blood imaging (FBI)*:
  - Magnetic resonance imaging technique that allows for the direct visualization of flowing blood without the use of a contrast medium
  - FBI uses a series of techniques to capture the MR signal from flowing blood, including 3D ultrafast spin echo acquisition, prospective ECG synchronization, and inversion pulse magnetization preparation.

Technique of FBI:
- Utilizes an ECG-gated FSE sequence
- Acquire images in both the systolic and diastolic phases of the cardiac cycle.
- Fast systolic arterial flow is differentiated from slower diastolic flow
- Subtraction technique is used to produce angiographic images

Advantages of FBI:
- FBI is a simple and effective technique that does not use toxic heavy metals like gadolinium. It can also be faster than other imaging techniques, such as TOF imaging, which can take up to 25 minutes to examine a whole leg
- It can also produce high-quality images with fewer artifacts and improved vessel-to-background contrast.

Limitations of Non-CE MRA

- Lower spatial resolution compared to contrast-enhanced methods, particularly for small vessels or complex anatomies. Imaging of distal calf and pedal arteries is still challenging
- *Longer acquisition times*: These techniques may take longer, requiring greater patient cooperation.
- *Flow artifacts*: Non-contrast techniques are more prone to artifacts in regions with turbulent flow or slow blood flow

Advances in MRA technique:
- *Higher field strength*:
  - Increased signal-to-noise-ratio
  - Higher spatial resolution (< 1 mm^3)
  - Increased T1 ↑ T1 relaxation time
    - Improved vessel vs. tissue contrast
    - higher sensitivity to T1-shortening CA
  - Increased anatomic coverage
- *Parallel imaging techniques (SMASH, SENSE, GRAPPA)*:
  - These are MRI acceleration techniques that use multiple receiver coils to acquire data from different spatial locations simultaneously, reducing the scan time.

- These techniques have revolutionized peripheral MRA by reducing scan times, improving image quality, and enabling high-resolution imaging across large fields of view.

- *Compressed sensing (CS)*:
  - CS enables significant reduction in scan time by acquiring less data, which is particularly beneficial in MRA where high spatial and temporal resolution is needed.
  - Scan times can be reduced by factors of 2–8× or more compared to conventional MRA without compromising image quality
- *Time-resolved angiography (TRICKS, TREAT, TWIST)*:
  - Time-resolved MRA sequences (also called 4D MRA) allows dynamic imaging of passage of contrast through the arterial and venous phases without compromising spatial or temporal resolution. This helps in evaluating vascular malformations, fistulas, or stenoses
- *Intravascular blood-pool contrast agents (BPA's)*
  - CCE-MRA with standard extracellular contrast material is well established for vascular imaging. Recently, introduction of blood pool contrast agents (BPA), which are retained in blood with a prolonged time-window of enhancement as compared to extracellular gadolinium chelates.
  - Bolus-injectable BPAs allow for first-pass CE-MRA similar to standard extracellular contrast media, but with higher relaxivity, allowing lower doses and reduced injection rates.
  - An additional feature of BPA is the steady-state phase with a broad time window enabling high-resolution angiography

Digital Subtraction Angiography[2,4]

Traditional first line imaging modality for many years, presently reserved for interventional purpose

Advantages:
- Easily interpretable complete arterial map of the lower limb
- Excellent spatial and temporal resolution
- Measurement of pressure gradients (hemodynamic significance)
- Can be performed as:
  - Non-selective overview DSA of pelvic and both lower limb arteries
  - Selective DSA of the most affected limb without option for immediate treatment

Disadvantages:
- Not easily available, costly, need expertise to perform
- Invasive procedure, requiring preparation and short stay ≥ 2 hours
- Access site complications (bleeding, arteriovenous fistula, pseudoaneurysm)
- *Check coagulation parameters*: INR < 1.5
- Stop vitamin K antagonists but no need to pause aspirin/clopidogrel
- *Radiation exposure 3.9 times greater than for MD-CTA*: 10– 30 mSv
- Risks due to the use of iodinated contrast agents
- Check of serum creatinine/GRF mandatory (< 1.5 mg/dL/> 60 mL/min)

Comparison of CTA/MRA with Digital Subtraction Angiography[2,4,11]

Refer to **Table 11**.

Image Analysis

MR/CT angiography images are analyzed in following manner:
- Evaluation of the ilio-femoral arterial anatomy from 2 cm above the aortic bifurcation to the level of the ankle joint on a segmental basis
- Images should be assessed for:
  - Extent of the disease
  - Level of occlusion
  - Number of segments involved
  - Distal reformation
  - Degree of collateralization
  - Distal run off (0, 1, 2, 3 vessels)
- Findings of the angiography should be depicted in schematic representation for easy understanding to the clinician.

TABLE 11: Comparison of CTA/MRA with digital subtraction angiography.

Computed tomography angiography (CTA)/magnetic resonance angiography (MRA)	Digital subtraction angiography (DSA)
Less invasive	Invasive
Fast	Short admission and postprocedure care
Minimal complications (contrast reactions)	Complication rate (2–3%)
Can be used in patients with extensive aortoiliac disease	Technically difficult in these group
Provide road map prior to interventions	Gold standard, now used mainly for intervention purpose
Overestimation of stenotic lesions, venous contamination	No such problem
Dynamics cannot be assessed	Pressure gradients can be assessed

Schematic Representation of CTA/ MRA Findings

Refer to **Figure 9**.

Summary of Imaging Strategy in Peripheral Arterial Disease

Refer to **Figure 10**.

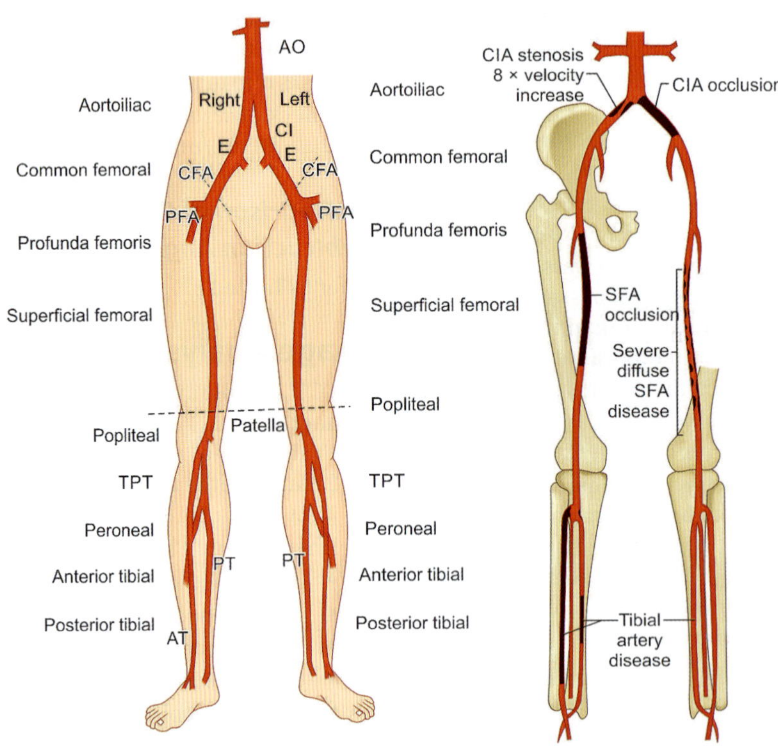

FIG. 9: Schematic representation of CTA/MRA findings.

(CFA: common femoral artery; CIA: common iliac artery; CTA: computed tomography angiography; MRA: magnetic resonance angiography; PFA: profunda femoral artery; SFA: superficial femoral artery; TPA: tibio-peroneal trunk)

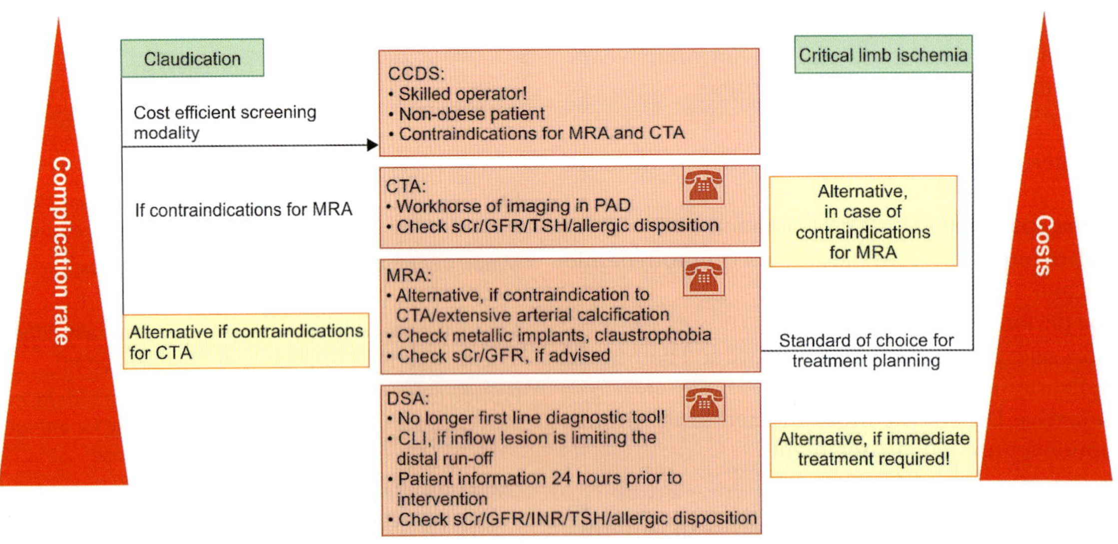

FIG. 10: Imaging strategies in peripheral arterial disease (PAD).

(CCDS: color coded doppler sonography; CTA: computed tomography angiography; DSA: digital subtraction angiography; GFR: glomerular filtration rate; INR: international normalized ratio; MRA: magnetic resonance angiography; PVD: peripheral vascular disease; TSH: thyroid stimulating hormone)

Endovascular Interventions in Peripheral Arterial Disease

Treatment Guidelines[8,11,25]

- Interventional treatments are increasingly being recognized as the first-line management strategy for PAD, whenever clinically feasible.
- Endovascular treatment provides a lower risk substitute to conventional surgery in many patients with multiple co-morbidities.
- Advances in interventional technology during the past few years have widened the choices for handling PAD percutaneously.
- Trans-Atlantic Inter-Society Consensus guidelines aimed to provide guidance on treatment decisions relating to the optimal revascularization strategy (endovascular vs. surgical) based on the anatomic and clinical status of the patient **(Fig. 11)**.
- TASC has classified the PAD diseases into A to D categories for each arterial segments (aortoiliac, femoropopliteal, and below knee segments).
- These categories are used for treatment guidance regarding the optimal revascularization strategy (endovascular vs. surgical) based on the complexity and location of the anatomic disease.
  - Endovascular therapy is the treatment of choice for TASC A lesions.
  - Endovascular treatment is preferred for TASC B.
  - Surgery is preferred for TASC C lesions.
  - Surgery is the treatment of choice for TASC D lesions.
- The endovascular technique is better for treating the short lesions and stenosis. Long diffuse lesions, occlusions, and circumferential calcification may require surgery.
- Noninvasive tests (ankle-brachial index) and arterial mapping (CT/MR angiography) done, prior to an endovascular treatment, help in localization of the disease and planning the procedure **(Fig. 12)**

Treatment Protocol[8,26-29]

- The primary goal of PAD management is to improve symptoms (rest pain, healing of ulcers), enhance quality of life, and prevent major amputation and also cardiovascular events.
- Management strategies include a combination of medical therapy, physical exercise, lifestyle modifications, and revascularization procedures
- Medical management is aimed at relieving symptoms, preventing disease progression, and reducing the risk of cardiovascular events
  - Antiplatelet therapy: To reduce the risk of cardiovascular events and major lower limb events
  - Cilostazol: A phosphodiesterase inhibitor used to improve walking distance in patients with intermittent claudication. It increases blood flow and has vasodilatory effects
  - Pentoxifylline: To reduce blood viscosity and improve microcirculation
  - Statin therapy: All patients with PAD should be on a high-intensity statin (e.g., atorvastatin, rosuvastatin) to lower LDL cholesterol levels and reduce cardiovascular risk.
  - Antihypertensive therapy: Blood pressure control is critical to reduce cardiovascular complications. The target BP is <130/80 mm Hg for most patients.
  - Glycemic control in diabetic patients: Optimal glycemic control (HbA1c <7%) helps in reducing the progression of PAD and microvascular complications.

Physical exercise: Supervised exercise therapy is a cornerstone in the management of PAD, particularly for improving functional status and reducing symptoms of intermittent claudication.

Risk factor modification: Lifestyle changes are essential to halt the progression of PAD and reduce cardiovascular risk.

- Smoking cessation
- Dietary modifications
- Weight management
- Glycemic control

Revascularization Procedures

Refer to **Table 12**.

Endovascular Procedures (Flowchart 1)[26-29]

Treatment Decisions[26-29]

- The scheduling and necessity for revascularization depends upon the clinical settings.
- *Three different clinical situations include*:
  i. Intermittent claudication
  ii. Critical limb ischemia
  iii. Acute limb ischemia
- Most of the patients with intermittent claudication are managed by exercise and medical therapy.
- Interventional procedures are reserved in circumstances, when these methods fail to improve quality of life and limb function
- In contrast, critical limb ischemia and acute limb ischemia pose an immediate threat to the limb, necessitating more urgent revascularization.

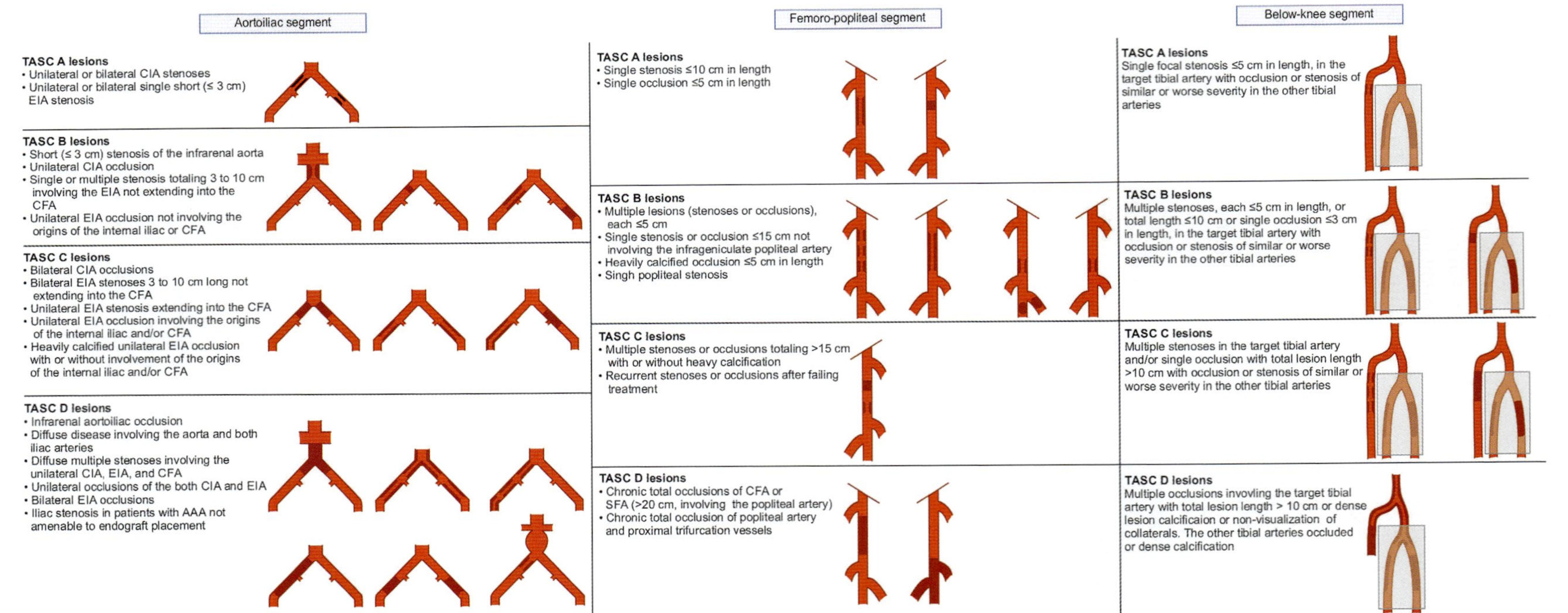

FIG. 11: TASC anatomic classification showing various patterns of disease based on extent of the disease at different segments of arterial tree. Used for treatment guidance regarding the optimal revascularization strategy (endovascular vs. surgical) based on the complexity and location of the anatomic disease.

Note: TASC—II recommendation

- *Type A*: Endovascular therapy is the treatment of choice.
- *Type B*: Endovascular treatment is the preferred treatment.
- *Type C*: Endovascular preferred treatment for high-risk patients, otherwise surgery.
- *Type D*: Surgery is the treatment of choice for type D lesions.

(AAA: abdominal aortic aneurysm; CFA: common femoral artery; CIA: common iliac artery; EIA: external iliac artery; SFA: superficial femoral artery; TASC: Trans-Atlantic Inter-Society Consensus)

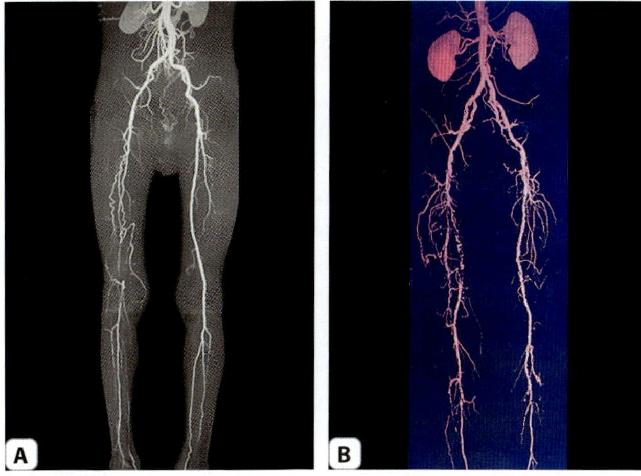

FIGS. 12A AND B: Computed tomography angiography [maximum intensity projection (MIP) and volume rendered technique (VRT)] images (A and B) of vascular mapping of bilateral lower limbs showing location of lesion and extent of the disease, important for planning the endovascular treatment.

TABLE 12: Revascularization procedures.

Treatment	Advantages	Disadvantages
Angioplasty and stenting	Minimally invasive, quicker recovery, less hospital stays	Risk of restenosis, requires long-term antiplatelet therapy
Bypass surgery	Effective for long-segment or complex occlusions	More invasive, longer recovery, higher surgical risk
Atherectomy	Removes calcified plaque, can be used for complex lesions	Limited availability, higher cost, risk of vessel injury
Endarterectomy	Direct removal of plaque, avoids grafts or stents	Limited to certain arterial locations, risk of infection

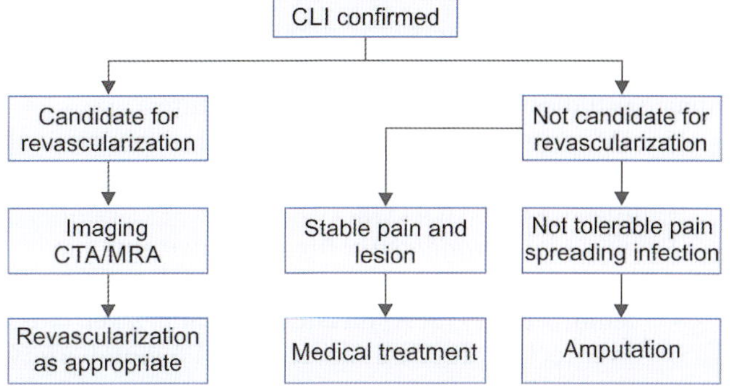

FLOWCHART 1: Algorithmic approach to endovascular procedures.
(CLI: critical limb ischemia; CTA: computed tomography angiography; MRA: magnetic resonance angiography)

Types of Endovascular Procedures, Results, Follow-up and Surveillance

- Balloon angioplasty and stenting are the key revascularization techniques.
- Latest advances in interventional treatments include, drug-eluting balloons, drug-eluting stents, plaque debulking devices (atherectomy devices) for crossing tight chronic total occlusions.
- In general, interventional therapies have better long-term durability for aortoiliac disease than femoral popliteal disease.
- Infrapopliteal revascularization has poor long-term results and is generally reserved for critical and acute limb ischemia.
- Patients receiving any form of interventional revascularization measures need a planned surveillance strategy for follow-up care.
  - Rigorous treatment of cardiovascular risk factors to avert myocardial infarction and stroke
  - Limb observation targets to identify restenosis and fresh disease elsewhere in the treated segments.

Technique of Angioplasty[30-32]

- *Definition*: Percutaneous transluminal angioplasty (PTA) refers to deliberate opening (dilatation) of a vascular stenosis or occlusion using a balloon catheter.
- *Mode of action of PTA*: Angioplasty causes rupture of the atherosclerotic plaque and a limited split or dissection of the vessel wall. The split might spread in the vessel wall either in circumferential or longitudinal direction. Also, it may spread deep into the internal elastic lamina or into the media, keeping adventitial layer intact.
  - Concentric lesions have good response to PTA, since the plaque and the vascular wall layers are split in an even fashion,
  - Whereas eccentric vascular lesions, respond poor to balloon dilatation due to recoil of the normal elastic wall

Key points of Revascularization Procedures[30-32]

Refer to **Table 13**.

Preprocedural Work-up[8,26,30-32]

- A comprehensive clinical and medical history must be taken. History regarding claudication symptoms, pertinent past history of cardiac and renal disease, risk factors for vascular disease such as diabetes, smoking and hypercholesterolemia. Also, history of contrast allergy must be obtained

TABLE 13: Key points of revascularization procedures.

Aspect	Details
Vascular access	• *Preferred access site*: Common femoral artery (CFA) • *Alternative sites*: Brachial, radial, or pedal access depending on lesion location • Ultrasound guidance may be used to reduce complications during access
Vascular sheath	• Sheath size typically ranges from 5 to 7 F, depending on the vessel and intervention type • Hydrophilic-coated sheaths reduce friction and trauma to the vessel during insertion • Heparinized saline flush to maintain sheath patency and reduce clot formation
Balloons	• Balloon sizes are selected based on vessel diameter and lesion length • Semi-compliant balloons for initial vessel dilation • Non-compliant balloons for calcified or resistant lesions • Drug-coated balloons (DCB) may be used to reduce restenosis risk in certain lesions • A cutting balloon has got non-compliant balloon with fine fins fixed longitudinally on the outer surface of the balloon. These fins are devised to cut a lesion during balloon inflation, permitting a simpler angioplasty at lower inflation pressures. Cutting balloons are recommended for stenoses resistant to standard angioplasty
	• Stents are used when there is residual stenosis or vessel recoil after balloon angioplasty. Provide an internal support for the vascular lumen • Generally, bare-metal self-expandable or balloon mounted stents are used • Drug-eluting stents (DES) are preferred to reduce restenosis in long or complex lesions • Covered stents may be used in specific cases, such as aneurysms or arterial perforation
Anticoagulation	• Unfractionated heparin (UFH) is administered to achieve activated clotting time (ACT) >250 s • ACT monitoring throughout the procedure ensures adequate anticoagulation • Antiplatelet therapy (aspirin, clopidogrel) is continued post-procedure to prevent thrombosis

- Take history about present-day medication. Some of the medications may need to be stopped or modified prior to the procedure, such as, oral anticoagulants, antiplatelets and insulin
- Patients are advised to start antiplatelet medicines (clopidogrel 75 mg/day, and aspirin 160 mg/day) 3–5 days prior to the procedure, which will help to diminish thrombotic events during the procedure. Prophylactic antibiotics are not routinely advocated.
- Evaluate all the fresh imaging findings to choose the proper site and direction of vascular access, i.e., ipsilateral versus contralateral approach, antegrade versus retrograde puncture
- Review the appearance of the lesion on imaging that will help to plan the appropriate management, i.e., angioplasty versus stenting. In general, short segment narrowing/occlusions are likely to benefit satisfactorily to angioplasty
- If there is renal dysfunction, IV hydration must be commenced a day prior to the procedure. Usage of iso-osmolar contrast agents is recommended
- It is appropriate to discuss with the patient about treatment options (angioplasty versus surgery), results and the possible complications. Informed consent should be taken prior to the procedure.

Day of Procedure

- The patient reports to the vascular lab after fasting for 4–6 hours, however, clear fluids are allowed. The site of vascular access is cleaned and draped in a sterile manner
- Close monitoring of the vital statistics (pulse, BP, SPO_2) is done prior to the start of procedure and is continued till the procedure is completed

Vascular Access (Fig. 13)[32]

The site of vascular access is determined by the site of vascular lesion to be treated as determined by analysis of imaging studies prior to the start of procedure.

- For the lesions in iliac arteries (cranial to the inguinal ligament), an ipsilateral retrograde common femoral approach is preferred **(Fig. 13)**.
- *For the lesions caudal to the inguinal ligament*:
  - Common femoral artery (CFA) and superficial femoral artery (SFA) till adductor canal level, cross over techniques from contralateral femoral artery **(Fig. 13B)**
  - For distal SFA and beyond, the antegrade common femoral puncture is the preferred access route **(Fig. 13C)**

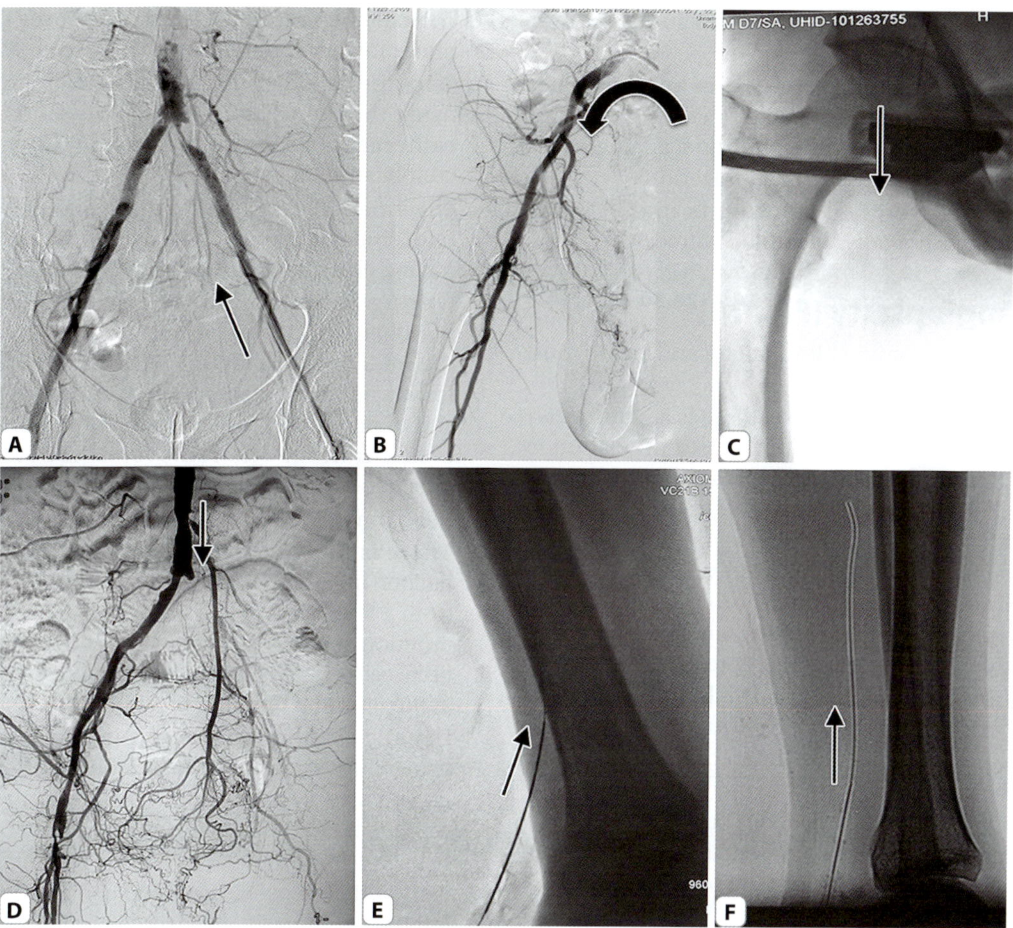

FIGS. 13A TO F: Digital subtraction angiography (DSA) spot images showing various types of vascular access. (A) Retrograde transfemoral approach. (B) Contralateral transfemoral access. (C) Antegrade transfemoral approach. (D) Brachial approach. (E) Anterior tibial approach. (F) Posterior tibial approach.

Other arterial access sites such as brachial artery **(Fig. 13D)**, the radial artery, the popliteal artery and the tibial arteries **(Figs. 13E and F)** may also be used to obtain vascular access.

Crossing of the Lesion[26]

- Appropriate size vascular sheath (preferably, 6F in common femoral access) is introduced into the access artery. If the contralateral approach is used, then crossover vascular sheath should be placed. The lesion is usually crossed using a combination of selective catheter and an atraumatic hydrophilic guidewire.
- *For Iliac and SFA crossing*: 0.032 hydrophilic soft tip wire and 5F catheter combination
- *For popliteal and below knee*: 0.014 or 0.018 low tip/medium tip/heavy tip load CTO guidewire and 4F catheter with microcatheter coaxial system combination

Lesion Crossing Techniques

1. Simple antegrade intraluminal crossing technique **(Fig. 14)**
2. Antegrade intimal plaque tracking
3. Upfront subintimal dissection
4. Limited antegrade subintimal tracking

- Low molecular weight heparin (3,000–7,000 IU) should be administered either in divided doses or as a single loading dose as per the institute practice
- After crossing the lesion with guidewire, the catheter is pushed over the guidewire and the guidewire is withdrawn. If the catheter tip is in true lumen, one should start seeing the free flow of blood coming from the catheter hub. It is always good idea to aspirate blood and/or inject contrast medium to check the catheter position within the lumen
- It is always important to ensure that the guidewire is long enough (use exchange guidewire of 260 cm) for exchanging the selective catheter, the balloon catheter or stent delivery system
- It is important to take care that the guidewire is of appropriate diameter, which is recommended for the lumen of the balloon catheter or stent delivery systems. For example, it is not feasible to introduce a stent

delivery system devised for a 0.018-inch guidewire over a 0.035-inch guidewire
- A choice of whether to treat the lesion by angioplasty alone or primary stenting could be made either prior to the start of procedure or after the initial angiographic images of the lesion location and appearance
- Occasionally, choice of stenting is made, when angioplasty fails or makes the lesion worse.

Balloon Angioplasty (Fig. 14)[26,30-32]

- A balloon catheter of suitable diameter and length must be chosen
- Regarding balloon catheter size, there is a controversy whether to use oversized balloon or not in relation to the normal artery diameter. Most of the interventionists choose balloon catheters 10–20% larger than the native artery diameter
- In case of uncertainty, it is a good idea to use a balloon catheter of lesser diameter than the artery as appreciated on a road map. This is to avoid selecting a balloon that is too big, which may cause vessel rupture
- Many interventionists choose the balloon catheter diameter using the "Eyeball technique" based on their clinical experience of the estimated diameter of the vessel to be treated
- Regarding the length of the balloon catheter, length must be sufficient to include the entire length of the lesion. If an undersized balloon is chosen for a considerably longer lesion, several dilatations may be needed to cover the full length of the lesion, which could be time consuming
- Proximal and distal radiopaque markers indicate the location of the balloon on the catheter

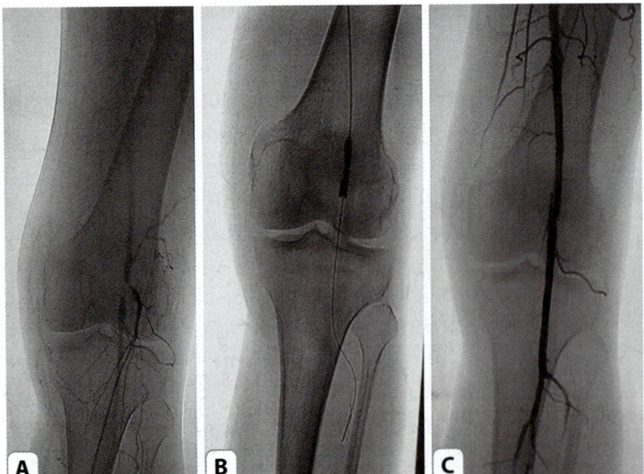

FIGS. 14A TO C: Image showing various steps of balloon angioplasty. Short segment occlusion of popliteal artery (A), crossed by the floppy end of hydrophilic guidewire followed by dilatation of the segment using balloon catheter (B). Final angiogram showing the opening of the occluded segment of popliteal artery (C).

- The balloon catheter is introduced over the guidewire under image guidance, steadily in smooth manner
- Once the balloon is placed accurately across the lesion using the radiopaque markers as guidance, balloon catheter is slowly inflated using diluted iodinated contrast media
- The inflation may be accomplished either by a 5 mL Luer-lock syringe or by mechanical inflation device having pressure measurement display
- During balloon inflation, expansion starts from periphery of the balloon and extends gradually toward the middle as the lumen gets dilated. Frequently, the lesion creates a central waist on the balloon at the site of maximum resistance resulting in an hourglass configuration. The removal of the waist suggests effective dilatation of the stenosis[22]
- Recommended balloon catheter sizes **(Table 14)**
- There is no agreement about the ideal duration of balloon inflation. Balloon inflation duration might range from a few seconds to a minute or more. However, the duration of balloon inflation does not matter in majority of cases. Generally, inflation for approximately 1 minute at the nominal pressure is optimum
- Usually, balloon dilatation is done from distal to proximal segments. At each station, after the balloon angioplasty, balloon should be fully deflated, so that it can be pulled easily to the next segment of narrowing
- Pain is an important factor during balloon inflation, and it should be closely observed. Generally, the balloon inflation produces some degree of pain due to stretching of the adventitia and this pain reduces following balloon deflation. However, when patient complains of continued pain following balloon deflation, one should suspect vessel rupture
- Once, the entire length of stenotic/occluded segment is dilated, the balloon catheter should be withdrawn carefully, while keeping the guidewire across the site of angioplasty. It is very important to remember because by mistake if the guidewire is pulled out and the lesion entails additional management due to unsatisfactory outcome or a complication (such as rupture/dissection), it may not be possible to go across the freshly treated lesion that may end in technical failure or a limb-threatening complication
- Once the balloon catheter is removed over the guidewire, the vascular sheath should be aspirated for removal of the clots (if any) present inside the sheath and sheath is flushed with heparinized saline. Post-angioplasty angiogram must be obtained to assess the technical

TABLE 14: Recommended balloon catheter sizes.

Iliac segments	7–8 mm
Femoral segments	6 mm
Popliteal segment	4–5 mm
Below knee	2–3 mm

outcome and to look for complications (such as dissection/rupture/distal migration of ruptured plaque).

- Post-angioplasty angiogram should include the distal run of vessels (e.g., trifurcation and tibial vessels) along with angioplasty site to look for distal vessel occlusion due to distal migration of plaque material from angioplasty site.
- Once the angiogram looks acceptable, the guidewire and vascular sheath are removed. Manual compression is applied at the puncture site to achieve hemostasis
- Sometimes, occlusion involves the origin of an artery (e.g., common iliac artery origin at the bifurcation), there is a hypothetical risk of creating an ostial stenosis of the contralateral vessel either by dissection or by dislodgment of plaque across the bifurcation. Hence, few interventionists ensure safety of the contralateral vessel by the placement of another balloon and is known as "kissing balloon technique" **(Fig. 15)**. This is debatable and several interventionists do not advocate the use of this technique for treating ostial lesions at bifurcations.
- Similarly, if stenting has to be done for the lesion at bifurcation due to unsatisfactory angioplasty result, some operators choose to place a stent in the contralateral artery based on similar justification and is called as kissing stent technique **(Fig. 16)**.[19,22]
- Angioplasty is preferred in below knee lesions. Stenting performed only in bailout situations

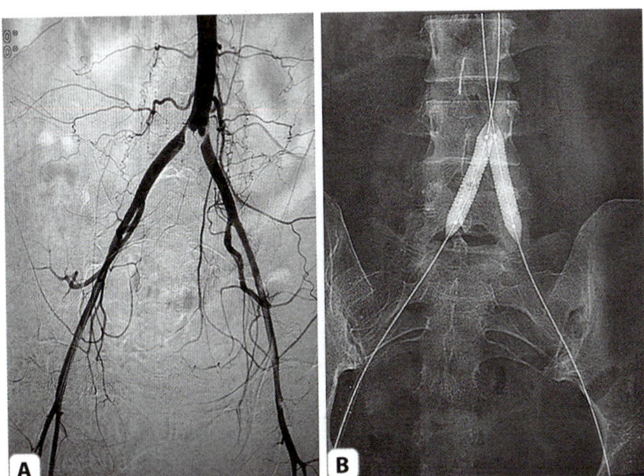

FIGS. 15A AND B: Kissing balloon technique: Digital subtraction angiography (DSA) spot images showing ostial stenosis of bilateral iliac artery (A), managed by kissing balloon technique (B).

How to decide the endpoint?[30-32]

The angioplasty site must be cautiously assessed on the check angiogram to guarantee that the vessel is effectively opened with residual stenosis <30% as measured by pressure measurement using manometers. PTA was considered technically successful if

- The arterial lumen after angioplasty has < 30% residual stenosis or
- The arterial lumen is at least > 50% diameter than its pretreatment calibre
- The pressure gradient across the residual stenosis is < 20 mm Hg.
- Another simple way of deciding the endpoint without pressure measurement is looking at the angiogram for disappearance of collaterals across the angioplasty site.

Subintimal Angioplasty (Fig. 17)[33,34]

- In case of true lumen angioplasty, narrowing is negotiated by passing a guidewire through the true lumen of the vessel
- Whereas in case of chronic tight occlusions, guidewire is intentionally negotiated through the wall of vessel (usually the subintimal space) rather than true lumen, and is known as subintimal angioplasty or also known as percutaneous intentional extraluminal recanalization (PIER)

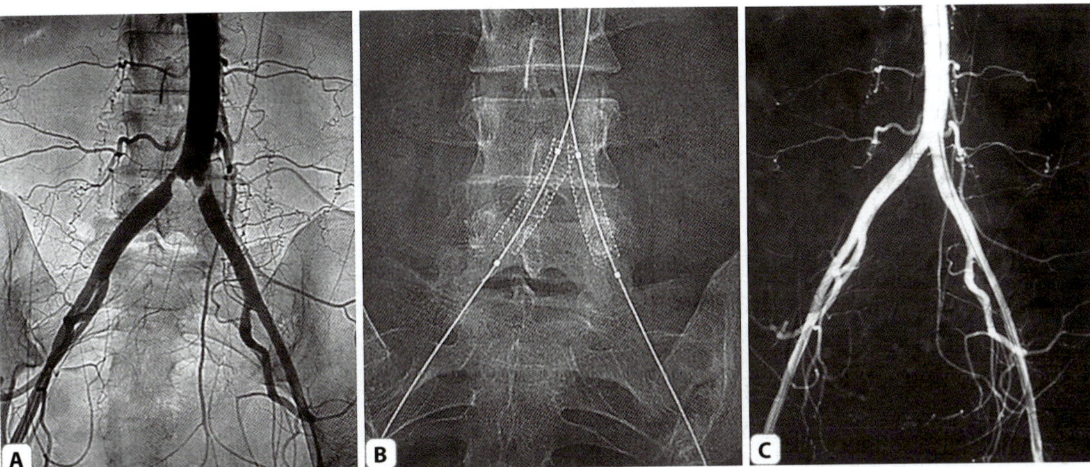

FIGS. 16A TO C: Digital subtraction angiography (DSA) images showing kissing stent technique in the management of bilateral iliac ostial stenosis.

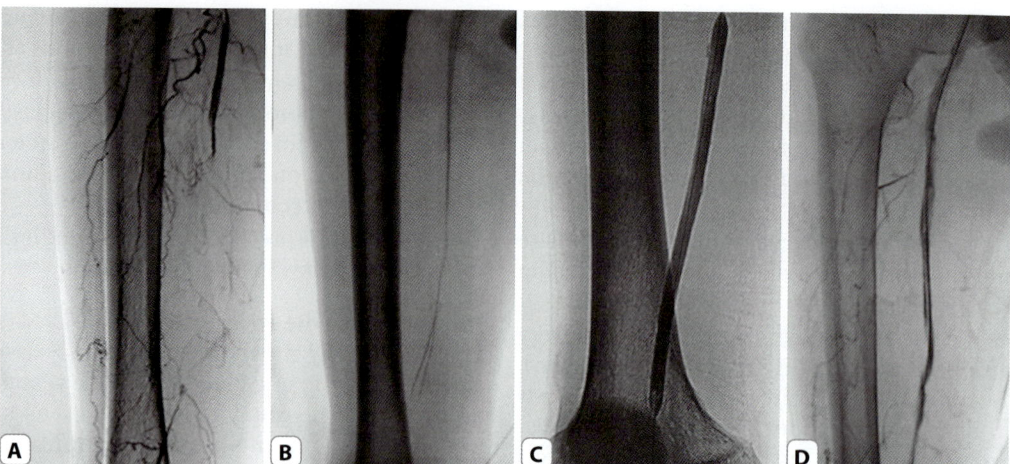

FIGS. 17A TO D: Digital subtraction angiography (DSA) spots images showing technique of subintimal angioplasty. Long segment occlusion of superficial femoral artery (A), which was crossed by a loop of floppy end of hydrophilic guidewire into the subintimal space (B) and subsequently dilated by balloon catheter (C). Final angiogram showing the opening of the occluded segment of superficial femoral artery (D).

- *Benefit of subintimal angioplasty*: Since we are doing angioplasty of the subintimal space, it provides a lumen that is free of atherosclerotic plaques as compared to true lumen angioplasty
- *Wire loop technique*: In this procedure, combination of angled catheter (such as Picard catheter) and J-tip hydrophilic catheter is used for intentional passage of the guidewire into subintimal space. Just proximal to the site of occlusion, this catheter and guidewire combination is brought and forcibly pushed against the site of occlusion. During this forcible attempt to cross the occlusion, a loop of guidewire is created. This loop has to be advanced further, so that this loop dissects the intima and enter the subintimal space. Once, the loop enters the subintimal space, catheter and guidewire are progressively advanced distally till the entire segment of occlusion is traversed.
- When the loop has crossed past the distal limit of the occlusion, pull the guidewire to shorten the length of the loop. Now push the guidewire forward by rapid backward and forwards movements, so that guidewire re-enters the true lumen
- Re-entry into the true lumen is complemented by sudden loss of resistance to passage of the guidewire
- If the catheter tip is in true lumen, one should start seeing the free flow of blood coming from the catheter hub. It is always good idea to aspirate blood and/or inject contrast medium to check the catheter position within the lumen
- Once the guidewire position within true lumen is confirmed after re-entry, the dissection plane is dilated with an angioplasty balloon of a suitable size.

Stenting[26-29,32]

- Stenting is performed when angioplasty is unsuccessful (>30% residual stenosis or >5 mm residual gradient) as well as in the case of complications due to flow-limiting dissection or vessel rupture.
- There are two types of stenting technique and the prevailing indications for stenting differ depending upon the site of lesion: Primary and secondary stenting
  i. In primary stenting, stenting is done without preceding angioplasty. It is encouraged/suggested in few locations, like stenosis involving ostium (renal artery stenosis, iliac artery stenosis) and malignant venous obstruction
  ii. In secondary stenting, stenting is done after the angioplasty especially when angioplasty results are poor due to elastic recoiling of wall or due to flow limiting dissection at angioplasty site
- Stents may comprise of only metal known as bare metal stent or may comprise of a metallic stent covered with graft material, which is known as a stent-graft
- Another method of classifying stents as balloon expandable and self-expandable, is based on their method of deployment
- Balloon-expandable stents are valuable at sites where stent has to be deployed with highest accuracy (i.e., ostial lesions) **(Fig. 18)**. They are preferred in severely calcified lesions and aortic bifurcation lesions.
- As compared to balloon expandable stents, self-expanding stents have smaller profiles, are more flexible and are available in longer lengths. Hence, these are used for treating long segment tortuous occlusions like SFA occlusions **(Fig. 19)**.

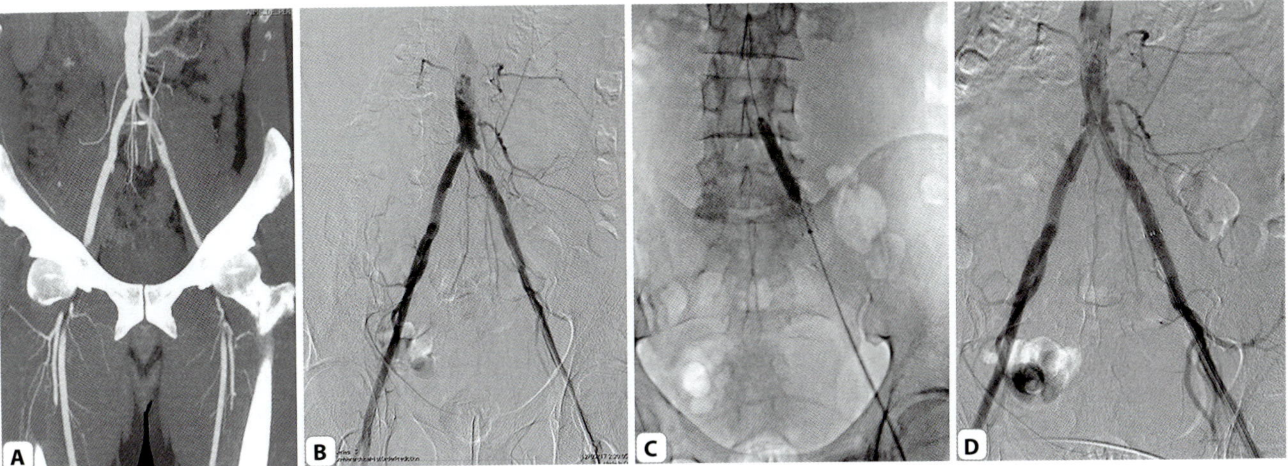

FIGS. 18A TO D: Images showing technique common iliac stenting using balloon mounted stent. Short segment occlusion of left common iliac artery involving the ostium (A and B), was initially crossed with floppy end of hydrophilic guidewire and subsequently managed by balloon mounted stent (C). Final angiogram showing the opening of the occluded segment of common iliac artery (D).

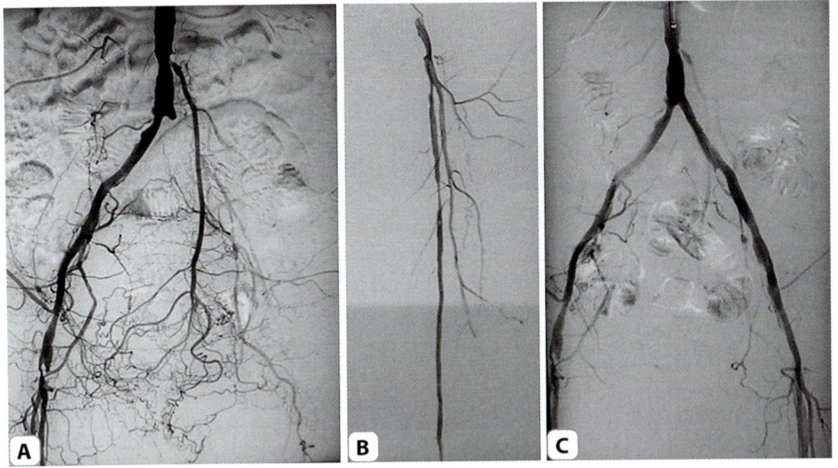

FIGS. 19A TO C: TASC type D lesion of left iliac segment managed by self-expandable stent. Long segment occlusion involving the left common iliac and external iliac arteries (A), with reformation of left common femoral and superficial femoral artery by collaterals (B), was subsequently managed by placing overlapping self-expandable stents across the occluded segment. Final angiogram showing the opening of the occluded entire segment of iliac artery (C).

- Occasionally, self-expanding stents may require additional dilatation using balloon catheter of the equal diameter after deployment to assist their expansion to their full diameter. This is not required in case of balloon expandable stent, since they are deployed by balloon dilatation.
- Stent placement should be avoided across the joints. Nevertheless, vasculomimetic stents may be placed in selected patients.

Complications[26,32]

Procedure related complications (peri-procedural or post-procedural) are not uncommon and are commonly seen in elderly patients with diffuse disease and other comorbidities.[28,34]

Most common complications are puncture site complications such as hematoma and pseudoaneurysm formation which are easily managed by manual compression. Occasionally, pseudoaneurysm needs to be managed by thrombin injection **(Fig. 20)**.

Most serious complications include arterial rupture and distal plaque embolization.

Arterial Rupture

- It is the most serious complications and is seen <1% cases. If the rupture occurs in the periphery (infrainguinal), it is usually self-limiting and bleeding is controlled by local tamponade effect of the surrounding soft tissues. However, if the arterial rupture occurs above the inguinal ligament, it may be fatal because there is no

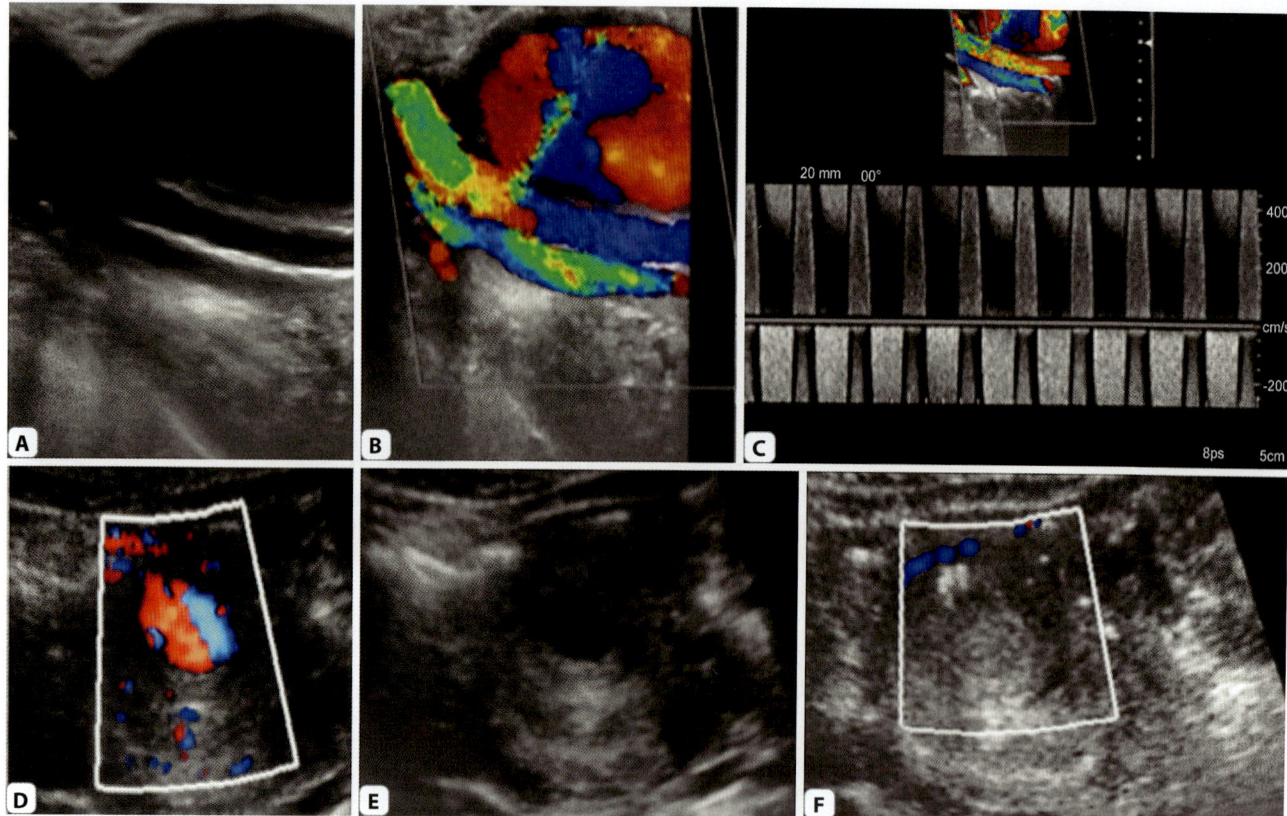

FIGS. 20A TO F: Postangioplasty pseudoaneurysm complication management: Sonography with color Doppler images showing narrow neck pseudoaneurysm arising from the common femoral artery at the puncture site (A and B) with Yin-Yang spectral wave form at the neck of pseudoaneurysm (C), which was subsequently managed by percutaneous thrombin injection into the pseudoaneurysm and achieving complete thrombosis of the pseudoaneurysm (D to F).

tamponade effect by the surrounding area. If the patient complaints of severe pain, which continues even after balloon deflation and is accompanied by hypotension and tachycardia, one should suspect vascular rupture.

- Vascular ruptures below the inguinal ligament are usually self-limiting and require no specific treatment except for manual compression. Whereas arterial rupture above inguinal ligament needs immediate attention. Instant balloon re-inflation at the site of rupture to stop bleeding, followed by either placement of stent-graft across the rupture or shift the patient to operation theatre for surgical repair **(Fig. 21)**.

Distal Plaque Embolization

- Distal plaque embolization is another serious complication, which may lead to acute limb ischemia, tissue necrosis and amputation of limb. Certain amount of distal embolization occurs in most of the angioplasty procedures, however the volume of plaque embolization is high in iliac angioplasty
- There is no specific treatment for this complication. Proper technique and careful patient selection are critical to circumvent this complication.

Stent-related Complications

- Stent migration during placement usually happens when the sizing of the stent is incorrect or due to faulty deployment technique
- Stent fracture usually happens when stents are deployed across the joints

Restenosis

Restenosis may occur following angioplasty alone or may occur within stents (in-stent restenosis). This restenosis may be due to disease progression or due to neointimal hyperplasia. This restenosis is managed either by repeat angioplasty or repeat stenting

TEACHING POINTS

- Doppler sonography is used as screening modality in suspected peripheral vascular disease
- CTA or MRA is needed to define disease extent and planning the treatment
- Endovascular treatments offer low-risk alternative to surgery in majority of the patients

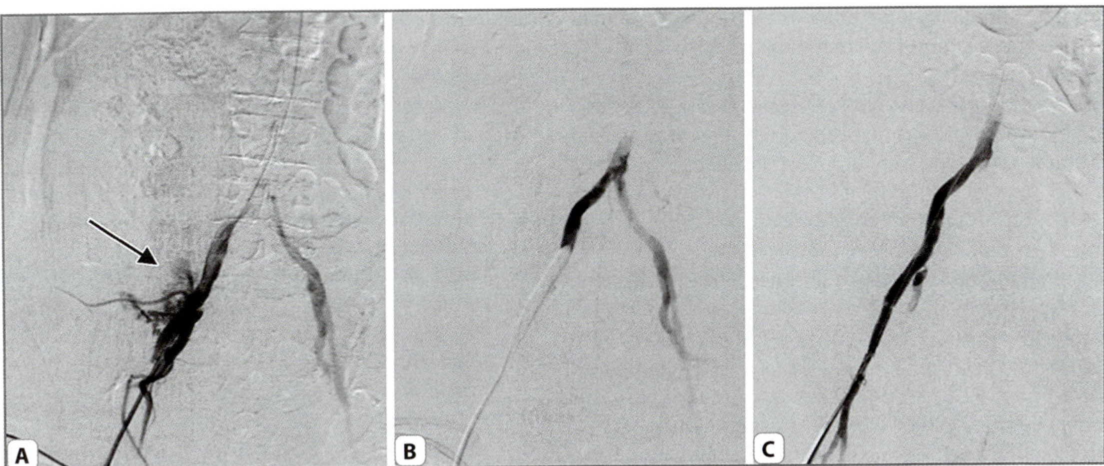

FIGS. 21A TO C: Postangioplasty complication of arterial rupture. Digital subtraction angiography (DSA) spot images showing rupture of the external iliac artery (arrow) following balloon angioplasty (A), which was subsequently managed balloon re-inflation for 10 minutes across the rupture site (B). Final angiogram showing the sealing of the ruptures site, maintaining the patency of external iliac artery (C).

- Angioplasty and stenting are the two most widely used treatment options
- Antegrade access is generally preferable to contralateral access for infrainguinal lesions. Never withdraw the guidewire back across the lesion before the procedure is finished
- Always check the run-off vessels at the end of the procedure for distal embolization
- Stents are usually indicated if angioplasty results are unsatisfactory or as bail out procedure
- Primary placement of stent is indicated in selected cases such as iliac artery occlusions and ostial renal artery stenoses
- Proper patient selection and technique are two most important factors, which can prevent most of the complications

REFERENCES

1. Selvin E, Erlinger TP. Prevalence of and risk factors for peripheral arterial disease in the United States: Results from the National Health and Nutrition Examination Survey, 1999-2000. Circulation. 2004;110(6):738-43.
2. Pollak AW, Norton PT, Kramer CM. Multimodality imaging of lower extremity peripheral arterial disease: Current role and future directions. Circ Cardiovasc Imaging. 2012;5(6): 797-807.
3. Lijmer JG, Hunink MG, van den Dungen JJ, Loonstra J, Smit AJ. ROC analysis of noninvasive tests for peripheral arterial disease. Ultrasound Med Biol. 1996;22(4):391-8.
4. Ota H, Takase K, Rikimaru H, Tsuboi M, Yamada T, Sato A, et al. Quantitative vascular measurements in arterial occlusive disease. Radiographics. 2005;25(5):1141-58.
5. Zemaitis MR, Boll JM, Dreyer MA. Peripheral Arterial Disease. [Updated 2023 May 23]. In: StatPearls [Internet]. Treasure Island (FL): StatPearls Publishing; 2024. Available from: https://www.ncbi.nlm.nih.gov/books/NBK430745/
6. Weinberg I, Weinberg MD. Non-atherosclerotic Arterial Disorders of the Lower Extremities. In: Lanzer P. (Eds) PanVascular Medicine. Springer: Berlin, Heidelberg; 2014. https://doi.org/10.1007/978-3-642-37393-0_113-1
7. Hiatt WR, Goldstone J, Smith SC Jr, McDermott M, Moneta G, Oka R, et al.; American Heart Association Writing Group 1. Atherosclerotic Peripheral Vascular Disease Symposium II: nomenclature for vascular diseases. Circulation. 2008;118(25):2826-9.
8. Gornik HL, Aronow HD, Goodney PP, Arya S, Brewster LP, Byrd L, et al; Peer Review Committee Members. 2024. ACC/AHA/AACVPR/APMA/ABC/SCAI/SVM/SVN/SVS/SIR/VESS Guideline for the Management of Lower Extremity Peripheral Artery Disease: A Report of the American College of Cardiology/American Heart Association Joint Committee on Clinical Practice Guidelines. Circulation. 2024;149(24):e1313-e1410.
9. Sibley RC 3rd, Reis SP, MacFarlane JJ, Reddick MA, Kalva SP, Sutphin PD. Noninvasive Physiologic Vascular Studies: A Guide to Diagnosing Peripheral Arterial Disease. Radiographics. 2017;37(1):346-57.
10. Leiner T, Carr JC. Noninvasive Angiography of Peripheral Arteries. In: Hodler J, Kubik-Huch R, von Schulthess G (Eds) Diseases of the Chest, Breast, Heart and Vessels 2019-2022. IDKD Springer Series. Springer: Cham; 2019. https://doi.org/10.1007/978-3-030-11149-6_20
11. Rooke TW, Hirsch AT, Misra S, Sidawy AN, Beckman JA, Findeiss LK. 2011 ACCF/AHA Focused Update of the Guideline for the Management of Patients With Peripheral Artery Disease (updating the 2005 guideline): a report of the American College of Cardiology Foundation/American Heart Association Task Force on Practice Guidelines. J Am Coll Cardiol. 2011;58(19):2020-45.

12. Ubbink DT, Fidler M, Legemate DA. Interobserver variability in aortoiliac and femoropopliteal duplex scanning. J Vasc Surg. 2001;33(3):540-5.
13. Kim ES, Sharma AM, Scissons R, Dawson D, Eberhardt RT, Gerhard-Herman M, et al. Interpretation of peripheral arterial and venous Doppler waveforms: A consensus statement from the Society for Vascular Medicine and Society for Vascular Ultrasound. Vasc Med. 2020;25(5):484-506.
14. Hwang JY. Doppler ultrasonography of the lower extremity arteries: anatomy and scanning guidelines. Ultrasonography. 2017;36(2):111-9.
15. American Institute of Ultrasound in Medicine (AIUM); American College of Radiology (ACR); Society of Radiologists in Ultrasound (SRU). AIUM practice guideline for the performance of peripheral arterial ultrasound examinations using color and spectral doppler imaging. J Ultrasound Med. 2014;33(6):1111-21.
16. Catalano C, Fraioli F, Laghi A, Napoli A, Bezzi M, Pediconi F, et al. Infrarenal aortic and lower-extremity arterial disease: Diagnostic performance of multi-detector row CT angiography. Radiology. 2004;231(2):555-63.
17. Schernthaner R, Stadler A, Lomoschitz F, Weber M, Fleischmann D, Lammer J, et al. Multidetector CT angiography in the assessment of peripheral arterial occlusive disease: Accuracy in detecting the severity, number, and length of stenoses. Eur Radiol. 2008;18(4):665-71.
18. Foley WD, Stonely T. CT angiography of the lower extremities. Radiol Clin North Am. 2010;48(2):367-96.
19. Rotzinger DC, Lu TL, Kawkabani A, Marques-Vidal PM, Fetz G, Qanadli SD. Computed Tomography Angiography in Peripheral Arterial Disease: Comparison of Three Image Acquisition Techniques to Optimize Vascular Enhancement-Randomized Controlled Trial. Front Cardiovasc Med. 2020;7:68.
20. Keddie D, Abdulrehman Y, Shiau G. Reporting lower extremity CT angiography for treatment planning. Diagn Interv Imaging. 2022;103(9):387-93.
21. Roditi G, Kusumawidjaja D. Magnetic resonance angiography and computed tomography angiography for peripheral arterial disease. Imaging. 2009;21(2):85-108.
22. Ward EV, Galizia MS, Usman A, Popescu AR, Dunkle E, Edelman RR. Comparison of quiescent inflow single-shot and native space for nonenhanced peripheral MR angiography. J Magn Reson Imaging. 2013;38(6):1531-8.
23. Hodnett PA, Koktzoglou I, Davarpanah AH, Scanlon TG, Collins JD, Sheehan JJ, et al. Evaluation of peripheral arterial disease with nonenhanced quiescent-interval single-shot MR angiography. Radiology. 2011;260(1), 282-93.
24. Amin P, Collins JD, Koktzoglou I, Molvar C, Markl M, Edelman RR, et al. Evaluating peripheral arterial disease with unenhanced quiescent-interval single-shot MR angiography at 3 T. AJR Am J Roentgenol. 2014;202(4):886-93.
25. Jaff MR, White CJ, Hiatt WR, Fowkes GR, Dormandy J, Razavi M, et al. An update on methods for revascularization and expansion of the TASC lesion classification to include below-the-knee arteries: A supplement to the inter-society consensus for the management of peripheral arterial disease (TASC II). Catheter Cardiovasc Interv. 2015;86(4):611-25.
26. Rholl KS, Durham JD, Sacks D, Cole PE, Matsumoto AH, Ray CE. Peripheral vascular interventions. In Darcy MD, Vedantham S, Kaufman JA. (Eds.), Society of Cardiovascular and Interventional Radiology (2nd ed., p. 391). SCVIR; 2001.
27. Pentecost MJ, Criqui MH, Dorros G, Goldstone J, Johnston KW, Martin EC, et al. Guidelines for peripheral percutaneous transluminal angioplasty of the abdominal aorta and lower extremity vessels: A statement for health professionals from a special writing group of the councils on cardiovascular radiology, arteriosclerosis, cardiothoracic and vascular surgery, clinical cardiology, and epidemiology and prevention, the American Heart Association. Circulation. 1994;89(1):511-31.
28. Khanna NN, Krishna V, Manjunath CN, Tyagi S, Jindal R, Chadha M, et al. The Indian Consensus Statement for the Management of Lower Extremity Peripheral Artery Disease. J Indian Coll Cardiol. 2023;13(Special Suppl 1):S1-S20.
29. Abola MTB, Golledge J, Miyata T, Rha SW, Yan BP, Dy TC, et al. Asia-Pacific Consensus Statement on the Management of Peripheral Artery Disease: A Report from the Asian Pacific Society of Atherosclerosis and Vascular Disease Asia-Pacific Peripheral Artery Disease Consensus Statement Project Committee. J Atheroscler Thromb. 2020;27(8):809-907.
30. Block PC, Myler RK, Stertzer S, Fallon JT. Morphology after transluminal angioplasty in human beings. N Engl J Med. 1981;305(7):382-5.
31. Bhat R, McBride K, Chakraverty S, Vikram R, Severn A. Primary cutting balloon angioplasty for treatment of venous stenoses in native hemodialysis fistulas: Long-term results from three centers. Cardiovasc Intervent Radiol. 2007;30(6):1166-70; discussion 1171-2.
32. Kaufman J, Lee M. Vascular and Interventional Radiology: The Requisites (2nd ed.). Saunders; 2013.
33. Bolia A. Percutaneous intentional extraluminal (subintimal) recanalization of crural arteries. Eur J Radiol. 1998;28(3): 199-204.
34. Reekers JA, Bolia A. Percutaneous intentional extraluminal (subintimal) recanalization: How to do it yourself. Eur J Radiol. 1998;28(3):192-8.

Amit Gupta, Krithika Rangarajan

CHAPTER 33

Role of Artificial Intelligence in Thoracic Imaging

INTRODUCTION

Artificial intelligence (AI) has emerged as a transformative force in thoracic imaging, offering potential solutions to longstanding challenges in diagnostics and workflow management. Various AI models have shown remarkable capabilities in automating complex tasks, including nodule detection, segmentation, and disease classification, while also paving the way for innovative applications such as predictive modeling and image reconstruction. This chapter explores the foundational principles of AI, its applications across key areas of thoracic imaging, and its role in improving diagnostic accuracy and clinical outcomes. It also highlights the challenges that hinder broader adoption and outlines future directions for integrating AI into routine clinical practice.

Basic Principles of Artificial Intelligence

Artificial intelligence refers to the ability of machines to perform tasks that typically require human intelligence, such as visual perception, speech recognition, and decision-making. At its core, AI involves algorithms that process data to achieve a specific goal, and it is broadly categorized into subsets based on the complexity and type of learning: machine learning (ML) and deep learning (DL).[1,2]

Machine learning is a subset of AI focused on developing algorithms that can learn from data without being explicitly programmed **(Fig. 1)**. The process involves providing the model with training data—pairs of inputs and their corresponding outputs—and allowing it to learn patterns that map inputs to outputs. For example, predicting patient survival based on tumor stage in a traditional program would require manually coding rules for each stage. In ML, the algorithm deduces these rules from training data, adapting dynamically to new information. ML models are categorized into supervised learning (trained on labeled data) and unsupervised learning (finding patterns in unlabeled data). This approach makes ML particularly suited for tasks involving large, complex datasets, such as medical imaging.

Deep learning, a specialized branch of ML, leverages deep neural networks (DNNs) to process data through multiple layers of computation. Each layer of a DNN performs specific calculations, extracting increasingly complex features of the input data. This structure allows DL models to excel in tasks like image classification, speech recognition, and natural language processing. Unlike traditional ML models, DL networks can handle vast amounts of data and learn intricate patterns, enabling groundbreaking advancements in areas such as radiology and genomics.

Neural networks are inspired by the structure of biological neurons. Each "neuron" in the network takes inputs, processes them through a mathematical function, and produces an output. When multiple neurons are arranged in layers—input, hidden, and output—they form a neural network. The "deep" in DNNs comes from having many hidden layers, allowing the network to model complex relationships. A specific type of neural network, the convolutional neural network (CNN), is particularly effective for image-related tasks. CNNs use mathematical operations called convolutions to extract features from images, such as edges or textures, which are then used to classify or interpret the data.

Transformers represent a recent innovation in AI. They are designed to process sequential data, such as text, using a mechanism called self-attention to focus on relevant parts of the sequence. Unlike CNNs, which excel at local feature extraction through convolutions, transformers are adept at capturing global relationships within data by attending to all input elements simultaneously. This makes transformers particularly powerful in scenarios where understanding long-range dependencies or complex spatial relationships

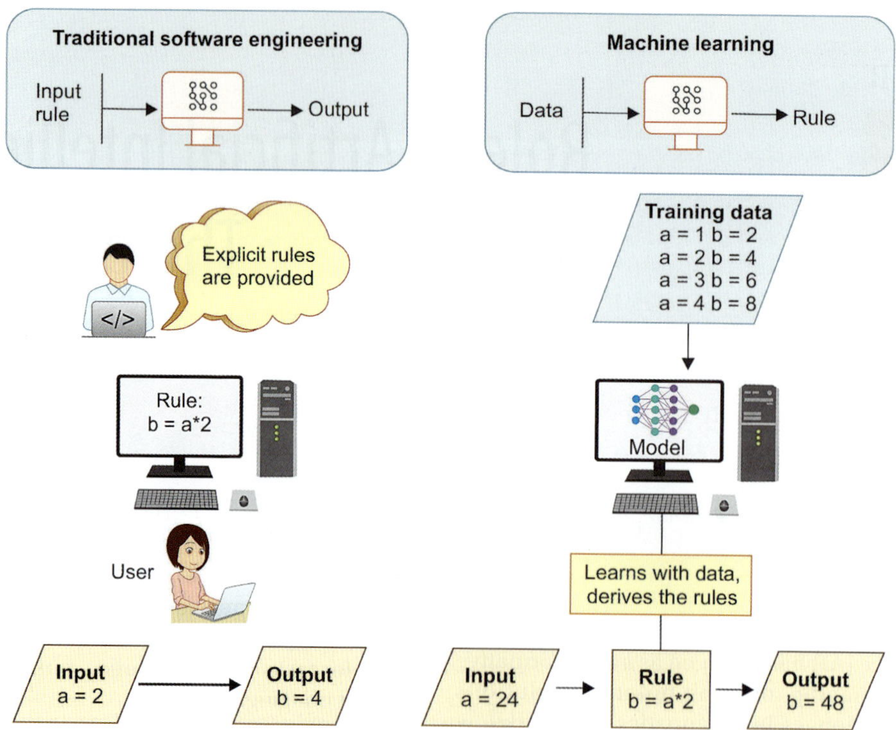

FIG. 1: Traditional software engineering versus machine learning: In traditional software engineering, predefined rules are programmed to generate outputs for given inputs. In contrast, machine learning systems derive rules by learning patterns from large training datasets to predict outputs.

is crucial. In medical imaging, transformers are increasingly applied for tasks such as image segmentation, classification, and predictive modeling.

Key Artificial Intelligence Task Categories in Thoracic Imaging

Classification involves assigning images to predefined categories, such as identifying whether a chest radiograph indicates COVID-19 pneumonia or normal findings. Training requires large, labeled datasets with input images and corresponding labels, often leveraging pre-trained models (like ResNet) through transfer learning. Models are evaluated using metrics like the area under the receiver operating characteristic curve (AUROC). Explored applications leveraging image classification in thoracic imaging include automated detection of pneumothorax on chest X-rays (CXRs) and prioritization of abnormal scans for review, streamlining workflow and reducing reporting delays.

Detection goes a step further by identifying and localizing lesions within an image, such as nodules or masses on chest CT. This task requires annotated datasets with bounding boxes around lesions and their labels, often involving models like Faster R-CNN and YOLO. Evaluation focuses on metrics like intersection over union (IoU) to measure the accuracy of localization. Potential applications include assisting radiologists in identifying lung nodules on CT scans and detecting abnormalities on radiographs, aiding early diagnosis and targeted interventions.

Segmentation focuses on classifying each pixel in an image, allowing for precise delineation of structures or lesions. Training involves datasets with pixel-level annotations, often created manually by experts. Segmentation models are evaluated using metrics like the Dice coefficient or IoU. Segmentation tools can facilitate tasks such as quantifying emphysema on CT scans or delineating tumor margins for radiotherapy planning, significantly reducing manual effort and ensuring consistency.

Image generation and reconstruction, powered by generative adversarial networks (GANs), create or enhance imaging data. Training often involves paired datasets, such as low-dose and high-resolution CT images, without requiring manual annotations. Evaluation is subjective, with human experts often assessing the quality of the generated images. GANs have shown potential to improve image resolution, reduce radiation dose, and simulate diverse pathologies for training, making them a valuable tool in both diagnostics and education.

Natural language processing (NLP) enables the processing of unstructured text data, such as extracting clinical details from radiology reports or automating report generation. Training involves corpuses of free-text reports, while evaluation assesses the accuracy and relevance of extracted data. In thoracic imaging, NLP can streamline the integration of data from electronic medical records (EMRs) and facilitate AI model training by converting unstructured information into usable datasets.

Predictive modeling, radiomics, and radiogenomics use AI to analyse imaging data for outcome prediction. These models often incorporate features extracted from images, such as texture or shape, to forecast therapy response, survival, or genetic mutations. Evaluation is done using metrics like AUROC. Potential applications of these tools include predicting EGFR mutation status in lung cancer patients, assessing the risk of disease progression, or forecasting therapy responses, paving the way for more personalized medicine.

The various tasks wherein AI has shown potential use in thoracic imaging are summarized in **Figure 2**.

Clinical Applications of Artificial Intelligence in Thoracic Imaging

- *Lung nodule and cancer:*
    - *Lung nodule detection:* AI has demonstrated significant potential in enhancing lung nodule detection, a critical task in thoracic imaging for early lung cancer diagnosis.[3,4] On CXR, detecting lung nodules is inherently challenging due to lower sensitivity compared to chest CT. Observer errors, particularly among less experienced radiologists, are a common cause of missed diagnoses. Traditional computer-aided detection (CADe) systems relied on hand-engineered methods and were limited by high false-positive rates and suboptimal performance. Recent advances in DL have leveraged public datasets, such as CheXpert and Chest X-ray14, to train models for nodule detection on CXRs. DL-based tools have shown diagnostic accuracy comparable to or surpassing radiologists, particularly for junior readers, improving sensitivity without significantly increasing false-positive rates. Commercially available DL tools have already demonstrated measurable improvements when used as second readers.

      On chest CT, lung nodule detection is a key focus, particularly in the context of lung cancer screening with low-dose CT (LDCT), which has been shown to reduce lung cancer mortality. DL-based CADe systems have become the preferred approach due to their ability to process large volumes of data and handle the complex 3D nature of CT images. These systems often employ two-step strategies: Detecting candidate nodules with high sensitivity followed by false-positive reduction. Using public datasets like LIDC-IDRI and NLST, these models have achieved sensitivities exceeding 90% for nodules above 5 mm, with fewer false positives compared to traditional CADe systems. Commercially available tools for lung nodule detection on CT have demonstrated higher detection rates than radiologists in screening settings, making them valuable as second or concurrent readers. Additionally, advancements in DL algorithms have improved the detection of subsolid nodules, which are clinically significant due to their higher malignancy risk. Despite these achievements, challenges remain in further reducing false-positive rates and ensuring

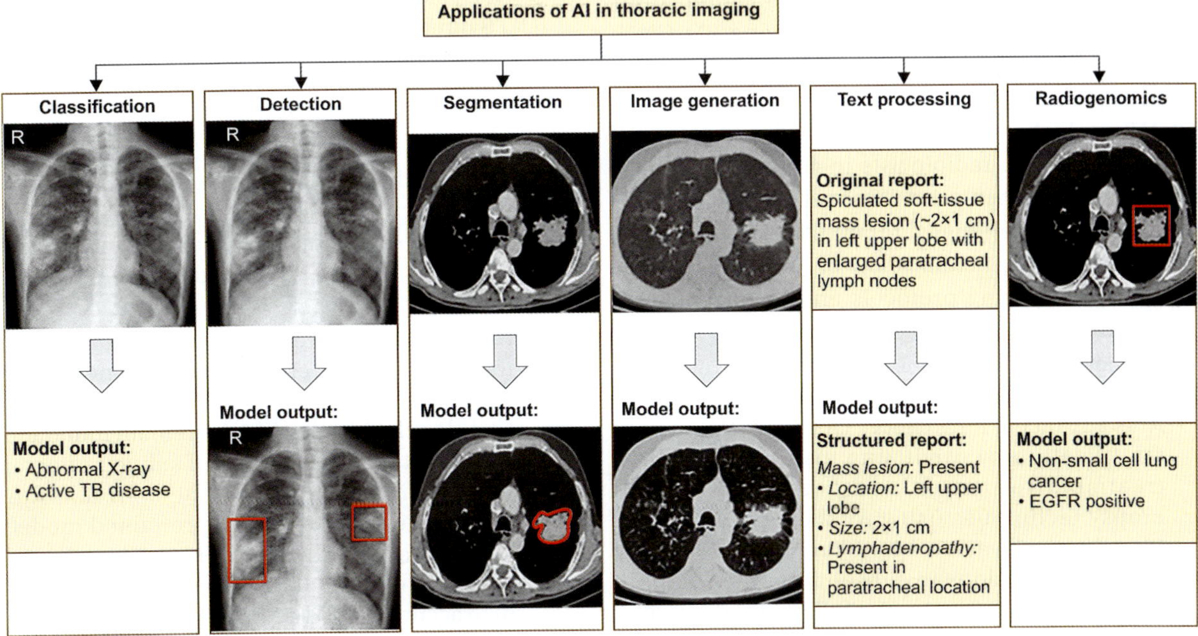

FIG. 2: Summary of key task categories performed by artificial intelligence (AI) models in thoracic imaging.

consistent performance in diverse imaging scenarios.

- *Lung nodule segmentation and characterization:* AI-driven segmentation and characterization of lung nodules have shown promise in automating critical aspects of nodule management, such as volume calculation and malignancy assessment. Accurate segmentation is vital for estimating nodule volume, which is essential for determining volume doubling times—a key parameter in nodule management. Manual segmentation is labor-intensive and prone to variability, highlighting the importance of automated methods. Traditional segmentation algorithms, which relied on thresholding and morphological processing, often struggled with irregularly shaped or subsolid nodules. In contrast, DL-based methods, particularly those employing encoder-decoder architectures like U-Net, have significantly improved segmentation performance, achieving dice similarity coefficients over 92%.

  Traditionally, characterization of lung nodules focuses on features such as size, morphology, and type (solid or subsolid), which are integral to clinical guidelines like those of the Fleischner Society and the British Thoracic Society. Guidelines increasingly recommend volumetric measurements, which offer greater accuracy than 2D diameter assessments. AI tools now enable not only automated segmentation but also integration with risk models, such as the Brock model, to estimate malignancy probabilities. Advanced AI systems can categorize nodules into risk categories, such as those outlined in lung-RADS, aiding clinical decision-making. DL-based classification tools now dominate this space, leveraging 3D CNN architectures and entire chest CT volumes to predict malignancy risk. Some DL models have shown AUCs as high as 0.955 in external validation datasets, outperforming radiologists in certain scenarios, particularly when prior CT scans are unavailable. However, challenges remain, particularly in ensuring the generalizability of AI models across different imaging protocols and reconstruction parameters, as these factors significantly impact segmentation and characterization performance.

- *Lung cancer characterization and classification:* AI is advancing lung cancer characterization and stratification by predicting histological types, treatment responses, and outcomes. Virtual biopsy techniques using AI show potential for identifying invasive adenocarcinomas versus preinvasive lesions in subsolid nodules, aiding decisions on surgery versus follow-up. Radiomic and deep-learning models have achieved AUCs exceeding 0.9 for malignancy differentiation and effective prediction of molecular markers like eGFR mutations and PD-L1 expression, which influence therapy decisions. AI has also been applied to predict immunotherapy response and stratify mortality risk in non-small cell lung cancer (NSCLC). DL models trained on pretreatment CTs have outperformed clinical models for 2-year survival prediction, leveraging features like the tumor-stroma interface. While promising, these tools currently complement rather than replace biopsy or traditional decision-making.

- *Tuberculosis:*
  - Chest X-rays, though widely used for tuberculosis (TB) screening, have limited diagnostic accuracy, with significant interobserver variability and only moderate sensitivity and specificity. DL has shown potential in addressing these challenges, with models such as AlexNet and GoogLeNet achieving AUCs as high as 0.99 for TB detection on CXRs.[5,6] These models have demonstrated global applicability by validating on datasets from diverse regions, though performance can vary due to differences in image acquisition and labeling practices. Recent developments include simpler DL models optimized for resource-limited settings, significantly reducing hardware requirements while maintaining competitive accuracy. Transfer learning, where pretrained models are fine-tuned for TB-specific tasks, has been particularly effective. Modality-specific retraining, which aligns models with the unique characteristics of CXRs, further enhances performance, delivering superior results in detecting TB-consistent findings.
  - AI has also been explored for advanced applications in TB management, such as detecting drug-resistant TB directly from radiographic patterns. While early models for drug-resistance classification achieved modest AUCs around 0.66, these results provide a foundation for further research. Ensemble approaches combining multiple AI models with human adjudication have achieved near-perfect sensitivity and specificity, underscoring the potential of AI to enhance TB diagnosis and improve outcomes, particularly in high-burden regions.

- *Pneumonia:*
  - AI has shown significant promise in improving the detection and classification of pneumonia on CXR, including both community-acquired and COVID-related cases.[7] CNNs remain foundational, enabling the identification of subtle radiographic patterns associated with pneumonia. Transfer learning techniques, using pretrained models on large datasets like ImageNet, have been particularly effective for pneumonia-specific tasks, achieving high accuracy with relatively small labeled datasets. Advanced ensemble learning methods, combining multiple models or architectures, further enhance

classification robustness and accuracy, with studies reporting performance metrics exceeding 98% for both COVID and non-COVID pneumonia detection.

- Recent innovations such as vision transformers (ViTs) have demonstrated competitive performance, with accuracies up to 99.39%, and show potential for replacing traditional CNNs in certain applications. Additionally, hybrid approaches incorporating clinical and laboratory data or leveraging advanced data augmentation techniques have improved model generalization and reduced overfitting. Beyond classification, AI tools are being used for segmentation and disease localization, enhancing interpretability by identifying regions of interest, which aids in explaining model predictions and increasing clinical trust.

- *Pneumoconiosis:* AI applications in pneumoconiosis have evolved from traditional approaches utilizing texture-based features and support vector machines (SVMs) to more advanced DL techniques.[8] Early methods relied on manually engineered features and classification models like SVMs to identify pneumoconiosis patterns in CXRs, often segmenting the lungs into subregions for localized analysis. Recent DL-based approaches employ architectures such as U-Net for segmentation and ResNet and DenseNet for classification, achieving improved accuracy over traditional methods. However, most studies are limited to private datasets with small sample sizes, highlighting the need for publicly available, diverse datasets to develop robust and generalizable models for pneumoconiosis detection and staging.
- *Multimodality cardiac imaging*:
  - *Cardiac CT*: AI has shown significant potential for advancement of cardiac CT by enhancing image quality, automating diagnostic workflows, and improving risk stratification.[9] AI-driven reconstruction techniques like deep learning reconstruction (DLR) outperform traditional methods by reducing radiation dose while maintaining high diagnostic accuracy. Automated coronary artery calcium (CAC) scoring and plaque analysis streamline risk assessment, with deep learning algorithms achieving expert-level accuracy in characterizing plaque morphology and stenosis. Fractional flow reserve CT (FFR-CT) combines anatomical and functional assessments, offering superior diagnostic accuracy for ischemia over traditional measures. AI's predictive capabilities extend to myocardial perfusion and prognosis, with machine learning models integrating clinical and imaging data to predict outcomes like major adverse cardiac events.
  - *Cardiac MRI*: In cardiac MRI, AI has improved the accuracy and efficiency of chamber quantification, functional assessments, and tissue characterization.[10] Automated segmentation algorithms provide rapid and reproducible measurements of ventricular volumes and ejection fraction, matching or surpassing manual methods. AI tools for tissue characterization, such as late gadolinium enhancement (LGE) segmentation, enable detailed assessment of myocardial fibrosis and scar burden, crucial for prognostic stratification. Emerging techniques like cardiac magnetic resonance fingerprinting (cMRF) allow for simultaneous quantification of multiple tissue properties, holding promise for broader clinical applications.
  - *Echocardiography*: AI applications in echocardiography focus on automating chamber quantification, strain measurements, and disease detection. Algorithms for ejection fraction (EF) and longitudinal strain calculation have demonstrated excellent correlation with manual methods while significantly reducing analysis time. Automated valvular assessment tools improve precision in evaluating valve morphology and function, aiding in preprocedural planning for interventions like transcatheter aortic valve replacement (TAVR). AI-driven disease detection models can identify conditions such as hypertrophic cardiomyopathy and pulmonary hypertension with high accuracy, enhancing early diagnosis and management in routine and resource-limited settings.
- *Emergency applications:*
  - AI has demonstrated transformative potential in emergency thoracic imaging by prioritizing critical cases and supporting accurate diagnoses.[11] Worklist prioritization tools, such as those for pneumothorax detection, have significantly reduced reporting times. AI algorithms developed for critical findings like pneumothorax achieve high sensitivity and specificity, outperforming traditional triage systems. For example, systems like HealthPNX have cut diagnosis times from over an hour to mere minutes. Similarly, CNN-based tools for CXR triage have reduced reporting delays for critical studies by several days, showcasing the impact of AI in streamlining emergency workflows.
  - In addition to prioritization, AI has been instrumental in enhancing diagnostic accuracy for conditions like pneumothorax, heart failure, pleural effusion, and pulmonary embolism. For pneumothorax, segmentation models using U-Net and ResNet architectures have achieved dice scores above 0.88 and sensitivities exceeding 90%, aiding in volume estimation and management planning. For heart failure, DL models like CardioNet have provided near-instantaneous cardiac size measurements with high precision, supporting swift decision-making in emergencies. Furthermore, models for pulmonary embolism detection have employed advanced techniques like multitask learning and U-Net-based architectures, achieving scan-level sensitivities of

up to 93% while enhancing diagnostic accuracy. These models have demonstrated their potential in distinguishing acute and chronic emboli, supporting timely and effective management in emergency settings.

- *Other AI applications:* AI applications in thoracic imaging extend beyond traditional diagnostic tasks to emerging areas such as disease quantification and advanced image reconstruction. Automatic quantification tools, e.g., enable precise assessment of conditions like emphysema, diffuse lung diseases, and coronary calcium scoring.[12] Besides cardiac imaging, deep learning reconstruction (DLR) algorithms have also been explored to improve lung CT image quality while significantly reducing radiation doses.[13] Besides this, DLR may also enhance lesion detection, preserve image texture at low doses, and offer superior visualization for conditions like interstitial lung disease and emphysema, compared to traditional image reconstruction techniques. While these applications show great potential, further research is necessary to validate their integration into routine clinical practice.

CURRENT CHALLENGES AND FUTURE DIRECTIONS

- *Dataset limitations and biases:* The lack of diverse, high-quality, and large-scale datasets severely limits the generalizability and reliability of AI models in thoracic imaging. Many datasets are region-specific, condition-specific, or biased due to nonrepresentative patient populations or imaging protocols, leading to skewed predictions and reduced accuracy. Furthermore, data imbalance exacerbates overfitting, especially in multiclass classification tasks. To address these limitations, efforts should focus on creating multicentric, standardized datasets that represent diverse populations and imaging scenarios. Collaboration among institutions to develop publicly available, annotated datasets for underrepresented conditions like pneumoconiosis or pediatric imaging can significantly enhance model performance and reliability.
- *Handling large image sizes and computational costs:* Processing high-resolution CXR and CT images poses computational challenges, even with advanced hardware, often necessitating image resizing that can compromise diagnostic accuracy. Training with large images remains time-intensive and resource-heavy, making cloud-based solutions an attractive yet underutilized alternative due to privacy and ethical concerns. Addressing these issues requires optimized algorithms that balance computational efficiency and diagnostic precision. Federated learning and privacy-preserving frameworks can facilitate cloud-based processing while safeguarding sensitive data, enabling broader adoption of resource-efficient AI solutions.
- *Challenges in multimodal data integration and limited labeling:* AI models predominantly rely on imaging data, overlooking the valuable insights that clinical, genetic, and laboratory information could provide. The limited availability of expert-annotated datasets further hampers AI development, as accurate labeling is resource-intensive and error-prone. Complex conditions with overlapping manifestations, such as TB and silicotuberculosis, exacerbate these issues. Future AI systems should prioritize integrating multimodal data streams for a more holistic diagnostic approach. Automated annotation tools and active learning strategies can alleviate the bottlenecks of manual labeling, while fostering collaboration with domain experts ensures accurate and comprehensive data.
- *Generalizability and interoperability:* AI models often struggle to generalize across institutions and patient populations due to variations in imaging protocols and equipment. This lack of interoperability restricts clinical adoption and limits the scalability of AI applications. Enhancing model robustness requires techniques such as domain adaptation, federated learning, and reconstruction algorithms that reduce dependency on site-specific features. Furthermore, cross-institutional validation and harmonization of imaging practices are essential to ensure consistent model performance across diverse clinical environments.
- *Interpretability and explainability gaps:* The "black-box" nature of many deep learning models undermines trust among clinicians, as these systems lack transparency in their decision-making processes. The limited adoption of standardized explainable AI (XAI) techniques further compound this issue. Developing intuitive, human-interpretable frameworks for AI decision-making can build confidence in these systems. Innovations such as Grad-CAM++ and standardized quantitative metrics for explainability are critical to bridging the gap between AI outputs and clinical understanding, ultimately fostering greater acceptance of AI tools in clinical practice.
- *Evaluation and benchmarking challenges:* The absence of standardized benchmarking datasets and evaluation metrics creates barriers to fair comparisons between AI models. Many studies lack external validation or direct comparisons with radiologists, raising concerns about reproducibility and clinical relevance. To overcome these challenges, future research should focus on creating comprehensive benchmarking datasets and standardizing performance metrics. Prospective multicenter trials and head-to-head evaluations with radiologists are necessary to establish the clinical efficacy of AI systems and support their integration into real-world workflows.

- *Adversarial vulnerabilities:* AI models in thoracic imaging are highly susceptible to adversarial attacks, where small input perturbations can lead to incorrect predictions, raising concerns about their reliability in critical clinical scenarios. Addressing these vulnerabilities requires the development of robust defence mechanisms such as adversarial retraining, noise injection, and denoising algorithms. Building resilient AI systems capable of maintaining performance under adversarial conditions will be key to ensuring their safe and effective deployment in clinical practice.
- *Ethical and legal concerns:* The integration of AI into clinical workflows raises unresolved ethical and legal questions, including accountability for errors, data privacy, and algorithmic fairness. Ambiguities in current frameworks impede widespread adoption and raise concerns about equitable healthcare delivery. Collaborative efforts between governments, industries, and healthcare organizations must define clear legal and ethical standards. Transparent frameworks addressing data privacy, accountability, and fairness are essential to foster trust in AI systems and ensure their responsible deployment in clinical settings.

CONCLUSION

Artificial intelligence has revolutionized thoracic imaging, enhancing diagnostics, workflow efficiency, and clinical decision-making. Despite challenges like dataset limitations, generalizability, and ethical concerns, advancements in multimodal integration, explainability, and robust evaluation promise a transformative future. Collaboration among clinicians, researchers, and policymakers will be key to unlocking its full potential for personalized and equitable healthcare.

REFERENCES

1. Ramachandran A, Bhalla D, Rangarajan K, Pramanik R, Banerjee S, Arora C. Building and evaluating an artificial intelligence algorithm: A practical guide for practicing oncologists. Artif Intell Cancer. 2022;3(3):42-53.
2. Bhalla D, Ramachandran A, Rangarajan K, Dhanakshirur R, Banerjee S, Arora C. Basic principles of AI simplified for a Medical Practitioner: Pearls and Pitfalls in Evaluating AI algorithms. Curr Probl Diagn Radiol. 2023;52(1):47-55.
3. Chassagnon G, De Margerie-Mellon C, Vakalopoulou M, Marini R, Hoang-Thi TN, Revel MP, et al. Artificial intelligence in lung cancer: current applications and perspectives. Jpn J Radiol. 2023;41(3):235-44.
4. de Margerie-Mellon C, Chassagnon G. Artificial intelligence: A critical review of applications for lung nodule and lung cancer. Diagn Interv Imaging. 2023;104(1):11-7.
5. Santosh KC, Allu S, Rajaraman S, Antani S. Advances in Deep Learning for Tuberculosis Screening using Chest X-rays: The Last 5 Years Review. J Med Syst. 2022;46(11):82.
6. Kulkarni S, Jha S. Artificial Intelligence, Radiology, and Tuberculosis: A Review. Acad Radiol. 2020;27(1):71-5.
7. Siddiqi R, Javaid S. Deep Learning for Pneumonia Detection in Chest X-ray Images: A Comprehensive Survey. J Imaging. 2024;10(8):176.
8. Akhter Y, Singh R, Vatsa M. AI-based radiodiagnosis using chest X-rays: A review. Front Big Data. 2023;6:1120989.
9. van den Oever LB, Vonder M, van Assen M, van Ooijen PMA, de Bock GH, Xie XQ, et al. Application of artificial intelligence in cardiac CT: From basics to clinical practice. Eur J Radiol. 2020;128:108969.
10. Xu B, Kocyigit D, Grimm R, Griffin BP, Cheng F. Applications of artificial intelligence in multimodality cardiovascular imaging: A state-of-the-art review. Prog Cardiovasc Dis. 2020;63(3):367-76.
11. Irmici G, Cè M, Caloro E, Khenkina N, Della Pepa G, Ascenti V, et al. Chest X-ray in Emergency Radiology: What Artificial Intelligence Applications Are Available? Diagn Basel Switz. 2023;13(2):216.
12. Vliegenthart R, Fouras A, Jacobs C, Papanikolaou N. Innovations in thoracic imaging: CT, radiomics, AI and x-ray velocimetry. Respirol Carlton Vic. 2022;27(10):818-33.
13. M OC, Pendem S, S PP, Chacko C, Priyanka, Kadavigere R. Influence of deep learning image reconstruction algorithm for reducing radiation dose and image noise compared to iterative reconstruction and filtered back projection for head and chest computed tomography examinations: a systematic review. F1000Research. 2024;13:274.

Index

Page numbers followed by *b* refer to box, *f* refer to figure, *fc* refer to flowchart, and *t* refer to table.

A

B

C

D

E

F

L

M

N

O

P

Q

R

S

T

U

V

W

X

Z